Hurwitz
CLINICAL
PEDIATRIC
DERMATOLOGY

Commissioning Editor: Claire Bonnett / Russell Gabbedy
Development Editor: Alexandra Mortimer
Editorial Assistant: Kirsten Lowson / Rachael Harrison
Project Manager: Jess Thompson
Design: Kirsteen Wright
Illustrator: Richard Prime
Marketing Manager(s) (UK/USA): Gaynor Jones/ Helena Mutak

FOURTH EDITION

Hurwitz CLINICAL PEDIATRIC DERMATOLOGY

A Textbook of Skin Disorders of Childhood and Adolescence

AMY S. PALLER MD

Walter J. Hamlin Professor and Chair of
Dermatology
Professor of Pediatrics
Feinberg School of Medicine
Northwestern University;
Attending Physician
Children's Memorial Hospital
Chicago, Illinois
USA

ANTHONY J. MANCINI MD

Professor of Pediatrics and Dermatology
Feinberg School of Medicine
Northwestern University;
Head, Division of Pediatric Dermatology
Children's Memorial Hospital
Chicago, Illinois
USA

ELSEVIER
SAUNDERS
Edinburgh, London, New York, Oxford, Philadelphia, St Louis, Sydney, Toronto 2011

ELSEVIER
SAUNDERS

SAUNDERS is an imprint of Elsevier Inc.

First edition 1981
Second edition 1993
Third edition 2006
Fourth edition 2011

Notices

Knowledge and best practice in this field are constantly changing. As new research and experience broaden our understanding, changes in research methods, professional practices, or medical treatment may become necessary. Practitioners and researchers must always rely on their own experience and knowledge in evaluating and using any information, methods, compounds, or experiments described herein. In using such information or methods they should be mindful of their own safety and the safety of others, including parties for whom they have a professional responsibility.

With respect to any drug or pharmaceutical products identified, readers are advised to check the most current information provided (i) on procedures featured or (ii) by the manufacturer of each product to be administered, to verify the recommended dose or formula, the method and duration of administration, and contraindications. It is the responsibility of practitioners, relying on their own experience and knowledge of their patients, to make diagnoses, to determine dosages and the best treatment for each individual patient, and to take all appropriate safety precautions.

To the fullest extent of the law, neither the Publisher nor the authors, contributors, or editors, assume any liability for any injury and/or damage to persons or property as a matter of products liability, negligence or otherwise, or from any use or operation of any methods, products, instructions, or ideas contained in the material herein.

Saunders
British Library Cataloguing in Publication Data

Hurwitz's clinical pediatric dermatology : a textbook of skin disorders of childhood and adolescence. – 4th ed.
  1. Pediatric dermatology.
  I. Paller, Amy.   II. Mancini, Anthony J., 1964-   III. Hurwitz, Sidney, 1925–Clinical pediatric dermatology.
  618.9′25–dc22

ISBN–13: 9781437704129

A catalogue record for this book is available from the British Library

Library of Congress Cataloging in Publication Data
A catalog record for this book is available from the Library of Congress

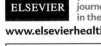

ELSEVIER   your source for books,
            journals and multimedia
            in the health sciences

www.elsevierhealth.com

Working together to grow
libraries in developing countries

www.elsevier.com | www.bookaid.org | www.sabre.org

ELSEVIER   BOOK AID   Sabre Foundation
            International

The
publisher's
policy is to use
paper manufactured
from sustainable forests

Printed in China
Last digit is the print number: 9 8 7 6 5 4 3 2 1

Contents

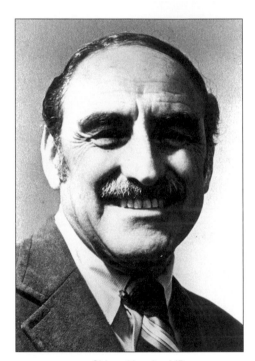

Sidney Hurwitz, MD

Foreword

After 15 years of practicing pediatrics and at 40 years of age, Dr. Sidney Hurwitz returned to Yale University School of Medicine to pursue a residency in dermatology, and subsequently, to embark upon a career dedicated to the advancement of research, knowledge and treatment of skin disorders in the young. During the next 25 years, Dr. Hurwitz became a legend in pediatric dermatology as Clinical Professor of Pediatrics and Dermatology at Yale University School of Medicine. He was a founder and President of both the Society for Pediatric Dermatology (U.S.) and the International Society of Pediatric Dermatology, and an author of more than 100 articles on childhood skin diseases and two single-authored textbooks, *The Skin and Systemic Disease in Children*, and *Clinical Pediatric Dermatology*, first published in 1981. According to Dr. Hurwitz, the first edition took six years of nights, weekends and holidays, and the second edition four years. He dedicated the texts to his family: wife, Teddy, and three daughters Wendy, Laurie, and Alison.

Dr. Hurwitz died of overwhelming viral pneumonia at the age of 67 in November 1995, during his tenure as Honorary President of the International Society of Pediatric Dermatology. In a tribute to him at their International Congress, it was noted: "Professor Sidney Hurwitz was truly a giant among men – a dedicated and learned physician, an outstanding clinician, a medical pioneer, noted author, exceptional teacher, and superb humanitarian. His contributions to medicine and mankind have left an indelible mark upon the world. He mentored and encouraged younger pediatric dermatologists. He single-authored the textbook *Clinical Pediatric Dermatology*, recognized throughout the world as 'the classic' in our field. He found great joy in the love of his family – and in the love of learning, teaching, writing, and sharing with colleagues. He embraced us all with his ready smile, his warmth, his affection, and his friendship. Sidney Hurwitz was a role model for all of us."

Dr. Amy S. Paller was new to the field of pediatric dermatology when she met Dr. Sidney Hurwitz in 1980. It was Dr. Hurwitz who invited her to give her first lecture at the Society for Pediatric Dermatology meeting in 1983, and he served as President while Dr. Paller was Secretary-Treasurer to the new Section on Pediatric Dermatology of the American Academy of Pediatrics that they co-founded. As a leader in pediatric dermatology, he inspired her research into the knowledge and treatment of difficult and challenging pediatric skin diseases. Dr. Paller became the head of the Division of Pediatric Dermatology at Children's Memorial Hospital in Chicago in 1988, following in the footsteps of her teacher and mentor, Dr. Nancy B. Esterly. She is currently Walter J. Hamlin Professor and Chair of Dermatology and Professor of Pediatrics at Northwestern University. True to the example set by Dr. Hurwitz, she has served as Secretary-Treasurer and then President of the Society for Pediatric Dermatology and President of the Society for Investigative Dermatology. She has been or is currently a Director for these organizations, as well as the American Academy of Dermatology (AAD), the Women's Dermatological Society, the American Dermatological Association, and the American Board of Dermatology. As both an NIH-funded bench scientist and clinical investigator, in addition to her almost 30 years of practice in pediatric dermatology, Dr. Paller has contributed to the specialty through a busy international and national lectureship schedule and publication of almost 300 papers, 60 chapters, and four textbooks, among them *Clinical Pediatric Dermatology*. In common with Dr. Hurwitz, Dr. Paller relishes her years of working with young pediatric dermatologists. She has been honored for her mentorship skills and has helped to launch the careers of more than 80 pediatric dermatologists.

Dr. Anthony J. Mancini first learned of the field of pediatric dermatology as a fourth year medical student. As a pediatrics intern at Stanford, he was introduced to Dr. Alfred T. Lane, who would become his role model and primary mentor. After completing his dermatology and pediatric dermatology training, Dr. Mancini accepted a position at Children's Memorial Hospital and Northwestern University Feinberg School of Medicine, where he ultimately became Head of the Division of Pediatric Dermatology in 2004. Following in the footsteps of his mentors, he has dedicated his career to pediatric and dermatology education, as well as patient care and clinical research. Dr. Mancini is currently Professor of Pediatrics and Dermatology at Northwestern, where he also directs the pediatric dermatology fellowship program, established in 1983 as the first fellowship program in the county. He is serving his second 5-year term as Secretary-Treasurer of the Society for Pediatric Dermatology, has served as an elected member to the Executive Committee of the Section on Dermatology of the American Academy of Pediatrics (AAP), and has held numerous posts within both the AAP and the AAD. Dr. Mancini, who lectures extensively at the national and international levels, has published over 140 scientific papers, abstracts and chapters, as well as 3 textbooks, including *Clinical Pediatric Dermatology* and the pediatric dermatology guide published by the AAP, for which he serves as Co-Editor. One of his greatest senses of accomplishment is that of mentoring his trainees in the fellowship program, including both U.S.-trained and international fellows who come from abroad, and the pediatric residents at his institution, who have recognized Dr. Mancini with the "Faculty Excellence in Education" award for 13 of the last 15 years. As such, he too embraces Dr. Hurwitz's love of the specialty and his philosophy in the care of children with skin diseases.

It is fitting that Drs. Paller and Mancini, authors of the third and now fourth edition of *Clinical Pediatric Dermatology*, continue to immortalize Dr. Hurwitz's legacy.

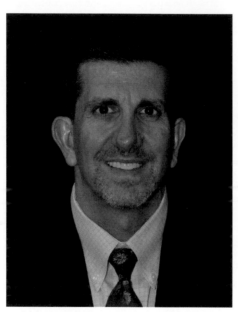

Anthony J. Mancini, MD

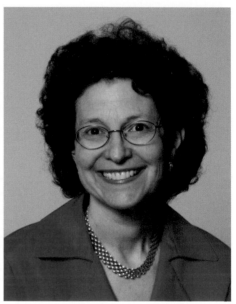

Amy S. Paller, MD

Preface

We were truly honored when asked to consider updating *Hurwitz Clinical Pediatric Dermatology.* Dr. Hurwitz was a true icon of our specialty, and one of its founding fathers. Thanks to Dr. Hurwitz, the widely recognizable book sits on many a shelf, and has educated and enlightened pediatricians, dermatologists, family practitioners, medical students, residents, nurses and other allied pediatric care providers for decades. It is our hope that this tradition will continue, and we have made every effort to maintain the practicality, relevance and usability of the text.

What lies between these covers will be familiar, but many additions have been made. The field of pediatric dermatology has exploded during the past decade. The molecular bases for many established skin diseases, as well as syndromes with cutaneous features, have been elucidated. Several new disease and syndrome associations have been recognized and described. The therapeutic armamentarium for cutaneous disease has broadened, with further elucidation of mechanisms of disease and, as a result, several newer classes of drugs available to the clinician. We have strived to maintain a text that is a marriage between cutting edge review and practical clinical application, while keeping the look and flavor of Dr. Hurwitz's first two editions and our third edition, each of them a balance between narrative text, useful tables and enlightening clinical photographs.

Several new features have been added to this fourth edition, including access to the complete fully-searchable contents online, and over 370 new clinical images. We have reorganized our discussion of genetic disorders to include the new classifications of the ichthyoses, epidermolysis bullosa and ectodermal dysplasia, as well as mention of new disorders and our new understanding. We have noted the shift of attention in treating atopic dermatitis to defects in the epidermal barrier, and discussed evolving therapeutic advances for many common childhood skin disorders, from infantile hemangiomas to head lice. This edition includes many new tables and clinical photographs. The references have been extensively updated, and we have shifted all but some excellent reviews and landmark articles to our companion online edition, to allow for more complete textual content for our readers in the print version.

We are indebted to several individuals, without whom this work would not have been possible. First and foremost, we must thank Dr. Sidney Hurwitz, whose vision, dedication and enthusiasm for the specialty of pediatric dermatology lives on as a legacy in this text, initially published in 1981. To Teddy Hurwitz, his wife, who entrusted to us the ongoing tradition of this awesome project. To Dr. Alvin Jacobs, a "father" of pediatric dermatology who kindled the flame of the specialty in both of us through his teaching at Stanford. To Dr. Nancy B. Esterly, the "mother" of pediatric dermatology, whose superb clinical acumen and patient care made her the perfect role model for another female physician who yearned to follow in her footsteps. And to Dr. Alfred T. Lane, who believed in a young pediatric intern and mentored him through the process of becoming a mentor himself.

To the staff at Elsevier, most notably Claire Bonnett and Alex Mortimer, who worked tirelessly to meet the many demands of two finicky academicians;

To our patients, who continue to educate us on a daily basis and place their trust in us to provide them care;

To the clinicians who referred many of the patients seen in these pages;

To our pediatric dermatology fellow and photographer, Daniela Russi M.D., who contributed enormously through maintaining our photography archival system;

And to our families, whose understanding, sacrifice, support and unconditional love made this entire endeavor possible.

Dedicated to

Our Families:

Etahn	Nicki
Josh	Mallory
Max	Chris
&	Mack
Ben	&
	Alex

whose patience, understanding, support and
personal sacrifice enabled us to
complete this project.

And to the memory of

Sidney Hurwitz, MD
A role model par excellence

An Overview of Dermatologic Diagnosis

Accurate diagnosis of cutaneous disease in infants and children is a systematic process that requires careful inspection, evaluation, and some knowledge of dermatologic terminology and morphology to develop a prioritized differential diagnosis. The manifestations of skin disorders in infants and young children often vary from those of the same diseases in older children and adults. The diagnosis may be obscured, for example, by different reaction patterns or a tendency towards easier blister formation. In addition, therapeutic dosages and regimens frequently differ from those of adults, with medications prescribed on a per kilogram (/kg) basis and with liquid formulations.

Nevertheless, the same basic principles that are used to detect disorders affecting viscera apply to the detection of skin disorders. An adequate history should be obtained, a thorough physical examination performed, and, whenever possible, the clinical impression verified by appropriate laboratory studies. The easy visibility of skin lesions all too frequently results in a cursory examination and hasty diagnosis. Instead, the entire skin should be examined routinely and carefully, including the hair, scalp, nails, oral mucosa, anogenital regions, palms, and soles, because visible findings often hold clues to the final diagnosis.

The examination should be conducted in a well-lit room. Although natural daylight is the most effective type of illumination for an examination, fluorescent or incandescent lighting of adequate intensity may be satisfactory. A properly sequenced examination requires initial viewing of the patient at a distance in an effort to establish the overall status of the patient. By this overall evaluation, distribution patterns and clues to the appropriate final diagnosis frequently can be recognized. This initial evaluation is followed by careful scrutiny of primary and subsequent secondary lesions in an effort to discern the characteristic features of the disorder.

Although not always diagnostic, the morphology and configuration of cutaneous lesions are of considerable importance to the classification and diagnosis of cutaneous disease. Unfortunately, a lack of understanding of dermatologic terminology frequently poses a barrier to the description of cutaneous disorders by clinicians who are not dermatologists. Accordingly, a review of dermatologic terms is included here (Table 1.1). The many examples to show primary and secondary skin lesions refer to specific figures in the text that follows.

Configuration of lesions

A number of dermatologic entities assume *annular*, *circinate*, or *ring* shapes and are interpreted as 'ringworm' or superficial fungal infections. Although tinea is a common annular dermatosis of childhood, other disorders that must be included in the differential diagnosis of ringed lesions include pityriasis rosea, seborrheic dermatitis, nummular eczema, lupus erythematosus, granuloma annulare, psoriasis, erythema multiforme, erythema annulare centrifugum, erythema migrans, secondary syphilis, sarcoidosis, urticaria, pityriasis alba, tinea versicolor, lupus vulgaris, drug eruptions, and cutaneous T-cell lymphoma.

The terms *arciform* and *arcuate* refer to lesions that assume arc-like configurations. Arciform lesions may be seen in erythema multiforme, urticaria, pityriasis rosea, and bullous dermatosis of childhood.

Lesions that tend to merge are said to be *confluent*. Confluence of lesions is seen in childhood exanthems, *Rhus* dermatitis, erythema multiforme, tina versicolor and urticaria.

Lesions localized to a dermatome supplied by one or more dorsal ganglia are referred to as *dermatomal*. Herpes zoster occurs in a dermatomal distribution.

Discoid is used to describe lesions that are solid, moderately raised, and disc-shaped. The term has largely been applied to discoid lupus erythematosus, in which the discoid lesions usually show atrophy and dyspigmentation.

Discrete lesions are individual lesions that tend to remain separated and distinct. *Eczematoid* and *eczematous* are adjectives relating to eczema and suggest inflammation with a tendency to thickening, oozing, vesiculation, and/or crusting.

Grouping and *clustering* are characteristic of vesicles of herpes simplex or herpes zoster, insect bites, lymphangioma circumscriptum, contact dermatitis, and bullous dermatosis of childhood.

Guttate or drop-like lesions are characteristic of flares of psoriasis in children and adolescents that follow an acute upper respiratory tract infection, usually streptococcal.

Gyrate refers to twisted, coiled, or spiral-like lesions, as may be seen in patients with urticaria and erythema annulare centrifugum.

Iris or target-like lesions are concentric ringed lesions characteristic of erythema multiforme.

Keratosis refers to circumscribed patches of horny thickening, as seen in seborrheic or actinic keratoses, keratosis pilaris, and keratosis follicularis (Darier disease). Keratotic is an adjective pertaining to keratosis and frequently refers to the horny thickening of the skin seen in chronic dermatitis and callus formation.

The *Koebner phenomenon or isomorphic response* refers to the appearance of lesions along the site of injury. The linear lesions of warts and molluscum contagiosum, for example, occur from autoinoculation of virus from scratching; those of *Rhus* dermatitis (poison ivy) result from the spread of the plant's oleoresin. Other examples of disorders that show a Koebner phenomenon are psoriasis, lichen planus, lichen nitidus, pityriasis rubra pilaris, and keratosis follicularis (Darier disease).

Lesions in a *linear* or band-like configuration appear in the form of a line or stripe and may be seen in epidermal nevi, Conradi's syndrome, linear morphea, lichen striatus, striae, *Rhus* dermatitis, deep mycoses (sporotrichosis or coccidioidomycosis), incontinentia pigmenti, pigment mosaicism, porokeratosis of Mibelli, or factitial dermatitis.

Table 1.1 Glossary of dermatologic terms

Lesion	Description	Illustration	Examples
Primary lesions			
The term *primary* refers to the most representative, but not necessarily the earliest, lesions; it is distinguished from the cutaneous features of secondary changes, such as excoriation, eczematization, infection, or results of previous therapy.			
Macule	Flat, circumscribed change of the skin. It may be of any size, although this term is often used for lesions <1 cm. A macule may appear as an area of hypopigmentation or as an area of increased coloration, most commonly brown (hyperpigmented) or red (usually a vascular abnormality). It is usually round, but may be oval or irregular; it may be distinct or may fade into the surrounding area.		Freckle or ephelide (Fig. 11.38); lentigo (Fig. 11.41); flat nevus (Fig. 9.1), and tinea versicolor (Fig. 17.28).
Patch	Flat, circumscribed lesion with color change that is >1 cm in size.		Mongolian spot (Fig. 11.58); port-wine stain (Fig. 12.54); nevus depigmentosus (Fig. 11.21); larger café au lait spot (Figs 11.37, 11.46), and areas of vitiligo (Figs 11.1–11.9).
Papule	Circumscribed, non-vesicular, non-pustular, elevated lesion that measures <1 cm in diameter. The greatest mass is above the surface of the skin. When viewed in profile it may be flat-topped, dome-shaped, acuminate (tapering to a point), digitate (finger-like), smooth, eroded, or ulcerated; it may be covered by scales, crusts, or a combination of secondary features.		Elevated nevus (Fig. 9.2); verruca (Fig. 15.18); molluscum contagiosum (Fig. 15.37); perioral dermatitis (Fig. 8.21), and individual lesions of lichen planus (Fig. 4.39).
Plaque	Broad, elevated, disk-shaped lesion that occupies an area of >1 cm. It is frequently formed by a confluence of papules.		Psoriasis (Fig. 4.4); lichen simplex chronicus (neurodermatitis) (Fig. 3.33); granuloma annulare (Fig. 9.51); nevus sebaceus (Figs 9.34–9.37), and lesions of lichen planus (Fig. 4.42).

Table 1.1 Continued

Lesion	Description	Illustration	Examples
Nodule	Circumscribed, elevated, usually solid lesion that measures 0.5–2 cm in diameter. It involves the dermis and may extend into the subcutaneous tissue, with its greatest mass below the surface of the skin.	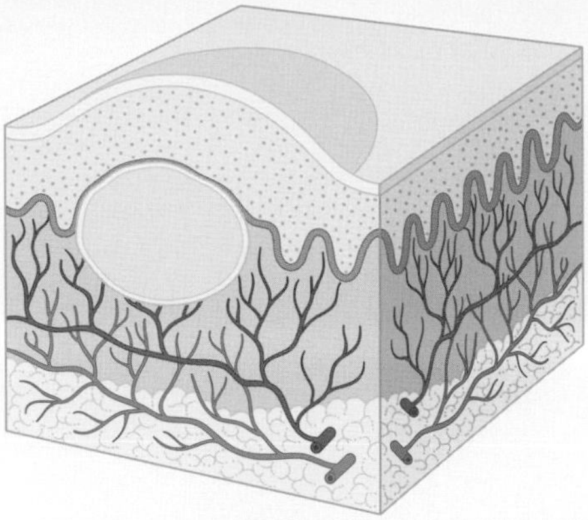	Neurofibroma (Fig. 11.49); pilomatricoma (Fig. 9.41); subcutaneous granuloma annulare (Fig. 9.52), and nodular scabies (Fig. 18.9).
Tumor	Deeper circumscribed solid lesion of the skin or subcutaneous tissue that measures >2 cm in diameter. It may be benign or malignant.	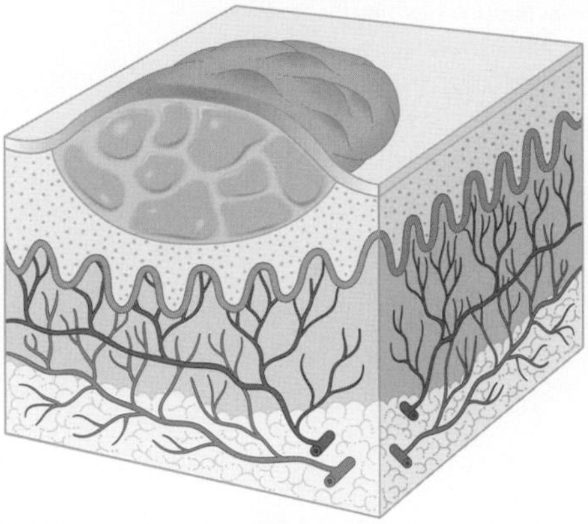	Deep hemangioma (Fig. 12.8) and sarcoma (Fig. 10.22).
Wheal	Distinctive type of elevated lesion characterized by local, superficial, transient edema. White to pink or pale red, compressible, and evanescent, they often disappear within a period of hours. They vary in size and shape.	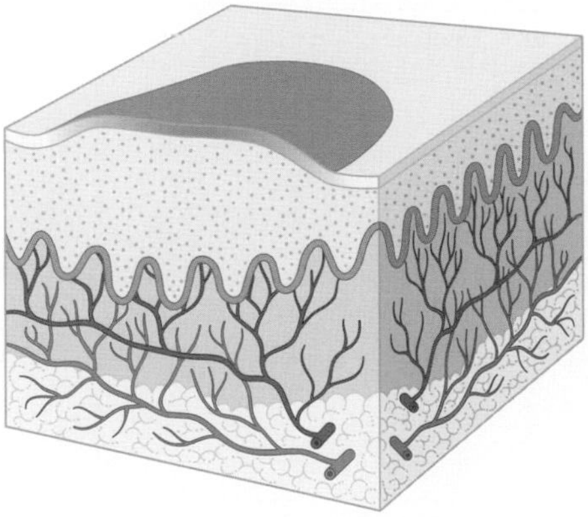	Darier's sign of mastocytosis (Fig. 9.45); urticarial vasculitis (Fig. 21.14), and various forms of urticaria (Fig. 20.1).
Vesicle	Sharply circumscribed, elevated, fluid-containing lesion that measures 1 cm in diameter or less.	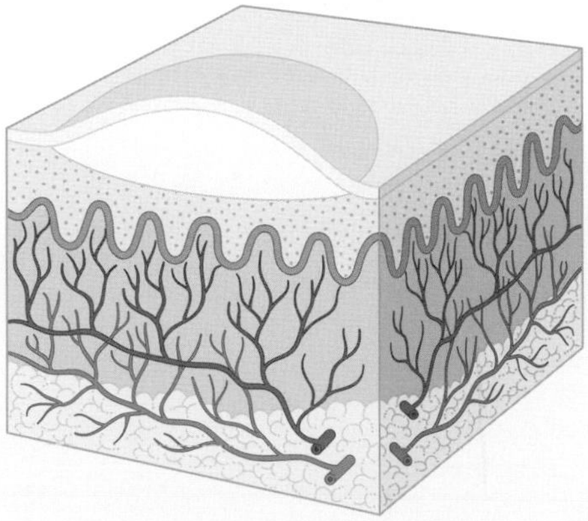	Herpes simplex (Figs 2.41, 15.17); hand-foot-and-mouth disease (Fig. 16.38); pompholyx (Fig. 3.38); varicella (Fig. 16.2), and contact dermatitis (Fig. 3.51).

Table 1.1 Continued

Lesion	Description	Illustration	Examples
Bulla	Larger circumscribed, elevated fluid-containing lesion that measures >1 cm in diameter.		Blistering distal dactylitis (Fig. 14.17); bullous pemphigoid (Fig. 13.23); chronic bullous disease of childhood (Fig. 13.26); bullous systemic lupus erythematosus (Fig. 13.30), and epidermolysis bullosa (Fig. 13.4).
Pustule	Circumscribed elevation <1 cm in diameter that contains a purulent exudate. It may be infectious or sterile.		Folliculitis (Fig. 14.8); transient neonatal pustular melanosis (Figs 2.5 and 2.16); pustular psoriasis (Fig. 4.18), and infantile acropustulosis (Fig. 2.17).
Abscess	Circumscribed, elevated lesion >1 cm in diameter, often with a deeper component, and filled with purulent material.		Staphylococcal abscess (in a neonate, Fig. 2.5; in a patient with hyperimmunoglob-ulinemia E, Fig. 3.31).
Other primary lesions			
Comedone	Plugged secretion of horny material retained within a pilosebaceous follicle. It may be flesh-colored (as in closed comedone or whitehead), or slightly raised brown or black (as in open comedone or blackhead). Closed comedones, in contrast to open comedones, may be difficult to visualize. They appear as pale, slightly elevated small papules without a clinically visible orifice.		Acne comedones (Figs 8.2, 8.3); nevus comedonicus (Fig. 9.38).
Burrow	Linear lesion produced by tunneling of an animal parasite in the stratum corneum.		Scabies (Fig. 18.3) and cutaneous larva migrans (creeping eruption, Fig. 18.37).

Table 1.1 Continued

Lesion	Description	Illustration	Examples
Telangiectasia	Persistent dilatation of superficial venules, capillaries, or arterioles of the skin.		Spider angioma (Fig. 12.80); periungual lesion of dermatomyositis (Fig. 22.23), and Goltz syndrome (Fig. 6.13).

Secondary lesions

Secondary lesions represent evolutionary changes that occur later in the course of the cutaneous disorder. Although helpful in dermatologic diagnosis, they do not offer the same degree of diagnostic aid as that afforded by primary lesions of a cutaneous disorder.

Lesion	Description	Illustration	Examples
Crust	Dried remains of serum, blood, pus, or exudate overlying areas of lost or damaged epidermis. Crust is yellow when formed by dried serum, green or yellowish green when formed by purulent exudate, and dark red or brown when formed by bloody exudative serum.		Herpes simplex (Fig. 15.4); weeping eczematous dermatitis (Fig. 3.1) and dried honey-colored lesions of impetigo (Figs 3.22 and 14.1).
Scale	Formed by an accumulation of compact desquamating layers of stratum corneum as a result of abnormal keratinization and exfoliation of cornified keratinocytes.		Seborrheic dermatitis (greasy and yellowish, Figs 3.4 and 3.34); psoriasis (silvery and mica-like, Fig. 4.2); pityriasis alba (fine and barely visible, Fig. 3.29), and lamellar ichthyosis (large and adherent, Fig. 5.10).
Fissure	Dry or moist, linear, often painful cleavage in the cutaneous surface that results from marked drying and long-standing inflammation, thickening, and loss of elasticity of the integument.		Angular cheilitis (Fig. 17.33), and the perianal lesions of streptococcal dermatitis (Fig. 14.16).

Table 1.1 Continued

Lesion	Description	Illustration	Examples
Erosion	Moist, slightly depressed vesicular or bullous lesions in which part or all of the epidermis has been lost. Since erosions do not extend into the underlying dermis or subcutaneous tissue, healing occurs without subsequent scar formation.	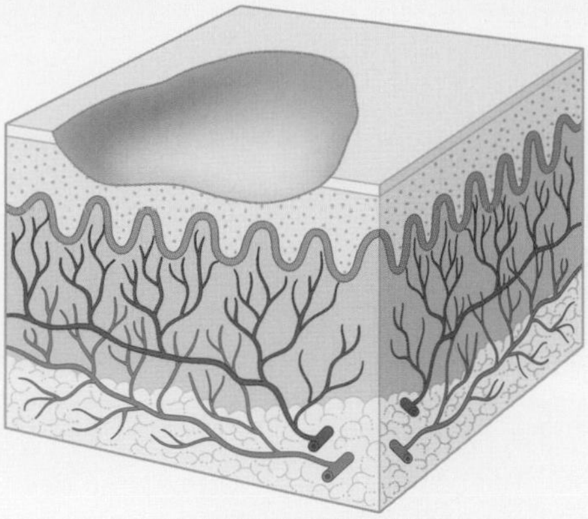	Herpes simplex (Figs 3.25, 15.1); epidermolytic ichthyosis in a neonate (Fig. 5.4); and acrodermatitis enteropathica (Fig. 2.25).
Excoriation	Traumatized or abraded (usually self-induced) superficial loss of skin caused by scratching, rubbing, or scrubbing of the cutaneous surface.	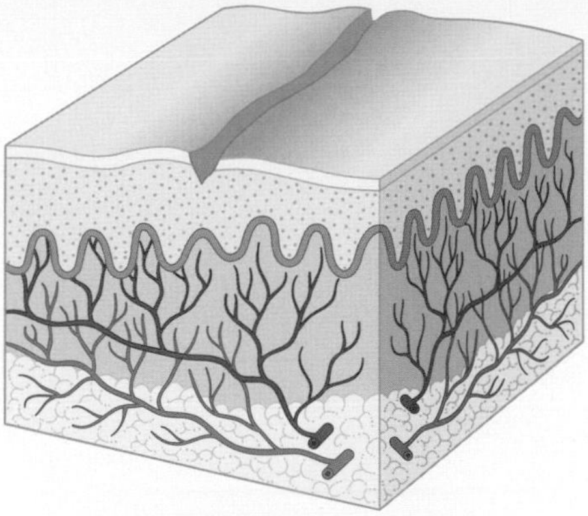	Atopic dermatitis (Fig. 3.21), and acne excoriée (Fig. 8.19).
Ulcer	Necrosis of the epidermis and part or all of the dermis and/or the underlying subcutaneous tissue.	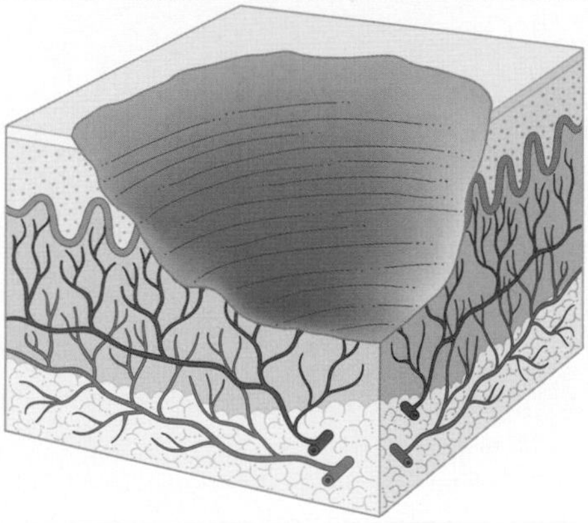	Pyoderma gangrenosum (Fig. 25.26) and ulcerated hemangioma of infancy (Figs 12.14, 12.23).
Atrophy	Cutaneous changes that result in depression of the epidermis, dermis, or both. Epidermal atrophy is characterized by thin, almost translucent epidermis, a loss of the normal skin markings, and wrinkling when subjected to lateral pressure or pinching of the affected area. In dermal atrophy the skin is depressed.	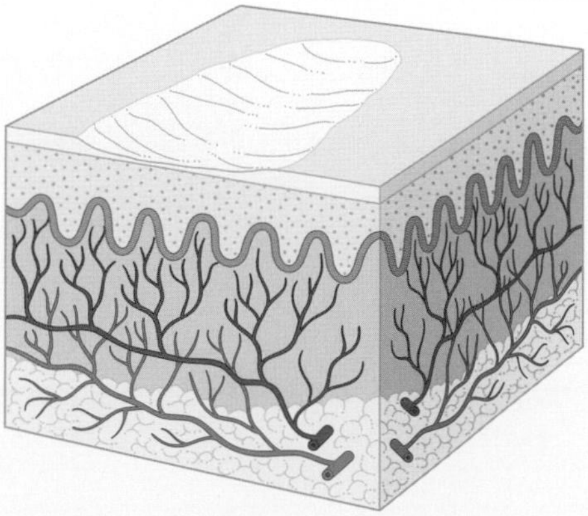	Anetoderma (Fig. 22.54); morphea (Fig. 22.47); steroid-induced atrophy (Fig. 3.28), and Goltz syndrome (Fig. 6.15).

	Table 1.1 Continued		
Lesion	**Description**	**Illustration**	**Examples**
Lichenification	Thickening of the epidermis with associated exaggeration of skin markings. Lichenification results from chronic scratching or rubbing of a pruritic lesion.		Atopic dermatitis (Fig. 3.14); chronic contact dermatitis (Fig. 3.46), and lichen simplex chronicus (Fig. 3.33).
Scar	A permanent fibrotic skin change that develops after damage to the dermis. Initially pink or violaceous, scars are permanent white, shiny and sclerotic as the color fades. Although fresh scars often are hypertrophic, they usually contract during the subsequent 6–12 months and become less apparent. Hypertrophic scars must be differentiated from keloids, which represent an exaggerated response to skin injury. Keloids are pink, smooth, and rubbery and are often traversed by telangiectatic vessels. They tend to increase in size long after healing has taken place and can be differentiated from hypertrophic scars by the fact that the surface of keloidal scars tends to proliferate beyond the area of the original wound.		Keloid (Fig. 9.71); healed areas of recessive dystrophic epidermolysis bullosa (Fig. 13.17); acne scarring (Fig. 8.8), acne keloidalis (Fig. 7.28), and amniocentesis scars (Fig. 2.4).

Moniliform refers to a banded or necklace-like appearance. This is seen in monilethrix, a hair deformity characterized by beaded nodularities along the hair shaft.

Multiform refers to disorders in which more than one variety or shape of cutaneous lesions occurs. This configuration is seen in patients with erythema multiforme, early Henoch–Schönlein purpura, and polymorphous light eruption.

Nummular means coin-shaped and is usually used to describe nummular dermatitis.

Polycyclic refers to oval lesions containing more than one ring, as frequently is seen in patients with urticaria.

A *reticulated* or net-like pattern may be seen in erythema ab igne, livedo reticularis, cutis marmorata, cutis marmorata telangiectatica congenita, and lesions of confluent and reticulated papillomatosis.

Serpiginous describes the shape or spread of lesions in a serpentine or snake-like configuration, particularly those of cutaneous larva migrans (creeping eruption) and elastosis perforans serpiginosa.

Umbilicated lesions are centrally depressed or shaped like an umbilicus or navel. Examples include lesions of molluscum contagiosum, varicella, vaccinia, variola, herpes zoster, and Kaposi's varicelliform eruption.

Universal (universalis) implies widespread disorders affecting the entire skin, as in alopecia universalis.

Zosteriform describes a linear arrangement along a nerve, as typified by lesions of herpes zoster, although herpes simplex infection can also manifest in a zosteriform distribution.

Distribution and morphologic patterns of common skin disorders

The regional distribution and morphologic configuration of cutaneous lesions are frequently helpful in dermatologic diagnosis.

Acneiform are those having the form of acne, and an acneiform distribution refers to lesions primarily seen on the face, neck, chest, upper arms, shoulders, and back (Figs 8.2–8.13).

Sites of predilection of *atopic dermatitis* include the face, trunk, and extremities in young children; the antecubital and popliteal fossae are the most common sites in older children and adolescents (Figs 3.1–3.12).

The lesions of *erythema multiforme* may be widespread but have a distinct predilection for the hands and feet (particularly the palms and soles) (Figs 20.33–20.37).

Lesions of *herpes simplex* may appear anywhere on the body but have a distinct predisposition for the areas about the lips, face, and genitalia (Figs 15.1–15.12). *Herpes zoster* generally has a dermatomal or nerve-like distribution and is usually but not necessarily unilateral (Figs 15.13, 15.14). More than 75% of cases occur between the second thoracic and second lumbar vertebrae. The fifth cranial nerve frequently is involved, and only rarely are lesions seen below the elbows or knees.

Lichen planus frequently affect the limbs (Figs 4.37–4.40). Favorite sites include the lower extremities, the flexor surface of the wrists, the buccal mucosa, the trunk, and the genitalia.

The lesions of *lupus erythematosus* most frequently localize to the bridge of the nose, the malar eminences, scalp, and ears, although they may be widespread (Figs 22.3–22.7). Patches tend to spread at the border and clear in the center, with atrophy, scarring, dyspigmentation, and telangiectases. The malar or butterfly rash is neither specific for nor the most frequent sign of lupus erythematosus; telangiectasia without the accompanying features of erythema, scaling, or atrophy is never a marker of this disorder.

Molluscum contagiosum is a common viral disorder characterized by dome-shaped skin-colored to erythematous papules, often with a central white core or umbilication (Figs 15.35–15.44). These papules most commonly localize to the trunk and axillary areas. Although molluscum lesions can be found anywhere, the scalp, palms and soles are infrequent sites of involvement.

Photodermatoses are cutaneous disorders caused or precipitated by exposure to light. Areas of predilection include the face, ears, anterior 'V' of the neck and upper chest, the dorsal aspect of the forearms and hands, and exposed areas of the legs. The shaded regions of the upper eyelids, subnasal, and submental regions tend to be spared. The major photosensitivity disorders are lupus erythematosus, dermatomyositis, polymorphous light eruption, drug photosensitization, and porphyria (see Ch. 19).

Photosensitive reactions cannot be distinguished on a clinical basis from lesions of photocontact allergic conditions. They may reflect internal as well as external photoallergens, and may simulate contact dermatitis from air-borne sensitizers. Lupus erythematosus can be differentiated by the presence of atrophy, scarring, hyperpigmentation or hypopigmentation, and the presence of periungual telangiectases. Dermatomyositis with swelling and erythema of the cheeks and eyelids should be differentiated from allergic contact dermatitis by the heliotrope hue and other associated changes, particularly those of the fingers (periungual telangiectases and Gottron's papules).

Pityriasis rosea begins as a solitary round or oval scaling lesion known as the herald patch in 70–80% of cases, often misdiagnosed as tinea corporis (Figs 4.32–4.35). After an interval of days to 2 weeks, affected individuals develop a generalized symmetrical eruption that involves mainly the trunk and proximal limbs. The clue to diagnosis is the distribution of lesions, with the long axis of these oval lesions parallel to the lines of cleavage in what has been termed a *Christmas-tree pattern*. A common variant, inverse pityriasis rosea often localizes in the inguinal region, but the parallel nature of the long axis of lesions remains characteristic.

Psoriasis classically consists of round, erythematous, well-marginated plaques with a rich red hue covered by a characteristic grayish or silvery-white mica-like (micaceous) scale, which, on removal, may result in pinpoint bleeding (Auspitz sign) (Figs 4.1–4.10). Although exceptions occur, lesions generally are seen in a bilaterally symmetrical pattern with a predilection for the elbows, knees, scalp, and lumbosacral, perianal, and genital regions. Nail involvement, a valuable diagnostic sign, is characterized by pitting of the nail plate, discoloration, separation of the nail from the nail bed (onycholysis), and an accumulation of subungual scale

(subungual hyperkeratosis). A characteristic feature of this disorder is the Koebner or isomorphic response in which new lesions appear at sites of local injury.

Scabies is an itchy disorder in which lesions are characteristically distributed on the wrists and hands (particularly the interdigital webs), forearms, genitalia, areolae, and buttocks in older children and adolescents (Figs 18.1–18.11). Other family members may be similarly affected or complain of itching. In infants and young children, the diagnosis is often overlooked because the distribution typically involves the palms, soles, and often the head and neck. Obliteration of demonstrable primary lesions (burrows) due to vigorous hygienic measures, excoriation, crusting, eczematization, and secondary infection is particularly common in infants.

Seborrheic dermatitis is an erythematous, scaly or crusting eruption that characteristically occurs on the scalp, face, and postauricular, presternal, and intertriginous areas (Figs 3.34–3.36). The classic lesions are dull or pinkish yellow or salmon colored, with fairly sharp borders and overlying yellowish greasy scale. Morphologic and topographic variants occur in many combinations and with varying degrees of severity, from mild involvement of the scalp with occasional blepharitis to generalized, occasionally severe erythematous scaling eruptions. The differential diagnosis may include atopic dermatitis, psoriasis, various forms of diaper dermatitis, Langerhans cell histiocytosis, scabies, tinea corporis or capitis, pityriasis alba, contact dermatitis, Darier disease, and lupus erythematosus.

Warts are common viral cutaneous lesions characterized by the appearance of skin-colored small papules of several morphologic types (Figs 15.16–15.33). They may be elevated or flat lesions and tend to appear in areas of trauma, particularly the dorsal surface of the face, hands, periungual areas, elbows, knees, feet, and genital or perianal areas. Close examination may reveal capillaries appearing as punctate dots scattered on the surface.

Changes in skin color

The color of skin lesions frequently assists in making the diagnosis. Disorders of brown hyperpigmentation include post-inflammatory hyperpigmentation, pigmented and epidermal nevi, café-au-lait spots, incontinentia pigmenti, fixed drug eruption, photodermatitis and phytophoto-dermatitis, chloasma, acanthosis nigricans, and Addison disease. Blue coloration is seen in mongolian spots, blue nevi, nevus of Ito and nevus of Ota, and cutaneous neuroblastomas. Cysts, deep hemangiomas, and pilomatricomas often show a subtle blue color, whereas the blue of venous malformations and glomuvenous malformations is often a more intense, dark blue. Yellowish discoloration of the skin is common in infants, related to the presence of carotene derived from excessive ingestion of foods, particularly yellow vegetables containing carotenoid pigments. Jaundice may be distinguished from carotenemia by scleral icterus. Localized yellow lesions may be juvenile xanthogranulomas, nevus sebaceous, xanthomas, or mastocytomas. Red lesions are usually vascular in origin, such as superficial hemangiomas, spider telangiectases, and nevus flammeus, or inflammatory, such as the scaling lesions of atopic dermatitis or psoriasis.

Localized lesions with decreased pigmentation may be hypopigmented or depigmented (totally devoid of pigmentation); Wood's lamp examination may help to differentiate depigmented lesions, which fluoresce a bright white, from hypopigmented lesions. Localized depigmented lesions may be seen in vitiligo, Vogt–Koyanagi syndrome, halo nevi, chemical depigmentation, piebaldism, and Waardenburg syndrome. Hypopigmented lesions are more typical of post-inflammatory hypopigmentation, pityriasis alba, tinea versicolor, leprosy, nevus achromicus, tuberous sclerosis, and the hypopigmented streaks of pigment mosaicism. A generalized decrease in pigmentation can be seen in patients with albinism, untreated phenylketonuria, and Menkes syndrome. The skin of patients with Chediak–Higashi and Griscelli syndromes takes on a dull silvery sheen and may show decreased pigmentation.

Racial variations in the skin and hair

The skin of African-American and other darker-skinned children varies in several ways from that of lighter-skinned children based on genetic background and customs.[1,2] The erythema of inflamed black skin may be difficult to see, and likely accounts for the purportedly decreased incidence of macular viral exanthems such as erythema infectiosum. Erythema in African-American children frequently has a purplish tinge that can be confusing to unwary observers. The skin lesions in several inflammatory disorders, such as in atopic dermatitis, pityriasis rosea, and syphilis, frequently show a follicular pattern in African-American children.

Post-inflammatory hypopigmentation and hyperpigmentation occur readily and are more obvious in darker-skinned persons, regardless of racial origin. Pityriasis alba and tinea versicolor are more commonly reported in darker skin types, perhaps because of the easy visibility of the hypopigmented lesions in marked contrast to uninvolved surrounding skin. Lichen nitidus is more apparent and reportedly more common in African-American individuals; lichen planus is reported to be more severe, leaving dark post-inflammatory hyperpigmentation. Vitiligo is particularly distressing to patients with darker skin types, whether African-American or Asian, because of the easy visibility in contrast with surrounding skin.

Although darker skin may burn, in general sunburn and chronic sun-induced diseases of adults such as actinic keratosis and carcinomas of the skin induced by ultraviolet light exposure (e.g., squamous cell carcinoma, keratoacanthoma, basal cell carcinoma, and melanoma) have an extremely low incidence in African-Americans and Hispanics. Congenital melanocytic nevi also tend to have a lower tendency to transform to malignancy in darker-skinned individuals. Café-au-lait spots are more numerous and seen more often in African-Americans, although the presence of six or more should still raise suspicion about neurofibromatosis. Dermatosis papulosa nigra commonly develop in adolescents, especially female, of African descent. Mongolian spots occur more frequently in persons of African or Asian descent. Physiologic variants in children with darker skin include increased pigmentation of the gums and tongue, pigmented streaks in the nails, and Voight–Futcher lines, lines of pigmentary demarcation between the posterolateral and lighter anteromedial skin on the extremities.

Qualities of hair may also differ among individuals of different races. African-American hair tends to tangle when dry and becomes matted when wet. As a result of its naturally curly or spiral nature, pseudofolliculitis barbae is more common in African-Americans than in other groups. Tinea capitis is particularly common in prepubertal African-Americans; the tendency to use oils because of hair dryness and poor manageability may obscure the scaling of tinea capitis. Pediculosis capitis, in contrast, is relatively uncommon in this population. Prolonged continuous traction on hairs may result in traction alopecia, particularly with the common practice of making tight corn row braids. The use of other hair grooming techniques, such as chemical straighteners, application of hot oils, and use of hot combs, increases the risk of hair breakage and permanent alopecia. Frequent and liberal use of greasy lubricants and pomades produces a comedonal and sometimes papulopustular form of acne (pomade acne).

Keloids form more often in individuals of African descent, often as a complication of a form of inflammatory acne, including nodulocystic acne and acne keloidalis nuchae. Other skin disorders reportedly seen more commonly are transient neonatal pustular melanosis, infantile acropustulosis, impetigo, papular urticaria, sickle cell ulcers, sarcoidosis, and dissecting cellulitis of the scalp. Atopic dermatitis and Kawasaki disease have both been reported most frequently in children of Asian descent.

Key References

1. Laude TA, Kenney JA Jr, Prose NS, et al. Skin manifestations in individuals of African or Asian descent. *Pediatr Dermatol.* 1996;13:158–168.
2. Dinulos JG, Graham EA. Influence of culture and pigment on skin conditions in children. *Pediatr Rev.* 1998;19:268–275.

2 Cutaneous Disorders of the Newborn

Neonatal skin

The skin of the infant differs from that of an adult in that it is thinner (40–60%), is less hairy, and has a weaker attachment between the epidermis and dermis.[1] In addition, the body surface area-to-weight ratio of an infant is up to five times that of an adult. The infant is therefore at a significantly increased risk for skin injury, percutaneous absorption, and skin-associated infection. Premature infants born prior to 32–34 weeks' estimated gestational age may have problems associated with an immature stratum corneum (the most superficial cell layer in the epidermis), including an increase in transepidermal water loss (TEWL). This increased TEWL may result in morbidity because of dehydration, electrolyte imbalance, and thermal instability. Interestingly, in the majority of premature infants, an acceleration of skin maturation occurs after birth such that most develop intact barrier function by 2–3 weeks of life.[2] However, in extremely low-birthweight infants, this process may take significantly longer, up to 4–8 weeks.[3] In light of the elevated TEWL levels seen in premature infants, a variety of studies have evaluated the use of occlusive dressings or topical emollients in an effort to improve compromised barrier function.[4–7]

The risk of percutaneous toxicity from topically applied substances is increased in infants, especially those born prematurely.[8,9] Percutaneous absorption is known to occur through two major pathways: (1) through the cells of the stratum corneum and the epidermal malpighian layer (the transepidermal route) and (2) through the hair follicle-sebaceous gland component (the transappendageal route). Increased neonatal percutaneous absorption may be due to the increased skin surface area-to-weight ratio, as well as the stratum corneum immaturity seen in premature neonates. Although transdermal delivery methods may be distinctly advantageous in certain settings, extreme caution must be exercised in the application of topical substances to the skin of infants, given the risk of systemic absorption and potential toxicity. Table 2.1 lists some compounds reported in association with percutaneous toxicity in the newborn.

Skin Care of the Newborn

The skin of the newborn is covered with a grayish-white greasy material termed *vernix caseosa*. The vernix represents a physiologic protective covering derived partially by secretion of the sebaceous glands and in part as a decomposition product of the infant's epidermis. Although its function is not completely understood, it may act as a natural protectant cream to 'waterproof' the fetus *in utero*, while submerged in the amniotic fluid.[10] Some studies suggest that vernix be left on as a protective coating for the newborn skin and that it be allowed to come off by itself with successive changes of clothing (generally within the first few weeks of life).

The skin acts as a protective organ. Any break in its integrity, therefore, affords an opportunity for initiation of infection. The importance of skin care in the newborn is compounded by several factors:

1. The infant does not have protective skin flora at birth.
2. The infant has at least one, and possibly two, open surgical wounds (the umbilicus and circumcision site).
3. The infant is exposed to fomites and personnel that potentially harbor a variety of infectious agents.

Skin care should involve gentle cleansing with a non-toxic, non-abrasive neutral material. During the 1950s, the use of hexachlorophene-containing compounds became routine for the skin care of newborns as prophylaxis against *Staphylococcus aureus* infection. In 1971 and 1972, however, the use of hexachlorophene preparations as skin cleansers for newborns was restricted because of studies demonstrating vacuolization in the central nervous system of infants and laboratory animals after prolonged application of these preparations.[11] At the minimum, neonatal skin care should include gentle removal of blood from the face and head, and meconium from the perianal area, by gentle water rinsing. Ideally, vernix caseosa should be removed from the face only, allowing the remaining vernix to come off by itself. However, the common standard of care is for gentle drying and wiping of the newborn's entire skin surface, which is most desirable from a thermoregulatory standpoint. For the remainder of the infant's stay in the hospital nursery, the buttocks and perianal regions should be cleansed with water and cotton or a gentle cloth. A mild soap with water rinsing may also be used at diaper changes if desired.

There is no single method of umbilical cord care that has been proven to limit colonization and disease. Several methods include local application of isopropyl alcohol, triple dye (an aqueous solution of brilliant green, proflavine, and gentian violet), and antimicrobial agents such as bacitracin or silver sulfadiazine cream. The routine use of povidone-iodine should be discouraged, given the risk of iodine absorption and transient hypothyroxinemia or hypothyroidism. A safer alternative is a chlorhexidine-containing product.[12]

Physiologic phenomena of the newborn

Neonatal dermatology, by definition, encompasses the spectrum of cutaneous disorders that arise during the first 4 weeks of life. Many such conditions are transient, appearing in the first few days to weeks of life, only to disappear shortly thereafter. The appreciation of normal phenomena and their differentiation from the more significant cutaneous disorders of the newborn is critical for the general physician, obstetrician, and pediatrician, as well as for the pediatric dermatologist.

At birth, the skin of the full-term infant is normally soft, smooth, and velvety. Desquamation of neonatal skin generally takes place

Table 2.1 Reported hazards of percutaneous absorption in the newborn

Compound	Product	Toxicity
Aniline	Dye used as laundry marker	Methemoglobinemia, death
Mercury	Diaper rinses; teething powders	Rash, hypotonia
Phenolic compounds		
Pentachlorophenol	Laundry disinfectant	Tachycardia, sweating, hepatomegaly, metabolic acidosis, death
Hexachlorophene	Topical antiseptic	Vacuolar encephalopathy, death
Resorcinol	Topical antiseptic	Methemoglobinemia
Boric acid	Baby powder	Vomiting, diarrhea, erythroderma, seizures, death
Lindane	Scabicide	Neurotoxicity
Salicylic acid	Keratolytic emollient	Metabolic acidosis, salicylism
Isopropyl alcohol	Topical antiseptic	Cutaneous hemorrhagic necrosis
Silver sulfadiazine	Topical antibiotic	Kernicterus, argyria
Urea	Keratolytic emollient	Uremia
Povidone-iodine	Topical antiseptic	Hypothyroidism, goiter
Neomycin	Topical antibiotic	Neural deafness
Corticosteroids	Topical anti-inflammatory	Skin atrophy, adrenal suppression
Benzocaine	Mucosal anesthetic	Methemoglobinemia
Prilocaine	Epidermal anesthetic	Methemoglobinemia
Methylene blue	Amniotic fluid leak	Methemoglobinemia

Reprinted with permission from Siegfried EC. Neonatal skin care and toxicology. In: Eichenfield LF, Frieden IJ, Esterly NB, eds.Textbook of neonatal dermatology. Philadelphia: WB Saunders; 2001:62–72.

24–36 h after delivery and may not be complete until the third week of life. Desquamation at birth is an abnormal phenomenon and is indicative of postmaturity, intrauterine anoxia, or congenital ichthyosis.

The skin at birth has a purplish-red color that is most pronounced over the extremities. Except for the hands, feet, and lips, where the transition is gradual, this quickly changes to a pink hue. In a great number of infants, a purplish discoloration of the hands, feet, and lips occurs during periods of crying, breath holding, or chilling. This normal phenomenon, termed *acrocyanosis*, appears to be associated with an increased tone of peripheral arterioles, which in turn creates vasospasm, secondary dilatation, and pooling of blood in the venous plexuses, resulting in a cyanotic appearance to the involved areas of the skin. The intensity of cyanosis depends on the degree of oxygen loss and the depth, size, and fullness of the involved venous plexus. Acrocyanosis, a normal physiologic phenomenon, should not be confused with true cyanosis.

Cutis Marmorata

Cutis marmorata is a normal reticulated bluish mottling of the skin seen on the trunk and extremities of infants and young children (Fig. 2.1). This phenomenon, a physiologic response to chilling with resultant dilatation of capillaries and small venules, usually disappears as the infant is rewarmed. Although a tendency to cutis marmorata may persist for several weeks or months, this disorder bears no medical significance and treatment generally is unnecessary. In some children cutis marmorata may tend to recur until early childhood, and in patients with Down syndrome, trisomy 18, and the Cornelia de Lange syndrome, this reticulated marbling pattern may be persistent. When the changes are persistent (even with rewarming) and are deep violaceous in color, *cutis marmorata telangiectatica congenita* (Fig. 2.2; see also Ch. 12) should be considered. In some infants a white negative pattern of cutis marmorata (*cutis marmorata alba*) may be created by a transient hypertonia of

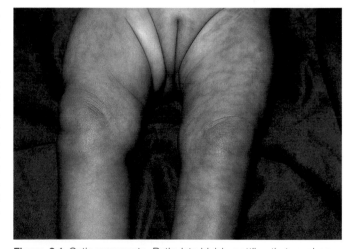

Figure 2.1 Cutis marmorata. Reticulate bluish mottling that resolves with rewarming.

the deep vasculature. Cutis marmorata alba is also a transitory disorder and appears to have no clinical significance.

Harlequin Color Change

Harlequin color change, not to be confused with harlequin ichthyosis (see Ch. 5), is occasionally observed in full-term infants but usually occurs in premature infants. It occurs when the infant is lying on his or her side and consists of reddening of one half of the body with simultaneous blanching of the other half. Attacks develop suddenly and may persist for 30 s–20 min. The side that lies uppermost is paler, and a clear line of demarcation runs along the midline of the body. At times, this line of demarcation may be incomplete; and when attacks are mild, areas of the face and genitalia may not be involved.

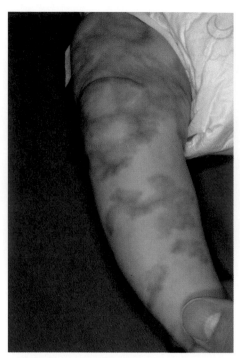

Figure 2.2 Cutis marmorata telangiectatica congenita. Violaceous, reticulate patches with subtle atrophy. These changes did not resolve with rewarming, and were associated with mild ipsilateral limb hypoplasia.

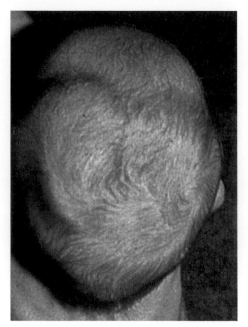

Figure 2.3 Cephalohematoma. Note the sharp demarcation at the midline.

This phenomenon appears to be related to immaturity of hypothalamic centers that control the tone of peripheral blood vessels and has been observed in infants with severe intracranial injury as well as in infants who appear to be otherwise perfectly normal. Although the peak frequency of attacks of harlequin color change generally occurs between the second and fifth days of life, attacks may occur anywhere from the first few hours to as late as the second or the third week of life.[13]

Bronze Baby Syndrome

The bronze baby syndrome is a term used to describe infants who develop a grayish-brown discoloration of the skin, serum, and urine while undergoing phototherapy for hyperbilirubinemia. Although the exact source of the pigment causing the discoloration is not clear, the syndrome usually begins 1–7 days after the initiation of phototherapy, resolves gradually over a period of several weeks after phototherapy is discontinued, and appears to be related to a combination of photoisomers of bilirubin or biliverdin or a photoproduct of copper-porphyrin metabolism.[14–16] Infants who develop bronze baby syndrome may have modified liver function, particularly cholestasis, of various origins.[17] The disorder should be differentiated from neonatal jaundice, cyanosis associated with neonatal pulmonary disorders or congenital heart disease, an unusual progressive hyperpigmentation (universal-acquired melanosis, the 'carbon baby' syndrome),[18] and chloramphenicol intoxication (the 'gray baby' syndrome), which is a disorder in infants with immature liver function, who are unable to conjugate chloramphenicol characterized by elevated serum chloramphenicol levels, progressive cyanosis, abdominal distention, hypothermia, vomiting, irregular respiration, and vasomotor collapse.[19] A distinctive purpuric eruption on exposed skin has also been described in newborns receiving phototherapy, possibly related to a transient increase in circulating porphyrins.[20] This condition, however, is unlikely to be confused with bronze baby syndrome.

Cephalohematoma

A cephalohematoma is a subperiosteal hematoma overlying the calvarium. These lesions are more common following prolonged labor, instrument-assisted deliveries, and abnormal presentations. They usually develop over the first hours of life and present as subcutaneous swellings in the scalp. They do not cross the midline (Fig. 2.3), as they are limited to one cranial bone, which helps to distinguish them from caput succedaneum (see below). Occasionally, a cephalohematoma may occur over a linear skull fracture. Other potentially associated complications include calcification (which may persist radiographically for years), hyperbilirubinemia, and infection. Although infected lesions (which are rare) may require aspiration,[21] most lesions require no therapy, with spontaneous resorption and resolution occurring over several months.

Caput succedaneum

Caput succedaneum is a localized edema of the newborn scalp related to the mechanical forces involved in parturition. It is probably related to venous congestion and edema secondary to cervical and uterine pressure, and as such, is more common with prolonged parturition and seen most often in primigravidas. Caput presents as a boggy scalp mass, and may result in varying degrees of bruising and necrosis in addition to the edema, at times with tissue loss. In distinction to cephalohematoma, caput succedaneum lesions often cross the midline. These lesions tend to resolve spontaneously over 48 h, and treatment is generally unnecessary. One possible complication in cases of severe caput succedaneum is permanent alopecia. 'Halo scalp ring' refers to an annular alopecia that presents in a circumferential ring around the scalp in infants with a history of caput.[22] It represents a pressure necrosis phenomenon, and the hair loss may be transient or, occasionally, permanent.

Complications from fetal and neonatal diagnostic procedures

Fetal complications associated with invasive prenatal diagnostic procedures include cutaneous puncture marks, scars or lacerations, exsanguination, ocular trauma, blindness, subdural hemorrhage, pneumothorax, cardiac tamponade, splenic laceration, porencephalic cysts, arteriovenous or ileocutaneous fistulas, digital loss (in 1.7% of newborns whose mothers had undergone early chorionic villus sampling), musculoskeletal trauma, disruption of tendons or ligaments, and occasionally gangrene. Cutaneous puncture marks, which occur in 1–3% of newborns whose mothers had undergone amniocentesis, may be seen as single or multiple 1–6 mm pits or dimples on any cutaneous surface of the newborn (Fig. 2.4).[23,24]

Fetal scalp monitoring can result in infection, bleeding, or fontanelle puncture, and prenatal vacuum extraction can produce a localized area of edema, ecchymosis, or localized alopecia. The incidence of scalp electrode infection varies from 0.3% to 5.0%, and although local sterile abscesses account for the majority of adverse sequelae, *S. aureus* or Gram-negative infections, cellulitis, tissue necrosis, subgaleal abscess, osteomyelitis, necrotizing fasciitis, and neonatal herpes simplex infections may also occur as complications of this procedure (Fig. 2.5) .[25–27]

Transcutaneous oxygen monitoring (application of heated electrodes to the skin for continuous detection of tissue oxygenation) and pulse oximetry may also result in erythema, tissue necrosis, and first- or second-degree burns. Although lesions associated with transcutaneous oxygen monitoring generally resolve within 48–60 h, persistent atrophic hyperpigmented craters may at times be seen as a complication. Frequent (2- to 4-h) changing of electrode sites and reduction of the temperature of the electrodes to 43°C, however, can lessen the likelihood of this complication.[28,29]

Anetoderma of prematurity refers to macular depressions or outpouchings of skin associated with loss of dermal elastic tissue seen in premature infants. Reports suggest that these cutaneous lesions may correlate with placement of electrocardiographic or other monitoring electrodes or leads.[30,31]

Calcinosis cutis may occur on the scalp or chest of infants or children at sites of electroencephalograph or electrocardiograph electrode placement, as a result of diagnostic heel sticks performed during the neonatal period, or following intramuscular or intravenous administration of calcium chloride or calcium gluconate for the treatment of neonatal hypocalcemia. Seen primarily in high-risk infants who receive repeated heel sticks for blood chemistry determinations, calcified nodules usually begin as small depressions on the heels. With time, generally after 4–12 months, tiny yellow or white papules appear (Fig. 2.6), gradually enlarge to form nodular deposits, migrate to the cutaneous surface, extrude their contents, and generally disappear spontaneously by the time the child reaches 18–30 months of age. Although calcified heel nodules are usually asymptomatic, children may at times show signs of discomfort with standing or with the wearing of shoes. In such instances, gentle cryosurgery and curettage can be both diagnostic and therapeutic. Calcinosis cutis following electroencephalography or electrocardiography is more likely to be seen in infants and young children or individuals where the skin has been abraded and usually disappears spontaneously within 2–6 months. It can be avoided by the use of an electrode paste that does not contain calcium chloride and, like calcified heel sticks, may be treated by gentle cryosurgery and curettage.[32,33]

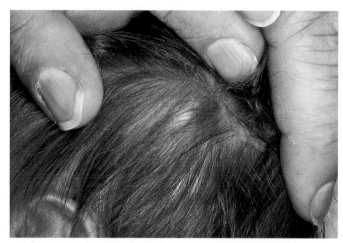

Figure 2.5 Staphylococcal scalp abscess. Fluctuant, erythematous nodule on the scalp of this 9-day-old infant as a complication of intrauterine fetal monitoring.

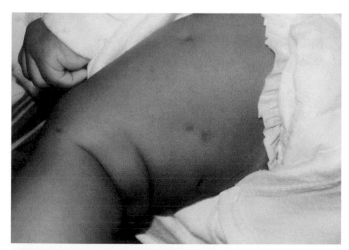

Figure 2.4 Amniocentesis scars. Multiple depressed scars on the thigh of an infant born to a mother who had amniocentesis during pregnancy. (Courtesy of Lester Schwartz MD.)

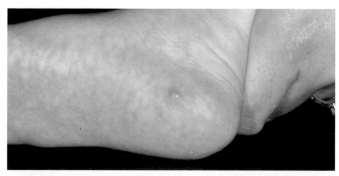

Figure 2.6 Heel stick calcinosis. Firm, white-yellow papules on the plantar and lateral heel in an infant who had multiple heel sticks as a newborn.

Abnormalities of subcutaneous tissue

Skin turgor is generally normal during the first few hours of life. As normal physiologic dehydration occurs during the first 3 or 4 days of life (up to 10% of birthweight), the skin generally becomes loose and wrinkled. Subcutaneous fat, normally quite adequate at birth, increases until about 9 months of age, thus accounting for the traditional chubby appearance of the healthy newborn. A decrease or absence of this normal panniculus is abnormal and suggests the possibility of prematurity, postmaturity, or placental insufficiency.

Sclerema neonatorum and subcutaneous fat necrosis are two disorders that affect the subcutaneous fat of the newborn. Although there is considerable diagnostic confusion between these two entities, there are several distinguishing features that enable a clinical differentiation (Table 2.2). Sclerema neonatorum seems to occur with significantly less frequency than subcutaneous fat necrosis.

Sclerema Neonatorum

Sclerema neonatorum is a diffuse, rapidly spreading, waxlike hardening of the skin and subcutaneous tissue that occurs in premature or debilitated infants during the first few weeks of life. The disorder, usually associated with a serious underlying condition such as sepsis or other infection, congenital heart disease, respiratory distress, diarrhea, or dehydration, is characterized by a diffuse non-pitting woody induration of the involved tissues. The process is symmetrical, usually starting on the legs and buttocks, and may progress to involve all areas except the palms, soles, and genitalia.[34] As the disorder spreads, the skin becomes cold, yellowish white, mottled, stony hard, and cadaver-like. The limbs become immobile, and the face acquires a fixed mask-like expression. The infants become sluggish, feed poorly, show clinical signs of shock, and in a high percentage of cases die.

Although the etiology of this disorder is unknown, it appears to represent a nonspecific sign of severe illness rather than a primary disease. Infants with this disorder are characteristically small or premature, debilitated, weak, cyanotic, and lethargic. In 25% of cases the mothers are ill at the time of delivery. Exposure to cold, hypothermia, peripheral chilling with vascular collapse, and an increase in the ratio of saturated to unsaturated fatty acids in the triglyceride fraction of the subcutaneous tissue (because of a defect in fatty acid mobilization) have been hypothesized as possible causes for this disorder but lack confirmation.[35]

The histopathologic findings of sclerema neonatorum consist of edema and thickening of the connective tissue bands around the fat lobules. Although necrosis and crystallization of the subcutaneous tissue have been described, these findings are more characteristically seen in lesions of subcutaneous fat necrosis.

The prognosis of sclerema neonatorum is poor, and mortality occurs in 50–75% of affected infants. In those infants who survive, the cutaneous findings resolve without residual sequelae. There is no specific therapy, although steroids and exchange transfusion have been used.[34]

Subcutaneous Fat Necrosis

Subcutaneous fat necrosis (SCFN) is a benign self-limited disease that affects apparently healthy full-term newborns and young infants. It is characterized by sharply circumscribed, indurated, and nodular areas of fat necrosis (Fig. 2.7). The etiology of this disorder remains unknown but appears to be related to perinatal trauma, asphyxia, hypothermia, and, in some instances, hypercalcemia.[36,37] Although the mechanism of hypercalcemia in SCFN is not known, it has been attributed to aberrations in vitamin D or parathyroid homeostasis. Birth asphyxia and meconium aspiration seem to be frequently associated. In one large series, 10 out of 11 infants with SCFN had been delivered via emergency cesarean section for fetal distress, and 9 of the 11 had meconium staining of the amniotic fluid.[38] The relationship between subcutaneous fat necrosis, maternal diabetes and cesarean section, if any, is unclear. SCFN following icebag application for treatment of supraventricular tachycardia has been reported.[39]

The onset of SCFN is generally during the first few days to weeks of life. Lesions appear as single or multiple localized, sharply circumscribed, usually painless areas of induration. Occasionally, the affected areas may be tender and infants may be uncomfortable and cry vigorously when they are handled. Lesions vary from small erythematous, indurated nodules to large plaques, and sites of predilection include the cheeks, back, buttocks, arms, and thighs. Many lesions have an uneven lobulated surface with an elevated margin separating it from the surrounding normal tissue. Histologic examination of SCFN reveals larger than usual fat lobules and an

Sclerema neonatorum	Subcutaneous fat necrosis
Premature infants	Full-term or postmature infants
Serious underlying disease (sepsis, cardiopulmonary disease, diarrhea, or dehydration)	Healthy newborns; may have history of perinatal asphyxia or difficult delivery
Wax-like hardening of skin and subcutaneous tissue	Circumscribed, indurated, erythematous nodules and plaques
Whole body except palms, soles	Buttocks, thighs, arms, face, shoulders
Poor prognosis; high mortality	Excellent prognosis; treat associated hypercalcemia, if present

Table 2.2 Features of sclerema neonatorum and subcutaneous fat necrosis

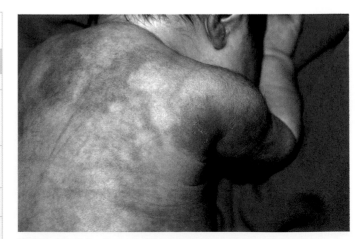

Figure 2.7 Subcutaneous fat necrosis. Indurated, erythematous plaques on the shoulders and back of this 1-week-old boy.

extensive inflammatory infiltrate, needle-shaped clefts within fat cells, necrosis, and calcification. Magnetic resonance imaging (MRI) reveals decreased T1 and increased T2 signal intensity in affected areas.[40]

The prognosis for SCFN is excellent. Although lesions may develop extensive deposits of calcium, which may liquefy, drain, and heal with scarring, most areas undergo spontaneous resolution within several weeks to months. Hypercalcemia is a rare association, and infants with this finding may require low calcium intake, restriction of vitamin D, and/or systemic corticosteroid therapy. Etidronate therapy has been reported for treatment of recalcitrant SCFN-associated hypercalcemia.[41] Infants should be followed for several months following delivery, as the onset of hypercalcemia can be delayed for several months.[38,42] Other rare systemic complications may include thrombocytopenia, hypoglycemia and hypertriglyceridemia, all of which tend to be mild and/or self-limited.

Miscellaneous cutaneous disorders

Miliaria

Differentiation of the epidermis and its appendages, particularly in the premature infant, is frequently incomplete at birth. As a result of this immaturity, a high incidence of sweat-retention phenomena may be seen in the newborn. Miliaria, a common neonatal dermatosis caused by sweat retention, is characterized by a vesicular eruption with subsequent maceration and obstruction of the eccrine ducts. The pathophysiologic events that lead to this disorder are keratinous plugging of eccrine ducts and the escape of eccrine sweat into the skin below the level of obstruction (see Ch. 8).

Virtually all infants develop miliaria under appropriate conditions. There are two principal forms of this disorder:

1. *Miliaria crystallina* (sudamina), which consists of clear superficial pinpoint vesicles without an inflammatory areola
2. *Miliaria rubra* (prickly heat), representing a deeper level of sweat gland obstruction, and characterized by small discrete erythematous papules, vesicles, or papulovesicles (Fig. 2.8).

The incidence of miliaria is greatest in the first few weeks of life owing to the relative immaturity of the eccrine ducts, which favors poral closure and sweat retention. A pustular form of miliaria rubra

has been observed in association with pseudohypoaldosteronism during salt-losing crises.[43]

Therapy for miliaria is directed toward avoidance of excessive heat and humidity. Light-weight cotton clothing, cool baths, and air conditioning are helpful in the management and prevention of this disorder. Avoidance of emollient overapplication (i.e., in infants with atopic dermatitis) should also be recommended, especially in warm, humid climates or in the winter when infants are bundled under heavy clothing.

Milia

Milia, small retention cysts, commonly occur on the face of newborns. Seen in 40–50% of infants, they result from retention of keratin within the dermis. They appear as tiny 1–2 mm pearly white or yellow papules. Particularly prominent on the cheeks, nose, chin, and forehead, they may be few or numerous and are frequently grouped (Fig. 2.9). Lesions may occasionally occur on the upper trunk, limbs, penis, or mucous membranes. Although milia of the newborn may persist into the second or third month, they usually disappear spontaneously during the first 3 or 4 weeks of life and, accordingly, require no therapy. Persistent milia in an unusual or widespread distribution, particularly when seen in association with other defects, may be seen as a manifestation of hereditary trichodysplasia (Marie-Unna hypotrichosis), dystrophic forms of epidermolysis bullosa, Bazex or Rombo syndromes, or the oral-facial-digital syndrome type I.

Bohn's Nodules and Epstein's Pearls

Discrete, 2–3 mm round, pearly white or yellow, freely movable elevations at the gum margins or midline of the hard palate (termed *Bohn's nodules* and *Epstein's pearls*, respectively) are seen in up to 85% of newborns. Clinically and histologically, the counterpart of facial milia, they disappear spontaneously, usually within a few weeks of life, and require no therapy.

Sebaceous Gland Hyperplasia

Sebaceous gland hyperplasia represents a physiologic phenomenon of the newborn manifested as multiple, yellow to flesh-colored tiny

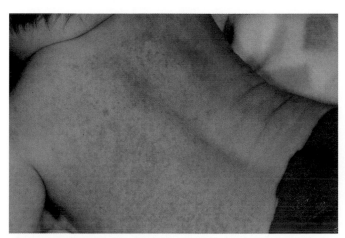

Figure 2.8 Miliaria rubra. Multiple, erythematous, pinpoint macules and papules, especially prominent on the occluded surface of the back. This infant was being followed for the segmental infantile hemangioma present on her lower back.

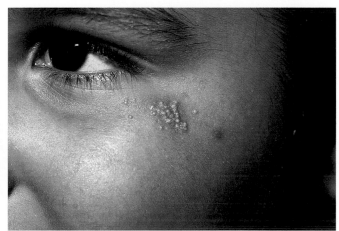

Figure 2.9 Milia. Clustered, small white papules on the lateral cheek.

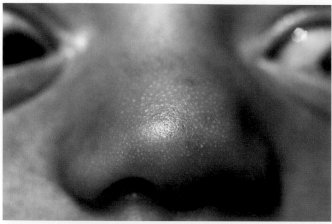

Figure 2.10 Sebaceous gland hyperplasia. Yellow-white, pinpoint papules on the nasal tip of this 2-day-old boy.

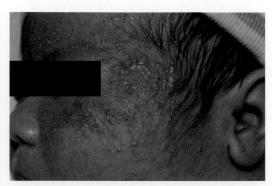

Figure 2.12 Neonatal cephalic pustulosis. This 1-week-old male had numerous small and large pustules on the forehead, cheeks and chin. They cleared rapidly with ketoconazole cream.

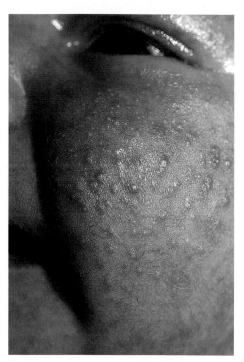

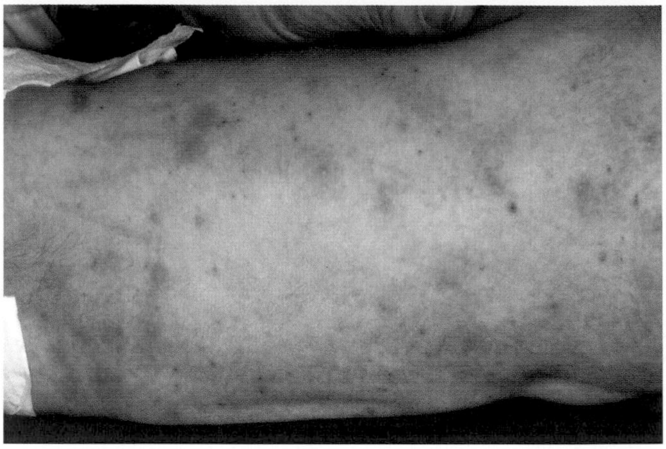

Figure 2.11 Acne neonatorum. Erythematous papules and papulopustules on the cheek.

Figure 2.13 Erythema toxicum neonatorum. Blotchy, erythematous macules and edematous papules.

papules that occur on the nose (Fig. 2.10), cheeks, and upper lips of full-term infants. A manifestation of maternal androgen stimulation, these papules represent a temporary disorder that resolves spontaneously, generally within the first few weeks of life.

Acne Neonatorum

Occasionally infants develop a facial eruption that resembles acne vulgaris as seen in adolescents (Fig. 2.11). Although the etiology of this disorder is not clearly defined, it appears to develop as a result of hormonal stimulation of sebaceous glands that have not yet involuted to their childhood state of immaturity. In mild cases of

acne neonatorum, therapy is often unnecessary; daily cleansing with soap and water may be all that is required. Occasionally, mild keratolytic agents or topical antibiotics may be helpful (see Ch. 8). Unusually severe or recalcitrant cases of acne neonatorum warrant investigation for underlying androgen excess.

A facial acneiform eruption in infants has been associated with the saprophytic *Malassezia* species, and has been termed *neonatal cephalic pustulosis*. Lesions consist of pinpoint papules, papulopustules, or larger pustules, and they are located on the cheeks, (Fig. 2.12), chin, and forehead. A correlation may exist between the clinical severity of lesions and the colonization with this fungal saprophyte.[44,45] In these infants, topical antifungal agents may lead to more rapid resolution of lesions.

Erythema Toxicum Neonatorum

Erythema toxicum neonatorum (ETN), also known as toxic erythema of the newborn, is an idiopathic, asymptomatic, benign self-limiting cutaneous eruption of full-term newborns. Lesions consist of erythematous macules, papules, and pustules (Fig. 2.13), or a combination of these, and may occur anywhere on the body, especially the forehead, face, trunk, and extremities. The fact that these lesions (which histologically reveal follicular-centered eosinophils) frequently tend to spare the palms and soles may be explained by the absence of pilosebaceous follicles in these areas.

ETN often initially appears as a blotchy, macular erythema that then develops firm 1–3 mm, pale-yellow or white papules and pustules. The erythematous macules are irregular or splotchy in appearance, varying from a few millimeters to several centimeters in diameter. They may be seen in sharp contrast to the surrounding unaffected skin, may blend into a surrounding erythema, or may progress to a confluent eruption.

Although ETN appears most frequently during the first 3–4 days of life, it has been seen at birth and may be noted as late as 10 days of age.[46] Exacerbations and remissions may occur during the first 2 weeks of life, and the duration of individual lesions varies from a few hours to several days. The etiology of ETN remains obscure. One study suggested that it represents an immune response to microbial colonization of the skin at the hair follicle.[47] ETN incidence data are variable. Some authors report an incidence as low as 4.5%; others report incidences varying from 31% to 70% of newborns.[48] The incidence of ETN clearly appears to increase with increasing gestational age of the infant.[49] No sexual or racial predisposition has been noted.

ETN is usually diagnosed clinically. Skin biopsy, which is rarely necessary, reveals a characteristic accumulation of eosinophils within the pilosebaceous apparatus. The diagnosis can be rapidly differentiated from other newborn pustular conditions by cytologic examination of a pustule smear that, with Wright's or Giemsa staining, reveals a predominance of eosinophils. Affected infants may have a peripheral eosinophilia. Although the eosinophilic response has led some observers to attribute the etiology of this disorder to a hypersensitivity reaction, specific allergens have never been implicated or confirmed.

Since erythema toxicum is a benign self-limiting asymptomatic disorder, no therapy is indicated. Occasionally, however, it may be confused with other pustular eruptions of the neonatal period, including transient neonatal pustular melanosis, milia, miliaria, and congenital infections including candidiasis, herpes simplex, or bacterial processes. Of these, the congenital infections are the most important diagnostic considerations because of the implications for possible systemic involvement. Table 2.3 lists the differential diagnosis of the newborn with vesicles or pustules.

Eosinophilic Pustular Folliculitis

Eosinophilic pustular folliculitis (EPF) is an idiopathic dermatosis that occurs in both adults and infants, and when occurring in neonates or young infants, it may be clinically confused with other vesiculopustular disorders. Lesions consist of follicular pustules, most commonly occurring on the scalp and the extremities. They tend to recur in crops, in a similar fashion to acropustulosis of infancy (see below), and some suggest that these conditions may be related.[50,51] As opposed to the adult form of EPF, the infancy-associated type does not reveal lesions grouped in an annular arrangement.

Histologic evaluation reveals an eosinophilic, follicular inflammatory infiltrate, and peripheral eosinophilia may be present. EPF of infancy appears to be distinct from classic (adult) and HIV-associated EPF, although an HIV-infected infant with EPF has been reported.[52] Importantly, infantile EPF may occasionally be the presenting sign of hyperimmunoglobulinemia E syndrome (HIES) (see Ch. 3). Treatment for EPF is symptomatic, including topical corti-

Table 2.3 Differential diagnosis of vesicles or pustules in a newborn

Clinical disorder	Comments
Acrodermatitis enteropathica	Periorificial erosive dermatitis common
Acropustulosis of infancy	Recurrent crops of acral pustules
Eosinophilic folliculitis	Scalp and extremities most common sites
Epidermolysis bullosa	Trauma-induced blistering; bullae, and erosions
Erythema toxicum neonatorum	Blotchy erythema, evanescent
Incontinentia pigmenti	XLD; linear and whorled patterns

Infectious
  Bacterial
    Group A or B streptococci
    Staphylococcus aureus
 	
    Listeria monocytogenes
    Pseudomonas aeruginosa
    Other Gram-negatives
  Fungal
    Candidiasis
 	
  Viral
    Herpes simplex
 	
    Varicella zoster
    Cytomegalovirus
 	
  Spirochetal
    Syphilis
	
	Superficial blisters rupture easily
	
	Palms and soles involved; nail changes
	
	3 types: SEM, CNS, disseminated
	
	'Blueberry muffin' more common
	
	Red maculos, papules; palm and sole scaling

Langerhans cell histiocytosis	Crusting, erosions, palms and soles, LAD
Miliaria	Especially intertriginous, occluded sites
Neonatal Behçet's	
Pustular psoriasis	
Scabies	Crusting, burrows
Transient neonatal pustular melanosis	Mainly blacks; pigment persists for months
Urticaria pigmentosa	Stroking leads to urtication (Darier's sign)

XLD, X-linked dominant; SEM, skin-eyes-mouth; CNS, central nervous system; LAD, lymphadenopathy.

costeroids and antihistamines, with eventual spontaneous resolution by 3 years of age in the majority of patients.

Impetigo Neonatorum

Impetigo in newborns may occur as early as the second or third day or as late as the second week of life. It usually presents as a superficial vesicular, pustular, or bullous lesion on an erythematous base. Vesicles and bullae are easily denuded, leaving a red, raw, and moist surface, usually without crust formation. Blisters are often wrinkled, contain some fluid, and are easily denuded. Lesions tend to occur on moist or opposing surfaces of the skin, as in the diaper area, groin, axillae, and neck folds. *S. aureus pustulosis* (or *neonatal pustulosis*) is a characteristic manifestation of cutaneous *S. aureus* infection in the neonate or infant. Patients present with small pustules on an erythematous base (Fig. 2.14A), often distributed in the diaper region. The lesions denude easily upon swabbing (Fig. 2.14B), and culture is positive for *S. aureus*. In term or late pre-term neonates with localized involvement, and without fever or systemic symptoms, evaluation for serious bacterial illness is generally not required, and treatment in the outpatient setting is often sufficient.[53]

The term *pemphigus neonatorum* is an archaic misnomer occasionally applied to superficial bullous lesions of severe impetigo widely distributed over the surface of the body. However, a transient neonatal form of pemphigus vulgaris does exist, and is caused by transplacental passage of antibodies from a mother with the same disease (see Ch. 13).

Sucking Blisters

Sucking blisters, presumed to be induced by vigorous sucking on the affected part *in utero*, are seen in up to 0.5% of normal newborns as 0.5–2 cm oval bullae or erosions on the dorsal aspect of the fingers, thumbs, wrists, lips, or radial aspect of the forearms. These lesions, which must be differentiated from bullous impetigo, epidermolysis bullosa, and herpes neonatorum, resolve rapidly and without sequelae.

Transient Neonatal Pustular Melanosis

Transient neonatal pustular melanosis (TNPM) is a benign self-limiting disorder of unknown etiology characterized by superficial vesiculopustular lesions that rupture easily and evolve into hyperpigmented macules (Fig. 2.15). This disorder is seen in <1% of newborns,[54] and occurs most commonly in infants with black skin. Lesions begin as superficial sterile pustules (Fig. 2.16) that rupture easily to leave a collarette of fine white scale around a small hyperpigmented macule. Although the distribution may be diffuse, common areas of involvement include the inferior chin, forehead, neck, lower back, and shins. Rarely, vesicles that do not progress to pigmented macules may be detected on the scalp, palms, and soles.

Wright-stained smears of the pustules of TNPM, in contrast to lesions of erythema toxicum neonatorum, demonstrate variable numbers of neutrophils, few or no eosinophils, and cellular debris. Histopathologic evaluation is usually unnecessary.

TNPM is a benign disorder without associated systemic manifestations, and therapy is unnecessary. The pustular lesions usually

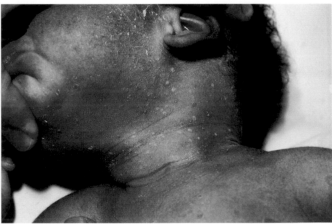

Figure 2.15 Transient neonatal pustular melanosis. Papules and papulopustules which rupture to leave a collarette of fine scales and eventual hyperpigmentation. (Courtesy of Nancy B. Esterly MD)

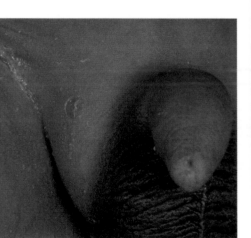

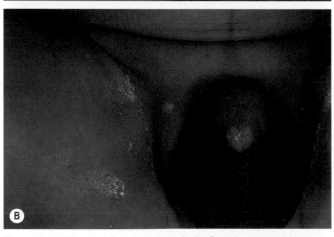

Figure 2.14 Neonatal *S. aureus* pustulosis. Pustule on a red base in the groin of a 6-day-old male (A). Note easy denudation and superficial erosion following skin swabbing (B). The culture was positive for *Staphylococcus aureus*.

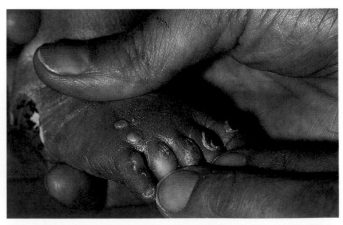

Figure 2.16 Transient neonatal pustular melanosis. Tense pustules and collarettes of scale at sites of older lesions.

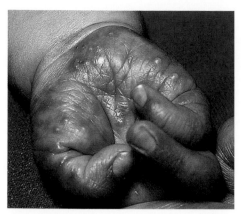

Figure 2.17 Acropustulosis of infancy. Multiple tense erythematous papules and pustules on the palm of this 4-month-old girl.

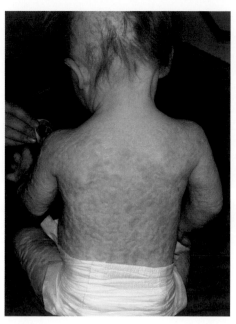

Figure 2.18 Congenital erosive and vesicular dermatosis healing with reticulated supple scarring. Generalized, supple, reticulated scarring. Note also the associated scalp alopecia.

disappear within 24–48 h, leaving behind hyperpigmented macules that fade gradually, usually over several weeks to months.

Acropustulosis of Infancy

Acropustulosis of infancy, also known as infantile acropustulosis (IA), is an idiopathic pustular disorder with onset usually between birth and 2 years of age. It is characterized by recurrent, pruritic vesiculopustular lesions that recur every few weeks to months. The lesions begin as pinpoint erythematous papules and enlarge into well-circumscribed discrete pustules.[55] They are concentrated on the palms (Fig. 2.17) and soles and appear in lesser numbers on the dorsal aspect of the hands, feet, wrists, and ankles. Occasional lesions may occur on the face and scalp.

The differential diagnosis of IA includes dyshidrotic eczema, pustular psoriasis, erythema toxicum neonatorum, transient neonatal pustular melanosis, scabies, impetigo, and subcorneal pustular dermatosis. However, the characteristic presentation and course of IA is usually distinctive enough to render a clinical diagnosis. A smear of pustule contents (or histologic evaluation) reveals large numbers of neutrophils, and occasionally eosinophils.[55–58] Although the etiology of IA remains unclear, several authors have noted a possible association with preceding scabies infestation.[59–61]

Patients with IA experience fewer and less intense flares of their lesions with time, and the entire process usually subsides within 2–3 years. Pruritus, however, may be severe early in the course, making therapy desirable. Possible associations include irritability, sleeplessness, excoriation, and secondary bacterial infection. Systemic antihistamines, usually in high doses, may relieve pruritus. High-potency topical corticosteroids are quite effective for this condition,[59] and given the limited distribution of lesions, the epidermal thickness at affected (acral) sites, and the periodicity of flares, concerns regarding systemic absorption of these medications should be minimal. Dapsone has long been a recommended therapy for severe cases, but the risk-to-benefit ratio of this agent is not generally justified in patients with IA.

Congenital Erosive and Vesicular Dermatosis

Congenital erosive and vesicular dermatosis healing with reticulated supple scarring is an uncommon disorder characterized by erosive and bullous lesions that, as the name implies, are present at birth and heal with characteristic scarring. Although its cause is unknown, it appears to represent a non-hereditary intrauterine event, such as infection or amniotic adhesions, or perhaps an unusual healing defect of immature skin. The disorder generally involves skin of the trunk, extremities, scalp, face, and occasionally the tongue, with sparing of the palms, and soles.

Congenital erosive and vesicular dermatosis occurs most often in premature infants, and patients present with extensive cutaneous ulcerations and intact vesicles that develop crusting and then heal during the first month of life. Occasionally, blistering may continue to occur beyond infancy.[62] Generalized, supple reticulated scars occur with alternating elevated and depressed areas (Fig. 2.18). Up to 75% of the cutaneous surface may be involved, and the skin lesions have been described as having depressed hypopigmented regions alternating with normally to hyperpigmented zones.[63,64] Scars on the trunk and head, which often have a cobblestone-like appearance, may be oriented along the cutaneous lines of cleavage; on the limbs they tend to follow the long axes of the extremities.[64–66] Although the eyebrows are usually normal, alopecia may be noted on the scalp. Nails may be absent or hypoplastic, and affected areas on the tongue may manifest scarring and absence of papillae. Hyperthermia, especially in warm weather or after exertion, is common and although sweating is absent in scarred areas, compensatory hyperhidrosis in normal-appearing skin may be noted. Chronic conjunctivitis is a major continuing problem for these patients, and corneal scarring may occur.[62,63] Some patients have also been found to have neurologic defects, including mental and motor retardation, hemiparesis, cerebral palsy, and seizures.[63]

Seborrheic Dermatitis

Seborrheic dermatitis is a common, self-limiting condition of the scalp, face, ears, trunk, and intertriginous areas characterized by greasy scaling, redness, fissuring, and occasional weeping. It appears to be related to the sebaceous glands and has a predilection for so-called 'seborrheic' areas where the density of these glands is high. It usually presents in infants with a scaly dermatitis of the scalp termed *cradle cap* (Fig. 2.19), and may spread over the face,

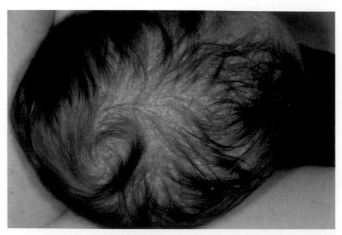

Figure 2.19 Seborrheic dermatitis of the scalp (cradle cap). Erythema and greasy yellow scales involving the scalp of an infant male, who also had similar changes in the eyebrows.

Table 2.4 Differential diagnosis of diaper dermatitis
Chafing dermatitis
Irritant contact dermatitis
Diaper candidiasis
Seborrheic dermatitis
Psoriasis
Intertrigo
Jacquet's dermatitis
Perianal pseudoverrucous papules and nodules
Miliaria
Folliculitis
Impetigo
Scabies
Nutritional deficiency (i.e., acrodermatitis enteropathica, cystic fibrosis, biotin deficiency)
Allergic contact dermatitis
Atopic dermatitis
Granuloma gluteale infantum
Langerhans cell histiocytosis
Burns
Child abuse
Epidermolysis bullosa
Congenital syphilis
Varicella/herpes
Tinea cruris
Chronic bullous dermatosis of childhood
Bullous mastocytosis

including the forehead, ears, eyebrows, and nose. Other areas of involvement include the intertriginous zones, umbilicus, and anogenital region. (For a more detailed discussion of seborrheic dermatitis and its therapy, see Ch. 3.)

Leiner Disease

The term *Leiner disease* refers to a shared phenotype for a number of nutritional and immunologic disorders, characterized by severe seborrheic dermatitis with exfoliation, failure to thrive, and diarrhea. The disorder may occur during the first week of life but generally starts around 2–4 months of age. Patients are particularly prone to recurrent yeast and Gram-negative infections. Among disorders that may show this phenotype are: deficiency or dysfunction of complement, Bruton's hypogammaglobulinemia, severe combined immunodeficiency, and HIES.[67–71]

Diaper Dermatitis

Diaper dermatitis is perhaps the most common cutaneous disorder of infancy and early childhood. The term is used to describe an acute inflammatory skin reaction in the areas covered by the diaper. The incidence of diaper dermatitis is estimated to be between 7% and 35%, with a peak incidence at 9–12 months of age.[72–74]

The term *diaper rash* is frequently used as a diagnosis, as though the diverse dermatoses that may affect this region constitute a single clinical entity. In actuality, diaper dermatitis is not a specific diagnosis and is best viewed as a variable symptom-complex initiated by a combination of factors, the most significant being prolonged contact with urine and feces, skin maceration, and, in many cases, secondary infection with bacteria or *Candida albicans*. Although diaper dermatitis may frequently be no more than a minor nuisance, eruptions in this area may not only progress to secondary infection and ulceration, but may become complicated by other superimposed cutaneous disorders or represent a manifestation of a more serious disease.

The three most common types of diaper dermatitis are chafing dermatitis, irritant contact dermatitis, and diaper candidiasis. However, the differential diagnosis of diaper dermatitis is broad (Table 2.4). In patients in whom a response to therapy is slow or absent, alternative diagnoses should be considered and appropriate diagnostic evaluations performed. The following is a brief discussion of several potential causes of diaper dermatitis. Many of these entities are discussed in more detail in other chapters.

Chafing dermatitis

The most prevalent form of diaper dermatitis is the chafing or frictional dermatitis that affects most infants at some time. Generally present on areas where friction is the most pronounced (the inner surfaces of the thighs, the genitalia, buttocks, and the abdomen), the eruption presents as mild redness and scaling and tends to wax and wane quickly. This form responds quickly to frequent diaper changes and good diaper hygiene.

Irritant contact dermatitis

Irritant contact diaper dermatitis usually involves the convex surfaces of the buttocks, the vulva, perineal area, lower abdomen, and proximal thighs, with sparing of the intertriginous creases (Fig. 2.20). The disorder may be attributable to contact with proteolytic enzymes in stool and irritant chemicals, such as soaps, detergents, and topical preparations. Other significant factors appear to be excessive heat, moisture, and sweat retention associated with the warm local environment produced by the diaper.

The etiology of irritant contact diaper dermatitis is multifactorial, and past hypotheses have included potential roles for ammonia, bacteria, and bacterial products and urine pH. In 1921, when Cooke demonstrated that an aerobic Gram-positive bacillus (*Bacillus ammoniagenes*) was capable of liberating ammonia from urea, this organism was pinpointed as the etiologic agent of most diaper dermatoses.[75] More recent studies, however, have refuted the role of urea-splitting bacteria in the etiology of this disorder and incriminate a combination of wetness, frictional damage, impervious diaper coverings, and increase in skin pH. It is suggested that urinary wetness increases the permeability of the skin to irritants as well as the pH of the diaper environment, thus intensifying the activities of the fecal proteases and lipases, the major irritants responsible for this disorder.[76,77]

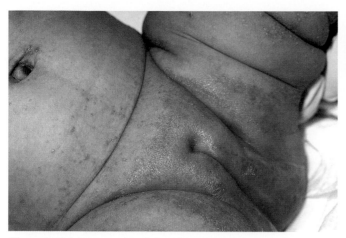

Figure 2.20 Irritant contact diaper dermatitis. Erythema of the vulva, buttocks, and medial thighs. The inguinal creases were relatively spared.

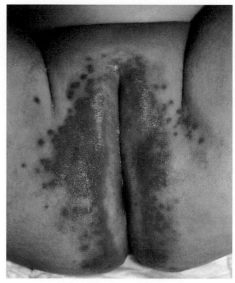

Figure 2.21 Diaper candidiasis. Beefy-red, erythematous plaques with multiple red satellite papules and papulopustules.

Several technological innovations in the design of disposable diapers and other diapering products have aimed to reduce moisture and irritancy in this environment, thus decreasing the risk of irritant dermatitis. The introduction of absorbent gelling materials into diaper technology was one such breakthrough, and has been shown to result in less diaper dermatitis than conventional cellulose core disposable diapers.[78] Other recent innovations include non-irritating disposable diaper wipes and diapers designed to deliver petrolatum-based formulations to the skin.[79]

Diaper candidiasis

Candidal (monilial) diaper dermatitis is a commonly overlooked disorder and should be suspected whenever a diaper rash fails to respond to usual therapeutic measures. Cutaneous candidiasis is a possible sequela of systemic antibiotic therapy and should be considered in any diaper dermatitis that develops during or shortly following antibiotic administration.[80]

Candidal diaper dermatitis presents as a widespread, beefy red erythema on the buttocks, lower abdomen, and inner aspects of the thighs. Characteristic features include a raised edge, sharp marginization with white scales at the border, and pinpoint pustulovesicular satellite lesions (the diagnostic hallmark) (Fig. 2.21). Although cutaneous candidiasis frequently occurs in association with oral thrush (Fig. 2.22), the oral mucosa may be uninvolved. Infants harbor *C. albicans* in the lower intestine, and it is from this focus that infected feces present the primary source for candidal diaper eruptions.

If necessary, the diagnosis of candidal diaper dermatitis may be confirmed by microscopic examination of a potassium hydroxide preparation of skin scrapings, which reveals egg-shaped budding yeasts and hyphae or pseudohyphae. Growth of yeast on Sabouraud's medium implanted with skin scrapings can also confirm the diagnosis, usually within 48–72 h.

Seborrheic dermatitis

Seborrheic dermatitis of the diaper area may be recognized by the characteristic salmon-colored, greasy plaques with a yellowish scale and a predilection for intertriginous areas (see above). Coincident involvement of the scalp, face, neck, and postauricular and flexural areas helps to establish the diagnosis.

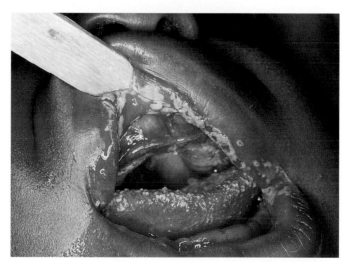

Figure 2.22 Oral candidiasis (thrush). Gray-white, cheesy patches and plaques of the buccal mucosa, tongue, and gingiva.

Psoriasis

Psoriasis of the diaper area must also be considered in persistent diaper eruptions that fail to respond to otherwise seemingly adequate therapy (Fig. 2.23). The sharp demarcation of lesions suggests diaper area psoriasis, but the typical scaling of psoriasis may be obscured because of the moisture of the diaper region. The presence of nail changes and red, well-marginated plaques with silvery mica-like scales on the trunk, face, axillae, umbilicus, or scalp may help confirm this diagnosis (see Ch. 4), although affected infants may have involvement limited to the diaper area.

Intertrigo

Intertrigo (see Ch. 17) is a common skin eruption in the diaper area, particularly in hot weather or when infants are overdressed. It usually involves the inguinal creases, the intergluteal area, and the thigh creases (especially in chubby babies), and presents as bright red erythema often with a mild white-yellow exudate.

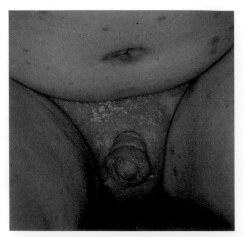

Figure 2.23 Psoriasis (diaper). Sharply demarcated, erythematous, scaly plaques involving the genitals and suprapubic region in this infant male.

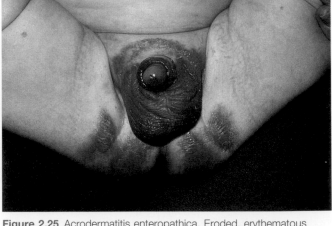

Figure 2.25 Acrodermatitis enteropathica. Eroded, erythematous patches and plaques in this 4-month-old boy with zinc deficiency. Note the associated balanoposthitis.

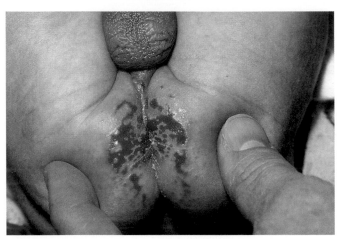

Figure 2.24 Jacquet's dermatitis. Severe diaper area erythema with ulcerated papules and islands of re-epithelialization.

Nondiapered areas of involvement include the anterior neck fold and the axillae.

Jacquet's dermatitis

The term *Jacquet's dermatitis* is used to describe a severe erosive diaper eruption with ulcerated papules or nodules (Fig. 2.24). In male infants, erosion and crusting of the glans penis and urinary meatus may result in painful or difficult urination.

Perianal pseudoverrucous papules and nodules

An eruption composed of verrucous (wart-like) papules has been observed to occur in children with incontinence of stool or urine. These patients present with verrucous papules and nodules of the perianal and suprapubic regions, possibly representing a distinct reaction to severe irritant diaper dermatitis. Reported patients had a history of delayed ileoanal anastomosis for Hirschsprung disease, encopresis, or urinary incontinence.[81–83] The importance of this diagnosis lies in differentiating it from condylomata acuminata or other more serious dermatoses.

Acrodermatitis enteropathica

Acrodermatitis enteropathica, a disorder of zinc deficiency, may mimic a severe irritant contact dermatitis in the diaper area (see Ch.

24). Patients present with a periorificial erosive dermatitis, which is often most accentuated in the diaper region (Fig. 2.25) but also may involve the perioral face. Erythema and pustules may involve intertriginous or acral sites, and diarrhea, failure to thrive, and alopecia are frequently present.

Langerhans cell histiocytosis

Lesions of Langerhans cell histiocytosis (LCH; see Ch. 10) may also have a predilection for the diaper area. This eruption, which often presents in a seborrheic dermatitis-like fashion, classically involves the groin, axillae, and retroauricular scalp. Palms and soles may also be involved. Characteristic lesions consist of yellowish to red-brown papules, often with concomitant erosive or purpuric qualities (Fig. 2.26). LCH should be considered in any infant with a recalcitrant or hemorrhagic seborrheic dermatitis-like eruption and/or flexural papules with erosions. Lymphadenopathy is common, and multi-organ involvement (especially bones, liver, lung, mucosa, and middle ear) is possible. Skin biopsy with special stains for Langerhans cells is diagnostic.

Treatment of diaper dermatitis

Prior to any consideration for therapy of diaper dermatitis, the appropriate etiology must be identified. Educating parents that diaper dermatitis is often recurrent is vital in an effort to prevent perceived management failure. The primary goals in preventing and treating diaper dermatitis include keeping the skin dry, protected, and infection-free.[84]

The primary goal in irritant or chafing dermatitis is to keep the area as clean and dry as possible. Frequent diaper changes, gentle cleansing with a moistened soft cloth or fragrance-free diaper wipe, exposure to air whenever possible, and the judicious use of topical therapy may be sufficient in most cases. Zinc oxide and petrolatum-based formulations tend to be most effective in forming a barrier to further skin contact with urine and feces. These products should be applied at every diaper change when acute dermatitis is present. Parents should be taught that diaper area cleansing is necessary only when stool is present, as overwashing in itself can lead to irritation. A low-potency, non-fluorinated topical corticosteroid (i.e., 1% hydrocortisone) applied two to three times daily is appropriate until improvement is noted. Stronger steroids and combination antifungal-corticosteroid preparations should be avoided, given risks of local cutaneous side-effects and, more important, systemic

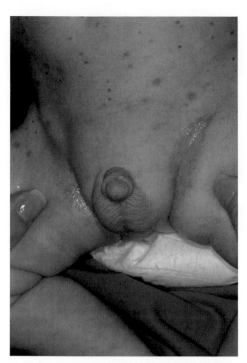

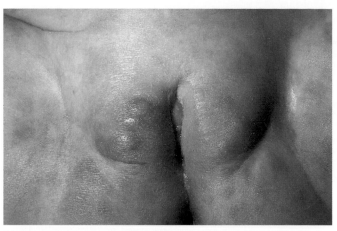

Figure 2.27 Granuloma gluteale infantum. Erythematous to violaceous papulonodules on the labia majora of this infant with a history of potent topical corticosteroid use in the diaper region.

Figure 2.26 Langerhans cell histiocytosis. Red-brown, purpuric eroded papules in a 3-month-old male. Note intertrigo-like erythema of the inguinal creases with superficial erosions.

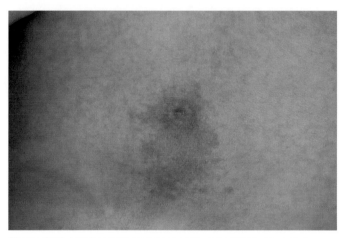

Figure 2.28 Lumbosacral port-wine stain associated with occult spinal dysraphism. Note the associated central depression in this boy who also had an underlying tethered spinal cord.

absorption because of increased skin penetration from occlusion effect.

Secondarily infected (bacterial) dermatitis should be treated with the appropriate systemic antibiotic. Candidal infection requires the use of a topical antifungal agent (i.e., nystatin, clotrimazole, econazole, miconazole). If there is evidence of *Candida* in the mouth (i.e., thrush) as well as the diaper area, topical therapy may be supplemented by oral nystatin. Oral fluconazole is useful for severe cutaneous candidiasis. Although gentian violet has been used for decades for the treatment of oral and diaper candidiasis, reports of bacterial infection and hemorrhagic cystitis, in addition to the staining associated with its use, suggest that gentian violet be avoided.[85,86] A newer combination product (0.25% miconazole nitrate, 15% zinc oxide, and 81.35% white petrolatum) is also available.

Granuloma Gluteale Infantum

Granuloma gluteale infantum is a benign disorder of infancy characterized by purple-red nodules in the skin of the groin (Fig. 2.27), lower abdomen, and inner thighs. Patients have usually received preceding therapy with topical corticosteroids. Although the appearance of these lesions may suggest a malignant process, granuloma gluteale infantum seems to represent a unique response to local inflammation, maceration, and possibly secondary infection (usually *C. albicans*). A similar eruption has been observed in elderly adults.[87] Histologic evaluation of granuloma gluteale infantum reveals a nonspecific inflammatory infiltrate, sometimes with giant cells.[88,89]

Lesions of granuloma gluteale infantum resolve completely and spontaneously within a period of several months after treatment of the initiating inflammatory process. Although intralesional corticosteroids or steroid-impregnated tape have been used, such therapy is not recommended.

Developmental abnormalities of the newborn

Skin Signs of Occult Spinal Dysraphism

Spinal dysraphism is a spectrum of disorders defined by absent or incomplete fusion of the midline bony elements and may include congenital spinal cord anomalies.[90] Because occult spinal dysraphism (OSD) can lead to irreversible neurologic complications, early recognition is desirable. Cutaneous or subcutaneous stigmata may be the presenting sign of OSD, and as such, a working knowledge of potentially associated lesions is vital. Lumbosacral skin lesions that may be associated with OSD and spinal cord defects include hypertrichosis (the classic 'faun tail' or finer, lanugo hair), lipomas, vascular lesions (infantile hemangioma, port-wine stain) (Fig. 2.28), prominent sacral dimples, sinuses, appendages (skin tag, tail), aplasia cutis congenita, and melanocytic nevi.[91] Gluteal cleft asymmetry or deviation is another useful finding. The presence of multiple findings increases the risk of OSD.[92] In one study, 11 of 18 patients with two or more congenital midline skin lesions has OSD, and the most common midline cutaneous lesion to be associated with OSD was lipomas (either isolated or in combination with other lesions).[93]

The majority of simple midline dimples are not associated with OSD. Atypical dimples (>5 mm in size, further than 2.5 cm from the anus, associated with other lumbosacral lesions), on the other hand, have a significant risk of associated OSD.[92] The association of nevus simplex (small dull-pink vascular malformation, most commonly seen on the occipital scalp, glabella, or eyelids) of the sacrum and OSD is unclear, although most agree that these lesions, when occurring alone, do not predict an increased risk of underlying malformations. Cervical OSD is significantly less common, and in those cases associated with cutaneous stigmata, more than one lesion is usually present.[94] It is important to remember that an isolated nevus simplex ('stork bite') of the posterior nuchal or occipital region is *not* an indicator of underlying OSD.

When OSD is being considered, radiographic imaging must be performed. Magnetic resonance imaging is the diagnostic modality of choice, especially with higher-risk cutaneous findings. Ultrasound screening may be considered in infants younger than 4 months (before ossification of the vertebral bodies is complete), with the advantages being that it is non-invasive and does not require sedation. However, ultrasonography is limited in that small cord lesions (i.e., lipoma or dermal sinus tracts) may be missed,[92] and the overall sensitivity is quite dependent on the experience of the ultrasonographer. In infants with low-risk lesions such as simple dimples or gluteal cleft deviation, without other higher-risk findings (i.e., hypertrichosis, skin tags, lipoma or other mass), the need for imaging is unclear. If it is performed, however, ultrasound may provide a reliable screening when interpreted by an experienced pediatric radiologist.[95] Early neurosurgical referral is indicated if underlying defects are diagnosed.

Drug-induced Fetal Skin Malformations

There are numerous drugs, including alcohol, hydantoin, valproic acid, warfarin, aminopterin, and isotretinoic acid, that, when taken by pregnant women, produce an adverse effect on the fetus and newborn. Exposure to these drugs *in utero* may result in a variety of organ malformations, although specific skin malformations are rare. Teratogenic risks as they relate to skin have most frequently focused on antithyroid drugs, especially methimazole (MMI), and their possible role in causing the congenital skin defect known as *aplasia cutis congenita* (ACC, see below).

Congenital Hemihypertrophy

Idiopathic congenital hemihypertrophy is a developmental defect in which one side of the body is larger than the other. Although differences in symmetry are often detectable during the newborn period, they usually become more striking with growth of the child. The cutaneous findings most often associated with hemihypertrophy are hyperpigmentation, telangiectasia, abnormal nail growth, and hypertrichosis (Fig. 2.29). Body temperature and sweating differences have also been reported in patients with this disorder.[96]

Of particular significance is the fact that about 50% of persons with hemihypertrophy may have associated anomalies, including Wilms' tumor, aniridia, cataracts, ear deformities, internal hemangiomas, genitourinary tract anomalies, adrenocortical neoplasms, and brain tumors. Patients who exhibit congenital hemihypertrophy, therefore, should be evaluated for potentially associated conditions. Associated tumors most commonly involve the kidney, adrenal gland, and liver.[97] In patients with hemihypertrophy combined with cutaneous vascular malformations (i.e., port-wine stain), the possibility of Klippel–Trenaunay or Proteus syndrome should be considered (see Ch. 12).

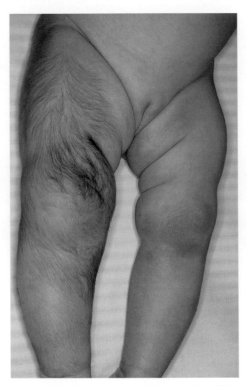

Figure 2.29 Congenital hemihypertrophy with hypertrichosis. (From Hurwitz S, Klaus SN. Congenital hemihypertrophy with hypertrichosis. *Arch Dermatol* 1971;103:98–100. © 1971 American Medical Association. All rights reserved.)[96]

Aplasia Cutis Congenita

Aplasia cutis congenita (ACC) is a congenital defect of the skin characterized by localized absence of the epidermis, dermis, and at times, subcutaneous tissues. Although ACC generally occurs on the scalp, it may also involve the skin of the face, trunk, and extremities. The diagnosis of ACC is usually a clinical one, and the histologic picture varies. Although most cases appear to be sporadic, a variety of potential associations, including teratogens, limb abnormalities, epidermal nevi, underlying embryologic malformations, epidermolysis bullosa, malformation syndromes, and infections, have been proposed.[98]

ACC classically presents as solitary or multiple, sharply demarcated, weeping or granulating, oval to circular, stellate defects ranging from 1 to 3 cm in diameter. Some 70% of scalp lesions are isolated, 20% are double, and in 8% of patients three or more defects may be present.[99] The most common location for ACC is the scalp, and in those cases, 80% occur in close proximity to the hair whorl.[100] Although aplasia cutis may also affect the occiput, the postauricular areas, and the face, involvement of these areas appears to be relatively uncommon. Whereas most scalp defects are small, larger lesions may occur and can extend to the dura or the meninges. Although treatment is generally unnecessary, large scalp lesions (i.e., >4 cm²) may require surgery with grafting to prevent the potential complications of hemorrhage, venous (sagittal sinus) thrombosis, and meningitis.

At birth, the skin defect may vary from an ulceration with a granulating base (Fig. 2.30) to a superficial erosion or even a well-formed scar. As healing of open lesions occurs, the defect is replaced by smooth, hairless scar tissue (Fig. 2.31), although sometimes raised and keloidal. Some lesions may present as a translucent, glistening membrane ('membranous aplasia cutis'), and when

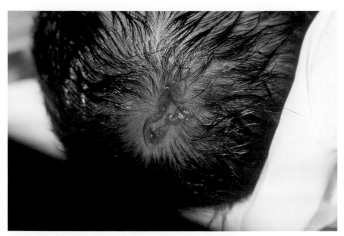

Figure 2.30 Aplasia cutis congenita. Sharply demarcated ulceration on the scalp of an infant with this disorder.

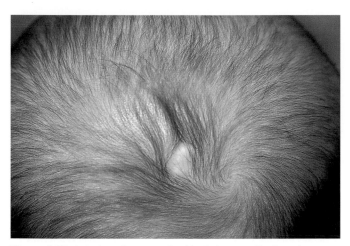

Figure 2.31 Aplasia cutis congenita. Healed scar with alopecia near the hair whorl in this 8-month-old girl.

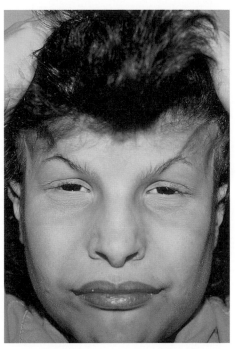

Figure 2.32 Setleis syndrome. A child with bilateral depressed oval areas on the temples, upwardly slanting eyebrows, narrowed palpebral fissures, and large lips. (Courtesy of Seth Orlow, MD.)

surrounded by a ring of long, dark hair (the 'hair collar sign'), may represent a form fruste of a neural tube defect.[101]

Although most infants with ACC are otherwise well, defects that may occasionally be present include cleft lip and palate, ophthalmologic defects, limb reduction defects, cardiac anomalies, gastrointestinal tract malformations, spinal dysraphism, hydrocephalus, defects of the underlying skull, congenital midline porencephaly, spastic paralysis, seizures, mental retardation, and vascular anomalies.[98] *Adams–Oliver syndrome*, an autosomal dominant malformation syndrome, is the association of ACC with transverse limb defects and cardiac and central nervous system abnormalities.[102,103] Up to 50% of patients with *trisomy 13* may have scalp ACC, and it may also occur with increased frequency in patients with *4p- syndrome*. Therefore, any patient presenting with scalp ACC and congenital anomalies warrants chromosomal evaluation. *Oculocerebrocutaneous (Delleman) syndrome* is the association of orbital cysts, cerebral malformations, and focal skin defects including ACC-like lesions and skin tags.[104,105] Other findings in this syndrome include central nervous system malformations, clefting, and microphthalmia/anophthalmia.

The etiology of aplasia cutis congenita remains unknown. Although most cases are sporadic, familial case reports have suggested autosomal dominant inheritance with reduced penetrance.

Incomplete closure of the neural tube or an embryologic arrest of skin development has been suggested as an explanation for midline lesions. This hypothesis, however, fails to account for lesions of the trunk and limbs. In such instances, vascular abnormality of the placenta, with a degenerative rather than an aplastic or traumatic origin, has been postulated as the cause of the cutaneous defects.[106] Antithyroid drugs, most notably methimazole (MMI), have long been hypothesized as causative teratogens in some cases of ACC. Although causality remains unproven, there are multiple reports of affected infants born to mothers treated with MMI during pregnancy, both as an isolated manifestation and as part of the presentation of 'MMI embryopathy', which includes dysmorphism, gastrointestinal tract malformations, and developmental delay.[107] Propylthiouracil has been recommended as the first-line agent in the management of hyperthyroidism during pregnancy, given its equal effectiveness and lack of reports of teratogenic ACC.[108]

Recognition of ACC and differentiation of it from forceps or other birth injury will help prevent possible medicolegal complications occasionally encountered with this disorder. In patients with localized sporadic lesions, aside from cutaneous scarring, the prognosis of ACC is excellent. With conservative therapy to prevent further tissue damage and secondary infection, most small defects of the scalp heal well during the first few weeks to months of life. With aging of the child, most scars become relatively inconspicuous and require no correction. Those that are large and obvious can be treated with plastic surgical reconstruction.

Setleis syndrome

Setleis syndrome was initially described in 1963 by Setleis and colleagues, who described five children of three families, all of Puerto-Rican ancestry, who presented with unique characteristic clinical defects confined to the face.[109] Patients present with atrophic skin at the temples (historically likened to 'forceps marks'), coarse facial appearance, absent or duplicated eyelashes, eyebrows that slant sharply upward and laterally, and periorbital puffiness (Fig. 2.32).

Lips may be large with an inverted 'V' contour. Although traditionally believed to have normal intelligence, patients with Setleis syndrome may have associated developmental delay.[110]

Reports of Setleis syndrome have suggested both autosomal recessive and autosomal dominant modes of inheritance,[110,111] and variable expressivity and reduced penetrance may be observed.[112] Setleis syndrome is considered by some to be a form of *focal facial dermal dysplasias* (see Ch. 6).[113]

Other Developmental Defects

A congenital *dermal sinus or dermoid cyst* is a developmental epithelium-lined tract (or cyst) that extends inward from the surface of the skin. Since midline fusion of ectodermal and neuroectodermal tissue occurs at the cephalic and caudal ends of the neural tube, the majority of such defects are seen in the occipital and lumbosacral regions. Dermoids, however, can occur anywhere.

Dermal sinus openings may be difficult to visualize, particularly in the occipital scalp region where they may be hidden by hair. A localized thickening of the scalp, hypertrichosis, or dimpling in the midline of the neck or back should alert the physician to the possibility of such an anomaly. These sinuses are of clinical importance as portals for infection that may give rise to abscesses, osteomyelitis, or meningitis.

Dermoid cysts most commonly occur on the orbital ridge, presenting as a non-tender, mobile subcutaneous nodule in the eyebrow/orbital ridge region (Fig. 2.33). In this location, there is no association with deep extension. About 3% of dermoids are located in the nasal midline[91] (including glabella, nasal dorsum, and columella), and recognition of these lesions is vital because of the potential for deep extension and CNS communication. Congenital midline nasal masses may represent not only dermoids, but also cephaloceles, gliomas, hemangiomas, and a variety of less common neoplasms or malformations. It is vital to consider the diagnostic possibilities carefully when a child presents with a nasal midline mass, given the potential for intracranial connection seen with some of these disorders. Invasive diagnostic procedures should never be performed until radiologic evaluation has been completed.

In midline nasal dermoid cysts or dermal sinuses, an overlying sinus ostium may be present, sometimes with a white discharge or protruding hairs (Fig. 2.34). Presence of such a pit may indicate a higher likelihood of intracranial extension.[114] Magnetic resonance (MR) or computed tomographic (CT) imaging of suspicious areas should be performed to evaluate for an underlying tract and CNS connection. Management of dermal sinuses and dermoid cysts consists of surgical excision, in an effort to prevent local infection and, in the case of intracranial extension, meningitis and/or abscess formation. Lesions of the lateral forehead or orbital ridge do not require radiographic imaging prior to surgical excision.

A *cephalocele* is a herniation of cranial contents through a defect in the skull. Cephaloceles develop as a result of faulty separation of neuroectoderm from surface ectoderm in early gestation, and occur most commonly at the occiput, followed by the dorsal nose, orbits, and forehead. These lesions present as a compressible mass that transilluminates with light.[91] Occasionally, an overlying blue hue may be present, which at times can suggest the incorrect diagnosis of deep hemangioma. A useful diagnostic feature is the enlargement of the lesion that may be seen with any maneuver that results in increased intracranial pressure (such as crying or straining). This temporary change is due to the patent connection between a cephalocele and the CNS. Hypertelorism, facial clefting, and brain malformations may be seen in conjunction with a cephalocele.[115] Surgical resection is the treatment of choice, and multidisciplinary care (plastic surgery, neurosurgery) may be indicated.

A *nasal glioma* represents ectopic neuroectoderm from early development, and may occur in extranasal (60%) or intranasal (30%) locations, and less commonly in both extranasal and intranasal sites. This lesion presents as a firm, non-compressible flesh-colored nodule, sometimes with a blue-red hue, and most often situated at the root of the nose. Hypertelorism may result, and no fluctuation in size is seen, as these lesions have no intracranial connection. Intranasal lesions present as a protruding mass from the nose, simulating a nasal polyp. *Heterotopic brain tissue* is a term that

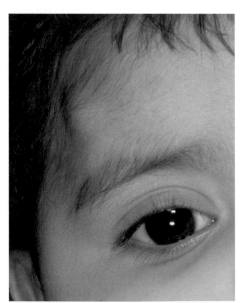

Figure 2.33 Dermoid cyst. This mobile, non-tender, subcutaneous nodule was present at birth in this 5-month-old girl. The lateral mid-forehead distribution is slightly higher than most dermoids, which present most often in the lateral eyebrow region.

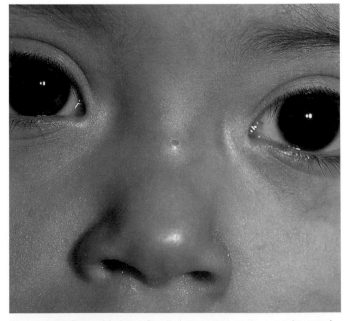

Figure 2.34 Dermoid sinus. Small sinus ostium at the superior nasal bridge. This patient had no intracranial extension.

has been used to similarly describe a rare developmental anomaly that occurs most often on the head and neck, especially in the nasal area, and usually without intracranial communication.[116,117] Surgical excision is the treatment of choice for these lesions.

Congenital fistulas of the lower lip (congenital lip pits) may be unilateral or bilateral and may be seen alone or in association with other anomalies of the face and extremities. They are characterized by single or paired, circular or slit-like depressions on either side of the midline of the lower lip at the edge of the vermilion border. These depressions represent blind sinuses that extend inward through the orbicularis oris muscle to a depth of ≥0.5 cm. They may occasionally communicate with underlying salivary glands. Excision of lip pits is unnecessary unless mucous gland secretions are problematic.

Congenital lip pits may be inherited as an autosomal dominant disorder with penetrance estimated at 80%. They may be seen alone or, in 70% of patients, in association with cleft lip or cleft palate. Other associated anomalies include clubfoot, talipes equinovarus, syndactyly, and the popliteal pterygium syndrome (an autosomal dominant disorder with clefting, filiform eyelid adhesions, pterygium, genitourinary anomalies, and congenital heart disease).[118]

Skin dimpling defects (depressions, deep pits, or creases) in the sacral area and over bony prominences may be seen in normal children and infants with diastematomyelia (a fissure or cleft of the spinal cord), congenital rubella or congenital varicella-zoster syndromes, deletion of the long arm of chromosome 18, and Zellweger (cerebrohepatorenal), Bloom, and Freeman-Sheldon (craniocarpotarsal dysplasia, 'whistling face') syndromes.

Amniotic constriction bands may produce congenital constriction deformities, and congenital amputation of one or more digits or extremities of otherwise normal infants may occur. The deformities are believed to result from intrauterine rupture of amnion with formation of fibrous bands that encircle fetal parts and produce permanent constriction of the underlying tissue.[119] *Acquired raised bands of infancy* (also known as *raised limb bands*) are linear skin-colored plaques which develop postnatally on the extremities of infants (Fig. 2.35), without constrictive defects. They may also occasionally occur on the trunk. Although some argue that these findings are distinct from amniotic constriction bands[120], co-existence with congenital constriction bands[121] and prenatal ultrasound observation of amniotic bands[122] in reported patients suggests a potential overlap of these two conditions.

Preauricular pits and *sinus tracts* may develop as a result of imperfect fusion of the tubercles of the first two branchial arches. Unilateral or bilateral, these lesions present as small skin pits that may become infected or result in chronic preauricular ulcerations (Fig. 2.36), retention cysts, or both, necessitating surgical excision. *Accessory tragi* are fleshy papules, with or without a cartilaginous component, that contain epidermal adnexal structures. Usually seen in the preauricular area, they may also occur on the neck (anterior to the sternocleidomastoid muscle). Accessory tragi may be solitary or localized (Fig. 2.37A) or multifocal, occurring along the embryologic migration line extending from the preauricular cheek to the mouth angle (Fig. 2.37B). Although generally seen as an isolated congenital defect, they may be associated with other branchial arch syndromes (i.e., oculoauriculovertebral or Goldenhar syndrome). The prevalence of preauricular pits and tags is estimated at around 0.5–1.0%.[123,124]

An important consideration with preauricular pits and tags is that of potential associations, the most common concerns being those of hearing or genitourinary defects. Several studies have demonstrated an increased incidence of hearing impairment in the setting of isolated pits or tags, thus suggesting that hearing assessment should be performed in any newborn with these lesions.[125,126] The

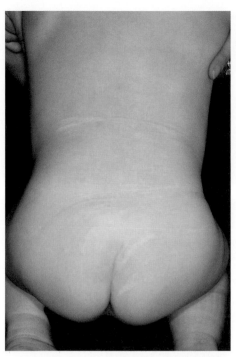

Figure 2.35 Acquired raised bands of infancy. Numerous linear raised bands on the back of an infant who had similar bands on the extremities. (Courtesy of Sarah L. Chamlin MD.)

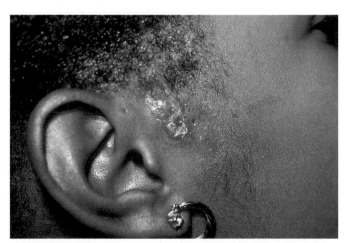

Figure 2.36 Preauricular sinus with ulceration. This lesion was prone to recurrent inflammation and infection, and ultimately was surgically excised.

data regarding genitourinary malformations are more controversial, with studies both supporting and refuting an association with preauricular pits or tags.[124,127] It appears that when these preauricular lesions occur in the absence of other dysmorphic or syndromic features, such associations seem less likely.

Branchial cleft cysts and sinuses, formed along the course of the first and second branchial clefts as a result of improper closure during embryonic development, are generally located along the lower third of the lateral aspect of the neck near the anterior border of the sternocleidomastoid muscle. Lesions may be unilateral or bilateral and may open onto the cutaneous surface or may drain into the pharynx. Although these lesions may present in childhood, they more commonly come to medical attention during adulthood because of recurrent inflammation. Treatment consists of complete

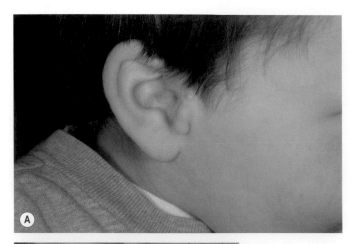

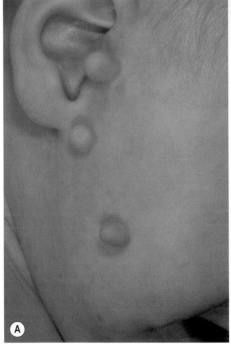

Figure 2.37 Accessory tragi. These fleshy papules may present in a solitary/localized fashion (A) or in a multifocal form, occurring along the embryologic migration line extending from the preauricular cheek to the mouth angle (B).

surgical removal or marsupialization (exteriorization, resection of the anterior wall, and suturing of the cut edges of the remaining cyst to the adjacent edges of the skin).

Thyroglossal cysts and sinuses are located on or near the midline of the neck, and may open onto the skin surface, extend to the base of the tongue, or drain into the pharynx. Clinically, they present as a midline neck cyst that moves with swallowing. These lesions represent persistence of the embryonic structure associated with normal thyroid descent, and occasionally may contain ectopic thyroid tissue. Although surgical excision is the treatment of choice, care must be exercised to preserve aberrant thyroid tissue to prevent postsurgical hypothyroidism.

Bronchogenic cysts present early, usually at birth, as a nodule or draining pit, usually over the suprasternal notch. These lesions may develop from ectopic elements of the tracheobronchial tree, or may represent ectopic branchial cleft cysts. Surgical excision is the treatment of choice. Figure 2.38 shows the locations of several types of congenital neck cysts.

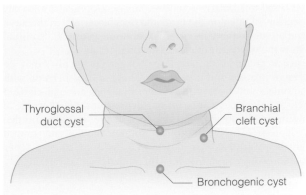

Figure 2.38 Congenital sinuses of the neck.

Congenital cartilaginous rests of the neck (also known as *wattles*) occur as small fleshy appendages on the anterior neck or over or near the lower half of the sternocleidomastoid muscle. Treatment consists of surgical excision with recognition of the fact that these cutaneous appendages may contain cartilage. *Pterygium colli*, congenital folds of skin extending from the mastoid region to the acromion on the lateral aspect of the neck, may be seen in individuals with the Turner, Noonan, Down, LEOPARD, or multiple pterygium syndrome, trisomy 18, short-limbed dwarfism, and combined immunodeficiency disease.

Supernumerary nipples (polythelia), present at times in males as well as females, are manifested as small brown or pink, concave, umbilicated or elevated papules along or slightly medial to the embryologic milk line. They are most common on the chest or upper abdomen, and occasionally seen in other sites including the face, neck, shoulder, back, genitals, or thighs. Although much has been written about a relatively high incidence of renal malformation in patients with supernumerary nipples, current studies suggest that this anomaly in an otherwise apparently normal individual does not appear to be a marker of urinary tract malformation.[128–130]

There is a variety of developmental anomalies that may occur in the umbilical region. *Urachal cyst or sinus* is a lesion that represents persistence of the embryonic urachus, a fibrous cord that develops from the urogenital sinus. A midline nodule near the umbilicus may result, and at times, urine drainage may be seen from a fistula connecting the umbilicus to the bladder. *Vitelline (omphalomesenteric duct) remnant* may present as an umbilical polyp or an umbilicoileal fistula that drains feces onto the skin surface. Complete excision is the treatment of choice for these anomalies.

Congenital infections of the newborn

Viral, bacterial, and parasitic infections during pregnancy can be associated with widespread systemic involvement, serious permanent sequelae, and a variety of cutaneous manifestations in the newborn. This section discusses the most significant of these: congenital rubella, congenital varicella-zoster syndrome, neonatal varicella, neonatal herpes, congenital syphilis, cytomegalic inclusion disease, and congenital toxoplasmosis.

Congenital Rubella

Congenital rubella syndrome (CRS) was initially identified in 1941 by Norman Gregg, an Australian ophthalmologist who observed an unusual form of congenital cataracts in babies of mothers who had had rubella during pregnancy.[131] It occurs following maternal rubella infection during the first 16 weeks of pregnancy, and only rarely when infection is acquired later in gestation. Earlier gestation directly correlates with the likelihood of CRS. Overall, the incidence of CRS in the USA has declined notably in parallel with the decline in rubella cases since licensure of the rubella vaccine in 1969. In 2008, only 11 cases of rubella were confirmed in the USA, and all were imported or related to an importation.[132] Occasional rubella outbreaks, such as those that occurred during the 1990s, have been related to a variety of factors, including occurrence in settings in which unvaccinated adults congregate, in unvaccinated foreign-born adults, and among children and adults in religious communities with low levels of vaccination coverage.[133,134] Studies suggest that young Hispanic women represent a population at elevated risk for delivering a CRS-affected infant, and thus, this population needs to be targeted specifically for immunization.[134,135]

Clinical manifestations of CRS are characterized by the classic triad of congenital cataracts, deafness, and cardiac defects (especially patent ductus arteriosus). *In utero* growth restriction may occur during the last trimester of pregnancy. CNS involvement may result in microcephaly, meningoencephalitis, and mental retardation. Other features include pigmentary retinopathy, hepatosplenomegaly, jaundice, radiolucent bone lesions in metaphyses, and thrombocytopenia.[136] Some infants with CRS may show few manifestations at birth or may be asymptomatic, but findings usually manifest over subsequent months. Occasionally, CRS findings may not become manifest until the second year of life.[137]

The most distinct cutaneous feature of CRS is a diffuse eruption composed of blue-red infiltrative papules and nodules and occasionally smaller purpuric macules, measuring 2–8 mm in diameter, representing so-called *blueberry muffin* lesions (Fig. 2.39). Blueberry muffin lesions are usually present at birth or within the first 24 h, and new lesions rarely appear after 2 days of age. They may be observed in association with a variety of disorders, usually either infectious or neoplastic (Table 2.5). Histologic evaluation reveals extramedullary hematopoiesis, characteristic of viral infection of the fetus, and not unique to infants with CRS but also seen in patients with congenital toxoplasmosis, cytomegalovirus infection, erythroblastosis fetalis, congenital leukemia, and twin transfusion syndrome. Other cutaneous manifestations in CRS may include a generalized nonspecific maculopapular eruption,

reticulated erythema of the face and extremities, hyperpigmentation, and recurrent urticaria. Vasomotor instability, manifested by poor peripheral circulation with generalized mottling and acral cyanosis, may also occur.

The diagnosis of CRS should be suspected in infants with one or more characteristic findings, including congenital cataracts, pigmentary retinopathy, cardiac defects, deafness, thrombocytopenia, hepatosplenomegaly microcephaly, or blueberry muffin lesions. The diagnosis may be confirmed by isolation of rubella virus from respiratory secretions, urine, cerebrospinal fluid, or tissue. Neonatal IgM rubella-specific antibodies or IgG antibodies that persist beyond a period of time expected for passively transferred immunity are also diagnostic.

There is no specific therapy for CRS apart from supportive therapy and recognition of potential disabilities. Because of the high incidence of ophthalmic complications, regular ophthalmologic examinations are indicated. Congenitally infected infants may shed virus in urine and the nasopharynx for several months to 1 year, and should be considered contagious until that time. The majority of infants who acquire CRS early in gestation will have permanent neurological and audiological sequelae, and long-term multidisciplinary care is indicated. A long-term follow-up study of 50 Australian patients with CRS revealed aortic valve disease in 68%, and increased incidences of diabetes, thyroid disorders, early menopause, and osteoporosis compared with the general population.[138]

Congenital rubella can be effectively prevented by immunization with live rubella virus vaccine, and universal vaccination is recommended. Current efforts focus on immunizing high-risk populations with two doses of rubella vaccine, with a special effort to vaccinate populations at increased risk including college students, military recruits, and healthcare and daycare workers.[137] Because of the high risk of fetal damage, women known to have contracted maternal rubella during the early months of pregnancy may consider abortion. Although limited data suggest that administration of immune globulin to the mother may reduce the amount of viremia and damage when given as early as possible after exposure, it does not appear to prevent congenital infection.

Congenital Varicella Syndrome

Congenital varicella syndrome, also known as fetal varicella syndrome, refers to a spectrum of congenital anomalies that may be

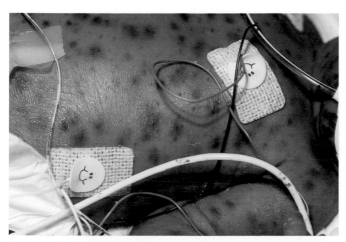

Figure 2.39 Congenital rubella with blueberry muffin lesions. Multiple violaceous, infiltrative papules and nodules in this newborn with congenital rubella.

Table 2.5 Differential diagnosis of the newborn with 'blueberry muffin' lesions

Dermal (extramedullary) hematopoiesis
Congenital infection
Toxoplasmosis
Rubella
Cytomegalovirus
Enterovirus
Parvovirus B19
Erythroblastosis fetalis
Inherited hemolytic diseases
Twin–twin transfusion
Neoplastic
Neuroblastoma
Leukemia
Histiocytosis
Alveolar rhabdomyosarcoma

seen in neonates born to women who contract varicella during the first 20 weeks of gestation. Overall it is quite rare, probably relating to the fact that primary varicella infection during pregnancy is uncommon since the majority of women have acquired immunity by child-bearing age.[139] The incidence of congenital varicella syndrome following maternal infection is estimated at around 0.4–1%, and the highest risk seems to be when infection is acquired between 13 and 20 weeks of gestation.[140,141] Although there are rare reports of fetal sequelae in infants born to mothers who develop herpes zoster infection (shingles) during pregnancy, this association is extremely rare.[140,142]

Congenital varicella syndrome may present with various findings, including low birthweight, ophthalmologic defects (including microphthalmia, Horner syndrome, cataracts, and chorioretinitis), neurologic defects (including mental retardation, seizures, cortical atrophy, encephalomyelitis, and developmental delay), limb hypoplasia with flexion contractures and malformed digits, and gastrointestinal and genitourinary defects.[139] Cutaneous findings include vesicles and/or scarring in a dermatomal distribution, although several affected newborns have been reported with cutis aplasia-like absence of skin.

Because the risk of fetal malformation in an infant born to a mother exposed to varicella-zoster virus during pregnancy is so slight, therapeutic abortion is not necessarily indicated. In fact, the majority of women who contract varicella during pregnancy have children with no evidence of the syndrome. Studies to date are inconclusive with regard to the utility of serologic or PCR-based testing of fetal blood or amniotic fluid.[143] Studies suggest that the use of varicella-zoster immune globulin (VZIG) may clearly modify or prevent disease in the exposed susceptible mother, but the potential benefit to the fetus is less clear. Treatment of mothers with severe varicella with acyclovir or valacyclovir may be considered. Most important is screening of women of child-bearing age without a history of varicella for antibody, and offering vaccination when indicated. Susceptible females who are already pregnant should be counseled about avoiding contact with individuals who have chickenpox and about the availability of VZIG should it become necessary.

Neonatal varicella is a varicella infection of the newborn that occurs when a pregnant woman develops chickenpox during the last few weeks of pregnancy or the first few days postpartum. In such instances, the timing of the onset of disease in the mother and her newborn is critical. If the disease onset in the mother is ≥5 days before delivery or in the newborn during the first 4 days of life, the infection tends to be mild. In contrast, if the onset in the mother is within 5 days before delivery to 2 days after delivery, or in the newborn between 5 and 10 days of birth, the infant's infection is often severe and disseminated (Fig. 2.40), with pneumonia, hepatitis, or meningoencephalitis and severe coagulopathy, and a mortality rate of around 30%. In an effort to prevent neonatal varicella infection, VZIG should be given as soon as possible after delivery to all infants in whom the mother has the onset of varicella within 5 days before or within 48 h after delivery, and these infants are also candidates for intravenous acyclovir therapy.[144]

Neonatal Herpes

Neonatal herpes simplex virus (HSV) infection may range from a mild, self-limited illness to one with devastating neurologic consequences or even death. It affects an estimated 1500 to 2200 infants per year in the USA.[145] Up to 70% of neonatal HSV infections are caused by type 2 ('genital') HSV, and the disease is acquired either by ascending *in utero* infection or by spread during delivery through an infected birth canal (perinatal transmission). Infection of the

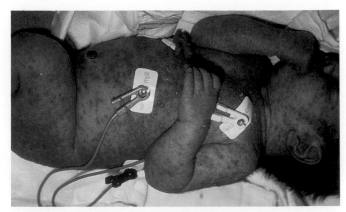

Figure 2.40 Neonatal varicella. Disseminated, erythematous papules, vesicles, and erosions.

Table 2.6 Clinical presentations of neonatal herpes

Type	Frequency[a] (%)	Skin vesicles (%)	Comment
SEM disease	45	80–85	May progress to more severe infection, especially without early therapy
CNS disease	30	60–70	Clinical overlap with neonatal bacterial sepsis
Disseminated	25	75–80	Respiratory collapse, liver failure and DIC common

Adapted from Kimberlin (2005)[149] and Kimberlin (2007) © 2007.[159]
[a]Approximate frequency out of all neonatal herpes patients. SEM, skin, eyes, and/or mouth; CNS, central nervous system; DIC, disseminated intravascular coagulopathy.

newborn may also be acquired by intrauterine infection because of maternal viremia with transplacental spread or by postnatal hospital or household contact with other infants or persons with oral HSV infection.[146–148] Of infants with neonatal HSV, 85% acquire their infection during birth, 10% postnatally, and 5% from *in utero* exposure.[149] *Congenital herpes*, which is not the focus of this section, is a rare disorder (approximately 5% of all neonatal HSV disease) resulting from intrauterine infection, and characterized by skin vesicles or scarring, chorioretinitis, microphthalmia, microcephaly, and abnormal brain CT findings.[150]

The risk of neonatal HSV infection in an infant born vaginally to a mother with primary genital infection is high (40–50%), whereas the risk to an infant born to a mother with recurrent infection is much lower, around 2–5%. The lower rate of transmission with recurrent maternal disease may reflect decreased viral load and partial protection of the fetus by transplacentally acquired antibodies.[151] Most babies with neonatal HSV become infected from mothers who are asymptomatic.

The clinical presentation of neonatal HSV has traditionally been divided into three separate patterns: *skin, eyes, and/or mouth (SEM) disease; central nervous system disease; and disseminated disease*. These presentations are summarized in Table 2.6. The exact frequency of the various forms is unclear, given partial overlap of patterns in some patients and potential delays in the appearance of CNS disease. Most infants affected with neonatal HSV become sick during the first 4 weeks, and in two-thirds, during the first week of life. SEM disease appears to be the least severe and associated with the most favorable prognosis. However, although most infants present with SEM disease, 60–70% will progress to more diffuse involvement.[152]

Presenting features of neonatal HSV include skin lesions, fever, respiratory distress, and central nervous system dysfunction. The latter includes seizures, lethargy, poor feeding, irritability, and hypotonia. The skin eruption may vary from erythematous macules to individual or grouped vesicles (Fig. 2.41) or a widespread generalized vesicobullous eruption affecting the skin and buccal mucosa. The vesicles of neonatal HSV may become pustular after 24–48 h, and eventually becomes crusted or ulcerated. Other skin findings may include purpuric, petechial, or zosteriform lesions, as well as large bullae with skin denudation similar to those seen in epidermolysis bullosa.[153] Skin lesions occur most often on the scalp and face, and in breech deliveries have a predilection for the presenting part. Occasionally, the scalp of the infant may reveal diffuse edematous swelling resembling that seen in caput succedaneum. Rather than resolving spontaneously during the first week, this swelling may become necrotic with resultant drainage and eschar formation and irregularly grouped herpetic vesicles. Fetal scalp monitoring is a risk factor for HSV, as the virus more readily gains entry into the lacerated scalp. Eye involvement, seen only in around 5% of affected infants, may present with conjunctivitis or pathognomonic keratitis.

The disseminated form of neonatal HSV may affect several organs, especially the liver, adrenal glands, and lungs, and the central nervous system. This form is associated with the highest mortality, up to 60%. In the absence of skin lesions or other pathognomonic features, disseminated disease may be difficult to diagnose and should always be considered in the neonate who presents with risk factors for HSV, with possible sepsis (especially if a lack of response to antimicrobial therapy is noted), with unexplained pneumonitis (especially in the first week of life), or with unexplained nonspecific findings such as thrombocytopenia, coagulopathy, hepatitis, or fever.[152] In addition, infants with an unexplained CSF pleocytosis (usually lymphocytic) merit consideration for the diagnosis of HSV.

The diagnosis of HSV infection in the newborn can be confirmed in a variety of ways. In the presence of skin lesions, a Tzanck smear can be performed on scrapings from the base of an unroofed vesicle and microscopically reveals multinucleated cells and nuclear inclusions. The Tzanck smear, however, is highly operator-dependent and thus may have a relatively low sensitivity; it is also not specific. Direct fluorescent antibody study of skin lesion scrapings has a high sensitivity (80–90%), excellent specificity,[154] and readily available results. The gold standard for diagnosis of HSV infections remains viral culture, which can be taken from skin (especially vesicular fluid), eyes, mouth, CSF, rectum, urine, or blood.[152] Serologic studies generally are not useful in diagnosing neonatal HSV infection, related to the slow serologic response of the newborn and the potential confounding factor of transplacental antibody. Polymerase chain reaction (PCR) studies have been a major advance in the diagnosis of neonatal HSV infection, and are especially useful for diagnosing CNS infection. Skin biopsy is rarely indicated, but if performed reveals characteristic intraepidermal vesicle formation with ballooning degeneration and multinucleation.

Other laboratory findings that may be suggestive of neonatal HSV infection include abnormal coagulation studies, thrombocytopenia, and elevated liver transaminases. Evaluation of CSF in those with CNS or disseminated disease often reveals a lymphocytic pleocytosis and elevated protein, although these findings may be absent in early disease and are not specific for HSV.[155] Electroencephalography and neuroimaging with MRI should also be performed.[155]

The outcome of neonatal HSV infection is quite variable. Prospective data on outcomes were gathered by the Collaborative Antiviral Study Group and revealed that the following were risk factors for mortality: CNS and disseminated disease, decreased level of consciousness at start of therapy, and prematurity. In those with disseminated disease, pneumonitis and disseminated intravascular coagulopathy were important risk factors.[146] Morbidity was greatest in infants with encephalitis, disseminated infection, seizures, or infection with HSV-2 (vs HSV-1).

Education is vitally important in the prevention of HSV (and therefore neonatal HSV) during pregnancy. Studies have shown that women at greatest risk of acquiring the infection during pregnancy are those who are seronegative and whose partners are HSV-positive. It appears that acquisition of infection with seroconversion completed before labor does not affect the outcome of the pregnancy, whereas infection acquired near the time of labor is associated with neonatal HSV and perinatal morbidity.[156] Overall, 70% of infants with neonatal HSV are born to mothers who do not manifest any sign or symptom of genital infection at the time of delivery. Cesarean delivery should be offered to women with active HSV lesions at the time of labor, although not all cases of neonatal HSV can be prevented.[150] The use of acyclovir during pregnancy is controversial, although it may shorten the period of active lesions in the mother. In instances where there is a known history of maternal HSV, use of fetal scalp electrodes should be avoided whenever possible. Viral cultures in mothers with suspected genital HSV during the last few weeks before delivery and routine prophylactic cesarean section for asymptomatic women have not been demonstrated useful and are not routinely recommended.

Newborns with vesicular lesions or suspected HSV should be isolated (contact precautions), evaluated thoroughly for systemic infection, and treated with empiric antiviral therapy. Ophthalmologic evaluation should be performed, and prophylactic topical ophthalmic preparations such as idoxuridine, vidarabine, or trifluorothymidine solution should be initiated. In addition to antiviral therapy, supportive measures are frequently indicated, including management of seizures, respiratory distress, hemorrhage, and metabolic aberrations. Women with active HSV infection may handle and feed their infants, provided they use careful hand-washing techniques and wear a disposable surgical mask or dressing to cover

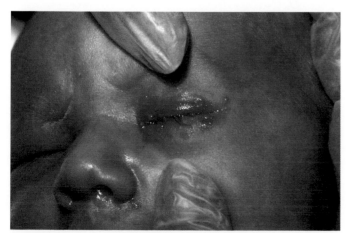

Figure 2.41 Neonatal herpes simplex infection. Clustered vesicles on an erythematous base in this newborn with congenital herpes simplex infection, SEM type (see text).

the lesions until they have crusted and dried. There is no unequivocal evidence that HSV is transmitted by breast milk or that breast-feeding by a mother with recurrent HSV infection poses a risk to the infant. It therefore appears that if the above precautions are utilized, breast-feeding by a mother with recurrent HSV may be acceptable. After hospital discharge, affected infants should be followed closely as 5–10% will develop a recurrent infection requiring therapy within the first month of life.[157]

Both vidarabine and acyclovir have been demonstrated effective in the treatment of neonatal HSV. However, because of its safety profile, acyclovir is the treatment of choice.[143] Early studies suggested a dose range of 15–30 mg/kg per day for affected infants, but it was subsequently demonstrated that higher dosages are more effective. The survival rate for patients with disseminated HSV treated with high-dose acyclovir (60 mg/kg per day) was significantly higher, with a borderline significant decrease in morbidity.[158] Toxicity was limited to transient neutropenia during therapy, suggesting the importance of monitoring absolute neutrophil counts. Treatment recommendations are for 14 days for SEM disease and 21 days for CNS and disseminated disease.[155,159]

Congenital Parvovirus B19 Infection

Human parvovirus B19, the same virus that causes erythema infectiosum (fifth disease), may be transmitted by a gravid female to the fetus and may result in anemia, hydrops fetalis, and even intrauterine fetal demise. The cellular receptor for B19, a virus that lytically infects erythroid precursor cells, is globoside or P-antigen, which is found on erythroblasts and megakaryocytes.[160] Overall, up to 65% of pregnant females are immune to B19 and therefore not at risk,[161] and the majority of infants born to B19-infected mothers are delivered at term and asymptomatic. The greatest risk appears to be when infection is acquired prior to 20 weeks' gestation, and the overall incidence of fetal loss is between 1% and 9%.[162–164] Fetal B19 infection may result in severe anemia, high-output cardiac failure, generalized edema, pleural effusions, and polyhydramnios. Although skin findings are not a major feature of congenital B19 infection, 'blueberry muffin' lesions have been described.[165]

In infants who survive congenital B19 infection, there appears to be no increased risk of congenital anomalies or developmental aberrations. Pregnant women exposed to B19 should be reassured regarding the relatively low potential risk, and offered serologic testing. Detection of B19 antigens in amniotic fluid or B19 DNA via PCR are other methods available for diagnostic confirmation.[166] If acute B19 infection is confirmed, serial fetal ultrasonography should be performed to assess for signs of *in utero* infection. Management of severely afflicted fetuses includes fetal digitalization and *in utero* blood transfusions.

Congenital Syphilis

As a result of advances in the detection and treatment of syphilis during the years following the Second World War, the incidence of neonatal syphilis dropped to relatively insignificant levels by the mid-1950s. Since 1959, however, the incidence of primary and secondary syphilis has increased, with a resultant resurgence in the incidence of congenital syphilis. Surveillance data reported to the CDC by 50 states and the District of Columbia from 1992 to 1998 revealed 942 deaths among 14 627 cases of congenital syphilis, resulting primarily from untreated, inadequately treated, or undocumented treatment of syphilis during pregnancy.[167] In the UK, the number of babies reported with congenital syphilis increased from two in 1996 to 14 in 2005.[168] Such data highlight that congenital syphilis still represents a public health problem.

Congenital syphilis is a disorder in which the fetus becomes infected with the spirochete *Treponema pallidum*, usually after the 16th week of pregnancy. The risk of fetal transmission is estimated to be 70–100% for untreated early syphilis.[169] The widely varied manifestations of congenital syphilis are determined in part by the stage of maternal syphilis, stage of the pregnancy at the time of infection, rapidity of maternal diagnosis, and treatment and immunologic reaction of the fetus.[170] Up to 40% of fetuses with congenital syphilis are stillborn, and among affected live newborns, two-thirds are symptom-free at birth.

The clinical manifestations of congenital syphilis are divided into lesions of *early congenital syphilis* (appearing prior to 2 years of age) and *late congenital syphilis* (occurring after 2 years of age). Skin lesions of early congenital syphilis are generally infectious and, since there is no primary stage, may resemble those of acquired secondary syphilis. They differ from those of the second stage of syphilis in that the fetal lesions are generally more widely distributed, more severe, and of longer duration. Lesions of late congenital syphilis represent either a hypersensitivity reaction on the part of the host or scars and deformities that are direct consequences of infection.

Early congenital syphilis

Fetal infection with *T. pallidum* results in multisystem involvement with considerable variation in clinical expression. Although infants with congenital syphilis frequently exhibit no external signs of disease at the time of birth, many present clinical manifestations within the first month. Those with florid manifestations at birth appear to be more severely infected, are often premature, and usually have a poor prognosis.

The most common clinical manifestations of early congenital syphilis are summarized in Table 2.7. *Rhinitis* (snuffles) is commonly the first sign of congenital syphilis. *Cutaneous lesions* of congenital syphilis are seen in one-third to one-half of affected infants, and may be quite varied. Most common is a diffuse papulosquamous eruption that includes the palms and soles, comparable with the rash seen in secondary syphilis in older patients. Vesiculobullous lesions are relatively rare but, when involving the palms and soles, are highly diagnostic of congenital syphilis. The palms and soles are often fissured, erythematous, and indurated with a dull red, shiny appearance (Fig. 2.42). Concomitant with these changes, desquamation in large dry flakes may occur over the entire body

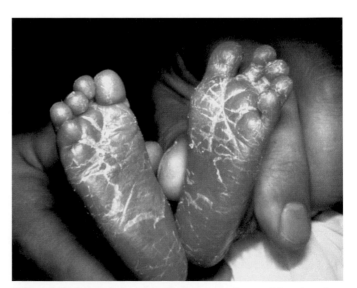

Figure 2.42 Congenital syphilis. Erythema, scaling, and fissuring of the plantar surfaces in early congenital syphilis.

Table 2.7 Manifestations of early congenital syphilis

System	Specific features	Comment
Constitutional	Fever, wasting	
Nasal	Snuffles (nasal discharge)	Commonly the first sign 2–6 weeks of life Ulceration of nasal mucosa If deep, may involve cartilage and result in 'saddle-nose deformity'
Hematologic	Hemolytic anemia Thrombocytopenia	
Lymphoid	Lymphadenopathy	Epitrochlear nodes highly suggestive
Visceral	Hepatosplenomegaly	50–75% of patients Icterus, jaundice, ascites associated
Mucocutaneous	Papulosquamous lesions	Diffuse eruption Palms and soles red, fissured (Fig. 2.42) Bright pink-red, fades to coppery brown Rare vesiculobullous lesions Eventual widespread desquamation
	Condylomata lata	Flat, wart-like lesions in moist areas (especially anogenital, nares, mouth angles)
	Mucous patches	Present in 30–35% Weeping, fissuring at mucocutaneous junctions Extend out from lips in radiating fashion When deep, may leave scars ('rhagades') of perioral region
Osseous	Osteochondritis	15% of patients, especially long bones of extremities; often focal Usually asymptomatic, but severe involvement may lead to subepiphyseal fracture and painful 'pseudoparalysis of Parrot'
	Periostitis	Most pronounced 2nd–6th months of life Usually diffuse Calcification and thickening of cortex may lead to permanent deformity (i.e., frontal bossing, anterior bowing of tibia or 'saber shins')
	Dactylitis	Affects small bones of hands/feet
CNS	CSF abnormalities	Increased protein, mononuclear pleocytosis, (+) CSF VDRL

CNS, central nervous system.

surface area. Flat, moist, wart-like lesions (*condylomata lata*) commonly appear in moist areas of skin in infants with congenital syphilis, and are extremely infectious. Intractable diaper dermatitis is occasionally present. *Mucous patches*, which present as fissures at mucocutaneous junctions, are among the most characteristic and most infectious of the early lesions seen in congenital syphilis.

Necrotizing funisitis, spiral zones of red and blue umbilical cord discoloration interspersed with streaks of chalky white (hence the term *barber-pole umbilical cord*), has been described as a frequently overlooked, early diagnostic feature of congenital syphilis. The external smooth surface of the umbilical cord without evidence of exudation apparently differentiates necrotizing funisitis from acute bacterial funisitis, an inflammation of the umbilical cord seen in newborns with acute bacterial infection.[171]

Hepatomegaly, when present, is frequently associated with icterus and, occasionally, ascites, splenomegaly, and generalized lymphadenopathy. The jaundice, together with anemia, edema, and cutaneous changes, produces a peculiar dirty, whitish brown (café au lait) appearance to the skin. Hemolytic anemia and occasional thrombocytopenia are common features of early congenital syphilis. When occurring with hepatosplenomegaly, jaundice, and large numbers of nucleated erythrocytes in the peripheral circulation, an erroneous diagnosis of erythroblastosis fetalis maybe be made. Nephrotic syndrome and pneumonitis are occasionally present.

Although only 15% of infants with congenital syphilis show clinical signs of osteochondritis at birth, 90% will show radiologic evidence of osteochondritis and/or periostitis after the first month of life. Syphilitic osteochondritis may occur in any bone but is found most frequently in the long bones of the extremities. Radiographic findings consist of increased widening of the epiphyseal line with increased density of the shafts, spotty areas of translucency and a resultant moth-eaten appearance. In most cases, the bony lesions are asymptomatic, but in some infants, severe involvement may lead to subepiphyseal fracture with epiphyseal dislocation and extremely painful pseudoparalysis of one or more extremities (so-called 'pseudoparalysis of Parrot'). Dactylitis, a rare form of osteochondritis of the small bones of the hands and feet that usually appears between 6 months and 2 years of age, may also occur.

Periosteal lesions are seldom present at birth. Periostitis of the frontal bones of the skull, when severe, may contribute to the flat overhanging forehead that persists as a stigma of children severely infected in infancy. The radiologic changes of periostitis are usually most pronounced between the second and sixth months of life and rarely persist beyond the age of 2 years. Lesions are usually diffuse (in contrast to the localized involvement characteristic of lesions of osteochondritis) and frequently extend the entire length of the involved bone. First seen as a thin, even line of calcification outside the cortex of the involved bone, the lesions progress and additional layers of opaque tissue are laid down, with the resulting 'onion-peel' appearance of advanced periostitis. This eventually produces calcification and thickening of the cortex and, when severe, a permanent deformity. In the tibia, this results in an anterior bowing referred to as saber shins. In the skull it is seen (in 30–60% of patients) as frontal or parietal bossing.

Even although clinical evidence of CNS involvement is a relatively uncommon finding, cerebrospinal fluid abnormalities may be detected in 40–50% of infants with congenital syphilis. Recently, IgM immunoblotting and PCR assay on serum or cerebrospinal fluid were shown to be most predictive of CNS infection.[172] Clinical evidence of meningitis with a bulging fontanelle, opisthotonos, and convulsions generally portends a poor prognosis. Low-grade syphilitic meningitis may result in a mild degree of hydrocephalus, and children with central nervous system involvement continuing beyond the period of infancy may go on to demonstrate marked residua with varying degrees of physical and mental retardation.

Late congenital syphilis

Late congenital syphilis refers to the findings that persist beyond 2 years of age. It also includes varying signs and stigmata of congenital syphilis in individuals in whom the diagnosis was overlooked or in those patients who were inadequately treated early in the course of the disease. Signs of late congenital syphilis are summarized in Table 2.8, and a few are discussed in more detail here.

Perhaps the most pathognomonic signs of late congenital syphilis are the dental changes. The deciduous teeth are prone to caries but show no specific abnormalities characteristic of this disorder. The term *Hutchinson's incisors* is applied to deformities of the permanent upper central incisors characterized by central notching with tapering of the lateral sides toward the biting edge (so-called screwdriver teeth). The simultaneous appearance of interstitial keratitis, Hutchinson's incisors, and eighth nerve deafness is termed *Hutchinson's triad*. Although described as a time-honored sign of congenital syphilis, owing to the relative infrequency of eighth nerve deafness, this triad is actually extremely uncommon and rarely observed. The *mulberry molar* is a malformation of the lower first molars. The mulberry appearance is created by poorly developed cusps crowded together on the crown. Since these teeth are subject to rapid decay, mulberry molars are rarely seen past puberty. When present, however, they are pathognomonic of congenital syphilis.

Higouménakis' sign refers to unilateral thickening of the inner third of the clavicle and is frequently described as a manifestation of late congenital syphilis. Since fracture of the middle third of the clavicle is the most common fracture occurring at birth, consequent healing and thickening of the involved bone often produces a clinical picture similar to that seen with Higouménakis' abnormality. This finding should therefore not be considered a reliable stigma of late congenital syphilis.

Paroxysmal cold hemoglobinuria is characterized by shaking chills and dark urine within 8 h following cold exposure, and it may also occur as a manifestation of late congenital syphilis. It is usually seen in patients with late congenital syphilis who did not receive treatment, and although not pathognomonic, is highly suggestive of late congenital or untreated acquired syphilis.

Diagnosis and Treatment of Congenital Syphilis

Determination of the maternal serologic status for syphilis is standard of care in hospitals, and no newborn infant should be discharged without this information being known.[173] All infants born to seropositive mothers require a thorough clinical and laboratory examination, namely a quantitative non-treponemal syphilis test (i.e., VDRL, RPR), and preferably the same as that performed on the mother so that the titers can be compared. Further evaluation of the infant should occur if the mother received no therapy, inadequate therapy, therapy <1 month before delivery, therapy without the expected drop in antibody titer, or therapy before pregnancy with insufficient serologic follow-up.[173] Confirmation of a reactive non-treponemal test is accomplished with a specific treponemal test, such as the fluorescent treponemal antibody absorption (FTA-ABS) test and the microhemagglutination test for *T. pallidum* (MHA-TP). Placental changes may be a useful adjunct in the diagnosis of congenital syphilis, and include necrotizing funisitis (see above), villous enlargement, and acute villitis.[174] Diagnosis may be confirmed by positive darkfield examination from the umbilical vein or from moist lesions of the skin or mucous membranes.

Serologic tests in the newborn must be interpreted with caution since their results may be due to passive transfer of nontreponemal and treponemal antibodies from the mother and their antibody response may be delayed. A serologic titer in the newborn higher than that of the mother, however, is diagnostic. Additionally, since maternal IgM antibodies do not cross the placenta, detection of IgM in the infant indicates active infection.[168] If no other indications of active infection are evident, with serologic titers equal to or lower than the maternal titer, infants should be followed closely, with repeated titers taken at appropriate intervals. In cases of passive transfer of antibody, the neonatal titer should not exceed that of the mother and should revert to negative within 4–6 months. In cases in which the mother is infected late in pregnancy, both mother and child may be non-reactive at delivery. In such instances, clinical signs and rising titers during the ensuing weeks will confirm the diagnosis.

Evaluation of the infant suspected of having congenital syphilis should include a thorough physical examination, serologic studies, cerebrospinal fluid VDRL and cellular/protein analysis, long bone radiographs, complete blood cell and platelet count, and other tests as clinically indicated (i.e., chest radiograph, liver function studies).[173]

Parenteral penicillin G is the treatment of choice for all forms of syphilis. Once the diagnosis of congenital syphilis is confirmed, treatment should commence immediately with aqueous crystalline penicillin G in a dosage of 100 000–150 000 units/kg per day intravenously, divided every 12 h during the first 7 days of life and every 8 h thereafter, for a total of 10 days. Procaine penicillin G in a dosage of 50 000 units/kg per dose administered intramuscularly once daily for 10 days is an alternative. Treated infants should be followed closely, with evaluations at 1, 2, 3, 6, and 12 months of age and non-treponemal tests at 2–4, 6, and 12 months after

---

Table 2.8 Signs of late congenital syphilis

Clutton's joints (knee effusions)
Eighth cranial nerve deafness[a]
Frontal bossing
Gummas (skin, subcutaneous, and bone inflammation and ulceration)
Higouménakis' sign (thickening of inner third of clavicle)
Hutchinson's teeth[a] (peg-shaped upper central incisors)
Hydrocephalus
Interstitial keratitis[a]
Mental retardation
Mulberry molars
Ocular changes (retinitis, optic nerve atrophy)
Paroxysmal cold hemoglobinuria
Rhagades (perioral fissuring)
Saber shins
Saddle nose
Short maxillae

[a]Hutchinson's triad.

conclusion of treatment or until results become non-reactive or the titer has decreased four-fold.[173]

Infants with evidence of central nervous system involvement should receive crystalline penicillin G at a dose of 200000–300000 units/kg per day given every 4–6 h for 10–14 days. Since studies with benzathine penicillin suggest inadequate penetration of the central nervous system of newborns when serum penicillin levels are low, its use for congenital syphilis with central nervous system involvement is not recommended.

Cytomegalic Inclusion Disease

Cytomegalic inclusion disease in the newborn is a generalized infection caused by the cytomegalovirus (CMV), a DNA virus of the herpesvirus group. Congenital CMV infection occurs in 0.3–2.4% of all live births in developed countries,[175] and primary CMV infections are reported in 1–4% of seronegative pregnant women. The risk of viral transmission to the fetus is estimated at 30–40%.[176] CMV transmission has been reported far less frequently in association with non-primary maternal infection.[175] In infants with congenital infection, around 5–18% will be symptomatic at birth.[177] Although the majority of infected infants are asymptomatic, sequelae of congenital CMV infection in symptomatic patients may range from mild defects to severe or fatal disease.

CMV is generally transmitted from a pregnant mother with inapparent infection across the placenta to the fetus late in gestation, although it can also be transmitted by passage through an infected maternal genital tract at the time of delivery or by postnatal CMV-positive blood transfusion. Postnatal transmission may also occur following consumption of infected breast milk, and low birthweight and early postnatal virus transmission are risk factors for symptomatic infection in this setting.[178] Congenital infection is usually suspected based on fetal ultrasound findings, including hydrops, intrauterine growth restriction, microcephaly, ventriculomegaly, and periventricular calcifications. Prematurity occurs in up to 34% of infants with symptomatic congenital CMV infection.[179] Although maternal immunity to CMV was once believed to protect the fetus from infection, it is now known that symptomatic congenital infection can occur after a recurrent maternal infection.[180,181] Since most congenital CMV infections are asymptomatic, diagnosis is most commonly made in infants who manifest several features of the syndrome.

Clinical findings of congenital CMV infection include jaundice, hepatosplenomegaly, anemia, thrombocytopenia, protracted interstitial pneumonia, chorioretinitis, deafness, microcephaly, and eventual mental retardation. Cerebral calcifications (often paraventricular) may be noted on imaging studies. Cutaneous manifestations include petechiae and purpura, a generalized maculopapular eruption, and a generalized 'blueberry muffin' eruption similar to that seen in infants with congenital rubella and toxoplasmosis. Although extremely rare, vesicular lesions have also been reported in infants with this disorder. Most symptomatic cases of congenital CMV infection are fatal within the first 2 months of life. Those who survive frequently manifest severe neurologic defects, including microcephaly, mental retardation, deafness, spastic diplegia, seizure disorder, chorioretinitis, optic nerve atrophy, and blindness. In CMV-infected infants who do not manifest clinical symptoms at birth, 5–15% develop late-onset sequelae such as hearing loss, chorioretinitis, mental retardation, and neurologic defects.[182]

The gold standard for diagnosis of congenital CMV infection remains the detection of virus in saliva or urine during the first few weeks of life.[175] Viral recovery or a strongly positive serum IgM anti-CMV antibody is considered diagnostic. PCR is becoming increasingly popular in the diagnosis of CMV disease, and be applied to urine, blood, saliva and/or cerebrospinal fluid. It offers more rapid results and increased sensitivity. Later in infancy, differentiation between intrauterine and perinatal infection is difficult unless signs of intrauterine infection, such as chorioretinitis or ventriculitis, are present. When the diagnosis remains in doubt, persistent or rising complement-fixation titers may provide confirmatory evidence. Electron microscopic examination for viral particles in urine samples is a rapid diagnostic technique that can also be used, if available. Quantitative PCR exams on peripheral blood leukocytes can be used to monitor viral load in CMV-infected newborns.

Prenatal diagnosis should be reserved for pregnancies in which ultrasonographic findings suggest suspicion for CMV fetal infection.[177] Available methods include CMV isolation from amniotic fluid and identification of CMV DNA by PCR analysis. Demonstration of IgM anti-CMV antibody in percutaneous umbilical blood samples is also diagnostic, but this test is more difficult and has a lower sensitivity. Diagnosis of primary CMV infection in pregnant women is achieved with sensitive IgM and IgG avidity serologic assays, as well as conventional and molecular detection of virus in blood.[183]

There is no consistently effective therapy for congenital CMV infection, and prognosis for the patient with severe involvement is poor. Ganciclovir has been used, although large-scale studies are lacking. One phase II collaborative study of ganciclovir treatment in symptomatic congenital CMV revealed hearing improvement or stabilization in 16% of patients, but only a temporary decrease in CMV excretion in the urine.[184]

Congenital Epstein–Barr Virus Syndrome

Because the majority of young adults are Epstein–Barr virus (EBV) seropositive, primary infection during pregnancy is uncommon. Although features of congenital EBV infection such as micrognathia, cryptorchidism, cataracts, hypotonia, erythematous skin eruptions, hepatosplenomegaly, lymphadenopathy, and persistent atypical lymphocytosis have been reported, the low frequency of EBV infection in pregnancy makes it difficult to assess the full extent of this risk. A recent prospective study comparing women with serologic evidence of primary, recurrent or undefined infection to a control group found no differences in pregnancy outcome, birthweights, or incidence of congenital anomalies, suggesting that EBV infection during pregnancy does not represent a significant teratogenic risk.[185]

Congenital Toxoplasmosis

Toxoplasmosis is a parasitic disorder caused by *Toxoplasma gondii*, an intracellular protozoan that may invade multiple tissues, including muscle (including the heart), liver, spleen, lymph nodes, and central nervous system. Although up to 23% of adolescents and adults may have laboratory evidence of *T. gondii* infection, most are asymptomatic or associated with self-limited symptoms.[186] However, infections in pregnant women may result in serious infantile sequelae if transmitted to the fetus, most notably mental retardation, seizures, and blindness. Toxoplasmosis is transmitted to the fetus transplacentally, and the greatest risk of transmission (60–90%) is when acute infection occurs during the 3rd trimester. The severity of fetal infection tends to be greater when infection is acquired during the 1st trimester. Toxoplasmosis is postnatally transmitted to humans via consumption of raw or inadequately cooked meat (especially pork, lamb, mutton, and wild game) or inadvertent ingestion of oocysts from cat feces in litter or soil.[186] Most pregnant women with acute *T. gondii* infection are asymptomatic without any obvious signs.[187]

Fetal infection with *T. gondii* may result in stillbirth or prematurity. Signs and symptoms of congenital toxoplasmosis may be present immediately at birth or develop during the first few weeks of life, and include fever, malaise, vomiting and diarrhea, lymphadenopathy hepatosplenomegaly, microphthalmia, cataracts, microcephaly, pneumonitis, bleeding diathesis, and seizures. The classic triad of congenital toxoplasmosis consists of chorioretinitis, hydrocephalus, and intracranial calcifications. Up to 80% of patients develop visual or learning disabilities later in life.

Cutaneous findings of congenital toxoplasmosis include a generalized rubella-like maculopapular eruption that generally spares the face, palms, and soles. 'Blueberry muffin'-like lesions (representing extramedullary hematopoiesis) may be present, as may a scarlatiniform eruption or subcutaneous nodules. The skin eruption usually develops during the first weeks of illness, persists for up to 1 week, and may be followed by desquamation or hyperpigmentation.

Laboratory findings in patients with congenital toxoplasmosis are nonspecific and may reveal anemia, eosinophilia, thrombocytopenia, and at times, severe leukopenia. The cerebrospinal fluid may be xanthochromic and may contain leukocytes, erythrocytes, and an elevated level of protein. Skull radiographs of affected infants may reveal diffuse, punctate comma-shaped intracranial calcifications.

The diagnosis of congenital toxoplasmosis is made via the combination of clinical findings, serologic studies, and occasionally, parasite isolation. Identification of *T. gondii*-specific IgG and IgM antibodies are the most commonly used diagnostic modality, although the clinical significance of IgG antibodies is difficult to interpret during the first 6 months of life. Much attention has been focused on the prenatal diagnosis of toxoplasmosis, and in addition to maternal serologic studies, other available methods include IgG avidity studies, the Sabin–Feldman dye test, and PCR analysis of amniotic fluid. Cordocentesis for evaluation of fetal blood serologies is rarely utilized in the current era.

Most newborns with toxoplasmosis are asymptomatic or have only mild symptomatology, although many may have learning disabilities later in life. Because of the serious sequelae that may develop, even in asymptomatic infants, congenital toxoplasmosis should be treated whether or not the infection is clinically apparent. If fetal infection is confirmed, recommended treatments for the mother have included various combinations of sulfadiazine, pyrimethamine, folinic acid, and spiramycin.[188,189] Therapy for affected infants has not been well studied in controlled clinical trials, although combinations of the same agents have been suggested as effective. Corticosteroids may also result in more rapid improvement, especially with regard to chorioretinitis.

The prognosis for infants with toxoplasmosis is variable, although infants who have predominantly CNS involvement have a uniformly poor prognosis. Affected infants may suffer from chorioretinitis with subsequent blindness, microcephaly, hydrocephaly, or mental retardation.

Key References

 The complete list of 189 references for this chapter is available online at **www.expertconsult.com.**
See inside cover for registration details.

Centers for Disease Control and Prevention. Progress toward elimination of rubella and congenital rubella syndrome – the Americas, 2003–2008. *Morb Mortal Wkly Rep MMWR.* 2008;57(43):1176–1179.

Guggisberg D, Hadj-Rabia S, Viney C, et al. Skin markers of occult spinal dysraphism in children. A review of 54 cases. *Arch Dermatol.* 2004;140:1109–1115.

Fortunov RM, Hulten KG, Hammerman WA, et al. Evaluation and treatment of community-acquired *Staphylococcus aureus* infections in term and late-preterm previously healthy neonates. *Pediatrics.* 2007;120:937–945.

Frieden IJ. Aplasia cutis congenita: A clinical review and proposal for classification. *J Am Acad Dermatol.* 1986;14:646–660.

Malm G, Engman ML. Congenital cytomegalovirus infections. *Semin Fetal Neonatal Med.* 2007;12:154–159.

Smith CK, Arvin AM. Varicella in the fetus and newborn. *Semin Fetal Neonatal Med.* 2009;14(4):209–217.

Walker GJA, Walker DG. Congenital syphilis: A continuing but neglected problem. *Semin Fetal Neonatal Med.* 2007;12:198–206.

Eczematous Eruptions in Childhood

3

Eczematous eruptions are characterized as acutely inflamed papules and plaques, often in association with pruritus and serous discharge. The specific subtype of eczematous dermatitis is based upon the clinical morphology, distribution of lesions, and in many cases, the history of exposure. Biopsy of the skin in these conditions is usually not helpful, except to consider alternative diagnoses with distinct histopathologic features. In children, the most prevalent type of eczematous eruption, by far, is atopic dermatitis.

Atopic dermatitis

Atopic dermatitis (AD), one of the most common skin disorders seen in infants and children, begins during the first 6 months of life in 45% of children, the first year of life in 60% of affected individuals, and before 5 years of age in at least 85% of affected individuals.[1] Although the term 'eczema' is frequently used, atopic dermatits is a more precise term to describe this subset of dermatitis, or inflammation of skin. The concept of 'atopy' (derived from the *Greek atopia*, meaning 'different' or 'out of place') was originated by Coca and Cooke in 1923.[2] Although initially only asthma and allergic rhinitis were included in this category, Wise and Sulzberger in 1933 coined the term *atopic dermatitis*,[3] noting the association of this form of eczema with other atopic disorders.

Prevalence and Association with Other Atopic Disorders

The almost 20% prevalence of AD in the USA[4] supports the data from Scandinavia[5] and Japan[6] and represents a marked increase during the past several decades. Studies performed before 1960 estimated the prevalence to be up to 3%.[7] The subsequent steady increase has paralleled the increase seen in children with asthma, suggesting shared triggers and consistent with the frequent development of other atopic disorders in children with AD. In fact, AD is often the first manifestation of this 'atopic march' to asthma and allergic rhinitis. Asthma occurs in up to 50% of children who develop AD during the first 2 years of life; allergic rhinitis develops in 43–80% of children with AD.[8] In general, children showing more severe dermatitis have a higher risk of developing asthma, as well as sensitization to foods and environmental allergens.[9] AD occurs more frequently in urban areas than in rural areas, in smaller families, and in higher socioeconomic classes, suggesting that exposure to antigenic pollutants and lack of exposure to infectious agents or other antigenic triggers early in life may play a role in the development of the dermatitis. Some have classified AD into an IgE-associated form ('true' or 'extrinsic' AD) and a non-IgE-associated form ('nonatopic' or 'intrinsic' AD). However, ultimately 80% of patients will develop increased IgE levels and newer research suggests that IgE-mediated sensitization develops after the onset of disease, especially when the impaired epidermal barrier as a primary defect,[10] blurring the etiologic distinction between 'extrinsic' and 'intrinsic' forms (see below).[11]

Genetic Alterations

A role for causative genetic alterations is suggested by the concordance of 77% in monozygotic twins[12] and the greater probability of having AD if one or, even more so, if both parents are atopic.[13] AD has most highly been linked to genes of the epidermal differentiation complex (including encoding filaggrin),[14] and genes encoding Th2 and Th1 cytokines that are involved in the regulation of IgE synthesis (particularly interleukins-4, -5, -12, and -13).[11,15] Loss-of-function mutations in profilaggrin (*FLG*) cause ichthyosis vulgaris, a common genetic disorder characterized by dry, scaling skin and hyperlinear palms (see Ch. 5) that has long been known to be common in individuals with AD. Distinct mutations in *FLG* have been discovered in the European and Japanese populations, but all are strongly linked with AD, particularly of early onset.[16–20]

Pathomechanism

AD results from the complex interaction between immune dysregulation, epidermal barrier dysfunction, and environmental interactions with skin.[21–23] The 'inside-out' concept of pathogenesis focuses on immune abnormalities as being primary, while the 'outside-in' theory considers the epidermal barrier dysfunction (a form of 'innate immunity') as primary. Several immunologic abnormalities have been noted in individuals with AD. In the acute phase of AD, epidermal Langerhans cells are activated by binding allergens, such as food, aeroallergens, and microbial superantigens, activating T lymphocytes of the T helper 2 (Th2) type, leading to increased expression of interleukins-4, -5, and -13 that promote eosinophilia and IgE production. With chronic AD, a Th1 cytokine phenotype is seen (predominantly interferon-γ). The switch from the acute phenotype of Th2 cell cytokines to Th0/1 cell cytokines of chronic lesions involves the infiltration of epidermis by inflammatory dendritic epidermal cells (IDEC) and production of IL-12 and IL-18 as intermediaries. Thymic stromal lymphopoietin (TSLP) is a keratinocyte-derived cytokine that has been shown to drive both the initial Th2 cytokine response and the switch to the Th0/1 phenotype.[24,25] Mechanical injury (such as scratching or rubbing), microbes, and proinflammatory cytokines themselves further stimulate release of TSLP, thus perpetuating the inflammation. Recent studies suggest that systemic circulation of keratinocyte-derived TSLP is key in the development of allergic sensitization in both the gastrointestinal tract and the lungs.[26,27] Although IgE is elevated in most patients, the elevation is usually noted weeks to months after the dermatitis starts, and it is not thought to be a primary component.

Dysfunction of innate immunity also plays a major role in AD.[28] An intact epidermis is required for the skin to function as a barrier against water loss and ingress of foreign agents, such as microbes and allergens.[29] This barrier can be altered by decreased expression of a structural protein, such as filaggrin (as occurs in ichthyosis vulgaris, see Ch. 5), or by increased expression of proteases (especially kallikrein 5) that break down the barrier and increase TSLP.[30-32] Increases in pH, such as from soaps, can further increase protease activation. In addition, children with AD tend to have a decreased content of ceramides, extracellular lipids that are important for normal barrier function.[33] Barrier dysfunction leads to increased transepidermal water loss and dry skin, a hallmark of AD. Epidermal barrier dysfunction also allows the penetration of high molecular weight allergens, such as dust mite antigens, foods and microbes, to penetrate. For many patients with AD, changes in the skin barrier are primary (as suggested by mutations in *FLG*), with secondary immunologic changes elicited by the more facile penetration of immunologic triggers through an impaired epidermis. The linkage of AD and asthma, but not asthma alone,[34,35] with mutations of *FLG* supports the concept of the 'atopic march', in which AD is the initial atopic disease during infancy with the later occurrence of other atopic conditions dependent on early allergen exposure through the abnormal epidermis (see below). *FLG* mutations are identified in up to 30% of European patients with AD. Nevertheless, immunologic abnormalities further contribute to barrier abnormalities, since the expression of Th2 cytokines IL-4 and IL-13 is known to suppress filaggrin expression.

Toll receptors of the innate immune system of skin recognize pathogens or epidermal injury, and in response produce proinflammatory cytokines and antimicrobial peptides, such as beta-defensins and cathelicidin. In the skin of AD, unlike in normal or psoriatic skin, Th2 cytokines (IL-4 and IL-13) and IL-10 are produced and dampen the production of antimicrobial peptides, contributing to the propensity towards development of skin infection in patients with AD.[36] Vitamin D3 upregulates the expression of cathelicidin, including in the skin of individuals with AD.[37,38]

Clinical Features

Pruritus, its chronicity, and the age-specific morphology and distribution of lesions remain the most important features of AD (Table 3.1). Extent of involvement may range from mild and limited, e.g. of flexural areas, to generalized and severe. AD may be divided into three phases based on the age of the patient and the distribution of lesions. These arbitrary divisions may be referred to as the infantile, childhood, and adult forms of this disorder.

Table 3.1 Clinical criteria for AD

Essential feature
Pruritus (or parental reporting of itching or rubbing) in past 12 months
Plus must have at least three of the following:
History of generally dry skin in past year
Personal history of allergic rhinitis or asthma (or history in first-degree family member if child <4 years old)
Onset before 2 years of age (unless currently under 4 years of age)
History of skin crease involvement (antecubital or popliteal fossae; front of ankles; neck; periorbital)
Visible flexural dermatitis (if child <4 years, include cheeks or forehead, and extensor surface of limbs)

Modified from Brenninkmeijer EE, Schram ME, Leeflang MM, et al. Diagnostic criteria for atopic dermatitis: a systematic review. *Br J Dermatol* 2008;158:754–765. Copyright © 2008 by John Wiley & Sons, Inc. Reprinted by permission of John Wiley & Sons, Inc.[39]

The *infantile phase* of AD reflects the manifestations of AD from birth to 6 months of age. It is characterized by intense itching, erythema, papules, vesicles, oozing, and crusting. In infants, it usually begins on the cheeks, forehead, or scalp (Figs 3.1–3.4), and then may extend to the trunk or particularly the extensor aspects of the extremities in scattered, ill-defined, often symmetrical patches. Generalized xerosis is common. Exacerbation of facial dermatitis on the medial cheeks and chin is often seen concomitant with teething and initiating foods. This localization likely reflects exposure to irritating saliva and foods, although contact urticaria may contribute. By 8–10 months the extensor surfaces of the arms and legs often show dermatitis (Fig. 3.5), perhaps because of the role of friction associated with crawling and the exposure of these sites to irritant and allergenic triggers, such as in carpets. Although dermatitis of the antecubital and popliteal fossae, periorbital areas, and neck are more commonly involved in older children and adolescents, these sites may be affected in infants and young children as well (Fig. 3.6). Typically, lesions of AD spare the groin and diaper area during infancy (Fig. 3.7), which aids in the diagnosis. This sparing likely reflects the combination of increased hydration in the diaper area, protection from triggers by the diaper, and

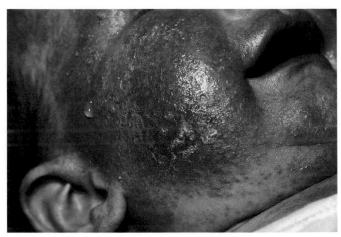

Figure 3.1 Acute atopic dermatitis on the cheek of an infant. Note the tremendous edema and exudation, typical of infantile atopic dermatitis.

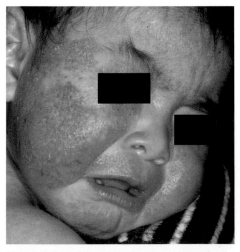

Figure 3.2 Atopic dermatitis on the face of a 9-month-old infant. This patient was rubbing the cheeks repeatedly on her mother's shirt and slept poorly.

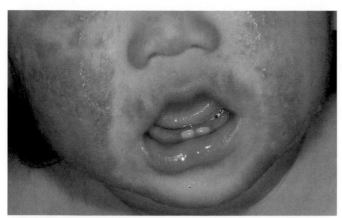

Figure 3.3 Atopic dermatitis and the headlight sign. Note the relative sparing of the midface and immediate perioral area.

inaccessibility to scratching and rubbing. The 'headlight sign' has been used to describe the typical sparing of the nose and medial cheeks in AD, even when there is extensive facial involvement elsewhere (Figs 3.2, 3.3).

Not uncommonly, infants initially present with seborrheic dermatitis, particularly during the first month or two of life. The associated pruritus and the dry (rather than greasier) scale suggest the combination of both disorders (Fig. 3.4); the seborrheic component usually clears by 6–12 months while the AD features persist. Alopecia may accompany the scalp involvement because of inflammation and chronic rubbing.

The childhood phase of AD may follow the infantile stage without interruption and usually occurs during the period from 2 years of age to puberty. Affected persons in this age group are less likely to have exudative and crusted lesions and have a greater tendency

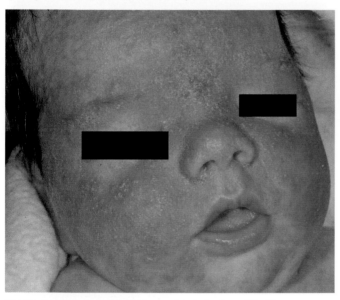

Figure 3.4 Atopic dermatitis and seborrheic dermatitis. The seborrheic dermatitis of this 2-month-old boy with AD cleared within a few months, but the facial dermatitis persisted and required topical immunosuppressive therapy.

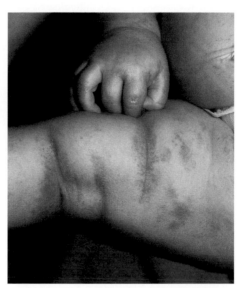

Figure 3.6 Atopic dermatitis. Although antecubital and popliteal fossa involvement is typical of the childhood and adult phases of atopic dermatitis, infants not uncommonly will show involvement at these fold areas. This infant is demonstrating his response to the pruritus.

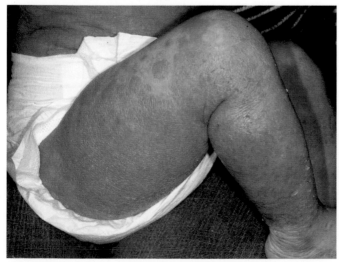

Figure 3.5 Atopic dermatitis. Involvement of the extensor surfaces of the legs and arms are commonly seen during the infantile phase of atopic dermatitis, beginning at about 8 months of age, concomitant with crawling and exposure to irritant and allergenic triggers.

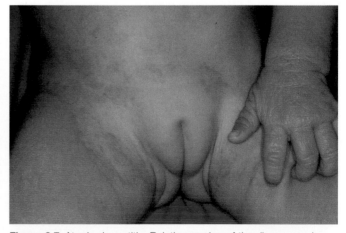

Figure 3.7 Atopic dermatitis. Relative sparing of the diaper area is typical in infants with atopic dermatitis, likely owing to the occlusion of this site and protection from scratching and rubbing, as well as from allergenic triggers.

toward chronicity and lichenification. Eruptions are characteristically more dry and papular and often occur as circumscribed scaly patches. The classic areas of involvement in this group are the wrists, ankles, hands, feet, and antecubital and popliteal regions (Fig. 3.8). Facial involvement switches from cheeks and chin to periorbital (Fig. 3.9) and perioral, the latter sometimes manifesting as 'lip-licker's dermatitis' (see Fig. 3.46). Dermatitis of the nipples (Fig. 3.10) occurs in some children and can be exacerbated by rubbing on clothing. Pruritus is frequently severe. Some children with AD show 'nummular' or coin-shaped lesions, with sharply defined oval scaly plaques on the face, trunk, and extremities (nummular dermatitis, see below). In African-American children, the lesions of AD are often more papular and follicular-based (Fig. 3.11). Although localization at flexural areas is more common, some children show an 'inverse' pattern with involvement primarily of extensor areas. Lymphadenopathy may be a prominent feature in affected children (Fig. 3.12), reflecting the role of lymph nodes in handling local infection and inflammation. Nail pitting or dystrophy may be seen when fingers are affected, indicating involvement of the nail matrix; children may show secondary staphylococcal or pseudomonal paronychia.

The *adult phase* of AD begins at puberty and frequently continues into adulthood. Predominant areas of involvement include the flexural folds (Fig. 3.13), the face and neck, the upper arms and back, and the dorsal aspect of the hands, feet, fingers, and toes. The eruption is characterized by dry, scaling erythematous papules and plaques, and the formation of large lichenified plaques from lesional chronicity. Weeping, crusting, and exudation may occur, but usually as the result of superimposed staphylococcal infection. Prurigo nodularis, well-circumscribed, usually hyperpigmented lichenified papules, most common on the lower extremities, is most commonly seen during adolescence (Fig. 3.14).

Regardless of the phase of AD, post-inflammatory hypopigmentation may be seen (Figs 3.13, 3.15). The pigmentary changes are transient and are reversible when the underlying inflammation is

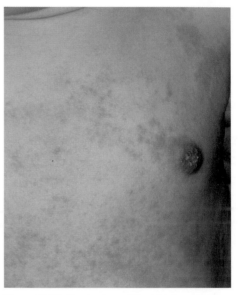

Figure 3.10 Atopic dermatitis. Nipple eczema occasionally occurs in children with atopic dermatitis and is exacerbated by the rubbing of clothes on the affected nipples.

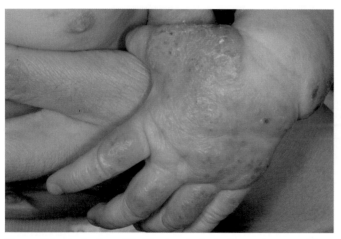

Figure 3.8 Atopic dermatitis. The hands, feet, elbows, knees, ankles, and wrists are commonly affected in children with atopic dermatitis. Note the edema, more common in infants and younger children, and mild crusting at sites of excoriation.

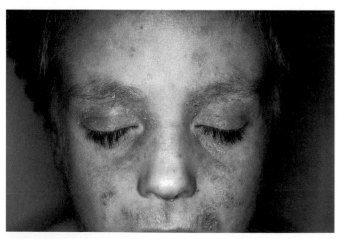

Figure 3.9 Atopic dermatitis. Facial atopic dermatitis in children and adolescents typically affects the periorbital and perioral areas.

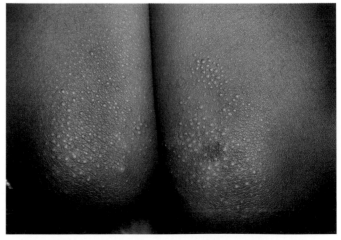

Figure 3.11 Atopic dermatitis. Papular atopic dermatitis is more commonly seen in African-American children with atopic dermatitis, and can be difficult to distinguish from lichen nitidus (see Fig. 4.44) and juvenile frictional lichenoid dermatosis (see Fig. 3.41).

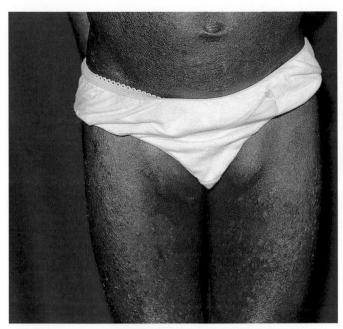

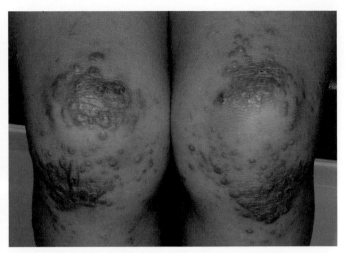

Figure 3.14 Prurigo nodularis. Well-circumscribed, usually hyperpigmented lichenified papules, most common on the lower extremities. Recurrent gouging of these intensely pruritic papules results in scarring.

Figure 3.12 Atopic dermatitis. Lymphadenopathy is a frequent accompanying feature of severe atopic dermatitis, especially when associated with infection.

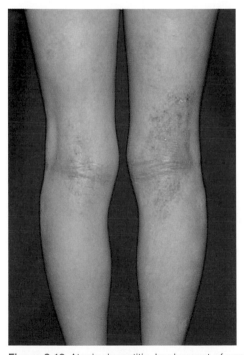

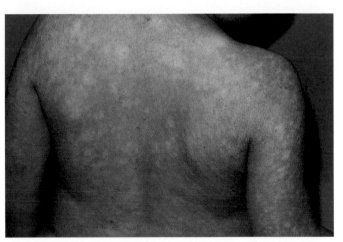

Figure 3.15 Post-inflammatory hypopigmentation of atopic dermatitis. Post-inflammatory hypopigmentation occurs as a sequela of the inflammation of atopic dermatitis, and is particularly prominent during summer months, when the surrounding, unaffected skin tans after exposure to ultraviolet light. The post-inflammatory hypopigmentation is not scarring, and tends to clear spontaneously after several months if further flares of dermatitis at the site are prevented.

Figure 3.13 Atopic dermatitis. Involvement of popliteal and antecubital areas is characteristic in children and adolescents with atopic dermatitis. Note the patches of post-inflammatory hypopigmentation on the legs.

controlled; however, 6 months or more may be required for repigmentation, and sun exposure will accentuate the differences between uninvolved and hypopigmented skin areas. Hyperpigmentation is predominantly noted at sites of lichenification, because the thickened epidermis, especially in darker skinned children, accumulates epidermal melanin pigment. Children with lichenification show accentuation of skin markings (Fig. 3.16). Parents may mistake the

post-inflammatory pigment change seen in some children for scarring or a toxicity of topically applied medications, and need reassurance. AD is not usually a scarring disorder, unless secondary infection or deep gouging of lesions occurs.

Other Clinical Signs

Several other clinical signs are seen with increased frequency in children with AD, although they may appear in children without AD as well. *Dermographism*, a manifestation of the triple response of Lewis that occurs in approximately 5% of the normal population, is characterized by a red line, flare, and wheal reaction. A red line develops within 15 s at the exact site of stroking, followed within 15–45 s by an erythematous flare (because of an axon-reflex vasodilatation of arterioles). The response finally eventuates in a

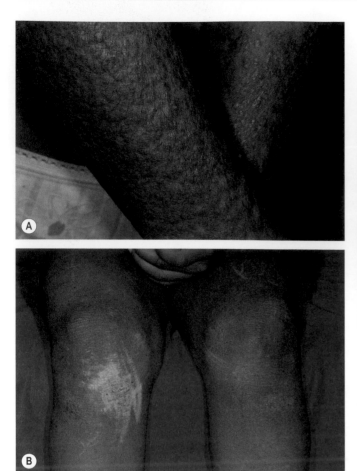

Figure 3.16 (A,B) Lichenification. Accentuation of skin markings are notable in thickened, lichenified skin of chronic atopic dermatitis. In darker-skinned individuals, hyperpigmentation tends to be associated with the lichenification. Note the 'ashy' color of scale (B) produced by scratching at the site.

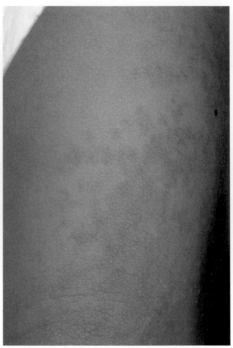

Figure 3.17 Keratosis pilaris. The fine follicular-based keratotic papules of keratosis pilaris are most prominently seen on the anterior thighs (as shown), the lateral aspect of the upper arms, and the lateral aspects of the face.

wheal (because of transudation of fluid from the injured capillaries in the original stroke line) 1 to 3 min later. Individuals with AD often demonstrate a paradoxical blanching of the skin termed *white dermographism*. The initial red line is replaced, generally within 10 s, by a white line without an associated wheal. Patients with AD may also show *circumoral pallor*, thought to relate to local edema and vasoconstriction.

Follicular hyperkeratosis or chicken-skin appearance, particularly on the lateral aspects of the face, buttocks, and outer aspects of the upper arms and thighs, is termed *keratosis pilaris* (Fig. 3.17) (see Ch. 7). Keratosis pilaris is not seen at birth, but is common from early childhood onwards, and often persists into adulthood. Each lesion represents a large cornified plug in the upper part of the hair follicles, often with surrounding inflammation and vasodilatation. Keratosis pilaris is more commonly associated with AD in children with ichthyosis vulgaris. Moisturizers alone tend to be insufficient as therapy for keratosis pilaris, and keratolytic agents, such as urea or α-hydroxy acids are required. Their use is limited, however, by the increased potential for irritation in children with AD. Treatment should be discouraged unless of significant cosmetic importance.

Lichen spinulosus manifests as round collections of numerous tiny, skin-colored to hypopigmented dry spiny papules (Fig. 3.18).[40] More common in African-American children, lichen spinulosus most commonly occurs on the trunk or extremities. Lesions tend to

be asymptomatic, and may respond to application of emollients and mild topical corticosteroids. Children with AD also show an increased incidence of *pityriasis alba, nummular dermatitis, dyshidrotic eczema*, and *juvenile plantar dermatosis* (see below).

Atopic individuals have a distinct tendency toward an extra line or groove of the lower eyelid, the so-called atopic pleat (Fig. 3.19). The atopic pleat, seen just below the lower lid of both eyes, is present at birth, or shortly thereafter, and is usually retained throughout life. This groove (frequently referred to as *Dennie-Morgan fold*) may result from edema of the lower eyelids and skin thickening; it represents a feature of the atopic diathesis rather than a pathognomonic marker of AD. The atopic pleat has been found with increased incidence in African-American children.[41] Slate-gray to violaceous infraorbital discolorations (*allergic shiners*), with or without swelling, are also seen in allergic patients and in patients with AD. Allergic shiners are thought to be a manifestation of vascular stasis induced by pressure on underlying venous plexuses by edema of the nasal and paranasal cavities; the swelling and discoloration become more prominent as a result of repeated rubbing of the eyes and post-inflammatory pigment darkening. Another clinical feature, an exaggerated linear nasal crease, is caused by frequent rubbing of the nasal tip (the so-called *allergic salute*). Although not a specific sign of AD, the nasal crease can also serve as a cutaneous clue to an atopic diathesis and allergic rhinitis.

Many atopic patients exhibit an increased number of fine lines and accentuated markings of the palms (Fig. 3.20). These accentuated palmar markings often are a clue to the concurrent diagnosis of ichthyosis vulgaris (see Pathomechanism above, and Ch. 5), a relatively common semi-dominant genetic disorder seen with increased frequency in children with AD. Although individuals with either AD or ichthyosis vulgaris may show accentuated markings on the palms and soles, the characteristic generalized scaling, with larger and more severe scaling on the lower extremities, worsening during winter months, and often positive family history of

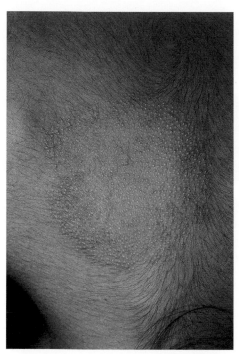

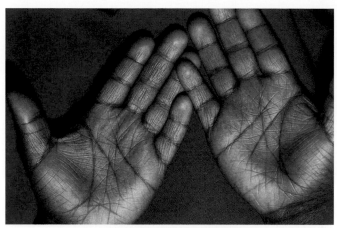

Figure 3.20 Accentuated palmar creases. Hyperlinearity of the palms is a sign of concurrent ichthyosis vulgaris (see Ch. 5), a genetic disorder of skin associated with an increased risk of atopic dermatitis.

Figure 3.18 Lichen spinulosus. Commonly seen in children with dry skin and sometimes with atopic dermatitis. The characteristic usually round collections of tiny, discrete flat-topped papules are usually asymptomatic.

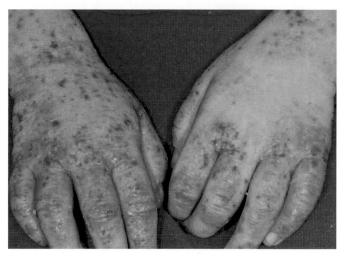

Figure 3.21 Staphylococcal infection in atopic dermatitis. Sites of excoriation on the dorsal aspects of the hand are oozing and crusted. Note the erythema and mild associated edema. Fissuring is often associated on the hands and feet, as seen on the right thumb. Both the dermatitis and the infection improved with oral administration of cephalexin, and the use of daily baths with sodium hypochlorite helped to maintain control, while minimizing crusting.

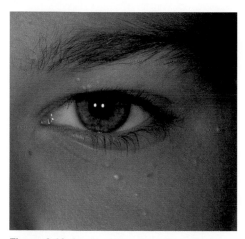

Figure 3.19 Atopic pleats. Accentuated lines or grooves (atopic pleats, Morgan's folds, Dennie's lines) are seen below the margin of the lower eyelids. This is a sign of the allergic diathesis, and is not specific to atopic dermatitis. Note that this child has numerous milia of the periorbital area, small inclusion cysts that are often a sign of chronic rubbing of the skin.

continuous rubbing of the eyes or as a degenerative change in the cornea. Onset is usually after adolescence.

Infectious Complications

Secondary infection, particularly due to *Staphylococcus aureus* and occasionally to *Streptococcus pyogenes*, is the most common complication seen in AD. The skin of patients with AD is inherently favorable for *S. aureus* colonization. In contrast to a prevalence of a carrier state in 5–20% of nonatopic individuals, *S. aureus* is recovered in ~90% of patients from lesions of AD, 76% from uninvolved (normal) skin, and ~80% from the anterior nares.[44,45] The increased adherence of *S. aureus* to the epidermal cells of individuals with AD[46] and a failure to produce endogenous antimicrobial peptides in the inflamed skin of patients with AD[47] may account for the high rate of *S. aureus* colonization and infection. The pyoderma associated with AD is usually manifested by erythema with exudation and crusting (Fig. 3.21), particularly at sites of scratching, and

patients with ichthyosis vulgaris further helps to distinguish these conditions.

Allergic keratoconjunctivitis, characterized by ocular pruritus and photophobia, has been described in up to 30% of children with AD.[42] *Posterior subcapsular cataracts* have been described in up to 13% of adult patients with severe AD.[43] Although rarely seen in children, these cataracts are usually asymptomatic. *Keratoconus* (elongation of the corneal surface) has been reported in about 1% of patients with AD and seems to develop independently of cataracts.[43] Keratoconus has been considered to be the result of occasionally by small pustules at the advancing edge (Fig. 3.22). This complication must be considered whenever a flare of chronic AD develops or fails to respond to appropriate therapy. *S. aureus* exacerbates the AD through: (1) release of superantigen toxins, which enhance T cell activation; (2) activation of superantigen-specific and allergen-specific T cells;[48] (3) expression of IgE antistaphylococcal antibodies;[49,50] and (4) increased expression of IL-31 which leads to pruritus.[51] Superantigen production also increases the expression of an alternative glucocorticoid receptor that does not bind to topical corticosteroids, leading to resistance.[52] These observations emphasize the role of *S. aureus* as an important trigger of AD and endorse therapies that decrease the numbers of bacteria on the skin (see below). Although methicillin-resistant *S. aureus* (MRSA) colonization and superinfection of AD is increasing, the majority of children with AD harbor methicillin-sensitive *S. aureus* (MSSA).[45,53] MRSA infection may manifest as abscesses (Fig. 3.23) or crusting that is indistinguishable clinically from MSSA infection.

Greater cutaneous dissemination of certain viral infections has also been noted in children with AD, and has been attributed to defects in the generation of antimicrobial peptide, and the relative deficiency of Th1 cytokine generation and cytotoxic T-cell function. *Molluscum contagiosum* is a cutaneous viral infection of childhood that most commonly affects the trunk, axillae, antecubital and popliteal fossae, and crural areas (Ch. 15). Lesions are usually small, dome-shaped papules that often show central umbilication. The often-extensive molluscum lesions tend to be most numerous at sites of active dermatitis and can induce pruritus as well as dermatitis around the molluscum papules ('molluscum dermatitis').

Eczema herpeticum (Kaposi's varicelliform eruption) describes the explosive development of a vesiculopustular eruption due to *Herpes simplex* virus in an atopic individual. Children with more severe AD and other atopic conditions are at greatest risk.[54] The clustering and often umbilication of the vesicles is characteristic (Figs 3.24, 3.25), with sites of the dermatitis most frequently affected. The diagnosis can be verified by direct fluorescent assay and viral culture. If these tests are not available, a Tzanck test can be performed by scraping

the floor of vesicles and, after staining the smear with Giemsa or Wright stain, searching for multinuclear virus 'giant cells' or balloon cells.

Eczema vaccinatum was a problem when smallpox vaccinations were compulsory, most frequently contracted by accidental contact

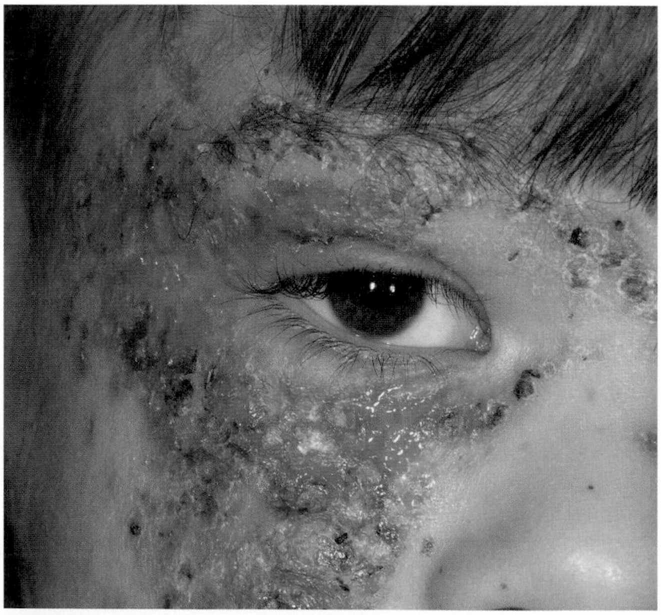

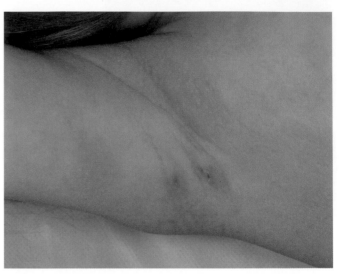

Figure 3.23 Methicillin-resistant *Staphylococcus aureus* infection in atopic dermatitis. Note the two resolving abscesses in the axillary area of this child with severe atopic dermatitis.

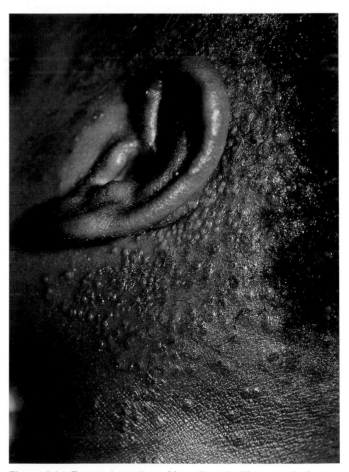

Figure 3.24 Eczema herpeticum (Kaposi's varicelliform eruption). Grouped vesiculopustular lesions on the face, retroauricular, and neck areas. Several of the pustules are beginning to show umbilication.

Figure 3.22 Staphylococcal infection in atopic dermatitis. Discrete non-grouped pustules and crusting overlying erythema and swelling of the periorbital area of a child with severe atopic dermatitis.

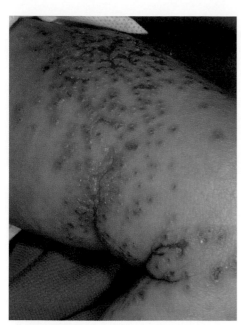

Figure 3.25 Eczema herpeticum. These small, round umbilicated vesicles and punched out erosions are typical lesions of *herpes simplex* infection.

with a recently vaccinated individual. The global threat of bioterrorism and consideration of smallpox vaccinations has again brought to attention the risk of eczema vaccinatum for patients, and particularly children, with AD.[55] Eczema vaccinatum is characterized by the widespread cutaneous dissemination of vaccinia viral lesions, characterized as firm, deep-seated vesicles or pustules that are all in the same stage of development (Ch. 15). Lesions may become umbilicated or confluent.

Reactivity to Malassezia has been blamed for recalcitrant AD of the head and neck in adolescents. Although there are no documented differences in Malassezia species colonization, patients with head and neck AD are more likely to have positive skin prick test results and Malassezia-specific IgE compared with healthy control subjects and patients with atopy without head and neck dermatitis. These patients may benefit from a 1- to 2-month course of daily itraconazole or fluconazole followed by long-term weekly treatment.[56]

Differential Diagnosis

AD is a chronic fluctuating disease. The distribution and morphology of lesions vary with age, but itching is the cardinal symptom of this disorder. Although many skin conditions may occasionally resemble AD, certain characteristics assist in their differentiation.

Seborrheic dermatitis is characterized by a greasy yellow or salmon-colored scaly eruption that may involve the scalp, cheeks, trunk, extremities, and diaper area. The major differentiating features include a tendency toward earlier onset, characteristic greasy yellowish or salmon-colored lesions with a predisposition for intertriginous areas, a generally well-circumscribed eruption, and a relative absence of pruritus (see below). Infants may show both atopic and seborrheic dermatitis (Fig. 3.4), with progression or persistence of the atopic lesions as the seborrheic dermatitis subsides.

Contact dermatitis can be divided into irritant contact dermatitis and allergic contact dermatitis. *Primary irritant dermatitis* is frequently seen in infants and young children. It is most commonly seen on the cheeks and the chin (owing in part to the irritation of

saliva), the extensor surfaces of the extremities (as a result of harsh soaps, detergents, or rough fabrics), and the diaper area (primarily from feces and vigorous cleansing). Primary irritant dermatitis is generally milder, less pruritic to asymptomatic, and not as eczematous and oozing as the eruptions seen in association with AD. Although irritant contact dermatitis to saliva and to exposure to harsh soaps and fabrics occurs more often in children with concomitant AD, irritant diaper dermatitis does not occur more frequently, with typical sparing of the diaper area in infants with AD. Irritant dermatitis may also result from bubble baths, personal care products, and in handling modeling clays.

Allergic contact dermatitis, although relatively uncommon in the first few months of life, can mimic almost any type of eczematous eruption and is characterized by a well-circumscribed pruritic, erythematous, papular, and vesicular eruption. Although such eruptions involute spontaneously on identification and removal of the cause, this disorder often requires a carefully detailed history and prolonged observation before the true causative agent is identified. Recent studies have found no difference in the rate of positive patch testing in atopic and nonatopic children.[57] Nevertheless, allergic contact dermatitis to nickel occurs frequently in children with AD and may be misdiagnosed as recalcitrant periumbilical AD. Patients with recalcitrant AD may have concomitant allergic contact reactions, particularly to nickel and less often to topically applied medications and emollients, suggesting the role for patch testing.[58] In recent studies, 6.2–22% of children with AD showed positive patch tests for potential allergens other than nickel.[57,59] In one study, half of these children showed reactivity to their emollient with a variety of individual ingredients found to the responsible (avena extract; wheat protein; calendula; lanolin). Others showed reactivity to topical antiseptic (chlorhexidine) and one to the topical steroid.[59]

Nummular dermatitis is a distinctive disorder characterized by coin-shaped lesions. Measuring 1 cm or more in diameter, lesions of nummular dermatitis develop on dry skin and are more often seen during dry winter months. The eruption is characterized by discrete erythematous round plaques formed by the confluence of papules and vesicles (Figs 3.26, 3.27). Nummular lesions tend to be more recalcitrant to topical therapy and, not uncommonly, become infected, so that comcomitant treatment of secondary staphylococcal infection and measures to limit staphylococcal overgrowth (such as dilute sodium hypochlorite baths) should be considered.

The lesions of *psoriasis*, another common skin disease of children, are bright red and topped with loosely adherent silvery micaceous scale (Ch. 4). Psoriatic lesions usually show a sharply delineated edge, and have a predilection for the extensor surfaces (particularly the elbows and knees), the scalp, the buttock, and the genital regions. Approximately 5% of children with psoriasis also show dermatitis, either as typical psoriasis and atopic dermatitis lesions or a psoriasiform dermatitis; these children often have a family history of both atopy and psoriasis.

Scabies in infants and children is commonly complicated by eczematous changes because of scratching and rubbing of involved areas or the application of harsh topical therapeutic agents. The diagnosis of scabies is best made by the history of itching, a characteristic distribution of lesions, the recognition of primary lesions (particularly the pathognomonic burrow when present), positive identification of the mite on microscopic examination of skin scrapings, and the presence of infestation among the patient's family or associates (Ch. 18).

Langerhans cell histiocytosis (LCH) most commonly occurs before 3 years of age (Ch. 10). In affected neonates, reddish brown, purpuric, crusted papules or vesiculopapules are typically present. In infants this skin eruption is often characterized as a scaly,

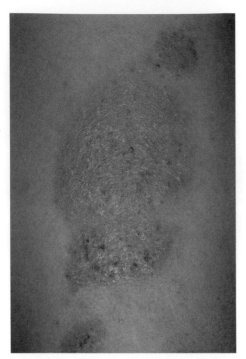

Figure 3.26 Nummular dermatitis. Characterized by well-defined, round (coin-shaped or nummular) plaques of vesiculopapules overlying erythema and edema. Oozing and secondary infection are common. Note that plaques can coalesce.

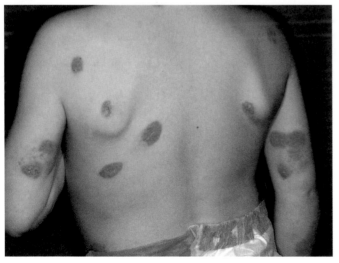

Figure 3.27 Nummular dermatitis. Some patients show multiple nummular plaques.

erythematous seborrheic eruption on the scalp, behind the ears, and in the intertriginous regions. On close inspection the presence of reddish brown, petechial or purpuric lichenoid papules, or vesicular or crusted papules, in infants is typical. Cutaneous biopsy and identification of CD1a+ Langerhans cells by immunostaining confirms the diagnosis of LCH.

Acrodermatitis enteropathica is an autosomal recessive disorder characterized by vesiculobullous eczematoid lesions of the acral and periorificial areas, failure to thrive, diarrhea, alopecia, nail dystrophy, and frequent secondary bacterial or candidal infection (see Chs 2 and 24). The characteristic distribution of lesions, accompanied by listlessness, diarrhea, failure to thrive, and low serum zinc levels, differentiate lesions of acrodermatitis enteropathica from those of AD. Usually a disorder in formula-fed babies with the hereditary form, acrodermatitis enteropathica may also occur in breast-fed babies owing to deficient zinc secretion into maternal breast milk.

Typical AD may be a feature of several forms of immuno-deficiency, most notably in *Wiskott–Aldrich syndrome* and the *hyperimmunoglobulinemia E syndrome* (HIES). These disorders are distinguished from AD by their recurrent noncutaneous infections and other characteristic features (e.g., thrombocytopenic purpura, bloody diarrhea, and purpuric lesions in Wiskott–Aldrich syndrome and facial and intertriginous staphylococcal abscesses in HIES).

Prognosis and Effect on Quality of Life

AD tends to clear in 43% of children by age 3, and in up to 70% of patients by puberty.[60,61] The quality of life in infants, children, and adolescents with moderate to severe dermatitis, however, is significantly reduced,[62] and having severe AD during childhood leads to delayed social development.[63] The disfigurement associated with moderate to severe AD, coupled with the reduction in sleep, restlessness and fatigue at school, and limitations in participation in sports, isolates the affected child and strains relationships with peers and with teachers. Infants with AD have been shown to be excessively dependent and fearful. The disorder also impacts the family both psychologically and financially. As a chronic disorder that requires frequent attention, the family carries a high financial burden of parental missed days from work for doctor visits and home care, lost wages owing to interruption of employment, expensive medications, and the costs of special or additional bedding, clothes, and food. The demonstrated average reduction by 1–2 h of parental sleep nightly also translates into increased parental stress[64] and the tendency of affected children to co-sleep with parents affects family dynamics.[65] These stressful psychological factors often exacerbate the AD, as may concurrent infectious illness or the stress of assignments at school. Stress-induced increases in the levels of eosinophils, subpopulations of T lymphocytes, and natural killer cells in patients with AD have been described, and have not been noted in healthy controls or individuals with psoriasis.[66]

The management of AD requires patient and parent education,[67] avoidance of irritants and allergic triggers, good moisturization, and use of anti-inflammatory medications[68] (Table 3.2). The National Eczema Association (NEA) offers a website for education and patient support (www.nationaleczema.org). Age-specific structured educational programs have improved objective and subjective severity scores,[69] and educational videos may improve severity beyond direct education.[70] Written action plans have been shown to improve adherence to therapy.[71]

Management

Use of emollients and bathing

In general, dryness is worse during cold months, when it is aggravated by heat in the house and low humidity. Although it is true that the dermatitis of xerotic individuals can be exacerbated by bathing because of evaporative loss, daily baths are considered an excellent means of hydrating the skin. Baths are also fun for infants and children, contribute to parent–child bonding, and remove surface bacteria and desquamated scale. Most experts recommend limitation of the bath to approximately 10 min to prevent loss of endogenous cutaneous lipids. Older children and adolescents should be instructed to avoid excessively warm baths and showers. Only mild soaps (such as Cetaphil, Dove or Basis) or soapless

	Table 3.2 Management of mild, moderate, and severe forms of AD	
Mild	**Moderate**	**Severe**
Bathing and barrier repair*	Bathing and barrier repair	Bathing and barrier repair
Avoidance of irritant and allergic triggers	Avoidance of irritant and allergic triggers	Avoidance of irritant and allergic triggers
Intermittent, short-term use of class VI or VII topical steroids (see Table 3.3) ± topical calcineurin inhibitors	Intermittent, short-term use of class III–V topical steroids (see Table 3.3) ± topical calcineurin inhibitors	Class II topical steroids for flares (see Table 3.3); class III–V topical steroids ± tacrolimus ointment for maintenance
Treat superinfection	Treat superinfection	Treat superinfection
	Oral antihistamines	Oral antihistamines
		Consider systemic antiinflammatory agents, ultraviolet light therapy

*Barrier repair may be accomplished by application of effective emollients or from 'barrier repair' agents.

cleansers (such as Cetaphil, Cerave or Aquanil) should be used, if a cleanser is felt to be needed. Bubble baths are contraindicated when severe involvement is present. Bath oils are only slightly beneficial and, since they tend to make the tub slippery, should be used sparingly and cautiously.

The key to maintaining hydration after bathing in patients with AD is application of a thick emollient within 3 min after exiting the bath, before evaporative loss occurs. Usually the thicker and greasier the emollient, the higher the content of oil relative to water and the more effective the emollient. In general, lotions with their water content higher than that of ointments or creams do not tend to be as effective as the thicker emollients for decreasing skin dryness. Nevertheless, non-ointment emollients, particularly ceramide-dominant creams, can be substituted when use of greasy ointment is objectionable, and may have inherent anti-inflammatory properties. A recent study suggests that application of an emollient with pH of ≤5 (normal skin surface pH is 5.5) may suppress inflammation.[72] 'Barrier repair' agents, such as N-palmitoylethanolamine (as in MimyX)[73], ceramide-dominant, physiological-lipid based cream (Epiceram)[74], and MAS063DP (Atopiclair)[75], also show mild anti-inflammatory properties and may be beneficial for children with mild to moderate AD.

The addition of dilute sodium hypochlorite (bleach) to the bath is helpful in controlling the dermatitis of children who with a history of skin infection.[45] The recent recognition that 38% of young children with mild disease have IgE antibodies against staphylococcal superantigen suggests that dilute bleach baths may be more universally helpful.[76] Children may complain about sitting in a tub bath because of stinging, particularly during acute exacerbations with raw skin and crusting. In such instances, the addition of 1 cup of salt may make the bath more tolerable until more aggressive therapy, including of secondary infection, leads to improvement. If a bath is not possible, wet compresses may be tolerated. Wet wraps of plain water can be applied at night, for example, after bathing and emolliation or after application of the topical antiinflammatory agent to decrease pruritus and the sensation of burning at night.[77–79] Short-term use (up to 14 days) of wet wraps over diluted topical

corticosteroids is more efficacious than over bland emollients alone but can be associated with transiently increased steroid absorption.[78] Although wet gauze bandage wraps (such as Kerlix or Kling) are often used in a hospital setting, dressing the young child at home in moist pajamas and socks that cling to the skin, topped by a dry layer to avoid excessive cooling, can be very soothing and promote sleep. Unna boots can also be loosely applied to the legs or arms at night (under self-adherent wraps) to decrease pruritus and protect from scratching.

Open wet compresses may be useful in children with weeping, oozing, or crusted lesions. Aluminum acetate (as in Burow's solution, 1:20 or 1:40) is germicidal and suppresses the weeping and oozing of acutely inflamed lesions. Burow's solution 1:40 is prepared by dissolving one packet or effervescent tablet (Domeboro) in a pint of cool or tepid tap water. These compresses are applied two to three times daily for 10–15 min for a period of up to 5 days, with a soft cloth such as a man's handkerchief or strips of bedsheeting. Washcloths and heavy toweling interfere with evaporation and therefore are not as effective. Compresses should be lukewarm, moderately wet (not dripping), and remoistened at intervals. Following the compress, the topical antiinflammatory agent may be applied.

Avoidance of irritant triggers

Many patients have problems with eccrine sweating and sweat retention during the summer months, leading to increased pruritus, especially in the face of lichenification and significant dermal inflammation. The increased vasodilatation of already inflamed skin from increased summer heat further contributes to pruritus and cutaneous warmth. Nevertheless, children with AD should be encouraged to participate as actively in sports as possible. Swimming is an excellent sport for children with AD if exposure to chlorinated pool water is tolerated. Children should be coated with a thick emollient (after sunscreen application) as a protectant against the high concentration of chlorine; rinsing immediately after swimming with application of emollient may decrease the risk of irritation. Air-conditioning is important during hot weather to decrease pruritus. Children should also be kept cool after application of the thick emollient or, if sweating is anticipated, a less occlusive moisturizer should be applied. The pruritus and erythematous papules of *miliaria rubra*, which can develop when sweating is prevented by application of a thick emollient (especially in infants), can be confused by parents with exacerbation of the dermatitis, setting up a cycle of worsening involvement from repeated application of the occlusive emollient. Recognition and education in decreasing the frequency of emollient application are vital in this situation.

Overdressing children during winter months should also be avoided to prevent overheating. The low humidity of winter months and use of indoor heating also increases skin xerosis and may promote dermatitis; humidifiers maybe useful, but may increase the exposure to mold allergens. Saliva is a major irritant for infants with AD and exposure to large amounts of saliva with teething and eating exacerbates the facial dermatitis. Protecting the face before meals or naptime with a thick, protective emollient may be helpful. Similarly older children with AD are at risk for lip-licker's dermatitis because of the irritant effects of saliva.

Attention to clothing is also important. Soft cotton clothing is recommended over wool or other harsh materials, which tend to precipitate itching and scratching. Fabrics that are designed to decrease bacterial colonization and prevent dust mite sensitization are currently under investigation.[80] Affected children should avoid use of harsh soaps and detergents, fabric softeners, products with fragrance, and bubble baths. Smoking of cigarettes in homes of children with AD should be avoided, since it can lead to an increase in irritation and pruritus, and may also increase the tendency toward subsequent development of asthma.[81]

Avoidance of triggering allergens

Potential allergen triggers can be identified by taking a careful history and doing selective allergy tests.[82] Most common are foods in infants and aeroallergens in children and adolescents. At 6 months of age, 83% of patients with severe dermatitis show IgE food sensitization to milk, eggs, and/or peanuts, and 65% of these children retain food sensitivity by 12 months of age. In comparison, 5% of 6-month-old infants and 11% of 12-month-old infants without atopy show IgE food sensitization.[83] The relationship between reactivity to foods and the dermatitis itself, however, is complex. Although food allergens have been noted to induce skin rashes in nearly 40% of children with moderate to severe AD,[84] many of these are urticarial or maculopapular in character and not dermatitic. Foods may also induce extracutaneous manifestations, particularly involving the gastrointestinal tract. It should be recognized that foods may act as irritants, especially citrus foods, and that reactions to chemicals in foods, such as tartrazine or other colorings, may occur.

Reactivity to food allergens (most commonly milk, eggs, soy, wheat, and peanuts) as shown by a wheal response after skin-prick testing or serum IgE testing serves as a guideline to consider the possibility that these foods may be triggering the dermatitis. Negative skin-prick tests or serum allergen-specific IgE levels are highly predictive at eliminating potential allergens; ImmunoCAP specific IgE levels have been found to correlate better than RAST and prick tests with clinically relevant food allergy to eggs, milk, peanut, and fish, based on both history and double-blind food challenges.[85,86] However, increased antigen-specific IgE levels are often elevated in children with AD, and their level does not necessarily predict a food that triggers the dermatitis.

Despite the frequency of reactivity, pediatric dermatologists estimate that up to 10–15% overall of children with moderate-to-severe AD have food allergies that may be relevant to their dermatitis, and these children tend to be the more severely affected children. Given the low accuracy of food allergy tests for predicting triggers in children with AD, these tests should be limited to moderate to severely affected children who are not responsive to traditional agents for treating the dermatitis or to those with suspected associated allergic conditions (e.g., allergic rhinitis or gastrointestinal involvement). Ideally, a relationship between certain foods and provocation of the AD should be suggested by clinical reactivity, not merely by positive prick, RAST tests, or ImmunoCAP specific IgE levels that may occur in children with AD, although basing food avoidance on clinical reactivity alone can be difficult. For children in whom food allergies are suspected to be relevant, co-management with a pediatric allergist is recommended.

Several older studies suggested that breast-feeding, extensively hydrolyzed casein formula (i.e., hypoallergenic), and elimination of the more highly allergenic foods (eggs, milk, and peanut) from the diets of infants and breastfeeding mothers (because protein passes into breast milk) may lower the risk of developing AD in at-risk families. The results of these studies, however, are controversial. A systematic review of nine randomized controlled trials of dietary exclusion found little benefit to elemental or other exclusion diets, except perhaps egg avoidance in infants with specific IgE to eggs.[87] The American Academy of Pediatrics has released several recommendations based on evidence-based studies. They conclude that: (1) exclusive breast-feeding for at least 4 months prevents or delays the occurrence of AD, but not asthma, in high-risk infants; (2) maternal dietary restrictions during pregnancy and lactation are not warranted in preventing atopic disease; (3) there is no clear evidence supporting the use of soy-based infant formulas to prevent allergy; (4) there is modest evidence that AD may be delayed or prevented by the use of extensively or partially hydrolyzed formulas in comparison to cow's milk formula in high-risk infants who are not exclusively breast-fed for 4–6 months; and (5) solid foods should not be introduced before 4–6 months of age, but delaying introduction, including of highly allergenic foods, beyond this time does not prevent the development of atopic disease.[88–91]

The most common food allergens frequently contaminate other foods and are difficult to avoid entirely. Restrictions in diet should not worsen the quality of the patient's and family's life more than the AD itself. Challenges of agents that may trigger IgE reactivity are best conducted under medical observation, since anaphylaxis has occasionally been reported. It should be remembered that excessively restrictive diets in atopic children may lead to weight loss, calcium deficiency, hypovitaminosis, and kwashiorkor, and proper nutritional counseling and supplementation should be included in management. After the first few years of life, the risk of significant reactivity to food diminishes (particularly with eggs, milk, soy, and wheat). Unless a careful dietary history suggests food sensitivity as a trigger, improvement through dietary manipulation in children >5 years is rarely noted.

In contrast to potential reactivity to foods, reactivity of children and adolescents with AD to aeroallergens increases with age. The most common aeroallergen triggers are house-dust mite (*Dermatophagoides pteronyssinus*), grass pollens, animal dander, and molds, particularly *Alternaria*. Plant pollens, particularly ragweed, also contain an oleoresin capable of producing sensitization and eczematous contact dermatitis. Air-borne dermatitis may involve the exposed surfaces of the face, neck, arms, legs, and 'V' area of the chest, but can be distinguished from photosensitivity, which results in sharper lines of demarcation between normal skin and eczematous skin. Exacerbation of facial dermatitis during pollen season or after children contact a pet, e.g., should alert parents to the possibility of allergy to an aeroallergen or contact allergen (see below). While pets certainly can be triggers of AD, a recent systematic review of 30 articles concluded that there was no clear evidence that telling families with young children to avoid pets is warranted in preventing the occurrence of AD;[92] nevertheless cat, but not dog allergy, was recently correlated with mutations in *FLG* and AD.[93]

Epicutaneous application of aeroallergens by atopy patch test on unaffected atopic skin shows reactivity as an eczematoid patch in 30–50% of patients with AD, but tends to be negative in patients with only respiratory allergy to these triggers or in healthy volunteers. However, these patch tests have not been standardized and their performance and interpretation vary widely. Mite allergen avoidance measures (encasing mattresses and pillows, washing bedding in hot water weekly, vacuuming living areas and bedrooms frequently, keeping only soft non-furry toys, cleaning carpets regularly or removing them, and eliminating pets) may lead to significant decreases in major dust mite allergens and severity of dermatitis.[94] Immunotherapy for food allergies or aeroallergens has long been controversial as treatment for AD, unlike its efficacy for treating allergic rhinitis and extrinsic asthma; recent double-blind, placebo-controlled studies, however, suggest some value of specific immunotherapy.[95] Sublingual immunotherapy is currently being studied as an alternative.[96–98]

Topical antiinflammatory medications

Topical corticosteroids have been the mainstay of treatment for AD (Table 3.2), and are available in a wide range of potencies from the weakest class VII corticosteroids (e.g., hydrocortisone acetate) to the ultrapotent class I steroids (Table 3.3). The use of more potent

Table 3.3 Relative potencies of topical corticosteroids (from most potent to weakest)

Class	Drug	Dosage form(s)	Strength (%)
I. Very high potency			
	Augmented betamethasone dipropionate	Ointment	0.05
	Clobetasol propionate	Cream, ointment, foam	0.05
	Diflorasone diacetate	Ointment	0.05
	Halobetasol propionate	Cream, ointment	0.05
II. High potency			
	Amcinonide	Cream, lotion, ointment	0.1
	Augmented betamethasone dipropionate	Cream	0.05
	Betamethasone dipropionate	Cream, ointment, foam, solution	0.05
	Desoximetasone	Cream, ointment	0.25
	Desoximetasone	Gel	0.05
	Diflorasone diacetate	Cream	0.05
	Fluocinonide	Cream, ointment, gel, solution	0.05
	Halcinonide	Cream, ointment	0.1
	Mometasone furoate	Ointment	0.1
	Triamcinolone acetonide	Cream, ointment	0.5
III–IV Medium potency			
	Betamethasone valerate	Cream, ointment, lotion, foam	0.1
	Clocortolone pivalate	Cream	0.1
	Desoximetasone	Cream	0.05
	Fluocinolone acetonide	Cream, ointment	0.025
	Flurandrenolide	Cream, ointment	0.05
	Fluticasone propionate	Cream	0.05
	Fluticasone propionate	Ointment	0.005
	Mometasone furoate	Cream	0.1
	Triamcinolone acetonide	Cream, ointment	0.1
V. Lower-medium potency			
	Hydrocortisone butyrate	Cream, ointment, solution	0.1
	Hydrocortisone probutate	Cream	0.1
	Hydrocortisone valerate	Cream, ointment	0.2
	Prednicarbate	Cream	0.1
VI. Low potency			
	Alclometasone dipropionate	Cream, ointment	0.05
	Desonide	Cream, gel, foam, ointment	0.05
	Fluocinolone acetonide	Cream, solution	0.01
VII. Lowest potency			
	Dexamethasone	Cream	0.1
	Hydrocortisone	Creams, ointments, lotions, solutions	0.25, 0.5, 1
	Hydrocortisone acetate	Creams, ointments	0.5–1

topical corticosteroids, particularly when applied to large surface areas, under occlusion or for long periods of time, may lead to adverse effects (Table 3.4). The face and intertriginous areas are the most susceptible sites, and may show local effects, even when weaker steroids are used for prolonged periods (Fig. 3.28). Because of their increased body surface area-to-weight ratio, small children have the greatest risk of systemic absorption of topically applied steroids. Concern about the use of topical steroids has led to 'steroid phobia' among families and even physicians.[99] As a result, compliance may be decreased and weak topical steroids insufficient for adequate control may be used.

In general, group I corticosteroids are not recommended for patients younger than the age of 12 years, should not be used in intertriginous areas or under occlusion, and require a rest period after 14 days of use. Use of this group of ultrapotent steroids is usually reserved for lichenified plaques and recalcitrant dermatitis of the hands and feet, and should be limited. Considering the widespread use of topical corticosteroids, few local adverse reactions occur when topical steroids are carefully chosen and used appropriately based on site of application and severity of the dermatitis.[100] As such, even potent topical corticosteroids may safely be used in small areas for short periods of time.

The choice of treatment will depend on the severity and localization of the dermatitis, the age of the pediatric patient, and the history of use of topical antiinflammatory agents. The least potent preparation that adequately controls the disease process should be

Table 3.4 Potential side-effects of topical corticosteriods

Local cutaneous side-effects
  Atrophy
  Striae
  Periorificial granulomatous dermatitis
  Acne
  Telangiectasia
  Erythema
  Hypopigmentation
Ocular effects
  Cataracts
  Glaucoma
Systemic side-effects
  Hypothalamic-pituitary-adrenal axis suppression

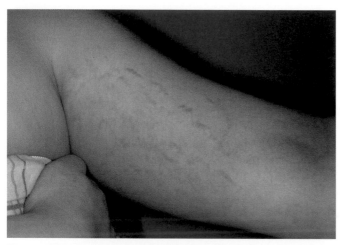

Figure 3.28 Steroid-induced atrophy. Although unusual, steroid-induced atrophy in this patient with atopic dermatitis resulted from the twice-daily application of a class III–IV topical steroid during a 1-year period. Note the excellent control of the dermatitis, but the obvious striae and prominence of veins because of atrophy of overlying skin.

used. For children with mild to moderate disease, intermittent use of a low strength topical steroid with emollient application to maintain clearance usually suffices. However, children with moderate to severe disease often show a cycle of rapid recurrent flaring when topical antiinflammatory suppression is discontinued. A commonly used regimen to maintain control in these children while minimizing the risk of chronic steroid application is to apply mid-potency to potent topical steroids for acute flares (e.g., for a few days to up to 2 weeks twice daily) followed by intermittent therapy with topical steroid[101] or, to avoid continuing steroid altogether, with a topical calcineurin inhibitor (see below). Studies have suggested that topical calcineurin inhibitors can be applied three times weekly to recurrently affected sites to retain control of the dermatitis once improved with the use of topical steroids.[102,103]

The potency of a topical corticosteroid is largely determined by vasoconstrictor assay, and is related to its vehicle as well as to its chemical formulation. Vasoconstrictor assays reveal that generic formulations tend to vary in their clinical activity and their vehicles may at times contain agents differing from those of brand name formulations. Thus, care must be taken in considering substitution of brand name corticosteroids by generic formulations. The concentration of each topical corticosteroid is only significant with respect to potency relative to other corticosteroids of the same chemical formulation. Accordingly, hydrocortisone acetate 2.5% is much weaker than triamcinolone acetonide 0.1%, which in turn is weaker than clobetasol propionate 0.05%, even though the concentrations would suggest the opposite. It also should be recognized that hydrocortisone acetate differs chemically from hydrocortisone butyrate, hydrocortisone probutate, and hydrocortisone valerate, which as mid-potency steroids are stronger than hydrocortisone acetate. Halogenated steroids are usually stronger than non-halogenated steroids.

Corticosteroid ointments afford the advantage of occlusion, more effective penetration, and in general greater efficacy than equivalent cream or lotion formulations. Ointments are particularly effective in the management of dry, lichenified, or plaque-like areas of dermatitis. Ointment formulations, however, may occlude eccrine ducts, inducing sweat retention and pruritus, and hair follicles, leading to folliculitis. As with emollients, formulations in ointments may not be as well tolerated during the summer months of increased heat, perspiration, and high humidity. On the other hand, creams often contain additives that may be irritating or sensitizing. Creams and lotions, however, are more cosmetically elegant, and afford the advantages of greater convenience and acceptability during hot weather and in intertriginous areas. Traditional gels and foams are not well tolerated in individuals with AD, but may be most effective in the management of acute weeping or vesicular lesions. Topical corticosteroids in emollient-based foam formulations and hydrocolloid gels (in contrast to the alcohol-containing foams and gels) are particularly useful for hairy areas, to avoid occlusion, and for cosmesis. Oil preparations are most commonly used for scalp dermatitis. Best applied to a wet scalp, oil formulations can be shampooed out after at least 1 hour to overnight. A fluocinolone acetonide oil preparation, however, has been shown to be helpful after the bath for children with extensive AD.[104]

Occlusion of treated areas with polyethylene film, such as Saran wrap, or the use of corticosteroid-impregnated polyethylene film (Cordran tape) enhances the penetration of corticosteroids up to 100-fold. This mode of therapy is particularly effective for short periods of time (8–12 h a day on successive days) for patients with chronic lichenified or recalcitrant plaques of dermatitic skin. Occlusive techniques, however, are contraindicated for prolonged periods of time, and are not recommended in infected or intertriginous areas. Given that the diaper is an occlusive dressing, application of steroids in the diaper area of infants should be avoided or limited to short-term use of low-strength topical steroids.

For sites of severely lichenified dermatitis, salicylic acid can be compounded into preparations with steroids to improve penetration. Tar (liquor carbonis detergens or crude coal tar) can be also be used as an adjunctive therapy in patients with chronic dermatitis in the form of tar baths (e.g., Cutar) or compounded with topical corticosteroids (e.g., compounding triamcinolone 0.1% with 6% salicyclic acid and 5–10% liquor carbonis detergens in Aquaphor ointment). The objectionable odor, staining properties, potential for irritation, risk of causing folliculitis, and low potential risk of later carcinogenesis make tar a choice only for only selected patients.

A variety of 'steroid-free' topical anti-inflammatory agents have been introduced to allow patients to decrease their application of topical steroids and thus associated risks. Topical calcineurin inhibitors (tacrolimus ointment 0.03% and pimecrolimus cream 1%) have been approved for the past decade as an alternative therapy for AD in children above 2 years of age.[105] Several studies and anecdotal reports have suggested good efficacy and safety for tacrolimus ointment 0.1% (above 2 years of age) and for tacrolimus 0.03% ointment and pimecrolimus cream in infants under 2 years of age, but their use is off-label.[106,107] Tacrolimus and pimecrolimus prevent the formation of a complex that includes calcineurin, a phosphatase.[108] Without this complex, the phosphate group from NF-AT (nuclear factor of activated T cells) cannot be cleaved, the NF-AT transcription factor cannot be transported to the nucleus, and production of cytokines associated with T-cell activation is inhibited. Tacrolimus and pimecrolimus also inhibit mediator release from mast cells and basophils and decrease IgE receptor expression on cutaneous Langerhans cells.[109]

To date, the only confirmed safety issue associated with the use of calcineurin inhibitors in children is burning or pruritus with application, described in the minority of affected children, particularly with active inflammation. This sensation has been shown to result from stimulation of TRPV1 receptors in skin with depletion of substance P.[110] Calcineurin inhibitors do not show the atrophogenic potential of the corticosteroids and can be safely used on the head, neck, and intertriginous areas. Furthermore, no adverse effects on the eyes have been found, allowing safe application in periorbital areas. No increase in cutaneous infections have been noted in children.[111,112] Tacrolimus ointment shows good efficacy in children with moderate to severe AD[113]; the efficacy of the 0.1% ointment is comparable to a midpotency topical corticosteroid,[114] while that of the 0.03% ointment to a low potency steroid. Pimecrolimus cream is also comparable to a low potency steroid and is indicated for pediatric patients with mild to moderate AD.[115,116] Assays of systemic absorption of tacrolimus and pimecrolimus have shown transient low levels in the blood, if at all, and no adverse effects on systemic immunity have been demonstrated.[113,117]

In 2006, the US Food and Drug Administration placed a black box warning on the class of calcineurin inhibitors based on the theoretical potential for topical calcineurin inhibitors to cause skin carcinogenesis and lymphoma. This theoretical risk was based on the known risk of malignancy (post-transplant lymphoproliferative disease and nonmelanoma skin cancer) in transplant patients who are profoundly immunosuppressed by systemically administered tacrolimus and animal studies when treated with 26–47 times the maximum recommended dosage. Since that time, task forces of the American College of Allergy, Asthma and Immunology, the American Academy of Allergy, Asthma and Immunology, and the American Academy of Dermatology found no evidence to support the issuance of a black box warning.[118,119] Furthermore, to date no evidence of an increased risk of the development of post-transplant lymphoproliferative disorder or non-melanoma skin cancer has been uncovered in children treated with topical calcineurin inhibitors. In fact, an increased risk of lymphoma has been linked to severe AD itself, but not to use of topical calcineurin inhibitors to date, including in children.[120,121] Nevertheless, pimecrolimus and tacrolimus are best used intermittently in rotation with topical steroids and patients need to be advised of these potential risks, at least until several additional years of further experience accrues, and to use sun protection while using these agents.

Several new 'non-steroidal' anti-inflammatory medical devices (also known as 'barrier repair agents'; see above) have also become available for mild to moderate dermatitis and may decrease the need for steroid application.[122]

Role of antihistamines

Reduction of the pruritus of AD is best achieved by application of topical antiinflammatory medications. Sedating antihistamines, such as hydroxyzine, diphenhydramine, and doxepin, may help itchy children fall asleep, although they have little direct effect on the pruritus itself. Non-sedating antihistamines may be valuable as treatment for other atopic conditions, such as allergic rhinitis, and have been shown to decrease the risk of urticaria, but their value in decreasing pruritus is unclear, since they are usually non-sedating.[123]

Long-term use in young children has not led to behavioral, cognitive, or psychomotor developmental abnormalities.[124] Regardless, many pediatric dermatologists use both sedating and non-sedating antihistamines as part of an overall atopic dermatitis treatment program, and attest to their clinical benefit. Application of diphenhydramine topically should be avoided, since it is a potential sensitizing agent; subsequent systemic administration of diphenhydramine can result in a systematized allergic contact reaction.

Treatment of secondary cutaneous infections

Antistaphylococcal antibiotics are important in the management of patients with heavy *S. aureus* colonization or infection because of the role of *S. aureus* overgrowth in triggering dermatitis. Topical antibiotics, such as mupirocin, or fusidic acid (not currently available in the USA), can be used for localized impetiginized lesions, but systemic antibiotics are required for more extensive involvement. Despite the increase in CA-MRSA nationally, most atopics still harbor MSSA 84–93%).[45,48] As a result, cephalexin is still used most commonly (and successfully) to empirically treat secondarily infected dermatitis. The chronic administration of systemic antistaphylococcal therapy for AD should be avoided in an effort to minimize the risk of the development of MRSA in the atopic population. The addition of dilute sodium hypochlorite (bleach) to the bathwater at least twice weekly ($\frac{1}{4}$–$\frac{1}{2}$ cup per full tub or a scant 2 tsp per gallon) markedly reduces the severity and extent of the dermatitis at submerged areas in children with moderate to severe AD who develop infections;[45] even daily maintenance dilute sodium hypochlorite baths are generally well tolerated, except when the skin is denuded. Intermittent application of mupirocin ointment to the nares and hands of patients and caregivers twice daily for five sequential days each month, and use of gentle antibacterial soaps[125] may also transiently decrease colonization.

Antiviral treatment of cutaneous herpes simplex infections is important in preventing widespread dissemination, which may be life threatening. Administration of oral acyclovir (100 mg tid to qid for children under 6 years of age; 200 mg qid for older children) for a week usually controls the infection. More extensive involvement may require hospitalization and intravenous acyclovir treatment, especially in younger children. For children with recurrent eczema herpeticum, a course of prophylactic administration of oral acyclovir once daily for 6 months or longer effectively suppresses the recurrences. Adjunctive therapies include topical compresses and concurrent administration of topical or systemic antibiotics if bacterial infection is also suspected. In general, topical corticosteroids can be continued during the course of systemic acyclovir therapy if the dermatitis is problematic without impacting clearance of the viral infection. Molluscum infections (see Ch. 15) can be managed by curettage after application of topical anesthetics[126] or, if available, by cantharidin application.[127] Children with atopic dermatitis and molluscum may show improvement in both their dermatitis and the molluscum lesions by treatment with high doses of oral cimetidine (40 mg/kg per day divided twice daily) for a 3-month course.[128,129] Imiquimod has not been found beneficial in double-blind, randomized trials.

Management of children with severe AD

Moderate to severe AD may be recalcitrant to topical corticosteroid and calcineurin therapy. However, secondary staphylococcal infection and poor compliance should always be considered to explain this situation. In one study with electronic cap monitoring to detect opening of tubes, mean adherence of patients with mild to moderate atopic dermatitis was 32%, increasing on or near office visit days.[130] Chronic, unresponsive dermatitis, especially involving the eyelids, hands, feet or vulva may result from allergic contact dermatitis,[57,131] and comprehensive patch testing (see below) should be undertaken. Systemic immunosuppressive therapy[132] or ultraviolet light treatment can be considered for patients with recalcitrant moderate to severe disease. For older children and adolescents, ultraviolet light therapy may be an option that avoids administration of systemic immunosuppressive therapy. Narrow band ultraviolet B light is most commonly used, and has been reported to cause at least moderate improvement in 89% of children and complete clearance in 40% over a median period of 3 months.[133] Nevertheless, the requirement for frequent treatments in a medical office (two to three times weekly), for holding still in a hot enclosed box while wearing protective goggles, and risk of long-term cutaneous damage from ultraviolet light preclude the use of this form of therapy for most pediatric patients.

Systemic corticosteroid therapy is effective for most patients with AD, but the rapid rebound after discontinuation of therapy and high risk of potential side-effects make its use impractical. Systemic administration of non-steroidal antiinflammatory medications to children with AD has largely replaced the use of systemic corticosteroids by pediatric dermatologists in the management of more recalcitrant severe AD. Cyclosporine is probably the most effective among these, but also has the highest risk of potential side-effects. Therapy is initiated with 5 mg/kg per day if Sandimmune or its generic formulation is used, or 2.5–3 mg/kg per day if the microemulsion form is used. Response may be seen within 1–3 months, but should be tapered once significant improvement is achieved; trough levels can be determined in patients without a sufficient response to determine if a higher dosage can be administered. Discontinuation of treatment usually leads to relapse flares, but low-dose continuing treatment or intermittent courses in children can be effective.[134–136] Renal function, blood pressure, and hepatic function must be carefully monitored. Azathioprine (2.5–3 mg/kg/d) has effectively suppressed severe, recalcitrant AD in 58% of children during a 3-month trial period.[137,138] Pre-treatment determination of thiopurine methyltransferase level can predict the risk of developing myelosuppression, and hepatic functions should also be monitored.

Mycophenolate mofetil has been found to cause at least 60% improvement in 91% of treated children with a dosage of 40–50 mg/kg per day for children and 30–40 mg/kg per day for adolescents with maximal effects at 8–12 weeks.[139] Complete blood counts and liver function testing should be performed. The use of methotrexate for AD in children has not been studied; however, an open-label trial in adults suggested the low dose methotrexate (0.3–0.5 mg/kg per week) may be beneficial as an alternative second-line therapy, especially for maintenance once control is achieved.[140] Complete blood counts should be followed weekly, and hepatic transaminases should be monitored at least monthly. Interferon-γ downregulates Th2 lymphocyte function, and treatment with recombinant interferon-γ (50 μg/m² daily or every other day) has led to improvement in some patients, including pediatric patients.[141–143] Clinical improvement correlates with decreases in peripheral eosinophilia, but not IgE levels. Flu-like symptoms are particularly common early in the treatment course. The high price and benefit for only a subset of individuals also limit the use of interferon-γ in severely affected children with AD. The available biologics used for patients with moderate to severe psoriasis have shown little benefit for treating AD.

Use of experimental or complementary treatment approaches

In one study, 42.5% of children with AD used at least one form of alternative medicine, particularly herbal remedies and homeopathy.[144] More than half reported no improvement, but tried the therapies based on recommendation from non-physicians, concern about the potential risks of topical steroids, and dissatisfaction with conventional treatment. Of concern is that these complementary approaches have potential side-effects, have not been adequately tested for safety and efficacy, and their use requires time and effort that might otherwise be directed towards use of physician-prescribed treatment.

Probiotics have recently received considerable attention as a means of prevention of AD, based on the hypothesis that lack of adequate microbial exposure at an early age predisposes to the development of AD. At this time, however, there is insufficient evidence to recommend probiotics to prevent AD or as part of standard management.[145,146] Although several trials have shown that probiotics may be effective in prophylaxis against AD in high-risk infants, more recent studies have not shown a beneficial effect. Prenatal administration may increase atopic sensitization[147] and the risk of developing wheezing and possibly allergic rhinitis.[148] Studies do not support the use of probiotics postnatally especially after the first years of life. It should be noted that there is strain specificity in the effect, with *Lactobacillus rhamnosus* (LGG) being the most effective strain.[149] Sepsis related to probiotic use has been reported, and antibiotic resistance and deleterious alterations in microbiota are theoretical risks.

Leukotriene antagonists, such as montelukast, which are used extensively in asthma prophylaxis have largely been ineffective.[150] Results of several studies have suggested that patients with AD benefit from treatment with traditional Chinese herbal therapy.[151] However, the demonstration of hepatic toxicity, cardiac adverse events, and idiosyncratic reactions from this therapy has raised concerns; furthermore, the discovery of glucocorticoid contamination in some preparations warns that these alternative agents be used with caution.[152] A more recent controlled trial failed to find benefit of Chinese herbal therapy for recalcitrant atopic dermatitis.[153] Massage therapy has been advocated as a means to improve the clinical signs of atopic dermatitis in young children, in addition to the psychological wellbeing of the patients and family members.[154] Psychological counseling, behavioral modification, hypnotherapy and biofeedback can also be helpful in decreasing scratching.[70] Psychological intervention for families can also be beneficial, since increased parental stress and depression correlate with higher levels of biological markers of inflammation.[155]

Pityriasis alba

Pityriasis alba is a common cutaneous disorder characterized by asymptomatic hypopigmented patches, usually on the face, neck, upper trunk, and proximal extremities.[156] Individual lesions vary from 1 cm or more in diameter and may show a fine scale (Figs 3.29, 3.30).

This disorder is thought to represent a nonspecific dermatitis with residual post-inflammatory hypopigmentation, and occurs more often in individuals with darker skin types.[157] Histologic evaluation shows normal numbers of melanocytes, but decreased epidermal melanosomes and melanocyte degeneration.[156] Most cases appear after sun exposure, because of the contrast that results between areas that can show a pigmentary response to ultraviolet light and the pityriasis alba areas that do not.

The differential diagnosis of the hypopigmented macules of pityriasis alba includes tinea versicolor, vitiligo, the white macules seen in association with tuberous sclerosis, nevus depigmentosus, cutaneous T-cell lymphoma, leprosy, and post-inflammatory hypopigmentation secondary to atopic dermatitis, psoriasis, tinea corporis,

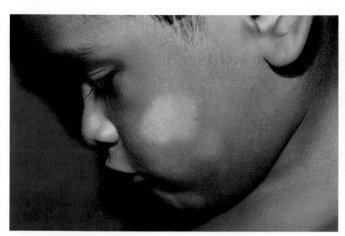

Figure 3.29 Pityriasis alba. Circumscribed scaly hypopigmented lesions on the cheek. These patches are thought to represent post-inflammatory hypopigmentation and are most easily visible in children with darker skin.

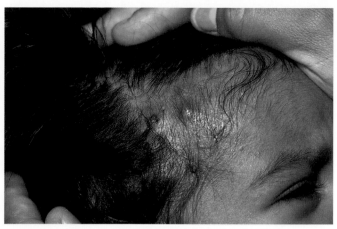

Figure 3.31 Hyperimmunoglobulinemia E syndrome. In addition to atopic dermatitis, most infants and children with hyperimmunoglobulinemia E syndrome show erythematous, slightly purulent 'cold abscesses,' shown here on the forehead and scalp. (From Bolognia et al. (2003),[284] Fig. 60.8.)

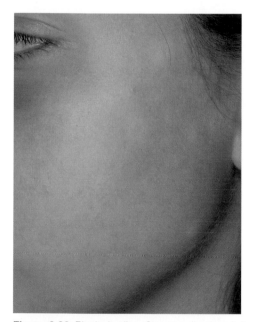

Figure 3.30 Pityriasis alba. Circumscribed scaly hypopigmented lesions on the cheek. The patches are much more subtle in a lighter-skinned patient, but tanning of the skin during summer may lead to cosmetic concerns.

or pityriasis rosea. Application of mild topical corticosteroids or calcineurin inhibitors for a few weeks, followed by frequent emolliation and protection of the sites and surrounding area from sun exposure, appears to diminish the dry skin and fine scaling, allowing repigmentation of involved areas. Patients and parents should be warned that, as with post-inflammatory hypopigmentation, repigmentation may take several months to years. Effective moisturization during drier months may help to prevent recurrence of the pityriasis alba in subsequent summers.

Hyperimmunoglobulinemia E syndrome (HIES)

HIES is a rare immunodeficiency disorder characterized by very high levels of IgE in association with atopic dermatitis and recurrent cutaneous and sinopulmonary infections.[158,159] Job's syndrome is a subgroup of HIES. The atopic dermatitis is seen in 100% of patients, usually within the first 6 months, and is of variable severity. Affected individuals also commonly present in the newborn or infantile period with pruritic papulopustules, especially on the face, that show eosinophilic folliculitis or eosinophilic dermatitis by biopsy of lesional skin.[160]

Infections often begin during the first 3 months of life. Cutaneous candidiasis may also be an early clinical feature (83%).[159] Cutaneous *S. aureus* infections may take the form of excoriated crusted plaques, pustules, furuncles, cellulitis, paronychia, lymphangitis, or abscesses, especially on the neck, scalp, periorbital areas, axillae, and groin (Fig. 3.31). The abscesses are slightly erythematous and tender, but not nearly to the degree expected for a normal individual. Although some patients demonstrate cutaneous manifestations only,[161] patients with HIES usually have recurrent bronchitis and pneumonias with resultant empyema, bronchiectasis and, in 77% of patients, pneumatocele formation. The pneumatoceles tend to persist and become the site of further infections with bacteria (pseudomonas) or fungi (aspergillus, scedosporium). Rarely, massive hemoptysis ensues. Other common sites of infection include the ears, oral mucosae, sinuses, and eyes. Visceral infections other than pneumonia are unusual.

Patients with HIES develop progressive facial coarseness,[158] probably reflecting both bony abnormalities and recurrent facial abscesses. Osteopenia is usually detected and patients have an increased risk of bone fractures, often because of unrecognized or minor trauma. Scoliosis occurs in 64% of patients 16 years of age or older, and hyperextensibility of joints has been reported in 70% of patients. Dental abnormalities associated with HIES syndrome include retention of primary teeth, lack of eruption of secondary teeth, and delayed resorption of the roots of primary teeth. Focal brain hyperintensities and an increased incidence of lymphoma are other features.

Autosomal recessive HIES is less common, and differs from the dominant form by the presence of unusual infection (mycobacterial and salmonella), viral infections (molluscum, herpes), neurologic changes (aneurysms and strokes), and an increased risk of autoimmune issues (anemia, thrombocytopenia, and vasculitis).[162]

The diagnosis of HIES is largely based on clinical findings[163] and the presence of very high levels of IgE. There are no specific tests to confirm the diagnosis, other than the finding of HIES-related muta-tions (see below). Patients have markedly elevated levels of poly-clonal IgE. Although levels of >2000 IU/mL are needed to consider the diagnosis in older children and adults, the normal levels of IgE in infants (0–50 IU/mL) are considerably lower than those in older children. A 10-fold increase in IgE levels above normal levels for age should trigger consideration of HIES, although these levels of IgE are more common in atopic dermatitis without HIES.[164] Affected individuals tend to have IgE antibodies directed against *S. aureus* and candida. Levels of IgE are not related to clinical course, and may decrease to normal in affected adults. Approximately 93% of patients have eosinophilia of the blood and sputum.[159] Abnormal polymorphonuclear leukocyte and monocyte chemotaxis has been noted, but is intermittent and not correlated with infection. Cell-mediated immunity (Th1-driven) is often abnormal as well, and may manifest as anergy to skin testing, altered responses in mixed leukocyte culture, and impaired blastogenic responses to specific antigens, such as *Candida* and tetanus. The decrease in memory (CD27+) B cells is markedly decreased in 80% of patients, in con-trast to individuals with atopic dermatitis and high levels of IgE.[165]

Most individuals with HIES have an autosomal dominant form that results from mutations in the gene encoding signal transducer and activator of transcription 3 (STAT3).[166,167] Not all patients, however, have STAT3 mutations, and a second locus has been mapped to chromosome 4q.[163] The clinical features of HIES have been attributed to abnormalities in STAT3 signaling and Th17 cell development, which leads to insufficient expression of IL-17 and IL-22 (decreased antimicrobial peptides and resultant *S. aureus* and candidal infections).[168] Homozygous mutations in tyrosine kinase 2, which activates STAT3, or in dedicator of cytokinesis (DOCK8), which regulates the actin cytoskeleton, have been found in auto-somal recessive HIES;[169,170] the additional clinical features have been ascribed to additional abnormalities in IL-12 and interferon α/β cytokine production.

HIES syndrome must be distinguished from a number of other disorders in which IgE levels may be elevated. Most common is atopic dermatitis, which shows similar inflammatory cutaneous fea-tures and often very high levels of IgE, especially if severe;[164] the concurrent presence of abscesses, coarse facies, noncutaneous infec-tions, and dental and bony abnormalities in HIES may enable differentiation. Wiskott–Aldrich syndrome (see below) can be dis-tinguished by thrombocytopenia with cutaneous petechiae and hemorrhagic episodes. Eosinophilia and elevations of IgE levels with dermatitis can also be seen in patients with DiGeorge syndrome, the Omenn syndrome type of severe combined immunodeficiency, graft-versus-host disease (GVHD), and selective IgA deficiency.

The mainstay of therapy for HIES is antistaphylococcal antibiotics, and patients are usually treated prophylactically with trimethoprim-sulfamethoxazole. When other bacterial or fungal infections develop, infections must be treated with appropriate alternative antibiotics. Recombinant interferon-γ has shown inconsistent efficacy. The cutaneous and pulmonary abscesses often require incision and drainage. The pneumatoceles should be removed surgically, especially if present for longer than 6 months, to prevent microbial superinfection. Therapy for atopic dermatitis as discussed above is also useful for HIES; omalizumab has improved the severe dermatitis of a recalcitrant patient with a rela-tively low level of IgE.[171]

Wiskott–Aldrich syndrome (WAS)

WAS is a rare X-linked recessive disorder, which in its classic form consists of recurrent pyogenic infections, bleeding because of thrombocytopenia and platelet dysfunction, and recalcitrant der-matitis.[172] Bleeding is the most common manifestation, but the presence of mild to severe atopic dermatitis distinguishes WAS from X-linked thrombocytopenia, which is allelic. The majority of patients are male, but full expression has been reported in girls.[173]

The dermatitis usually develops during the first few months of life, and fulfils criteria for the definition of atopic dermatitis (Fig. 3.32). Excoriated areas frequently have sero-sanguineous crust and often show petechiae or purpura. IgE-mediated allergic problems such as urticaria, food allergies, and asthma are also seen with increased frequency.

The hemorrhagic diathesis results from both quantitative and qualitative defects in platelets. Platelets from patients with WAS are small and structurally abnormal, with a reduced half-life, although megakaryocyte numbers are normal. Epistaxis and bloody diarrhea are often the initial manifestations. Mucocutaneous petechiae and ecchymoses (Fig. 3.32), spontaneous bleeding from the oral cavity, hematemesis, melena, and hematuria are common, but the severity varies.

Recurrent bacterial infections begin in infancy as placentally transmitted maternal antibody levels diminish and include staphylococcal impetigo, furunculosis, otitis externa and media, pneumonia, pansinusitis, conjunctivitis, meningitis, and septi-cemia. Infections with encapsulated bacteria such as pneumococ-cus, *Haemophilus influenzae*, and *Neiserria meningitidis* predominate. With advancing age, T-cell function progressively deteriorates and patients become increasingly susceptible to infections due to herpes and other viruses, and to *Pneumocystis jiroveci*.

Additional clinical features may be hepatosplenomegaly, lym-phadenopathy, and autoimmune complications. The most frequent autoimmune complication is hemolytic anemia, occurring in 36% of patients and usually before 5 years of age.[174] Other autoimmune disorders that clearly seem linked to WAS are auto-immune neutro-penia (25%), arthritis (29%), IgA nephropathy, and painful

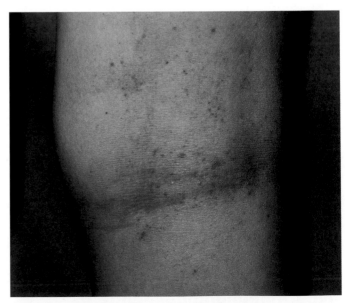

Figure 3.32 Wiskott–Aldrich syndrome (WAS). A bleeding diathesis owing to thrombocytopenia and platelet dysfunction, the most common manifestation of patients with WAS, may manifest as petechiae, ecchymoses, and purpuric patches. The dermatitis of patients with WAS is indistinguishable from atopic dermatitis.

cutaneous vasculitis (22%) that can appear as purplish induration of skin and soft tissues.

The clinical course of WAS is progressive, usually resulting in death by adolescence without transplantation. Overall, 40% of patients die of infection, 21% of hemorrhage (usually intracranial), and 25% of malignant neoplasia. Lymphoreticular malignancies occur overall in 13–22% of patients,[175] with an average age of onset of 9.5 years. Non-Hodgkin's lymphoma[175,176] is the most common malignancy, often linked to EBV infection, and extranodal and brain involvement predominate. Fewer than 5% who develop lymphoma survive more than 2 years.

Individuals with WAS have mutations in the gene that encodes WASP,[177] which is critical for cell movement, formation of immune synapses, T cell activation, and B cell homeostasis.[178] Pleatelet abnormalities result from defective migration in proplatelet formation, inherent platelet defects increasing fragility, and autoimmunity against platelets. T regulatory cell dysfunction has been blamed for the increased risk of autoimmune complications. The mechanism for the atopic dermatitis is not well defined, but Th2-skewed cytokines predominate with suppression of Th1 cytokine production. Langerhans cells show abnormal interactions with T cells and fail to move to lymph nodes after antigenic stimulation.

Laboratory studies show thrombocytopenia in 100% of patients, with platelets below about 80 000/mm^3 and often below 20 000/mm^3. Platelets tend to be small and aggregation is sometimes defective. Eosinophilia is common, but lymphopenia is not usually seen until after 6–8 years of age. Total serum gammaglobulin is usually normal, but levels of IgM are often low, with variable IgG levels and increased levels of IgA, IgE, and IgD. The number of T lymphocytes and response *in vitro* to mitogens may be normal in early life, but often decreases with advancing age. Delayed hypersensitivity skin test reactions are usually absent, and antibody responses to polysaccharide antigens are markedly diminished.

Several conditions may be confused with WAS. Many of the other immunodeficiencies are characterized by dermatitis, increased susceptibility to infections, and the development of malignancy, but do not share the bleeding diathesis. The clinical findings of hemorrhage, petechiae, and recurrent sinopulmonary infections in WAS help to differentiate WAS from atopic dermatitis.

Bone marrow transplantation with HLA-identical marrow is the treatment of choice. Full engraftment results in normal platelet numbers and functions, immunological status, and, if T lymphocytes engraft, clearance of the dermatitis.[177–180] Optimal survival occurs with matched sibling donors and allogeneic transplantation below the age of 5 years (87%). Despite the good result of matched unrelated donors in young children (71%), there is a higher risk of acute GVHD after transplant (56%) versus matched siblings (16%).[172,181] Mixed chimerism (i.e., engraftment of T cells but not myeloid or B cells) increases greatly the risk of chronic GVHD.

Appropriate antibiotics and transfusions of platelets and plasma decrease the risk of fatal infections and hemorrhage.[182] Intravenous infusions of gammaglobulin are also useful in patients. Topical corticosteroids may improve the dermatitis, and chronic administration of oral acyclovir is appropriate for patients with eczema herpeticum. Splenectomy has been used selectively for patients with severe platelet abnormalities; however, splenectomy increases the risk of infection by encapsulated organisms, markedly increasing the risk of mortality after transplantation. Children with WAS are unable to mount immune responses after administration of vaccines against encapsulated organisms. Rituximab has been used successfully in some children with EBV-induced lymphoma to prolong survival.[183]

Lichen simplex chronicus

Lichen simplex chronicus (circumscribed neurodermatitis) is a localized, chronic pruritic disorder characterized by patches of dermatitis that result from repeated itching, scratching, and rubbing of the involved area. The pruritus may begin in an area of normal-appearing skin or may be initiated in a preexisting lesion of atopic, seborrheic, or contact dermatitis, lichen planus, or psoriasis.

Lesions of lichen simplex chronicus generally occur in adolescents or adults, but may be seen in younger children. The disorder may develop at any location on the body, but the most common areas of involvement are those that are easily reached and may be scratched unobtrusively (particularly during periods of tension and concentration). These include the nape or sides of the neck, wrists, ankles, hands, and pretibial areas. Other common sites of involvement include the inner aspects of the thighs, vulva, scrotum, and perianal areas.

The clinical features of lichen simplex chronicus include single or multiple oval plaques with a long axis that usually measure up to 15 cm in diameter (Fig. 3.33). During the early stages, the skin is reddened and slightly edematous with exaggerated skin markings. Older, more typical lesions are characterized by well-circumscribed, dry, thickened, scaling, pruritic, often hyperpigmented plaques.

The diagnosis of lichen simplex chronicus is dependent on the presence of pruritic lichenified plaques in the characteristic sites of predilection. Lesions of tinea corporis may be differentiated by a lack of lichenification, by the presence of a scaly border (often with clearing in the center), by demonstration of hyphae on microscopic examination of skin scrapings, and by fungal culture. Psoriatic plaques generally may be differentiated by a characteristic thick, adherent white or silvery scale, their underlying deep red hue, and characteristic areas of involvement. Lesions of atopic dermatitis may be differentiated by history, more poorly demarcated lesions, the presence of atopic stigmata, and a tendency toward involvement in antecubital and popliteal areas.

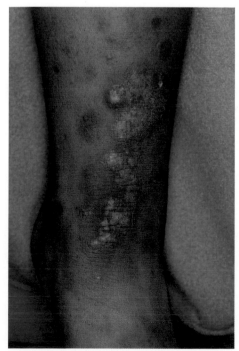

Figure 3.33 Lichen simplex chronicus. Localized plaques of dermatitis that result from repeated scratching and rubbing of the involved area.

The successful management of lichen simplex chronicus depends on an appreciation of the itch-scratch-itch cycle and the associated scratching and rubbing that accompany and perpetuate this disorder.[184] Topical application of potent corticosteroids, under occlusion if necessary, and the administration of systemic antihistamines (such as diphenhydramine or hydroxyzine) will usually induce remission of the pruritus and the eruption within a period of several weeks. Use of tap water compresses before application of the topical corticosteroid or compounding topical steroid with salicylic acid (e.g., 6% salicylic acid and 0.1% triamcinolone powder in hydrophilic ointment) may increase penetration of the topical anti-inflammatory agent. Other techniques include application overnight of flurandrenolide-impregnated tape, protection from scratching and rubbing by occluding with adherent dressings, and injection of intralesional triamcinolone acetonide (e.g., 5 mg/cc) in tolerant adolescents.

Seborrheic dermatitis

Seborrheic dermatitis refers to a self-limiting erythematous, scaly, or crusting eruption that occurs primarily in the so-called seborrheic areas (those with the highest concentration of sebaceous glands), namely the scalp, face, and postauricular, presternal, and intertriginous areas. Seborrheic dermatitis in the pediatric population is most commonly seen in infants and adolescents. The cause of seborrheic dermatitis is not well understood. Its predilection for areas of high sebaceous gland density and the correlation of activity with increased hormonal levels during the first year of life[185] and adolescence suggests a relation to sebum and sebaceous glands. Seborrheic dermatitis of adolescence and adulthood has been attributed to *Pityrosporum ovale* (*Malassezia ovalis*), a lipophilic yeast normally found in abundance on the human scalp.[186] However, the relationship between seborrheic dermatitis in infants and that of adolescents and adults is controversial, as is whether this organism plays an etiologic role in infants.[187,188] The observation that many infantile cases improve with topical ketoconazole suggests that this yeast infection may, at least in some instances, play a role in the pathogenesis of this disorder.

Seborrheic dermatitis appears in infancy between the second and tenth weeks of life (usually the third or fourth) and peaks in incidence at 3 months of age.[189] Infantile seborrheic dermatitis often begins with a non-eczematous erythematous scaly dermatitis of the scalp (termed cradle cap) or the diaper area and is manifested by thin dry scales or sharply defined round or oval patches covered by thick, yellowish brown greasy crusts. Although the condition is limited to the scalp in most affected infants, it may progress to the forehead, ears, eyebrows, nose, and back of the head (Figs 3.4, 3.34). Erythematous greasy, salmon-colored, sharply marginated scaly patches may also involve the intertriginous and flexural areas of the body, the postauricular areas, the trunk, umbilicus, anogenital areas, and groin (Fig. 3.35). Pruritus is slight or absent, and the lesions usually lack the dry, fine scaling character associated with atopic dermatitis. Overlap of seborrheic dermatitis and atopic dermatitis, however, may occur with the features of AD becoming more prominent as the seborrheic dermatitis subsides. In one study, 49% of 2–12-month-old infants with atopic dermatitis had a history of infantile seborrheic dermatitis, in contrast to 17% of controls.[190]

The differential diagnosis of seborrheic dermatitis during infancy includes atopic dermatitis, psoriasis, Langerhans cell histiocytosis, and the 'Leiner's phenotype' of immunodeficiency.[191] Lesions of atopic dermatitis are almost always pruritic, are poorly defined, and show dry fine scaling. In addition, the occluded diaper area is usually spared in atopic dermatitis, in contrast to the frequent diaper area involvement of seborrheic dermatitis. Psoriasis can be

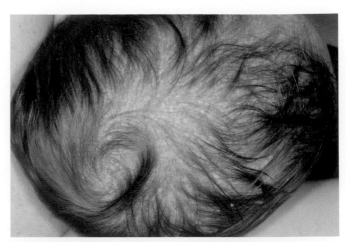

Figure 3.34 Seborrheic dermatitis. A self-limiting erythematous, scaling eruption that occurs primarily in the so-called seborrheic areas (those with the highest concentration of sebaceous glands), particularly on the scalp (shown), face (see Fig. 3.4), and postauricular areas.

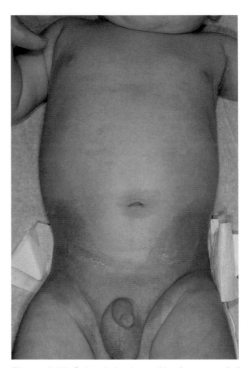

Figure 3.35 Seborrheic dermatitis. A cause of diaper rash in young infants, seborrheic dermatitis is difficult to distinguish clinically from infantile psoriasis, but tends to be less erythematous, to have thinner scaling, and to respond more quickly to topical antiinflammatory medications.

quite difficult to differentiate, as it can present in infants in a fashion very similar to that of seborrheic dermatitis with sharply marginated, brightly erythematous scaling patches. Psoriasis tends to show a slower response to topical corticosteroid therapy and can be distinguished, if necessary, by skin biopsy. Although Langerhans cell histiocytosis can at times be mistaken for seborrheic dermatitis, the presence of discrete 1–3 mm yellowish to red-brown crusted or eroded papules, purpuric lesions, hepatosplenomegaly or lymphadenopathy support the diagnosis of Langerhans cell histiocytosis; histopathologic and immunohistochemical examination of cutaneous lesions confirms the diagnosis of Langerhans cell histiocytosis. When the erythema and scaling of infantile seborrheic dermatitis becomes severe, generalized, and exfoliative, the diagnosis of immunodeficiency must be considered. The lack of constitutional findings (diarrhea, fever, weight loss), alopecia, associated infections, and the spontaneous clearance or rapid response to therapy of seborrheic dermatitis help to distinguish the conditions. Leiner's disease was once thought to be a distinct immunodeficiency disorder because of complement dysfunction that resembled severe seborrheic dermatitis. The Leiner's phenotype now describes a spectrum of immunodeficiency disorders, including C3 and C5 complement deficiencies, C5 dysfunction, hypergammaglobulinemia E syndrome, severe combined immunodeficiency (especially Omenn syndrome), and X-linked agammaglobulinemia.[192]

Between puberty and middle age, seborrheic dermatitis may appear on the scalp as a dry fine flaky desquamation, commonly known as dandruff. This seborrhea is an extreme form of normal desquamation in which scales of the scalp become abundant and visible, often overlying inflammation. Erythema and scaling of various degrees may also involve the supraorbital areas between the eyebrows and above the bridge of the nose, nasolabial crease (Fig. 3.36), lips, pinna, retroauricular areas, and aural canal. Blepharitis is a form of seborrheic dermatitis in which the eyelid margins are red and covered with small white scales. Seborrheic dermatitis may also involve the sideburns, beard, and moustache areas, with diffuse redness, greasy scaling, and pustulation. The severity and course of seborrheic eruptions of the eyelids and bearded areas are variable and have a tendency to chronicity and recurrence.

Occasionally an adolescent patient may have an eruption that has clinical features of both seborrheic dermatitis and psoriasis. Such eruptions may be termed sebopsoriasis. Lesions of seborrheic dermatitis can be differentiated from those of psoriasis by a lack of the characteristic vivid red hue or micaceous scale, a predisposition toward flexural rather than extensor aspects of the extremities, and the fact that lesions of seborrhea generally tend to remain within the confines of the hairline. Lesions of psoriasis (or sebopsoriasis) frequently extend beyond the hairline and, in general, are more resistant to standard antiseborrheic therapy.

The prognosis of infantile seborrheic dermatitis is excellent.[193] In some patients, the disorder clears within 3–4 weeks, even without treatment, and most cases clear spontaneously by 8–12 months of age. The condition generally does not recur until the onset of puberty, although mild scaling of the scalp, particularly at the vertex, can be seen in some affected children through pre-school years. Treatment of infantile scalp seborrheic dermatitis is best managed by frequent shampooing.[194] Although antiseborrheic shampoos including ketoconazole shampoo[195] may be useful, in infants or young children these products may be drying or irritating to the eyes. A gentle 'no tears' shampoo usually suffices. If the scales are thick and adherent, removal can be facilitated by the thin application of mineral or baby oil, followed by gentle scalp massage with a soft toothbrush and then shampooing. Antiseborrheic shampoos (see below) are alternatives if therapy with 'no tears' shampoo is not effective. If there is a significant inflammatory component, a topical corticosteroid lotion, oil or solution, with or without 3–5% precipitated sulfur or salicylic acid, may be applied once to twice daily. For involvement other than the scalp, a low-strength topical corticosteroid or topical antifungal agent is usually effective when applied once to twice daily.

Adolescents with seborrhea of the scalp may try a variety of antiseborrheic shampoos, tar shampoo, ketoconazole shampoo,[196] or 5% tea tree oil shampoo.[194,197] Antiseborrheic shampoos may contain selenium sulfide (e.g., Sebulex, Exsel, and Selsun), salicylic acid (e.g., T-sal), or zinc pyrithione (e.g., Head and Shoulders and DHS Zinc). If the scale is extremely thick and adherent, it can be loosened by warmed mineral oil massaged into the scalp or by the use of P&S Liquid (Baker Cummins), ideally left on overnight. Scales are then loosened by scrubbing gently with the fingers or a soft brush, and the scalp is shampooed. For patients with associated erythema or pruritus, topical corticosteroid lotions, gels, oils, or foams may be used. Seborrheic dermatitis of the face or intertriginous areas in adolescents usually responds quickly to the application of a mild corticosteroid calcineurin inhibitor or antifungal medication. If these are too greasy, a foam preparation of ketoconazole is available.[198]

Blepharitis may be managed by warm water compresses, gentle cleansing with a dilute solution of a non-irritating or baby shampoo, and mechanical removal of scales when necessary. Topical corticosteroids on the eyelids or eyelid margins should be used with caution, although calcineurin inhibitors (e.g., tacrolimus or pimecrolimus) may be used safely in this area.

Seborrheic dermatitis of the intertriginous or diaper areas occasionally may be complicated by secondary candidal or bacterial infection. Candidal infection is usually seen in the diaper areas as discrete erythematous scaling papules and sometimes pustules, especially at the periphery of the affected area. Secondary bacterial infection is more commonly seen as oozing at the neckfold and other intertriginous sites. In such instances, topical anticandidal and/or antibacterial agents are generally helpful. For patients refractory to topical treatment or for those with significant secondary bacterial infection, bacterial cultures and appropriate systemic antibiotics are necessary.

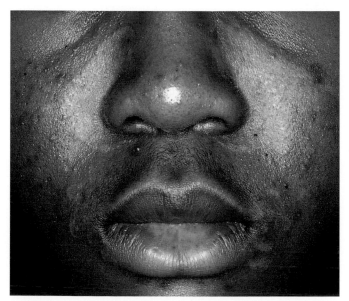

Figure 3.36 Seborrheic dermatitis. Facial seborrheic dermatitis in adolescents typically involves nasolabial folds and may result from overgrowth of lipophilic yeasts of the normal flora. In this patient, tinea faciei was considered less likely because of the bilaterally symmetrical distribution and the localization to perinasal and perioral sites; no fungi grew in cultures. Post-inflammatory hypopigmentation is a sequela of seborrheic dermatitis on patients with darker skin types.

Intertrigo

Intertrigo is a superficial inflammatory dermatitis that occurs in areas where the skin is in apposition (Figs 3.37; Fig. 17. 32). As a result of friction, heat, and moisture, the affected areas become

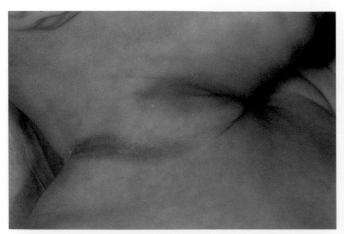

Figure 3.37 Intertrigo. A superficial inflammatory dermatitis that occurs at sites of skin apposition. Secondary bacterial or yeast infection is common.

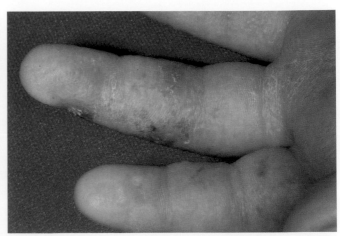

Figure 3.39 Pompholyx/dyshidrotic eczema. Superficial crusting and desquamation often replace the ruptured tiny vesicles of dyshidrotic eczema.

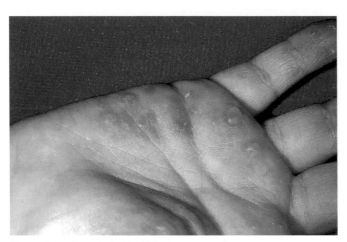

Figure 3.38 Pompholyx/dyshidrotic eczema. An acute recurrent or chronic eruption of the palms, soles, and lateral aspects of the fingers with deep-seated tapioca-like vesicles to large, tense bullae.

erythematous, macerated, and secondarily infected by bacteria or Candida, or in adolescents by dermatophytes (see Ch. 17). Treatment is directed toward elimination of the macerated skin. Open wet compresses, dusting powders (such as ZeaSorb), topical corticosteroid lotions, and when indicated, appropriate antibiotics or fungicidal agents may be used.

Dyshidrotic eczema

Dyshidrotic eczema (pompholyx) is an acute recurrent or chronic eczematous eruption of the palms, soles, and lateral aspects of the fingers.[199] Of unknown etiology, it is characterized by deep-seated, variously inflammatory lesions that range from tapioca-like vesicles to large, tense bullae (Figs 3.38, 3.39). The distribution of lesions generally is bilateral and somewhat symmetrical. Patients complain of considerable pruritus and/or burning. Hyperhidrosis is often associated. Attacks usually last a few weeks, but relapses are frequent, often several times per year.

Dyshidrotic eczema may be confused with contact dermatitis or tinea, disorders commonly unilateral or more localized. Allergic contact dermatitis (see below) on the feet or hands most commonly results from exposure to potassium dichromate (for tanning leather) or rubber, but occasionally is caused by paraphenylenediamine (PPD, in hair dyes), nickel, fragrance mix, or colophony (in glues and also in violin rosin), and potassium dichromate.[200,201] Fungal culture and patch testing can be performed to distinguish these disorders. 'Id' reactions and pustular psoriasis must also be considered in the differential diagnosis of this disorder and are most commonly bilateral. Juvenile plantar dermatosis is limited to the feet and tends to be bilateral. A reaction on the palms and soles resembling dyshidrotic eczema has also been described after IVIG therapy.[202,203]

The natural course of dyshidrotic eczema is one of frequent recurrence. Open wet compresses tend to open the vesicles, and application of moderate to potent topical corticosteroids, although not curative, helps to relieve the manifestations of this disorder. Topical tacrolimus 0.1% ointment has been used successfully as an alternative that allows rotational therapy.[204] When infection is present, antibiotics may be administered topically or systemically. Although not a disorder of eccrine glands *per se*, the use of topical aluminum chloride in concentrations of 12% (e.g., Certain Dri) to 20% (e.g., Drysol) may decrease the associated hyperhidrosis and help to control the disorder, if not too irritating. Hyperhidrosis can also be controlled by oral administration of glycopyrrolate, if topical application of drying agents is ineffective. For adolescents with recalcitrant hyperhidrosis, intradermal injections of botulinum toxin might be considered.[205] Phototherapy with either narrow band ultraviolet B or high doses of UVA1 light has also been used.[206]

Juvenile plantar dermatosis

Juvenile plantar dermatosis (dermatitis plantaris sicca, 'sweaty sock dermatitis') is a common dermatosis of infancy and childhood, most commonly localized to the distal aspect of the soles and toes, particularly the great toes, but sparing the interdigital spaces. Associated with hyperhidrosis and thought to represent a frictional irritant dermatitis, the disorder is manifested by a symmetrical, smooth, red, glazed, and fine scaling (Fig. 3.40). Similar changes have also been reported on the fingertips in up to 5% of patients with excessive perspiration. Untreated juvenile plantar dermatosis generally tends to persist for several years, and although there is no seasonal pattern, some patients report slight worsening of the condition during the summer and in cold weather.

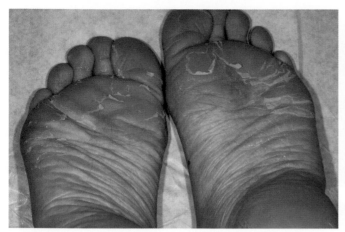

Figure 3.40 Juvenile plantar dermatosis. A characteristic smooth, glazed dermatosis with scaling on the skin of the toes and distal plantar surfaces of the feet of a child with juvenile plantar dermatosis ('sweaty sock dermatitis'). This patient also has ichthyosis vulgaris, which explains the hyperlinear soles and thicker desquamating scale.

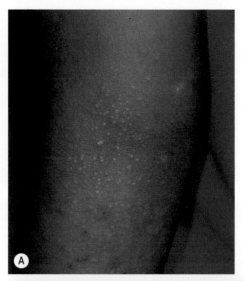

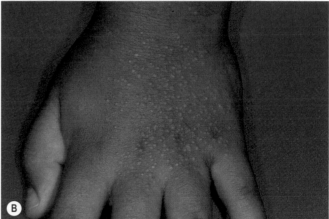

Figure 3.41 Frictional lichenoid dermatosis. Aggregates of lichenoid papules occur primarily on the (A) elbows, knees; (B) knuckles, and backs of the hands of children. Although the somewhat monomorphic appearance of the papules on the hand in this child is suggestive of lichen nitidus (see Ch. 4), the associated pruritus, localization, and concurrent presence of lichenoid papules of various sizes on the elbows allow the diagnosis to be made clinically.

The differential diagnosis of juvenile plantar dermatosis includes tinea pedis, palmoplantar psoriasis, pityriasis rubra pilaris, and shoe contact dermatitis. Tinea pedis can manifest as scaling and erythema of the plantar foot, but is more likely to involve the interdigital spaces. Associated pustulation of tinea may be mistaken for secondary staphylococcal infection. Potassium hydroxide scrapings and culture may be required to distinguish tinea pedis and juvenile plantar dermatosis. The plaques of psoriasis are often more brightly erythematous and thicker. Pityriasis rubra pilaris may closely resemble psoriasis, but often shows a salmon-orange coloration on the palms and soles. Both psoriasis and pityriasis rubra pilaris usually show lesions elsewhere. Contact dermatitis owing to a component of shoes is more commonly on the dorsum of the foot, but the plantar foot is occasionally involved (see below).

Although treatment is not always completely successful, children with hyperhidrosis of the feet should wear all-cotton socks and avoid occlusive footwear whenever possible, remove their shoes when indoors, change their socks whenever they are damp, dust an absorbent powder such as ZeaSorb into shoes and hosiery (to help lessen perspiration), and use an emollient cream as soon as the shoes and socks are removed. Use of a medium-strength to potent topical steroid is usually effective in diminishing the associated pruritus and inflammation. Low-strength topical steroids are often not effective, probably owing to the thick overlying stratum corneum of the plantar surface. Topical or systemically administered antistaphylococcal antibiotics may be needed if patients show crusting or pustulation suggesting secondary infection. Careful application of 'superglue' to fissured areas often provides relief from the associated discomfort.

Frictional lichenoid dermatitis

Frictional lichenoid dermatitis (frictional lichenoid eruption, juvenile papular dermatitis, recurrent summertime pityriasis of the elbows and knees) is a recurring cutaneous disorder affecting children, especially boys, between 4 and 12 years of age.[207] Most cases are seen in the spring and summer when outdoor activities are common, and many cases have been associated with playing in sandboxes (sandbox dermatitis) or on grass. Approximately half of the affected children have atopic dermatitis, allergic rhinitis or asthma.[208] The eruption is characterized by aggregates of discrete lichenoid papules, 1 or 2 mm in diameter, which occur primarily on the elbows, knees, and backs of the hands of children in whom such areas are subject to minor frictional trauma without protection of clothing (Fig. 3.41). Lesions may be hypopigmented, and associated pruritus is often severe, but may be absent. It tends to occur in children with a predisposition to atopy.

The differential diagnosis of this disorder includes psoriasis, atopic dermatitis, molluscum, flat warts, lichen nitidus, and the papular acrolocated syndrome (Gianotti–Crosti syndrome; see Ch. 16). The management of frictional lichenoid dermatitis includes avoidance of frictional trauma to the involved areas (as might occur with leaning on elbows and knees) and application of topical corticosteroids and emollient, especially to ease the associated pruritus.

Nummular dermatitis

Nummular dermatitis is characterized by discoid or coin-shaped plaques. The name is derived from the Latin word *nummulus* ('coin-like'), because of the shape and size of the lesions. The plaques of nummular dermatitis are composed of minute papules and vesicles, which enlarge by peripheral extension to form discrete, round or oval, erythematous, often lichenified and hyperpigmented plaques that measure ≥1 cm in diameter (Figs 3.26, 3.27). They usually occur on the extensor surfaces of the hands, arms, and legs as single or multiple lesions on dry or asteatotic skin. Pruritus is usually associated and may be intense. Occasionally the face and trunk may be involved. The surrounding skin may be xerotic, particularly in children with atopic dermatitis and nummular dermatitis, but in many patients is normal. Secondary staphylococcal infection is common and manifests as crusting and exudation.

Nummular dermatitis must be differentiated from allergic contact dermatitis, atopic dermatitis (which may be seen concurrently), psoriasis, and superficial dermatophyte infections of the skin. History of exposure, patch testing if appropriate, fungal culture, and biopsy of lesional skin can help to distinguish these conditions.

Effective therapy requires application of class II–IV topical corticosteroids, preferably in an ointment base or under occlusion. The combination of a refined tar preparation (liquor carbonis detergens 5–10%) in a strong corticosteroid used twice daily is an alternative means of treatment. Secondary staphylococcal infection should always be considered, especially in recalcitrant lesions, and commonly requires systemic administration of antibiotic (such as cephalexin). Therapy with a topical corticosteroid can be continued in the face of treated infection.

Winter eczema

Winter eczema, also known as asteatotic eczema, eczema craquelé, or xerotic eczema, is a subacute eczematous dermatitis characterized by pruritic scaly erythematous patches, usually associated with dryness and dehydration (asteatosis) of the epidermis. Generally seen on the extremities and occasionally on the trunk, these changes are most frequent during winter when the humidity is low, particularly in adults and adolescents who bathe or shower frequently with harsh or drying soaps. Frequent bathing with incomplete drying and resultant evaporation of moisture causes dehydration of the epidermis, with redness, scaling, and fine cracking that may resemble cracked porcelain (hence the term *eczema craquelé*). Treatment of winter eczema is centered in the maintenance of proper hydration of the stratum corneum and is dependent on the routine use of emollients, limiting the time and temperature of showers, use of mild soaps, and topical therapy with corticosteroids (preferably those in an ointment base) for individual lesions.

Lichen striatus

Lichen striatus is a self-limiting inflammatory dermatosis that follows Blaschko's lines, the path of ectodermal embryologic development of skin (Fig. 3.42).[209-211] Although not considered contagious or inherited, lichen striatus has been described in more than one family member.[212,213] It has followed viral infections, vaccination (e.g., HBV), and trauma, but its cause is unknown. The mean age of onset is 4 years of age, although older children may be affected. Girls appear to be affected two to three times more frequently than boys. In the largest series to date, 60 of 115 affected children were atopic.[210]

The eruption is usually asymptomatic, and reaches its maximum extent within a few weeks to months. Only 6% of affected children show more than one band. Lesions begin as 2–4 mm erythematous to hypopigmented, slightly scaling, flat-topped papules that rapidly coalesce to form the curvilinear band. The line of involvement tends

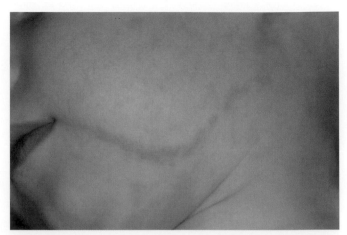

Figure 3.42 Lichen striatus. A self-limiting, usually unilateral curvilinear collection of small, erythematous, flat-topped papules that follows one of Blaschko's lines, lines of the embryologic development of skin.

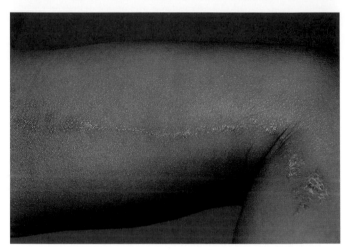

Figure 3.43 Lichen striatus. Linear collection of papules of lichen striatus, most commonly seen on the extremities. The erythema is more difficult to appreciate on darker skin, but the mild scaling may be more apparent.

to be narrow, but can range from several millimeters to 1 or 2 cm in width. Most commonly lichen striatus affects an extremity but occasionally, the face, neck, trunk, or buttocks is affected. Nail involvement is seen, typically by extension of an extremity lesion.[214] In dark-skinned or tanned individuals the eruption may appear as slightly scaly (Fig. 3.43) or as a band-like area of hypopigmentation (Fig. 3.44). Although the band is usually continuous, it may occasionally be interrupted by or interspersed with coalescent plaques several centimeters in diameter along a line of Blaschko.

The differential diagnosis of lichen striatus most commonly includes inflammatory linear verrucous epidermal nevus (ILVEN, which tends to be more psoriasiform (Fig. 3.45); see also Ch. 9) and blaschkitis[215] (more eczematous). In contrast to lichen striatus, blaschkitis is usually papulovesicular, pruritic, and predominantly truncal; it tends to last for about a month, and recurs frequently. Other acquired inflammatory lesions distributed along lines of Blaschko can include linear forms of lichen planus, linear lichen nitidus, lichenoid drug eruptions,[216] lichenoid chronic GVHD, lupus erythematosus, atopic dermatitis, and linearly arranged (koebnerized) lesions of verruca plana. When the diagnosis remains in doubt, histopathologic examination of a cutaneous biopsy specimen will help exclude other possible linear eruptions.

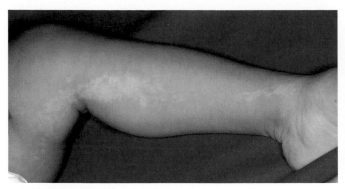

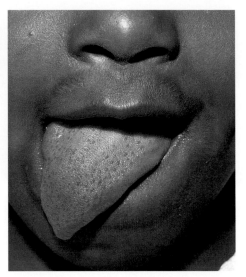

Figure 3.44 Lichen striatus. A darker-skinned child with hypopigmented linear streaks of lichen striatus. In this child, the erythematous papules can be seen, suggesting post-inflammatory hypopigmentation. In other children, only a hypopigmented streak is seen. The stripe of hypopigmentation can be a broad band, as seen on the thigh, or a narrow stripe.

Figure 3.46 Lip-licker's dermatitis. Chronic contact dermatitis with lichenification and hyperpigmentation in the shape of licking from the tongue.

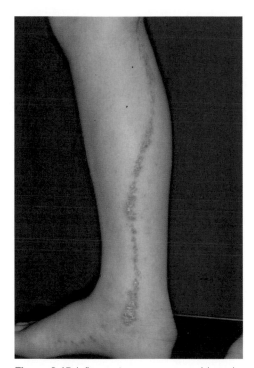

Figure 3.45 Inflammatory verrucous epidermal nevus (ILVEN). Lichen striatus must be differentiated from ILVEN, a persistent mosaic lesion that follows Blaschko's lines (Ch. 9). The papules of ILVEN tends to be more erythematous, less discrete, more scaly and more pruritic than those of lichen striatus, but biopsy or observation over 2–3 years may be necessary to determine the diagnosis.

Lichen striatus usually resolves spontaneously within 3–24 months (mean duration, 6 months),[210] but occasionally lasts longer (up to 3 years), and often leaves an area of hypopigmentation that subsequently disappears. Recurrences occur in 2% of children. Therapy is generally unnecessary, and topical corticosteroids do not tend to hasten resolution. Calcineurin inhibitors have been associated with lesional clearing, particularly on the face.[217,218]

Contact dermatitis

Contact dermatitis may be defined as an eczematous eruption produced either by local exposure to a primary irritating substance (*irritant contact dermatitis*) or by an acquired allergic response to a sensitizing substance (*allergic contact dermatitis*). A contact allergen can 'sensitize' but does not cause a reaction on first exposure. With continued or repeated exposure, the allergen may trigger a contact dermatitis based on a type IV allergic reaction. An irritant, on the other hand, may be defined as a substance that produces an eczematous response on the basis of irritation rather than by immunologic means, and can occur in anyone; allergens only can trigger contact dermatitis in susceptible individuals. Photocontact reactions (Ch. 19), such as phytophotodermatitis after contact with the juice or rinds of certain lemons and limes, occur only when the skin is exposed to ultraviolet light.

Primary Irritant Dermatitis

Common substances that produce primary irritant dermatitis include harsh soaps, bleaches, detergents, solvents, acids, alkalis, bubble baths, certain foods, saliva, urine, feces, and intestinal secretions. The severity of the dermatitis varies from person to person, or from time to time in the same person, as a result of the condition of the skin at the time of exposure, the strength of the irritant, the location of the eruption, the cumulative effect of repeated exposures to the irritating substance, and local factors such as perspiration, maceration, and occlusion.

In children, the lips and adjacent skin frequently become dry and, as a result of a licking habit, inflamed and scaly (lip-licker's dermatitis) (Fig. 3.46). Lip-licker's dermatitis must be distinguished from perioral granulomatous dermatitis, which is characterized by small erythematous papules of the perioral, and often suborbital, areas and is exacerbated by application of topical corticosteroids (Ch. 8). Saliva also frequently becomes trapped between the thumb and mouth of thumbsuckers, and a similar reaction is commonly seen in toddlers who continue to use pacifiers for long periods of time. In infants with atopic dermatitis, saliva is a significant irritant, associated with the extensive drooling from teething, and contributing to the dermatitis on the cheeks and chin. In the infant and young child, circumoral erythema may also represent a contact dermatitis in response to foods such as citrus foods, carrots, shrimp, and spinach. The dermatitis is caused by direct contact with the skin, not from ingestion of the offending food substances, although exposure is aggravated by regurgitation of food particles, dribbling of saliva, and rubbing of the involved areas.

Diaper dermatitis is the most common form of irritant contact dermatitis in infancy (see Ch. 2), with a peak age of incidence of 9–12 months of age. Allergic contact dermatitis in the diaper area is rare. Toddlers and younger children who use 'pull-up' diapers at night and children with enuresis not uncommonly show an irritant dermatitis of the buttocks region related to exposure to urine. Peri-anal dermatitis is often irritant, related to exposure to stool, but must be distinguished from perianal psoriasis (Ch. 4) and perianal streptococcal cellulitis (Ch. 14).

Juvenile plantar dermatosis has been linked to exposure to sweat, and is more commonly seen in children with plantar hyperhidrosis (see above). Excessive hand-washing, especially during winter months and in compulsive hand-washers, is the most common cause of dermatitis on the dorsum of the hands. The increased attention to handwashing as a means to decrease the spread of infectious disease has markedly increased the risk of developing irritant hand dermatitis in school-children.

A common form of irritant dermatitis occurs in the distribution of soccer and hockey shin guards on the anterior aspect of the lower legs of school-aged children. Many of these children have no history of atopic dermatitis, but recurrent or persistent dermatitis may become lichenified. Patch testing for 51 standard allergens, as well as samples of the shin pads themselves, has shown no evidence of allergic contact dermatitis in tested children. This testing further confirms the irritant nature of the dermatitis, likely related to friction and the trapping of sweat under the shin guards. Strategies to reduce friction, such as wearing a cotton sock under the guard and coating with absorbent powder or petrolatum before using the guards, together with topical antiinflammatory therapy for the dermatitis as needed, have been helpful.[219] Irritant reactions may also occur from exposure to fiberglass particles,[220] attached to clothes after exposure to fiberglass insulation panels or drapes. Because clothes washed in a washing machine in which fiberglass materials have been washed are also capable of inducing this cutaneous reaction, children whose parents have been exposed may also be affected. Fiberglass dermatitis presents as a pruritic, patchy follicu-litis or subacute dermatitis. Microscopic examination of skin scrap-ings of involved areas or suspected articles of clothing may reveal pale, greenish, granular rod-like fibers one to two times the width of a hair.[221] The use of methylphenidate transdermal patches in children with attention deficit hyperactivity disorder often leads to irritant reactions confined to the site of patch application; allergic contact dermatitis to the patch is rare.[200]

Avoidance of the irritant is key to improvement. Low-potency topical corticosteroids or calcineurin inhibitors are used to treat the dermatitis of face and intertriginous areas; medium-strength topical steroids, or even potent topical steroids for hands and feet, may be required. Moisturizing creams or ointments lubricate and protect the affected areas. The treatment of irritant diaper dermatitis is discussed in Chapter 2.

Allergic Contact Dermatitis

Allergic contact dermatitis may account for up to 20% of all derma-titis in childhood, and is likely to be underdiagnosed.[92,222,223] Reac-tions to *Rhus* family contact allergens (e.g., poison ivy) are the most common triggers in children. Several series have noted that patch testing in children is positive in up to 83%, with up to 77% of patch test reactions relevant.[224–228] Other major sources of contact allergy in children are metals (especially nickel and cobalt), preservatives, fragrances, topical antibiotics, and rubber products (Table 3.5). Girls are at greater risk for developing contact allergy, especially

during adolescence and on the face, because of their greater exposure to ear piercing (nickel), cosmetics (preservatives and fragrances), and hair products. Initial sensitization to common allergens and occasionally allergic contact dermatitis itself may occur during infancy.[229] Of tested children, 23–49% have atopic dermatitis, although it is unclear whether this high number repre-sents a referral bias or truly increased risk;[58,225–227] the greatest rel-evant reactivity in this group is to allergens in the emollients.[59] More recently recognized triggers in children are p-phenylenediamine (PPD) contaminating henna tattoos,[230] disperse dyes in clothing,[231] and cocamidopropyl betaine in 'no tears' shampoos and cleansers.[232]

Allergic contact dermatitis represents a type IV immunologic (delayed hypersensitivity or cell-mediated) reaction in which anti-genic contact with cutaneous Langerhans cells and T lymphocyte activation are key. After sensitization to the offending allergen, allergic contact dermatitis will develop upon re-exposure to the sensitizing substance. Sensitization may occur after only a few expo-sures to the offending substance or allergy may occur after years of contact. Once the area has become sensitized, however, re-exposure to the offending allergen may result in an acute dermatitis within a relatively brief period (generally 8–12 h following exposure to the sensitizing allergen).

The diagnosis of allergic contact dermatitis is based on the appearance and distribution of skin lesions, aided when possible by a history of contact with an appropriate allergen (Tables 3.5, 3.6). Appearance on exposed areas only, linearity, and sharp edges are also clues to a reaction to a contactant. For example, linearly distributed vesicles and bullae overlying erythema are typical of poison ivy reactions. Dermatitis on the eyelids, hands, feet, and leg are most frequently associated with positive reactions.[57] Eyelid der-matitis often results from preservatives in cosmetics, fragrances, or emollients applied to the hands. Shoe dermatitis (to the leather chromates, rubber or dyes) should be suspected if lesions occur on the dorsum of the foot. Subumbilical or earlobe dermatitis is typical of nickel contact allergy, and axillary vault dermatitis should lead to investigation of sensitivity to deodorant or fragrances, whereas if sparing the vault, axillary dermatitis may relate to clothing dyes. The histopathologic picture of allergic contact dermatitis usually does not allow differentiation from primary irritant dermatitis or atopic dermatitis.

The acute lesions of allergic contact dermatitis are characterized by intense erythema accompanied by edema, papules, vesiculation (sometimes bullae), oozing, and a sharp line of demarcation between involved and normal skin. In the subacute phase, vesicula-tion is less pronounced and is mixed with crusting, scaling, and thickening of the skin. Chronic lesions, conversely, are characterized by lichenification, fissuring, scaling, and little or no vesiculation.

Autosensitization dermatitis or id reaction

An *id reaction* (autosensitization dermatitis, autoeczematization) describes a hypersensitivity disorder characterized by the acute onset of small edematous papules or papulovesicles. Id reactions to nickel are found in up to 50% of patients,[233] and may appear on the trunk (Fig. 3.47), forearms, flexor aspects of the upper arms, the extensor aspects of the upper arms and thighs, and, less commonly, the face. The eruption is nearly always symmetrical but may dem-onstrate light sensitivity or an isomorphic response (the Koebner phenomenon), in which trauma elicits new lesions. Lesions are generally associated with moderate to severe pruritus. The disorder usually appears acutely over a few days and nearly always is pre-ceded by an exacerbation of the pre-existing dermatitis by infection, rubbing, or inappropriate therapy. The acute eruption may subside spontaneously in a few weeks if the primary dermatitis is controlled.

Table 3.5 Most common sensitizers in children and their sources

Group	Allergen	Sources	Typical distribution	Other comments
Plant	Urushiol	Poison ivy, sumac, oak	Extremities in linear streaks; face, genitals	Reaction to aerosolized can resemble angioedema
Metal	Nickel	Jewelry, snaps, buckles, eyeglasses, keys, coins, cell phones, orthodontics	Subumbilical, face, eyelids, earlobes, neck, wrists	Detect with glyoxime
Topical antibiotic	Neomycin	Antibiotic-containing ointments	Face, eyelids	Bacitracin can also sensitize
Fragrance/ Balsam of Peru	Fragrance mix	Cosmetics, perfumes, toothpaste, flavoring agents, lozenges	Face, eyelids, mouth, lips, neck	Cross-reacts with tomato and cinnamon
Preservative	Thimerosal	Creams, lotions, mascara, vaccines	Torso, face	Largely removed
Metal	Cobalt	Buttons, snaps, jewelry, cement, ceramics, vitamin B12	Umbilical, earlobes, neck, hands	Contaminant with nickel
Metal	Chromate	Leather (tanned), cement, paints, matches, green felt	Umbilical, hands, soles	
Rubber accelerant	Thiuram	Elastic (waistband, socks), gloves, shoes (soles and insoles), pesticides	Waistline, feet, hands	Bleach causes release
Emollient	Lanolin	Emollients, lip balms, soaps, waxes that prevent rusting	Hands, body	Sheep wool product
Preservative	Formaldehyde/ formaldehyde releasing	Lotions, cosmetics, shampoo, newsprint, wrinkle-resistant clothes	Hands, face, ears, trunk (sparing axillae)	
Oxidative chemical	Paraphenylenediamine	Hair dyes, printer ink, contaminant in henna tattoos (black)	Hairline, ears, hands, sites of tattoos	

Table 3.6 Distribution of dermatitis and possible triggers

Localization	Triggers
Eyelids	Cosmetics, emollients (hands), fragrances, hair dyes, metals, nail products
Hairline, postauricular, ear helix	Hair dyes, hair products
Earlobes, neck	Fragrance, metal jewelry
Periaxillary	Textile dyes, formaldehyde and formaldehyde releasers
Axillary vault	Deodorants
Subumbilical	Metal (snaps, belt buckles)
Extremities, linear streaks	Poison ivy and oak, phytophotodermatitis
Plantar aspect of feet	Adhesive, rubber in shoes
Dorsal aspect of feet	Leather (chromates, dyes), rubber, adhesive

Relapses, however, are common, particularly when the initial local lesion flares and is followed by a further disseminated eruption.

The diagnosis of id reaction is made clinically on the basis of a generalized papulovesicular eruption that develops in the wake of pre-existing eczematoid dermatitis. Treatment depends on the use of open wet compresses, antihistamines, and topical corticosteroid preparations. Control of the primary lesion is critical to prevent further or recurrent antigenic stimulation. Although seldom indicated, a 2–3-week course of systemic corticosteroids may at times be necessary in cases unresponsive to more conservative therapy.

Id reactions may also be seen in response to infectious agents, particularly in bacterial and dermatophyte infections. The tiny papules of the id reaction associated with tinea capitis most commonly are localized to the head and neck. Often, the id reaction of tinea capitis occurs after initiation of treatment with oral antifungal agents and is erroneously considered to be a drug reaction. Recognition of the underlying infection and continuing the antimicrobial treatment is critical for clearance.

Patch testing

Patch tests may be used to confirm the diagnosis of allergic contact dermatitis if a specific agent is suspected. Different panels of antigens for patch testing are available in Europe, the USA, and Japan, which has led to efforts to standardize testing internationally. In the USA, the T.R.U.E. TEST patch testing kit (Allerderm) is commercially available (Table 3.7). These kits test for reactivity against the most common contact allergens, but are not inclusive. The North American Contact Dermatitis Group (NACDG) screening allergen series is a more extensive set of test substances that has all agents in the T.R.U.E. TEST kit but thimerosal (removed because of its rare relevance). In one study, 39.5% of relevant contact allergens in children would have been missed if only the T.R.U.E. TEST had been used and 15.9% would have had at least one allergen missed with the use of both the T.R.U.E. and NACDG screening tests.[227] Of the top 15 allergens in children,[224] cocamidopropyl betaine (CAPB) disperse dyes, and topical steroids are not found in the T.R.U.E. TEST kit.

When patch testing is performed, patches should be placed on grossly normal, non-hairy skin, such as the back or volar forearm.[234] Distraction techniques, such as having the child watch a video, are very useful, particularly for testing smaller children.[235] Patch testing should be deferred in the presence of extensive active dermatitis; false-positive reactions may be obtained, and a strongly positive patch-test reaction may cause acute exacerbation of the dermatitis. Antihistamines affect type I reactions and not type IV reactions;

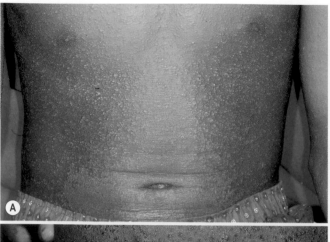

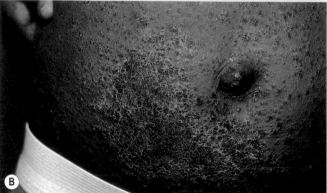

Figure 3.47 (A, B) Nickel contact dermatitis with id. Note the characteristic subumbilical (or periumbilical) hyperpigmented plaque of dermatitis in this patient with nickel contact dermatitis. The lichenification and hyperpigmentation indicate a chronic dermatitis. The tiny discrete papules seen around the plaque extend across the entire trunk and represent an id reaction to the dermatitis.

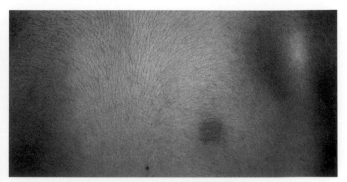

Figure 3.48 Patch testing. Positive patch test reaction to *p-tert*-butylphenol formaldehyde resin in a patient with shoe dermatitis because of reactivity to the glue (see Fig. 3.55).

removal of the patch (Fig. 3.48) to allow the skin to recover from the effects of pressure. The patch or its removal may produce mild transient erythema or a temporary blanching effect, resulting in false reactions. Reactions are graded based on redness, induration and presence of blistering. Unless testing for weak sensitizers (such as fabrics or cosmetics), a doubtful reaction (faint macular erythema only) is usually of no significance. A 1 plus (1+) reaction is characterized by erythema, infiltration, and possibly papules. The addition of vesicles to this response indicates a 2 plus (2+) reaction, and a bullous reaction is read as 3 plus (3+). A second reading of the patches should be performed at 72, 96, or 108 h after the patches are placed. This reading distinguishes irritant from allergic reactions, since irritant reactions often resolve after patches are removed, whereas allergic reactions increase in time. In addition, delayed reactions may be missed if a second reading is not done.

Occasionally, positive reactions may have no clinical significance. Similarly, the offending material may not give rise to a positive reaction at the site of the test but may show a positive test if carried out on an area of skin closer to the point of the previously existing dermatitis. The value of patch tests is corroborative and should be used only as a guide in an attempt to confirm a suspected allergen. Scratch and intracutaneous tests are not useful in contact allergic dermatitis.

Poison ivy (*Rhus* dermatitis)

In the USA, poison ivy, poison oak, and poison sumac produce more cases of allergic contact dermatitis than all other contactants combined. The plants causing poison ivy dermatitis are included under the botanical term *Rhus* and are *Toxicodendron* species. Poison ivy and poison oak are the principal causes of *Rhus* dermatitis in the USA. Regardless of the specific *Rhus* plant, the clinical appearance of the dermatitis may be identical. The *Rhus* group belongs to the family of plants known as Anacardiaceae, and cross-reactions may occur. These include furniture lacquer derived from the Japanese lacquer tree, oil from the shell of the cashew or Brazil nut, the fruit pulp of the gingko tree, and the marking nut tree of India, from which a black 'ink' used to mark wearing apparel is produced. The allergic contact dermatitis to this ink is termed *dhobi itch*. The rind of the mango also cross-reacts, and the possibility of contact dermatitis to *Rhus* should be considered in children with perioral dermatitis after eating mango (Fig. 3.49).

The poison ivy plant (Fig. 3.50) characteristically shows three leaflets notched at the edge. It grows luxuriantly as a tall shrub or woody rope-like vine in vacant lots, among grasses, and on trees or fences throughout all sections of the USA, except the extreme southwest. Poison sumac grows as a shrub or tree, never as a vine. It has 7–13 leaflets (arranged in pairs along a central stem), with a single

Table 3.7 Allergen components in the commercially available T.R.U.E. TEST kit

Balsam of Peru	Methylchloroisothiazolinone/methylisothiazolinone
Black rubber mix	Neomycin sulfate
Caine mix	Nickel sulfate hexahydrate
Carba mix	Quaternium-15
Cobalt chloride	Paraben mix
Colophony	p-Phenylenediamine base
Epoxy resin	Potassium dichromate
Ethylenediamine dihydrochloride	p-tert-Butylphenol formaldehyde resin
Formaldehyde	Thimerosal
Fragrance mix	Thiuram mix
2-Mercaptobenzothiazole	Wool alcohol (lanolin)
Mercapto mix	Negative control

thus, their administration is not a contraindication to patch testing. Systemic corticosteroid therapy might mask weak patch-test responses, and it is preferable that oral steroids be discontinued at least 1 week before patch testing. Potent topical steroids have also been shown to suppress patch test reactivity.[236]

Patch tests generally should be kept in place for 48 h, and a reading can be made after an interval of 20–60 min following

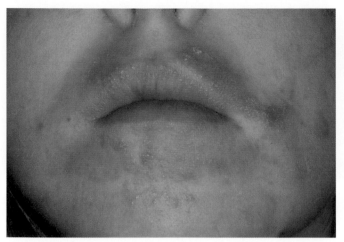

Figure 3.49 Mango dermatitis. Individuals who react to Rhus family plants may demonstrate a perioral dermatitis after eating mango, but only when in contact with the mango rind, not from the fruit itself.

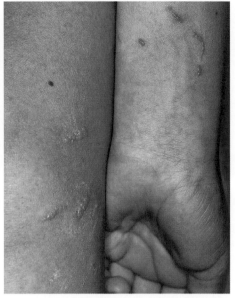

Figure 3.51 *Rhus* dermatitis with Koebner phenomenon. A characteristic linear vesicular eruption on the forearm of a young man with poison ivy (*Rhus*) dermatitis.

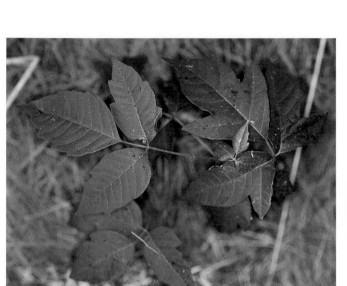

Figure 3.50 Poison ivy plant. A member of the *Rhus* family, showing three notched leaflets. (Courtesy of Dr Jon Dyer.)

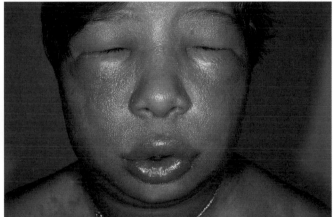

Figure 3.52 *Rhus* dermatitis. The entire face may become swollen with *Rhus* dermatitis, especially if exposed through aerosolization. The fine vesiculation distinguishes contact dermatitis from angioedema.

leaflet at the end, is relatively uncommon, grows less abundantly, and is found only in woody or swampy areas primarily east of the Mississippi River. Poison oak, conversely, grows as an upright shrub, is most prominent on the West Coast, and is not a problem in the eastern USA. Although *Rhus* dermatitis is more common in the summer, the eruption may occur at any time of year by direct contact with the sensitizing allergen from the leaves, roots, or twigs of the plants.

The eruption produced by poison ivy and related plants is a delayed contact hypersensitivity reaction to an oleoresin (urushiol) of which the active sensitizing ingredient is pentadecylcatechol. It is characterized by itching, redness, papules, vesicles, and bullae (Fig. 3.51). Although often irregular and spotty, a linear distribution is highly characteristic because of scratching and transfer of the urushiol oleoresin ('Koebner' reaction). When contact is indirect, such as from a pet that has the oleoresin on its fur, the dermatitis is often diffuse, thus making the diagnosis more difficult unless the

true nature of exposure is suspected. In the fall, when brush and leaves are burned, it must be remembered that the sensitizing oil may be vaporized and transmitted by smoke to exposed cutaneous surfaces, often presenting as a diffuse facial dermatitis with periorbital swelling (Fig. 3.52).

Rhus dermatitis usually first appears in susceptible, sensitized individuals within 1–3 days after contact with the sensitizing oleoresin; in highly sensitive individuals it may occur within 8 h of exposure. Such temporal differences are probably due to the degree of exposure, individual susceptibility, and variation in cutaneous reactivity of different body regions.

About 70% of the population of the USA would acquire *Rhus* dermatitis if exposed to the plants or the sensitizing oleoresin contained in its leaves, stems, and roots. The result is an acute eczematous eruption which, barring complications or re-exposure to the offending allergen, persists for 1–3 weeks. Since the sap from plants of the *Toxicodendron* species turns black when exposed to dry surfaces and skin, dramatic black lacquer- or enamel-like deposits on the skin and clothing of individuals exposed to poison ivy or other urushiol-containing plants may rarely be seen.[237]

The best prophylaxis, as with any type of allergic contact dermatitis, is complete avoidance of the offending allergen. Patients should be instructed in how to recognize and avoid members of the poison *Rhus* group. When poison ivy is present in the garden or children's play areas, chemical destruction or physical removal is indicated. Heavy-duty vinyl gloves should be used if the plants are uprooted, since the uroshiol is soluble in rubber and can penetrate latex gloves.[238] No topical measure is totally effective in the prevention of poison ivy dermatitis, but certain commercially available barrier preparations with quaternium-18 bentonite (organoclay) have been shown to diminish reactivity significantly (IvyBlock, Stokogard, Hollister Moisture Barrier, Hydropel).[239,240] Desensitization to the oleoresin of poison ivy by systemic administration of *Rhus* antigen is unreliable, and should be reserved only for extremely sensitive individuals who cannot avoid repeated exposure to the antigen. Systemic reactions are not uncommon with the use of hyposensitization procedures.

In an effort to minimize the degree of dermatitis, individuals with known exposure should wash thoroughly with soap and water as rapidly as possible so that removal of the oil is accomplished, preferably within 5–10 min of exposure. If the oleoresin is not carefully removed shortly after exposure, the allergen may be transmitted by the fingers to other parts of the body (particularly the face, forearms, or male genitalia) (Fig. 3.53). However, the fluid content of vesicles and bullae is not contagious and does not produce new lesions. Thus, unless the sensitizing antigen is still on the skin, the disorder is neither able to be spread on an individual nor contagious from one person to another.

Complete change of clothing is advisable and, whenever possible, contaminated shoes and clothing should be washed with soap and water or cold water mixed with alcohol to remove the urushiol. Harsh soaps and vigorous scrubbing offer no advantage over simple soaking and cool water. Thorough washing may not prevent a severe dermatitis in highly sensitive persons. It may, however, reduce the reaction and prevent spread of the oleoresin. When early washing is not feasible, it is worthwhile to wash at the first opportunity in an effort to remove any oleoresin remaining on the skin or clothing and thus prevent its transfer to other parts of the body.

In the management of mild *Rhus* dermatitis, treatment with an antipruritic 'shake' lotion such as calamine lotion is helpful. Topical preparations containing potential sensitizers such as diphenhydramine or benzocaine should be avoided. As in other acute eczematous eruptions, cool compresses with plain tap water or Burow's solution are soothing, help remove crusts, and relieve pruritus. Administration of potent topical corticosteroids and systemic use of antihistamines and antipruritic agents are helpful. Because the acutely involved areas tend to be vesicular and weeping, creams and lotion forms of topical steroids are more commonly used than occlusive ointments.

In severe, more generalized cases of *Rhus* dermatitis, short-term systemic corticosteroid treatment may be indicated. Systemic corticosteroid therapy may be initiated with dosages of 1 mg/kg per day of prednisone or its equivalent. Steroids should be tapered gradually over a period of 2–3 weeks. Premature termination of systemic corticosteroids may result in a rapid rebound, with return of the dermatitis to its original intensity.

Metal and metal salt dermatitis

The most common form of contact dermatitis to metal is that caused by sensitivity to nickel. Most objects containing metal or metal salts are combinations of several metals, some of which may have been used to plate the surface, thus enhancing its attractiveness, tensile strength, or durability. Nickel may be present in some white gold, 14-carat yellow gold, chrome, silver, bronze, and brass. Nickel is found with two other metal salts that may cause contact allergy, chromium and cobalt, added to increase the composite strength. Diethylenetriamine pentaacetic acid (chelator) cream can prevent nickel, chrome, and copper dermatitis.[240]

Nickel dermatitis is by far the most common cause of contact allergy in patch tested children, with a prevalence of 10.3–40% of tested children worldwide.[224,225,241] Ear piercing has repeatedly been shown to be a strong risk factor for both females[242] and males.[243] The current trend towards piercing of additional body areas, in both males and females, will likely further increase the numbers of nickel-sensitive individuals. A positive family history of nickel allergic contact dermatitis appears to be a risk factor.[233] Several studies have shown an increased risk of nickel sensitivity in girls (perhaps because of piercing).[244]

Earlobe dermatitis is a cardinal sign of nickel dermatitis. Prominent pruritic peri- and subumbilical papules should trigger consideration of contact allergy to nickel from the nickel-containing buttons on pants and belt buckles (Fig. 3.47), and may present as recalcitrant lichenified plaques in children with atopic dermatitis.[245] Circular erythematous scaling patches on the midline trunk of infants may signal reactivity to the metal snaps in baby clothes, and at least 6% of the fasteners in children's clothing have been shown to release nickel ion.[246] Other potential triggers are zippers, clothing hooks, the dorsal eyelets on shoes, nickel-containing eyeglass rims (Fig. 3.54), shoe buckles, musical instruments[247] and cell phones.[248,249] Restriction on the releasable nickel in products with potential skin contact to <0.5 mg/cm² per week by the European Union has reduced rates of sensitization;[250] to date, no limits have been legislated in the USA.[251] Although the concentration of nickel in orthodontic appliances is low and has not been found to sensitize against nickel, patients who are already nickel sensitive, usually from exposure through ear piercing, may rarely show gingival reactions induced by the appliance;[252] the prevalence of

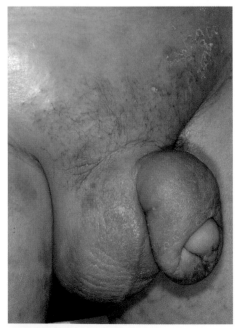

Figure 3.53 *Rhus* dermatitis. The oleoresin may be transmitted by the fingers to other parts of the body, including the male genitalia.

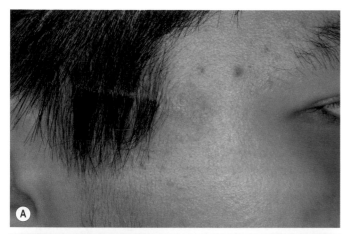

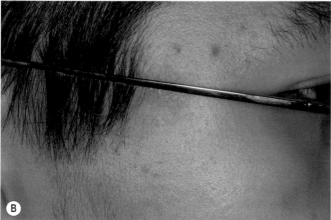

Figure 3.54 Nickel contact dermatitis. This postauricular dermatitis (A) represents a reaction to nickel-containing eyeglass frames (B).

reactions to orthodontic appliances was noted to be 0.03% in a recent survey.[253,254] Students should be aware of the presence of nickel in seats with metal studs, which may lead to patches on the posterior thighs, while metal ballet balance bars may lead to hand dermatitis. Hand dermatitis may also be associated with nickel allergy, as nickel may be present in the metal handles of scissors, keys, doorknobs, and the wheels of skateboards. Nickel coins in the USA no longer contain nickel, but small amounts are present in the 1- and 2-Euro coins, and reactions to coin rolling have been described. Patch testing for nickel sensitivity can be performed, but false negatives are not infrequent, and repeating testing may be helpful. If a substance is suspected of containing free nickel, application of a test solution of dimethylglyoxime in a 10% aqueous solution of ammonia (Allerderm Ni kit) to the suspected item will usually cause the suspected metal to turn pink.

Since piercing of ears or other sites is responsible for an increased tendency of sensitization to nickel and nickel products, piercing should be done with a stainless steel needle. Persons undergoing piercing should be advised to wear only stainless steel earrings or titanium earrings until the earlobes (or other sites) are completely healed, usually about 3 weeks. Although stainless steel contains up to 20% nickel, the nickel is bound tightly and usually causes no problems.

Once the presence of hypersensitivity to nickel has been established, the hypersensitivity usually lasts for years. Patients, therefore, must be taught how to avoid contact with nickel objects through the use of proper substitutes. If possible, wearing clothes with nickel

should be avoided, such as substitution of pants with elasticized waists for jeans with metal snaps and leather for metal belt buckles. Periodic coating of the offending metal with clear nail polish (including after each washing if laundered) may prevent loss of nickel, but sewing cloth over the nickel snap is not effective, since sweating encourages nickel to leach through the fabric into contact with skin. In general, watches with stainless steel backs should be worn; application of an adhesive moleskin on the back of a watch may be helpful. Sterling silver or platinum jewelry is usually tolerated. Nickel-free eyeglass frames are available. The majority of inexpensive earrings contain some nickel,[255] so that allergic individuals should wear only surgical stainless steel earrings, 'hypoallergenic' earrings with titanium (which looks like platinum) or earrings with plastic casings (Blomdahl, Simply Whispers). Vinyl gloves can be worn by nickel-sensitive patients to avoid hand contact with nickel. Mid-strength to potent topical steroids can be used to treat, but avoidance of nickel is required for full efficacy.

Chromates are an ingredient in the manufacture of many products, such as cement, mortar, leather, paints, and anticorrosives. They are used in the dye of the green felt fabric used for pool tables and the yellow-green pigment of tattoos and cosmetics. Dichromates are used to toughen the collagen in leather and allow it to resist wear, water, and changes because of heat. Most contact reactions in children that are due to chromates manifest as shoe dermatitis (see below).

Cobalt blue pigment is found in glass and pottery, and used in the blue and green of watercolor paints and crayons. It is inextricably linked to nickel in metal-plated objects and costume jewelry, and can be found in cosmetics, joint replacements and cement. Oral administration of vitamin B_{12}, which also contains cobalt, can cause intractable hand eczema and injection may lead to dermatitis at the injection site in cobalt-sensitive individuals.

Shoe dermatitis

Shoe dermatitis is an extremely common form of contact dermatitis in childhood that usually results from rubber products, especially given the increasing trend for athletic shoes. It is frequently misdiagnosed as tinea pedis, a disorder that occurs uncommonly in children prior to puberty. In one study, >50% of the children with foot dermatitis showed reactivity to suspected contact allergens.[256]

Shoe dermatitis usually begins over the dorsal surface of the base of the great toe. It may remain localized or spread to involve the dorsal surfaces of the feet and other toes. The thick skin of the plantar surfaces is generally more resistant, but may demonstrate dermatitis over the sole, ventral surface of the toes, instep, or even the entire plantar surface that may be confused with juvenile plantar dermatosis or psoriasis. Erythema, lichenification, and in severe cases, weeping and crusting are typical, but the interdigital spaces usually are spared. In contrast, maceration, scaling, and occasional vesiculation of the interdigital webs, particularly between the fourth and fifth toes, are usually seen with tinea pedis. Irritant dermatitis from friction and ill-fitting shoes may also sharply localize to the dorsal aspects of the toes.

Rubber components are the principal allergens;[257] these include accelerants (thiuram and carbamate) and rubber antioxidants. Rubber accelerants facilitate the transformation of liquid rubber to solid. Several components of the approved patch-test kit in the USA test for rubber, including the carba mix, the black rubber mix, mercaptobenzathiazole, mercapto mix, and the thiuram mix (see Table 3.6), but additional testing should be performed if shoe dermatitis is suspected but an agent is not found in this standard kit, as it is not fully inclusive. Rubber is a common component of the insoles of shoes and particularly of the box toes. Rubber cement may be using in joining show uppers, outer leather, and linings.

of dyes in light-colored clothing, and dark colors tend to 'bleed' more readily than dyes of lighter hue). Disperse dyes may be used in patch testing, but the garment can also be directly applied for patch testing. Children may also react to the epoxy resin in the adhesive holding a knee patch onto jeans, and elastic or rubber waist bands in underwear in which the rubber components are leached out after exposure to bleach.

Compositae dermatitis

Compositae is one of the largest plant families, and includes among its members chrysanthemum, ragweed, artichoke, sunflower, lettuce, spinach, chamomile, gingko, feverfew, parthenium, and dandelions. Contact allergy to compositae is well recognized in florists, gardeners and farmers, but only occasionally occurs in children.[282] Atopic dermatitis may be a significant risk factor,[283] suggesting that Compositae allergy may explain recalcitrant or recurrent dermatitis of the late spring and summer, particularly affecting the distal extremities and face.

Key References

Bieber T. Atopic dermatitis. *N Engl J Med.* 2008;358:1483–1494.

Cork MJ, Danby SG, Vasilopoulos Y, et al. Epidermal barrier dysfunction in atopic dermatitis. *J Invest Dermatol.* 2009;129:1892–1908.

Elias PM, Steinhoff M. 'Outside-to-inside' (and now back to 'outside') pathogenic mechanisms in atopic dermatitis. *J Invest Dermatol.* 2008;128:1067–1070.

Huang JT, Abrams M, Tlougan B, et al. Treatment of Staphylococcus aureus colonization in atopic dermatitis decreases disease severity. *Pediatrics.* 2009;123:e808–e814.

Krakowski AC, Eichenfield LF, Dohil MA. Management of atopic dermatitis in the pediatric population. *Pediatrics.* 2008;122:812–824.

Lee PW, Elsaie ML, Jacob SE. Allergic contact dermatitis in children: common allergens and treatment: a review. *Curr Opin Pediatr.* 2009;21:491–498.

Ong PY, Ohtake T, Brandt C, et al. Endogenous antimicrobial peptides and skin infections in atopic dermatitis. *N Engl J Med.* 2002;347(15):1151–1160.

Palmer CN, Irvine AD, Terron-Kwiatkowski A, et al. Common loss-of-function variants of the epidermal barrier protein filaggrin are a major predisposing factor for atopic dermatitis. *Nat Genet.* 2006;38:441–446.

Sandilands A, Terron-Kwiatkowski A, Hull PR, et al. Comprehensive analysis of the gene encoding filaggrin uncovers prevalent and rare mutations in ichthyosis vulgaris and atopic eczema. *Nat Genet.* 2007;39:650–654.

Taieb A, When and how to perform allergy tests in children and adults with AD. *Eur J Dermatol.* 2007;17:263–266.

Zug KA, McGinley-Smith D, Warshaw EM, et al. Contact allergy in children referred for patch testing: North American Contact Dermatitis Group data, 2001–2004. *Arch Dermatol.* 2008;144:1329–1336.

Papulosquamous and Related Disorders

4

Childhood psoriasis

Psoriasis is a common immune-mediated disorder that accounts for 4% of all dermatoses seen in children under 16 years of age and occurs at all ages in 2–3% of the population.[1,2] Presence of psoriasis at birth has been described.[3] A total of 31–45% of adults with psoriasis have noted the onset during the first two decades of life. As in the adult population, psoriasis occurs most frequently in Caucasian children. The severity of the condition may vary from a life-threatening neonatal pustular or exfoliative dermatosis to a mild localized disorder that causes no distress. Psoriasis usually follows an irregularly chronic course marked by remissions and exacerbations of unpredictable onset and duration.

Both complex genetic and environmental factors participate in the risk of psoriasis. Up to 70% of pediatric patients have a family history of psoriasis and the risk of occurrence in monozygotic twins is 2–3 times that of dizygotic twins.[4] The major genetic determinant is *PSOR1* (35–50% of patients), which is within the major histocompatibility complex on chromosome 6.[5] Early-onset psoriasis has been linked to HLA antigen Cw6, and 73.7% of patients with guttate psoriasis show HLA Cw6 antigen, in contrast to a frequency of 7.4% in the general population. At least eight additional susceptibility loci for psoriasis have subsequently been identified at other chromosomal locations, among them genes regulating IL23 function (IL23A, IL23R, IL12B), TNF-α activation of NF-κB (TN1P1, TNFAIP3), and Th2 cytokines (IL4 and IL-13).[5]

Evidence that psoriasis is an immune-mediated disorder is based on laboratory studies, clinical observation, and success of targeted therapy, such as cyclosporine, anti-CD4+ monoclonal antibodies, and inhibitors of TNF-α and interleukins (IL)-12 and -23. The majority of T cells in psoriatic plaques are CD45RO+ memory-effector T cells that migrate into skin exposed to an antigenic trigger. Th1 and Th17 cytokines predominate, in contrast to the largely Th2 cytokine response of the acute lesions of atopic dermatitis. The innate immune system plays a key role in psoriasis, initiating a cascade that involves activation of myeloid dendritic cells (by TNF-α, interferon-γ, interleukin (IL)-6 and IL-1β). The activated dendritic cells express IL-12 and IL-23, leading to Th1 and Th17 cell expression of TNF-α/interferon-γ and of IL-17/IL-22, respectively. These cytokines stimulate the keratinocyte to produce more IL-1β and IL-6, TNF-α, chemokines and antimicrobial peptides, further contributing to immune activation and cutaneous inflammation.[6] Skin injury and streptococcal infections[7] are well-known environmental triggers but the occurrence of psoriasis has also been linked to *S. aureus* infection[8] and Kawasaki disease,[9] suggesting a role for superantigens. Psoriasis has been triggered by growth hormone therapy and administration of interferon (e.g., for chronic hepatitis). Flares of psoriasis have also clearly been linked to psychological and physical stress.

Clinical Manifestations

Classic lesions of psoriasis consist of round, brightly erythematous, well-marginated plaques covered by a characteristic grayish or silvery-white (mica-like or 'micaceous') scale.[10] Psoriatic papules coalesce to form plaques that measure 1 cm or more in diameter (Figs 4.1–4.3).

The disorder may present as solitary lesions or countless plaques in a generalized distribution. Lesions are usually bilaterally symmetrical with a distinct predilection for the scalp, elbows, knees, and lumbosacral and anogenital regions. However, lesions may also be found in a flexural distribution with involvement of the axillae, groin, perineum, central chest, and umbilical region. This variant, termed inverse psoriasis (Figs 4.4, 4.5), may be seen without any extensor surface involvement in 2.8–6.0% of patients or in association with only regional involvement in 30% of patients. A peripheral white ring is often the first sign of involution (termed *Wernoff's ring*). However, when the central portions of the plaques resolve, the involuting lesions may appear nummular (small circles), annular (central clearing), gyrate, or arcuate (semi circular). A linear variant that courses along Blaschko's lines has also been described,[11] and may be associated with psoriatic arthritis.[12]

The hallmark of psoriasis is the micaceous scale, generally attached at the center rather than the periphery of lesions. Removal of this scale results in fine punctate bleeding points. This phenomenon (termed *Auspitz sign*) is highly characteristic and relates to rupture of capillaries high in the papillary dermis of lesions. The Koebner phenomenon (Fig. 4.6), seen in psoriasis as well as in verrucae, Rhus dermatitis, lichen planus, lichen nitidus, Darier's disease, and pityriasis rubra pilaris, describes the occurrence of skin lesions at sites of local injury. This valuable diagnostic sign of psoriasis represent a reaction to trauma (an isomorphic response) that may follow simple irritation such as a scratch or sunburn, a surgical scar, or a preexisting disease such as seborrheic or atopic dermatitis.

Facial psoriasis

Facial psoriasis is more common in children than in adults, and occurs without other involvement in 4–5% of patients. Involvement of the periorbital area is most typical, and lesions may be subtle, leading to confusion with atopic dermatitis (Fig. 4.7). The plaques of psoriasis tend to be more clearly delineated than patches of atopic dermatitis, are less pruritic, and may show an annular configuration. It should be noted, however, that approximately 5% of pediatric patients show an eczema/psoriasis overlap, either showing typical lesions of both atopic dermatitis and psoriasis or lesions that are intermediate (e.g., nummular and psoriasiform).[13] Almost all patients with the overlap have a family history of both atopic disease and psoriasis. Although mucosae do not tend to be affected

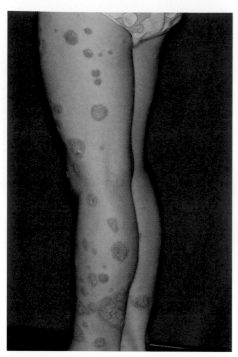

Figure 4.1 Psoriasis. Typical plaques of psoriasis with thick, micaceous scale overlying erythema.

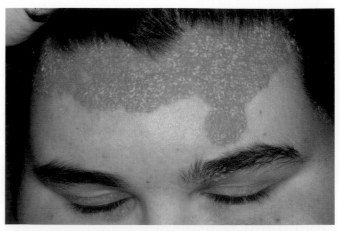

Figure 4.3 Psoriasis. Psoriasis often involves the forehead, particularly contiguous to the scalp. Note the eyelid and brow involvement. Given the yellowish scaling, this has been called 'sebopsoriasis'.

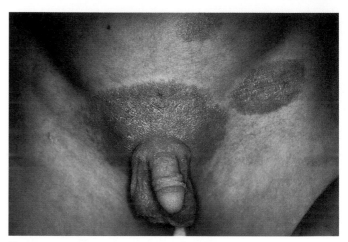

Figure 4.4 Psoriasis. Discrete, brightly erythematous plaques of inverse psoriasis in a 3-year-old boy. Note that the scaling tends to be thinner in an intertriginous area.

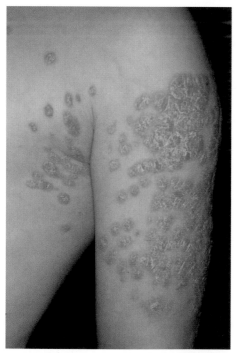

Figure 4.2 Psoriasis. Small erythematous plaques with moderately thick overlying scale.

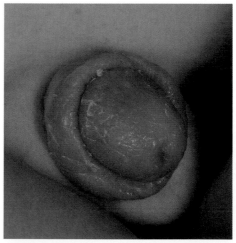

Figure 4.5 Psoriasis. In contrast to the relative sparing of the glans in the toddler in Figure 4.4, this boy's psoriasis of the genital region involved only the glans.

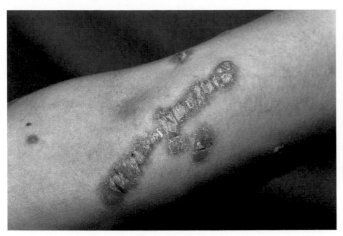

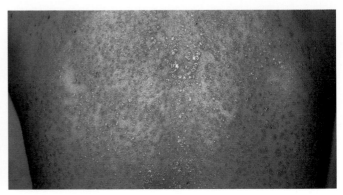

Figure 4.9 Guttate psoriasis. Tiny guttate (tear-drop) plaques after a streptococcal infection.

Figure 4.6 Psoriasis. This patient shows the Koebner phenomenon, with development of a linear plaque of psoriasis after trauma to the arm.

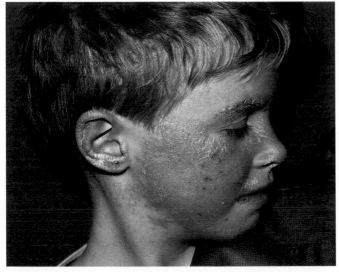

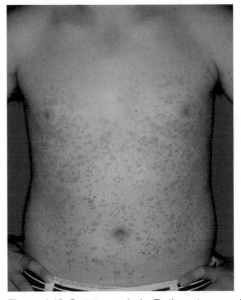

Figure 4.10 Guttate psoriasis. Erythematous, scaling plaques on the trunk that measure up to 1 cm in diameter.

Figure 4.7 Psoriasis. Facial psoriasis most commonly involves the periorbital area, but more extensive facial involvement can occur.

in psoriasis, geographic tongue is an often unrecognized feature of psoriasis in many children (Fig. 4.8).

Guttate psoriasis

Seen in up to 44% of pediatric patients, guttate psoriasis generally occurs in children and young adults and is often the first manifestation of psoriasis.[4] Lesions are drop-like (guttate), round or oval, measure from 2 mm to 6 mm in diameter (Figs 4.9, 4.10), and generally occur in a symmetrical distribution over the trunk and proximal aspects of the extremities (occasionally the face, scalp, ears, and distal aspects of the extremities). Guttate psoriasis is often, but not necessarily, triggered by group A streptococcal infection of the oropharynx or perianal area.[14] Two-thirds of patients with guttate psoriasis give a history of an upper respiratory tract infection 1–3 weeks before the onset of an acute flare of the disorder.[15,16] Although guttate psoriasis may clear spontaneously, 40% of affected children progress to the plaque type.[17] In general, suppressive therapy with antibiotics does not ameliorate psoriasis,[18] but some patients with refractory psoriasis have been shown to improve following tonsillectomy for the treatment of chronic and recurring streptococcal infection.[19]

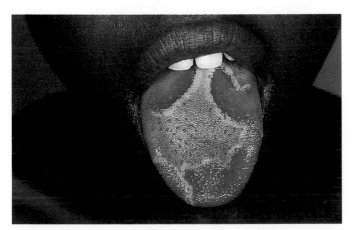

Figure 4.8 Psoriasis. Geographic tongue can be seen as the most common mucosal manifestation of patients with psoriasis.

Scalp psoriasis

The scalp is frequently the initial site of psoriatic involvement (20–40%). Most typical are well-demarcated erythematous plaques with thick adherent silvery scales (Fig. 4.11), similar in appearance to those on other parts of the body. However, psoriatic lesions of the scalp, eyebrows, and ears (the superior and postauricular folds and external auditory meatus) may instead be greasy and more salmon-colored, suggesting a diagnosis of seborrheic dermatitis. In this variant, often termed *sebopsoriasis*, lesions may present with features of both seborrhea and psoriasis. Whereas lesions of seborrheic dermatitis generally remain within the hairline, lesions of psoriasis frequently extend beyond the confines of the hairline onto the forehead (Fig. 4.3), preauricular, postauricular, and nuchal regions. Rapid response to therapy further distinguishes seborrhea from psoriasis. Another scaling disorder of the scalp that may be a variant of psoriasis is *pityriasis amiantacea* (asbestos-like) (Fig. 4.12).[20] This disorder has also been called *tinea amiantacea*, but is unrelated to dermatophyte infection. It more commonly occurs in pediatric patients without other signs of psoriasis. The disorder is characterized by large plates of scale firmly adherent to the hair and scalp. Focal hair loss and secondary infection may be associated. Pityriasis amiantacea usually begins in school age children and adolescents, and progresses to more typical psoriasis in 2–15% of pediatric patients.

Diaper area psoriasis

Psoriatic diaper rash (Fig. 2.23) with or without dissemination, is the presenting manifestation in 13% and 4% of patients, respectively.[13] This form of psoriasis must be differentiated from infantile seborrheic dermatitis (Ch. 3) and other forms of diaper dermatitis when localized (Ch. 2). The sharply defined plaques, bright red coloration, shininess, and larger, drier scales of psoriasis help to differentiate it from seborrheic dermatitis. Many infants with diaper area psoriasis also show psoriasiform lesions elsewhere (Fig. 4.13). Because of the increased moisture of the occluded diaper region, scale may not be visible clinically, but can be revealed by scraping the area gently. The frequency of psoriasis in the diaper area during infancy probably reflects the Koebner phenomenon, triggered by trauma from exposure to stool and urine, and resolves when toilet trained. Nevertheless, boys and girls out of diapers may also show genital area involvement. Of prepubertal girls presenting with a genital region complaint, 17% had psoriasis,[21] particularly involving the vulva, perineum, and natal cleft.

Nail involvement

Although statistics vary, the nails appear to be affected in 25–50% of pediatric patients with psoriasis, more commonly during the second decade of life (Figs 4.14–4.16). Pitting is most characteristic, manifesting as small, irregularly spaced depressions measuring <1 mm in diameter (Fig. 4.14). Larger depressions or punched-out areas of the nail plate may also be noted. These pits are thought to represent small intermittent psoriatic lesions in the nail matrix region that forms the superficial layers of the nail plate. Psoriatic pitting may be indistinguishable from nail pitting seen in alopecia areata (Ch. 7) and atopic dermatitis (Ch. 3), although other features assist in differentiating these disorders. Discoloration, onycholysis (separation of the distal and lateral nail plate edges), and subungual hyperkeratosis (lifting of the nail plate with nail thickening) (Fig. 4.16) are also commonly seen. Secondary bacterial, candidal, and

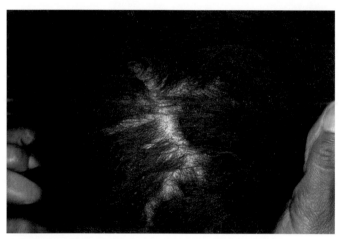

Figure 4.11 Scalp psoriasis. Thick discrete scaling overlying erythema on the scalp.

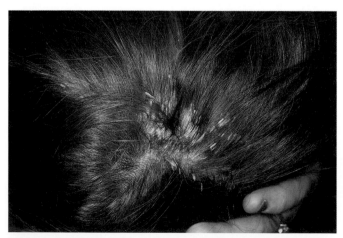

Figure 4.12 Pityriasis (tinea) amiantacea. In this severe form of psoriasis of the scalp the scales are strongly adherent (asbestos-like).

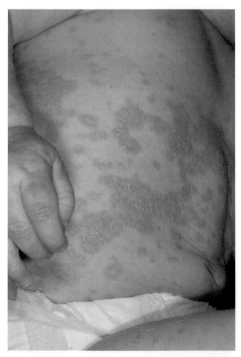

Figure 4.13 Psoriasis in an infant. In addition to diaper area involvement, this infant showed disseminated plaques of typical psoriasis.

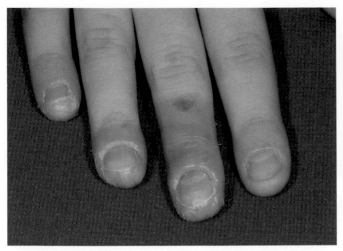

Figure 4.14 Nail psoriasis. Nail pitting is seen, particularly on the index finger. In this child, the fingers show periungual edema, erythema and desquamation, but most children with nail involvement have no cutaneous lesions of the digits.

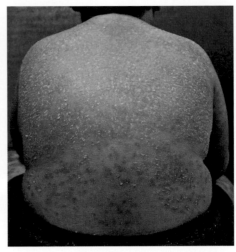

Figure 4.17 Erythrodermic psoriasis. Bright underlying erythema topped with exfoliative scaling involving most of the back and chest.

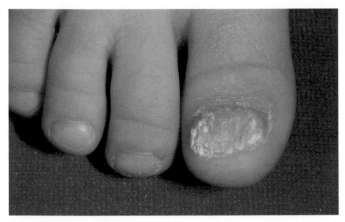

Figure 4.15 Nail psoriasis. Dystrophy, discoloration, and crumbling of the nail plate. Having just a few nails involved is common.

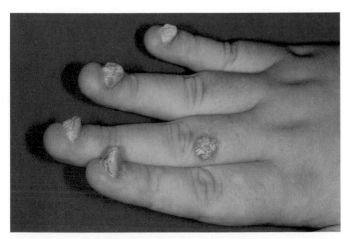

Figure 4.16 Nail psoriasis. Extensive subungual hyperkeratosis in a teenager. Note the isolated small plaque on one finger.

occasionally dermatophyte infections occur with increased frequency.

Pustular psoriasis and **erythrodermic (exfoliative) psoriasis** are the most severe variants of childhood psoriasis,[22] but occur in ~1% of pediatric patients with psoriasis.[4] Patients with extensive pustular or erythrodermic psoriasis usually require hospitalization, and courses are not uncommonly complicated by cutaneous infection and bacterial septicemia. Erythrodermic or exfoliative psoriasis occurs occasionally in adults and, on rare occasions, in children with psoriasis (Fig. 4.17). More than 90% of the skin shows intense erythema, massive exfoliation, and associated abnormalities of temperature and cardiovascular regulation. Affected children may show failure to thrive.

Pustular psoriasis has been described as early as the first week of life.[23] It usually occurs as *generalized pustular psoriasis*, but can be limited to the palms and soles (*pustulosis palmaris et plantaris*) or to fold areas.[24] Pustular psoriasis may be associated with sterile lytic lesions of bone (*chronic recurrent multifocal osteomyelitis*, or *SAPHO syndrome*: synovitis, acne, palmo-plantar pustulosis and psoriasis, hyperostosis, osteitis), usually affecting the bones of the lower limb, pelvis, and clavicle.[25,26] Fever, malaise and anorexia are typically associated with generalized pustular psoriasis.

The course of generalized pustular psoriasis tends to be explosive. On previously quiescent psoriatic plaques or normal skin, erythematous halos develop and rapidly become studded with superficial pinpoint to 2–3 mm pustules (Fig. 4.18). Sheets of erythema and pustulation can involve the flexures, genital regions, webs of the fingers, and periungual areas. The nails often become thickened or separated by subungual lakes of pus. Mucous membrane lesions in the mouth and tongue are not uncommon. The cutaneous inflammation typically progresses from discrete sterile pustules to crusts and ultimately to generalized exfoliative dermatitis. The lesions of generalized pustular psoriasis in children show an annular morphology in 60% of patients.[23,27] The disease is cyclic and associated with complete clearance of the pustular phase and unexplained exacerbations that span decades. Relapses are common and become progressively more severe, often with a poor prognosis. In contrast to the frequency of pustular psoriasis in adults known to have psoriasis, pustular psoriasis is often the first manifestation of psoriasis in affected infants and children. The cause of pustular psoriasis in children is unknown. The recent description of pustules beginning in the neonatal period that resemble pustular psoriasis clinically

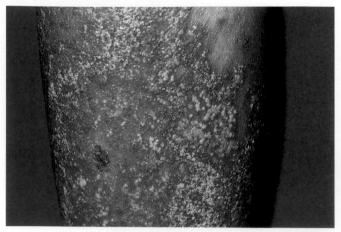

Figure 4.18 Pustular psoriasis. Collections of small pustules, some with an annular configuration, overlying bright erythema.

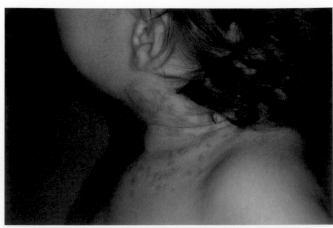

Figure 4.19 Localized pustular psoriasis in an infant. In infants, pustular psoriasis may be localized to intertriginous areas, particularly the neckfold, and be confused with dermatitis or infection. This form is difficult to treat and may eventuate in generalized pustular psoriasis.

and histologically due to mutations in interleuklin-1 receptor antagonist (see Differential Diagnosis, below) raises the possibility of increased activation of interleukin-1 signaling.

Pustulosis palmaris et plantaris (*pustulosis of the palms and soles*) is a bilaterally symmetric, chronic pustular eruption on the palms and soles, sometimes in association with psoriasis elsewhere on the body. This localized form of pustular psoriasis is characterized by deep-seated 2–4 mm sterile pustules that develop within areas of erythema and scaling on the palms and/or soles. Within several days the pustules resolve and leave a yellow-brown scale that is generally shed within 1–2 weeks. Phases of quiescence and exacerbation are characteristic, and exfoliating crusted lesions may be seen concurrently with newly developing pustules. The predominant histologic feature on biopsy is the large intraepidermal unilocular pustules containing polymorphonuclear leukocytes (the spongiform pustules of Kogoj), with little if any surrounding spongiosis or inflammation. Although staphylococcal infection may at times occur as a secondary complication, bacterial cultures of these abscesses usually remain sterile.

Onset of localized pustular psoriasis during infancy has recently been described, and protends greater recalcitrance to therapy and a tendency to progress to more widespread disease.[24] Patients typically have initial involvement of the neckfold that may be confused with dermatitis, bacterial or candidal infection (Fig. 4.19). Biopsy allows the diagnosis of localized pustular psoriasis to be made, particular given that many lesions may appear more papular than pustular. Other fold areas may be affected, and dissemination to generalized pustular psoriasis is not uncommon.

Extracutaneous involvement

Arthritis and uveitis are noncutaneous features of childhood psoriasis and occur only occasionally. A recent study of 211 children with moderate to severe psoriasis, however, found that 9% of affected children claim to have joint disease,[28] suggesting that inquiry about pain, joint swelling or limping as well as examination of the joints should be part of the routine evaluation. Psoriatic arthritis is now considered a form of juvenile idiopathic arthritis, and criteria have been established by the International League of Associations for Rheumatology (ILAR).[29,30] These include arthritis with psoriasis, or arthritis and: (1) a family history of confirmed psoriasis in a parent or sibling; (2) dactylitis;[31] or (3) nail pitting or onycholysis;[31] the diagnosis is excluded if the patient has a positive

rheumatoid factor titer or signs of systemic disease (daily fever, evanescent erythematous eruption, generalized adenopathy, hepatomegaly or splenomegaly, or serositis). The early presence of ankle/toe arthritis, HLA-DRB1* 11/12 status, and onset after 6 years of age may also distinguish juvenile psoriatic arthritis from oligoarthritis or polyarthritis JIA subtypes.[32]

The occurrence of pediatric psoriatic arthritis is biphasic. Younger children affected by psoriatic arthritis tend to be female with dactylitis and small joint involvement that is more likely to progress and persist. The swelling often includes the juxta-articular tissue, resulting in a blunt 'sausage-shaped' appearance of the involved fingers or toes. With long-standing disease, flexure deformities and severe bone destruction may occur with osteoporosis, shortening and tapering of the involved distal phalanx. On radiologic examination, this resembles a sharpened pencil (the so-called pencil-in-cup or pencil-and-goblet deformity) at the metatarsophalangeal and metacarpophalangeal joints. Arthritis in older children is characterized by more enthesitis and axial joint disease.[29] The psoriatic skin lesions in patients who develop arthritis are identical to those seen in patients who do not manifest joint disease, and there is no relationship between the severity of the cutaneous disease and the development of joint disease. Either skin disease or arthritis may develop initially, and in most patients, flares of joint and skin disease do not correlate.

The asymmetric anterior uveitis of psoriasis has been found in 14–17% of children with juvenile psoriatic arthritis. The cutaneous lesions of psoriasis may develop several years after the onset of persisting uveitis.[33]

More recently, moderate to severe plaque type psoriasis in adults has been clearly linked to an increased risk of metabolic syndrome and cardiovascular disease.[34,35] Studies in pediatric patients suggest that the risk of obesity and, most likely, cardiovascular complications, begins in childhood and adolescence. The mean body mass index (BMI) of pediatric patients with moderate to severe psoriasis was at the 87th percentile with 37% having a BMI of >95th percentile.[28,36] Juvenile psoriasis is associated with ~2–4 times the rate of comorbidity from hyperlipidemia, hypertension, diabetes and Crohn's disease versus unaffected children and adolescents.[37] These data suggest that early intervention with lifestyle modification and possibly systemic antiinflammatory therapy may decrease the long-term metabolic risk for these children.

Diagnosis of Psoriasis

The diagnosis of psoriasis can usually be made on the basis of clinical findings alone. Biopsy can be performed if the diagnosis is in question. Biopsy sections show epidermal thickening (acanthosis with elongation of the rete ridges), retention of nuclei in the stratum corneum (parakeratosis), and a mononuclear infiltrate. Focal collections of neutrophils in the stratum corneum or subcorneal layer (Munro's microabscesses) are an additional feature in biopsies from patients with pustular psoriasis.

Course

The course of psoriasis is typically prolonged, chronic, and unpredictable. In most patients the disease is not severe and remains confined to localized cutaneous regions. Remissions and exacerbations are the rule in most patients, with a marked tendency to improvement in summer, particularly during long periods of sun exposure. In some patients the disease may undergo spontaneous improvement; in others exacerbations may occur without apparent cause. Although sunlight generally is beneficial, sunburns can elicit the Koebner phenomenon and lead to exacerbation. Despite the chronicity of the disorder for most patients, satisfactory control of the disease is possible in a majority of patients with appropriate therapy.

Differential Diagnosis (Table 4.1)

Guttate psoriasis and *plaque psoriasis* are most commonly confused with other papulosquamous disorders described in this chapter, especially pityriasis rosea or pityriasis lichenoides chronica. Pityriasis rubra pilaris is the hardest to differentiate, especially when involving largely the palms, soles, elbows, and knees. The follicular accentuation, focal areas of sparing, and sometimes more salmon coloration of pityriasis rubra pilaris can help to distinguish the conditions clinically; biopsy sections of pityriasis rubra pilaris may show perifollicular inflammation. A plaque-type psoriasiform eruption and less often a generalized or annular pustular psoriatic eruption may follow Kawasaki disease (Ch. 21).[38–40] Generalized and localized forms of *pustular psoriasis* can be differentiated from infectious causes of pustulosis by cultures and non-infectious conditions, such as eosinophilic folliculitis or infantile acropustulosis (see Ch. 2) by biopsy. Psoriasis-like pustules during the neonatal period or in association with other features, such as joint swelling and pain, sterile multifocal osteomyelitis or periostitis, oral stomatitis, or pyoderma gangrenosum, may be seen in patients with deficiency of interleukin-1 receptor antagonist (DIRA).[41] Skin biopsies show features similar to those seen in pustular psoriasis, with intraepidermal collections or neutrophils and psoriasiform epidermal hyperplasia.[42] The distribution of pustules may be widespread or grouped and more localized. In addition to the early onset, the poor response to standard therapy for psoriasis is a clue to this autosomal recessive disorder. Patients respond rapidly to subcutaneous administrations of anakinra 1–2 mg/kg per day. The possibility of alterations in IL1RN in children with pustular psoriasis is currently under investigation. Psoriasiform dermatitis may also be seen in boys with *IPEX syndrome*. The disorder results from mutations in FOXP3 at Xp11.23, leading to absent or dysfunctional regulatory T-cells and self-reactive T-cell activation and proliferation. Failure to thrive, diabetes, thyroiditis, autoimmune cytopenias alopecia, food allergies and high levels of IgE and eosinophils are associated.[43,44] Atypical cases of *psoriatic arthritis* must be differentiated from rheumatoid arthritis or systemic lupus erythematosus. Compared with rheumatoid arthritis, the

Table 4.1 Differential diagnosis of psoriasis

Guttate and plaque psoriasis	Scalp psoriasis
Pityriasis rubra pilaris	Tinea capitis
Pityriasis rosea	Seborrheic dermatitis
Parapsoriasis	
Psoriasiform dermatitis	**Pustular psoriasis**
Lichen planus	Staphylococcal pustulosis
Drug eruptions	Candidal pustulosis
Widespread dermatophytosis	*Herpes simplex* infection
Facial psoriasis	Acute generalized exanthematous pustulosis (viral, drug)
Discoid lupus erythematosus	Extensive eosinophilic folliculitis
Seborrheic dermatitis	Interleukin-1 receptor antagonist deficiency
Diaper area psoriasis	
Seborrheic dermatitis	**Palmoplantar pustular psoriasis**
Irritant dermatitis	Candidasis
Candidal diaper dermatitis	Infantile acropustulosis
Nail psoriasis	**Erythrodermic psoriasis**
Trauma	Extensive pityriasis rubra pilaris
Onychomycosis	Congenital ichthyosiform erythroderma
Lichen planus	Erythrokeratodermia variabilis

onset of psoriatic arthritis is generally, but not invariably, monoarticular and subacute. It tends to be less painful, and flexural deformity (rather than ulnar deviation) is characteristic of this disease.

Therapy of Pediatric Psoriasis

Education is a key component of therapy of psoriasis. Patients and parents must understand the chronicity of the disorder and the tendency for spontaneous remissions in 38% of pediatric patients, lasting for variable time periods.[45] Most patients respond well to therapeutic measures currently available, but response is much slower than with dermatitis.[46–48] The approach to medication should be made as simple as possible, since therapy is time consuming, burdensome, and easily rejected. Patients and family members of the patient should understand the rationale for treatment, and the older children and adolescents should be empowered to maintain their own therapeutic routine with parental guidance.

The concept that injury to skin may exacerbate psoriasis (Koebner phenomenon or isomorphic response) should also be explained (Table 4.2). Removal of potential trigger factors, including medications (e.g., other systemic steroids, lithium, antimalarials, and beta-blockers) and, most importantly, infection (especially streptococcal) should also be explored. Above all, therapy should be as conservative as is appropriate for the type of psoriasis and its severity with careful information imparted to parents about the potential side effects of prescribed therapy.

Topical therapy

The topical therapies most commonly used in children include topical corticosteroids, topical calcineurin inhibitors, calcipotriene and calcitriol, tar preparations, and anthralin (short-contact therapy) (Table 4.3). Emollients are used as adjunctive agents to decrease the associated scaling and dryness, but should not replace medications when inflammation is present. In plaque psoriasis, the mainstay of treatment remains *topical corticosteroids* (see Ch. 3, Table

3.3), which frequently produce dramatic resolution of lesions as monotherapy. Application up to twice daily of class II–IV midpotency topical steroids is most useful for lesions on the trunk and extremities. Ointments tend to penetrate the psoriatic scale better and are preferred. If individual thick plaques fail to respond, a course of ultrapotent topical steroid ointment (such as clobetasol, halobetasol, or augmented betamethasone dipropionate) can be initiated, but should be restricted to no >2 weeks because of the risk for developing striae (especially in the preadolescent/adolescent population) and local atrophy. 'Weekend therapy' regimens combine class I steroids (used on weekend days only) and topical calcipotriene/calcitriol (see below), and should be administered by a dermatologist familiar with the use of these regimens.[49] Use of keratolytic agents to enhance penetration, such as 6% salicylic acid compounded into steroid ointment with or without tar (see below) or alone (e.g., Keralyt gel), occlusion, or steroid impregnated tapes are alternative treatments for more hyperkeratotic, resistant lesions. Use of halogenated and more potent steroids should be avoided in the diaper area, intertriginous areas, and on the face. Topical calcipotriene/calcitriol and tacrolimus ointment, combined or as monotherapy, are steroid-sparing alternatives (see below). Once the acute lesions are under control, treatment can be tapered to lower potency steroids and/or emollients.

Tar is a time-honored and effective adjunct to the topical treatment of psoriasis that is both anti-inflammatory and antiproliferative. Tar (in the form of 1–10% crude coal tar or 5–10% liquor carbonis detergens) can be compounded into preparations with topical steroids and/or salicylic acid, and applied overnight or before ultraviolet light exposure. Tar as a single agent is available in several over-the-counter preparations (e.g., Estar Gel®, Fototar®). Tar preparations, however, stain skin and clothing, have an odor that is often objectionable to children and adolescents, and increase the risk of developing folliculitis. Tar may also be administered in the

---

Table 4.2 Prevention of psoriasis in pediatric patients

Site of potential psoriasis	Preventative behavior
Creases and folds	Minimize friction by maintaining appropriate weight
	Avoid irritating underarm deodorants
Face	Avoid irritating soaps and burning from exposure to ultraviolet light
Genital and perianal regions	Avoid irritation from tight garments and exposure to accumulated feces and urine
Hands and feet	Minimize excessive sweating and exposure to irritants such as harsh soaps
	Avoid tight shoes
Nails	Avoid long fingernails or toenails, trauma to nails in play situations, excessive use of nail polish and remover, and wearing tight shoes
	Hydrate nails before trimming and avoid manipulation of cuticles
Scalp	Avoid vigorous brushing, combing, or scratching of scalp

---

Table 4.3 Treatment of psoriasis in children

Medication	Use in children	Potential side-effects and comments
Topical preparations		
Emollients	Useful in mild disease; adjunct	None
Topical steroids	First-line therapy	Local side-effects: esp. atrophy, striae.
		Systemic side-effects: impaired growth, adrenal suppression, cataracts, tachyphylaxis
Tar	Thicker plaques	Irritation, staining, folliculitis
Anthralin	Short contact application	Less staining than tar
Calcipotriol	Usually adjunct with steroids	Irritation
Tazarotene gel	Usually adjunct with steroids	Irritation
Tacrolimus/pimecrolimus	Face, intertriginous areas	Burning with initial applications
Phototherapy		
Ultraviolet B (UVB) light	Widespread plaques	Costly, inconvenient; risks include premature aging, skin cancer.
Psoralens-UVA	Rarely indicated	The same as for UVB; cataracts with systemic psoralens.
Systemic therapy		
Methotrexate	Recalcitrant psoriasis, all types	Bone marrow suppression and hepatotoxicity.
Cyclosporine	Recalcitrant psoriasis, all types	Renal and hepatic toxicity, hypertension, hypertrichosis, immunosuppression, UVB-induced skin cancer.
Acetretin	Especially for pustular psoriasis	Cheilitis, hyperlipidemia, musculoskeletal pain, hair loss, skin fragility, bone toxicity if used long-term, teratogenicity.
Etanercept	Effective for plaque psoriasis	Increased risk of mycobacterial infection and possibly lymphoma
Other biologic agents	Only anecdotal reports in children	Increased risk of mycobacterial/salmonella (IL12/23) infection and possibly lymphoma

form of a tar bath (e.g., Cutar bath oil®, Doak Oil Forte®, Balnetar®).

An alternative to tar therapy is *short-contact anthralin therapy*, formulated in a temperature-sensitive vehicle that releases the active medication at skin surface temperature.[50] Anthralin is available in a 1% preparation. It is applied for 5 min initially, with gradually increasing times of exposure as tolerated and needed for efficacy. Discoloration of skin or clothing is significantly less than that with tar therapy. Contact with face, eyes, and mucous membranes should be avoided.

Calcipotriene and *calcitriol*, analogues of vitamin D3, are formulated as 0.05% cream and ointment and 0.003% ointment, respectively. They are most effective when combined with topical steroids, but serve as steroid-sparing agents that may be efficacious in children as monotherapy as well.[51,52] These vitamin D3 analogues are best applied twice daily, but the onset of action is slow (often 6–8 weeks). Combination therapy of betamethasone dipropionate (0.064%) and calcipotriene (0.005%) ointment and a scalp solution of calcipotriene are also available. Irritant dermatitis, particularly on the face and intertriginous areas, occurs in up to 20% of patients. The topical retinoid *tazarotene* is available in 0.05% and 0.1% strength creams and gels. Tazarotene is best applied once a day in combination with once daily application of a medium to potent topical steroid, but even with the topical steroid is often too irritating for use in childhood psoriasis.

Calcineurin inhibitors, particularly *tacrolimus ointment 0.1%* are useful with twice daily application for 1–2 months for facial and intertriginous psoriasis.[53] Although not found to be useful in double-blind trials in adults, topical tacrolimus ointment is sometimes useful outside of the facial and intertriginous areas for childhood psoriasis with thinner plaques.

Treatment of scalp lesions

Psoriatic scalp lesions are a frustrating and sometimes recalcitrant component of psoriasis. Topical corticosteroids may be applied in the form of oils, solutions, or foams. Removal of scales can be facilitated by softening scales through application of oil-based medications. For example, fluocinolone solution in a peanut and mineral oil base (DermaSmoothe-FS) under shower cap occlusion can be applied for a few hours to overnight to the wet, affected scalp, followed by washing with shampoos containing tar, steroid (0.01% fluocinolone, Capex), zinc, or keratolytic agents. Alternatively, a phenol and saline (Baker's P&S) solution with a shower cap for occlusion can be applied overnight. In the morning, one can shampoo, followed by application of a steroid solution.

Treatment of nail psoriasis

Psoriatic nails are extremely distressing to the patient, respond slowly to therapy, and are difficult to treat topically because of the failure of topical agents to penetrate the nail plate. Instillation of class I steroid solutions into the subproximal nail fold area can be successful, but application nightly of flurandrenolide-impregnated tape (Cordran) to the base of the nail for approximately 6 months tends to yield better results. Injections of triamcinolone acetonide suspension (10 mg/mL) into the nail fold of the abnormal nail with a 30-gauge needle every 4–6 weeks is painful, even with the use of topical anesthetic creams, and should be reserved for the motivated older child or adolescent who fails topical application. More recently, nightly application of tazarotene 0.05% or 0.1% gel under occlusion, if tolerated, has been shown to cause improvement.[54]

Compresses for pustular psoriasis

Local applications of wet dressings with Burow's solution 1:40 or potassium permanganate 1:5000 (one crushed 65 mg tablet into 250 mL of water) frequently help relieve acute flares of the pustular aspect of palmoplantar or generalized pustular psoriasis).

Ultraviolet light

Most psoriatic patients benefit from exposure to sunlight and, accordingly, are frequently better during the summer months. However, sunburn precautions must be taken with sunscreens, avoidance during hours of most intense sunlight, and sun-protective clothing, since sudden overexposure may result in sufficient epidermal injury to cause exacerbation of the disorder. For those who can arrange exposure to sunlight on a regular basis, this can be an important aspect of therapy, alone or in combination with topical therapies. Although natural sunlight is easier for children and less aggressive than artificial ultraviolet therapy, ultraviolet treatments under professional supervision may also be used as therapy,[55,56] especially when psoriasis involves more than 15–20% body surface area or involves the palms and soles, and is recalcitrant to topical therapy. Response to phototherapy is enhanced by pre-exposure application of oil or ointment.[56]

Narrowband ultraviolet B (UVB) (~311 nm) has a higher ratio of therapeutic to toxic wavelengths than broadband UVB light (290–320 nm), and is considered at least as efficacious. The UVB is best initiated in a light-box at a dermatology office as outpatient therapy. Once patients and parents know how to increase the doses of UV light gradually, judge the effects of the daily treatment, and practice preventive eye care, home light-box therapy can be initiated. Home light-boxes are ultimately less invasive to the mainstream activities of a family and more cost-effective than alternative treatment sites. In general, ultraviolet light therapy is started at 70–75% of the minimal erythema dose and increased by about 10–20% with each treatment as tolerated. A minimum of three treatments per week is required to clear psoriasis. Although rarely used in young children, phototherapy may be administered to young children who are accompanied by parents in the light unit. Tricks such as use of singing together or listening to a radio or CD player with earphones can be used to distract the child during treatment. Acutely, UVB therapy is associated with skin darkening, a chance of skin burning, and, not infrequently, with early pruritus. Although long-term data are lacking in children with psoriasis, recurrent exposure to UVB could theoretically increase the long-term risk of the development of skin cancer and premature aging.

The excimer laser (~308 nm) is fiber-optically targeted UVB that can treat localized plaques of psoriasis without exposing normal skin to unnecessary radiation. Although its use in children has been limited to date, it is painless and offers safety advantages over nbUVB.[57,58] Psoralens and ultraviolet A light (PUVA) (320–400 nm) are used rarely in children because of the ocular toxicity, generalized photosensitivity, and the risk of later development of actinic changes and cutaneous carcinomas.[59] If PUVA is used for severe psoriasis, 8-methoxypsoralen (0.6 mg/kg) or topical both PUVA is administered. Protective eyewear and clothing as appropriate must be worn in patients receiving ultraviolet light treatments. With PUVA therapy and systemically-administered psoralen, protective eyewear must be worn for 24 h after each exposure because of the risk of cataract development. The use of topical psoralens and ultraviolet A light in a hand/foot box has proven effective in adolescents and older children with psoriasis of the hands and feet.

Systemic therapy

Oral medications for treating psoriasis have potentially harmful side-effects and should be reserved for children with erythrodermic and pustular forms of psoriasis, or with severe plaque-type psoriasis recalcitrant to topical therapies.[60] In general, systemic corticosteroids should be avoided. Although occasionally effective, steroids are often ineffective or lead to flares of psoriasis, including triggering of pustular psoriasis, when withdrawn. Before considering more toxic therapy, some practitioners will prescribe a course of *antistreptococcal antibiotics*, especially for patients with recent flares of guttate or plaque psoriasis. Examination for the possibility of pharyngitis or perianal cellulitis should be performed, and culture for β-hemolytic streptococcus obtained as appropriate. Antibiotics should be prescribed if the culture is positive, although recurrent positive cultures may signal a carrier state. Although important for treating streptococcal infections, trials of antibiotic therapy are usually not helpful.[18] Uncontrolled studies have suggested that *tonsillectomy* is superior to antibiotic administration in the clearance of psoriasis in children,[19] but controlled trials have not been performed. Regardless, many pediatric dermatologists still utilize systemic antibiotics as part of the treatment approach for children with acute guttate psoriasis.

Methotrexate is indicated for severe unresponsive psoriasis, exfoliative erythrodermas, pustular psoriasis, and psoriatic arthritis. Although effective for nail psoriasis, its profile of potential side effects makes it inappropriate for patients with isolated nail involvement. Methotrexate has antimitotic, antichemotactic, and antiinflammatory activities. After appropriate screening tests (blood counts, hepatic testing) and testing for pregnancy in female patients of child-bearing age, oral methotrexate is initiated at an oral (or intramuscular) dosage of 0.3 mg/kg per week, and can be increased to 0.6 mg/kg per week if needed for efficacy.[60–62] The most common side-effects are nausea, fatigue, headaches, and anorexia. The most significant is bone marrow suppression. Concurrent administration of folic acid 1–5 mg/day diminishes the risk of nausea, mucosal ulcerations, and macrocytic anemia.[63] Although optimal dosing of folic acid has not been determined, a common practice is to administer the folic acid on the 6 days when methotrexate is not given, since it antagonizes the efficacy of the methotrexate. In young children, two children's chewable multivitamins usually provide the necessary amount of daily folic acid supplementation. Liver and bone marrow function should be monitored by blood testing; liver biopsy is unnecessary in children, and hepatic toxicity is rare. During childhood, live vaccines such as measles, mumps, and rubella (MMR) and poliovirus vaccines may not be given to a child taking weekly methotrexate. Improvement is generally seen within 3–6 weeks after initiation of treatment, but several months may be required for clearance. Once clearing is achieved, the methotrexate should be gradually lowered (e.g., 2.5 mg/month) during the subsequent months.

Cyclosporine has been used in young patients with severe unresponsive psoriasis, exfoliative erythrodermas, or pustular psoriasis.[60,64] Its mechanism of action involves inhibition of cytokine production by T-lymphocytes. Cyclosporine is usually initiated orally at a dosage of 4–5 mg/kg per day (and 3 mg/kg per day if microemulsion) and maintained for a 3–4-month period followed by gradual downward titration and discontinuation. The potential complications are hypertension, renal and hepatic toxicity, and hypertrichosis; however, concerns about future leukemias, lymphomas, cutaneous carcinomas, and other oncogenic risks are heightened with childhood use. Live vaccines (e.g., MMR and poliovirus) cannot be used in patients on cyclosporine therapy.

Retinoids tend to be less effective than methotrexate or cyclosporine as a single agent for treating plaque-type psoriasis, but can be quite effective for exfoliative erythrodermas and for pustular psoriasis that does not respond to more conservative therapy, including compresses and topical corticosteroids.[65] Oral retinoids are often used more successfully in combination with topical ointments, ultraviolet light treatment, methotrexate, or cyclosporine. Acitretin normalizes epidermal differentiation and has an antiinflammatory effect.

The usual regimen is oral administration at a dosage of 0.5–1.0 mg/kg per day, although the dosage can be titrated, depending on patient response and laboratory results.[49] Complications related to retinoid usage are most commonly dryness of the skin and mucous membranes and elevation of serum triglyceride levels. The potential for skeletal toxicity (premature epiphyseal closure and hyperostosis), although rare, must be monitored clinically and, if appropriate, radiographically during infancy, childhood, and puberty in patients administered retinoids long term. Screening tests include blood counts, fasting lipid profiles, and hepatic studies. Retinoids cause severe teratogenicity and should be avoided in sexually active adolescent girls. Isotretinoin may be an alternative retinoid for female adolescents with pustular psoriasis because of its much more rapid clearance, but generally it is not as effective as acitretin.

Biological agents fall into three classes (antibodies, fusion proteins, and recombinant cytokines). Several biological agents have successfully treated moderate to severe psoriasis in adults. Currently available targeted therapies can be divided into two major therapeutic classes: T-cell targeted therapies (alefacept) and anticytokine therapies.[66] The anticytokine therapies can be directed against TNF-α (adalimumab, etanercept, infliximab) or against interleukin-12 and interleukin-23 (ustekinumab; anti-p40 antibody).[67–70] All of these agents have shown efficacy in treating adult patients; of them, etanercept has been used the most in children and as young as infancy.[71] Etanercept is also the only agent tested in a double-blind, randomized trial in children.[28] In this trial of 211 pediatric patients with moderate to severe plaque type psoriasis, 57% achieved 75% improvement by 12 weeks of therapy with 0.8 mg/kg etanercept; only 11% of patients treated with the vehicle control achieved this degree of improvement. The long-term risks of biologic therapy in children are unknown, although to date serious adverse events are rare. Because these therapies are more targeted than other immunosuppressants, the global risk of infection is lower. Nevertheless, patients may be at risk for mycobacterial and salmonella infections[72] and baseline PPD$_i$ with annual re-evaluation is recommended. Adverse effects on the development of the immune system in young children and an increased risk of lymphoma are theoretical concerns. Etanercept is approved in Europe for treatment of pediatric psoriasis in children 8 years of age and above, but is not yet FDA-approved for children in the USA.

Therapy for Psoriatic Arthritis

Many patients with psoriatic arthritis require only nonsteroidal antiinflammatory drugs, maintenance of joint position, functional splinting, and physiotherapy. The combination of methotrexate and a biologic agent is now most commonly used for more recalcitrant cases. Occasionally arthroscopic synovectomy or joint replacement is required.

Psychosocial and Educational Support

The National Psoriasis Foundation (www.psoriasis.org) is available as a support group for patients and families of patients and provides superb educational material about psoriasis.

Reactive arthritis

Reactive arthritis (Reiter syndrome) is a reactive disorder that has been described in children as young as 9 months of age. The disorder most commonly occurs in young men between 20 and 40 years of age, but has been reported in almost 100 children, usually boys.[73] In affected adults, Reactive arthritis usually occurs after sexually transmitted infection, particularly *Chlamydia*, or gastrointestinal infection, and has been associated with HIV infection.[74] In children, it is most likely to develop after an acute enteric infection, particularly one caused by *Shigella flexneri*, *Salmonella typhimurium*, or *Yersinia*. Diarrhea is initially present in 90% of affected children but in only one-third of adults with this disorder. Fever, anorexia, weight loss, and malaise may be other early signs. Several weeks may pass between the onset of fever and diarrhea and the clinical findings of reactive arthritis.

The classic triad of reactive arthritis includes nonbacterial conjunctivitis, urethritis, and arthritis. However, the complete triad is rarely seen at onset, may take several weeks to develop, and is incomplete in the majority of affected children. Conjunctivitis is the most common ocular manifestation and occurs overall in 50% of children. It tends to be bilateral, is self-limited with clearance in weeks, and ranges in severity from mild injection to mucopurulent inflammation. Acute, painful anterior uveitis, iritis, keratitis, corneal ulceration, and optic neuritis have rarely been described. The arthritis typically is asymmetric and involves more than one joint, most commonly large weight-bearing joints, such as the hip, knee, and ankle. However, other large or small joints can be affected and involvement occasionally is symmetric. In contrast to the pattern in affected adults, the sacroiliac joint is rarely involved in pediatric cases. Many children will also show enthesitis, a typical feature of reactive arthritis characterized by focal tenderness at sites where ligament and tendon insert into bone. The arthritis and enthesitis tend to resolve after a few months, but occasionally persist or recur. The urethritis in children is usually asymptomatic, and detection of sterile pyuria may be the only evidence of urethral inflammation. Less commonly, inflammation of the meatus may be clinically detectable or urethral discharge may be noted.

The cutaneous manifestations of reactive arthritis may develop in association with, or independently of, the other features of the disorder. Most classic are the circinate balanitis/vulvitis and *keratoderma blenorrhagica*. The circinate balanitis/vulvitis occurs in 15–75% of affected children[75,76] and presents as well-defined erosions on the glans penis in uncircumcised males and on the vulva in females; circumcised male patients often show inflamed hyperkeratotic plaques on the shaft and scrotum. The keratoderma blenorrhagica occurs in 8–25% of children,[73,75] and appears as psoriasiform scaling, inflammatory papules, pustules, and plaques on pressure or weight-bearing areas of the palms and soles (Fig. 4.20).

Psoriasiform papules and plaques have also been described on the extensor surfaces of the extremities and the dorsal aspects of the feet and hands. Oral lesions consist of painless erythema, shallow erosions, and small pustules that may occur on the buccal mucosa, gums, lips, palate, and tongue. Oral lesions generally resolve spontaneously after a period of several days. Lesions on the tongue, particularly when thickly coated, may simulate a geographic tongue.

Diagnosis of the disorder is made based on the constellation of clinical features and is supported by nonspecific laboratory findings. Rheumatoid factor is negative, but most affected children show HLA-B27 antigen. Sterile pyuria and significant elevation of erythrocyte sedimentation rate are usually found. Mild anemia with leukocytosis may be present as well. If performed early, stool cultures may yield the triggering bacterial organism. Although biopsy of the skin lesions may be helpful, it does not distinguish the cutaneous lesions of reactive arthritis from those of psoriasis. Reactive arthritis must be differentiated from other seronegative arthropathies, including psoriatic arthritis,[77] juvenile idiopathic arthritis, infectious arthropathies (especially gonococcal and Lyme disease), Kawasaki disease,[78] Behçet syndrome, and rheumatic fever.

Reactive arthritis is almost always self-limiting in children and clears without sequelae. A few children have died, but the prognosis

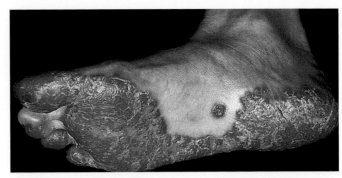

Figure 4.20 Keratoderma blennorrhagicum, showing thickened, psoriasiform papules and plaques on the foot of a patient with reactive arthritis. (Reprinted with permission from Schachner LA and Hansen RC, eds. Pediatric dermatology, Edinburgh: Mosby; 2003:Fig. 15.16.)

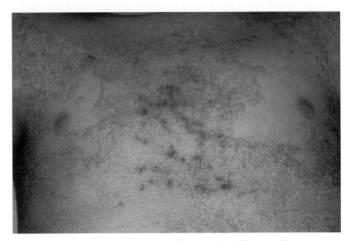

Figure 4.21 Pityriasis rubra pilaris. Symmetric, diffuse, well-circumscribed salmon-colored plaques, representing the coalescence of follicular-based papules. The discrete papules can be seen at the borders. Note the 'skip areas'.

in children is considered much better than that in adults.[74] A minority of children show recurrent or chronic arthritis. Treatment consists primarily of bed rest and administration of non-steroidal antiinflammatory drugs. The cutaneous lesions may respond to topical corticosteroids. Ophthalmologic consultation is appropriate for patients with ocular manifestations. Occasionally, intra-articular injection of corticosteroids or administration of systemic medication is required. Sulfasalazine, methotrexate, acitretin, cyclosporine, and infliximab[79] have been used for patients with severe unresponsive disease.

Pityriasis rubra pilaris

Pityriasis rubra pilaris (PRP) is a chronic skin disorder characterized by small follicular papules, disseminated yellowish-pink scaly plaques surrounding islands of normal skin, and hyperkeratosis of the palms and soles (Figs 4.21–4.25). Small, follicular-based keratotic papules are an important diagnostic feature, but are not always present. Although most pediatric cases are acquired without a family history of the disorder, PRP may be inherited as an autosomal dominant disorder.[80] Hereditary and acquired forms may be indistinguishable clinically and histologically, although in general patients with the autosomal dominant form tend to have less severe disease with onset from birth to early childhood. PRP must

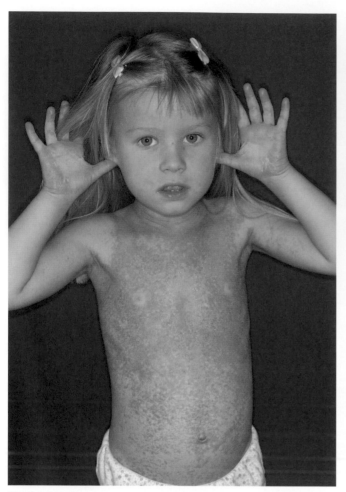

Figure 4.22 Pityriasis rubra pilaris. This patient's eruption began on the face and extended in a caudad distribution. Note the salmon-colored palmar erythema, spared areas, and keratoderma.

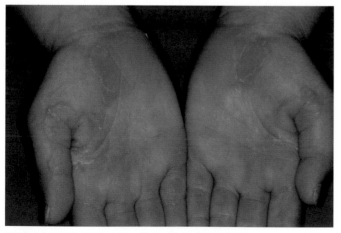

Figure 4.23 Pityriasis rubra pilaris. Note the well-circumscribed palmar erythema.

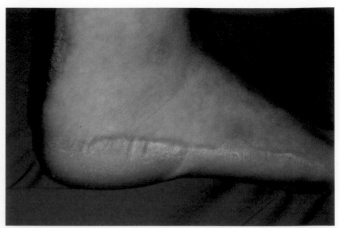

Figure 4.24 Pityriasis rubra pilaris. The keratodermic sandal of a patient with type IV PRP.

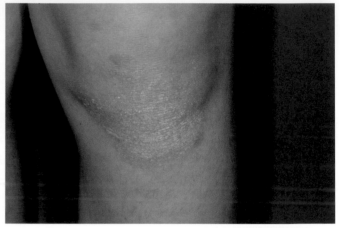

Figure 4.25 Pityriasis rubra pilaris. Salmon-colored scaling plaque on the knee, a common site.

be distinguished from psoriasis and disorders of cornification, especially the erythrokeratodermias; it is a rare manifestation of dermatomyositis.[81]

The cause of PRP is unclear, although it is known to represent a disorder of abnormal keratinization. Skin lesions, both clinically and histologically, are suggestive of those seen in phrynoderma (vitamin A deficiency), but vitamin A levels tend to be normal. The association of previous infection in some affected patients has led to speculation about a role for bacterial superantigens as triggers.[82]

Keratoderma of the palms and soles develops in the majority of affected children, and can be present prior to or after the appearance of other features.[83] When seen on the soles, this has been referred to as a 'keratodermic sandal' (Fig. 4.24). The keratoderma shows a sharply demarcated border, sometimes extending to involve the dorsum of the hands and feet. The salmon color and associated edema help to distinguish the keratoderma from psoriasis, ichthyosis, hereditary palmoplantar keratoderma, and erythrokeratodermias (see Ch. 5). Thickening of the elbows, knees (Fig. 4.25), ankles, and Achilles tendon is seen in most affected children.

The most characteristic clinical feature is the 1 mm follicular papule with a central keratotic plug, often surrounded by salmon-colored erythema (see edges of coalescent scale, Fig. 4.21). Initially discrete, the papules usually coalesce into hyperkeratotic plaques with sharply marginated patches and thickened psoriasiform plaques with a coarse texture similar to the surface of a nutmeg grater. The plaques are generally symmetrical and diffuse and contrast sharply with islands of normal skin that occur within the affected areas. Despite their frequency in affected adults, the distinct follicular-based papules on the dorsal aspect of the fingers are found in the minority of affected children.[83]

More than 40% of pediatric patients show cephalic involvement, often extending from the face to the neck and onto the upper trunk in a capelike configuration with sharp borders (Fig. 4.22). Scalp scaling may be extensive, with large, adhesive scales and underlying salmon-colored erythema. Although perioral and periorbital areas may show the keratotic papules and erythema, the mucosae are spared. Ectropion has been described in children with extensive PRP.

The nails are dystrophic in 13% of patients and can show thickening, onycholysis, transverse striations, and subungual debris (Fig. 4.26). The characteristic pitting of nails seen in psoriasis, however, is not a feature of this disorder. The Koebner phenomenon, a hallmark of psoriasis, has been described in approximately 10% of children with PRP. Pruritus is only occasionally a feature, but may occur in children with diffuse disease.

The onset of PRP in children may be acute, as is more typical of adults, appearing and spreading during a few days. Alternatively, the eruption may begin on the scalp and forehead and extend gradually. Exfoliative, rapidly progressive dermatitis with associated malaise, chills, and fever is rarely described in children. Biopsy of a follicular-based papule can aid in diagnosis if it shows the characteristic follicular keratosis, as well as epidermal parakeratosis and dermal mononuclear infiltrates, particularly surrounding the hair follicle.

The disorder has been classified by Griffiths into five types based on the age of onset (types I and II in adults; types III–V in children)

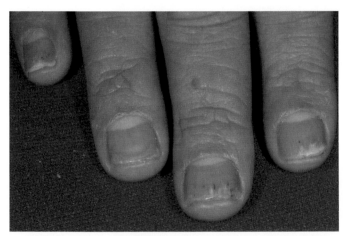

Figure 4.26 Pityriasis rubra pilaris. Unusual nail changes in a girl with extensive PRP. Note the onycholysis and splinter hemorrhages. Her skin disease was more typical of PRP than psoriasis.

and clinical features (Table 4.4).[84] Type IV PRP is the most common type in pediatric patients. Most patients develop their first manifestations during teenage years, although the disorder can occur during the first year or two of life; the mean age in prepubertal children is 4.4 years.[85] Patients with type IV PRP usually present at 12 years of age or earlier, but with a mean age of onset of 6.3 years.[85] Many children cannot easily be fit into any of these classifications because of overlap. Children have also been shown to present originally as one type and to evolve into another type. An alternative system of classification of five types has been proposed based on the presentation and courses of 104 children. This newer classification adds a new type I that shows only palmoplantar keratoderma without follicular plugging (20% of children), but combines Griffiths' types I and III into a single classification that includes all ages.[83]

The clinical course of pityriasis rubra pilaris is variable. In a review of 29 pediatric cases, 52% showed clearance within 6 months (mean 2.7 months) and an additional 11% by 1 year after onset.[85] In another study of 30 children, 43% showed 90–100% clearing, an additional 23% showed at least 30% clearing, and 17% showed a poor outcome.[86] However, in a more recent study of 28 patients, two-thirds of patients with type III and IV juvenile PRP (e.g., most of the patients) had a protracted course lasting >3 years.[87] The prognosis does not correlate with acute versus gradual onset or extent of involvement. The course at times is characterized by spontaneous remissions and exacerbations; some children evolve into a phenotype more typical of psoriasis than PRP.

Patients with PRP may respond to emollients, topical corticosteroids, tazarotene[88] and keratolytic agents (e.g., formulations containing urea, salicylic acids, or α-hydroxy acid, particularly those with milder disease. Calcineurin inhibitor therapy may clear facial lesions.[89]

Non-responders with more extensive disease are best treated with systemic retinoid therapy. Although other patients have been treated with ultraviolet B light and tar or systemic therapy with high-dose vitamin A (>100 000 U/day), methotrexate, cyclosporine, or azathioprine, the response with isotretinoin has been far superior to these treatment regimens in children.[86] Adequate therapeutic trials of retinoids require at least 4–6 months. The usage of oral retinoids requires careful monitoring by a dermatologist familiar with their many potential risks. Extensive extraspinal hyperostosis has been described in a child with PRP after long-term administration of oral retinoid therapy.[90] Given the self-limited nature of the disorder in many affected children, retinoids should be tapered and discontinued as tolerated after several months of continuous therapy. The combination of etanercept and acitretin has also been used in a recalcitrant patient,[91] and infliximab has been used for adult-onset disease.[92]

Table 4.4 Classification of pityriasis rubra pilaris in adults and children[84]

Type		Frequency	Clinical features
I	Classic adult	Most adults	Follicular keratotic papules, first on face and extending caudally; progresses to generalized keratoderma with islands of sparing; palms and soles usually involved; generally clears within 3 years
II	Atypical adult	Rare	More ichthyosiform scaling; coarse palmoplantar keratoderma; long duration
III	Classic juvenile	14–35% of children	Same as type I
IV	Circumscribed juvenile	Most common type in children	Thick plaques on knees, elbows; palms and soles involved
V	Atypical juvenile	Rare, familial. Onset in first years of life	'Sclerodermatous' changes on palms and soles; follicular hyperkeratosis

Pityriasis lichenoides

Pityriasis lichenoides (formerly called parapsoriasis) is a spectrum of cutaneous eruptions that has been subdivided into two forms:[93] (1) an acute form (pityriasis lichenoides et varioliformis acuta; PLEVA; Mucha–Habermann disease); and (2) a chronic form (pityriasis lichenoides chronic; PLC). A total of 19–38% of cases occur in pediatric patients,[94,95] commonly during the first decade of life, and the condition has been described at birth.[96] Some children show clinical and/or histological features of both acute and chronic form, suggesting considerable overlap and confirming the concept that these groups represent a spectrum of disease. As a result, a newer classification is based on distribution into diffuse, central (neck, trunk, and extremities), and peripheral (acral) forms, rather than the morphology of lesions.[97] Acral involvement, including of the face, is more common in children than in adults, and the disorder persists longer before spontaneous remission in children as well.[98]

PLEVA is a polymorphous eruption that usually begins as asymptomatic to pruritic symmetrical 2–3 mm, oval or round, reddish brown macules and papules. The papules occur in successive crops and rapidly evolve into vesicular, necrotic, and sometimes purpuric lesions (Fig. 4.27). These develop a fine crust and gradually resolve, with or without a varioliform scar. Lesions may involve the entire body but are often most pronounced on the trunk, proximal thighs, and upper arms, especially the flexor surfaces. The face, scalp, mucous membranes, palms, and soles are frequently spared or may be involved to a lesser degree. Transient hypopigmentation or hyperpigmentation may result. The course usually lasts for periods of a few weeks to several months. Patients occasionally have associated fever and constitutional symptoms. A rare variant, the febrile ulceronecrotic form, is characterized by large, coalescing, ulceronecrotic nodules and plaques associated with high fever; 50% of reported cases have been children.[99]

PLC may begin de novo or may evolve from PLEVA; overall it affects 37.5% of pediatric patients with pityriasis lichenoides.[92] The course of PLC is variable and may last for periods of 6 months to several years. Lesions characteristically appear as scaling papules and plaques (Figs 4.28, 4.29) that resolve with dyspigmentation but no scarring.

In the early stages, pityriasis lichenoides may be mistaken for chickenpox, arthropod bites, impetigo, vesicular pityriasis rosea, vasculitis, or scabies; chronic forms may be confused with psoriasis, lichen planus, pityriasis rosea, and secondary syphilis. The duration of the eruption (often in crops), the presence of macules and papules interspersed with vesicular, crusted, or hemorrhagic lesions with or without varioliform scarring, and subsequent hypopigmentation or hyperpigmentation help to differentiate pityriasis lichenoides from other conditions. When the diagnosis remains in doubt, histopathologic examination of a skin biopsy specimen will often substantiate the proper diagnosis, showing heavy mononuclear cell perivascular infiltration and, in more acute lesions,

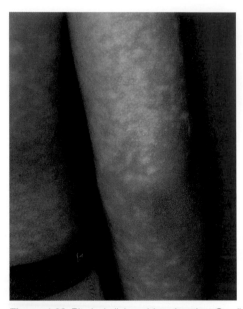

Figure 4.28 Pityriasis lichenoides chronica. Small, erythematous papules with numerous residual macules of post-inflammatory hypopigmentation.

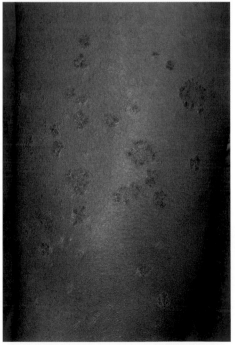

Figure 4.29 Pityriasis lichenoides chronica. Annular scaling plaques with associated hyperpigmentation in an African-American patient.

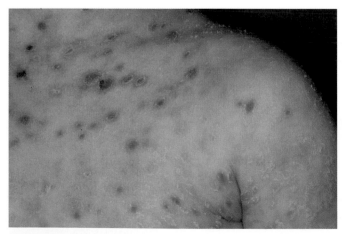

Figure 4.27 Pityriasis lichenoides et varioliformis acuta (PLEVA). Symmetrical oval and round reddish brown macular, papular, necrotic, and crusted lesions on the chest and abdomen of a 9-year-old boy.

erythrocyte extravasation into the dermis, intraepidermal vesicle formation, and epidermal necrosis.

The cause of pityriasis lichenoides is unknown. However, studies demonstrating T-cell clonality[100,101] suggest that pityriasis lichenoides is a benign lympho-proliferative process in which a vigorous host immune reaction prevents the condition from evolving into lymphoma. The frequent temporal association of preceding viral exposure in many children implicates an abnormal immune response to a viral antigenic trigger.[92] These results are consistent with rare reports of cutaneous T-cell lymphoma occurring in patients with clinical manifestations or a history of PLEVA or PLC.[102–104] CD30+ T cells in the biopsy specimens of a few patients with pityriasis lichenoides[105] shows overlap with lymphomatoid papulosis (see below) and suggests a spectrum of lymphoproliferative disorders from benign (PLEVA, PLC) to lymphomatoid papulosis to T-cell lymphoma.

Pityriasis lichenoides does not tend to improve with topical corticosteroids or oral antihistamines, although the associated pruritus may decrease. Up to 70% of children show a partial to full response to administration of systemic antibiotics,[94] particularly erythromycin, azithromycin,[106] or tetracyclines. A 1–2 month trial is sufficient. If successful, antibiotics can be tapered, but continued, administration at low to full dosage may be required for sustained clearance. Tetracyclines should not be administered to children younger than 8 years of age (depending on the status of eruption of secondary teeth) or to pregnant women. Ultraviolet light is the most effective therapy,[107] and most children show clearance of sun-exposed areas.[108] The improvement from exposure to ultraviolet light may also explain the common onset during autumn or winter months. Ultraviolet light exposure through light boxes can be used for pediatric patients who are unresponsive to antibiotics, do not have exposure to natural sunlight, and are significantly bothered by the pityriasis lichenoides.[55] Methotrexate[109] and cyclosporine[110] have resulted in improvement in persistent cases, but are only appropriate to consider for severely affected children, such as those with the febrile ulceronecrotic form.

Lymphomatoid papulosis

Lymphomatoid papulosis is a benign, recurrent self-healing dermatosis with histologic features suggesting lymphoma.[111–113] It is considered to be within the spectrum of lymphoproliferative disorders that ranges from pityriasis lichenoides to cutaneous T-cell lymphoma, and has been included as a separate group in classifications of lymphomas.[114]

The disorder is manifested by numerous reddish brown papules or less frequently vesiculopustules, most commonly noted on the trunk and proximal extremities, but occasionally on the hands and feet, scalp, and genitalia (Fig. 4.30).[115] Regional distribution has been described in children, although more generalized spread may occur after several years.[116] Lesions characteristically develop hemorrhagic necrotic centers and crusting, which gradually involute with residual hyperpigmentation or hypopigmentation. Occasionally, varioliform scars or large ulcerating nodules (Fig. 4.31), plaques, or non-ulcerating papules occur. Although individual lesions evolve over a period of several weeks to 1 month or more, tend to appear in crops, and sometimes disappear spontaneously within a few weeks to months, the entire course of the disorder may be prolonged and last for years. The disorder is generally asymptomatic.

Lymphomatoid papulosis must be distinguished clinically and histopathologically from arthropod bites, PLEVA, pseudolymphoma, and lymphoma. The classic histopathologic picture of lymphomatoid papulosis in children is characterized by a heavy

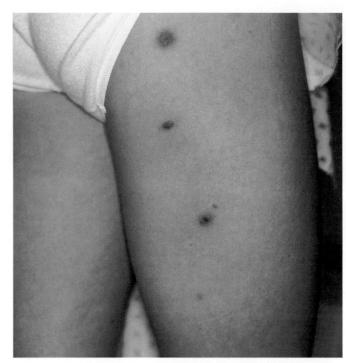

Figure 4.30 Lymphomatoid papulosis. Reddish-brown papules, most commonly noted on the proximal extremities and trunk. This picture shows lesions in different stages of evolution from development of necrotic centers and crusting to resolution.

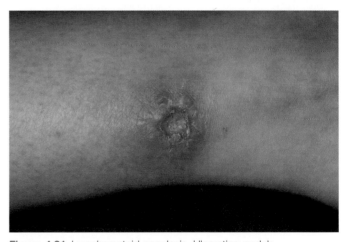

Figure 4.31 Lymphomatoid papulosis. Ulcerating nodule.

infiltrate of scattered large CD-30+ CD15− cells that resembles Hodgkin disease in a background of inflammatory cells (type A), although variants resembling mycosis fungoides (type B), anaplastic large T-cell lymphoma (type C), and mixtures of these lymphomas have been described.

In 10–20% of adult patients, malignant lymphoma develops, and adults with lymphomatoid papulosis are also at increased risk for developing nonlymphoid malignancies.[117] In a report of 35 pediatric patients with lymphomatoid papulosis, 9% of them developed non-Hodgkin lymphoma during a mean follow-up period of 9 years,[113] emphasizing the need for long-term surveillance. Treatment is generally unnecessary, except for cosmetic reasons, because of the asymptomatic nature and tendency toward spontaneous clearance. The sometimes aggressive nature of lymphomatoid papulosis may lead to the misdiagnosis of lymphoma and chemotherapeutic treatment.[114] Application of ultrapotent topical corticosteroids twice daily for 2–3 weeks followed by weekly pulses has resulted in near clearance.[118] Other described therapies in children have included systemic steroids, systemic antibiotics, and PUVA and UVB light. None of these treatments led to sustained complete remission.

Pityriasis rosea

Pityriasis rosea is an acute benign self-limiting disorder that affects male and female patients equally.[119,120] Approximately 50% of cases occur before 20 years of age, especially in adolescents. Only 4% of cases occur before 4 years of age. Most patients are otherwise well; however, a prodrome of headache, malaise, pharyngitis, lymphadenopathy and mild constitutional symptoms is present in approximately 5% of affected patients, particularly in association with more florid involvement. The etiology of pityriasis rosea remains controversial. A viral disorder is suggested by the occasional presence of prodromal symptoms, the course of the disease, epidemics with seasonal cluster, occasional reports of simultaneous occurrence in closely associated individuals, and a tendency to lifelong immunity in 98% of cases. There is evidence both to support and refute the idea that PR is a reaction to human herpesvirus (HHV)-6 and/or -7.[121]

Some 70% of cases start with a single isolated lesion, the so-called herald patch (Fig. 4.32), which is found most commonly on the trunk, upper arm, neck, or thigh. This characteristic initial lesion presents as a sharply defined oval area of scaly dermatitis (2–5 cm in diameter), with a finely scaled, slightly elevated border that gradually expands. After an interval of 2–21 days, a secondary generalized eruption of smaller (0.2–1 cm) papules appears in crops, characteristically sparing the face (in 85% of individuals), scalp, and distal extremities. In about 25% of cases, itching, particularly of secondary lesions, may be noted. The orientation of the long axis of these lesions is most characteristic. The typically ovoid lesions run parallel to the lines of skin cleavage, leading to a pattern resembling a 'Christmas-tree' on the back, wrapping around the trunk horizontally at the axillary area and suprapubic areas, and following inguinal folds. The smaller lesions also show a 'collarette of scale' that surrounds the lesions (Fig. 4.33). Although the truncal distribution is most common, some patients, particularly children, show an 'inverse' distribution of lesions on the face, axillae, and groin (Figs 4.34, 4.35). This atypical form of pityriasis rosea may be particularly difficult to diagnose if there is no history of a herald patch and if the characteristic morphology of lesions goes unrecognized. The face and neck are more frequently involved in children than in

adults, particularly in African-American children. Pityriasis rosea has also been found to be more extensive, more often papular (34%), and associated with residual dyspigmentation in affected African-American children.[122]

Occasionally, lesions may be predominantly round papular lesions, particularly in young children and African-Americans (Fig. 4.36). Vesicular, pustular, urticarial, and hemorrhagic variants have also been described. The herald patch occasionally is the only manifestation. Involvement of the oral mucous membranes occurs in up to 16% of patients as asymptomatic erythematous patches that rarely appear erosive, hemorrhagic, or bullous.

The secondary eruption peaks within a few days to a week. Clearance usually occurs within 6 weeks, initially in the lesions that appeared earliest, but may require as long as 5 months. The disorder is rarely recurrent.[121] Post-inflammatory hypopigmentation or hyperpigmentation may frequently be noted, particularly in dark-skinned individuals, and may persist for weeks to months after clearance of the pityriasis rosea.

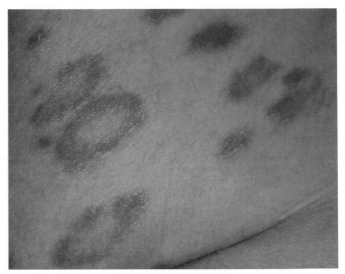

Figure 4.33 Pityriasis rosea. The collarette of scale can be subtle.

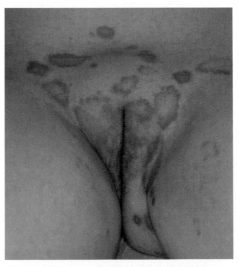

Figure 4.34 Pityriasis rosea. Inverse pattern showing the distribution along skin lines. Scaling may be more difficult to appreciate in intertriginous areas.

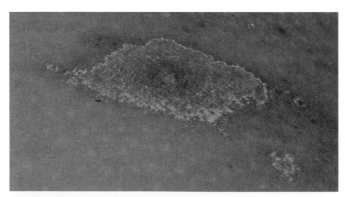

Figure 4.32 Herald patch (pityriasis rosea). Oval lesion with finely scaled elevated border, occasionally misdiagnosed as tinea corporis.

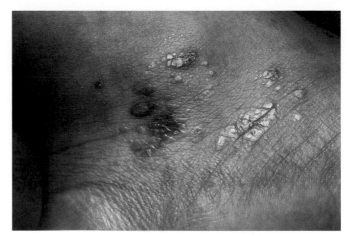

Figure 4.37 Lichen planus. The shiny flat-topped polygonal violaceous papules of lichen planus may be linear in orientation, suggesting the Koebner phenomenon after scratching. Note the intense residual hyperpigmentation and subtle overlying reticulated scaling.

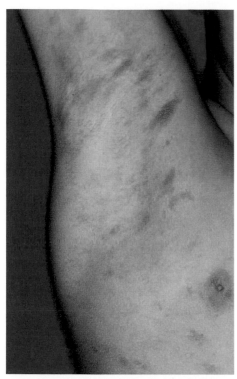

Figure 4.35 Pityriasis rosea. The axillary area is a good site to look for orientation along skin lines that facilitates the diagnosis.

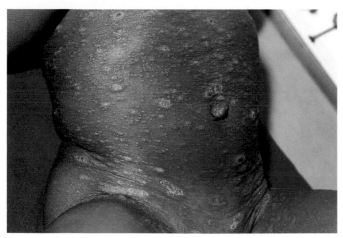

Figure 4.36 Pityriasis rosea. Truncal involvement with larger plaques and predominantly round papular lesions, most commonly see in young children and African-Americans. Note the peripheral scale and distribution along skin lines.

The diagnosis of pityriasis rosea depends on recognition of the distribution of lesions and the characteristic appearance of the oval lesions with their fine peripheral or 'collarette' scales. The histologic features of pityriasis rosea are not diagnostic and resemble those of a subacute or chronic dermatitis. The herald patch may be mistaken for tinea corporis, and the full-blown eruption must be differentiated from widespread tinea infection, drug eruption, PLEVA, seborrheic dermatitis, nummular eczema, psoriasis (particularly the guttate variety), and importantly, secondary syphilis. The latter must be considered in sexually-active individuals who show involvement of the palms and soles, an unusual (but occasional) site for lesions

of pityriasis rosea. The hemorrhagic form of pityriasis rosea must also be distinguished from vasculitis, including Henoch–Schönlein purpura, and viral disorders with thrombocytopenia.

Most patients require no treatment beyond reassurance as to the nature and prognosis of the disorder. Pruritus, if present, usually responds to topical antipruritics (calamine lotion, lotions containing menthol and/or camphor, lotions with pramoxine), oral antihistamines, colloidal starch or oatmeal baths, and mild topical corticosteroid formulations. Exposure to ultraviolet light or sunshine tends to hasten resolution of lesions, and in the summertime it is not uncommon to see patients with pityriasis rosea under covered areas with little to no evidence of the eruption on sun-exposed regions. Although a preliminary study suggested that early administration of oral erythromycin could shorten the course of the disorder, subsequent studies have shown no benefit or either oral erythromycin or azithromycin.[123,124]

Lichen planus

Lichen planus is a relatively common subacute or chronic dermatosis that occurs in persons of all ages. Although 66–85% of cases occur in adults above 30 years of age, the disorder has also been recorded in an infant 3 weeks of age. Of reported cases, 2–11% occur in children and adolescents.[125] The etiology of lichen planus is unknown, but current evidence suggests a cell-mediated autoimmune response and in some patients, a genetic predisposition. Familial cases are rare, but have an earlier age at onset, increased severity, a greater likelihood of chronicity, and an increased incidence of erosive, linear, ulcerative, and hypertrophic forms. Several cases in children have been described after hepatitis B vaccination.[126,127,128] The association of lichen planus with hepatitis C, as seen in adults,[129] has not been noted in children.[126,130] Lesions resembling lichen planus are a common manifestation of chronic graft-versus-host disease (see Ch. 25).

The primary lesion is a small shiny flat-topped polygonal reddish or violaceous papule (Figs 4.37, 4.38). Individual papules vary from 2 mm to 1 cm or more, and may be closely aggregated or widely dispersed. Lichen planus is generally mildly to intensely pruritic, but the lesions are often non-pruritic in affected children.[125] The disorder is usually limited to a few areas, with the lower legs the

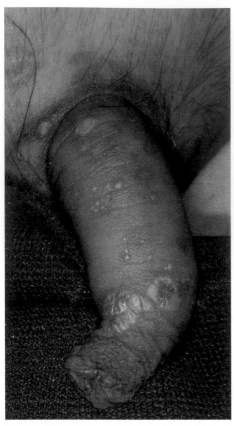

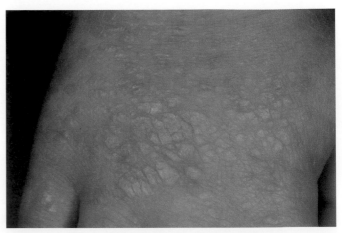

Figure 4.39 Lichen planus. The shiny flat-topped polygonal violaceous papules of lichen planus on the dorsal aspect of the hands. Note the pinker color on fair skin.

Figure 4.38 Lichen planus. Typical violaceous lesions of lichen planus on the penile shaft, a common site.

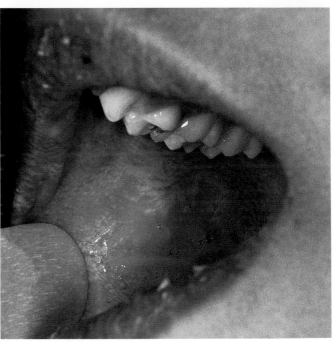

Figure 4.40 Oral lichen planus. Wickham's striae on the buccal mucosa.

most common site;[126] lichen planus also often affects the flexural surfaces of the ankles and wrists, the genitalia (Fig. 4.39), and the lower back.

At times, one may detect characteristic small grayish puncta or streaks that form a network over the surface of papules. These delicate white lines, termed Wickham's striae, become more visible under magnification with a hand lens or by wetting the lesion with an alcohol swab or a drop of oil, which renders the horny layers of lesions more transparent. Occasionally, lesions may coalesce to form plaques or a linear configuration (the Koebner phenomenon) over sites of minor trauma, such as scratch marks (Fig. 4.37).

Mucous membrane involvement is seen in up to 40% of pediatric patients, and is much less common than in adult patients (50–70% of adult patients).[125,127] When present, lesions usually appear as pinhead-sized white papules forming annular or linear lace-like patterns on the inner aspects of the cheeks (Fig. 4.40).[131,132] Lesions on the palate, lips, and tongue are less characteristic and, except for their reticulated appearance, may easily be mistaken for areas of leukoplakia. On the lips, the papules are more often annular, sometimes with adherent scaling reminiscent of that seen in lupus erythematosus. Although the typical reticulated mucosal lesions of lichen planus are asymptomatic, painful ulcerative lesions have been found on the tongue, oral mucous membranes, and mucosal surfaces of the pharynx, esophagus, gastrointestinal tract, vulva, and vagina.

Up to 10% of adult patients with lichen planus demonstrate involvement of one to all nails, but nail involvement appears to be less common in affected children; one study, however, noted nail involvement in 19% of 100 children.[125,126] Violaceous lines or papules in the nail bed may occasionally be seen through the nail

plate. The nail dystrophy consists of loss of luster, thinning of the nail plate, longitudinal ridging or striation, splitting or nicking of the nail margin, atrophy, overlapping skin folds (pterygia), marked subungual hyperkeratosis, lifting of the distal nail plate, red or brown discoloration, and, at times, complete and permanent loss of the nail (Fig. 4.41).[133] Some children with 20-nail dystrophy (see Ch. 7) may have lichen planus, but biopsy of the nail matrix would be needed to confirm the diagnosis in the absence of cutaneous changes.[134]

Although lichen planus is considered to be papulosquamous, many variations in morphology and configuration may be noted. These variations include vesicular, bullous, actinic, annular, hypertrophic (Fig. 4.42), atrophic, linear, erythematous, and follicular forms (Table 4.5). *Lichen planus pemphigoides* is a rare autoimmune blistering disease, in which the typical lichen planus lesions evolve

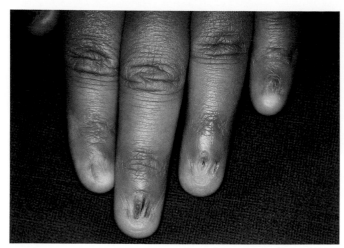

Figure 4.41 Lichen planus of the nails. Anonychia and pterygium formation.

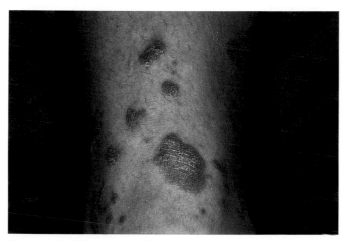

Figure 4.42 Lichen planus. The plaques of lichen planus may be hypertrophic, but show the characteristic violaceous coloration and intense hyperpigmentation.

Table 4.5 Variants of lichen planus (LP)

Variant type	Characteristics
Bullous[135]	Bullae develop on existent LP lesions
LP pemphigoides[136]	LP + bullous pemphigoid with autoimmune reactivity, usually against type XVII collagen (bullous pemphigoid 180 antigen)[137]
Actinic	Onset during spring, summer; primarily sun-exposed surfaces (face, neck, dorsum of arms and hands); often annular configuration; most commonly in children and young adults
Annular	Occur in 10% of patients, often scattered amidst typical lesions of LP
Hypertrophic	Pruritic, thick hyperkeratotic plaques, especially on the legs and dorsal regions of the feet; persistent
Atrophic	May represent a resolving phase in which larger plaques become centrally depressed with residual hyperpigmentation
Hemorrhagic/ purpuric	Shows non-blanching component on diascopy
Linear[138]	LP occurring spontaneously along the lines of Blaschko; presumably reflects somatic mosaicism
Erosive/ulcerative	Intensely painful ulcerations on the palms and soles; chronic lesions may evolve into squamous cell carcinoma; erosive lesions may occur on mucosal surfaces
LP-lupus erythematosus	Overlapping features of lupus and LP; lesions are usually acral and patients may show high titers of ANA
Lichen planopilaris (LPP)	Follicular LP; keratotic plugs surrounded by violaceous erythema, especially on scalp but can affect any hair-bearing area; usually results in cicatricial alopecia

into bullous lesions with a mean lag time of 8 weeks (see Ch. 13).[136] The extremities are most commonly involved and approximately half of the affected children show palmoplantar lesions. Direct and indirect immunofluorescence shows the presence of circulating antibodies, and patients often respond to topical corticosteroid and oral dapsone therapy, but systemically administered steroid may be required.

Many drugs may produce an eruption that resembles lichen planus (lichenoid drug eruption). Most commonly implicated are antihypertensives (captopril, enalapril, labetalol, and propranolol), diuretics (especially hydrochlorothiazide), antimalarials (especially hydroxychloroquine and quinidine), metals (especially gold salts), and penicillamine. Among other agents rarely implicated but used often in children and adolescents, are griseofulvin, tetracycline, carbamazepine, phenytoin, and non-steroidal antiinflammatory drugs. In contrast to other drug eruptions, in which the latent period between introduction of the drug and the reaction is within 1 month, the latent period with lichenoid drug eruptions is typically several months to years after initiation of a medication. Similarly, the time to clearance after discontinuation of the medication is also prolonged and can take several weeks to months. The lichenoid lesions of lichenoid drug eruptions tend to be more eczematous, psoriasiform, or pityriasis rosea-like than the typical papules of lichen planus. Lesions occur much less commonly on oral mucosae than on skin.[139] In addition, they uncommonly show Wickham's striae and are frequently photodistributed, particularly on the extensor forearms. The histologic picture resembles lichen planus, but shows more eosinophils.

The diagnosis of lichen planus depends on the recognition of the typical purple, polygonal, pruritic papules and plaques. When the diagnosis is in doubt, histopathologic examination of a cutaneous lesion can confirm the proper diagnosis. Characteristic changes are destruction of the basal cell layer (liquefactive degeneration), sawtoothing of the rete pegs, and a band-like lymphocytic infiltrate that hugs and invades the lower epidermis. Although cases of lichen planus occasionally clear in a few weeks, two-thirds of affected individuals with acute forms display spontaneous resolution within 8–15 months. In most patients, the lesions tend to flatten but are often replaced by an area of intense hyperpigmentation that may persist for months or years (Fig. 4.43). Occasionally, lichen planus itself may persist for years, and 10–20% of patients suffer one or more recurrences of their disorder.

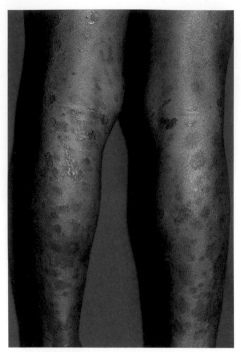

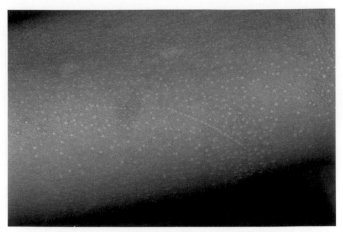

Figure 4.44 Lichen nitidus. Sharply demarcated, pinpoint to pinhead sized monomorphic, round, usually flesh-colored lesions. Lesions may be distributed in a linear configuration after trauma to the site (Koebner phenomenon).

Figure 4.43 Lichen planus. Intense residual post-inflammatory hyperpigmentation.

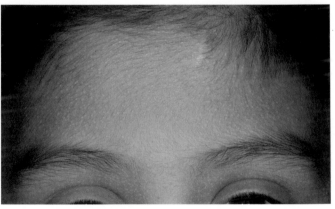

Figure 4.45 Lichen nitidus. Note the even distribution of these pinpoint to pinhead sized round lesions on the upper face.

The standard therapy for lichen planus in pediatric patients involves administration of class II–IV topical steroids and oral antihistamines. Pruritus may require 3 weeks of therapy to subside and the lesions themselves 6 weeks to begin to flatten.[126] Topical tacrolimus has been effective in cases recalcitrant to topical steroids.[140] For more extensive or recalcitrant cases, the addition of a 2- to 6-week course of systemic corticosteroids (1 mg/kg per day) is usually helpful in ameliorating the associated pruritus and hastening clearance.[141] Hypertrophic lichen planus lesions may respond to application of class I topical steroids under occlusion, flurandrenolide-impregnated tape, or intra-lesional injections of triamcinolone. When traditional forms of therapy fail, metronidazole,[142] griseofulvin,[143] dapsone,[125] PUVA or UVB light therapy,[125] oral retinoids,[141] cyclosporine,[144] and thalidomide[145] have been shown to be effective in selected cases. If drug-induced lichen planus is considered, medications should be discontinued whenever possible. Mucous membrane lesions should be treated if symptomatic, eroded, or ulcerated. Topical anesthetics such as diphenhydramine elixir, viscous lidocaine, topical corticosteroids (such as Kenalog in Orabase), or topical tacrolimus ointment[146] may be beneficial. Since erosive forms of oral lichen planus may have an increased risk of malignant transformation, patients with oral lesions should avoid carcinogenic factors (such as tobacco) and receive periodic follow-up examinations and biopsy of suspicious lesions.[147] Nails may respond to administration of systemic corticosteroids, but local application of potent steroids under occlusion or flurandrenolide-impregnated tape at the nail base can be used if the disorder is largely limited to the nail.[133]

Lichen nitidus

Lichen nitidus is a relatively uncommon benign dermatosis that affects individuals of all ages, but is most commonly seen in children of preschool and school age. Although the etiology remains unknown, association with lichen planus has been reported[148] and some authorities consider lichen nitidus to be a variant of lichen planus. Familial cases have rarely been described.[149,150]

The individual papules of lichen nitidus are sharply demarcated, pinpoint to pinhead sized, round or polygonal, and usually flesh-colored (Figs 4.44, 4.45). The surface of each lesion is flat, shiny, and slightly elevated, sometimes with a central depression. The eruption is arranged in groups, primarily located on the trunk, genitalia, abdomen, and forearms of affected individuals, but may be generalized.[151] Linear lesions in lines of trauma (Koebner reaction) are common. Minute grayish flat papules on the buccal mucous membrane and nail changes (thickening, ridging, pitting, onycholysis) have occasionally been noted.[152] Lichen nitidus occasionally clears spontaneously after a period of several weeks to months, but more frequently lasts much longer (occasionally years) with little or no response to treatment. As with lichen planus, significant post-inflammatory pigmentary changes may persist.

Biopsy can confirm the diagnosis, and characteristically shows claw-like projections of the rete ridges encircling an inflammatory infiltrate of lymphocytes, histiocytes, and occasionally giant cells, resembling a hand clutching a ball. Topical corticosteroids or calcineurin inhibitors occasionally clear the lesions, but more often are not effective. However, the usually asymptomatic nature and tendency for spontaneous healing make intervention less critical.

Keratosis lichenoides chronica

Keratosis lichenoides chronica is a rare, chronic, progressive, dermatosis that is much more common in adults than in pediatric patients.[153] Lesions may be present from birth or appear during infancy, and are sometimes pruritic in children.[154] Familial occurrence (probably autosomal recessive) is more common in pediatric cases than in adults. The characteristic erythematous lichenoid papules and scaling verrucous lesions show a linear or reticulated pattern. The eruption tends to be symmetric, particularly on the limbs and less commonly the abdomen and buttock. Pediatric patients often have facial involvement, with well-defined scaling erythematous papules that may appear purpuric or resemble seborrheic dermatitis. Forehead, eyebrow and eyelash alopecia may be noted. The palms and soles may show keratoderma, and nails may be discolored with thickening and longitudinal ridging. Occasionally, mucosae are affected; painful ulcerations or keratoses of the oropharyngeal or genital mucosae, hoarseness, and keratoconjunctivitis have been described. Biopsy sections resemble those of lichen planus.

Keratosis lichenoides chronica may persist for decades and is unresponsive to topical therapy, including topical corticosteroid therapy. Ultraviolet light exposure, PUVA therapy, and oral administration of retinoids, however, alone or in combination, may at times be beneficial.

Key References

 The complete list of 154 references for this chapter is available online at **www.expertconsult.com**.
See inside cover for registration details.

Bowers S, Warshaw EM. Pityriasis lichenoides and its subtypes. *J Am Acad Dermatol*. 2006;55(4):557–572; quiz 573–576.

Browning JC. An update on pityriasis rosea and other similar childhood exanthems. *Curr Opin Pediatr*. 2009;21(4):481–485.

Cordoro KM. Systemic and light therapies for the management of childhood psoriasis: part II. *Skin Therapy Lett*. 2008;13(4):1–3.

Ersoy-Evans S, Altaykan A, Sahin S, Kölemen F. Phototherapy in childhood. *Pediatr Dermatol*. 2008;25(6):599–605.

Ersoy-Evans S, Greco MF, Mancini AJ, et al. Pityriasis lichenoides in childhood: a retrospective review of 124 patients. *J Am Acad Dermatol*. 2007;56(2):205–210.

Kanwar AJ, De D. Lichen planus in childhood: report of 100 cases. *Clin Exp Dermatol*. 2010;35(3):257–262

Nair RP, Duffin KC, Helms C, et al. Genome-wide scan reveals association of psoriasis with IL-23 and NF-kappaB pathways. *Nat Genet*. 2009;41(2):199–204.

Nestle FO, Kaplan DH, Barker J. Psoriasis. *N Engl J Med*. 2009;361(5):496–509.

Paller AS, Siegfried EC, Langley RG, et al. Etanercept treatment for children and adolescents with plaque psoriasis. *N Engl J Med*. 2008;358(3):241–251.

Yang CC, Shih IH, Lin WL, et al. Juvenile pityriasis rubra pilaris: report of 28 cases in Taiwan. *J Am Acad Dermatol*. 2008;59(6):943–948.

5 Hereditary Disorders of Cornification

The hereditary disorders of cornification, or the ichthyoses, are characterized by impairment in desquamation with hyperkeratosis and/or scaling.[1-3] The ichthyoses are largely distinguished by their clinical, and in some cases, histologic and ultrastructural features. The discovery of the underlying molecular basis of most of the forms of ichthyosis has not only further refined classification, but has also facilitated our understanding of the interactions among epidermal proteins and the role of epidermal lipids in normal epidermal function. Desquamation is the end result of proteolytic degradation of corneodesmosomes (the intercellular junctions within the stratum corneum), abetted by friction and cell hydration. Desquamation requires normal epidermal differentiation and depends on a gradient of pH, the presence of protease inhibitors, and the generation of hygroscopic molecules within the stratum corneum cells. Abnormalities in desquamation and differentiation usually result from abnormal corneocyte shedding (retention hyperkeratosis) or from increased epidermal cell proliferation (epidermal hyperplasia).

The epidermal barrier consists of stacked corneocytes (cells of the stratum corneum) and surrounding highly hydrophobic lipid layers (lamellae) formed by the secretion of lamellar body contents at the interface of the stratum granulosum and the stratum corneum. Most of the mutations that lead to ichthyosis affect lipid metabolism or epidermal proteins, leading to barrier dysfunction and resulting in increased transepidermal water loss and decreased water-holding capacity.[4,5] Many of the features of ichthyosis are thought to be continuous compensatory attempts to restore the barrier (e.g., upregulated epidermal lipid synthesis, epidermal hyperproliferation, and inflammation). This homeostatic response likely allows survival of affected individuals. In 2009, an international group of experts on the ichthyoses met to discuss a new classification based on the known clinical, histological, biochemical and genetic features of forms of the ichthyoses. This chapter's discussion on ichthyosis follows this new classification scheme.[6]

Non-syndromic forms of ichthyosis

Four major forms of non-syndromic ichthyosis have been delineated, based largely on clinical and genetic characteristics.[7] These are the most common forms of ichthyosis:

1. Ichthyosis vulgaris, the most common ichthyosis, transmitted as an autosomal semi-dominant trait
2. Recessive X-linked ichthyosis (RXLI), expressed only in males and transmitted as an X-linked recessive trait
3. Keratinopathic ichthyosis, autosomal dominant (most common, epidermolytic ichthyosis)
4. Autosomal recessive congenital ichthyosis or ARCI (most collodion babies; the lamellar ichthyosis/congenital ichthyosiform erythroderma spectrum).

Ichthyosis Vulgaris

Ichthyosis vulgaris is by far the most common genetic form of ichthyosis, and the majority of individuals affected by the disorder are undiagnosed (Table 5.1). This disorder, which is not present at birth, may be noted after the first 2 months of life and often not until later in childhood. Ichthyosis vulgaris generally improves with age, in summer, and in warm moist environments. Scales are most prominent on the extensor surfaces of the extremities, and are most severe in cold and dry weather. Scales on the pretibial and lateral aspects of the lower leg are large and plate-like, resembling fish scales (Fig. 5.1A); the flexural areas are characteristically spared. In other areas small, white, bran-like scales may be seen. Scales tend to be darker on dark-skinned individuals. Scaling of the forehead and cheeks, common during childhood, generally diminishes and clears with age, but hyperlinearity and mild to moderate thickening of the palms and soles is characteristic (Fig. 5.1B). Discrete hyperkeratosis may occur on the elbows, knees, and ankles.

Patients with ichthyosis often reveal an atopic background with a tendency toward atopic dermatitis, asthma, and/or allergic rhinitis.[8] The diagnosis of ichthyosis vulgaris should be considered in patients with atopic dermatitis who show large scales, particularly on the extensor aspects of the extremities; examination of the palms and soles shows the hyperlinearity. The presence in a parent of hyperlinear palms and dry skin, especially on the lower extremities, may be helpful in confirming this diagnosis. Keratosis pilaris, which is frequently associated with ichthyosis vulgaris and atopy[9] (see Ch. 3, Fig. 3.17 and Ch. 7, Figs 7.22 and 7.23), is most predominant on the upper arms, buttocks, and thighs.

A reduced or absent granular layer in skin sections may help to differentiate ichthyosis vulgaris from other forms of ichthyosis. Given that filaggrin is the major protein of the granular layer, it is not surprising that mutations in the gene encoding for profilaggrin, the precursor of filaggrin, are responsible.[10] In fact, almost 10% of all Northern Europeans were found to harbor these mutations in at least one allele of profilaggrin.[9,10] Ichthyosis vulgaris is now known to be a semi-dominant condition, in contrast to the previous assumption of dominant inheritance (i.e., manifestations are seen with a mutation on one allele, 1:10; but are worse if both alleles are mutated, 1:400).

The cleaved product of profilaggrin, filaggrin, plays an important role in linking a protein (involucrin) and lipids (ceramides) in the corneocyte envelope (see Ch. 3). In addition, filaggrin breaks down to amino acid metabolites that increase skin hydration ('natural moisturizing factor'). Without filaggrin, the epidermis cannot provide normal barrier function; transepidermal water loss is increased, leading to xerosis, and the ingress of foreign substances (such as allergens and pathogens) occurs more readily, thereby increasing the risk of exposure to triggers of atopy. In fact, mutations in profilaggrin are strongly linked to the risk of atopic dermatitis and secondary asthma, regardless of the ethnicity or specific

Table 5.1 Comparison among the most common types of ichthyosis

	Ichthyosis vulgaris	X-linked recessive ichthyosis	Keratinopathic ichthyosis,[a] epidermolytic ichthyosis	ARCI: Classic lamellar ichthyosis	ARCI: Classic congenital ichthyosiform erythroderma
Incidence	1:250	1:2000–6000 males	1:300 000	1:300 000	1:300 000
Inheritance	Autosomal semi-dominant	X-linked recessive	Usually autosomal dominant	Usually autosomal recessive	Autosomal recessive
Onset	2 months and beyond	17% at birth; 83% by 1 year	Birth, with superficial blistering	Birth, as collodion baby	Birth, as collodion baby
Character of scales	Fine white to larger scales, esp. on legs	Large, brown	Verrucous scale, superficial blisters	Large, platelike scales	Fine white scaling overlying erythema
Localization	Can be generalized; relative sparing of flexures; hyperlinear palms	Accentuation at neck and behind ears; relative sparing of flexures	Generalized; esp. at flexures and overlying joints	Generalized; ectropion, occ. alopecia, nail dystrophy	Generalized; ectropion; occ. alopecia
Distinct histologic features	Often shows decreased granular layer	None	Epidermolytic hyperkeratosis	Massive orthokeratosis; moderate acanthosis	More acanthosis
Molecular basis	Mutations in profilaggin (FLG); worse if both alleles	Deletions in ARSC1 (=arylsulfatase C)	Mutations in KRT1 and 10; Superficial form with mutations in KRT2	Mutations in TGM1; NIPAL4; ALOX12B; ABCA12; other loci	Mutations in ALOXE3; ALOX12B; NIPAL4; ABCA12; CYP4F22; TGM1; other loci
Comments	Increased risk of atopic dermatitis and keratosis pilaris	Accumulation of cholesterol sulfate; FISH analysis to detect deletion; Genital abnormalities rare; asymptomatic corneal opacities Contiguous gene deletion: with retardation, anosmia (Kallman syndrome) and/or chondrodysplasia punctata	Superficial form shows more superficial blistering and much less thickening; secondary Staphylococcus aureus infection	Transglutaminase activity can be measured in skin samples	May be associated with neurologic abnormalities

[a]Previously known as bullous congenital ichthyosiform erythroderma and ichthyosis bullosa of Siemens. ARCI, autosomal recessive congenital ichthyosis.

profilaggrin mutation. The risk is highest in individuals with two mutated alleles. Overall, up to 30% of patients with atopic dermatitis of a Northern European background and >20% of Japanese with atopic dermatitis[11] have ichthyosis vulgaris. Signs of atopic dermatitis may be seen before other clinical signs of ichthyosis vulgaris, and many individuals with ichthyosis vulgaris never show evidence of atopic dermatitis. Nevertheless, the incredibly strong link of null mutations in profilaggrin and atopic dermatitis support an important role of the epidermal barrier as a primary issue in many patients with atopic dermatitis (see Ch. 3).

Although rare in children, 'acquired' ichthyotic scaling has been described in patients with nutritional disorders such as hypovitaminosis or hypervitaminosis A, hypothyroidism, sarcoidosis, dermatomyositis, leprosy, tuberculosis, HIV infection, and neoplastic disorders, particularly lymphomas. It should be noted that these forms were described before the availability of testing for profilaggrin mutations; given the many undiagnosed patients, it is possible

that the underlying condition served as a trigger for increased cutaneous inflammation or dryness that led to increased expressivity of the gene mutation. Pityriasis rotunda, a rare variant of acquired ichthyosis, is characterized by asymptomatic, circular or oval, brown scaly patches on the trunk or extremities. Seen primarily in individuals of Japanese, African, and West Indian origin, its occurrence in Caucasians is extremely rare. The condition may at times be associated with an underlying disorder (see above), may follow pregnancy, or may be familial. In contrast to ichthyosis vulgaris, pityriasis rotunda is chronic, is resistant to treatment, and tends to improve only when the underlying disorder is treated.

Recessive X-Linked Ichthyosis (RXLI)

RXLI occurs in 1:2500–5000 males, and results from mutation (and usually a complete deletion) in the ARSC1 gene that encodes steroid sulfatase, also known as arylsulfatase C (Table 5.1). The disorder

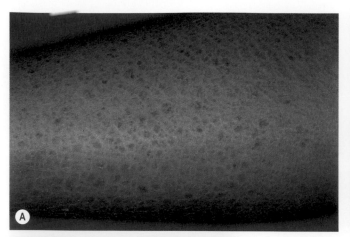

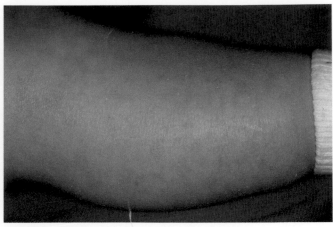

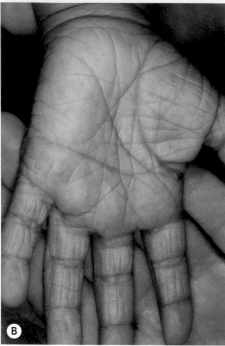

Figure 5.2 Recessive X-linked ichthyosis. Scaling may be subtle, particularly in younger infants. This 6-month-old boy was diagnosed *in utero* by increased maternal estradiol levels and then FISH analysis of chorionic villus samples.

Figure 5.1 Ichthyosis vulgaris. Scales are most prominent on the extensor surfaces of the extremities, especially the lower extremities and may be large and plate-like (A). The palms and soles are thickened with increased palmar markings (B).

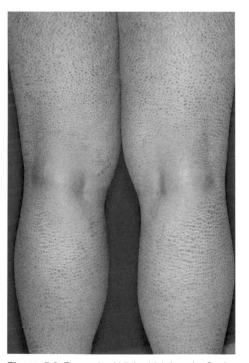

Figure 5.3 Recessive X-linked ichthyosis. Scales may be large and hyperpigmented, especially in darker skinned individuals. The popliteal and antecubital areas are typically spared.

has rarely been described in females who have Turner syndrome or carry the mutation on both alleles. Female carriers do not tend to show ichthyosis because the affected gene is located at the distal tip of the X chromosome, a location that escapes X-inactivation. Thus, rather than having random inactivation of one of the X chromosomes as dictated by the Lyon hypothesis, both of the alleles are expressed in every cell, providing sufficient enzyme. Steroid sulfatase normally is concentrated in lamellar bodies and secreted into the spaces between stratum corneum cells. It degrades cholesterol sulfate, generating cholesterol for the epidermal barrier. Cholesterol sulfate itself is an epidermal protease inhibitor, so that steroid sulfatase deficiency prevents normal degradation of the stratum corneum desmosomes and leads to corneocyte retention.[12] Low placental production of estrogens and elevated sulfated steroid levels have been described in the urine of mothers of boys with RXLI, associated with a difficult or prolonged labor and failure to have cervical dilatation. Deletion of both *ARSC1* and a contiguous

gene (up to 10% of patients) results features of ichthyosis and *Kallmann syndrome* (associated with mental retardation, hypogonadism, and anosmia) and/or X-linked recessive chondrodysplasia punctata (bone dysplasia with stippled epiphyses; see below).[13]

RXLI usually manifests within the first 3 months of life. Approximately 17% of affected individuals show scaling at birth, often in the form of a mild collodion-like membrane. Most develop scaling during the first 6 months of life. The severity of the scaling can range from mild (Fig. 5.2) to severe (Fig. 5.3). This form of ichthyosis generally involves the entire body with accentuation on the neck, abdomen, back, front of the legs, and feet, but sparing the palms, soles, central face, and flexural areas (Fig. 5.3). Scales may be small to large and tend to be brown in coloration, darker in darker-skinned patients. The sides of the neck often appear dark and unwashed. Patients may shed or molt their scales episodically, particularly in the spring and fall.

Boys with X-linked ichthyosis rarely have hypogonadism and/or cryptorchidism; testicular cancer has been described in one patient.[16] Deep corneal opacities may be found in ~50% of affected adult males and less often in female carriers of this disorder. The opacities, easily detectable by slit lamp examination, are discrete and diffusely located near Descemet's membrane or deep in the corneal stroma. Although a marker for the disorder in older patients, these opacities do not affect vision.

X-linked ichthyosis is often suspected prenatally because fetal steroid sulfatase (STS) deficiency leads to low maternal serum and urinary estriol levels; FISH analysis (fluorescent *in situ* hybridization for the STS gene) shows deletion of the gene, which is found in 90% of patients. RXLI can also be confirmed by reduced arylsulfatase C activity in leukocytes. Elevated blood levels of cholesterol sulfate and increased mobility of β-lipoproteins have also been seen.[17]

The features of RXLI may be seen in patients with the autosomal recessive *multiple sulfatase deficiency*, a syndromic form of ichthyosis characterized by features of mucopolysaccharidoses, metachromatic leukodystrophy, X-linked recessive chondrodysplasia punctata and RXLI. The disorder results from mutations in Sulfatase Modifying Factor 1 (SUMF1), which encodes α-formylglycine generating enzyme, required for post-translation modification of sulfatases.[14,15] Progressive neurologic deterioration, a feature of the metachromatic leukodystrophy, usually leads to death during infancy.[17]

Keratinopathic Ichthyoses

The new classification of the ichthyoses has renamed the group of epidermolytic forms of ichthyosis associated with keratin gene mutations as 'keratinopathic'. The major subgroups are *epidermolytic ichthyosis* (formerly called bullous congenital ichthyosiform erythroderma, Brocq type) and *superficial epidermolytic ichthyosis* (formerly called ichthyosis bullosa of Siemens). The designation 'epidermolytic hyperkeratosis' is a histologic description that is not specific to this group of disorders, although it traditionally referred to epidermolytic ichthyosis.

Mutations are usually point mutations that lead to an abnormal, but full-length keratin that incorporates into the keratin filament. The resultant keratin network functions poorly, leading to skin cell collapse and clinical blistering, especially in response to trauma. The thickening of skin is thought to be compensatory to protect against blistering, but has also been linked to abnormal lamellar body secretion.[18] Virtually all forms are inherited in an autosomal dominant manner, although epidermolytic ichthyosis may rarely be autosomal recessive.[19,20] Epidermolytic ichthyosis results from mutations in *KRT1* or its partner in intermediate filament formation, *KRT10*; both are expressed throughout the suprabasal layers of epidermis. Superficial epidermolytic ichthyosis is caused by mutations in *KRT2*, which is only expressed in more superficial epidermis and also partners with keratin 10.[21–24]

Epidermolytic ichthyosis (EI) affects approximately 1 in 300 000 individuals, and 50% of patients have new mutations. The skin is red and may be tender at birth. Superficial bullae generally appear within the first week of life (often within a few hours after delivery; Fig. 5.4A) and may be confused with those of epidermolysis bullosa (see Ch. 13) or with staphylococcal scalded skin syndrome (see Ch. 14); skin thickening often appears from the third month on (Fig. 5.4B), but subtle thickening may be detectable during the first month of life, especially over the elbows and knees, and may be

useful in suggesting the diagnosis. The blisters occur in crops and vary from 0.5 cm to several centimeters in diameter. They tend to heal quickly, consistent with their superficial location. When ruptured, they discharge clear fluid and leave raw denuded areas. Secondary bacterial infection, especially with *Staphylococcus aureus*, is commonly associated with this disorder.

Verruciform grayish-brown scales eventually cover most of the skin surface; the flexural creases and intertriginous areas show particularly marked involvement (Fig. 5.5).[25] Palms and soles have varying degrees of thickening and scaling (Fig. 5.6), but more marked involvement often occurs in individuals with mutations in *KRT1*, since keratin 9 expression in the palms and soles can compensate for abnormal keratin 10 expression, but expression of *KRT1* (which is the partner for both keratins 9 and 10) remains critical.[22,25] Facial involvement may occur, but ectropion does not; although scalp involvement may result in nit-like encasement of hair shafts, the hair, eyes, teeth, and nails are normal. A disagreeable body odor is frequently associated with severe forms of this disorder owing to the thick, macerated scale and overgrowth of bacteria. Skin biopsy specimens show marked hyperkeratosis with lysis of the epidermal cells above the basal cell layer ('epidermolytic hyperkeratosis'), leading to the bullae.[26] Keratolytic agents are often poorly tolerated in keratinopathic forms of ichthyosis and can increase skin fragility.

Mutations in *KRT1* and *KRT10* can lead to other ichthyotic phenotypes as well. Mutations in either can lead to an annular variant (*annular EI*).[27] Annular erythematous polycyclic scaling plaques on the trunk and extremities slowly enlarge, resolve, and later recur. Ichthyosis with confetti, a dominant disorder in which islands of normal-appearing skin replace congenital erythroderma early in life, has been shown to result from revertant mutations in which loss of heterozygosity in *KRT10* results from mitotic recombination.[28]

Ichthyosis Curth–Macklin (formerly called ichthyosis hystrix) has its onset of manifestations during early childhood as progressively worsening diffuse or striate palmoplantar keratoderma that can be associated with deep fissuring, flexural contracture, and digital constriction. Affected individuals develop characteristic 'porcupine quill-like' verrucous yellow-brown scaling, especially on hands and feet, and overlying the large joints. Binuclear cells and pathognomonic concentric perinuclear 'shells' of aberrant keratin are characteristic ultrastructural findings.[29] Keratin 1 mutations have been described[30,31] but keratin gene mutations are more commonly excluded.

The *epidermolytic hyperkeratotic form of epidermal nevus* shows a histologic appearance identical to that of epidermolytic hyperkeratosis (see Ch. 9). This form of nevus represents a mosaic condition in which the affected skin, but not the normal intervening skin, carries a mutation in *KRT1* or *KRT10*.[32] Individuals with more extensive forms of the epidermolytic hyperkeratotic form of epidermal nevus can have offspring with generalized epidermolytic hyperkeratosis, reflecting germline mutations. Prenatal diagnosis can be performed to in at-risk families.[33]

Superficial epidermolytic ichthyosis shows milder thickening and more superficial blistering. Palms and soles are minimally thickened if at all. Although large, tense bullae can occur intermittently, in general the appearance of blisters has been likened to molting ('Mauserung phenomenon') (Fig. 5.7) because of the superficial location of the cleavage plane. Accordingly, less hyperkeratosis is seen in sections of skin biopsies, and the lysed areas of epidermis only begin halfway up the stratum spinosum. Affected individuals may be misdiagnosed as mild epidermolytic ichthyosis clinically, but the limited localization of the epidermolysis histologically and the finding of mutations in *KRT2* by molecular genetic testing can distinguish the disorders.[34,35]

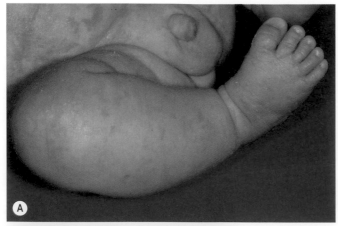

Collodion Baby

The collodion baby is a descriptive term for infants who are born with a membrane-like covering resembling collodion (Fig. 5.8). The collodion baby is not a disease entity but is a phenotype common to several forms of ichthyosis. At least 65% of collodion babies have autosomal recessive congenital ichthyosis (ARCI, see below), a group of genetically distinct forms of ichthyosis with overlapping clinical features; some infants in this group (5–6%) shed their collodion membranes and show apparently normal skin (self-healing collodion baby, SHCB).[36,37] Less often, collodion babies shed their membranes and show features of Conradi syndrome, trichothiodystrophy (Ch. 7), or recessive X-linked ichthyosis.

Collodion babies are often born prematurely.[38] At birth they are completely covered by a cellophane or oiled parchment-like membrane that, owing to its tautness, may distort the facial features and extremities. Thus, peripheral edema with digital constriction, flattened ears, and bilateral eversion of the eyelids, lips, and at times the vulva frequently cause affected infants to resemble one another

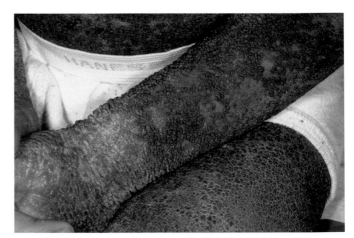

Figure 5.5 Epidermolytic ichthyosis. Thick verrucous scale on the arm of a 6-year-old boy. Note the areas of mild thickening between areas of dramatic thickening, a characteristic finding of children with epidermolytic hyperkeratosis.

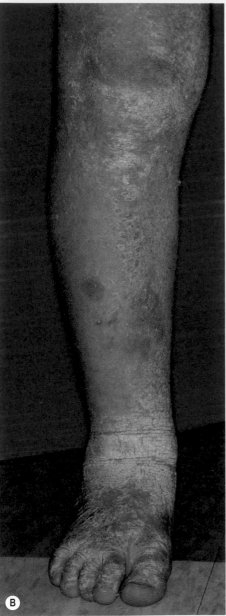

Figure 5.4 Epidermolytic ichthyosis. In the neonate superficial blisters predominate and may be mistaken for epidermolysis bullosa (A). At 3 years of age, the same leg continues to show superficial blistering, but now much more erythema and overlying verrucous scaling (B).

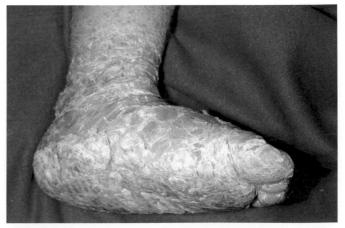

Figure 5.6 Epidermolytic ichthyosis. The marked hyperkeratotic sole in this child virtually assures that the underlying gene defect involves *KRT1*.

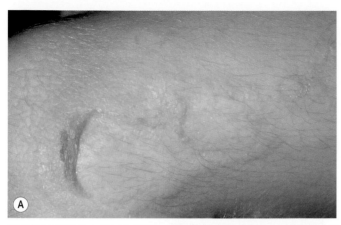

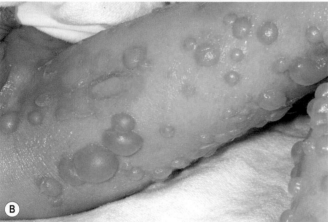

Figure 5.7 (A) Superficial epidermolytic ichthyosis. Note the milder hyperkeratosis and the 'molting' appearance of desquamation of superficial scale. (B) Occasionally, affected individuals may show tense bullae that resemble bullous pemphigoid (see Ch. 13). The bullae arose when he developed a viral exanthema.

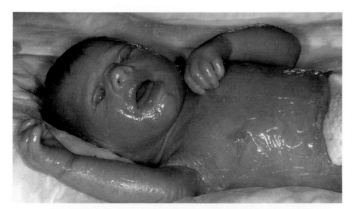

Figure 5.8 Collodion baby. Note the shiny thickened skin, mild ectropion, mild eclabium, and ear deformity. In this 5-day-old baby, the 'membrane' is starting to crack and desquamate.

during the first few days of life. Among the problems facing these infants are an inability to suck properly, respiratory difficulty due to restriction of chest expansion by the thick membrane, cutaneous and systemic infection, and aspiration pneumonia. Despite the thickening of the stratum corneum, this 'membrane' is a poor barrier, leading to excessive transcutaneous fluid and electrolyte

loss,[39] hypernatremic dehydration, increased metabolic requirements, and temperature instability.

Supportive care is of primary importance in the management of collodion babies. They are best managed in a humidified incubator, with special attention given to the prevention of temperature instability, sepsis, and fluid and electrolyte imbalance. Systemic antibiotic therapy should be initiated if infection is detected, but not prophylactically. Desquamation is encouraged by the application of emollients, rather than manual debridement; given the poor cutaneous barrier and potential toxicity, use of keratolytic agents should be avoided.

Autosomal Recessive Congenital Ichthyosis (ARCI)

ARCI encompasses a wide range of clinical phenotypes that range from classic harlequin ichthyosis (HI) and non-bullous congenital ichthyosiform erythroderma (CIE) to classic lamellar ichthyosis (LI).[40] The same individual may show a range of overlapping clinical features; e.g., retinoid treatment may decrease the lamellar scaling, but increase erythroderma.[41] Failure to thrive is a feature of ARCI, especially if severe, and short stature may ensue.[42] Overall, ARCI occurs in approximately 1 in 100 000–300 000 live births. The diagnosis is based on clinical findings; biopsy is not helpful, except if needed to exclude alternative diagnoses. The features of the ARCI group of disorders usually persist throughout the affected individual's lifetime. Many affected individuals complain of associated pruritus. Owing to the obstruction of eccrine glands by the overlying hyperkeratosis, severely affected patients tend to experience hyperpyrexia, heat intolerance, difficulty with perspiration, and heat exhaustion during periods of warm or hot humid weather and vigorous physical exercise.

Mutations in six known genes have been shown to result in the ARCI phenotype, and most of these mutated genes have been related to both LI and CIE phenotypes (Table 5.1). A few cases of autosomal dominant LI have been described,[43] but the underlying gene defect(s) have not been identified. The discovery of the underlying genetic basis in families with ARCI has facilitated the prenatal diagnosis based on genotyping, rather than the riskier diagnosis by fetal skin biopsy.[44] Up to 55% of individuals with ARCI have mutations in the gene encoding transglutaminase 1 (*TGM1*), particularly patients with the LI phenotype.[45] Transglutaminase-1 crosslinks several proteins to form the cornified envelope surrounding corneocytes. In patients missing transglutaminase, transglutaminase activity is undetectable in frozen skin specimens.[46,47] HI has been shown to result from nonsense mutations in the gene encoding the ABCA12 transporter.[48,49] Deficiency of ABCA12 leads to perturbation of lipid transport, leading to a paucity of lamellar bodies, the upper epidermal lamellar structures that provide intracellular lipids to the stratum corneum,[49,50] and to premature terminal differentiation of keratinocytes. ABCA12 also has been shown to be important for protease function.[51,52] Mutations in *ABCA12* that lead to the LI or CIE phenotype tend to be missense mutations,[53] so that some gene product is present for function, leading to the milder phenotype. Other genes found to be mutated in ARCI encode proteins of the hepoxilin pathway, including ALOXE3 (lipoxygenase-3), ALOX12B (12(R)-lipoxygenase),[54,55] NIPAL4 (ichthyin)[56,57,58] and CYP4F22. In addition to their disruption of stratum corneum lipid synthesis, these enzymes (or receptors) within the lipoxygenase pathway may also disrupt the processing of profilaggrin to filaggrin.[59]

The clinical features of the *classic LI* phenotype may range from very mild to severe. Individuals who show the greatest severity of LI have large lamellar plate-like scales with relatively mild underlying erythroderma, ectropion (eversion of an edge or margin of the eyelid resulting in exposure of the palpebral conjunctiva) (Fig. 5.9), and mild eclabium (eversion of the lips) (Table 5.1). Lamellar scales are large, quadrangular, yellow to brown-black, often thick, and centrally adherent with raised edges resembling armor plates (hence the term lamellar ichthyosis) (Fig. 5.10). Scales are most prominent over the face, trunk, and extremities, with a predilection for the flexor areas. Cheeks are often red, taut, and shiny; more scales appear on the forehead than on the lower portion of the face. The palms and soles are almost always affected in LI; severity varies from increased palmar markings to a thick

keratoderma with fissuring. The scalp is often scaly with scarring partial hair loss (especially with *TGM1* mutations). Involvement of the nails is variable. They may be stippled, pitted, ridged, or thickened, often with marked subungual hyperkeratosis.

Variant forms of LI from mutations in *TGM1* manifest in a more limited distribution of lesional skin. Patients with *bathing suit ichthyosis* (BSI) are born with a full collodion membrane and transition to LI, but within the first months of life, the scaling on the extremities clears (Fig. 5.11). The residual LI on warmer skin areas (axillae, trunk, scalp, neck) has been linked to temperature-sensitive mutations in *TGM1*.[2,60] Mutations in *TGM1* that encode proteins sensitive to hydrostatic pressure can result in the *self-healing collodion baby* (SHCB). Affected neonates show either a generalized or acral[61] collodion membrane at birth, which clears entirely as the baby transitions to the 'dry' environment postnatally.[36] The *TGM1* mutations in both BSI and SHCB phenotypes are missense mutations that are predominantly in the catalytic core domains.[62] ALOX12B and ALOX3B mutations have also been described with SHCB.[37,63]

Classic non-bullous congenital ichthyosiform erythroderma (CIE) is characterized by a much more prominent erythrodermic component, which may first become apparent as the collodion membrane is shed; some patients show CIE at birth without a classic collodion membrane. Affected individuals show fine white scales on the face, scalp, and trunk, although scaling may be more platelike scales on the extensor surfaces of the legs (Fig. 5.12). The degree of ectropion is variable, but often milder than with LI, and there is less palmoplantar keratoderma. Cicatricial alopecia is possible, and nails may show thickening and ridging. Some patients with CIE show intrauterine growth retardation and/or failure to thrive, although nutritional deficiency and gastrointestinal abnormalities are uncommon.[64] Patients with CIE may have associated neurologic abnormalities.

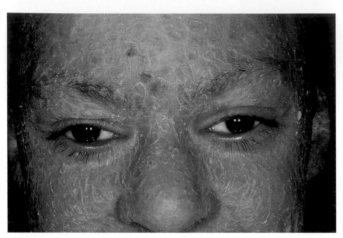

Figure 5.9 Lamellar ichthyosis phenotype of ARCI. Large plate-like scaling on the forehead and cheeks. This patient shows moderate ectropion.

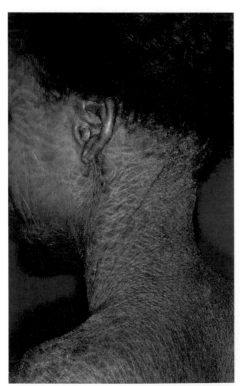

Figure 5.10 Lamellar ichthyosis phenotype of ARCI. Large plate-like scaling on the neck and trunk. The face appears less involved, because this teenager selectively applied tazarotene, a topical retinoid, to the face.

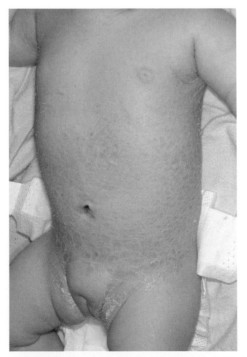

Figure 5.11 Bathing suit distribution, lamellar ichthyosis phenotype of ARCI. This distribution of the ichthyosis, largely involving the trunk and intertriginous areas with sparing of the face and limbs, signals a temperature-sensitive mutation in TGM1, encoding transglutaminase 1. This baby was born with a full collodion membrane.

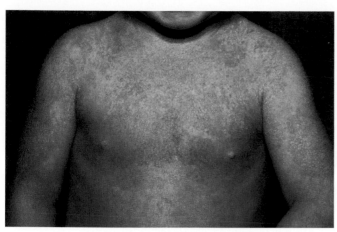

Figure 5.12 Congenital ichthyosiform erythroderma phenotype of ARCI. Marked erythroderma underlying fine white scaling.

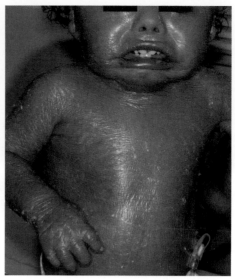

Figure 5.14 Harlequin ichthyosis. This boy survived the neonatal period without retinoid intervention and is thriving. Note the severe erythroderma with scaling, persistent eclabium and residual deformities of the fingers.

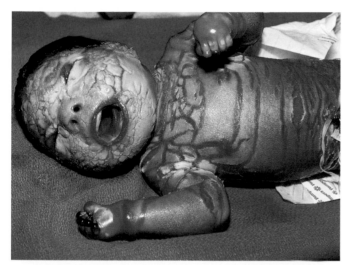

Figure 5.13 Harlequin ichthyosis. Profoundly thickened, armor-like skin with fissuring, leading to the polygonal, triangular, or diamond-shaped plaques that simulate the costume of a harlequin. Note the severe ectropion, eclabium, and the digital infarction. (Courtesy of Sylvia Suarez, MD.)

Harlequin ichthyosis is the most severe form of ARCI. At birth, the disorder manifests as profoundly thickened, armor-like skin that is fissured into polygonal, triangular, or diamond-shaped plaques that simulate the traditional costume of a harlequin (Fig. 5.13). Rigidity of the skin results in marked ectropion, everted O-shaped lips with a gaping fishmouth deformity, and a distorted, flattened, and undeveloped appearance to the nose and ears. The skin rigidity can restrict respiratory movements, sucking, and swallowing. The hands and feet are ischemic, hard, and waxy, often with poorly developed digits and an associated rigid and claw-like appearance. Flexion deformity of the limb joints is common, and the nails may be hypoplastic or absent. *Restrictive dermopathy* (see Ch. 6) shows congenital contractures, tight skin, ectropion and intrauterine growth retardation and can thus sometimes be confused with HI, but shows no hyperkeratosis or scaling.

Initiation of aggressive intervention for babies with HI is controversial. With the administration of systemic retinoids or spontaneous clearance of the armor-like scaling, the optimal outcome resembles that of severe CIE (Fig. 5.14). Thus, the decision to initiate systemic retinoids requires careful consideration. Physicians often reserve initiation for babies who survive the first few weeks, since most infants are stillborn or die during the neonatal period (usually during the first few hours or days of life). Death is usually associated with prematurity, pulmonary infection (associated with hypoventilation due to thoracic rigidity), poor feeding, excessive fluid loss, poor temperature regulation, or sepsis as a result of cutaneous infection. The severity may be variable, however, and prolonged survival has been achieved by intensive supportive measures, emollients and, in some cases, oral administration of systemic retinoids.[65] Surgical procedures may improve the cicatricial ectropion.[66] Prenatal diagnosis of harlequin ichthyosis has been suspected based on ultrasound-based discovery of distal arthrogryposis[67] and can be performed definitively by molecular analysis.[68]

Other Forms of Non-Syndromic Ichthyosis

Loricrin keratoderma

Loricrin keratoderma (also called Camisa, variant of Vohwinkel keratoderma) is an autosomal dominant disorder with ichthyosis and palmoplantar keratoderma.[69] Mutations occur in the gene encoding loricrin, a protein that is linked by transglutaminase-1 to involucrin and other proteins of the corneocyte envelope, thereby participating in barrier function and normal epidermal maturation.[70,71] Affected individuals may be born with a collodion membrane and later show a mild, non-erythrodermic generalized ichthyosis with flexural accentuation. The PPK is initially noted during the first weeks of age and shows a honeycomb pattern, resembling the Vohwinkel PPK caused by connexin 26 mutations (see below). Pseudoainhum (constricting bands of the digits) may occur, but usually not until adolescence or even adulthood; the starfish-shaped keratoses of Vohwinkel's are not seen with loricrin keratoderma. Alopecia is occasionally seen, but not other ectodermal abnormalities or hearing impairment. Parakeratosis on routine skin biopsy is a characteristic histologic feature. Nevertheless, the phenotype may be heterogeneous; termination mutations in the C-terminus have recently been linked to milder palmoplantar keratoderma without pseudoainhum and without parakeratosis on affected skin biopsy.[72]

Erythrokeratodermia variabilis

Erythrokeratodermia variabilis (EKV) is a dominantly inherited ichthyosis characterized by two distinct types of lesions: (1) Sharply marginated, pruritic or burning areas of erythema with finer scaling that are often figurate in configuration and undergo changes in size, shape, and distribution during a period of days to weeks; and (2) Hyperkeratotic plaques with thick, yellow-brown scales that usually overlie erythema (Fig. 5.15). Lesions are most often symmetrically distributed on the limbs, trunk, and buttock with relative sparing of the face, scalp, and flexures. In contrast to the chronic but remitting appearance of these plaques and figurate lesions, plaques on the knees, elbows, Achilles tendons, and soles of the feet are often persistent. Palmoplantar keratoderma has been described in 50% of affected families.

Although lesions are usually noted at birth or shortly thereafter during the first year of life, in a few individuals the onset has been noted during late childhood or early adulthood. The disorder may partially regress at puberty and tends to improve in summer. Patients usually tend to respond well to systemically administered retinoids.[73]

EKV is known to result from mutations in genes that both map to chromosome 1p35.1 and encode interacting connexins: *GJB3* encoding connexin 31[74] and *GJB4* gene encoding connexin 30.3.[75,76]

Progressive symmetric erythrokeratodermia

Progressive symmetric erythrokeratodermia (PSEK; Darier-Gottron syndrome) is a dominant disorder that tends to have its onset during infancy, tends to stabilize after 1 or 2 years, and may partially regress at puberty. It has been distinguished from EKV by the absence of the migrating red patches, the typical sparing of the chest and abdomen with scaling plaques limited to the extremities, buttocks, and face (Fig. 5.16), and a higher incidence of palmoplantar keratoderma (~50% of cases). Nevertheless, PSEK shares many clinical features with EKV, particularly the fixed, slowly progressive well-delineated keratotic plaques, and a G12D missense mutation in connexin 30.3 has been shown to cause both disorders.[77] A PSEK locus has also been found at chromosome 21q11, suggesting genetic heterogeneity,[78] although the manifestations in the affected family were atypical.[79]

Peeling skin syndrome

Peeling skin syndrome (PSS) or keratolysis exfoliativa congenita is an unusual autosomal recessive disease characterized by life-long, spontaneous superficial peeling of the skin that may be persistent or periodic.[80–82] The Nikolsky sign tends to be positive. The desquamation has been associated with increased stratum corneum and serum kallikrein levels. Two generalized types have been described. Type B results from loss of corneodesmin,[83] found in the corneum and hair follicle. The underlying genetic basis of type A is unclear. The desquamation is generalized, other than the palms and soles, which may be mildly thickened. Seasonal variation with worsening during summer months has been described.

In type A, the onset may be at birth, but commonly begins in early childhood (by 6 years of age). These patients are asymptomatic. Skin biopsy shows a thickened stratum corneum with an intracorneal or subcorneal separation. In type B, the condition always begins at birth. Patients show erythematous migratory peeling patches and complain of associated pruritus or burning. Patients with the type B form may show short stature and easily removable anagen hairs.[80] Biopsy specimens reveal psoriasiform thickening of the epidermis and a subcorneal split.

An acral form of hereditary PSS is characterized by life-long painless peeling of the hands and feet in superficial sheets[84] and exacerbation during summer months with increased sweating.[85] A facial variant has recently been described.[86] The acral form is caused by mutations in *TGM5* encoding transglutaminase-5,[87,88] which crosslinks epidermal proteins. Mutations in *TGM5* have not been found in the generalized forms,[87] and it is unclear why the manifestations of acral PSS are localized to the dorsal aspect of the hands and feet, given the widespread distribution of transglutaminase-5.

Keratosis linearis-ichthyosis congenital-keratoderma

Keratosis linearis-ichthyosis congenital-keratoderma (KLICK) is a rare, autosomal recessive disorder characterized by distinctive striate hyperkeratosis in the flexures (perpendicular to the fold) and palmoplantar keratoderma. It has been mapped to 13q, but the gene mutations have not been determined.[89,90]

Syndromic forms of ichthyosis

Syndromic forms of ichthyosis may be associated with a variety of extracutaneous abnormalities, most commonly involving the hair (e.g., Netherton, IFAP, and IHSC syndromes; ichthyosis with

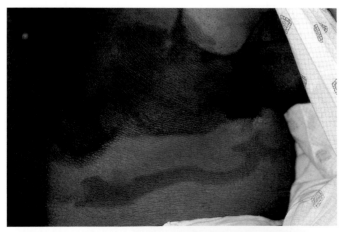

Figure 5.15 Erythrokeratodermia variabilis. This girl shows the fixed plaque form with thick hyperkeratotic plaques that overlie erythema. In darker skinned individuals, the plaques can be intensely hyperpigmented.

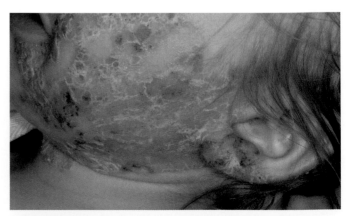

Figure 5.16 Progressive symmetric erythrokeratodermia. Well-demarcated erythematous scaling plaque on the face of a child. Thick erythematous plaques were also noted on the knees and dorsal aspect of the hands.

hypotrichosis; trichothiodystrophy) and neurologic system (e.g., Sjögren-Larsson, Refsum, CEDNIK and MEDNIK syndromes). Some syndromic disorders are lethal in the neonate (e.g., Neu-Laxova), infant (e.g., Gaucher disease type 2, ARC syndrome, multiple sulfatase deficiency) or child (e.g., CEDNIK syndrome).

Neutral Lipid Storage Disease with Ichthyosis

Neutral lipid storage disease with ichthyosis, or Chanarin–Dorfman syndrome, is a rare autosomal recessive disorder seen primarily in individuals of Middle Eastern or Mediterranean descent.[91] The clinical phenotype can variably include liver steatosis with hepatomegaly, muscle weakness/myopathy, ataxia, neurosensory hearing loss, subcapsular cataracts, nystagmus, strabismus, and mental retardation, but ichthyosis of the CIE phenotype is an almost constant finding. Patients are often born as collodion babies, occasionally with ectropion and eclabium. Skin biopsies show skin thickening with foamy keratinocyte cytoplasm owing to prominent neutral lipid droplets in the basal cells and eccrine glands seen best on oil red O-stained frozen sections. Serum lipids are normal, although the triglyceride content of lymphocytes, macrophages, and fibroblasts in culture is 2–20 times that of normal cells. Muscle and liver enzymes may be elevated two- to three-fold. The diagnosis is confirmed by a peripheral blood smear, which shows lipid droplets in granulocytes ('Jordan's anomaly') that are also seen in the leukocytes of heterozygous carriers of Chanarin–Dorfman syndrome. Mutations have been identified in the *ABHD5* or *CGI-58*,[92] a gene that encodes an enzyme expressed during differentiation in lipid transporting lamellar granules of epidermis[93] that is required for triglyceride degradation and normal barrier function.[94,95]

CHIME Syndrome

Individuals with CHIME syndrome (also called Zunich neuroectodermal syndrome) show a combination of *c*oloboma, *h*eart defects, *i*chthyosiform dermatosis, *m*ental retardation, and *e*ar anomalies, including conductive hearing loss.[96,97] The cause of the disorder is unknown. The skin is notably thickened and dry at birth, with pruritus often developing during the first months of life (Fig. 5.17). The colobomas are usually retinal, although choroidal colobomas have been described. Several heart defects, including pulmonic stenosis, ventricular septal defect, transposition of the great vessels, and tetralogy of Fallot, have been associated. Patients show a typical facies, with hypertelorism, a broad flat nasal root, upslanting palpebral fissures, epicanthic folds, a long columella but short philtrum, macrostomia, full lips, and cupped ears with rolled helices. All patients show brachydactyly. The hair may be fine and sparse, and trichorrhexis nodosa has occasionally been described. Some patients have renal or urologic anomalies, and cleft palate has been described in association.

KID Syndrome

KID syndrome is a rare autosomal dominant disorder characterized by *k*eratitis, congenital *i*chthyosis, and neurosensory *d*eafness.[98,99] Patients are usually born with erythematous skin, which progressively becomes more thickened and leathery during the first months of life. Generalized, tiny stippled papules are characteristic, and 90% of patients develop well-defined verrucous plaques, especially on the face and limbs. Alopecia may be congenital (25%) and ranges from sparse hair to total alopecia (Fig. 5.18); a thick yellow scale may cover the scalp at birth. Most patients show palmoplantar keratoderma with a stippled or leathery pattern. Nails tend to be dystrophic, and sweating may be diminished.

The hearing loss is congenital, neurosensory, and nonprogressive; it can be detected by brainstem auditory-evoked potential testing. In contrast, ocular features are rarely seen at birth, but progress and become evident by childhood or early adolescence. Photophobia may be the earliest sign, and the characteristic corneal vascularization and keratoconjunctivitis sicca lead to pannus formation and marked reduction in visual acuity.[100] KID syndrome must be distinguished from IFAP syndrome (Ch. 7), an ichthyotic condition in which patients have total alopecia, thickened skin with spiny projections, palmoplantar keratoderma, and photophobia with decreased visual acuity.

Almost half of KID patients have recurrent infections of the skin, eyes, and ear canals, with bacterial and candidal infections predominating.[98,101] Some patients have demonstrated abnormal chemotaxis and impaired lymphocyte proliferative responses to *Candida albicans*. The follicular occlusion syndrome (including hidradenitis suppurativa) has been described in some patients, may lead to scarring alopecia, and may require surgical intervention.[102] More than 10% of patients develop squamous cell carcinoma of the skin or tongue,[98,103] occasionally during childhood, and follicular

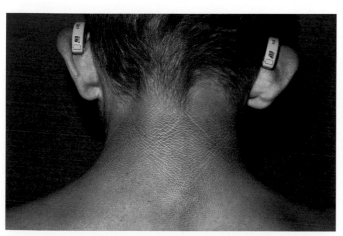

Figure 5.17 CHIME syndrome. Thickened skin on the back of the neck. Note the hearing aids because of conductive hearing loss.

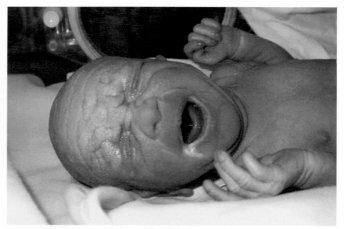

Figure 5.18 KID syndrome. Markedly thickened skin with fine stippling on the cheeks and perioral skin. Note the total alopecia in this patient who was found to have a mutation in *GJB2*, which encodes connexin 26. (Courtesy of Amy Theos, MD.)

tumors have also been described.[104,105] Dandy-Walker malformation has been described in several affected individuals.[106]

The disorder results from mutations in one of two connexins (proteins critical in intercellular communication), either connexin 26[107] or connexin 30 (GJB6).[108,109] The latter connexin is also mutated in patients with Clouston syndrome, which shares the alopecia, nail dystrophy, palmoplantar keratoderma, and sometimes photophobia of KID syndrome (see Ch. 7). Therapy is largely supportive. Chronic administration of fluconazole has improved the verrucous plaques of cutaneous candidiasis.[110] Cochlear implants and corneal transplants have been used to correct the sensorineural hearing loss and corneal vascularization, respectively.[100,111–113]

Netherton Syndrome

Netherton syndrome (NS) is an autosomal recessive condition that combines ichthyosis, atopy, and hair shaft deformities. Netherton syndrome presents during the neonatal or early infantile period with generalized scaling erythroderma, but not a collodion baby phenotype. Neonates with Netherton syndrome are usually born prematurely, and develop the eruption *in utero* or during the first weeks of life. Failure to thrive is often profound, requiring hospitalization for nutritional support and correction of the hypernatremic dehydration that may be associated.[114]

Patients may have diarrhea, associated with intestinal villus atrophy, and the majority experience sepsis, upper and lower respiratory infections, and cutaneous *S. aureus* infection.[115] Adults with Netherton syndrome are also at risk for extensive papillomavirus infection,[116] usually involving the genital region. A variety of immunologic abnormalities have been described, suggesting that Netherton syndrome should be considered a primary immunodeficiency disorder. These include reduced memory B cells, defective response to vaccination, impaired antibody amplification and class switching, decreased natural killer (NK) cell cytotoxicity, a skewed Th1 phenotype, and increased proinflammatory cytokine levels.[115] Treatment with intravenous immunoglobulin may cause an increase in NK cell cytotoxicity and clinical improvement.[115]

Ichthyosis linearis circumflexa, the characteristic skin change associated with NS, is characterized by migratory, polycyclic scaly lesions with a peripheral double-edged scale (Fig. 5.19). Although most commonly seen in association with NS, patients may show only the ichthyosis linearis circumflexa without the hair shaft abnormalities or other features of NS. Ichthyosis linearis circumflexa is not generally seen before 2 years of age, and occurs eventually in only 70% of patients. The ichthyosiform erythroderma that is the typical manifestation in the neonatal and infantile periods tends to improve with increasing age. Partial remissions have been noted and spontaneous fluctuation is common, but there is little tendency to spontaneous resolution. Routine histologic examination of skin biopsy sections is not helpful, but electron microscopic studies have revealed features that are specific to NS.[117,118]

The classic hair shaft abnormality, trichorrhexis invaginata ('bamboo hairs', 'ball-and-socket deformity'), is thought to result from a defect in keratinization of the internal root sheath. The hair defect results in easy hair breakage and hair that is poorly manageable, dry, and lusterless (Fig. 5.20; see also Ch. 7, Fig. 7.5). Multiple hairs from different areas should be examined, since only 20–50% of hairs may be affected. Examination of hairs from the eyebrow region often is most fruitful, and dermoscopy facilitates visualization of the 'matchstick' hair defect.[119,120] Finding the hair shaft disorder is particularly difficult in the affected neonate.

NS results from mutations in *SPINK5*, which encodes lymphoepithelial Kazal-type-related inhibitor (*LETKI*), a serine protease inhibitor.[121] Immunohistochemical studies show absent or reduced expression of LEKTI.[122,123] The increase in serine protease activity (kallikrein 5) leads to decreases in desmosomal proteins (desmoglein 1 and desmocollin 1) with premature degradation of corneocyte desmosomes and excessive desquamation).[124–126] Approximately two-thirds of patients show pruritic atopic-like dermatitis, food allergies, urticaria, angioedema, asthma, and/or anaphylaxis. In addition, most patients have increased levels of circulating eosinophils and IgE. These atopic manifestations likely result from the unregulated kallikrein 5 activity, which activates PAR-2 and TSLP (as in atopic dermatitis, see Ch. 3), as well as other cytokines,[127] and contributes to both the very poor skin barrier and the cutaneous inflammation. The marked impairment in barrier function can lead to significant absorption of topically applied medication, necessitating careful monitoring of serum levels or adrenal suppression. Application of hydrocortisone 1% ointment caused Cushing syndrome in an 11-year-old boy, and immunosuppressive serum levels may be detectable after application of tacrolimus ointment.[128] Nevertheless, several patients have responded well to application of topical calcineurin inhibitors without detectable absorption.[129,130]

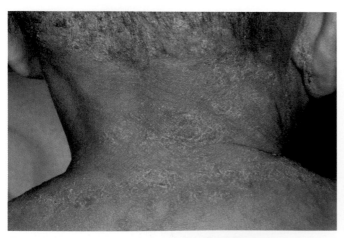

Figure 5.19 Netherton syndrome. Polycyclic scaling lesions, many showing the scale edge. Note the underlying erythroderma, scalp involvement and short hair.

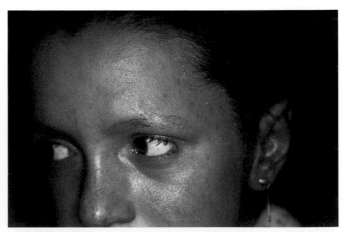

Figure 5.20 Netherton syndrome. Dry lusterless hair that breaks and thus remains short and unmanageable. Note the eyebrow alopecia and facial erythroderma.

Netherton syndrome should be distinguished from other forms of ichthyosis with abnormal hair. *Trichothiodystrophy* shows a variety of hair shaft defects under light microscopy, but a characteristic 'tiger tail' appearance under polarized microscopy. Patients with trichothiodystrophy and ichthyosis may also have brittle hair, impaired intelligence, decreased fertility, short stature, and photosensitivity (Ch. 7).[131] Hypotrichosis and ichthyosis are features of two recently described autosomal recessive disorders: *ichthyosis hypotrichosis syndrome* (*IHS*, also called *autosomal recessive ichthyosis with hypotrichosis* or *ARIH syndrome*) and *ichthyosis-hypotrichosis-sclerosing cholangitis* (*IHSC* or *NISCH*) *syndrome*.[132,133] Diffuse non-scarring alopecia of the scalp, eyelashes, and eyebrows is present at birth in IHS, but tends to improve with time to sparse, unruly hair during adolescence and merely recession of the frontal hair line by adulthood.[134,135] Patchy follicular atrophoderma and hypohidrosis may be associated. The congenital lamellar ichthyosis tends to be generalized, but tends to spare the face, palms and soles. Patients may show photophobia from corneal abnormalities, blepharitis, and dental abnormalities.[136] Microscopic evaluation may show pili torti or pili bifurcati. IHS results from mutations in *ST14*, leading to a deficiency of matriptase and defective processing of profilaggrin.[135,137] IHSC (also called NISCH syndrome) manifests at birth or shortly thereafter with generalized xerosis and fine to polygonal scaling, predominantly on the limbs and abdomen, but sparing the skinfolds, palms and soles.[132,138] The hair tends to be coarse and curly with frontotemporal cicatricial alopecia. Neonatal jaundice with hepatomegaly is often seen from congenital paucity of bile ducts or sclerosing cholangitis. Most patients show oligodontia and enamel dysplasia, and small eosinophil and keratinocyte vacuoles without lipid contents have been noted.[138] IHSC results from mutations in *CLDN1*, the gene encoding claudin, a structural protein of the tight junctions of epidermis.[133]

Refsum Disease

Refsum disease is an autosomal recessive neurocutaneous disorder caused by deficiency in oxidation of phytanic acid, a branched, long-chain fatty acid derived from dietary chlorophyll.[139,140] The clinical features usually develop in late childhood or early adult life and progress slowly during months to several years. Neurological manifestations are most prominent and include sensorineural deafness, anosmia, failing vision, night blindness due to retinitis pigmentosa and a progressive weakness, foot drop, and loss of balance due to a mixed sensorimotor neuropathy and cerebellar involvement. Delayed diagnosis may result in severe neurological impairment, wasting, and depression. The associated ichthyosis, which can either coincide or postdate the neurological features, resembles ichthyosis vulgaris or, in severe untreated cases, lamellar ichthyosis. Accentuated palmoplantar markings are associated.

Refsum disease results from mutations in one of two genes, either PHYH (also named PAHX), which encodes the peroxisomal enzyme phytanoyl-CoA hydroxylase, or PEX7, which encodes the PTS2 (peroxisomal targeting signal 2) receptor.[141] Phytanic acid cannot be synthesized by humans and is mainly derived from plant chlorophyll. Normally serum levels are undetectably low, but in Refsum disease may account for up to 30% of serum lipids. The accumulation of phytanic acid disturbs the cholesterol balance and may alter lipid degradation. Histology shows variably sized vacuoles in the epidermal basal and suprabasal cells, corresponding to the lipid accumulation seen with lipid stains of frozen sections. The diagnosis is based on the demonstration of increased levels of phytanic acid in the patient's serum, tissue, or urine. Therapy consists of a chlorophyll-free diet and avoidance of phytanic acid-containing foods.

Sjögren–Larsson Syndrome

The ichthyosis of the autosomal recessive disorder, Sjögren–Larsson syndrome (SLS), usually manifests in the neonatal period as fine, white scaling, accentuated in flexural areas.[142] Erythema is occasionally present at birth, but clears within months. Presentation as a collodion baby is rare. By 1 year of age, the ichthyosis of Sjögren–Larsson syndrome is not erythrodermic, but shows generalized velvety lamellar thickening (often with a yellowish hue), particularly on the trunk and neck, with minimal desquamation (Fig. 5.21), palmoplantar keratoderma, and relative sparing of the face.[143,144] The skin is characteristically pruritic, and most patients are hypohidrotic. The degree of scaling varies from mild to severe (Fig. 5.22), and does not change with increasing age.[145] Hair and nails are normal. The neurologic disease usually becomes within the first year with failure to reach normal developmental milestones

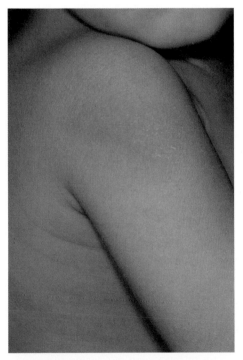

Figure 5.21 Sjögren–Larsson syndrome. The skin shows velvety lamellar thickening with a yellowish hue and minimal desquamation.

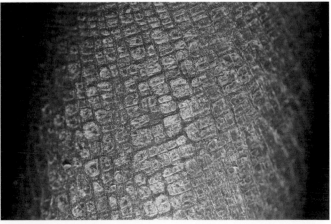

Figure 5.22 Sjögren–Larsson syndrome. Thick lamellar scaling in an adolescent with severe retardation.

and the onset of spasticity. Phenotypic variability is seen, and some patients have been described with mild neurologic features of SLS without associated skin disease.[146] Spasticity and muscle paresis is most pronounced in the legs,[145] and most affected persons become dependent on a wheelchair for mobility. Most patients have learning disability to a variable degree and a speech disorder, and some show seizures, short stature, kyphosis, and enamel hypoplasia. The pathognomonic retinal 'glistening dots' are not present in all patients, but photophobia is common.

SLS results from mutations in the fatty aldehyde dehydrogenase gene (*FALDH* or *ALDH3A2*), a component of fatty alcohol: nicotinamide adenine dinucleotide oxidoreductase (FAO), which converts fatty alcohol to fatty acid.[147] Epidermal cells in affected individuals show abnormal lamellar bodies and lipid droplets, consistent with defective lipid metabolism.[148] Prenatal diagnosis of SLS is possible by measurement of FAO activity in cultured amniocytes or chorionic cells, histologic analysis, and/or analysis of fetal DNA if the gene defect is known. The ichthyosis is treated with topical keratolytic agents and retinoids;[145] dietary supplementation with medium-chain fatty acids are generally not helpful.[143] The leukotriene inhibitor zileuton may decrease the associated pruritus,[149] but no therapy to date has been found to slow the progressive neurologic deterioration.

Ichthyosis Prematurity Syndrome

Ichthyosis prematurity syndrome (IPS) is an autosomal recessive disorder in which affected babies are born more than 6 weeks prematurely in association with polyhydramnios and opaque amniotic fluid because of the extensive shedding of epidermal cells.[150,151] Typically, neonates show respiratory distress (which may be lethal) and generalized thick spongy desquamating skin that resembles vernix caseosa, accentuated on the scalp and eyebrows. During the neonatal period, the scaling may resemble cobblestones overlying moderate erythroderma. Although the marked thickening clears in survivors, xerosis with follicular keratosis persists, and patients often show atopic dermatitis, dermographism, asthma, and eosinophilia. Mutations have been identified in SLC27A4, the fatty acid transport protein 4 gene, which encodes a fatty acid transporter and leads to defective stratum corneum lipid homeostasis.

Some autosomal recessive forms of ichthyosis are associated with a high risk of early death. Neu–Laxova syndrome is characterized by severe intrauterine growth retardation, an edematous appearance, microcephaly, and abnormal brain development with lissencephaly and agenesis of the corpus callosum.[152–155] The ichthyosis tends to be present at birth, but ranges in severity from mild ichthyosis to a harlequin ichthyosis appearance. Patients tend to show typical facies, including protuberant eyes with a flattened nose, slanted forehead, micrognathia, deformed ears, and a short neck. Some affected neonates show microphthalmia or cleft palate. Syndactyly, limb or digital hypoplasia, and limb contractures are common, and X-rays often show poor bone mineralization. These craniofacial and limb defects have been seen in a variety of syndromes with reduced intrauterine movement (fetal akinesia/hypokinesis sequence).

Gaucher Syndrome Type 2

Gaucher syndrome type 2 results from an absence of lysosomal β-glucocerebrosidase, which hydrolyzes glucosylceramide to ceramide. The neonate with type 2 Gaucher (acute infantile cerebral form) may present as a collodion baby,[156,157] with the onset during infancy of neurologic signs and hepatosplenomegaly.[158] Glucosylceramide and ceramide are critical components of the intercellular

bilayers of the stratum corneum and play a role in epidermal barrier function.[159] The absence of glucocerebrosidase leads to abnormal skin thickening and increased transepidermal water loss. Even when the skin appears normal clinically in affected patients, ultrastructural abnormalities in lamellar membranes may be seen.[160] Despite enzyme replacement therapy, non-neurologic manifestations of Gaucher disease may progress.[161]

Cerebral dysgenesis-neuropathy-ichthyosis-palmoplantar keratoderma (CEDNIK) syndrome first manifests between 5 and 11 months of age, with progressive neurologic deterioraton.[162] Affected infants show a generalized mild LI phenotype with sparing of skin folds but palmoplantar thickening. The hair tends to be fine and sparse. Microcephaly, neuropathy, cerebral dysgenesis, sensorineural deafness, optic nerve atrophy, neurogenic muscle atrophy, and cachexia are associated, and affected individuals usually die within the first decade of life. Patients with CEDNIK syndrome have mutations in *SNAP29*, a component of the secretory (SNARE) pathway that is important for vesicle fusion and lamellar granule maturation and secretion. In CEDNIK syndrome, glucosylceramide and kallikrein-containing granules are abnormally retained in the stratum corneum, leading to retention hyperkeratosis and an abnormal epidermal barrier.

Mental Retardation–Enteropathy–Deafness–Neuropathy–Ichthyosis–Keratoderma (MEDNIK) Syndrome

MEDNIK syndrome is an autosomal recessive disorder that shows manifestations at birth or within the first weeks of life.[163,164] Among the ichthyoses, it most closely resembles erythrokeratodermia variabilis and, in fact, has also been called EKV3. Nail thickening and mucosal involvement may be associated. Patients show congenital sensorineural deafness, psychomotor and growth retardation, mental retardation and peripheral neuropathy. The severe congenital chronic diarrhea is life threatening. MEDNIK syndrome results from mutations in *AP1S1*, encoding a subunit (1A) of an adaptor protein complex (AP-1) that is involved in the organization and transport of proteins during skin and spinal cord development.

Arthrogryposis–Renal Dysfunction–Cholestasis (ARC) Syndrome

ARC syndrome presents with generalized desquamative lamellar scaling within the first days to weeks of life, but not at birth.[165–167] Ectropion and mild scarring alopecia may be present. The distinguishing features are the associated arthrogryposis (contractures of the limbs, particularly of the knee, hip and wrist; rocker bottom feet; talipes equinovarus), renal tubular degeneration with metabolic acidosis, and intrahepatic bile duct hypoplasia with cholestasis. Patients may also show cerebral malformations, hypothyroidism, deafness, dysmorphic features and large, dysfunctional platelets. Death ensues during the first year of life. ARC syndrome results from mutations in VPS33B, which regulates SNARE protein-mediated fusion of membrane vesicles required for lamellar body secretion. Incomplete ARC syndrome has been described without the arthrogryposis.[168]

Conradi Syndrome

The key clinical features of Conradi–Hünermann–Happle (CHH) syndrome (also called X-linked dominant chondrodysplasia punctata type II) are linear ichthyosis, chondrodysplasia punctata, cataracts, and short stature. Neonates tend to show severe ichthyosiform erythroderma with patterned yellowish markedly hyperkeratotic plaques. After the first 3–6 months of life the erythroderma and scaling resolve, leaving erythema and later follicular atrophoderma in a distribution that follows Blaschko's lines, hypo- and hyperpigmented streaks, particularly on the trunk (Fig. 5.23), and circumscribed cicatricial alopecia of the scalp and eyebrows (Fig. 5.24). Patients may show persistent psoriasiform lesions in intertriginous areas (ptychotropism) (Fig. 5.25). In addition to the cutaneous findings, patients with CHH show asymmetric skeletal involvement with punctate calcification of the epiphyseal regions that usually results in an asymmetric shortening of the long bones (especially the humeri and femora) and sometimes in severe kyphoscoliosis, facial dysplasia, and hip dislocation. Unilateral or bilateral sectorial cataracts, patchy coarse lusterless hair, nasal bone dysplasia with saddle-nose deformity (Fig. 5.24), and a high-arched palate further characterize the disease. The bony abnormalities, but not the skin lesions of CHH syndrome, have been described in association with teratogenic exposures to medications and infections, and maternal autoimmune diseases.[169]

X-chromosomal inactivation explains the distribution of skin lesions along Blaschko's lines, the sectorial cataracts, and the asymmetric skeletal abnormalities. Abnormal cholesterol synthesis/metabolism has been detected in patients with CHH, and mutations have been identified in *EBP*, which encodes 3β-hydroxysteroid-Δ8, Δ7-isomerase (emopamil binding protein), a key component in cholesterol biosynthesis. Abnormal lamellar granules and malformed intercellular lipid layers have been detected ultrastructurally,[170] and plasma sterol analysis shows markedly elevated levels of 8(9) cholesterol and 8-dehydrocholesterol.[171]

Child Syndrome

The CHILD syndrome is a congenital disorder characterized by *c*ongenital *h*emidysplasia, *i*chthyosiform erythroderma, and *l*imb *d*efects. Also known as unilateral congenital ichthyosiform erythroderma, the hallmark of the disorder is the sharp midline demarcation and its largely unilateral cutaneous and skeletal features (Fig. 5.26). This X-linked dominant condition occurs almost exclusively in girls, and is presumed to be lethal in affected males. The only

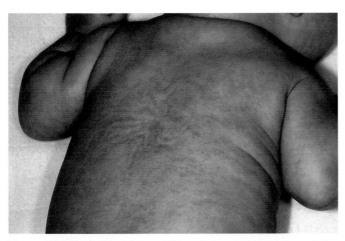

Figure 5.23 Conradi syndrome. Mild erythema and hyperpigmentation in a distribution that follows Blaschko's lines in this infant after clearing her congenital scaling.

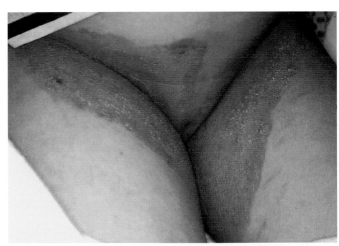

Figure 5.25 Conradi syndrome. Bilateral ptychotropism with psoriasiform plaques.

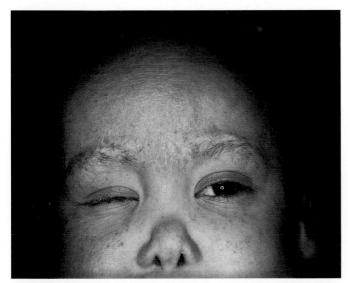

Figure 5.24 Conradi syndrome. Cicatricial alopecia of the eyebrows. Approximately half of her scalp hair was replaced by cicatricial alopecia as well. Note the deformity of the nose.

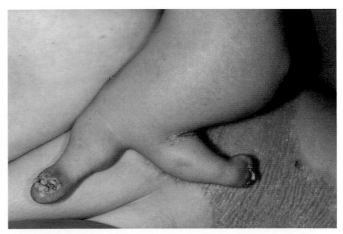

Figure 5.26 CHILD syndrome. Unilateral congenital ichthyosiform erythroderma with marked deformity of the arm. This girl's ipsilateral leg was also markedly shortened and required amputation.

case in a boy is thought to represent early postzygotic mosaicism.[172] The inflammatory ichthyosiform skin lesions of CHILD syndrome may be present at birth or develop during the first few months of life. They are characterized by yellow and waxy scaling and/or streaks of inflammation and scaling that is often patchy but may follow Blaschko's lines. Similarly, streaks of normal skin may be interspersed within the area of the CHILD nevus. Unilateral alopecia and severe nail dystrophy with claw-like nails have been described. The face is typically spared. With increasing age, lesions may improve or even clear spontaneously, but lesions in intertriginous areas (ptychotropism) tend to persist and be the most severely affected sites.[173] Rarely a localized hyperkeratotic plaque with a sharp demarcation at the midline is the sole manifestation of the CHILD syndrome ('CHILD nevus') (Fig. 5.27). A mild form of CHILD syndrome has been described in three generations,[174] suggesting genetic control of the skewing of X inactivation.[175]

Ipsilateral skeletal hypoplasia, ranging in severity from hypoplasia of the fingers to complete agenesis of an extremity, is an important feature of CHILD syndrome. As with the skin changes, unilaterality is not absolute, and slight changes may be present on the contralateral side. Punctate epiphyseal calcifications may be demonstrable by radiography, but tend to disappear after the first few years of life. Cardiovascular and renal abnormalities are the major visceral manifestations of CHILD syndrome, although anomalies of other viscera have been described. Biopsy of skin lesions shows epidermal thickening with characteristic infiltration of the papillary dermis of histiocytes showing foamy cytoplasm ('verruciform xanthoma'). Inactivating mutations have been identified in the *NSDHL* gene encoding a 3β-hydroxysteroid dehydrogenase,[176] which functions upstream of EBP in the cholesterol synthesis pathway. Treatment with keratolytic agents and retinoids is poorly

tolerated, but topical application of 2% lovastatin/2% cholesterol has led to dramatic improvement.

Treatment of Lesional Skin of Non-Syndromic and Syndromic Ichthyoses

Treatment of patients with most forms of ichthyosis involves topical application of keratolytic agents and topical or systemic administration of retinoids.[3] FIRST, the Foundation for Ichthyosis and Related Skin Types (www.firstskinfoundation.org), is a support group for patients and families with disorders of cornification. In additional to educational materials, FIRST provides information about commercially available treatment options. Several other foundations worldwide support families with ichthyosis and have educational websites as well (e.g., www.ichthyosis.org.uk and www.ictiosis.org).

The management of all types of ichthyosis consists of retardation of water loss, rehydration and softening of the stratum corneum, and alleviation of scaliness and associated pruritus. Daily to twice daily baths using a superfatted soap or a soapless cleanser, followed immediately by application of the emollient to moist skin, can be helpful for all forms. Shorter baths are preferred for patients with ichthyosis vulgaris, especially with associated atopic dermatitis. However, many patients with LI or EI have found long baths to be particularly helpful. Ichthyosis vulgaris and recessive X-linked ichthyosis can be managed quite well by topical application of emollients and the use of keratolytic agents to facilitate removal of scales from the skin surface. α-Hydroxy acid preparations, such as lactic and glycolic acids, are the most commonly used as agents to desquamate excessive scale and increase hydration. Urea, in concentrations of 10–20%, has a softening and moisturizing effect on the stratum corneum and is helpful in the control of dry skin and pruritus. Propylene glycol (40–60% in water), applied overnight under plastic occlusion, hydrates the skin and causes desquamation of scales. Salicylic acid is another effective keratolytic agent and can be compounded into petrolatum at concentrations between 3% and 6% to promote shedding of scales and softening of the stratum corneum. When it is used to cover large surface areas for prolonged periods, however, patients should be monitored for salicylate toxicity, most commonly complaints of tinnitus. The combination of 6% salicylic acid in propylene glycol may be particularly helpful for keratoderma of the palms and soles, especially when used under occlusive wraps. The lamellar ichthyosis phenotype of ARCI generally requires more potent keratolytic agents; individuals with milder forms of LI often respond well to the topical application of the retinoid, tazarotene (Fig. 5.28).[177,178] As the skin normalizes, the risk of irritation from tazarotene increases, often requiring therapy to be intermittent. In contrast, the skin of EI is quite fragile, and patients generally will tolerate intermittent use of keratolytic agents only for short periods, if at all. Similarly, individuals with Netherton syndrome and CHILD syndrome tolerate topically applied keratolytic agents poorly. It should be remembered that individuals with ichthyosis usually have a barrier abnormality that can lead to increased percutaneous absorption. Although topical antiinflammatory medications may be used for associated dermatitis or to decrease intense pruritus, the risk of detectable levels of corticosteroids or calcineurin inhibitors must be kept in mind. For example, topical tacrolimus ointment has been found to be helpful for individuals with Netherton syndrome, but toxic levels have sometimes been detected,[128] emphasizing the need for careful monitoring.[179]

Oral retinoids (isotretinoin, acitretin) have led to dramatic improvement in some pediatric patients with the ichthyoses, but should be used with caution because of their many potential side-effects that limit long-term therapy, particularly bone toxicity.[180]

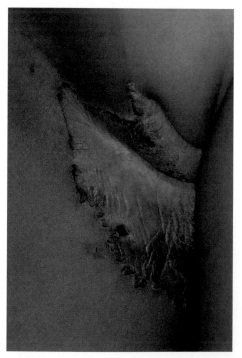

Figure 5.27 CHILD nevus. The ptychotropism of a sharply demarcated thickened plaque of the inguinal area that ends abruptly at the midline. This girl showed mild thickening and hyperpigmentation involving only the right side of her body, but no limb deformities or hemidysplasia.

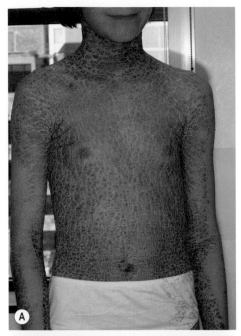

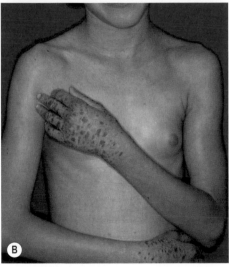

Figure 5.28 (A,B) Clearance of the lamellar phenotype of ichthyosis with topically applied tazarotene. After 2 months of nightly application of tazarotene 0.1% cream, this girl experienced remarkable improvement in her ichthyosis.

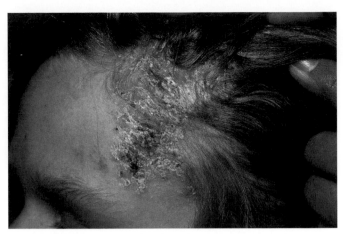

Figure 5.29 Darier disease. Thickened, warty plaques on the forehead and temples are characteristic and tend to be symmetrically distributed.

5–10 cc per 3.8 liters; one-half cup per full standard tub) or baking soda (1 cup) into the bath water. Dermatophyte infections often require administration of systemic antifungal medications.

Sweating is often inadequate in patients with ichthyosis owing to the occlusion of eccrine ducts. Affected individuals should be guarded against overheating during winter months, and kept in air-conditioning during warmer months, with frequent wetting of the skin or even cooling suits (see Ch. 7) during sports activities. The ectropion of patients with ARCI exposes the conjunctivae and cornea, resulting in irritation. Bland moisturizing drops can be administered several times daily to provide protective moisture, and patients may benefit from wearing eye patches at night if the eyes cannot close entirely. Some physicians recommend plastic surgery to correct the ectropion, since damage to the cornea may impair vision, but this surgery is complex, often unsuccessful, and should be discouraged. Periorbital application of small amounts of tazarotene 0.05% cream can be helpful.

In countries without significant dietary supplementation with vitamin D3, children must have adequate exposure to ultraviolet B light to prevent the development of rickets. Ichthyosis, and particularly the epidermolytic and lamellar forms, has been associated with an increased risk of the development of rickets.[185–188] The increased risk may relate to decreased ultraviolet light exposure, failure of UVB to penetrate the thickened scale, and/or an abnormality in processing of vitamin D3 in response to UVB. Nevertheless, vitamin D3 supplementation should be considered.

Other disorders of differentiation

Darier Disease

Darier disease (keratosis follicularis, Darier–White disease; acral form, acrokeratosis verruciformis of Hopf) is an autosomal dominant disorder that most commonly first manifests between 8 and 15 years of age, as flesh-colored papules that become covered with a yellow, waxy scaling crust (Figs 5.29, 5.30).[189] Lesions often coalesce to form thickened, warty plaques that are malodorous. Sites most often affected include the forehead, temples, ears, nasolabial folds, scalp, upper chest and back, in the so-called 'seborrheic' distribution. Isolated scalp involvement has been reported, and may be the presenting sign.[190] Linear streaks of Darier disease along Blaschko's lines have been attributed to gene mosaicism.[191] Localized congenital Darier disease has been described and likely

Liarozole, a retinoic acid metabolism blocking agent (RAMBA),[181] has shown the efficacy of acitretin with fewer retinoic acid-related adverse events.[182–184] These systemic agents are generally reserved for use in adolescents and adults with more severe ichthyotic disorders that do not show a satisfactory response to topical agents.

Patients with the ichthyoses tend to be more susceptible to cutaneous infection, particularly dermatophyte and staphylococcal infections. Secondary infection should be considered when patients with ichthyosis (particularly ARCI and EI) develop a new eruption. The accumulation of scale predisposes to overgrowth of bacteria and an odor, which in addition to the significant cosmetic ramifications of these disorders, may lead to additional problems in social acceptance by peers. Patients with thick scale may benefit from use of mild antibacterial soaps (e.g., Lever 2000 or Cetaphil antibacterial soap) or use of antibacterial washes if not too irritating. Many patients benefit from the addition of bleach (1–2 tsp per gallon or

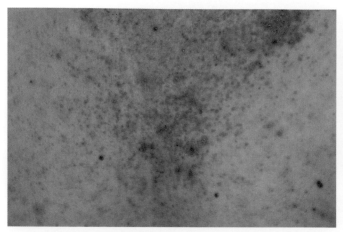

Figure 5.30 Darier disease. The discrete keratotic papules of Darier syndrome have led to the alternative name of keratosis follicularis.

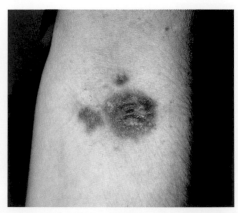

Figure 5.31 Hailey–Hailey disease. Crusted, erosive plaques that are symmetrically distributed, especially at fold areas.

represents type 2 mosaicism.[192] Lesions of Darier disease are often worsened by exposure to ultraviolet radiation, heat, friction, and other forms of trauma. Secondary bacterial or herpes simplex virus infection is common.[193]

Punctate keratoses on the palms and soles, either raised or with a central pit, occur in most patients. Keratoses resembling flat warts may be found on the dorsal aspects of the hands (acrokeratosis verruciformis). In some patients, these acral keratotic lesions are the only manifestation. The nails are easily broken and often show a characteristic V-shaped scalloping of the free edge (see Ch. 7, Fig. 7.62). Subungual thickening with streaks of discoloration and subungual hemorrhage may be seen. White, centrally depressed-papules or verrucous white plaques simulating leukoplakia are often seen on the mucosae of the cheeks, palate, and gums[194] and may involve the rectum and vulva. Neuropsychiatric problems including mental handicap, schizophrenia, bipolar disorder, and/or seizures are seen in approximately 5% of patients,[195] and bone cysts may be associated with Darier disease as well.[196]

The characteristic histopathologic changes of Darier disease include intraepidermal suprabasal clefts or lacunae and the formation of acantholytic 'corps ronds' (cells with a basophilic nucleus surrounded by a clear halo) and 'grains' (small dark cells with a pyknotic nucleus) in the stratum corneum. Mutations responsible for Darier disease involve ATP2A2, which encodes the sarco/endoplasmic reticulum calcium ATPase type 2 (SERCA2).[197] Epidermal differentiation requires elevations in calcium levels for intercellular junction assembly, and the affected enzyme participates in the calcium pump system.[198–202] and systemic[203,204] administration of retinoids has resulted in significant improvement in affected individuals.[205] Topical application of 5-fluorouracil[206,207] and tacrolimus ointment[208] have more recently been reported to be helpful. Recalcitrant areas have been treated successfully with carbon dioxide, erbium:YAG and pulsed dye lasers.[209–211]

Hailey–Hailey Disease (Familial Benign Pemphigus)

Hailey–Hailey disease is an autosomal dominant genodermatosis characterized by recurrent vesicles and erosions, which most commonly appear on the sides and back of the neck, in the axillae, in the groin, and in the perianal regions (Fig. 5.31).[212] The disorder is not seen before puberty and usually has its onset in the late teens or early 20s. Most cases have a fairly constant course. The primary

lesions are small vesicles that occur in groups on normal or erythematous skin. The vesicles may enlarge to form bullae and rupture easily, leaving an eroded base; they exude serum and develop crusts resembling impetigo. The Nikolsky sign may be present. Lesions tend to spread peripherally, with an active, often serpiginous border, and central resolution with peripheral extension often results in circinate lesions. In the intertriginous area lesions tend to form erythematous plaques with dry crusting and soft, flat, and moist granular vegetations. Burning or pruritus is common and, particularly in the intertriginous areas, lesions tend to become irritating, painful, and exceedingly uncomfortable. As with Darier disease, mosaic forms of Hailey–Hailey have been described and course along lines of Blaschko;[213] streaks of Hailey–Hailey disease may present during childhood in individuals with genomic ATP2C1 mutations who develop a second mutation in the normal allele (type 2 mosaicism).[214]

Mucosal involvement is uncommon, but papular lesions of the oral mucosa, esophagus, vagina, and conjunctivae have been described. Patients may experience spontaneous improvement, with exacerbations and remissions.

Skin sections from the advancing border of a lesion show a suprabasal vesicle with acantholysis of epidermal cells, resembling a 'dilapidated brick wall'. Mutations have been identified in ATP2C1, encoding a secretory Ca^{++}/Mn^{++}-ATPase pump of the Golgi apparatus.[215]

The cutaneous lesions of familial benign pemphigus are induced by several external stimuli, particularly heat, humidity, friction from ill-fitting clothing, exposure to ultraviolet light, and bacterial or candidal infection. Intervention includes avoidance of these precipitating factors through wearing lightweight clothing, avoiding friction and overheating, and treatment with topical or systemic antimicrobials as required for colonization or infection. Topical application of corticosteroids or calcineurin inhibitors[216] has been the mainstay of treatment for most patients; topical calcitriol has led to improvement as well.[217] Topical application of gentamicin led to lesional clearance in a patient with an ATP2C1 premature stop mutation, attributed both to the antibacterial effect and to the ability of aminoglycoside therapy to induce readthrough of a pathogenic nonsense mutation;[218] oral antibiotics are used for recurrent secondary infections. Because of the role of sweating as an exacerbation, botulinum toxin type A injections have been useful for selected patients.[219] In persistent and disabling cases, oral retinoids,[220] photodynamic therapy,[221] ablative laser therapy, dermabrasion, or excision of involved regions followed by split thickness skin grafts have been used.

Porokeratoses

The porokeratoses are a group of hyperkeratotic disorders characterized by a thread-like raised hyperkeratotic border that shows a typical thin column of parakeratosis, or cornoid lamella, on histological examination of lesional tissue. The cornoid lamella can be more easily seen clinically by dermoscopy.[222] The porokeratoses may appear in several forms:[223]

1. Classic porokeratosis of Mibelli
2. Linear porokeratosis
3. Porokeratotic adnexal ostial nevus (PAON)
4. Punctate porokeratosis
5. Porokeratosis palmaris et plantaris disseminata
6. Disseminated superficial actinic porokeratosis.

Porokeratosis of Mibelli may appear as one, a few, or many annular lesions that usually appear during childhood, enlarge over years, and persist indefinitely (Figs 5.32, 5.33).[224] Boys are affected more commonly than girls. The disorder has a predilection for the face, neck, forearms, and hands, but also may affect the feet, ankles, buccal mucosa, and glans penis. Porokeratosis on the scalp may be associated with alopecia. The initial lesion begins as a crateriform hyperkeratotic papule that gradually expands to a plaque of circinate or irregular contour measuring from a few millimeters to several centimeters in diameter. If several lesions are present, they are usually unilateral. The diagnostic feature of this disorder is the raised hyperkeratotic peripheral ridge, which has been compared to the 'great wall of China'. Lesions are commonly mistaken for tinea corporis, warts or granuloma annulare.

Linear porokeratosis presents in infancy or childhood as one to several collections of porokeratotic lesions that resemble porokeratosis of Mibelli but follow the lines of Blaschko, similar to epidermal nevi.[225] They likely represent a mosaic form. Ulcerated forms of linear porokeratosis have been described.[226]

Porokeratotic adnexal ostial nevus (*PAON*) could be considered a form of linear porokeratosis, except that the porokeratosis involves adnexal structures, specifically the eccrine ostia and ducts and hair follicles.[227] The thread-like elevated rims seen so easily in linear porokeratosis and correlating with the cornoid lamellae are not as easily visualized in PAON, and the lesions of PAON outside of acral areas have a delicate cribriform appearance, rather than the spiny, scalier character of lesions of linear porokeratosis. PAON includes the previously termed *porokeratotic eccrine ostial and dermal duct nevus* and the *porokeratotic eccrine and hair follicle nevus*. The nevus may be present at birth and, if not, usually appears during the first years of life and occasionally during adulthood. Lesions present as multiple

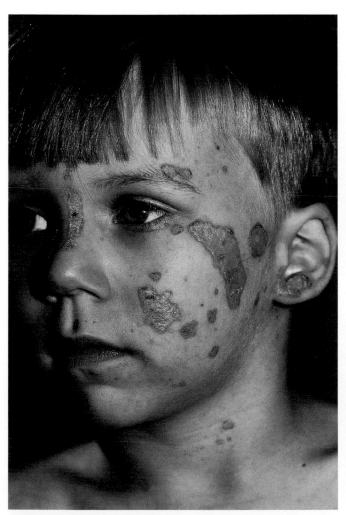

Figure 5.32 Porokeratosis. Multiple erythematous annular lesions surrounded by a wall-like ridge of scaling.

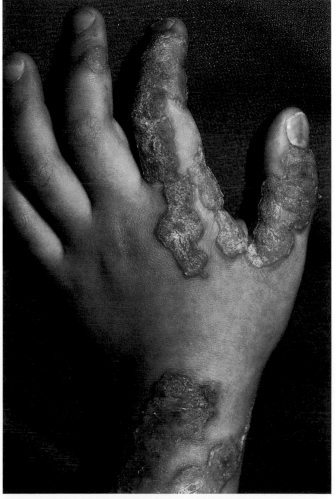

Figure 5.33 Porokeratosis. Annular lesions with a hyperkeratotic peripheral wall-like ridge.

asymptomatic hyperkeratotic sometimes spiny papules and plaques, and punctate pits, often filled with a comedo-like keratin plug. The collections of papules tend to be distributed along Blaschko's lines, particularly on the distal extremities, although lesions have been described on the face, trunk and proximal extremities. Lesions may be erythematous and eroded, especially during the neonatal period. Biopsy sections show a dilated eccrine acrosyringium and, in some cases hair follicle, with an overlying cornoid lamella. In most patients, the lesions are static, but progressive extension has been described. Spontaneous improvement of lesions on the extremities has been noted, while lesions on the palms and soles tend to persist. PAON has been associated with unilateral breast hypoplasia.

Punctate porokeratosis presents as 1–2 mm punctate papules of the palms and soles during adolescence or adulthood. The peripheral raised rim may be difficult to appreciate, and differentiation from keratoderma punctata, Darier disease and Cowden disease may require biopsy.

Porokeratosis palmaris et plantaris disseminata is an autosomal dominant variant of punctuate porokeratosis that occurs more often in males. Small 'seed-like' keratotic papules with a slightly elevated peripheral rim first develop during childhood or adolescence on the palms and soles. Lesions subsequently disseminate to other areas of the body, including parts not exposed to sunlight and the mucous membranes. Lesions may be asymptomatic to pruritic.

Disseminated superficial actinic porokeratosis (DSAP) is the most common form of porokeratosis, but rarely presents in its disseminated form during childhood and only occasionally during late adolescence. Women are more often affected than men. An autosomal dominant disorder, most cases are sporadic and first show manifestations during the third or fourth decade of life. Lesions appear on sun-exposed areas of the skin, particularly on the lower legs and forearms, and are usually multiple, with most patients having >50 lesions. Most lesions measure 0.5–1.0 cm, with a range from 0.1 to 4.5 cm in diameter, and are asymptomatic to mildly pruritic. In contrast to the borders of the lesions of porokeratosis of Mibelli, the ridges are only slightly elevated above the cutaneous surface. Several individuals have been described with both DSAP and linear porokeratosis. Linear porokeratosis may be present during childhood in patients with DSAP as type 2 mosaicism with mutation in the normal allele (loss of heterozygosity), leading to an earlier and more severe lesion distributed along a line of Blaschko.[228–230] Disseminated superficial porokeratosis is also autosomal dominant and has its onset during the third or fourth decade of life. Lesions primarily occur on the extremities and are bilaterally symmetric, but do not spare sun-protected areas, as occurs in DSAP.

Although its underlying pathomechanism is unclear, porokeratosis is thought to be a disorder of dysregulated keratinization, with epidermal cell hyperproliferation and premature apoptosis of keratinocytes.[231] Recent gene profiling suggests a role for T-cell mediated immunity and keratinocyte activation.[232] Ultraviolet light exposure and immunosuppression (HIV infection, organ transplantation) are triggers.[233] Several gene loci have been linked to DSAP, and two candidate genes with mutations have been found.[234–236] The locus at chromosome 12q24.1–24.2 in both DSAP and porokeratosis palmaris et plantaris disseminata[237] suggests that these disorders are allelic.

Lesions of porokeratosis are slowly progressive and relatively asymptomatic, but may require intervention for cosmesis. The development of squamous cell carcinoma or Bowen's disease within lesions has occasionally been reported with all forms, except the punctuate form, but the risk is highest with long-standing lesions. A variety of therapies have been used, many unsuccessfully, to destroy the abnormal clone of keratinocytes. Among these are keratolytics, topical retinoids, topical imiquimod, topical 5-fluorouracil, cryotherapy, electrodesiccation, laser ablation, photodynamic therapy with methyl aminolevulinate cream,[238,239] dermabrasion, curettage, and excision. Diclofenac sodium 3% gel has improved the appearance of DSAP.[240] Oral retinoids have been used for more extensive lesions, for example, systematized linear porokeratosis.[241]

Palmoplantar keratodermas

Palmoplantar keratoderma (PPK, palmar and plantar hyperkeratosis, keratoderma of the palms and soles) describes a diffuse or localized thickening of the palms and soles that may occur as part of a genetic disorder or as an inflammatory disorder, such as pityriasis rubra pilaris, psoriasis, or Reactive arthritis (see Ch. 4).[242] Genetic forms of palmoplantar keratoderma may appear alone or as part of a more generalized disorder such as epidermolysis bullosa simplex and Kindler syndrome (Ch. 13), lamellar ichthyosis, epidermolytic ichthyosis, Sjögren–Larsson syndrome, Conradi syndrome, pachyonychia congenita (Ch. 7), or hidrotic ectodermal dysplasia (Ch. 7). Several classification systems have been proposed for the inherited forms of PPK, the simplest of which is diffuse, focal, or punctate PPK. The identification of the underlying molecular defect allows further classification. Finally, a classification by functional subgroup has also been proposed and includes abnormalities in structural proteins (keratins), cornified envelopes (loricrin), cell–cell communication (connexins), cohesion (desmoplakin 1, desmoglein 1, plakophilin), and transmembrane signaling (cathepsin C).[243]

Hereditary forms of PPK often first manifest when the affected child starts to walk, and are usually symmetrical. Diffuse forms may initially appear focal, but the more extensive involvement is notable within the first few years of life.

Diffuse Keratodermas

Epidermolytic palmoplantar keratoderma (EPPK; Vörner type) is an autosomal dominant disorder characterized by sharply circumscribed congenital thickening of the palms and soles (Fig. 5.34). Most patients have hyperhidrosis, which may lead to maceration and fissuring. The waxy hyperkeratosis, limited to the palms and soles, is surrounded by an erythematous border. Transgrediens (to the dorsal surface) may be seen, and some patients show thickened skin over the joints (knuckle pads).[244,245] Mild thickening over the elbows

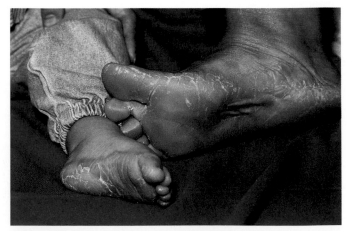

Figure 5.34 Epidermolytic palmoplantar keratoderma. Waxy thickening is limited to the palms and soles and usually surrounded by an erythematous border. This is an autosomal dominant disorder, as shown in mother and daughter.

and knees may occur. Hyperhidrosis is often present, and may promote skin fissuring and maceration. An associated odor suggests secondary bacterial or fungal infection. Biopsy sections will often show epidermolytic hyperkeratosis, similar to that seen in epidermolytic ichthyosis, although more than one sample may be required to demonstrate the epidermolysis. Blistering, however, is not usually seen except the increased fragility that can occur with retinoid therapy. The disorder results from mutations in keratin 9, a form of keratin protein expressed only in the palms and soles.[246]

Diffuse non-epidermolytic palmoplantar keratoderma (NEPPK; Unna type) is an autosomal dominant genodermatosis that clinically is indistinguishable from epidermolytic PPK other than tending to be milder, but does not show epidermolysis in biopsy sections. This form of PPK has been attributed largely to mutations in noncritical regions of the gene that encodes keratin 1 and to mutations in *KRT6a* or *16*.[247] *Greither syndrome*, with transgrediens involvement in a glove-and-sock distribution, is considered a more severe form of diffuse NEPPK and mutations have been found in *KRT1*.[248] Diffuse NEPPK is a component of *Naegeli–Franceschetti–Jadassohn syndrome* and *dermatopathia pigmentosa reticularis*, allelic disorders resulting from mutations in *KRT14* that are also characterized by abnormal sweating, reticulate hyperpigmentation, absence of dermatoglyphics and other ectodermal anomalies (Ch. 7).[249,250]

Palmoplantar keratoderma associated with hearing loss occurs in individuals with *Vohwinkel syndrome*, an autosomal dominant mutilating keratoderma characterized by extensive PPK with a distinct 'honeycomb' pattern and constrictions (pseudoainhum) that may lead to amputation of distal digits.[251] In some cases, distinctive hyperkeratotic 'starfish'-like plaques are present over the elbows, knees and sometimes the knuckles. Sensorineural deafness is a common accompanying feature. Mutations in the *GJB2* gene encoding connexin 26 underlie Vohwinkel syndrome with deafness, and are also responsible for KID syndrome, non-mutating PPK with deafness, knuckle pads, and leukonychia (Bart–Pumphrey syndrome).[252,253] Knuckle pads can also be a feature of other forms of palmoplantar keratoderma[243,244,254] and occur as an isolated entity (Fig. 5.35).[255] The ichthyotic variant of Vohwinkel syndrome also shows PPK with a honeycomb appearance and pseudoainhum, but

has associated ichthyosis and no deafness (see Loricrin Keratoderma, above).

Clouston syndrome (hidrotic ectodermal dysplasia) is an autosomal dominant condition that results from mutations in the *GJB6* gene encoding connexin 30 (see Ch. 7).[256] Keratoderma (hyperkeratosis) of the palms and soles is common and may be diffuse or focal. It occasionally extends to involve the sides and dorsal aspects of affected hands and feet. Nails grow slowly and may appear thickened or thinned, striated, discolored, brittle, or hypoplastic. The tips of the digits show pseudoclubbing (see Ch. 7, Fig. 7.20), and hyperpigmentation may overline digital joints. Paronychial infections are common and may result in partial to complete destruction of the nail matrix. Body hair may be sparse; eyebrows and eyelashes may be thinned or absent, and the skin has a smooth texture. Scalp hair, generally normal during infancy and childhood, may become thin, fragile, or sparse to absent following puberty.

Mal de Meleda (keratosis palmoplantaris transgrediens) is an autosomal recessive form of diffuse PPK, associated with inflammatory keratotic plaques that extend to the dorsal aspects of the hands and feet and may overlie joints (Fig. 5.36).[257] Hyperhidrosis, superinfection, and occasionally perioral erythema, brachydactyly, and nail abnormalities may be associated. Female carriers may show mild palmoplantar keratoderma with interdigital fissures and keratotic papules.[258] Flexion contractures and spontaneous amputation of the digits occurs in severe cases. Mal de Meleda is due to mutations in *ARS component B*, which encodes SLURP-1.[259,260] The role of SLURP-1 in epidermal homeostasis and TNF-α inhibition explains the hyperproliferative and inflammatory phenotype.

Olmsted syndrome (mutilating palmoplantar keratoderma with periorificial plaques) is a rare, autosomal dominant disorder characterized by the progressive development of mutilating, painful plaques of keratoderma on the palms and soles that begins during infancy to early childhood (Fig. 5.37).[261,262] The borders of the

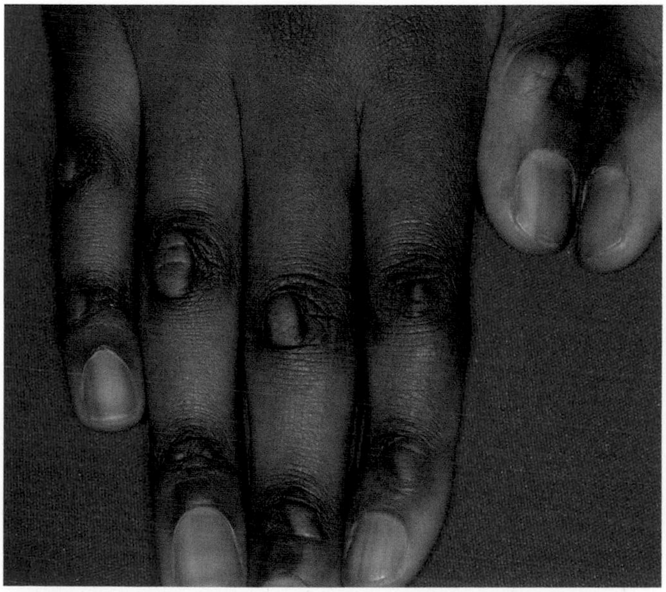

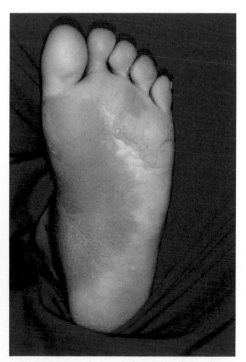

Figure 5.35 Knuckle pads. These hyperkeratotic plaques can be seen as an isolated entity, but may be associated with palmoplantar keratoderma.

Figure 5.36 Mal de Meleda palmoplantar keratoderma. Diffuse plantar keratoderma overlying erythema that extends to the dorsal aspects of the feet and hands. The Mal de Meleda type is one of the few autosomal recessive forms of hereditary palmoplantar keratoderma.

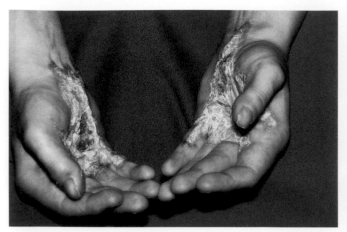

Figure 5.37 Olmsted syndrome. Mutilating, painful plaques of keratoderma on the palms and soles begin during infancy to early childhood.

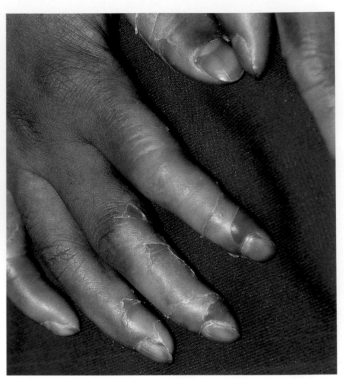

Figure 5.38 Huriez syndrome. Palmoplantar keratoderma is associated with sclerodactyly. Affected individuals have a high risk of developing local squamous cell carcinoma.

keratoderma tend to be erythematous, and hyperkeratotic plaques may affect intertriginous folds. Contractures and autoamputation from progressive constriction of the digits are common. Periorificial areas become thickened and fissured to varying degrees. Patients often show alopecia, corneal defects and nail dystrophy. The risk of cutaneous squamous cell carcinoma is increased. The affected gene is unknown. In addition to oral retinoids, EGFR inhibitors have been shown to improve the PPK.[263] Full thickness excision of plaques with skin grafting has been successful in several patients.[264]

Sclerotylosis (Huriez syndrome, PPK with scleroatrophy) is an autosomal dominant PPK that presents at birth with a diffuse, symmetric keratoderma of the palms and soles. The fingers have a pseudosclerodermatous appearance with scleroatrophy (Fig. 5.38),[265] often with contractures and sometimes with reticulate erythema on the dorsal surface. Raynaud phenomenon is not associated. Nail abnormalities, including longitudinal ridging, hypoplasia, and clubbing, have been reported. Patients show an increased risk of developing squamous cell carcinoma of the palms or soles during the third and fourth decades,[266] and bowel cancer has been described. The gene has not yet been identified, but is mapped to 4q23.[267] Sclerodactyly and PPK with an increased risk of squamous cell carcinoma are also features of *Micali syndrome*,[268,269] an autosomal recessive disorder which results from mutations in *RSPO1*, mapped to 1q34 and encoding R-spondin 1.[270,271] Deficiency of R-spondin 1 in males results in PPK and the risk of SCCs alone, but in 46XX female individuals leads to sex reversal with the development of ambiguous genitalia, hypospadias, hypoplastic testes, and low testosterone levels. R-spondin 1 has recently been shown to be critical in ovarian differentiation,[272] and its deficiency both prevents the development of female genitalia and eradicates keratinocyte expression of β-catenin and the ability to differentiate.[273] Variable features include chronic periodontal disease with early loss of teeth, bilateral cataracts and optic nerve colobomata, and hypertriglyceridemia.

Naxos disease (keratosis palmoplantaris with arrhythmogenic cardiomyopathy) is an autosomal recessive form of PPK associated with an early risk of sudden death from cardiac arrhythmia. The keratoderma is diffuse rather than striate (vs *Carvajal syndrome*, see below) and is associated with woolly hair. The prominent cardiac abnormalities, including EKG changes, ventricular arrhythmias, and right ventricular structural alterations, may not become clinically apparent until the middle of the second decade of life. The disorder results from mutations in *JUP*, which encodes the desmosomal component plakoglobin.[274]

The *Papillon–Lefèvre syndrome* and its variant, Haim–Munk syndrome, are autosomal recessive disorders that usually first show erythema and diffuse to localized psoriasiform hyperkeratosis of the palms and especially the soles during infancy or early childhood, coinciding with the timing of eruption of the primary teeth.[275-277] The keratoderma often extends to the dorsal aspects of the hands and feet. Psoriasiform lesions occur on the knees and elbows. Rapidly progressive periodontitis and periosteal changes of the alveolar bone result in loss of both deciduous and permanent teeth (Fig. 5.39). Gingival involvement may manifest as early as 1 year of age, and tends to be present by 5 years of age; both the deciduous and permanent teeth are lost prematurely and patients are usually edentulous by 15 years. Although an increased risk of acral lentiginous melanoma has been suggested, the reports are primarily in the Japanese population, which has a high frequency.[278] Haim–Munk syndrome (in individuals descended from Cochin, India) has the additional features of arachnodactyly, acroosteolysis, and onychogryphosis, but not the calcification of the falx cerebri or susceptibility for bacterial infection described in some patients with Papillon–Lefèvre syndrome.[279]

Both disorders result from mutations in the *CTSC* gene, encoding cathepsin C, leading to impaired innate immune responses and desquamation from activation of serine proteases.[280,281] Diffuse NEPPK and chronic periodontal disease with loss of teeth are also a feature of *Micali syndrome* (see below).

Focal Keratodermas

Pachyonychia congenita (PC) describes a group of autosomal dominant conditions characterized most prominently by a characteristic nail dystrophy (see Ch. 7; Figs 7.56–7.58). Mutations occur in one of four keratins: *KRT6a*, *KRT6b*, *KRT16*, and *KRT17*.[282] The historical

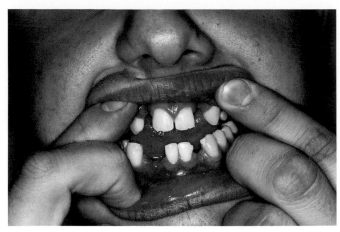

Figure 5.39 Papillon–Lefevre syndrome. Focal plaques of palmoplantar keratoderma are associated with the progressive periodontitis and periosteal changes of the alveolar bone that begins during infancy or early childhood and result in loss of both deciduous and permanent teeth.

terms PC-1 (Jadassohn–Lewandowsky syndrome) and PC-2 (Jackson–Lawlor syndrome) should be abandoned since cysts often occur in PC-6a in addition to PC6b and PC-17. The pachyonychia may be accompanied by focal painful PPK, follicular keratoses, and oral leukokeratosis, which can be mistaken during infancy for candidal infection. Presentation with focal PPK alone with minimal or no nail changes occasionally is due to mutations in *KRT16*, but has been described in mutations in *KRT6c*.[283]

Striate palmoplantar keratoderma is an autosomal dominant condition characterized by focal keratoderma on the soles that often develops during infancy. Focal or characteristic streaks of keratoderma may develop on the palmar surface, especially if traumatized. Plantar involvement is nummular, not linear. The condition results from mutations in the gene encoding either desmoplakin or desmoglein-1[284–288] and affects the ability of keratin filaments to attach to the cell membrane.

Dilated cardiomyopathy with keratoderma (Carvajal syndrome) results from mutations in desmoplakin, but is autosomal recessive.[289] Patients show curly woolly hair at birth and striate keratoderma at around 1 year of age. Patients progressively develop striated lichenoid keratoses of the flexural areas and follicular keratoses of the knees and elbows. Premature death from cardiac failure and left ventricular cardiomyopathy is not uncommon during teenage years, and cardiac signs are rarely present in the first year decade.[290] The focal nature of the PPK and the presence of left, rather than right, ventricular cardiomyopathy serve to distinguish Carvajal syndrome from Naxos disease; however, a patient has recently been reported with focal PPK and biventricular cardiomyopathy.[291]

PPK and deafness due to mutations in the mitochondrial genome occur in the mitochondrial tRNA encoding the *MTTS1* gene. The focal PPK is typically first seen at 5–15 years of age.[292] Most prevalent over the plantar surface, keratotic plaques may also develop on the palm and at other pressure sites including the knees and elbows, Achilles tendons, and the dorsal surface of the toes. Palmar involvement is most pronounced in adults who are manual workers. Hearing loss occurs in approximately 60%, and the PPK in approximately 30%.

Richner–Hanhart syndrome (tyrosinemia type II) is an autosomal recessive disorder caused by a deficiency of hepatic tyrosine aminotransferase (mutations in the TAT gene)[293] and resulting in accumulation of tyrosine.[294] The early cutaneous lesions may be seen during childhood as sharply demarcated, yellowish keratotic papules of the palmar and plantar surfaces, and sometimes occur during the late teenage years. The lesions become more erythematous, erosive, and painful with time. Nail dystrophy may be associated. Photophobia and bilateral tearing commonly occur within the first 3 months of life, and progress to corneal erosions; herpetic ulceration is often erroneously diagnosed. Mildly affected individuals have been described, and may have just focal PPK with mild or no ocular manifestations.[295,296] The treatment of choice is dietary restriction of tyrosine with a low phenylalanine, low tyrosine diet.

Howel–Evans syndrome (tylosis with esophageal cancer) is a late-onset form of autosomal dominant focal PPK, associated with the development of mucosal squamous cell carcinoma in 95% of affected patients by the age of 65 years, particularly of the esophageal mucosa (38-fold increased risk).[297] The PPK is most prominent on pressure areas on the soles and is usually fully penetrant with the onset between 6 and 12 years of age. Palmar involvement is most prominent in manual laborers. Frictional hyperkeratosis may occur at other areas of trauma such as the elbows and knees, and oral leukokeratosis is often seen. Follicular hyperkeratoses are common and may be the initial manifestation in younger patients. The condition maps to 17q25, but the mutated gene has not been discovered.[298]

Keratosis punctata palmaris et plantaris is an autosomal dominant disorder, characterized by discrete keratoses of the palms and soles.[299–301] Confined to the palmoplantar creases and volar aspects of the fingers, the central keratinous plug may be lost or can be picked out, leaving a shallow depressed pit with a keratotic base. Lesions can be particularly painful when walking or from pressure on the hands in persons who perform manual labor. Punctate papules of the palms and soles are also a feature of porokeratosis punctata palmaris et plantaris (see above), Cole disease (in association with guttate hypopigmentation),[302] keratosis punctata of the palmar creases, Darier disease (see above), and Cowden syndrome (Ch. 9).[303] Although the underlying molecular mechanism is not known, the gene has been mapped to chromosomes 8q24 and 15q22.[304]

The treatment of all forms of hyperkeratosis of the palms and soles is generally palliative and consists of application of keratolytic formulations, such as 10–20% salicylic acid in a thick emollient cream (under occlusion at night if tolerated), intermittent use of Keralyt Gel or 40% salicylic acid (Mediplast) plasters, periodic soaking of the affected area in water, and gentle removal of excessive keratinous material by a pumice stone, scalpel, or single-edged razor blade. Painful fissures can be treated by a formulation of 30% tincture of benzoin in zinc oxide, or cryoglycate (Superglue) prior to the application of a keratolytic formulation. Patients should wear comfortable shoes, and avoid pressure or friction to affected areas. Although oral retinoids are helpful, they are recommended only for short-term use for the temporary relief of individuals with significant disability.

Hereditary papulotranslucent acrokeratoderma is a rare autosomal dominant disorder characterized by persistent, asymptomatic whitish papules and plaques that are most prevalent at the margins and pressure areas on the palms and soles.[305] The condition usually begins during adolescence. Fine hair and an atopic diathesis have been associated. The disorder must be distinguished from *aquagenic wrinkling of the palms* (also called acquired aquagenic palmoplantar keratoderma, aquagenic syringeal acrokeratoderma, and transient aquagenic palmar hyperwrinkling), a transient and recurrent keratoderma of the palms and lateral fingers induced by exposure to water.[306–308] Exposure to water elicits a whitening of the wet palm within a few minutes and visible thickening ('hand in the bucket sign'), often associated with a tight, tingling, pruritic or even painful

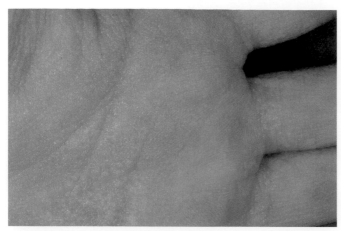

Figure 5.40 Aquagenic wrinkling of the palms. The palm becomes whitened and thickened within a few minutes after exposure to water.

sensation (Fig. 5.40). The lesions disappear within about 30 min after drying. This condition also often begins at puberty and is often accompanied by palmar hyperhidrosis. Unilateral involvement has been described in a child.[309] In contrast to the hereditary, fixed form, biopsy of aquagenic wrinkling shows dilated eccrine ostia with only mild hyperkeratosis. The cause is thought to be influx of water across an osmotic gradient into eccrine ducts.

Aquagenic wrinkling of the palms was originally described in patients with cystic fibrosis,[310,311] is most obvious in patients with the DeltaF508 mutation,[312] and may be a cutaneous sign of carriers of cystic fibrosis.[313] Tobramycin can induce aquagenic wrinkling without exposure to water.[314] Aquagenic wrinkling can also be seen in individuals with increased sweat chloride levels, but without cystic fibrosis.[315] Palmar injection of botulinum toxin has been used for symptomatic patients.[316]

Key References

Arin MJ. The molecular basis of human keratin disorders. *Hum Genet.* 2009;125(4):355–373.

Brecher AR, Orlow SJ. Oral retinoid therapy for dermatologic conditions in children and adolescents. *J Am Acad Dermatol.* 2003;49(2):171–182; quiz 183–186.

Elias PM, Williams ML, Holleran WM, et al. Pathogenesis of permeability barrier abnormalities in the ichthyoses: inherited disorders of lipid metabolism. *J Lipid Res.* 2008;49(4):697–714.

Itin PH, Fistarol SK. Palmoplantar keratodermas. *Clin Dermatol.* 2005;23(1):15–22.

Kundu RV, Garg A, Worobec SM. Lamellar ichthyosis treated with tazarotene 0.1% gel. *J Am Acad Dermatol.* 2006;55(Suppl):S94–S95.

Katugampola RP, Finlay AY. Oral retinoid therapy for disorders of keratinization: single-centre retrospective 25 years' experience on 23 patients. *Br J Dermatol.* 2006;154(2):267–276.

Oji V, Traupe H. Ichthyosis: clinical manifestations and practical treatment options. *Am J Clin Dermatol.* 2009;10:351–364.

Oji V, Tadini G, Akiyama M, et al. Revised nomenclature and classification of inherited ichthyoses: Results of the First Ichthyosis Consensus Conference in Soreze 2009. *J Am Acad Dermatol.* 2010, in press.

Schmuth M, Gruber R, Elias PM, et al. Ichthyosis update: towards a function-driven model of pathogenesis of the disorders of cornification and the role of corneocyte proteins in these disorders. *Adv Dermatol.* 2007;23:231–256.

Smith FJ, Irvine AD, Terron-Kwiatkowski A, et al. Loss-of-function mutations in the gene encoding filaggrin cause ichthyosis vulgaris. *Nat Genet.* 2006;38(3):337–342.

Vahlquist A, Ganemo A, Virtanen M. Congenital ichthyosis: an overview of current and emerging therapies. *Acta Derm Venereol.* 2008;88(1):4–14.

Hereditary Disorders of the Dermis

6

Several hereditary disorders of the skin primarily manifest as disorders of the dermis. Clinical manifestations range from laxity of skin to infiltrated papules, and rigidity to thinning of dermis. Disorders of mucopolysaccharides are reviewed in Chapter 24.

Ehlers–Danlos syndrome

Ehlers–Danlos syndrome (EDS) consists of a group of inherited disorders of collagen characterized by increased cutaneous elasticity, hyperextensibility of the joints, and fragility of the skin, with formation of pseudotumors and large gaping scars.[1] The newest classification (Villefranche), proposed in 1997,[2] consolidates Ehlers–Danlos into six main subgroups (Table 6.1), including autosomal dominant and autosomal recessive forms, although many patients have overlapping features. The prevalence of EDS, including the mild forms, may be as high as 1:5000 individuals.[3] The spectrum of severity of EDS ranges from almost imperceptible findings to severe, debilitating disease. Most common is the classical type. The vascular type tends to be most devastating. The kyphoscoliosis, arthrochalasia, and dermatosparaxis types are considerably less common than other forms. The effect on quality-of-life can be considerable, and three-quarters of affected individuals report fatigue, which may be impacted by pain, sleep disturbance, difficulty with concentration, and diminished social functioning.[4]

Infants with Ehlers–Danlos syndrome are prone to premature birth because of early rupture of membranes. Pre-term delivery occurs in 40% of pregnancies with affected neonates and 21% of pregnancies of affected mothers.[5–8] The skin of individuals with the *classic type* is velvety, soft, and has a doughy consistency. After being stretched, it returns to its normal position as soon as released, in contrast to the lax skin of cutis laxa. Skin hyperextensibility should be tested at a site not subjected to mechanical forces or scarring, such as the volar surface of the forearm (Fig. 6.1). In contrast to 10% of apparently normal individuals, approximately 50% of patients with Ehlers–Danlos can touch the tip of their nose with their tongue (Gorlin's sign) (Fig. 6.2). In addition, the skin of the hands, feet, and at times the elbows tends to be lax and redundant, thus resulting in a loose-fitting glove-or moccasin-like appearance. A number of patients have pressure-induced herniation of subcutaneous fat on the wrists or on the medial or lateral aspect of the heels, evident when the patient is standing (piezogenic pedal papules).

In addition to abnormal elasticity, the skin of patients with the classical (but not the hypermobile) form of Ehlers–Danlos syndrome is extremely fragile, and minor trauma may produce gaping 'fishmouth' wounds (Fig. 6.3). It has poor tensile strength and cannot hold sutures properly. This leads to frequent dehiscence, poor healing, and the formation of wide, papyraceous, wrinkled hernia-like scars, particularly over areas of trauma (such as the forehead, elbows, knees, and shins). Blood vessels are fragile, resulting in hematomas and a chronic bruise-like appearance, particularly

on the anterior aspect of the lower extremities (Fig. 6.4). The resolution of hematomas is accompanied by fibrosis, which produces soft subcutaneous nodules (pseudotumors) and calcified subcutaneous nodules, especially on the shins and forearms (spheroids). Hyperextensible joints may result in 'double-jointed' fingers or frequent subluxation of larger joints (Fig. 6.5). This may occur spontaneously or follow slight trauma. Generalized hypermobility is determined by a score of ≥5 in the 9-point scale established by Beighton and colleagues[2] (Table 6.2). Sprains, dislocations or subluxations, and pes planus occur as complications, and patients complain of chronic joint and limb pain, despite normal skeletal radiographs.[9] Muscle hypotonia and delayed gross motor development have been described. Hiatal hernia, postoperative hernias, and anal prolapse have been noted as manifestations of the tissue hyperextensibility and fragility.[10] Anomalies of the heart and dissecting aortic aneurysms have been described, primarily in individuals with the arterial form; premature deaths have occurred from gastrointestinal bleeding, rare bowel perforation, and rupture of cardiovascular defects. Mitral valve prolapse is a common manifestation, but aortic root dilatation is uncommon; both can be assessed by echocardiography, CT, or MRI examinations.[10]

Patients with the *hypermobility type* show extensive joint hypermobility and dislocations, particularly of the shoulder, patella and temporomandibular joints. The skin is often soft and velvety, but heals well and only occasionally shows hyperextensibility. Given that up to 40% of school-age children may show a score of ≥5/9 using the Beighton criteria, the diagnosis of hypermobility type EDS may be difficult.[11] It is also hard to distinguish from benign joint hypermobility syndrome,[12] and the term 'joint hypermobility syndrome' has been suggested to encompass any child with symptomatic joint hypermobility,[11,13] including with hypermobility type EDS.

The *vascular type* of EDS is characterized by extensive bruising and often thin, translucent skin that is not hyperextensible.[10,14,15] Joint hypermobility is usually limited to the digits, and only 17% meet Beighton criteria.[16] The facial appearance is often typical, with sunken eyes, a thin upper lip, and decreased facial fat. Spontaneous rupture of arteries, particularly mid-sized arteries, may occur during childhood, although its peak age of incidence is the 3rd or 4th decade of life. Arterial or intestinal rupture often presents as acute abdominal or flank pain, and intracranial aneurysms may be associated with cerebrovascular accidents.[17] Arterial rupture is the most common cause of death. Pregnancies may be complicated by pre-and postpartum arterial bleeding, and by intrapartum uterine rupture. Vaginal and perineal tears from the delivery heal poorly, and pneumothorax occurs in 11% of affected individuals. In one series, 94% of patients with vascular EDS showed blue sclerae.[16] Vascular EDS may be confused with periodontal EDS (see below) and Loeys–Dietz syndrome. The latter is an autosomal dominant disorder characterized by joint hypermobility with dislocations, soft velvety skin, arterial tortuosity and widespread vascular aneurysm and dissection.[18] The disorder has been divided into Loeys–Dietz

Table 6.1 Classification of Ehlers–Danlos syndrome (EDS)

Type	Mutations	Skin findings	Joint changes	Inheritance	Old type	Other
Classic	*COL5A1*, *COL5A2*	Hyperextens-ibility, bruising, velvety skin, widened atrophic scars, molluscoid pseudotumors, spheroids	Hypermobility and its complications, joint dislocations	AD	Type I; Type II	
EDS/OI overlap	*COL1A1*	Overlap of classic EDS, OI. May have late arterial rupture		AD		
Cardiac valvular	*COL1A2*	EDS with severe cardiac valve issues as adult		AR		
'Classic-like'	*TNXB*	Hyperextensibility, bruising, velvety skin	Hypermobility	AR		
Hypermobility	*TNXB* (5%); *COL5A*	Mild hyperextens-ibility, scarring, textural change	Hypermobility, chronic joint pain, recurrent dislocations	AD	Type III	Deficiency of tenascin X or type V procollagen
Vascular	*COL3A1*	Thin, translucent skin, bruising, early varicosities, acrogeria	Small joint hypermobility	AD	Type IV (arterial-ecchymotic)	Abnormal type III collagen secretion. Rupture of bowel, uterus, arteries. Typical facies. Pneumothorax
Kyphoscoliosis	*PLOD* (deficient lysyl hydroxylase)	Soft, hyperextens-ible, bruising, atrophic scars	Hypermobility	AR	Type VI	Severe muscle hypotonia, congenital kyphoscoliosis, scleral fragility and rupture, marfanoid, osteopenia
Arthrochalasis	Exon 6 deletion of *COL1A1* or *COL1A2*	Hyperextensible, soft skin with or without abnormal scarring	Marked hypermobility with recurrent subluxations	AD	Type VIIA; Type VII B	Congenital hip dislocation; arthrochalasis multiplex congenital; short stature
Dermatosparaxis	Type I collagen N-peptidase *ADAMTS-2*	Severe fragility; sagging, redundant skin			Type VIIC	Also occurs in cattle
Other						
Progeroid	Galactosyl-transferase I					Facial features

OI, osteogenesis imperfecta.

type 1 and type 2. Type 1 patients have a marfanoid habitus (but do not fulfill Ghent criteria for Marfan syndrome), craniofacial abnormalities, and mutations in TGFBR1 (TGF-beta1 receptor), while type 2 patients have no craniofacial or skeletal anomalies, and result from mutations in TGFB2R.[18]

The *kyphoscoliotic type* is characterized by generalized joint laxity with severe muscle hypotonia at birth, which leads to gross motor delay, and congenital progressive scoliosis.[19] The severe hypotonia is predominant during infancy, and patients are thought to have congenital muscular dystrophy or myopathies. By the second or third decade of life, patients tend to lose the ability to ambulate. The skin may be fragile, and heals with atrophic scars. Easy

bruisability and arterial rupture have been described. Patients often show a Marfanoid habitus, osteopenia, and scleral fragility with rupture of the ocular globe. The *spondylocheirodysplastic form* of EDS resembles the kyphoscoliotic form, but lacks the severe muscular hypotonia from birth and progressive kyphoscoliosis. In contrast to the kyphoscoliotic form, the spondylocheirodysplastic form shows moderate short stature, wrinkled palms with thenar and hypothenar atrophy, blue sclerae but no other eye abnormalities, and a variety of bone abnormalities.[20]

Patients with the *arthrochalasia type* show generalized joint hypermobility with recurrent subluxations and congenital bilateral hip dislocation. The skin may be hyperextensible, fragile, and easy to

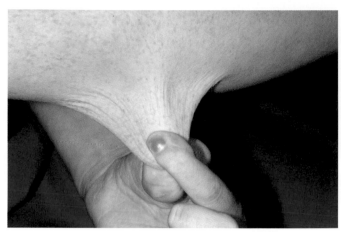

Figure 6.1 Ehlers–Danlos syndrome. Skin hyperextensibility over the lower extremities.

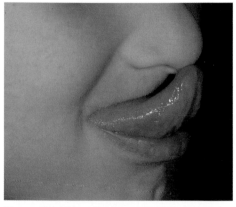

Figure 6.2 Ehlers–Danlos syndrome. Gorlin sign is five times more common than in normal individuals.

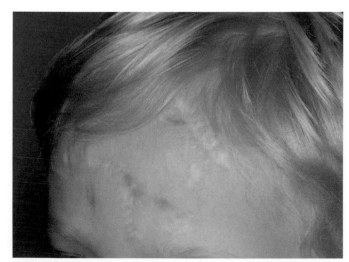

Figure 6.3 Ehlers–Danlos syndrome. Recurrent minor trauma to this boy's fragile forehead skin poorly healed 'fishmouth' scars.

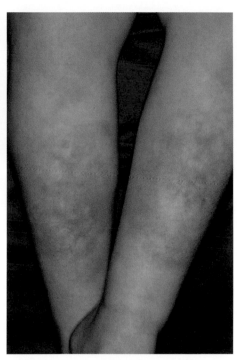

Figure 6.4 Ehlers–Danlos syndrome. Blood vessels are fragile, resulting in hematomas and chronic discoloration of the anterior aspect of the lower extremities.

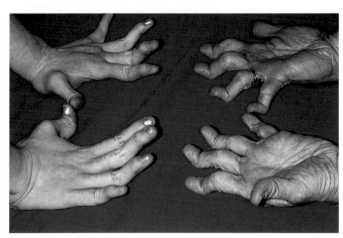

Figure 6.5 Ehlers–Danlos syndrome. Hyperextensible joints may result in 'double-jointed' fingers, as seen in this affected mother and daughter.

Table 6.2 Beighton scale for generalized joint hypermobility (≥5/9 meets criteria)

Finding	Negative	One side	Both sides
Passive flexion of thumb to forearm	0	1	2
Passive dorsiflexion of fifth finger >90°	0	1	2
Hyperextension of elbows >10°	0	1	2
Hyperextension of knees >10°	0	1	2
Touching the floor with palms open and knees fully extended (Present = 1)			

bruise. Muscle hypotonia, kyphoscoliosis, and mild osteopenia have been described. The *dermatosparaxis form* is characterized by severe skin fragility with sagging, redundant skin;[21] wound healing leads to wide atrophic scars, especially past infancy.[22] The skin may be soft and doughy in texture, with easy bruisability. Characteristic facies, gingival hyperplasia, large umbilical and inguinal hernias, delayed closure of the fontanelles, postnatal growth failure, and premature rupture of the fetal membranes may be seen.

Two of the 'other' types of EDS deserve mention. The *periodontal type* was formerly type VIII. The periodontal type is associated with periodontitis, a marfanoid body habitus, prominent eyes and a short philtrum.[23,24] It is now considered a variant of the classic type of EDS. Although the procollagen III gene shows no mutations, types I and III collagen may be reduced.[25] Patients with progeroid EDS (PEDS) exhibit loose, wrinkled facial skin, fine curly hair, sparse eyebrows and eyelashes, downslanting palpebral fissures, developmental delay, skeletal abnormalities, as well and cutaneous findings typical of EDS.[26]

The diagnosis of EDS is a clinical one. Routine histopathologic examination of skin from patients with EDS is usually normal, but electron microscopy demonstrates various abnormalities in the appearance of collagen fibrils. Studies of platelet function and coagulation are usually normal, despite a tendency for bruising and increased bleeding, further implicating the defective structural integrity of skin and blood vessels. Measurement of total urinary hydroxylysyl pyridinoline and lysyl pyridinoline cross-links is a biochemical test for the kyphoscoliosis type.[19] Electrophoretic demonstration of procollagen $\alpha1(I)$ or $\alpha2(I)$ chains from collagen or cultured fibroblasts is seen with the arthrochalasia and dermatosparaxis forms.

The genetic and clinical characteristics of the major subtypes of Ehlers–Danlos are reviewed in Table 6.1.[1,27-43] The underlying molecular defect for at least 50% of patients with the classical form of EDS is mutations in the $\alpha1$ or $\alpha2$ chain of type V collagen, often leading to haploinsufficiency.[27,35] Type V collagen is a minor fibrillar collagen that regulates collagen fibril diameter. Patients with mutations in COL1A1 at non-glycine site (mutations at glycine sites lead to osteogenesis imperfecta) may exhibit features of classic EDS or EDS/osteogenesis imperfecta overlap.[29] Some children with non-glycine substitutions in type I collagen have classic EDS, but develop spontaneous arterial rupture during adulthood.[36] A 'classic-like' AR form of EDS is caused by tenascin-X deficiency; these patients show typical EDS, but normal wound healing.[38] Approximately 40% of patients with the hypermobility form exhibit abnormal skin findings similar to classical EDS without the atrophic scarring.[1] The vascular form of EDS has been associated with mutations in type III collagen (COL3A1), resulting in a reduced amount of type III collagen in dermis, vessels, and viscera.[39]

Management is mainly supportive and should include genetic counseling. The possibility of premature birth should be discussed,[44] and cutaneous, skeletal, cadiovascular, and ocular difficulties (possible retinal detachment and abnormalities of the lens) should be emphasized. Children with skin fragility should use protective pads on the shins, knees, and forehead to decrease the risk of laceration and bruising. Ongoing rheumatologic and orthopedic care may be required to prevent progressive joint disease in certain patients. Low-impact sports (such as swimming) are preferable to contact sports and weight training in patients with hypermobility. Children with significant hypotonia or motor developmental delay should be referred for appropriate physical therapy to improve muscular strength and coordination.

Surgical procedures present problems because tissues are friable and difficult to suture. Edges of wounds, therefore, should be approximated without tension by closely-spaced sutures in two layers (absorbable and retained), adhesive reinforcement (e.g., Steri-Strips), and pressure bandages to aid healing, diminish scarring, and lower the risk of hematoma and pseudotumor formation. Sutures should be kept in place for at least twice as long as for normal skin, and use of absorbable suture material without removal has been proposed. Prophylactic antibiotics after injury and close monitoring for postoperative infection are important to minimize postoperative complications. Ascorbate is a co-factor that stimulates prolyl hydroxylase and lysyl hydroxylase, enzymes that catalyze the formation of hydroxyproline and hydroxylysine to promote collagen deposition. Doses of 2–4 g/day have been administered to patients with the kyphoscoliosis type to improve wound healing and decrease the bleeding tendency.[45] Antiinflammatory drugs may improve the musculoskeletal pain associated with EDS but those interfering with platelet function should be avoided in patients with significant bruising. Dental procedures require extra precautions as well, because of increased bleeding.[46]

Patients who have mitral valve prolapse and regurgitation should be given prophylactic antibiotics to prevent bacterial endocarditis. Baseline echocardiograms are recommended before 10 years of age, with measurement of the aorta and follow-up studies if abnormal. The use of beta-blockers is currently under investigation For individuals with vascular EDS, invasive vascular procedures should be avoided if elective because of the risk of vascular rupture and intraoperative tissue fragility, although they have been performed safely.[47] Prenatal diagnosis is possible by genetic and biochemical analyses. The Ehlers–Danlos National Foundation (at: www.ednf.org) is a national support group.

Marfan syndrome

Marfan syndrome is an autosomal dominant disorder that occurs in 1:5000 persons and affects primarily the skeletal, ocular, and cardiovascular systems.[48–50] Mutations occur in the *FBN1* gene that encodes fibrillin-1 (66–91%), while others occur in TGFβR1 or TGFβR2, the genes also associated with Loeys–Dietz syndrome (see above). Fibrillin-1 is secreted into the extracellular matrix and polymerizes to form microfibrils of the zonular fibers of the lens and associated with elastic fibers in the aorta and skin.[51] The microfibrils stabilize latent transforming growth factor-β (TGF-β)-binding proteins (LTBPs), which bind to and maintain TGF-β in an inactive state.[50] Deficiency of fibrillin-1 thus leads to TGF-β activation. About 27% of cases occur by spontaneous mutation; recurrence as a result of parental germline mosaicism has been described.[52] Early diagnosis is critical because of the potentially fatal complications, but the clinical features evolve with advancing age and diagnosis is difficult. Family history is also important, but manifestations may not be evident until adolescence and expressivity is variable, so that generations appear to be skipped. The Ghent criteria (Table 6.3) were devised in 1996,[52] and have been adapted for inclusion of mutations in the most commonly affected gene, *FBN1*, as a major criterion. Nevertheless, they are unreliable in children,[48,49] and care should be made to avoid branding children unnecessarily with Marfan syndrome, given the potential stigma and lifestyle restrictions. Diagnosis is best made by clinical examination (particularly measurement of body proportions), echocardiography, slit-lamp ophthalmologic examination, and radiographs or imaging as needed to find criteria. Examinations should be repeated every 3–5 years until adulthood if the diagnosis is unclear.[49]

Patients are often tall with long extremities ('marfanoid habitus') (Fig. 6.6). The arm span characteristically is greater than the height, and after puberty, the upper segment (vertex to pubis) to lower

Table 6.3 Ghent criteria for Marfan syndrome and their frequency in children

System[a]	Criterion[b]	
Skeletal	Major:	Pectus carinatum or excavatum requiring surgery (26%; 31%)
		Dolichostenomelia (48%; 58%)
		Positive wrist and thumb signs (79%; 81%)
		Scoliosis>20° or spondylolisthesis (35%; 52%)
		Reduced elbow extension (<170°) (11%; 12%)
		Pes planus (46%; 55%)
		Protrusio acetabulae (6%; 12%)
	Minor:	Pes excavatum (not requiring surgery) (32%; 31%)
		Joint hypermobility (68%; 67%)
		High arched palate with dental crowding (61%; 73%)
		Characteristic facies (52%; 55%)
Ocular	Major:	Lens dislocation (ectopia lentis) (63%; 55%)
	Minor:	Flat cornea
		Myopia (increased axial length of globe) (44%; 44%)
		Hypoplastic iris or ciliary muscle
Cardiovascular	Major:	Dilatation of the aortic root 66%; 68%)
		Dissection of the ascending aorta (1%; 1%)
		Other dilatation of dissection (1%; 2%)
	Minor:	Mitral valve prolapse (62%; 59%)
		Dilatation of the pulmonary artery (<40 y/o)
		Calcified mitral annulus (<40 y/o)
Pulmonary	Major:	None
	Minor:	Spontaneous pneumothorax (3%; 4%)
		Apical blebs (3%; 4%)
Skin	Major:	None
	Minor:	Striae (7%; 32%)
Dura	Major:	Lumbosacral dural ectasia (11%; 35%)
	Minor:	None

[a]If no family history, must have major involvement of at least two organ systems and minor involvement of a third system. If a FBN1 mutation or a family history, one major and one minor criterion is sufficient. With skeletal ≥4 major = 1 major system criterion.

[b]Major or minor criterion and, when information is available, percentage of children who show this feature who are <10 years old and 10–18 years old (in parentheses).

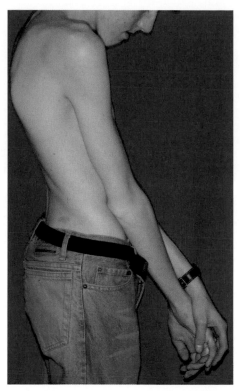

Figure 6.6 Marfan syndrome. The long arm span and decreased upper to lower body ratio are characteristic of the 'marfanoid habitus'.

segment (pubis to sole) ratio is <0.86. Arachnodactyly, hyperextensible joints, kyphoscoliosis, pectus excavatum, and flat feet are commonly seen in patients with this disorder. Lack of subcutaneous fat and the presence of striae, most prominent on the upper chest, arms, thighs, and abdomen, are the most common cutaneous

manifestations of Marfan syndrome. In addition, elastosis perforans serpiginosa (see below) occurs with increased frequency in patients with Marfan syndrome.

Joint laxity from capsular, ligamentous, and tendinous involvement may cause hyperextensibility and/or dislocation. Patellar dislocation is not uncommon; dislocation of the hip, often detected during the newborn period, may be the first sign of Marfan syndrome. The thumb sign (thumb extends well beyond the ulnar border of the hand when overlapped by fingers) and wrist sign (thumb overlaps the fifth finger as they grasp the opposite wrist) are screening tests for the joint hypermobility of Marfan syndrome.[53] Dural ectasia is occasionally seen in children, and imaging is performed largely to consider an additional Ghent criterion for diagnosis, but its presence is nonspecific.

The most common ocular abnormalities are lens displacement (ectopia lentis; the hallmark of ocular involvement, seen in at least 55% of affected children) and myopia (almost half of children). Retinal detachment, cataracts or glaucoma may impair vision and cause blindness. Cardiovascular abnormalities occur in almost 70% of children with Marfan syndrome. Dilatation of the aorta is the most common defect, generally greatest at the sinuses of Valsalva, and diffuse dilatation of the proximal segment of the ascending aorta with aortic regurgitation often occurs. Mitral valve prolapse occurs in approximately 60% of affected children and adolescents, especially pectus excavatum.[54] Left ventricular dilation may predispose to alterations of repolarization and fatal ventricular arrhythmias.[55] The most severely affected children, those with neonatal Marfan syndrome, almost always have aortic dilatation and severely impaired valves, leading to congestive heart failure, pulmonary hypertension, and a risk of early death. In a child diagnosed with Marfan syndrome, serial echocardiography at 6–12 month intervals is recommended, the frequency depending on the aortic diameter in relation to the body surface area and the rate of increase.

Conditions most often considered when patients present with cutaneous and other system concerns are Ehlers–Danlos syndrome vascular type (aortic root dilatation or dissection), Loeys–Dietz syndrome (aortic root dilation or dissection), homocysteinuria, and MASS (see below). Patients with Marfan syndrome do not have the translucent and velvety skin or easy bruising of Ehlers–Danlos or Loeys–Dietz syndrome. Neither type I nor type II Loeys–Dietz syndrome includes myopia or ectopia lentis, and craniosynostosis, hypertelorism and bifid uvula, features of Loeys–Dietz, are not features of Marfan syndrome.[50] Homocysteinuria is an autosomal recessive disorder due to mutations cystathionine β-synthase, in which patients also show ectopia lentis and a marfanoid habitus; the presence of retardation in patients with homocysteinuria is a distinguishing feature. A defect in cobalamin C, an essential co-factor for cystathionine β-synthase, similarly presents with marfanoid features, arachnodactyly, joint laxity and scoliosis, in addition to macrocytic anemia and developmental delay.[56] Perhaps hardest to distinguish is MASS (Mitral valve prolapsed and myopia, mild and non-progressive Aortic root dilatation, marfanoid Skeletal changes, or Skin features), a Marfan-like disorder due to FBN-1 mutations with a better prognosis; among the distinguishing features are a stable and mild aortic root dilatation (<2.5 SD) and lack of ectopia lentis. The prognosis depends on the extent and severity of cardiovascular defects. Death usually occurs in adulthood, but occasionally during childhood, as a result of cardiovascular sequelae, especially owing to complications related to dilatation of the aortic root.[57,58] A rare neonatal form of Marfan syndrome features the body disproportion of Marfan syndrome, lax skin, emphysema, ocular abnormalities, joint contractures, kyphoscoliosis, adducted thumbs, crumpled ears, micrognathia, muscle hypoplasia, and deficient subcutaneous fat over joints.[59] Severe cardiac valve insufficiency and aortic dilatation result in death during the first 2 years of life.

Children with Marfan syndrome should be excused from participation in physical education in order to avoid potentially harmful exertion, contact sports (to protect the aorta and lens), and isometric exercises (such as weightlifting), which might lead to further aortic root dilatation, aortic rupture or congestive heart failure. Scuba-diving should be avoided because of the risk of pneumothorax. Long-term propranolol therapy may decrease myocardial contractility,[60] thus decreasing the risk of aortic dilatation, but may not affect survival;[61] two recent trials have both suggested[62] and refuted[63] the value of beta-blockers in preventing aortic root dilatation. Based on mouse studies[64] showing rescue of the cardiovascular phenotype by losartan, an angiotensin II receptor antagonist, a small number of children with severe aortic dilatation have been treated with losartan, leading to significant reduction in the aortic root diameter, either when used alone or with beta-blockers.[65] Large, long-term randomized trials are underway. In another model, long-term treatment with doxycycline was shown to be more effective than a beta-blocker in preventing thoracic aortic aneurysm through its inhibition of matrix metalloproteinases-2 and -9.[66] Aneurysmal and valvular heart defects may require prosthetic replacement, but this should be postponed as long as possible to avoid recurrent prosthesis replacement, particularly in growing children. Prophylactic replacement of the aortic root to prevent aortic dissection has led to increased life expectancy. Early and regular ophthalmologic examinations are required to detect correctable amblyopia and retinal detachment. The ectopia lentis and even complete luxation may be tolerated for decades, but lens extraction may be required to treat diplopia, glaucoma, cataracts, or retinal detachment. Repair of the pectus excavatum is indicated if cardiopulmonary compromise

occurs, but should be delayed until skeletal maturation is nearly complete to prevent recurrence and should employ internal stabilization. Scoliosis may be lessened in adolescent girls by estrogen therapy, but this therapy may also produce an overall decrease in height. Bracing, physical therapy, and vertebral fusion may all be necessary to prevent severe scoliosis. The website for the National Marfan Foundation is: www.marfan.org.

Osteogenesis imperfecta

Osteogenesis imperfecta (OI) refers to a group of inherited disorders of bone fragility in which the skin may be thin, atrophic and somewhat translucent.[67–70] The easy bruisability and bone fractures may raise the possibility of child abuse. Wound healing may be normal, but scars are frequently atrophic or hypertrophic. Patients often show hyperlaxity of ligaments and hypermobility of joints, but joint dislocation does not occur. Blue sclerae are distinctive features in ~90% of patients, but can also be seen in Marfan and Ehlers–Danlos syndromes; the thinned sclera from defects in scleral collagen permits scattering of light by normal pigment within the orbit. Otosclerosis with hearing loss may begin during adolescence (50% of the common type I by adulthood), and fragile, discolored teeth are particularly common in the more unusual forms (dentinogenesis imperfecta). Patients may show mitral and aortic valve dilatation and regurgitation, and cystic medionecrosis of the aorta. Clinically, patients with OI have been subdivided into eight subtypes of variable clinical features, severity, prognosis, and underlying genetic defects (Table 6.4). At least 50% of affected individuals have type I OI, which is by far the mildest form.

Most patients have mutations in type I collagen, which is composed of two alpha1 (COLIA1) and one alpha2 (COLIA2) polypeptide chains, forming a triple helical structure. However, OI results from mutations in CRTAP, LEPRE1 (encoding P3H1), or peptidyl-prolyl isomerase B, in 5% of patients;[71,72] these proteins form a complex required for hydroxylation of proline 986 in the helical domains of both type I collagen alpha1(I) and type II collagen alpha1(II) chains.[73] Supportive orthopedic therapy includes physical therapy to prevent contractures and immobility-induced bone loss, orthoses to protect the lower limbs, and in more severe cases, bisphosphonates.[74] Although oral bisphosphonate therapy increased bone mass density and decreases fractures, intravenous administration also markedly decreases chronic bone pain and improves mobility.[67,70]

Cutis laxa

Cutis laxa (generalized elastolysis) results from mutations in elastin, leading to abnormal elastic fibers[75] or absence of elastin (Table 6.5).[75–77] Cutis laxa can be acquired or congenital, with the genetic forms inherited as autosomal dominant or autosomal recessive forms, the latter usually being more severe.[78] An X-linked form (occipital horn syndrome; formerly Ehlers–Danlos type IX) is now classified as a copper transport disease caused by a mutation in the copper transporting ATPase, alpha-polypeptide ATP7A. Most dominant cases result from heterozygous mutations in the gene encoding elastin. Patients with cutis laxa present a striking picture of loose inelastic redundant skin that sags and hangs in pendulous folds, as if it were too large for the body. The drooping and ectropion of the eyelids, together with the sagging facial skin and accentuation of the nasal, labial, and other facial folds, help produce the 'bloodhound' or aged appearance (Fig. 6.7). The autosomal dominant form may appear at any age and presents as a cosmetic problem with few systemic changes. The skin in cutis laxa is extensible but,

Table 6.4 Classification of osteogenesis imperfecta

Type	Frequency/ inheritance	Gene	Clinical features
I	50%/AD	COL1Al, COL1A2	Fractures, blue sclerae, hearing loss, normal statues, rarely DI
II	AD[a]	COL1Al, COL1A2l Glycine substitutions	Perinatal lethal. Multiple fractures, severe rib and long bone deformities, frog leg positioning, blue-gray sclerae, small for gestational age
III	AD	COL1Al, COL1A2l Glycine substitutions	Severe deformities. Multiple fractures with progressive deformities, short stature with severe scoliosis, marked osteopenia, non-ambulatory. Triangular face, adolescent onset hearing loss, may have DI
IV	AD	COL1Al, COL1A2l Glycine substitutions	Milder than OI III. Moderately short, mild to moderate scoliosis, typically ambulatory. DI common, adult onset hearing loss, normal to gray sclerae
V	4–5%/AD	?	Mild to mod. fractures and short stature, dislocation of radial head; white sclerae, no DI
VI	4% of mod. severe/?	?	Similar to type III, moderately short, scoliosis, white sclerae, no DI; abnormal bone mineralization
VII	<10% for types VII and VIII/AR	CRTAP (cartilage-associated protein	Moderately deforming, overlap with types II and III, but milder forms documented. Rhizomelic shortening of humerus and femur, coxa vara, 'popcorn epiphyses'. White sclerae, no DI
VIII	AR	LEPRE1 (prolyl-3-hydroxylase-1)	Moderately deforming, overlap with types II and III, but milder forms documented. Rhizomelic shortening of humerus and femur, coxa vara, 'popcorn epiphyses'. White sclerae, no DI
IX	AR	PPIB (peptidyl-prolyl isomerase B)	Fractures with generalized osteopenia, wide anterior fontanelle. Moderate growth deficiency, gross motor delay. No rhizomelia or DI. White sclerae.

DI, dentinogenesis imperfecta; ?=unknown.
[a]Usually new mutation; parental germline mosaicism in 2–6% of cases.

Table 6.5 Most common features of cutis laxa

- Autosomal dominant or autosomal recessive forms
- Autosomal recessive forms subdivided into those with cardiovascular features (ARCL-1), those with developmental delay (ARCL-2), and those with developmental delay, athetosis and corneal clouding (ARCL-3). A variety of underlying molecular bases for each group have been discovered (Table 6.6)
- Skin
  - Loose, inelastic skin
- Most common other
  - Facial dysmorphism
  - Aortic dilation
  - Pulmonary artery stenosis
  - Pulmonary emphysema
  - Diverticulae: gastrointestinal, genitourinary
  - Uterine or rectal prolapse
  - Ventral, hiatal, inguinal hernias

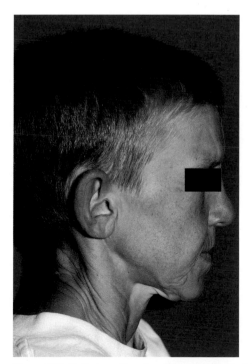

Figure 6.7 Cutis laxa. Sagging skin in an affected 8 year old.

in contrast to that of Ehlers–Danlos syndrome, does not spring back to place on release of tension. Special stains for elastic tissue (Verhoeff–van Gieson stain) of skin biopsy specimens demonstrate significantly decreased or absent dermal elastic fibers.

Systemic manifestations caused by weakened supportive tissue include aortic dilatation, pulmonary artery stenosis, pulmonary emphysema, diverticulae of the gastrointestinal tract or urinary bladder, uterine or rectal prolapse, and ventral, hiatal, or inguinal hernias. In patients with the severe autosomal recessively inherited disease, the disorder is gradually progressive and death from pulmonary complications related to emphysema may occur early in infancy or, in many instances, in the 2nd to 4th decades of life.

The autosomal recessive forms have traditionally been divided into three subgroups based on clinical characteristics, ARCL-1, -2,

and -3 (Table 6.6).[79–91] During the past decade, several of the gene mutations underlying ARCL have been discovered, and the group is quite heterogeneous. All patients tend to have cutis laxa with hernias (umbilical, inguinal, diaphragmatic) and facial dysmorphism. ARCL-1 is characterized by severe cardiopulmonary lesions,

Table 6.6 Genetic and clinical characteristics of autosomal recessive cutis laxa (ARCL)

	ARCL-1	ARCL-2	ARCL-3
Gene change(s)	*Fibulin 4, fibulin 5*	*ATP6V0A2, SCYL1BP1, PYCR1*	Unknown, *PYCR1*
Gene function	Elastic fiber assembly	Glycoprotein glycosylation and secretion	Mitochondrial proline metabolism
Hernias	+++	+++	+
Facial dysmorphism	+++	+++	+++
Joint laxity	+	+++	+++
Congenital hip dislocation	+	++	−
Hypotonia	+	+++	−
Emphysema	+++	−	−
Cardiovascular problems	+++	+	−
Bladder diverticula	+++	−	−
Delayed development	−	+++	+++
Mental retardation	−	++	++
IUGR	−	+++	+++
Large anterior fontanel	−	+++	++
Microcephaly	−	+++	++
Seizures	−	++	+++
Eye anomalies	−	+++	+++
Intracranial anomalies	−	++	?
Corneal clouding	−	−	+++
Athetoid movements	−	−	+++

including infantile emphysema and cardiac defects, and bladder diverticulae. Fibulin-5 deficiency has been associated with supravalvular aortic stenosis. Fibulin-4 deficiency may be associated with mild to moderate cutis laxa and has been linked to arachnodactyly, tortuous vessels with aneurysm, joint laxity, microcephaly, bone fractures, and pulmonary artery occlusion (Fig. 6.8). Fibulins 4 and 5 are critical in elastic fiber assembly in the skin and other elastic tissues. Patients with ARCL-2 (which includes 'wrinkly skin syndrome' and gerodermia osteodysplastica) have mild cutis laxa with growth, distinct facial features, and developmental delay without prominent vascular lesions or emphysema, in contrast to ARCL-1.[84] ARCL-3 or de Barsy syndrome[91] can be distinguished from ARCL-2 by athetoid movements and corneal opacities, but otherwise there is overlap between ARCL-2 and ARCL-3.[91–93]

Cutis laxa is also a component of several additional syndromes.[94–98] Best recognized among these are Costello syndrome and Lens–Majewski hyperostotic dwarfism.[95] Costello syndrome is an autosomal dominant disorder, characterized by soft, loose skin of the neck, hands, and feet, with excessive wrinkling and deep creases, resembling cutis laxa.[94,99,100] The digits tend to be hyperextensible with loose skin and characteristic ulnar deviation at the wrist (Fig. 6.9). Affected children develop papillomata around the nares, mouth (Fig. 6.10), and anal areas, and acanthosis nigricans. Although prenatal overgrowth and polyhydramnios occur, patients tend to have postnatal failure to thrive and a distinctive appearance, with craniofacial findings that resemble those of lysosomal storage disorders. The facies are coarse with thick lips, macroglossia, and relative macrocephaly. Severe short stature, mental retardation, and hypertrophic cardiomyopathy are other associated manifestations. Costello syndrome results from activating mutations in HRAS[101–103] and is associated with a 15% lifetime risk for malignancy, most commonly rhabdomyosarcoma.[104] Cutis laxa has also been described in children with Lenz–Majewski hyperostotic dwarfism in association with generalized hyperostosis, proximal symphalangism, syndactyly, brachydactyly mental retardation, hypertelorism,

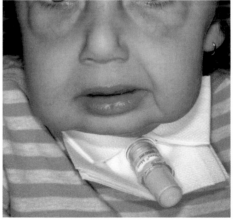

Figure 6.8 Cutis laxa syndrome. This 2-year-old girl with fibulin 4 deficiency shows the sagging infraorbital and cheek skin of cutis laxa.

and enamel hypoplasia.[95] Cutis laxa is a component of MACS syndrome (macrocephaly, alopecia, cutis laxa, and scoliosis), an autosomal recessive disorder which has recently been found to result from deficiency of RIN2, a protein that interacts with Rab5 in regulating endocytosis.[70] RIN2 deficiency leads to decreased fibulin-5 and microfibrils. Deficiency of transaldolase (TALDO) presents with liver failure and cirrhosis, in association with dysmorphic features, hypertrichosis, cutis laxa, hemolytic anemia, thrombocytopenia and genitourinary malformations;[105] patients may die *in utero* with hydrops fetalis. Cutis lax has recently been described in a child with typical Kabuki make-up syndrome.[106]

Cutis laxa can also be an acquired condition, in either a generalized or a localized form.[107] In *type I acquired cutis laxa*, ill-defined areas of loose skin appear insidiously but progressively, usually first on the face and then progressing in a cephalocaudad direction. The

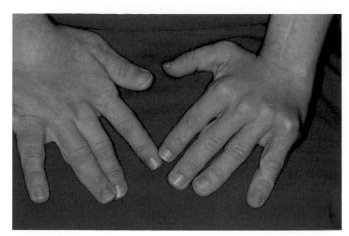

Figure 6.9 Costello syndrome. Note the loose, hyperextensible skin of the digits.

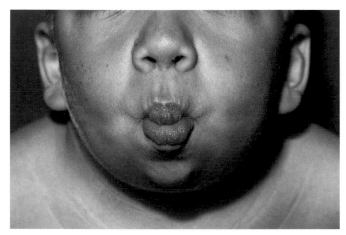

Figure 6.10 Costello syndrome. In addition to their hyperextensible joints and loose skin, affected children develop papillomata around the nares and mouth. The facies are coarse with thick lips, macroglossia, and relative macrocephaly.

Table 6.7 Most common features of pseudoxanthoma elasticum
• Autosomal recessive
• Skin
– Yellow papules and plaques (*peau d'orange*, 'plucked chicken skin')
• Ocular
– Angioid streaks
– Retinal epithelial mottling (*peau d'orange*)
– Loss of central vision
• Vascular calcifications, hemorrhage
– Gastrointestinal bleeding
– Hypertension
– Cerebrovascular accidents
– Claudication, myocardial infarction

development of cutis laxa is often preceded by an urticarial eruption. Emphysema, aortic aneurysms with subsequent rupture, and gastrointestinal and genitourinary diverticulae have been associated. Although most affected children have not had systemic evidence of acquired cutis laxa, aortic dilatation, emphysema, and severe tracheobrachiomegaly have led to the demise of children with acquired cutis laxa. Children may develop type I cutis laxa after drug exposure to penicillin, D-penicillamine,[108] or isoniazid. Elastosis perforans serpiginosa may be related[109] (see below). *Type II acquired cutis laxa* is a post-inflammatory elastolysis characterized by well-demarcated, non-pruritic erythematous plaques that appear in crops during a period of days to weeks, often in association with fever, malaise, and peripheral eosinophilia. Several children have developed the cutis laxa after Sweet's syndrome,[110] with areas of cutis laxa occurring at sites of previous inflammation.[111] Acquired cutis laxa has recently been described in a child with extensive cutaneous mastocytosis.[112] Systemic involvement is rare, but fatal aortitis has been described. Interestingly, a child with acquired cutis laxa following *Toxocara* infestation was found to have compound heterozygous mutations in elastin and a fibulin-5 mutation on one allele, suggesting that environmental factors may trigger acquired cutis laxa in genetically predisposed individual.[80]

Therapy for cutis laxa is limited. Surgery can correct diverticulae, rectal prolapse, or hernias, and plastic surgery can make a dramatic improvement in patients, inevitably with important psychological benefit.[113] Unlike patients with Ehlers–Danlos syndrome, patients with cutis laxa have no vascular fragility and heal well, enabling repeated facelift procedures. Pulmonary function studies may aid in the early detection of emphysema.

Pseudoxanthoma elasticum

Pseudoxanthoma elasticum (PXE) is a genetic disorder of the elastic tissue that involves the skin, eyes, and cardiovascular system (Table 6.7).[114] Approximately 1/60 000 individuals are affected.[115] PXE has been linked to mutations in the ATP-binding cassette subfamily C member 6 (*ABCC6*) gene, which encodes a transmembrane ATP-binding cassette (ABC) transporter.[116,117] Most of the demonstrated gene mutations would be predicted to lead to autosomal recessive inheritance patterns, although pseudodominant inheritance due to familial consanguinity has been described. PXE demonstrates marked phenotypic heterogeneity, even among patients from the same family.[118]

Lesions often develop prepubertally, especially on the lateral aspects of the neck, but may be overlooked because they are small and asymptomatic.[119–121] Most commonly, the diagnosis becomes apparent when the patient reaches the second or third decade of life. The severity may range from extensive flexural cutaneous elastic tissue involvement with severe retinal and cardiovascular complications, frequently resulting in early blindness and coronary artery disease, to primarily skin changes, milder eye findings, and rarely vascular disease. No evidence to date suggests a worse prognosis with earlier onset of cutaneous signs. The cutaneous lesions are characterized by soft, yellowish (xanthoma-like) papules and polygonal plaques on the neck (Fig. 6.11), below the clavicles, in the axillae, antecubital fossae, and periumbilical areas, and on the perineum and thighs. They vary from several papules to linear plaques resembling plucked chicken skin, morocco leather, or orange skin (*peau d'orange*). The skin becomes more redundant with advancing age and tends to show progressive calcification at affected sites. Oral, anal, and vaginal mucosal lesions may occur, most commonly infiltration of the lip mucosa. Skin lesions that are similar clinically and ultrastructurally to PXE have been described in patients with β-thalassemia,[122] sickle cell anemia[123] or as a complication of D-penicillamine use,[124] but these are rare in children.

The characteristic angioid streaks are slate-gray to reddish-brown linear bands, resembling vasculature, radiating from the optic

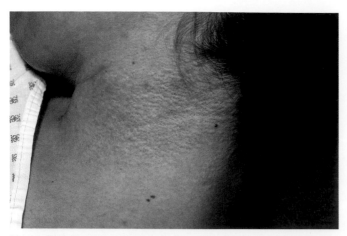

Figure 6.11 Pseudoxanthoma elasticum. Xanthoma-like papules and plaques on the neck have been likened to plucked chicken skin.

papilla. Seen ultimately in 87% of patients, angioid streaks represent visualization of the choroid through tears in the calcified and brittle elastic lamina of Bruch's membrane.[125] Angioid streaks usually do not appear until the third decade of life, but have been described in children as young as 10 years of age. Characteristic irregular retinal epithelial mottling (*peau d'orange*), resulting from degenerated elastic tissue, are frequently detected in children with PXE and usually precede angioid streaks.[120] Loss of central vision (due to retinal hemorrhage and choroidal neovascularization with scarring, not to the angioid streaks per se) is the most frequent disability and may develop in >70% of patients with this complication.[126] These retinal changes are not pathognomonic, since they may also be found in patients with sickle cell anemia, Paget's disease of the bone, idiopathic thrombocytopenic purpura, acromegaly, Ehlers–Danlos syndrome, and lead poisoning.[127] Carriers uncommonly may experience ophthalmologic complications.[128]

Calcification of degenerated elastic tissue of the internal lamina of blood vessels with subsequent hemorrhage is a common and potentially serious complication of PXE. The mid-sized arteries of the extremities, gastrointestinal tract and renal vasculature are sites of early manifestations of this degenerative damage. Both hypertension from resultant renal artery stenosis and gastrointestinal bleeding may occur during adolescence. Late vascular sequelae in PXE include cerebrovascular accidents, intermittent claudication, and myocardial infarction. Severe coronary artery disease has been noted in adolescents with PXE, and may respond to bypass surgery. In addition, an infant with *ABCC6* mutations and a brother with typical manifestations of PXE since adolescence died of generalized arterial calcification, leading to extensive arterial stenosis and myocardial ischemia.[129] Early evidence suggests that carriers of ABCC6 loss-of-function mutations have an increased risk of coronary artery disease, so that parents should be counseled about preventive intervention.[130]

The diagnosis of pseudoxanthoma elasticum is based on the clinical findings and on histopathologic evidence of calcification in elastic tissue and basophilic degeneration of the elastic tissue in the middle and deeper zones of the dermis. Elastic tissue degeneration also affects connective tissue elements of the aorta and medium-sized muscular arteries in the heart, kidneys, gastrointestinal tract, and other organs.

PXE is now recognized to be a metabolic disease, rather than a primary disease of elastic tissue.[131,132] ABCC6 is expressed primarily in the liver and kidneys, and at low levels if at all in tissues affected by PXE. ABCC6 is thought to distribute to the dermis a reduced

form of vitamin K. The form of vitamin K is a co-factor of matrix gla-protein, an inhibitor of ectopic calcification, suggesting a reason for the dermal calcification.[115] Interestingly, a disorder that resembles severe PXE (with pendulous PXE-like skin changes that usually start during adolescence and only spares the face, hands and feet) results from deficiency of an enzyme that activates matrix gla-protein. This matrix gla-protein activator (γ-glutamyl carboxylase or GGCX) is also important for vitamin K-dependent clotting, leading to cerebral aneurysms and a bleeding diathesis in addition to PXE-like changes.[133–137]

Patients with PXE should be advised to protect their eyes from even mild trauma, and about the potential for future visual loss. Intravitreal injection and inhibitors of vascular endothelial growth factor appear promising, and laser and photodynamic therapeutic options are being investigated.[125,137,138] Because of the potential risk to eyes and calcified vessels when traumatized, contact sports and high-intensity cardiovascular exercise should be prohibited for persons with PXE. Avoidance of high cholesterol foods and smoking, control of blood pressure, and safe aerobic exercises are always appropriate because of the vascular risks. Serial cardiac evaluation (careful auscultation and echocardiographic monitoring) to detect mitral valve prolapse and ophthalmologic examinations are important. Early studies suggest that patients who ingested dairy products extensively, rich in calcium and phosphate, had more severe later disease. Subsequently, clinical and histologic improvement in skin lesions has been described in 50% of patients treated systemically with aluminum hydroxide.[139] The recent demonstration that increased dietary intake of magnesium prevents connective tissue mineralization in a mouse model of PXE suggests a new dietary manipulation for affected patients.[140] Plastic surgery may improve the appearance of sagging skin, although extrusion of calcium particles through the surgical wound may result in delayed healing and unsightly scars.[141] Gastrointestinal bleeding can usually be managed conservatively. Two support groups, the National Association for Pseudoxanthoma Elasticum (at: www.napxe.org) and PXE International, Inc (at: www.pxe.org), are available.

Elastosis perforans serpiginosa

Elastosis perforans serpiginosa (perforating elastoma) is a disorder of elastic tissue characterized by an annular, arciform, or linear arrangement of keratotic papules.[142] The individual papules measure 2–4 mm in diameter, but collectively can lead to lesions as long as 15–20 cm in overall length. The papules are generally capped by a distinctive keratotic plug, which, when forcibly dislodged, reveals a bleeding crateriform lesion. Biopsy shows elongated tortuous channels within the epidermis, perforated by abnormal and degenerated elastic tissue extruded from the dermis. Lesions show a predilection for distribution on the posterolateral aspects of the neck (Fig. 6.12) and occasionally the chin, cheeks, mandibular areas of the face, antecubital fossae, elbows, and knees.[143]

This cutaneous disorder primarily affects young persons, especially those in the second decade of life, and generally disappears spontaneously within 5–10 years. Up to 44% of the reported cases have been seen in association with Down syndrome, osteogenesis imperfecta, Ehlers–Danlos syndrome, pseudoxanthoma elasticum, cutis laxa, Rothmund–Thomson syndrome, acrogeria, morphea, or Marfan syndrome, or as a complication of penicillamine therapy.[144–147] Thorough history and physical examination should suffice to consider underlying causes.[147] Treatment with stripping of the surface keratinous material by repeated application of Scotch tape, cryosurgery, laser, and use of keratolytic agents or imiquimod[148] may result in improvement of some lesions, but recurrences are common if therapy is effective.

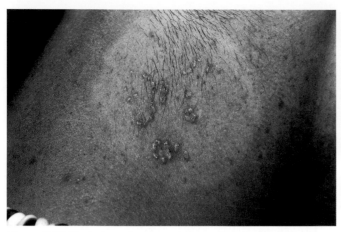

Figure 6.12 Elastosis perforans serpiginosa. Annular, arcuate and linear arrangement of erythematous keratotic papules on the posterolateral aspects of the neck. (Courtesy of Annette Wagner, MD.)

Table 6.8 Most prominent features of focal dermal hypoplasia (Goltz syndrome)
• X-linked dominant, 10% of patients are male
• Linear or reticular patterns of:
– Thinned dermis
– Focal fat herniation
– Hyper- or hypopigmentation
– Papillomas
– Ulcerations
• Ectodermal abnormalities
– Sparse hair
– Thin nails
– Hypodontia, enamel hypoplasia
• Skeletal abnormalities, especially digital anomalies
• Ocular colobomas, strabismus, microphthalmia
• Diagnosis
– Clinical features
– Osteopathia striata (plain radiography)

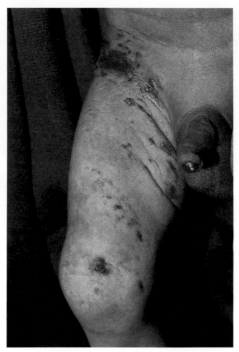

Figure 6.13 Goltz syndrome (focal dermal hypoplasia). Linear streaks of dermal hypoplasia with visible telangiectasia in an affected boy. The condition is presumed to be lethal in male individuals, suggesting that this boy's manifestation reflects post-zygotic mosaicism.

Focal dermal hypoplasia

Focal dermal hypoplasia (Goltz syndrome) is characterized by linear streaks of dermal hypoplasia (Table 6.8). The condition is X-linked dominant, and thought to be lethal in homozygous males; 90% of patients are female. The disorder results from mutations in PORCN, which encodes a protein that is critical for the secretion of Wnt, critical for the development of skin and bones.[149-151] In general, the disorder reflects mosaicism of the mutated PORCN gene in male individuals.[152,153] (Fig. 6.13).

Many of the cutaneous manifestations of focal dermal hypoplasia are present from birth.[154,155] These include the widely distributed linear areas of hypoplasia of the skin, often with associated telangiectasia (Fig. 6.14); soft, yellow, reddish-yellow, or yellowish-brown nodular outpouchings, often in a linear distribution (caused by herniation of the subcutaneous fat through the thinned dermis); and sometimes large cutaneous ulcers (due to congenital absence of skin) that gradually heal with atrophy. Patients often show streaky hyper- or hypopigmentation, and erythematous papillomas of the affected skin or mucosae of the oral, anal, or genital region may develop. Paper-thin nails, sparseness of hair, and hypodontia with enamel hypoplasia have been described. Skeletal abnormalities are most commonly digital abnormalities (adactyly, syndactyly,

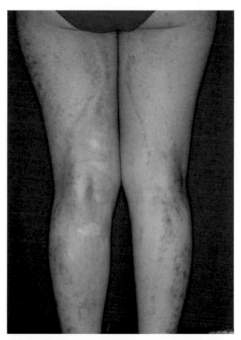

Figure 6.14 Goltz syndrome. Streaks of dermal hypoplasia with visible telangiectasia that follow Blaschko's lines. The white patches are scar tissue after healing of sites of cutis aplasia.

and 'lobster claw' deformities) (Fig. 6.15). Associated ocular abnormalities include colobomas, strabismus, and microphthalmia of the eyes. Other associated abnormalities include umbilical or inguinal hernia, cleft lip and/or cleft palate, and, in some affected individuals, microcephaly and mental retardation.

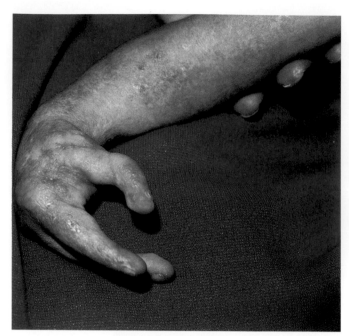

Figure 6.15 Goltz syndrome. Skeletal deformities are common, especially involving the hand.

Focal dermal hypoplasia should not be confused with *focal facial dermal dysplasia* (FFDD), characterized by bitemporal, round, scar-like lesions that resemble forceps marks. Both autosomal dominant (type I) and recessive (types II and III) inheritance have been described. Patients with Brauer syndrome (types I and II FFDD) have no other associated anomalies.[78,156] Only affected individuals with Setleis syndrome (type III FFDD, see Ch. 2) show the bitemporal lesions of focal facial dermal hypoplasia in association with a coarse facial appearance, anomalies of the eyelashes and lateral eyebrows,[157,158] dysplastic low-set ears, and a characteristic mouth with large lips and an inverted 'V' contour with downturned corners.[159] Setleis syndrome results from mutations in *TW15Tc*, a transcription factor important for development. Focal dermal hypoplasia must also be distinguished from *microphthalmia with linear skin defects* (MLS) syndrome, an X-linked dominant developmental defect with microphthalmia and other eye abnormalities, in association with linear, jagged skin defects typically involving the face, scalp, neck and occasionally the upper trunk.[160] Other typical features can include short stature, developmental delay, structural brain abnormalities, seizures, diaphragmatic hernia, and congenital heart defects. Mutations in mitochondrial holocytochrome c-type synthase (HCCS) at chromosome Xp22 are responsible.[161]

Virtually all cases of focal dermal hypoplasia reveal fine parallel linear striations in the metaphyses of long bones at or near epiphyseal junctions on radiographs. Although striations can be seen with other bony abnormalities, this linear change in the metaphyseal regions of the long bones (termed *osteopathia striata*) is a very useful index for the diagnosis of this disorder. The diagnosis can be further confirmed by biopsy of an affected area of skin, which shows hypoplasia of dermal connective tissue with upward extension of the subcutaneous fat tissue, almost to the normal epidermis. Even mildly affected females (from mosaicism or skewed X-inactivation) or males (mosaics) require genetic counseling, because of the risk of having severely affected offspring.[154,162] Surgical intervention can ameliorate the developmental defects, such as syndactyly or polydactyly, and remove papillomas of the skin or mucous membranes. Pulsed dye laser therapy can reduce telangiectasia, and dental care

can dramatically improve the hypodontia and enamel dysplasia.[163] Families can find support resources internationally through the National Foundation for Ectodermal Dysplasias (see: www.nfed.org).

Werner syndrome

Werner syndrome (progeria of the adult) is a rare autosomal recessive disorder that results from mutations in the *WRN* gene, which encodes Werner protein, a DNA helicase enzyme that maintains genomic stability.[164–167] Patients usually develop and appear normal until adolescence, when they lack the pubertal growth spurt. Premature graying of hair at the temples may be seen then, and patients develop progressive alopecia, short stature, birdlike facies, and an apparent aged appearance. Cutaneous features include sclerodermoid changes of the skin of the extremities and, to a lesser degree, the face and neck; telangiectasias; mottled or diffuse pigmentation; keratoses; and indolent ulcers over pressure points, particularly on the soles and ankles.

Patients with Werner syndrome develop severe, often generalized vascular disease; diabetes mellitus (71%); hypogonadism (80%); osteoporosis (91%); cataracts (100%); loss of subcutaneous tissue and severe muscle wasting in the legs, arms, feet, and hands with large abdominal fat deposits (leading to a body habitus of a stocky trunk with spindly extremities); soft tissue calcification; a high-pitched voice or hoarseness; and a predisposition to neoplastic disease (hepatoma, thyroid adenocarcinoma, ovarian carcinoma, fibrosarcoma, osteogenic sarcoma, and carcinoma of the breast).[168] The mean age of death is 54 years. 'Atypical Werner syndrome' affects about 15% of patients clinically diagnosed with Werner syndrome, but is related to mutations in *LMNA* (see Progeria, below), rather than *WRN*. Therapy for Werner syndrome is supportive, but a recent study in a mouse model of Werner syndrome suggests that vitamin C supplementation may reverse aging abnormalities and lengthen the lifespan.[169]

Progeria

Progeria (Hutchinson–Gilford progeria syndrome, HGPS) is a rare disease that most often results from a specific mutation (1824C>T; G608G) on one allele of *LMNA*, which encodes lamin A, a component of the nuclear lamina.[170–172] Although this common mutation does not even change an amino acid, it does activate a cryptic splice site, so that mutant lamin A precursor, or progerin, lacks a series of 50 missing amino acids and is thus permanently modified by lipid farnesylation. Farnesylation of progerin prevents its proper insertion into the nuclear lamina and leads to progressive deformities in the nuclei of patients with HGPS. It is unclear if non-farnesylated progerin also has toxicity.[173] Interestingly, progerin has also been shown to accumulate with aging in normal cells.[174] Although the mutations in HGPS are dominant negative, an autosomal recessive form with homozygous *LMNA* mutations (R527C) has been described.[175] Affected children showed features of HGPS but additional gastrointestinal and skeletal abnormalities, and carrier parents are asymptomatic. Atypical progeroid syndrome may result from missense *LMNA* mutations other than G608G that lead to nuclear abnormalities but are not rescued by farnesyltransferase inhibitors.[176]

HGPS first manifests at 6–18 months of age with cutaneous alterations: perioral and nasolabial cyanosis, dyspigmentation, and localized sclerodermatous changes.[177] Patients progressively develop additional signs of premature aging, including alopecia of the scalp, eyebrows and lashes, early skin wrinkling, osteopenia with fractures, and atherosclerosis.[178] Other characteristics are reduced birthweight with postnatal growth retardation;[179] profound midfacial hypoplasia and micrognathia, but the appearance of hydrocephalus because upper head size is minimally reduced; and generalized atrophy of muscle and subcutaneous tissue with a beaked nose and a bird-like appearance. Veins are particularly prominent on the alopecic scalp and thighs (Fig. 6.16). The teeth become crowded, irregular in form, or deficient in number, and deciduous dentition is often retained.[180] Speech becomes high pitched and squeaky, and intelligence is generally normal. The chest becomes narrow and the abdomen protuberant; owing to a mild flexion of the knees, a 'horse-riding' stance becomes apparent.

Cardiac murmurs frequently occur after the age of 5 years and are soon followed by atherosclerosis-induced hypertension, cardiomegaly, angina, myocardial infarction, and congestive heart failure. Death usually occurs at a mean age of 13.4 years, usually owing to the coronary artery disease.[181] Growth hormone treatment increases weight by ~50% and linear growth by only ~10%.

In progeria mouse models, farnesyltransferase inhibitor treatment reverses the nuclear distortion and prevents the progression of cardiovascular disease.[182] Trials of farnesyltransferase inhibitors[183] and a statin and bisphosphonate[184] are ongoing.

Late-onset progeria has also been called atypical Werner syndrome, and is now known to result from heterozygous missense mutations in LMNA.[185] Affected individuals start to show aging as young adults but show an accelerated rate compared to patients with Werner syndrome, and usually have no diabetes or cataracts. Progeria should be distinguished from scleroderma, and from Werner, Hallermann–Streiff, Cockayne, Bloom, and Rothmund–Thomson syndromes.

Restrictive dermopathy

Restrictive dermopathy is a rare, fatal, autosomal recessive disorder characterized by taut, translucent, thin skin with erosions and fissures.[186,187] The intrauterine course is characterized by polyhydramnios with reduced fetal movements, beginning at about 31 weeks' gestational age.[188,189] Clavicular hypoplasia is a consistent *in utero* characteristic.[190] Affected neonates show a dysmorphic facies (fixed round open mouth with micrognathia, a small pinched nose,

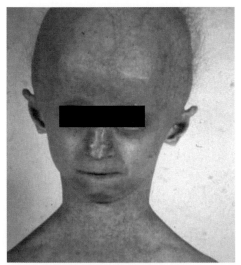

Figure 6.16 Progeria. Alopecia, subcutaneous atrophy, prominent scalp veins, and bird-like facies. (Courtesy of Schachner LA, Hansen RC, eds. Pediatric dermatology, 3rd edn. New York: Elsevier.)

hypertelorism, enlarged fontanelles, and widened sutures) and flexion contractures. Death usually occurs shortly after birth owing to pulmonary atelectasis, but affected babies have survived as long as months with respiratory and nutritional support. Biopsy sections show a flat epidermal junction and a thin dermis with compact collagen fibers, sparse elastic fibers, and rudimentary skin appendages. Restrictive dermopathy most commonly results from mutations in both alleles of *ZMPSTE24*, and occasionally from dominant negative mutations in *LMNA*.[191–194] ZMPSTE24 is an important metalloproteinase that processes lamin A; in the face of ZMPSTE24 deficiency, prelamin A accumulates and leads to nuclear membrane toxicity.

Stiff skin syndrome

In patients with the stiff skin syndrome (also called congenital fascial dystrophy), cutaneous and subcutaneous induration first develops between the neonatal period and early childhood, and is most severe on the legs, thighs, buttocks, and overlying joints.[195–198] Congenital fascial dystrophy is considered a subset.[199] Joint stiffness begins during early childhood, can significantly limit movement, and can be progressive, although the skin induration is relatively stable. Hypertrichosis may be associated, but viscera are not affected. Biopsies show thickening of the dermis and fascia with fibroblasts in the subcutaneous tissues and deposition of hyaluronic acid, but no inflammation.[200] The condition needs to be distinguished from scleredema neonatorum, subcutaneous fat necrosis, and scleroderma.[201] Systemic administration of corticosteroids and other immunosuppressive agents has caused no improvement. Management is through physical therapy.

Winchester syndrome

This autosomal recessive disorder has been described in fewer than a dozen patients;[202] in the reported cases, parents have been consanguineous. It is characterized by short stature, coarse facies, corneal opacities, thickened leathery and hypertrichotic skin, hypertrophic lips and gingivae, generalized osteolysis and progressive painful arthropathy with joint stiffness and contractures of distal phalanges.[203] Osteolysis may first be detectable after 1 year of age and can be progressive. Symmetrical restrictive banding has been reported to develop in early adulthood.[204] The disorder has been attributed to mutations in both alleles of matrix metalloproteinase 2 (MMP2).[205,206] Nodulosis-arthropathy-osteolysis (NAO) and Torg syndromes are allelic.[206,207]

Buschke–Ollendorff syndrome

Buschke–Ollendorff syndrome is an autosomal dominant disorder, which, when fully expressed, manifests as elastomas and osteopoikilosis.[208–212] The estimated incidence is estimated at 1 : 20 000.[213] It results from loss of function mutations in the LEMD3 gene, which leads to enhanced TGF (transforming growth factor)-β signaling.[214,215] Defects in LEMD3 have also been detected in cases of isolated osteopoikilosis. In some affected individuals, dermal lesions are absent;[216] in others, the radiographic changes are not seen.[217]

The connective tissue nevi appear as collections of subtle 3 mm, skin-colored to yellow papules or plaques (dermatofibrosis lenticularis disseminata) on the buttocks, proximal trunk, and limbs. Most patients first develop lesions in early childhood. Histopathologic examination of lesional skin usually shows increased amounts of

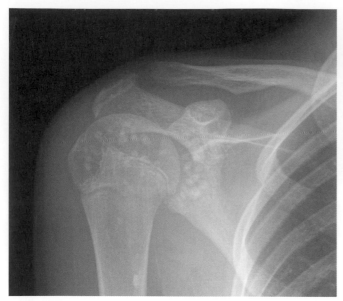

Figure 6.17 Buschke–Ollendorff syndrome. An oncology consultation was recommended because the small round radiodensities on X-rays of this boy with Buschke–Ollendorff syndrome were not recognized to be osteopoikilosis.

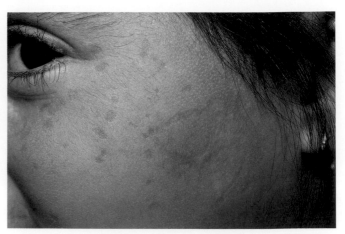

Figure 6.18 Lipoid proteinosis. Linear or varioliform scars develop after clearance of the vesicular, crusted lesions of childhood; the papular lesions characteristic of lipoid proteinosis do not tend to appear until late childhood.

elastic tissue (elastoma).[218,219] The bony lesions most frequently appear after 15 years of age. They are discrete spherical areas of increased radiodensity, most frequently noted in the epiphyses and metaphyses of long bone, pelvis, scapulae, carpal and tarsal bones (Fig. 6.17). The osteopoikilosis causes no clinical problems, but in the absence of cutaneous changes may be misdiagnosed as bony metastases. Other skeletal abnormalities, including short stature, otosclerosis, spinal stenosis,[209] and supernumerary vertebrae and ribs have been described. Connective tissue nevi (with increased collagen), papular elastorrhexis,[220] morphea, and PXE are the most frequent disorders considered in the differential diagnosis. The lesions of papular elastorrhexis resemble dermatofibrosis lenticularis disseminata, but show decreased, fragmented elastic fibers rather than elastomas. Although usually sporadic, papular elastorrhexis has been described as familial with an autosomal dominant mode of inheritance.[221] No therapy is available or necessary.

Lipoid proteinosis

Lipoid proteinosis (hyalinosis cutis et mucosae) is an autosomal recessive disorder characterized by hoarseness beginning in infancy, and the later appearance of yellowish, beaded papules and nodules in the skin.[39,222–224] Both the hoarseness and the cutaneous lesions result from the abnormal deposition of hyaline material at the dermal-epidermal and microvascular basement membranes and papillary dermis.[225] The underlying molecular basis of lipoid proteinosis is mutations in extracellular matrix protein 1 (ECM1), a secreted protein that may play roles in skin adhesion and protein interactions near the basement membrane.[226,227] Interestingly, ECM1 is an autoantigen in lichen sclerosus (Ch. 22).[228]

Hoarseness secondary to vocal cord involvement is a clinical feature in virtually every case, and adolescents and adults with this disorder can be recognized instantly because of their husky voice and thickened eyelids. The voice may be hoarse from birth or within the first few years of life and becomes progressively worse during early childhood. Young children most commonly show vesicles or bullae that rapidly erode and become crusted.[229] Ultrastructural analysis of these lesions and cultured keratinocytes shows 'free-floating' intact desmosomes, consistent with the role of ECM1 in cell–cell adhesion.[230]

Peculiar linear or discrete varioliform scars develop, particularly on the face, trunk, and upper extremities (Fig. 6.18). Herpes simplex infection, impetigo, or epidermolysis bullosa may be considered as alternative diagnoses.

Patients first develop the typical discrete or confluent 2–3 mm yellowish-white to yellowish-brown papules in later childhood. These papules are found most frequently on the face, eyelids, neck, and hands. In about 50% of individuals, a string of bead-like papules, often followed by a loss of cilia, appears on the free eyelid margins. The flexural areas often show a yellow waxy appearance with diffuse thickening of the skin. Many adults with lipoid proteinosis have hyperkeratotic plaques on elbows, knees, and palms, with infiltrative plaques at sites of trauma.

Also characteristic in patients with extensive manifestations are eversion of the lips (with their surfaces studded with tiny yellow nodules), hypertrophic or vegetative lesions at the corners of the mouth, round papules just below the lip on the midline of the chin, and radiating fissures at the corners of the mouth. Partial alopecia of the scalp, eyebrows, eyelashes, or bearded area is common by later childhood. Other features that have been described are hypohidrosis; hypertrichosis; hypoplasia or aplasia of permanent teeth; parotid pain and recurrent parotid swelling as a result of obstruction of Stensen's duct; and impaired nail growth.

Because of hyaline deposition, the tongue becomes thick, firm, and woody, is bound to the floor of the mouth, and is difficult to extrude; the soft palate, tonsils, uvula, and undersurface of the tongue show extensive irregular yellow-white infiltrations. Dysphagia caused by pharyngeal infiltration and respiratory obstruction as a result of severe laryngeal involvement can complicate the disorder. Central nervous system involvement has been associated with attacks of rage and psychomotor or grand mal seizures. Usually, however, the central nervous system involvement is restricted to asymptomatic calcification (seen in 70% of patients older than 10 years of age), which can be seen on radiographic examination as bilateral bean-shaped opacities above the sella turcica.

Diagnosis is aided by a history of hoarseness from early childhood; thickening, stiffening, and difficulty in extrusion of the tongue; an impaired ability to swallow; characteristic involvement of the skin and mucous membranes; and histopathologic examination of involved tissue. Histologic features consist of thick homogeneous bands of eosinophilic, periodic acid-Schiff-positive, hyaline-like amorphous material in the upper dermis, with an associated patchy distribution surrounding blood vessels, sweat glands, and arrector pili muscles.

Lipoid proteinosis has a chronic but relatively benign course. Treatment is chiefly symptomatic and consists of surgical or laser removal of laryngeal nodules or tracheostomy for laryngeal obstruction, and cosmetic measures such as laser resurfacing or dermabrasion for unappealing cutaneous lesions on the face or other exposed surfaces. Acitretin markedly improved the hoarseness in a patient, but not the skin lesions.[231]

Infantile systemic hyalinosis and juvenile hyaline fibromatosis

Infantile systemic hyalinosis (ISH) and juvenile hyaline fibromatosis (JHF) are similar autosomal recessive conditions that represent allelic variants, resulting from mutations in the gene that encodes capillary morphogenesis protein 2 (CMP2).[232–234] The histologic and ultrastructural features of ISH and JHF are similar. Hyaline deposition occurs in multiple organ systems.

ISH represents the most severe end of the spectrum,[235] with manifestations present within the first few weeks of life, although intrauterine growth retardation and reduced fetal movements have been described. The predominant cutaneous findings of ISH are diffusely thickened skin, small nodules of the perianal region, ears, and lips, and a reddish-blue to hyperpigmented discoloration overlying bony prominences.[236–238] The joint contractures and osteopenia lead to the frog-leg position and virtual immobility that are typical of affected infants.[239] Patients with ISH also develop malabsorption and a protein-losing enteropathy, leading to diarrhea and failure to thrive. Oral manifestations include thickening of the oral mucosa, extensive overgrowth of the gingival tissue, marked curvature of the dental roots, and replacement of periodontal ligament by hyaline fibrous material. These oral findings may cause difficulty in feeding and compound the nutritional deficiency resulting from malabsorption. Thyroid dysfunction has also been described.[240] The condition is usually fatal by 2 years of age because of recurrent pulmonary infections and diarrhea.

Juvenile hyaline fibromatosis (JHF), also known as juvenile systemic hyalinosis, encompasses mild to moderate disease within the spectrum of CMP2 mutations.[241] JHF is characterized by joint contractures, gingival hypertrophy, generalized osteopenia, and papular and nodular skin lesions, typically on the scalp, perianal and perinasal areas (Fig. 6.19), palms, and trunk.[242,243] JHF has a later onset and patients survive into adulthood.

There is no satisfactory treatment at this time, although administration of interferon α-2B led to remarkable improvement in skin nodules, gingival hypertrophy, and joint mobility in a girl with JHF.[244] Early dental intervention is important, and gingivectomy may be required[245] with careful anesthetic management.[246,247]

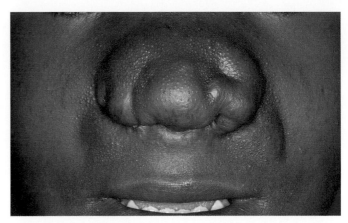

Figure 6.19 Juvenile hyaline fibromatosis. Note the nodules on the nose and the gingival hypertrophy. Fine papules can be seen on the nose and perinasal area; the patient had dozens of visible 1–2 mm papules on the chin as well.

Key References

The complete list of 247 references for this chapter is available online at **www.expertconsult.com**.
See inside cover for registration details.

Beighton P, De Paepe A, Steinmann B, et al. Ehlers-Danlos syndromes: Revised nosology, Villefranche, 1997. Ehlers-Danlos National Foundation (USA) and Ehlers-Danlos Support Group (UK). *Am J Med Genet.* 1998;77(1):31–37.

Callewaert B, Malfait F, Loeys B, De Paepe A. Ehlers-Danlos syndromes and Marfan syndrome. *Best Pract Res Clin Rheumatol.* 2008;22(1):165–189.

Dean JC. Marfan syndrome: clinical diagnosis and management. *Eur J Hum Genet.* 2007;15(7):724–733.

Maas SM, Lombardi MP, van Essen AJ, et al. Phenotype and genotype in 17 patients with Goltz-Gorlin syndrome. *J Med Genet.* 2009; 46(10):716–720.

Merideth MA, Gordon LB, Clauss S, et al. Phenotype and course of Hutchinson-Gilford progeria syndrome. *N Engl J Med.* 2008;358(6): 592–604.

Mitchell AL, Schwarze U, Jennings JF, Byers PH. Molecular mechanisms of classical Ehlers-Danlos syndrome (EDS). *Hum Mutat.* 2009;30(6):995–1002.

Naouri M, Boisseau C, Bonicel P, et al. Manifestations of pseudoxanthoma elasticum in childhood. *Br J Dermatol.* 2009;161(3):635–639.

Ramirez F, Dietz HC. Marfan syndrome: from molecular pathogenesis to clinical treatment. *Curr Opin Genet Dev.* 2007;17(3):252–258.

Ringpfeil F. Selected disorders of connective tissue: pseudoxanthoma elasticum, cutis laxa, and lipoid proteinosis. *Clin Dermatol.* 2005;23(1):41–46.

Uitto J, Li Q, Jiang Q. Pseudoxanthoma elasticum: molecular genetics and putative pathomechanisms. *J Invest Dermatol.* 2010;130(3): 661–670.

Disorders of Hair and Nails

Hair

Hair is a protein by-product of follicles distributed everywhere on the body surface except the palms, soles, vermilion portion of the lips, glans penis, penile shaft, nail beds, and sides of the fingers and toes. Although hair is of minimal functional benefit to humans, the psychological effects of disturbances of hair growth are frequently a source of great concern to children, adolescents, and their parents.

In the human fetus, groups of cells appear in the epidermis at about the 8th week of gestation. These differentiate to form the hair follicles, and hair begins to develop between the 8th and 12th weeks of fetal life. This growth continues throughout fetal development. Although there are indications that some hair is lost during gestation and at the time of birth, the majority of hairs on the newborn are 5–6 months old.

Lanugo hairs are fine, soft, unmedullated, and poorly pigmented hairs, seen only in fetal and neonatal life, except in the rare hereditary syndrome hypertrichosis lanuginosa. They appear as a fine dense growth over the entire cutaneous surface of the fetus. Lanugo hair is normally shed *in utero* in the 7th or 8th month of gestation, but may cover the entire cutaneous surface of the premature newborn infant. Postnatal hair may be divided into *vellus* and *terminal* types. Vellus hairs are the fine, lightly pigmented hairs seen on the arms and faces of children. Terminal hairs are the mature thick darker hairs on the scalp, eyebrows, eyelashes, and areas of secondary sexual hair distribution. The number and distribution of individual hair follicles are genetically determined and constant from birth. As the infant's skin grows, however, the density of hair follicles reduces from $1135/cm^2$ at birth to $615/cm^2$ by adulthood.

The average human scalp contains 100 000 hairs. The average growth rate of terminal hair is approximately 2.5 mm/week (1 cm/month). The hair shaft represents the equivalent of the stratum corneum of skin, with the follicular keratinocytes dictating the characteristics of the shaft. The hair root is characterized by three definable cyclic stages of growth-anagen (Fig. 7.1A), catagen, and telogen (Fig. 7.1B; Table 7.1). The human hair follicle has a fairly long phase of regular growth (the anagen phase), which lasts 2–6 years, with an average of 3 years. The hairs then undergo a period of partial degeneration (the catagen phase), lasting up to 3 weeks, followed by a resting (telogen or club) phase. The telogen phase of the follicle lasts for about 3 months. At the end of this time, new growth is initiated. As new hairs grow, they push out the old telogen hairs that have remained in the resting follicles. In healthy individuals, 80–90% of the scalp is in the actively growing anagen stage, and 5% is in the brief transitional (catagen) stage; 10–15% is in the resting or telogen stage, with an average of 50–100 hairs shed and simultaneously replaced each day.

Neonatal hair

The first crop of terminal scalp hair is in the actively growing anagen phase at birth, but within the first few days of life there is a physiologic conversion to the telogen phase. Consequently, a high proportion of neonatal scalp hairs are shed during the first 4 months of life (Fig. 7.2). This telogen shedding (*telogen effluvium of the newborn*) may occur as a sudden hair loss or, more commonly, as gradual hair loss; hair loss may range from barely perceptible to almost complete alopecia. Whether sudden or gradual, replacement of the first terminal hairs is generally completed before the first 6 months of life. The neonatal hairline frequently extends along the forehead and temples to the lateral margin of the eyebrows. These terminal hairs gradually convert to vellus hairs during the first year of life. Premature infants are frequently covered by lanugo hairs, which are more densely distributed on the face, limbs, and trunk. This is probably related to the cyclic activity *in utero* and the normal shedding of telogen vellus hairs in the fetus during the last few weeks of gestation.

Alopecias

Hair loss disorders can be divided into non-scarring (non-cicatricial) or scarring (cicatricial) types. Causes of non-scarring alopecia include alteration of the hair growth cycle, inflammatory cutaneous disease, and structural abnormalities of the hair.[2,3] Some traumatic disorders, such as traction alopecia, pressure alopecia or trichotillomania, can scar if severe, but often resolve without clinical evidence of scarring. Evaluation typically involves gentle traction on the hair (pull test) to determine if hair comes out easily (as in loose anagen syndrome, alopecia areata or telogen effluvium) and microscopic evaluation of hair shafts to seek hair shaft abnormalities.

Non-scarring alopecias with hair shaft abnormalities

Hair Shaft Abnormalities with Increased Fragility

Variations in the structure of the hair shaft are a common occurrence and, at times, may provide clues to other pathologic abnormalities. Because each hair shaft anomaly has a distinctive morphology, the diagnosis frequently can be established in the office by dermatoscopy[4] or by microscopic examination of snipped hairs.[2] Other than reduction of trauma to reduce breakage, there is no effective treatment for this group of disorders.

Trichorrhexis nodosa

Trichorrhexis nodosa, the most common hair shaft anomaly, is a distinctive disorder manifested by increased fragility.[2,5] Grayish-white nodules may be seen on the hair (Fig. 7.3), which under a light microscope, have the appearance of two interlocking brushes or brooms, the result of segmental longitudinal splitting of fibers without complete fracture. The disorder features dry lusterless short

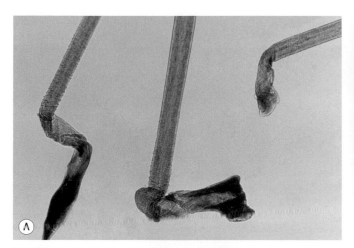

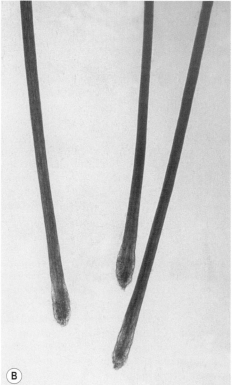

Figure 7.1 Stages of growth of the hair root. Anagen hairs are the growing hairs that comprise 90% of hair at any time and persist for several years. The anagen hairs shown here are distorted at their root (A), which can occur from vigorous plucking but are the cardinal microscopic feature of the hair of children with loose anagen syndrome. Telogen hairs (B) are in a resting phase that persists for 3 months. Note the small bulb and lack of sheath. (Reprinted with permission from Bolognia et al. (2003).[1])

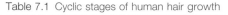

Table 7.1 Cyclic stages of human hair growth

1. Anagen phase (active growth phase) lasts 2–6 years (average 3 years)
2. Catagen phase (stage of partial degeneration) lasts 10–14 days
3. Telogen phase (resting stage) lasts 3–4 months.

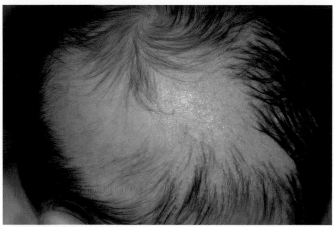

Figure 7.2 Telogen shedding of the newborn. This 4-month-old boy shows generalized thinning of scalp hair, reflecting telogen effluvium. He also had suction, leading to caput succedaneum and 'halo alopecia'.

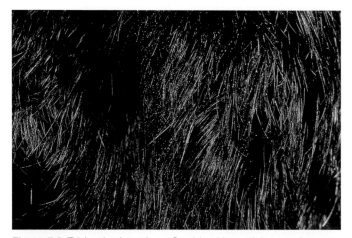

Figure 7.3 Trichorrhexis nodosa. Grayish-white nodules may be seen on the hair, which resemble two interlocking brushes or brooms by light microscopic examination.

hair that is easily fractured. Trichorrhexis nodosa usually occurs as an acquired form unassociated with other problems; however, the condition may be genetic and manifest during infancy. Infants with the autosomal dominant form show normal hair at birth, but the hair that regrows within a few months is abnormal; the hair defect tends to improve with advancing age. Trichorrhexis nodosa may also be a manifestation of children with the late-onset form of *argininosuccinic aciduria*, a condition that results from lack of argininosuccinase. In this condition, the hair is usually normal at birth and first becomes fragile at 1–2 years of age with a dull, matted appearance, especially at the occipital area. The hair defects are associated with psychomotor retardation, cerebellar ataxia, and a marked increase of argininosuccinic acid in the blood, urine, and cerebrospinal fluid.[6,7] Dietary treatment of the metabolic abnormality leads to normalization of the appearance and integrity of the hair. Similar clinical manifestations are found in infants with *citrullinemia*, caused by a deficiency of argininosuccinic acid synthetase. Trichorrhexis nodosa is the most common hair shaft abnormality, but pili torti has been described and hair bulbs may be atrophic. Some patients show an eruption that resembles acrodermatitis enteropathica. Trichorrhexis nodosa has also been described in oculo-dental-digital dysplasia (see below).[8,9] Trichorrhexis nodosa is the hair shaft defect in tricho-hepato-enteric syndrome, characterized by facial dysmorphism, immune defects, and severe diarrhea, requiring intravenous nutrition. Trichorrhexis nodosa is also one of the hair shaft abnormalities seen in trichothiodystrophy (below).

Usually seen in adolescents, acquired trichorrhexis nodosa most commonly occurs from trauma to the hair. The injury may result from the use of hot combs, excessively hot hairdryers, hair straighteners, or other chemical treatments, or from the cumulative cuticular damage from vigorous combing and brushing, repeated salt-water bathing, prolonged sun exposure, and frequent shampooing. Cream rinses and protein conditioners are helpful. If hair-straightening procedures, vigorous grooming habits, and thermal and chemical trauma to the hair are discontinued, the acquired form of trichorrhexis nodosa generally improves within 2–4 years.

Monilethrix

Monilethrix (beaded hair) is an autosomal dominant disorder characterized by variation in hair shaft thickness, with small node-like deformities that produce a beaded appearance, internodal fragility, breakage, and partial alopecia (Fig. 7.4). In individuals with this disorder, normal neonatal lanugo hairs are shed during the first few weeks of life. The regrown hair, which generally appears at about the 2nd month of life, is dry, lusterless, and brittle, and fails to grow to any appreciable length. In severe cases, the infant may remain bald or the scalp hair may be sparse, easily fractured, and stubble-like. Although generally a disorder of scalp hair, body hairs may

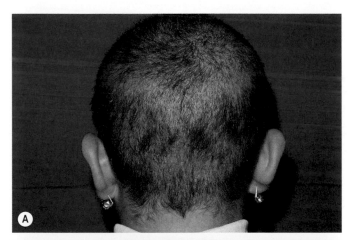

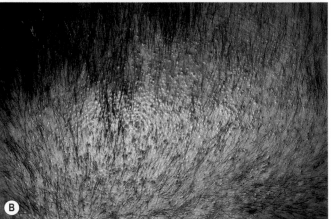

Figure 7.4 Monilethrix. (A) The hair is dry, lusterless, brittle, and fails to grow to any appreciable length. The occipital area is most frequently and most severely affected in most cases. (B) The follicles are prominent and often hyperkeratotic.

also be affected. The clinical findings are limited to the occiput and nape in more limited cases. Occasionally this disorder is not apparent during infancy, but becomes apparent later in childhood or during adult life. Follicular keratosis is associated in some pedigrees, and may affect the face, scalp, and extremities. Some patients show koilonychia. Spontaneous improvement or remission may occur at puberty or during pregnancy, suggesting a hormonal influence,[10] but the condition may persist unchanged throughout adulthood. Administration of oral retinoids can lead to clinical improvement.[11]

Monilethrix most commonly is autosomal dominant and results from mutations in hair keratins. Of the 26 known hair follicle-specific keratins, three have been associated with monilethrix and all are type II keratins.[12] Mutations in KRT81 and KRT86 are most common,[13] but a mutation in KRT83 has been reported. Because keratins provide structural integrity to hair, abnormalities in these keratins lead to hair fragility with breakage occurring at the internodal sites. Autosomal recessive monilethrix has been linked to mutations in DSG4, which encodes desmoglein 4, a transmembranous cell adhesion molecule of the cadherin family that is predominantly expressed in the hair cortex and upper cuticle.[14,15] Desmoglein 4 is thought to integrate keratin filaments into desmosomes.[16] Desmoglein 4 mutations may also manifest as *autosomal recessive hypotrichosis*, which resembles monilethrix but lacks the characteristic beaded appearance of the hair shaft under light microscopy.[17]

Pseudomonilethrix

Pseudomonilethrix was originally described as an autosomal dominant developmental defect of fragile hair with irregularly shaped nodes.[3,18] In fact, the hair changes are artifactual, and related to overlapping hairs under the pressure of an overlying glass slide.[19] Pseudomonilethrix is seen more commonly when fine hairs are handled by forceps.

Trichorrhexis invaginata

Trichorrhexis invaginata (bamboo hair) is characterized clinically by dry, lusterless, easily fractured, sparse, and short hair. Under light microscopy, the hairs show a peculiar intussusception or telescope-like invagination along the hair shaft, which microscopically resembles the ball-and-cup joints of bamboo.[2,20] Variations in trichorrhexis invaginata occur, most commonly the 'golf tee hair', presenting the expanded proximal end of an invaginate node.[21] The hair defect in trichorrhexis invaginata is thought to be abnormal keratinization of the hair shaft, which results in softening of the hair cortex and promotes intussusception of the distal portion of the hair shaft into the softer proximal portion.

Although trichorrhexis invaginata may occur as an isolated finding, this hair shaft abnormality is characteristic of Netherton syndrome (Fig. 7.5), an autosomal recessive genodermatosis that has recently been linked to mutations in SPINK5 (see Ch. 5).[22] Neonates with this disorder characteristically show generalized exfoliative erythroderma and failure to thrive, often associated with hypernatremic dehydration, recurrent infections, and sepsis. Severely affected neonates may show extremely sparse and even absent hair, making the diagnosis based on hair shaft examination difficult. However, the eyebrows are almost always short and broken (Fig. 7.5A); eyebrow hairs should be examined in cases in which the abnormality cannot be demonstrated from scalp hair, and dermoscopy can be helpful.[23,24] Beyond infancy, many affected individuals show a characteristic skin finding, ichthyosis linearis circumflexa, with walls of scale surrounding red patches, in addition to their dry, lusterless hair that breaks easily (Fig. 7.5B; see Figs 5.19, 5.20). Atopic conditions usually accompany the ichthyosis. Although spontaneous remission of the hair defect has been

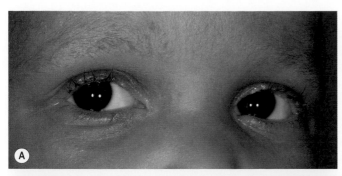

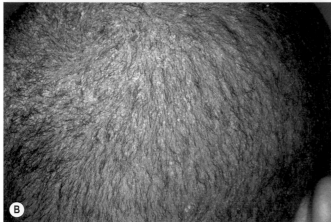

Figure 7.5 Netherton syndrome. (A) The characteristic microscopic features of Netherton hair (trichorrhexis invaginata) are often found in eyebrow hairs. Note the sparse, broken brows and lashes in this young girl who also shows the periorbital dermatitis. (B) Short, broken hair throughout the scalp. Note the desquamative scaling and excoriations.

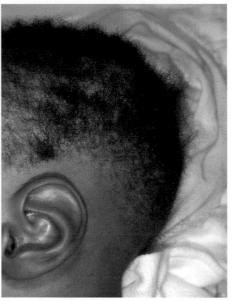

Figure 7.6 Menkes syndrome. The hair is fine, dull, hypopigmented compared with other family members, and stands on end. It looks and feels like steel wool.

described (generally between 6 and 15 years of age), the vast majority show persistence.

Pili torti

Pili torti hairs show three or four regularly spaced twists, which occur at irregular intervals along the hair shaft.[2,25] The hair shaft appears flattened at the site of the twist, which is almost always through 180°. The dry, fragile hair is often lighter in color than expected and shimmers in reflected light, the twisted feature often leading to a 'spangled' appearance. The hair tends to be short, especially in areas subject to trauma, and may extend out from the scalp. Pili torti must be distinguished from twisted hair, which has been described in association with anorexia nervosa.[26]

Pili torti may occur as an isolated phenomenon with onset at birth or early infancy. This genetic disorder shows both autosomal dominant and autosomal recessive inheritance patterns. The appearance of the hair in patients with pili torti may become more normal with time, although twisted hairs can still be found in the adult scalp; those who still manifest the disorder at puberty, however, are unlikely to show significant improvement with age. A late-onset, autosomal dominant form has also been described, in which brittle hair and patchy alopecia develop after puberty. Mental retardation has been noted in some pedigrees. Pili torti has been associated with several mitochondrial disorders (see below).

Menkes syndrome (trichopoliodystrophy) is an X-linked recessive neurodegenerative disorder that affects male infants. Classical Menkes syndrome affects 90–95% of patients, with a less common mild form associated with long survival and occipital horn

syndrome (previously called X-linked cutis laxa or Ehlers–Danlos syndrome type IX) showing largely connective tissue manifestations. Carrier females may exhibit pili torti. Classical Menkes syndrome is characterized by coarse facies, pili torti, temperature instability, seizures, psychomotor retardation, arterial intimal changes, soft doughy skin, joint laxity, low or absent plasma copper and ceruloplasmin levels, growth failure, increased susceptibility to infection, and death, generally by age 3 or 4 years.[27,28] Clinical features often include premature birth, hypothermia, and relatively normal development until 2–6 months of age, when drowsiness and lethargy are noted, intractable seizures begin, and growth and development cease. Usually the hair is fine, dull, sparse, and poorly pigmented in infancy; it stands on end, and looks and feels like steel wool (Fig. 7.6). Additional features include tortuosity of cerebral and other medium-sized arteries; osteoporosis; frequent subdural hematomas; widening of the metaphyses with spurring; and frequent fractures, at times simulating the radiologic findings characteristic of patients with the battered child syndrome. Although pili torti is generally a prominent feature of this disorder, other less frequently reported hair abnormalities include monilethrix and trichorrhexis nodosa.

Menkes syndrome results from mutations in *ATP7A*,[29] which encodes a copper transporting adenosine triphosphatase that incorporates copper into copper-dependent enzymes and maintains copper levels by removing excessive copper from the cytosol.[30] The combination of clinical features, bone abnormalities, and low plasma copper and ceruloplasmin levels establishes the correct diagnosis. Parenteral administration of copper histidine can prevent neurological degeneration and pigmentation if initiated in the neonatal or infantile period.[31]

Bazex–Dupre–Christol and *Rombo syndromes* are X-linked dominant traits characterized by congenital hypotrichosis with pili torti, number facial milia, trichoepitheliomas, vellus hair cysts and an increased risk of the early development of basal cell carcinomas.[20,32–35] Distinguishing features are follicular atrophoderma, hypohidrosis, comedones and facial and neck pigmentation in Bazex–Dupre–Christol syndrome, and atrophoderma vermiculatum and photosensitivity in Rombo syndrome. Females often do not show the hypotrichosis, with normal and pili torti hairs intermingled.[36] *Pili torti with hypotrichosis* occur in association with *macular dystrophy* and severe retinal dysfunction as an autosomal recessive disorder; the underlying mutation affects *CDH3*, which encodes P-cadherin.[37]

Crandall syndrome, an X-linked recessive disorder, consists of pili torti with alopecia, sensorineural deafness, and hypopituitarism.[38] *Björnstad syndrome* is characterized by sensorineural deafness, pili torti, and, occasionally, mental retardation. The syndrome is autosomal recessive, but families with an autosomal dominant pattern have been described.[39] The recessive form has more recently been linked to mutations in *BCS1L*, which encodes an ATPase needed to assemble complex III in the mitochondria. More severe defects in BCS1L markedly increase reactive oxygen species and are neonatal lethal with multisystemic involvement (complex II deficiency and GRACILE syndrome).[40]

Individuals with *mitochondrial enzyme abnormalities* have shown a wide variety of abnormalities, predominantly failure to thrive and neuromuscular changes; however, skin or hair abnormalities have been described in 10% of affected children.[41] Hair abnormalities range from alopecia to dry, thick brittle hair, to hypertrichosis, especially on the back. Syndromic disorders with hair abnormalities may also affect mitochondrial function (e.g., Bjornstad syndrome and cartilage-hair hypoplasia). Light microscopy examination of affected hair has shown a variety of hair shaft defects associated with increased fragility, including trichothiodystrophy, trichorrhexis nodosa, pili torti, and diffuse longitudinal grooving with flattened hair shafts.[41,42] Patchy erythematous lesions have been described and many of the patients with skin manifestations have shown mottled pigmentation.

Pili bifurcati

Pili bifurcati is an uncommon anomaly of hair growth characterized by intermittent bifurcation of the hair shaft in which affected hairs divide into two separate shafts that subsequently become rejoined along the hair shaft.[43,44] This bifurcation is repeated at intervals, and the anomaly appears to be transitory, with only a small percentage of hairs exhibiting the bifurcation. This disorder should not be confused with *pili multigemini*, a disorder in which multiple hairs project from a single hair follicle.

Trichothiodystrophy

Trichothiodystrophy (TTD) is a heterogeneous group of autosomal recessive disorders in which patients have dry, brittle, cysteine-deficient hair as an isolated finding or in association with often multisystemic disease.[45] To date, four genes have been linked to TTD: *ERCC2* (encoding XPD), *ERCC3* (XPB), *p8* or *GTF2H5* (TTDA), and *C7Orf11* (TTDN1). The function of TTDN1 is not well understood, but it likely regulates cell cycling and transcription efficiency.[46] The other three genes encode subunits of transcription/repair factor IIH (TFIIH), a multiprotein complex involved in transcription and nucleotide excision repair.[47,48] Unlike xeroderma pigmentosum, TTD is not prone to cancer, although squamous cell carcinoma has been described.[49]

Light microscopy of TTD hairs shows a wavy, irregular outline and a flattened shaft that twists like a folded ribbon. Two types of fracture may be seen: trichoschisis (clean transverse fracture) or an atypical trichorrhexis nodosa with only slight splaying of the cortical cells. Polarizing microscopy is critical to show the characteristic alternating light and dark bands, the 'tiger-tail' appearance.[50,51] While the severity of hair shaft defects is inversely proportional to the hair sulfur content, there is no association between the extent of systemic disease and percentage of abnormal hairs.[51] Sparse hair

is often associated with the shaft defect. Some patients have described cyclic hair loss with fever, which may reflect a mutation leading to thermosensitive XPD.

A recent review of 112 published cases of TTD described the abnormalities beyond hair defects.[52] Ichthyosis has been noted in 65% and clinical evidence of photosensitivity in 24% of these patients. The ichthyosis may resemble ARCI or ichthyosis vulgaris (see Ch. 5), and some patients show marked depletion of the granular layer in skin biopsy sections.[53] A total of 37% of the TTD patients with ichthyosis and 26% of all patients with TTD present at birth as a collodion phenotype.[52] Patients may also show xerosis, palmoplantar keratoderma, atopic dermatitis and/or follicular keratosis.[53] Nail abnormalities have been described in 63% of patients overall, especially dystrophy with thickening or yellow discoloration.

Among the most common non-cutaneous features are developmental delay/intellectual impairment (86%), short stature (73%), and ocular abnormalities (51%, especially cataracts). Facial dysmorphism is seen in 66% of patients, especially microcephaly, large or protruding ears, and micrognathia. Bone abnormalities are seen radiographically in 38%, particularly osteosclerosis and delayed bone age. Gonadal abnormalities were noted in 14% overall, most commonly hypogonadism and cryptorchidism. Recurrent infections have been noted in 46%, particularly involving the respiratory and gastrointestinal tracts and the inner ear, but associated immunodeficiency or neutropenia.[54,55] Overall, mortality in the first decade of life is increased 20-fold. Complications during pregnancy are noted in 26% of patients, most commonly intrauterine growth retardation.

Subgroups of TTD have been classified based on clinical characteristics (BIDS, IBIDS/Tay syndrome, PIBIDS). However, a new classification has been proposed that divides patients based on their mutations as Group I (mutations in genes encoding subunits of transcription/repair factor IIH (TFIIH) – XPD, XPB, p8), II (TTDN1) and III (no known molecular basis).[53] Group I includes patients with photosensitivity (either clinical or *in vitro*), 10% of non-photosensitive patients are in Group II, and currently unclassified but non-photosensitive patients (such as Pollitt and Sabinas syndromes),[56] are in group III. Using this classification, ichthyosis and the collodion baby phenotype are most highly correlated with group I, while hypogonadism has been found more in Groups II and III. Mild collodion babies, however, may have normal DNA repair.[53]

Marie-Unna hypotrichosis

Marie-Unna hypotrichosis is an autosomal dominant disorder manifested by almost complete congenital absence of scalp hair, eyebrows, and eyelashes at birth.[57,58] The hair regrows to normal density, but is coarse, flattened, and twisted (Fig. 7.7). Beginning at puberty the hair becomes progressively sparser, particularly on the vertex and scalp margins, resulting in a high frontal and nuchal hairline. By adulthood, only a sparse fringe of hair at the scalp margin may remain, and eyelashes, eyebrows, and body hair, including secondary sexual hair, tend to be sparse. Scattered follicular horny plugs may be associated. Other ectodermal structures are unaffected, except that 50% of affected individuals show exceptionally widely spaced upper incisor teeth. Mutations that cause Marie-Unna hypotrichosis affect *U2HR*, an open reading frame upstream of the hairless gene that inhibits hairless expression; as a result hairless expression and Wnt signaling are increased.[59,60]

Hypotrichosis simplex

Hypotrichosis simplex is a rare autosomal dominant form of non-syndromic, non-scarring alopecia in which patients are born with normal hair. Gradual loss of scalp hair begins in the middle of the

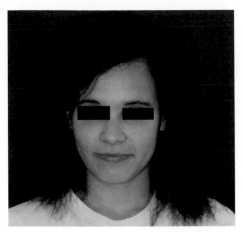

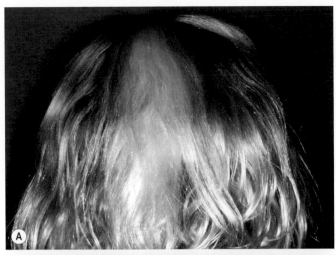

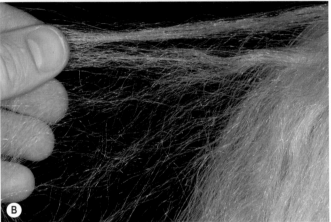

Figure 7.7 Marie-Unna hypotrichosis. This adolescent's hair is coarse and lusterless. Her hairline is receding at the frontal and nuchal areas, and she paints her sparse brows with eyeliner. Her progressive alopecia will leave her largely alopecic as an adult.

Figure 7.8 Woolly hair nevus. The affected hair is lighter (A), sometimes sparser, and more 'woolly' in consistency from the normal surrounding scalp hair (B).

first decade, and progresses to almost complete loss of scalp hair by adulthood. Graying has been reported to coincide with hair loss. Some individuals show sparse, fine, short hairs, especially at the crown, but hair on sites other than the scalp is normal. The disorder results form mutations in the gene encoding corneodesmin, a glycoprotein specifically of the corneocyte desmosomes and inner hair sheath (see Peeling skin syndrome, Ch. 5).[61]

Hair Shaft Abnormalities without Increased Fragility

Pili annulati

Pili annulati (ringed hair) is an autosomal dominant condition with onset shortly after birth. The hair looks shiny with attractive highlights, but alternating bright and dark bands are seen on close inspection. The bright areas are the result of light scattering from clusters of air-filled cavities within the cortex, which appear as dark areas under light microscopy, especially in more proximal hair regions.[62] There are no associated defects, but pili annulati has been reported to markedly improve or clear after the occurrence of alopecia totalis.[63] The gene mutated in pili annulati has been linked to chromosome 12q24.33, but to date no mutations in candidate genes in this region have been found.[64]

Pseudopili annulati is an unusual variant of normal hair in which bright bands are seen at intervals along the hair shaft. Secondary to periodic twisting or curling of the hair shaft, this banding is conspicuous only in blond hairs and represents an attractive optical effect due to reflection and refraction of light by flattened and twisted hair surfaces.

Woolly hair

Woolly hair describes a tight, curly hair usually present from birth and shows abnormalities under light microscopy.[2] The individual scalp hairs are fine and dry, light-colored, and corrugated at intervals, resembling the wool of sheep. Recognition of woolly hair is important because of the many associated abnormalities. The autosomal recessive disorders characterized by generalized woolly hair, keratoderma, and, in some kindreds, dilated cardiomyopathy have recently been linked to mutations in desmoplakin (Carvajal syndrome)[65,66] and plakoglobin (Naxos disease),[67] two desmosomal proteins (see Ch. 5). Diffuse woolly hair has also been associated with ocular abnormalities, keratosis pilaris atrophicans, keratosis

follicularis spinulosa decalvans,[68] giant axonal neuropathy, and primary osteoma cutis.

Woolly hair without associated systemic manifestations can be inherited as either an autosomal dominant or autosomal recessive trait. The entire scalp tends to be affected from birth, but other hair is normal. The hair grows slowly, is hypopigmented, and shows varying degrees of hypotrichosis. Plucked hair shows a dystrophic bulb and sometimes nonspecific shaft defects. The recessive forms have now been explained by mutations in two interacting genes, P2RY5 and LIPH (encoding lipase H).[69,70] Lipase H is a key enzyme in the synthesis of lysophosphatidic acid, which is involved in lipid and energy metabolism, and P2RY5 is thought to be a receptor for lysophosphatidic acid in the hair follicle.[71]

The *woolly hair nevus* is sporadic condition characterized by the development of one or more patches of hair different in color, shape, and consistency from the normal surrounding scalp hair (Fig. 7.8). The hairs on the affected area are usually smaller in diameter, lighter in color, and sparser than those on the rest of the scalp.[72] When examined under a dissecting microscope, the individual hairs are noted to twist about their long axis. The majority of reported cases of woolly hair nevus have been recognized during the first few months of life, but some have appeared in young adulthood.[73,74] In about 50% of cases, woolly hair nevus coexists with a linear epidermal nevus in the same area or elsewhere.[75,76] Ocular involvement has been described as an associated feature.

Acquired progressive kinking of the hair

Acquired progressive kinking of the hair is a rare disorder of scalp hair, with onset in adolescence or in young adulthood.[77] The condition is characterized by a rapid onset of extreme curliness of the hair (mainly on the frontoparietal region of the scalp and vertex), often in association with an increased coarse texture, diminished luster, and striking unruliness. More common in males than in females, the hair may become darker or remain unaltered in color, and the rate of growth may be decreased or unchanged.[78] Examination of abnormal hairs by light microscopy reveals alterations in hair shaft diameter, and partial twisting of the hair on its longitudinal axis.

Although the etiology of this disorder is unknown, it may follow treatment with systemic retinoids, including isotretinoin. The localization of hair kinking, frequent family history of androgenetic alopecia, pathologic features of affected scalp, and tendency to evolve into androgenetic alopecia suggest acquired kinking as a harbinger of androgenetic alopecia.[79] No therapy is effective, and application of topical minoxidil has not affected the progressive thinning of hair in the areas of kinking.[79] Spontaneous reversion to normal hair has been reported.[80]

Uncombable hair syndrome

The uncombable hair syndrome (pili trianguli canaliculi, spun glass hair syndrome) is a unique hair disorder characterized by very pale, silvery, blond, or straw colored hair that is dry, frizzy, and unruly, and does not lie flat on the scalp, thus making combing impossible (Fig. 7.9).[81,82] The syndrome is thought to be autosomal dominant with variable penetrance, although no associated gene mutations have been identified. The onset is usually during infancy or early childhood, and eyebrows, lashes, and body hair are normal. Affected children may have minor nail abnormalities[83] and some show both uncombable hair and loose anagen hair (see below).[84] The characteristic structural defect, the presence of canalicular depressions along the hair shaft, can be demonstrated by scanning electron microscopy[85] or by routine microscopy of hair in cross-section.[86] Cross-sectional microscopy shows a variety of shapes, including triangular, quadrangular, and reniform. The longitudinal grooving and abnormal shape in cross-section, however, are not specific for uncombable hair syndrome, and have been described in several other syndromes, among them Marie-Unna hypotrichosis, the ectodermal dysplasias with clefting, hypohidrotic ectodermal dysplasia, angel-shaped phalangoepiphyseal dysplasia, oral-facial-digital syndrome type I, and progeria. The clinical appearance of the spun glass hair requires a sizable proportion of abnormal hairs, and at least 50% of hairs are abnormal by scanning electron microscopy. The hair tends to become progressively more manageable by adolescence, and some patients have responded to biotin administration.[83]

Uncombable hair syndrome must be distinguished from extremely unruly hair, which is seen in 2% of individuals. Extremely unruly hair that tends to stand up from the area of the posterior parietal whorl toward the frontal hairline may be associated with microcephaly and is a potential indicator of abnormal brain growth and morphogenesis, similar to upsweep of anterior scalp hair and aberrant parietal whorl position.

Loose Anagen Syndrome

Loose anagen syndrome occurs in 10% of all children who present with alopecia[87] and is characterized by actively growing anagen hairs that are loosely anchored and can be easily and painlessly pulled from the scalp.[88] Although considered an autosomal dominant disorder, most cases are sporadic and occur in girls. A mutation in a hair keratin (KRT75, formerly called K6hf) has been found in some families, but its relevance is unclear since it does not reliably segregate with the loose anagen phenotype.[12] Most patients are blond girls above the age of 2 years (mean, 6 years of age). Affected children generally have sparse short scalp hairs that seldom require cutting. Examination shows patchy or subtle diffuse thinning with hairs of uneven length. The hair often appears to be limp and a matted texture has been noted, particularly of occipital hair. Some 80–100% of actively growing anagen hairs show ruffled cuticles and pigmented misshapen bulbs (Figs 7.1A, 7.10). Gentle pulling of hair tends to yield several hairs, allowing the diagnosis to be made by light microscopic examination of hair; forceful extraction of hairs may lead to misshaping of normal anagen hairs and thus should be avoided. Shedding of the hair is cyclic, and the inability to extract large amounts of hair by gentle pull test does not definitively rule out the diagnosis. Although no treatment is available for this disorder, it is reassuring for patients and their families to know that other abnormalities are not associated with this disorder and individuals with this condition tend to improve with time.

Loose anagen hair is also a feature of an autosomal recessive Noonan-like syndrome ('Noonan-like syndrome with loose anagen hair'),[89] which has been linked to mutations in SHOC2.[90] In addition to the fine, sparse hair, affected children show the Noonan syndrome facies and broad neck, macrocephaly, reduced growth with delayed bone age (often from growth hormone deficiency), variable cognitive defects, hyperactivity, hypernasal voice, darkly pigmented, thickened skin with dermatitis, and cardiac defects.

Non-scarring Alopecias without Hair Shaft Abnormalities[91]

Congenital/genetic disorders

Congenital triangular alopecia is characterized by an area of alopecia that, although sometimes notable at birth in babies with abundant scalp hair, is often first detected at 2 or 3 years of age (Fig. 7.11);[92] the initial appearance of triangular alopecia during adulthood has

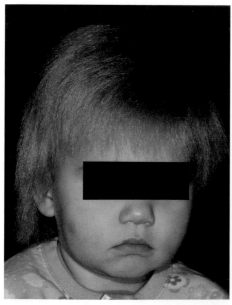

Figure 7.9 Uncombable hair syndrome. Blond hair that is dry and frizzy, and does not lie flat on the scalp, thus making combing impossible. (Courtesy of Sarah Chamlin, MD.)

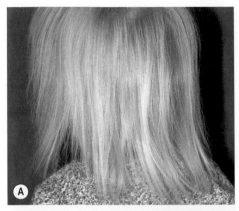

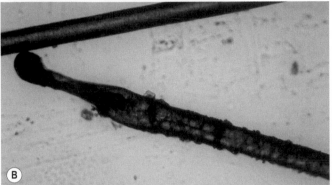

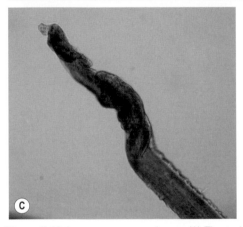

Figure 7.10 Loose anagen syndrome. (A) The typical patient is a blonde preschool girl whose hair comes out easily and has become lusterless, fine, and sparse. When viewed under light microscope, the hairs that are easily able to be removed without plucking, show a ruffled cuticle (B) and distorted bulb (C, and see Fig. 7.1A).

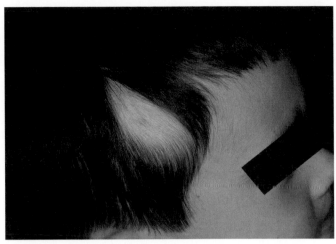

Figure 7.11 Congenital triangular alopecia. This usually unilateral triangular patch of alopecia may not appear until 2–3 years of age or even later, but then persists unchanged.

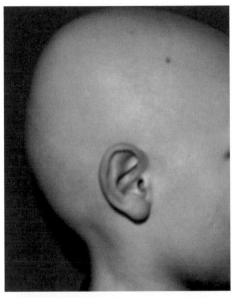

Figure 7.12 Congenital atrichia. This boy lost his hair during the first year of life and has never regrown it. A mutation in the *hairless* gene was demonstrated.

been described.[93] The area is triangular and overlies the frontotemporal suture, with the base of the triangle directed forward. The triangular patch may extend to the hairline, but often a fringe of hair may separate it from the forehead. Generally measuring 3–5 cm from base to apex, the area may be completely bald or partially covered by vellus hairs and remains unchanged throughout life. Dermoscopy of the affected shows normal follicular openings with vellus hairs, while dermoscopy of alopecia areata shows dystrophic and exclamation point hairs.[94] Although unilateral in 80% of affected individuals, it may be bilaterally symmetrical and, on rare occasions, similar triangular patches may be noted on the nape of the neck. The condition is almost always sporadic, although the association with developmental delay and seizures has been

described in a mother and daughter.[95] Hair transplants have been used to repopulate the area of triangular alopecia.[96] Bilateral congenital localized patches of alopecia of the parietal area that resemble the alopecia of congenital triangular alopecia have been seen in patients with *Gomez–Lopez–Hernandez syndrome* (cerebellotrigeminaldermal dysplasia). Although the alopecia classically affects the parietal area, other sites have been reported to show symmetrical alopecia.[97] Other features are skull defects (craniosynostosis with brachycephaly, midfacial hypoplasia), neurologic abnormalities, short stature, hypertelorism, and corneal opacities.[98]

Individuals who initially have hair, but lose it all with the first hair shedding shortly after birth, likely have *atrichia with papular lesions* (APL) due to mutations in the hairless gene, or *vitamin D-dependent rickets type IIA* (due to mutations in the vitamin D receptor).[99,100] Affected individuals never regrow scalp hair and tend to be nearly totally devoid of eyebrows, lashes, and axillary and pubic hair (Fig. 7.12). Follicular cysts and milia-like lesions may appear on the skin later in life (hence the nomenclature of 'with papular lesions'). Scalp biopsies show disintegration of the lower two-thirds of the hair follicle, often replaced by cysts. Patients with vitamin D-resistant rickets are clinically and histologically identical to patients with APL,[101] but show the additional manifestations of early-onset rickets, hypocalcemia, secondary hyperparathyroidism, and elevated 1,25-dihydroxyvitamin D_3.[102] The similarity in phenotype reflects the direct regulatory effect of the vitamin D receptor and hairless on each other via a transcriptional mechanism.[103,104] This group of patients is often misdiagnosed as having alopecia universalis, and they must be also be distinguished from patients with ectodermal dysplasia of the hair and nail type, in which neonates are born with the alopecia and severe nail dystrophy because of mutations in the gene encoding keratin 85.[105,106]

In the *Hallermann–Streiff syndrome* (oculomandibulo-dyscephaly), hypotrichosis of the scalp, eyebrows, and eyelids is associated with dwarfism, beaked nose, and brachycephaly. The alopecia is most prominent at the frontal and parietal areas and is especially marked along suture lines. Axillary and pubic hair may also be scant, and cutaneous atrophy, largely limited to the scalp and nose, may appear as thin taut skin and prominent underlying blood vessels. Other features include frontal and parietal bossing, mandibular hypoplasia, microphthalmia, low-set ears, thin and small lips, high-arched palate, atrophy of the skin of the face, congenital cataracts, blue sclerae, motor and, occasionally, mental retardation, and dental abnormalities.

Sensenbrenner syndrome or cranioectodermal dysplasia is a rare autosomal recessive disorder manifested by small stature, dolichocephaly, an unusual facies, and tubulointerstitial nephritis leading to early end-stage renal failure.[107] The typical facies show frontal bossing, hypertelorism, prominent epicanthal folds, antimongoloid palpebral fissures, eversion of the lip, and full-rounded cheeks. Patients have small, gray, widely spaced teeth, short, fine, hair, and hypohidrosis.[108]

The *cartilage-hair hypoplasia syndrome* is an autosomal recessive disorder that occurs primarily in inbred Amish or Finnish populations.[109,110] Patients have short limbs and sparse, fine scalp and body hair. Several patients with hyperextensible digits and soft, doughy skin, reflecting degenerated elastic tissue, have been described.[111] Defective cell-mediated immunity is seen in most patients, and results in relative anergy, altered T-cell responses, and increased susceptibility to severe viral infections, particularly varicella.[112] Patients may have infantile neutropenia, Diamond–Blackfan anemia, severe combined immunodeficiency, celiac syndrome, and/ or toxic megacolon. Mild to severe bronchiectasis has been noted in >50% of patients.[113] Approximately 10% develop malignancy, especially lymphoreticular; an increased prevalence of early basal cell carcinomas has also been described.[114] The disorder results from mutations in RNAase MRP, which cleaves RNA in mitochondria DNA synthesis and pre-rRNA in the nucleolus.[115]

Patients with the *Coffin–Siris* syndrome most commonly show a constellation of severe mental retardation, a characteristic coarse-appearing facies, scalp hypotrichosis with hypertrichosis of the eyebrows, eyelashes, face, and back, hypotonia, hypoplastic to absent fifth fingernails and distal phalanges, and feeding problems with postnatal growth deficiency.[116] Occurrence in siblings of unaffected parents suggests an autosomal recessive mode of inheritance.[116]

Trichorhinophalangeal syndrome I is an autosomal dominant disorder characterized by a distinctive facies with pear-shaped nose, elongated philtrum, thin upper lip, supernumerary incisors, and receding chin (Fig. 7.13); and skeletal abnormalities, including brachydactyly, deviation of the middle phalanges (Fig. 7.14), hip malformation, and short stature.[117,118] Most patients show fine, sparse,

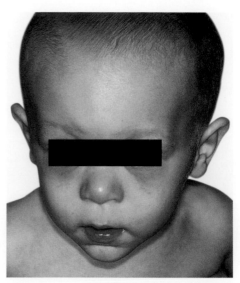

Figure 7.13 Trichorhinophalangeal syndrome, type I. This 9-month-old boy shows the distinctive facies, including the pear-shaped nose, elongated philtrum; thin upper lip, and receding chin, as well as the sparse hair. He had hip dysplasia as well.

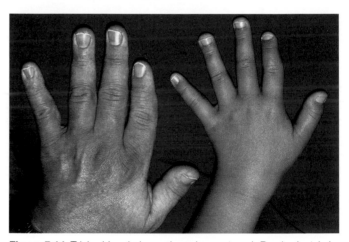

Figure 7.14 Trichorhinophalangeal syndrome, type I. Brachydactyly in an affected father and daughter with short stature and typical facies. Note the deviation of the middle phalanges.

slow-growing hair, but almost normal hair to complete baldness have been described. The underlying molecular basis is mutation in TRPS1, which encodes a transcription factor. Individuals with *trichorhinophalangeal syndrome II* (*Langer–Giedion syndrome*) have associated multiple cartilaginous exostoses. The diagnosis is made by the demonstration of cone-shaped epiphyses of the fingers seen on plain radiography. These findings may not be detectable until 3 years of age or older. The type II form is a contiguous gene syndrome, with deletion of both the *TRPS1* gene and the gene that is mutated in multiple exostosis type I (*EXT1*). Type III TRPS results from mutations in *TRPS1*, but manifests with much more severe short stature and generalized shortening of all phalanges and metacarpals than TRPS1.[119]

The *oral-facial-digital syndrome* type I (OFD1) is an X-linked dominant disorder limited to girls and thought to be lethal in boys.[120] Facial features occur in almost 70% of patients, and include hypoplasia of nasal cartilages, and hypertelorism with lateral

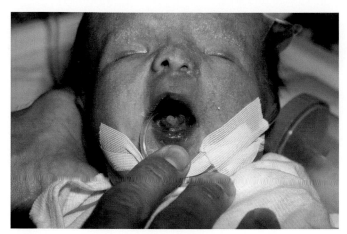

Figure 7.15 Oral-facial-digital syndrome, type I. This infant girl shows the asymmetric hypoplasia of nasal cartilages and lobulated cleft tongue. Note the many facial milia on the cheek and eyelids. The hair continues to be sparse and dry.

displacement of the inner canthi (dystopia canthorum)[121] (Fig. 7.15). Among the oral anomalies described are tongue hamartomas, lobulated cleft tongue, cleft lip and palate, maldeveloped frenula, asymmetry of the lips and tongue, and maxillary gingival swelling.[122] Associated hand malformations are common, and include brachydactyly, syndactyly, clinodactyly, and polydactyly. Almost half of affected individuals show CNS involvement, most commonly retardation or selective cognitive impairment. Cutaneous abnormalities occur in the minority of patients, but include numerous milia at birth,[123] and sparse fine or coarse, dry and lusterless hair to frank alopecia. Polycystic kidney disease with renal insufficiency is occasionally seen in children, but more often occurs with advancing age (>50% after age 36 years).[124] The disorder results from mutations in *OFD1*, which encodes a centrosomal protein of primary cilia. Other 'ciliopathies' share the CNS, skeletal and cystic renal abnormalities of OFD1.

Ectodermal dysplasias

Ectodermal dysplasias are a complex group of developmental disorders that were traditionally classified based on their sites of abnormalities (hair, teeth, nails and/or eccrine glands) and other ectodermal and non-ectodermal features.[125] A new classification of ectodermal dysplasias focuses on the molecular basis of these disorders, the function of the affected proteins, and the clinical features. As a result, ectodermal dysplasias are divided into two groups (Table 7.2).[126] The first group includes disorders in ectodermal derivatives fail to develop or differentiate because of the absence of reciprocal signals from the ectoderm to the mesenchyme. This group can be further divided into: (1) abnormalities of the tumor necrosis factor (TNF)-like/TNF receptor pathway (including hypohidrotic ectodermal dysplasias); (2) the nuclear factor-kappa-beta (NF-κβ), essential modulator (NEMO) and IκB molecules (such as HED with immunodeficiency); and (3) transcription factors, such as p63 and DLX3. Inductive signals for normal differentiation are preserved in the second group, but tissues become dysplastic because abnormal regulation of transcription or expression leads to altered cell-cell interactions or disorganization of the cytoskeleton. Abnormalities in Group 2 may affect nectin 1 (cleft lip/palate-ectodermal dysplasia syndrome), connexins (as in Clouston syndrome and oculodentodigital dysplasia), desmosomal proteins (such as plakophilin in ectodermal dysplasia/skin fragility

syndrome, also classified as a form of epidermolysis bullosa simplex, see Ch. 13), and molecules that interact with β-catenins (cadherins and WNT10A, as in odonto-onycho-dermal dysplasia).

Group 1 ectodermal dysplasia

Hypohidrotic ectodermal dysplasia Hypohidrotic ectodermal dysplasia (HED) or Christ–Siemens–Touraine syndrome (formerly termed *anhidrotic ectodermal dysplasia*), is characterized by the triad of reduced sweating, hypotrichosis, and defective dentition.[127] Individuals with mutations in *NEMO* or *IKBA* also have issues related to immunodeficiency. Identical developmental abnormalities of the hair and glands result from mutations in one of several genes:[128]

1. Ectodysplasin-A1 (*ED1* at Xq12–q13), by far the most common type
2. Ectodysplasin receptor (*EDAR* at 2q13)
3. EDAR-associated death domain (*EDARADD* at 1q42.2–q43)
4. NF-κβ essential modulator (*NEMO*/IKKγ at Xq28)
5. IκBα (*IKBA* at 14q13).

Most patients are male and show only ectodermal dysplasia as a result of mutations in *ED1*, leading to X-linked recessive form HED. Female carriers with an ectodysplasin mutation show random inactivation of the abnormal gene, and can show manifestations ranging from none to extensive dental defects, alopecia, and patchy hypohidrosis following the lines of Blaschko, which are lines of embryologic development of skin. Mutations in the receptor (*EDAR*) or the death domain (*EDARADD*) may be inherited in a recessive or dominant pattern.[126] The phenotype with recessive mutations closely resembles those in X-linked recessive HED, whereas dominant mutations tend to be less severe with respect to sweating and hair loss.[129] HED with immunodeficiency (HED-ID) is usually due to hypomorphic NEMO defects and affects males,[130] although HED-ID from hypermorphic mutations in *IKBA* is autosomal recessive. Features of hypohidrotic ectodermal dysplasia have been described in 77% of boys with NEMO mutations and immunodeficiency, and in 8% osteopetrosis and lymphedema are associated.[131] Boys with HED-ID occasionally show the clinical vesiculopapules and histologic features of incontinentia pigmenti, but the distribution is not blaschkoid, given the lack of mosaicism.[132] Female carriers of more severe NEMO mutations show features of incontinentia pigmenti (see Ch. 11).

Features of ectodermal dysplasia: Affected persons often appear more like each other than like their own siblings;[133] classic features are usually obvious by infancy. Most have a distinctive pathognomonic facies – a square forehead with frontal bossing, large conspicuous nostrils, wide cheekbones with flat malar ridges, a thick everted lower lip, and prominent chin. Ears may be small, satyr-like (pointed), low-lying, and anteriorly placed (Figs 7.16, 7.17).

Alopecia is often the first feature to attract attention but is seldom complete. The hair tends to be lightly pigmented, sparse, and short. The skin is soft, thin, and light-colored, but shows fine wrinkling and sometimes darkening of the periorbital areas. Many affected neonates are born with red, peeling skin, but collodion-like thickening has occasionally been described.[134,135] Atopic dermatitis and other atopic conditions occur with increased frequency, and periorbital dermatitis is particularly common. Nails tend to be normal.

The decreased capacity for perspiration often results in hyperthermia, and patients manifest with intermittent fevers, especially during hot weather or following exercise or meals. These recurrent fevers of unknown origin may be the presenting manifestation in affected infants. Hypoplastic lacrimal and mucous glands can lead to decreased tearing or epiphora, chronic nasal discharge, and to an increased risk of otitis media and respiratory tract infections.[136]

Table 7.2 Classification for ectodermal dysplasias

Disorder	Inheritance	Gene	Protein	Function
Group 1				
TNF/TNFR pathway				
Hypohidrotic ectodermal dysplasia	XLR	ED1	Ectodysplasin (EDA)	Membrane ligand
Hypohidrotic ectodermal dysplasia	AD, AR	EDAR	EDA receptor	Receptor of EDA
Hypohidrotic ectodermal dysplasia	AD, AR	EDARADD	EDAR-associated death domain	Adaptor molecule
NF-κβ inhibitors				
Hypohidrotic ectodermal dysplasia with immune deficiency (males) + osteopetrosis (males)	XLR	NEMO/IKKγ	NF-κβ essential modulator	NF-κβ inhibitor
Incontinentia pigmenti (females)	XLD	NEMO/IKKγ	NF-κβ essential modulator	NF-κβ inhibitor
Hypohidrotic ectodermal dysplasia with immune deficiency	AR	IκBα	IκBα	NF-κβ inhibitor
Transcription factors				
Ectrodactyly-ectodermal dysplasia-clefting syndrome	AD	p63	p63	Transcription factor
Rapp–Hodgkin syndrome	AD	p63	p63	Transcription factor
Ankyloblepharon-ectodermal dysplasia-clefting syndrome	AD	p63	p63	Transcription factor
Acro-dermato-ungual-lacrimal-tooth (ADULT)	AD	p63	p63	Transcription factor
Limb-mammary syndrome	AD	p63	p63	Transcription factor
Tricho-dento-osseous syndrome	AD	DLX3	DLX3	Transcription factor
Witkop syndrome	AD	MSX1	MSX1	Transcription factor
Ellis van Creveld syndrome	AR	EVC, EVC2	EVC, EVC2	Unknown
Group 2				
Clouston syndrome	AD	GJB6	Connexin 30	Intercellular junctions
Oculo-dental-digital dysplasia	AD	GJA1	Connexin 43	Intercellular junctions
Clefting-ectodermal dysplasia	AD	PVRL1	Nectin 1	Tight junction/ membrane stability
Ectodermal dysplasia: skin fragility syndrome (see Ch. 13)	AR	PKP1	Plakophilin 1	Desmosomal plaque/ stability
Ectodermal dysplasia, ectrodactyly, and macular dystrophy	AR	CDH3	Cadherin 3	Adhesion molecule for cell-cell binding
Odonto-onycho-dermal dysplasia	AR	WNT10A	Wnt10A	β-catenin-mediated signaling

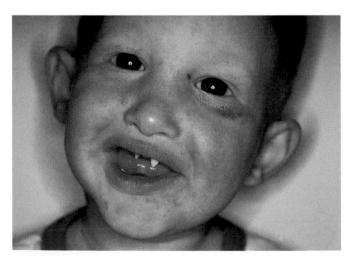

Figure 7.16 Hypohidrotic ectodermal dysplasia. This boy shows the short, sparse hair, large conspicuous nostrils, wide cheekbones with flat malar ridges, a thick everted lower lip, prominent chin, and low-lying, anteriorly placed, pointed ears. Note the conical incisors.

Dentition is generally delayed, and dental anomalies vary from complete to partial absence of teeth with peg-shaped or conical incisors.

Features of immunodeficiency: Boys with HED-ID usually present with recurrent infections. Serious pyogenic infections occur in 86% of affected individuals, and mycobacterial infections (especially atypical) in 44%.[133,137,138] Viral and fungal infections occur less often. Bacteremia or sepsis is common,[133,139] and the most frequent sites of infection are the lungs, sometimes leading to bronchiectasis, and the skin, sometimes with abscesses. Inflammatory colitis affects 21% of boys and presents as intractable diarrhea and/or failure to thrive. Some patients develop autoimmune hemolytic anemia. Natural killer cell dysfunction has been described in all patients, but otherwise a range of immune defects have been described, largely reflecting the functional impairment in CD40, IL-1, TNF-α, and toll receptor signaling.[133,140] Almost 60% of affected boys show hypogammaglobulinemia, with high levels of IgM in 15%. Hyper-IgM syndrome much more commonly results from mutations in CD40 ligand (CD40L),[141] and may manifest with CD40L deficiency as oral aphthae and warts.[142] Most mutations in NEMO that lead to HED-ID occur in exon 10 and affect the C-terminal zinc finger

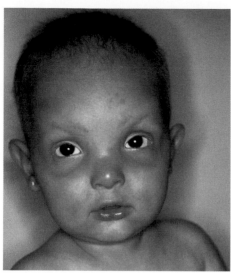

Figure 7.17 Hypohidrotic ectodermal dysplasia. This girl is a carrier for a mutation in ectodysplasin, but shows all of the characteristic facies features. Note her periorbital wrinkling as well. Girls with hypohidrotic ectodermal dysplasia may also have a mutation in a gene encoding the receptor for ectodysplasin, inherited as an autosomal disorder.

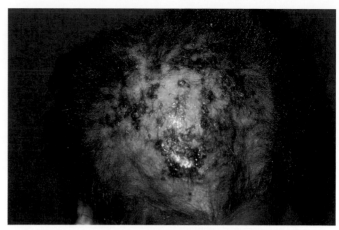

Figure 7.18 Ankyloblepharon-ectodermal dysplasia-clefting syndrome. Scalp dermatitis with secondary chronic staphylococcal infection is a chronic problem and leads to cicatricial alopecia.

domain, which is critical for normal dendritic cell immune stimulation.[143]

Therapy for patients with all forms of hypohidrotic ED is directed toward temperature regulation; cool baths and drenching with water, air conditioning, light clothing, cooling suits, and the reduction of the causes of normal perspiration are beneficial.[144] Lubricating eyedrops and nasal irrigation can compensate for the decreased glandular secretion. Dental intervention should begin by 2 years of age, and can include dental prostheses and dental implants in older adolescents and adults to improve mastication, encourage normal speech development, and reduce cosmetic disfigurement. In a dog model of X-linked HED, the administration of recombinant ectodysplasin postnatally improved dentition, lacrimation, sweating, and bronchopulmonary gland function.[145,146] The National Foundation for Ectodermal Dysplasias (NFED) provides excellent education materials on management of the hypohidrosis and dental abnormalities (www.nfed.org; info@nfed.org). Individuals with HED-ID are at high risk for early death from infections without transplantation.[147–150]

p63-related forms of ectodermal dysplasia Mutations in *p63*, a gene that plays a critical role in maturation of ectodermal, orofacial and limb development, lead to an autosomal dominant disorder with ectodermal dysplasia, orofacial clefting, and limb malformations as key characteristics. These clinical manifestations have traditionally been used to classify subtypes, but significant clinical and genotypic overlap is now recognized.[151–153] Included are *Rapp–Hodgkin syndrome* (clefts of the lip, palate, and/or uvula, small narrow dysplastic nails, hypodontia with small conical teeth, and maxillary hypoplasia);[154] *ankyloblepharon-ectodermal dysplasia-clefting* (*AEC* or *Hay–Wells syndrome*; ankyloblepharon or congenital fusion of the eyelids in association with facial clefting and midfacial hypoplasia);[155,156] *EEC syndrome* (ectrodactyly, ectodermal dysplasia, and cleft lip/palate); *limb-mammary syndrome* (ectrodactyly, cleft palate, and mammary gland abnormalities); *ADULT syndrome* (acro-dermato-ungual-lacrimal-tooth syndrome); and non-syndromic split hand/foot malformation.

The skin, hair, teeth, nails, and glands (eccrine, sebaceous, lacrimal, mammary) are abnormally developed.[157] The skin tends to be dry, itchy and hypopigmented. Extensive erosions have been described in 80% of neonates with the AEC phenotype. The hair is often sparse and wiry, and nails tend to be dystrophic. Scalp dermatitis and erosions with secondary chronic staphylococcal infection may be recurrent in the first few years of life, and lead to cicatricial alopecia, especially of the vertex and frontal scalp (Fig. 7.18). Teeth are often decreased in number with malformations and enamel hypoplasia.[158] Hypohidrosis may be present, tearing is often decreased, and nipple hypoplasia has been described. Patients may show split hand/foot malformations (lobster claw deformity; ectrodactyly) and/or syndactyly.[159] Short stature, poor weight gain and hypospadias are other commonly described characteristics.[160] The features of p63 mutation disorders overlap with autosomal dominant *CHAND syndrome*, in which patients are born with *c*urly *h*air at birth, and also have *a*nkyloplepharon, *n*ail *d*ysplasia and, variably, ataxia.[161,162]

The *tricho-dento-osseous syndrome* is an autosomal dominant disorder characterized by kinky, curly hair at birth that tends to become straighter during childhood; small, widely spaced, pitted, eroded, and discolored teeth with early caries as a result of defective enamel; thickness and splitting of the nails; dolichocephaly, frontal bossing, and a square jaw, giving affected persons a distinctive facies; normal physical development; and increased bone density, especially of the cranial bones. The condition results from mutations in *DLX3*, a crucial regulator of hair follicle differentiation and cycling.[163]

The *trichodental syndrome*, also known as Witkop syndrome or the tooth and nail syndrome, is an autosomal dominant disorder characterized by fine, dry, slow-growing lusterless hair; sparseness or absence of the lateral halves of the eyebrows; congenitally missing and small teeth; and slow-growing, small, spoon-shaped nails (especially toenails) (Fig. 7.19).[164,165] Mutations have been described in *MSX1*, which directs the formation of teeth and nails.[166] The other ectodermal dysplasia with mucocutaneous features included in Group 1 is *Ellis van Creveld syndrome*. This autosomal recessive disorder features nail dysplasia in association with chondrodysplasia, polydactyly, orofacial abnormalities and sometimes cardiovascular malformations.[167] The mutated genes, EVC and EVC2, localize to cilia and are thought to be involved in hedgehog signaling.[168]

Group 2 ectodermal dysplasia

Clouston syndrome (hidrotic ectodermal dysplasia) The most common hidrotic type of ectodermal dysplasia is *Clouston syndrome*,

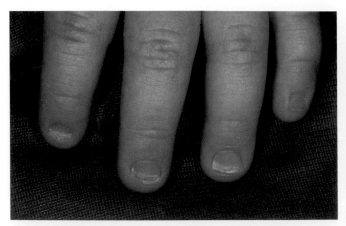

Figure 7.19 Trichodental syndrome (Witkop syndrome). Slow-growing, small, spoon-shaped nails are a characteristic feature, in addition to the slow-growing lusterless hair, sparse outer eyebrows and small, sometimes absent teeth.

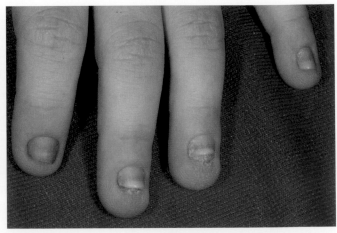

Figure 7.20 Hidrotic ectodermal dysplasia (Clouston syndrome). Nail dystrophy, accentuation of ridging on the digital tips, and bulbous swelling of the soft tissue surrounding the nail and at the finger pad are the most typical manifestations of this syndrome. The nails can be confused with pachyonychia congenita, but the hair changes of hidrotic ectodermal dysplasia help to distinguish the disorders.

an autosomal dominant disorder characterized by nail dystrophy, hyperkeratosis of the palms and soles, and hair defects.[169] Most cases have been reported in French-Canadian families. Unlike hypohidrotic ectodermal dysplasia, individuals with the hidrotic form have a normal facies and show no abnormality of sweating, although eccrine syringofibroadenomas have been described in association.[170] The teeth are normal developmentally, but are prone to caries. The predominant feature is nail dystrophy, which may be the only manifestation in about one-third of affected individuals. The nails are thickened or thinned, striated, and often discolored (Fig. 7.20). They grow slowly and frequently show chronic paronychial infections, which may result in partial to complete destruction of the nail matrix. Typically, the skin and soft tissue surrounding the nail and at the finger pad appear thickened and swollen. The palmoplantar keratoderma can extend to the dorsal aspects of the hands and feet. Hair may be normal during infancy and childhood, but thereafter often becomes sparse, fine, and brittle and may eventuate in total alopecia (Fig. 7.21). Body hair may be sparse; eyebrows and eyelashes may be thinned or absent. The skin may show a mottled hyperpigmentation with thickening and hyperpigmentation over the knees, elbows, and knuckles. Ocular abnormalities may be associated, including strabismus, conjunctivitis, and premature cataracts. Clouston syndrome has been attributed to mutations in *GJB6*,[171] encoding connexin 30, a structural component of the intercellular gap junction; mutations in both *GJB6* and *GJA1* (encoding connexin 43, see below) have also been described.[172] Mutations in *GJB6* have also been noted in patients with KID syndrome (see Ch. 5), who share the palmoplantar keratoderma and sometimes early alopecia with thickening of the scalp. The combination of tretinoin and minoxidil has reportedly caused hair growth in Clouston syndrome.[173]

Oculo-dental-digital dysplasia Oculo-dental-digital dysplasia (ODDD), an autosomal dominant disorder, results from mutations in *GJA1*, which encodes connexin 43.[8,9] In addition to abnormalities of the eyes, teeth and digits, patients show curly hair (sometimes with trichorrhexis nodosa), focal keratoderma, a characteristic facies with hypoplastic ala nasi, and neurologic, cardiac and hearing defects. *Cleft lip/palate-ectodermal dysplasia* features spoon-shaped, slow-growing finger and toenails and pili torti, mental retardation, malformed ears and partial syndactyly. It results from mutations in nectin 1, encoded by *PVRL1*.[174,175]

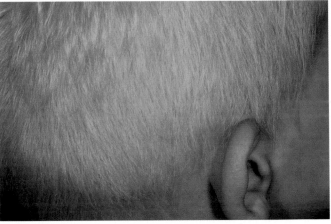

Figure 7.21 Hidrotic ectodermal dysplasia. This child shows the fine, sparse, brittle hair of Clouston hidrotic ectodermal dysplasia. Not uncommonly, the hair abnormality does not develop until after puberty.

Disorders of Follicular Plugging

Keratosis pilaris

Keratosis pilaris is a common skin condition characterized by keratinous plugs in the follicular orifices surrounded by a variable degree of erythema (see Ch. 3).[176] These small follicular-based papules are most commonly distributed on the cheeks (Fig. 7.22), extensor areas of the upper arms, and anterior thighs (Fig. 7.23, see also Fig. 3.17), but may be widespread. Children with keratosis pilaris tend to have xerosis and sometimes atopic dermatitis and/or ichthyosis vulgaris. Occasionally, facial keratosis pilaris overlies intense erythema (keratosis pilaris rubra)[177] and may also be pigmented (erythromelanosis follicularis faciei et colli).[178] Keratosis pilaris does not tend to be symptomatic, but may be cosmetically distressing, especially if quite inflammatory or extensive. Treatment is difficult, but usually requires application of keratolytic agents, such as creams or lotions containing lactic acid, glycolic acid, salicylic acid or urea, and gentle exfoliation by a pumice stone, wash-cloth, loofah sponge, or Buf-Puf. Responsive patients must maintain

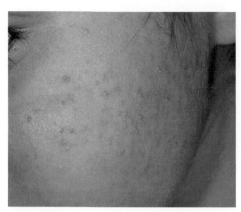

Figure 7.22 Keratosis pilaris. Keratotic, follicular-based plugs with variable associated erythema are common on the lateral cheeks of young children.

therapy to achieve continued remission or improvement. The intense erythema of keratosis pilaris rubra may be lessened by pulsed dye laser therapy;[179] the erythema is sometimes decreased by treatment with low strength topical steroids or calcineurin inhibitors.

Keratosis pilaris atrophicans

Numerous terms have been used to describe a group of interrelated syndromes characterized by inflammatory keratotic follicular papules and later by atrophy. Frequently described as atrophic variants of keratosis pilaris, these include ulerythema ophryogenes, atrophoderma vermiculata, and keratosis follicularis spinulosa decalvans (keratosis pilaris decalvans)[180,181] (Table 7.3).[182] This group of disorders has been attributed to abnormal keratinization of the follicular infundibulum, resulting in obstruction of the growing hair shaft, chronic inflammation, and scarring. No therapy is terribly effective,[183] although topical keratolytic and anti-inflammatory agents (topical corticosteroids and calcineurin inhibitors) may reduce the keratotic and inflammatory components, respectively. In general, systemic retinoids have not been helpful.

Ulerythema ophryogenes (keratosis pilaris atrophicans faciei) is characterized by persistent reticular erythema, small horny papules, atrophy, and scarring of the outer half of the eyebrows (Fig. 7.24). The disorder is more common in boys and usually starts in the first

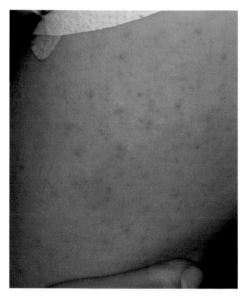

Figure 7.23 Keratosis pilaris. The anterior and lateral thighs are a common site.

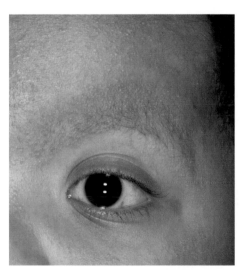

Figure 7.24 Ulerythema ophryogenes. Extensive keratosis pilaris with alopecia of the eyebrows in a boy with Noonan syndrome.

Table 7.3 Classification of keratosis pilaris atrophicans

	Atrophoderma vermiculata	Ulerythema ophryogenes	Keratosis follicularis spinulosa decalvans
Skin lesions	Erythematous papules, follicular plugs, horn cysts, atrophic	Follicular papules, plugging, scarring	Milia, thornlike follicular projections, atrophic scars
Sites	Cheeks, neck, limbs	Lateral eyebrows, extending medially	Scalp, eyebrows, eyelashes, cheeks, nose, neck, dorsal hands, fingers
Alopecia	Absent	Minimal eyebrows	Scarring alopecia of the scalp
Photophobia	Absent	Absent	Marked, corneal opacities
Inheritance	Sporadic or autosomal dominant	Sporadic or autosomal dominant	X-linked recessive or autosomal dominant

Reprinted with permission from Schachner and Hansen (2003).[182]

several months of life. Occasionally the disorder extends to include the adjacent skin, adjacent scalp, and cheeks. Ulerythema ophryogenes and keratosis pilaris have been described in patients with two similar but distinct disorders of the Ras-MAPK signaling pathway, the *cardio-facio-cutaneous* (CFC) syndrome and *Noonan* syndrome. Patients with CFC syndrome often show widespread keratosis pilaris-like lesions of the face, ears, scalp, and extensor surfaces of the extremities that may be more lichenoid and prominent than keratosis pilaris.[184] Sometimes patients with CFC and Noonan syndrome have alopecia of the eyelashes and eyebrows with follicular hyperkeratosis, but lack the atrophy and scarring of ulerythema ophryogenes. Both CFC and Noonan syndromes share features of short stature, congenital cardiac abnormalities (particularly pulmonary valve stenosis), retardation, macrocephaly, hypertelorism, a high forehead, pectus carinatum, curly hair and many pigmented nevi.[185] Lymphedema and a low posterior hairline are more typical features of Noonan syndrome. Patients with CFC often show hypoplastic supraorbital ridges, bitemporal constriction, and an anti-Mongoloid slant, features not described in Noonan syndrome.[184] The recent finding that the most commonly mutated genes in Noonan syndrome, *PTPN11* and *SOS1*,[186] are not mutated in patients with CFC syndrome (in which alterations in BRAF, KRAS, MEK1 and MEK2 are found) further distinguish the conditions.[187–189] Ulerythema ophryogenes has also been associated with Cornelia de Lange[190] and Rubenstein-Taybi[191] syndromes, as well as with woolly hair.[192]

Atrophoderma vermiculata (folliculitis ulerythema reticulata, atrophoderma vermicularis) is a variant of keratosis pilaris atrophicans that usually has its onset between 5 and 12 years of age and occasionally later.[180] This disorder is characterized by the formation of numerous tiny symmetric atrophic and, at times, erythematous pits on the cheeks, periauricular areas, and occasionally the forehead and eyebrows. These cribriform lesions generally measure 1–2 mm across and 1 mm deep, and are separated from each other by narrow ridges of normal-appearing skin. Laser and dermabrasion have been advocated to improve the cosmetic appearance of affected individuals when the condition is stable, which usually occurs after puberty.

Keratosis follicularis spinulosa decalvans (KFSD) is characterized by atrophic keratotic follicular papules of the scalp, eyebrows, and eyelashes that eventuate in scarring alopecia (Fig. 7.25). Associated features are palmoplantar keratoderma, photophobia, and atopy.[193] Although usually an X-linked recessive disorder, KFSD may be autosomal dominant in inheritance.[34,194] Female carriers of X-linked KFSD at most show milder manifestations. The initial signs are photophobia with tearing, ophthalmitis, and conjunctival and corneal inflammation, which occur in the first weeks or months of life; congenital glaucoma and cataracts have been noted in association. Extensive keratosis pilaris of the face, extremities and trunk tends to begin during early childhood, often in association with facial erythema. Cicatricial alopecia of the scalp begins around puberty and slowly progresses in association with follicular inflammation and fibrosis; eyebrows also tend to be affected. Some patients show palmoplantar keratoderma and marked xerosis. Acne keloidalis nuchae (see below) and tufted hair folliculitis has been described in several patients with KFSD.[195] X-linked KFSD results from mutations in spermidine/spermine N(1)-acetyltransferase, which leads to accumulation of putrescine.[196,197]

KFSD must be differentiated from *ichthyosis follicularis, congenital atrichia, and photophobia* (IFAP), most commonly an X-linked condition, in which affected neonates show keratotic follicular papules with a sandpapery feel to the skin, atrichia or severe hypotrichosis, and photophobia from birth (Fig. 7.26).[198–201] In contrast to KSFD, the alopecia of patients with IFAP does not scar. Mental retardation

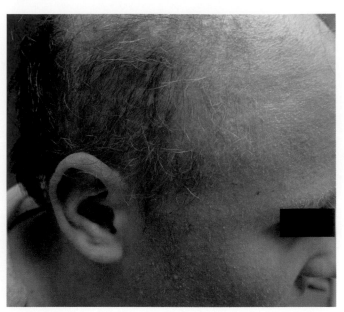

Figure 7.25 Keratosis follicularis spinulosus decalvans. This patient showed widespread spiny follicular-based keratosis, photophobia and abnormal hair with cicatricial alopecia.

and developmental delay have been described in both KSFD and IFAP syndromes. Other features of IFAP are gingival hyperplasia and angular stomatitis, psoriasiform plaques, and palmoplantar erythema with thickening. Ichthyosis in association with hair abnormalities may also be seen in ichthyosis hypotrichosis syndrome, ichthyosis-hypotrichosis-sclerosing cholangitis syndrome, Netherton syndrome (see Ch. 5) and trichothiodystrophy. IFAP has recently been shown to result from mutations in a zinc metalloprotease (MBTPS2) that is important for sterol homeostasis and cell differentiation.[202] Another disorder with non-scarring partial alopecia that must be distinguished is *hereditary mucoepithelial dysplasia*.[203] In addition to extensive keratosis pilaris and psoriasiform plaques, affected individuals show fiery red mucosal inflammation (hard palate, gingival, tongue, perianal and perineal), and ocular photophobia with keratitis, cataracts and corneal opacities.

The follicular scarring of these disorders should be distinguished from disorders of follicular atrophoderma without keratotic plugs. These include perifollicular atrophoderma of acne scarring (Ch. 8), Conradi-Hunermann syndrome (Ch. 5), Rombo syndrome and Bazex syndrome. Treatment of these disorders of follicular plugging is challenging, with most patients refractory to systemic and topical steroids, systemic antibiotics, dapsone, methotrexate, and systemic retinoids.[194,201]

Other Scarring Alopecias

Scarring or cicatricial alopecia is the end result of a wide number of inflammatory processes in and around the pilosebaceous units, resulting in irreversible destruction of tissue and consequent permanent scarring alopecia.[91,204] The scarring may be the result of a developmental defect (aplasia cutis) (see Figs 2.30, 2.31); inflammatory changes due to severe bacterial, viral, or fungal infection; physical trauma (halo alopecia from caput succedaneum,[205] (Fig. 7.2; see also Ch. 2); irradiation; trichotillomania practiced over a long period of time; thermal or caustic burns); neoplastic or infiltrative disorders (including severe alopecia mucinosa); various dermatoses (lichen planus, lupus erythematosus, localized or systemic

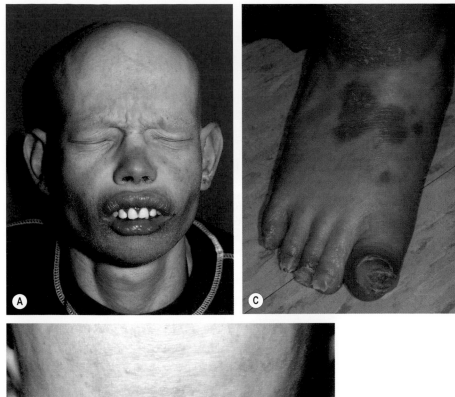

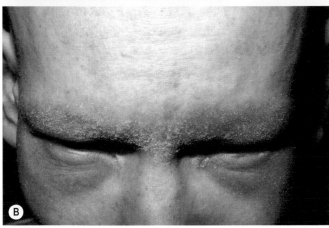

Figure 7.26 IFAP syndrome. (A) Note the total alopecia and the erythematous, scaling skin. (B) Note the spiny keratotic follicular papules of the eyebrows and lashes and the atrichia. His photophobia prevents him from looking at the camera, and has led to tearing. (C) Periungual erythema and marked nail yellowing and thickening; note the psoriasiform plaques at the ankle and on the dorsal aspect of the foot.

scleroderma (see Ch. 22)); keratosis pilaris atrophicans, a group of disorders of hair plugging; or various dermatologic syndromes, such as folliculitis decalvans, dissecting cellulitis of the scalp, acne keloidalis, and pseudopelade.

Alopecia mucinosa

Alopecia mucinosa (follicular mucinosis) is an inflammatory disorder characterized by sharply defined follicular papules or infiltrated plaques, with scaling, loss of hair, and accumulation of mucin in sebaceous glands and the outer root sheaths of affected hair follicles.[206–208] A relatively uncommon condition affecting children as well as adults, the disorder presents in three morphologic forms:

1. Flat rough patches consisting of grouped follicular papules
2. Scaly plaques formed through the coalescence of follicular papules
3. Nodular boggy infiltrated plaques with overlying erythema and scaling (Fig. 7.27).

Lesions usually measure 2–5 cm in diameter. Distributed primarily on the face, scalp, neck, and shoulders (occasionally the trunk and extremities), lesions are usually devoid of hair. Except in the scalp or eyebrows, this is generally not a conspicuous feature.

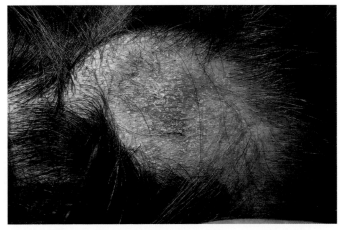

Figure 7.27 Alopecia mucinosa. An erythematous, mildly scaling, infiltrated hairless plaque. Biopsy shows mucin in the hair and sebaceous glands. Alopecia mucinosa tends to be a benign condition in children, but has been associated with cutaneous T-cell lymphoma in adults.

The cause of follicular mucinosis is unknown. In the majority of cases (in those <40 years of age) it is a benign idiopathic condition.[209] In persons older than age 40, however, the presence of boggy infiltrated plaques of alopecia mucinosa may be the first sign of cutaneous T-cell lymphoma. Cutaneous T-cell lymphoma has rarely been described in children with follicular mucinosis,[210] so affected children must be followed carefully.

Alopecia mucinosa must be differentiated from lichen spinulosus,[211] pityriasis rubra pilaris, tinea infection, pityriasis alba, granulomatous diseases, and the papulosquamous group of disorders. When the diagnosis remains in doubt, cutaneous biopsy of an affected area is generally confirmatory, showing accumulation of mucin within the hair and sebaceous glands.

In patients with solitary or few lesions, clearing usually occurs spontaneously within 2 years. In the chronic form, lesions are more numerous, more widely distributed, plaques. Destruction of follicles may give rise to permanent alopecia, and the disorder may persist, with new lesions continuing to appear over a period of many years. Although some cases appear to benefit from topical or intralesional corticosteroids, such claims are difficult to evaluate since spontaneous healing is the rule.

Folliculitis decalvans

Folliculitis decalvans is characterized by successive crops of patchy, painful folliculitis, leading to progressive hair loss and scarring.[212] The disorder must be distinguished by culture from bacterial folliculitis caused by *Staphylococcus aureus*, although the two forms often co-exist, leading to the hypothesis that folliculitis decalvans results from an abnormal host response to staphylococcal toxins.[213] Folliculitis decalvans may begin during adolescence in male patients, but is rarely seen in female patients before 30 years of age. Although the scalp is the most commonly affected site, hair-bearing areas of the trunk, axillae, and pubic region may be affected. Typical lesions show round to irregular bald, atrophic patches, each surrounded by crops of follicular pustules. Tufted folliculitis is a variant in which tufts of hair emerge from dilated follicular openings amidst areas of scarring.[213]

Treatment of folliculitis decalvans is difficult. Systemic antibiotics that penetrate the follicle well (tetracyclines, clindamycin, erythromycin) with or without rifampicin will often prevent disease extension, but continued administration is required to prevent relapse. Many individuals develop severe alopecia and scarring despite long-term and intensive therapy.

Dissecting cellulitis of the scalp

Dissecting cellulitis of the scalp, also termed *perifolliculitis capitis abscedens et suffodiens*, is characterized by painful fluctuant nodules and abscesses of the scalp connected by tortuous ridges or deep sinus tracts with cicatricial alopecia. The connection can often be demonstrated by applying pressure to one nodule and observing purulent drainage emerging from another. Lesions are usually first noted at the occipital area or vertex, but may progress to involve the entire scalp. The disorder occurs most commonly in African-American male teenagers and young adults.[214] An association with acne conglobata and hidradenitis suppurativa has been described ('follicular occlusion triad'), suggesting an inflammatory reaction to *Propionibacterium acnes*. Other pustular disorders of the scalp, including bacterial folliculitis and inflammatory tinea capitis (kerion), must be considered.[215]

The disorder has a chronic, relapsing course. Although use of oral tetracyclines or erythromycin with or without surgical drainage of lesions may be effective, many studies suggest systemic administration of isotretinoin to be the treatment of choice.[216] Laser ablation has also been advocated.[217]

Acne keloidalis

Acne keloidalis (folliculitis keloidalis) is a chronic scarring folliculitis and perifolliculitis of the nape and occipital scalp.[218,219] Initial lesions tend to be inflammatory papules and occasionally pustules that evolve into firm keloidal, often coalescent papules and plaques (Fig. 7.28). Severe cases may show abscesses and sinus formation. Patients may complain of pruritus and discomfort. The disorder is seen most frequently in postpubertal males, especially African-Americans between the ages of 14 and 25 years, but is occasionally described in females.[220]

Acute inflammation of the follicle is thought to be the primary pathologic process, followed by a granulomatous foreign body reaction to released hair, and subsequent fibrosis; a variety of triggers have been proposed, among them irritation from shirt collars or helmets, bacterial folliculitis, or ingrown hairs after a short haircut. Treatment of this disorder is difficult and consists of long-term systemic antibiotics and intralesional corticosteroids. Patients should avoid close 'clipper' haircuts and scratching of the area. Laser and excision with second-intention healing have been helpful for selected patients, especially with fibrotic nodules.[221,222]

Pseudofolliculitis barbae

Pseudofolliculitis barbae, commonly called 'razor bumps' or 'ingrown hairs,' is an inflammatory condition of hair follicles of the beard area that is particularly common in adolescent males of African ancestry with curly, coarse hair (see Ch. 14).[221,223,224] The condition can affect adolescent girls with tightly curled hair, however, especially if shaving on the face because of hirsutism, or because of hair removal elsewhere (waxing plucking or shaving of the axillae or pubic area). Erythematous, 2–4 mm flesh-colored or often hyperpigmented follicular-based papules are characteristic. The shape of the hair follicle, hair cuticle, and direction of hair growth predispose to the inflammatory response when hair is shaved or plucked.[225] A single-nucleotide polymorphism (SNP) in *KRT75*, encoding hair keratin 75, has been linked with a much greater tendency to develop pseudofolliculitis barbae. It is theorized that the pressure and traction exerted by close and regular shaving destabilizes the hair keratin.[226]

Pseudofolliculitis barbae is thought to represent a foreign body reaction around an ingrown hair. Therapy largely involves prevention, particularly by temporarily discontinuing shaving or other forms of hair removal and then instituting alternative techniques that decrease the closeness of the shave, such as use of an electric

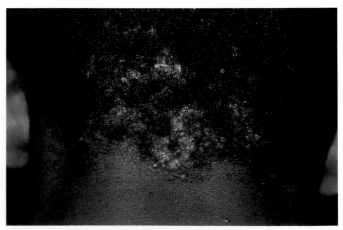

Figure 7.28 Acne keloidalis. Scarring folliculitis with keloidal scarring at the nape and occipital scalp in this 17-year-old black adolescent.

razor (avoiding the 'closest' shave setting), the 'Bumpfighter' razor (American Safety Razor Company, Staunton, VA),[227] or chemical depilatories. The condition tends to clear 4–8 weeks after discontinuation of triggers. Shaving should always be in the direction of hair growth, and pretreatment with an antibacterial soap or benzoyl peroxide wash may decrease the potential inflammation from bacterial overgrowth. Adjunctive topical agents are retinoids, low potency topical steroids, topical antibiotics and depigmenting agents. Non-laser epilation is not recommended and may exacerbate pseudofolliculitis barbae; however, the Nd:YAG 1064 nm and diode (800–810 nm) lasers have been used to epilate the curly hairs and can cause significant improvement.[228–230] Eflornithine cream, which inhibits hair growth, may also be helpful, but may be associated with the development of local irritation.

Pseudopelade

Pseudopelade is a nonspecific scarring form of slowly progressive alopecia of the scalp generally seen in adults, although it has been described rarely in children. It may represent the end result of discoid lupus erythematosus (see Ch. 22) or lichen planopilaris (see Ch. 4). It is characterized by multiple small, round, oval, or irregularly shaped hairless cicatricial patches of varying sizes. Affected areas are shiny, ivory white or slightly pink, and atrophic. Lesions frequently coalesce to form finger-like projections and have been compared to 'footprints in the snow'. Lesions generally appear at the vertex of the scalp. A few hair-containing dilated hair follicles may be interspersed between the patches. The condition tends to resolve spontaneously after several years, leaving the alopecia. Therapy is often unsuccessful, although intralesional injections of triamcinolone have temporarily benefited some patients. Cosmetic improvement has also been achieved by the multiple-punch autograft technique of hair transplantation.

Telogen effluvium

The normal cyclic pattern of anagen and telogen hair phases may be interrupted by a variety of different stimuli, resulting in *telogen effluvium*.[90] Telogen effluvium represents the most common type of alopecia in children and is characterized by diffuse thinning of scalp hair to varying degrees (Fig. 7.29). For most children, the condition is barely noticed and medical attention is not sought. Several stimuli are capable of producing an interruption in the anagen phase of the hair follicles (Table 7.4). Most common are acute illnesses, especially with fever, major trauma, surgery or childbirth. Initiation of medications (Table 7.5) or discontinuation of medications, particularly oral contraceptives, isotretinoin, anticonvulsants, cimetidine, and terbinafine, has also been implicated.[231,232] More chronic telogen effluvium has been associated with chronic illness, thyroid abnormalities, iron deficiency anemia, malabsorption (e.g., celiac disease), malnutrition (e.g., anorexia nervosa),[26] systemic lupus erythematosus,[233] and zinc deficiency. The proportion of follicles affected and the severity of the subsequent alopecia depend on the duration and severity of the trigger and individual variations in susceptibility.

The average individual who shampoos at least every other day loses 50–100 hairs per day. Twenty-five percent (25 000 hairs) must be shed before unmistakable thinning becomes apparent.[234–236] Telogen effluvium may be suggested by a history of a stressful event preceding the onset of alopecia by 6–16 weeks that shifts more hairs into telogen phase. The diagnosis may be confirmed by both counting the number of hairs shed each day and determining the percentage of telogen hairs in the scalp. Loss of an average of more than 100 intact hairs a day can be considered excessive.

Anagen hair roots can be recognized by their intact outer and inner hair sheaths, with or without a portion of the dermal papilla

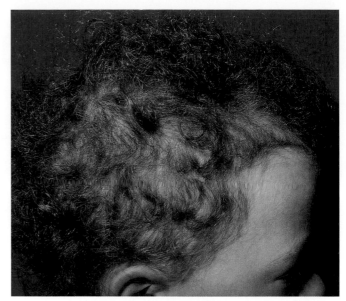

Figure 7.29 Telogen effluvium. Hair shedding is increased and, if a significant amount, a detectable increase in sparsity of hair may be noted. The loss is diffuse across the scalp, but tends to stabilize after a few months and usually returns to normal within about 6 months.

Table 7.4 Potential triggers of telogen effluvium
Emotional stress
Fever (high)
Medications (see Table 7.5)
Nutritional
Biotin deficiency
Dieting, crash; anorexia
Essential fatty acid deficiency
Iron deficiency
Hypervitaminosis A
Physiologic telogen effluvium of the newborn
Parturition
Severe chronic illness
Severe infection
Surgery
Thyroid disease (hyper- or hypo-)

Table 7.5 Pediatric medications that may be associated with telogen effluvium
Albendazole
Amphetamines
Angiotensin converting enzyme inhibitors (e.g., captopril, enalapril)
Anticoagulants (e.g., heparin, warfarin)
Anticonvulsants (e.g., valproic acid, carbamazepine)
Beta blockers (e.g., propranolol)
Cimetidine
Danazol
Interferon-α
Lithium
Oral contraceptions (during use or with discontinuation)
Retinoids (e.g., isotretinoin)

adherent to the tip of the root (Fig. 7.1A). Telogen hair roots have uniform shaft diameters, contain no pigment, and are club shaped (Fig. 7.1B), much like the tip of a cotton-tipped applicator. Telogen hair represents approximately 15% and anagen 85% of scalp hair. If 25% or more of gently pulled hairs are telogen, telogen effluvium can be diagnosed. Increased telogen hair loss can also be seen in children with *short anagen syndrome*, in which the short, fine hair does not require haircuts and is present from birth. The shortening of the anagen phase, despite a normal rate of growth, leads to the decrease in the maximal hair length and an increase in the number of hairs in telogen. The disorder tends to resolve spontaneously during puberty and adulthood.[237]

There is no effective treatment for telogen effluvium, but complete regrowth almost invariably occurs within months, unless the stressful event is repeated or the underlying trigger is sustained. Careful explanation of the cause of this disorder and its favorable prognosis, with careful instructions to the patient to avoid unnecessary manipulation, tends to suffice. Blood tests for underling disorders should be performed based on personal and family history and on examination, especially if no trigger is obvious. Adolescents predisposed to androgenetic alopecia may show incomplete regrowth after telogen effluvium with a residual pattern of hair loss consistent with androgenetic alopecia. Rarely, prolonged illness with high fevers destroys some follicles completely and only partial recovery ensues. Telogen effluvium occasionally occurs more than once in an individual, suggesting a predisposition to more significant hair loss with stress.

Anagen effluvium

In anagen effluvium, hair shaft production is markedly reduced, leading to tapering of the shaft and shedding. Given that >80% of scalp hair is in anagen phase, hair loss is usually profound. Anagen effluvium usually occurs in patients administered radiation or chemotherapy for malignancy. Most commonly implicated are cyclophosphamide, methotrexate, 6-mercaptopurine, doxorubicin, and vincristine.[231,232] In addition, anagen effluvium may be associated with exposure to colchicine and toxic levels of boric acid, lead, thallium, arsenic, bismuth, and warfarin.[231]

The clinical features of anagen effluvium depend on the degree of toxicity created by the causative agent. With lower doses of the toxic agent, only segmental thinning or narrowing may occur, without actual fracture of the hair shaft. Gentle hair pulls yield 'pencil point' dystrophic hairs with proximal tips tapered to a point.[235] With extensive anagen effluvium, the remaining hairs are telogen, and the hair plucks late in the course may show as many as 100% telogen hairs. A careful history, documented evidence of hair loss, microscopic examination of spontaneously shed and manually epilated hairs, and appropriate physical and toxicologic examinations help to establish the correct diagnosis. Cessation of the responsible drug or toxin generally results in regrowth of hair.

Alopecia areata

Alopecia areata, a common disorder that affects 0.1–0.2% of the population, is characterized by the sudden appearance of sharply defined round or oval patches of hair loss.[238,239] Although the condition occurs at all ages, 24–65% of patients experience their first episode before 16 years of age.[240] The condition has been described in neonates and young infants.[241] Familial occurrence is reported in 8–52% of children, with an estimated lifetime risk of 7.1% in siblings, 7.8% in parents and 5.7% in offspring.[242] Occurrence in both identical twins is 55%, emphasizing the importance of environmental as well as genetic factors.

The hair follicle is considered a site of immune privilege, with active suppression of natural killer cells and downregulation of major histocompatibility complex MHC class I expression.[243]

Alopecia areata is thought to be a tissue-restricted autoimmune disorder with an attack by T lymphocytes on the follicle after loss of immune privilege.[244,245] Haplotype mapping has recently implicated both innate and adaptive immunity, showing significant association with gene regions controlling T regulatory cells, cytotoxic T lymphocyte-associated antigen 4, interleukins, the HLA region and the hair follicle.[246] Single nucleotide polymorphisms in *AIRE* (mutated in APECED syndrome, see differential diagnosis)[247] and *PTPN22* (a phosphatase)[248] have been linked to alopecia areata as well. Loss of function mutations in *FLG* (encoding filaggrin) have been associated with a more severe course and associated atopy, but not a higher risk.[249] Although associated autoimmune disorders in affected children are quite rare, a family history of other autoimmune disorders, especially thyroiditis, is common and autoantibodies may be detected in patient sera.[250] An increased incidence has also been noted in patients with trisomy 21. A stressful event precedes the onset of alopecia areata in 9.5–58% of patients.[251,252] Stress may trigger release of substance P and collapse of the MHC class I-based immune privilege.[253]

The typical clinical picture of alopecia areata generally consists of a sudden (overnight or several days) appearance of one or more round or oval well-circumscribed, clearly defined patches of hair loss (Fig. 7.30). Occasionally, the initial patches may lack a regular outline and, at times, may demonstrate scattered long hairs within the bald areas. In other instances, the initial loss may be diffuse, with discrete patches of alopecia being apparent only after 1 or 2 weeks, if at all. The primary patch may appear on any hairy cutaneous surface but usually occurs on the scalp. The skin is smooth, soft, and almost totally devoid of hair. Rarely, slight erythema or edema may be found at an early stage. Depigmented or hypopigmented hair shafts, simulating poliosis, may be seen before hair loss or with early hair regrowth (Fig. 7.31). Discrete islands of hair loss sometimes are separated by completely uninvolved or partially involved scalp. Around the margins of patches of alopecia, pathognomonic 'exclamation-mark' hairs may be detected (Fig. 7.32). These loose hairs, with attenuated bulbs and short stumps, are easily plucked out of the scalp. Examination of such hairs under a low-power microscope reveals an irregularity in diameter and a poorly pigmented hair shaft that tapers to an attenuated bulb. The hair bulb represents the dot of the exclamation point. Dermoscopic evaluation of affected scalp can be very helpful, showing the tapered hairs and sometimes yellow perifollicular dots, demarcating the hyperkeratotic follicular plugs.[254,255]

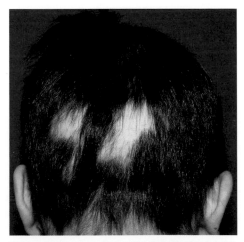

Figure 7.30 Alopecia areata. Individuals with this common hair disorder suddenly develop one or more round or oval well-circumscribed, clearly defined patches of hair loss.

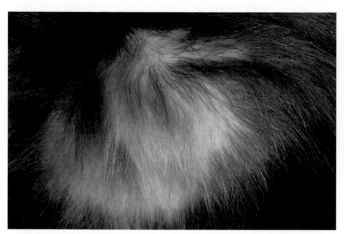

Figure 7.31 Alopecia areata. Re-growing hair may initially appear hypopigmented or depigmented, and is eventually replaced by normally pigmented hair. Loss of hair pigment may also precede alopecia.

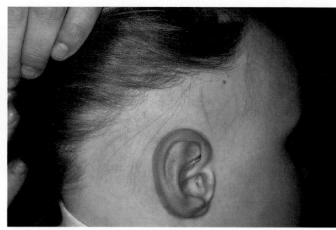

Figure 7.33 Alopecia areata. The ophiasis pattern involves hair loss in a band extending from the occiput bilaterally along the hair margin toward the region above the ear and sometimes circling to the anterior scalp.

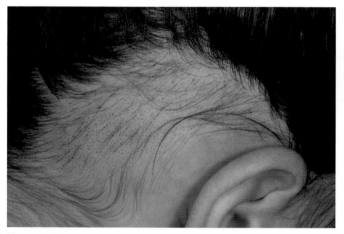

Figure 7.32 Alopecia areata. 'Exclamation point hairs' in a girl with an *ophiasis pattern* of hair loss. Under the microscope, these hairs demonstrate a tapered shaft to an attenuated bulb (the 'dot' of the exclamation point).

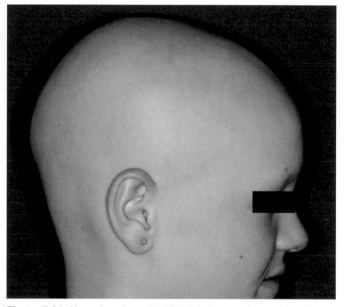

Figure 7.34 Alopecia universalis. All hair is lost on the scalp and elsewhere. This is associated with a much poorer prognosis for hair regrowth.

The *ophiasis* pattern of hair loss begins as a bald spot on the posterior occiput and extends anteriorly and bilaterally in a 1–2-inch wide band encircling the posterior scalp, usually extending above the ear, but occasionally to the anterior aspect of the scalp (Fig. 7.33). The ophiasis pattern occurs in <5% of children, and is generally associated with a poor prognosis.[256] *Alopecia totalis* (loss of all scalp hair) may ultimately develop in 5% of cases of partial alopecia. Progression to the totalis form occurs more slowly, but more frequently, in children than in adults. Complete or virtually complete loss of body hair may also occur and is termed *alopecia universalis* (Fig. 7.34). Alopecia may involve any hair; eyebrows and eyelashes may be lost with or without patches of hair loss on the scalp (Fig. 7.35). Overall, 83% of children have mild to moderate disease (<50% hair loss).

Nail defects are seen in 10–20% of cases. Although it is true that the more extensive the disease, the more likely the possibility and severity of nail involvement, some patients may have gross nail dystrophy with little hair change. The most characteristic nail abnormality is a fine grid-like stippling, regularly arranged in horizontal and/or vertical rows with smaller and shallower pits than those seen in patients with psoriasis (Fig. 7.36). Proximal shedding (onychomadesis), longitudinal ridging (trachyonychia), opacification, serration of the free edges, and severe dystrophy (Fig. 7.37), although less common, appear to be more likely in patients with alopecia totalis and universalis.

The diagnosis of alopecia areata is based on its clinical picture. The sudden appearance and circumscribed non-scarring, patterned nature of hair loss will frequently distinguish it from other disorders of alopecia. Trichotillomania is typically associated with bizarre, irregular patches of hair loss, with areas of broken hairs of different lengths. The absence of signs of inflammation and scaling will generally help distinguish this disorder from that of tinea capitis. When the diagnosis is in doubt, microscopic examination of hairs, potassium hydroxide mounts, fungal cultures, and cutaneous punch biopsy will frequently establish the proper diagnosis. Alopecia universalis beginning in infants must be distinguished from atrichia

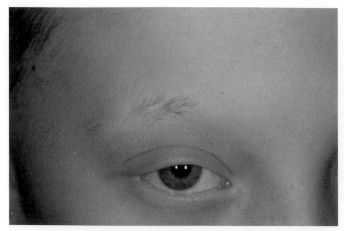

Figure 7.35 Alopecia areata. The alopecia may involve the eyebrows and eyelashes, even without hair loss on the scalp; in this situation, trichotillomania must also be considered.

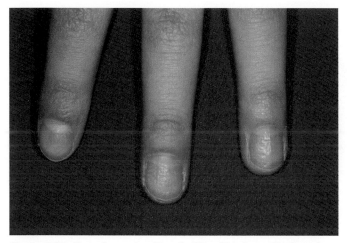

Figure 7.36 Alopecia areata with nail pitting. This boy with alopecia areata shows punctate depressions result from alterations in the proximal matrix.

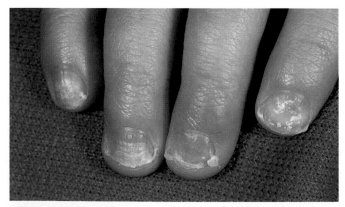

Figure 7.37 Alopecia universalis. Proximal shedding (onychomadesis), Beau's lines (horizontal dells), mild longitudinal ridging (trachyonychia), opacification, and serration of the free edges are all seen in the nails of this young girl with alopecia universalis.

with papules.[257] The alopecia areata spectrum can be a feature in 33% of children with autoimmune polyendocrinopathy-candidiasis-ectodermal dystrophy (APECED, see Ch. 23) syndrome, due to mutations in *AIRE*.[258]

The course of alopecia areata is variable and difficult to predict. New patches of hair loss may appear for 4–6 weeks and, occasionally, for several months. Spontaneous regrowth may occur. In general, when the process is limited to a few patches, the prognosis is good, with complete regrowth occurring within 1 year in 34–50% of patients,[259] while 15–43% will progress to total loss of scalp hair[259] from which full recovery is unusual (<10%). About 30% of patients overall will have future episodes of alopecia areata once regrown. The earlier the onset, the poorer the prognosis. Other prognostic indicators of a worse outcome are family history of autoimmune disease, personal history of atopy, and nail abnormalities. Therapy for alopecia areata at best controls the condition, but does not cure it or prevent development of new areas.[260–262] Because of the chronic nature of the condition and the slow growth of hair, any trial of a treatment modality requires at least 4 months. The sudden hair loss, cosmetic ramification, and unpredictable course make alopecia areata a frightening disorder for affected families; psychological support and counseling are required for all patients and parents. Adequate camouflage of alopecic areas may be achieved by hats, headbands, or hairstyle changes. In children with severe involvement, wigs can be helpful. Locks of Love is an organization that provides hair prostheses to financially disadvantaged children under the age of 18 years (www.locksoflove.org).[263] The National Alopecia Areata Foundation (PO Box 150760, San Rafael, CA; www.alopeciaareata.com) is a national support group for affected children and their families. Given the high percentage of children with patchy alopecia areata who show spontaneous remission within a year, some physicians prescribe no therapy for this condition. In general, patients with more extensive alopecia areata, or with limited involvement unresponsive to topical corticosteroids, should be referred to a dermatologist.

The most commonly used therapy for more limited alopecia areata in children is topical corticosteroids, with or without occlusion (such as may be achieved under a wig, bathing cap, or Saran Wrap); class II (potent) steroids are usually administered. Because the regrowth rate without medications is high, it has been hard to demonstrate clear evidence of the efficacy of steroids. If a class I (ultrapotent) steroid is employed, its use should be limited to intermittent pulse therapy; longer use may result in significant local atrophy and systemic absorption. Intradermal corticosteroid injections frequently result in regrowth in tufts at injection sites within 4–6 weeks, but are too uncomfortable for most children, even with the use of topical anesthetic creams. When an intralesional corticosteroid is used, a syringe with a 30-gauge needle or jet-injection is best. Triamcinolone acetonide is injected in concentrations of 2.5 mg/mL (eyebrow area) to 10 mg/mL (scalp). Dosage should be limited to 0.1 mL per site, spaced at least 1 cm apart, with injections at intervals of at least 4–6 weeks.[239] Transient local atrophy may occur. Efficacy appears to be greatest in those who have <75% hair loss and with a relatively short duration of hair loss.

Minoxidil has been shown to stimulate follicular DNA synthesis. Although largely used for androgenetic alopecia, 2–5% topical minoxidil solution has been shown to cause cosmetically acceptable hair regrowth in approximately 20–45% of patients when used twice daily for 2 months.[264] Best results occur in patients with limited hair loss and when used concurrently with topical corticosteroids or anthralin. Cutaneous side-effects may include local irritation, allergic contact dermatitis, and hypertrichosis, especially on the forehead. Although quite rare, three children treated with topical minoxidil developed tachycardia, palpitations and dizziness.[265] Prostaglandin F2α analogues (e.g., latanoprost, bimatoprost, travoprost) have not been helpful for alopecia of the eyelashes or brows,[266] but have been linked to periorbital hyperpigmentation.[267]

Anthralin cream is an alternative therapy that seems to elicit hair growth by nonspecific immunostimulation. The 1% cream is usually applied as short-contact therapy, initially for 30 min with a gradual increase in exposure as tolerated to a maximum of 2 h prior to shampooing of the scalp. A mild dermatitis is often required for regrowth, so concurrent use of topical corticosteroids is not recommended. New hair growth is usually seen in 3 months, but 6 months or more may be required for an acceptable response. Scalp irritation, folliculitis, and staining of the skin or clothes are potential adverse effects.

Excimer laser therapy twice weekly is painless and has recently been shown to cause hair regrowth in 60% of recalcitrant patches of alopecia areata in children; only 22% of responders relapsed after 6 months.[268]

Treatment of more extensive alopecia areata (>50%), alopecia totalis and alopecia universalis is very difficult. Generally, application of topical corticosteroids is not helpful, but anthralin has shown greater responses. Topical immunotherapy has been useful for patients with chronic, severe alopecia areata. Patients are initially sensitized to the contact allergen (2%), then increasing concentrations of the allergen (usually beginning at 0.001%) are applied to the scalp until mild erythema and scaling develop. Squaric acid dibutyl ester and diphenylcyclopropenone are used most commonly in children, because they are effective, but not mutagenic or carcinogenic. Excessive contact dermatitis with vesiculation and regional lymphadenopathy are the risks of this therapy.[269,270] In patients with >50% involvement, approximately 30–45% respond, but relapse occurs in 81% of responders.[271,272] In atopics with extensive alopecia areata, the addition of oral fexofenadine to the contact allergen treatment may increase the response.[273] Although PUVA (photochemotherapy with systemic psoralen followed by ultraviolet A) and cyclosporine therapy have been successful in some adults with this disorder, their efficacy and safety have not been established in children.

Although not recommended for general use, systemic corticosteroids may be considered for carefully selected patients with severe involvement and rapidly progressive hair loss who are psychologically handicapped by their disorder. In such instances, prednisone may be administered in dosages of 0.5–1 mg/kg per day for 4 weeks until hair loss ceases, then tapered to alternate-day therapy for a few months. It must be emphasized that close follow-up evaluation is indicated in such cases and that the potential side effects associated with systemic corticosteroid therapy must be explained to the patient and parents. Pulse therapy with intravenous methylprednisolone has also been administered at a dosage of 250 mg twice daily for three sequential days with cessation of hair loss,[274] but the long-term outcome after corticosteroid therapy is poor.[275] Continuing application of topical minoxidil after a steroid taper has been shown to decrease hair loss. Trials with biologics have been disappointing.[276,277]

Androgenetic alopecia

Androgenetic alopecia occurs in both males (common balding or male-pattern baldness) and females (hereditary thinning or female-pattern hair loss), and is the most common cause of hair loss in adults. In many cases, it begins in teenage years with onset as young as 7 years;[278,279] in general, the earlier the onset, the more profound the subsequent alopecia. The disorder is characterized by patterned, progressive hair loss from the scalp and results from the effects of circulating androgens in genetically susceptible individuals.

Dihydrotestosterone is the primary androgen implicated, converted from testosterone by the enzyme 5-α-reductase. These androgens gradually decrease the size of scalp hair follicles, resulting in miniaturized hairs. In addition, the anagen growth phase is shortened, leading to more hairs in telogen phase. The condition is inherited as a polygenic trait influenced by both maternal and paternal genes; thus, a history of baldness on either the maternal or paternal side should be determined.[280]

Most patients with androgenetic alopecia note thinning of scalp hair rather than shedding, although shedding may occur early in the course and be confused with telogen effluvium. Androgenetic alopecia in females is generally less severe than that seen in males. The frontal hairline is relatively unaffected, with only slight recession. Most commonly, the hair is thinned from the frontal scalp to the vertex (Fig. 7.38), with relatively normal density of hairs of the occiput and sides of the head. Widening of the central hair part is often seen, leading to scalp visibility (Fig. 7.39). The mildest and

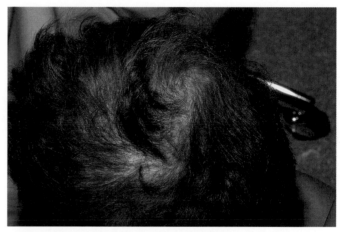

Figure 7.38 Androgenetic alopecia. The scalp hair is thinned progressively, but most notably between the frontal region of the scalp and the vertex.

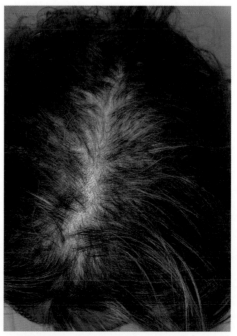

Figure 7.39 Androgenetic alopecia. Widening of the central hair part is often seen, leading to scalp visibility.

often earliest form of androgenetic male-pattern alopecia in males is seen as a symmetrical triangular recession of the hairline in the frontoparietal and occasionally frontal scalp margins. Androgenetic alopecia in teenage boys can also first be seen at the vertex region (Fig. 7.38), and in 20% follows a female pattern with a decrease in hair density and tapered hair diameter, and not the bitemporal recession commonly seen in adult males.[279]

The diagnosis of androgenetic alopecia can be suspected by the patterning of the scalp hair loss; if confirmation is required, especially in female patients, hair plucks may be performed and will show an increased ratio of telogen:anagen hairs in the frontal region in contrast to the occipital and parietal areas of the scalp. Scalp biopsies show the miniaturized follicle with an underlying collapsed connective tissue sheath that can be diagnostic. Whereas no further evaluation in young men is needed, hormonal evaluation and endocrinologic consultation for female patients should be considered, especially in the presence of menstrual irregularities, moderate to severe acne, and evidence of virilization, such as hirsutism. Laboratory evaluation should include testing for thyroid disease and anemia, free and total testosterone, DHEA-S, and if appropriate 17-OH-progesterone and prolactin levels.

The occurrence of androgenetic alopecia during teenage years can be quite disturbing to both young men and women. Careful examination and repeated reassurance are required to discourage expensive and ineffective therapeutic regimens. Without treatment, androgenetic alopecia is progressive; the aim of treatment is to retard the further thinning of the hair and to promote hair growth. Topical minoxidil has been shown to promote hair growth and decrease hair loss in large controlled trials of both male and female patients when applied twice daily.[281-283] Moderate to dense growth is appreciated in about one-third of patients. The mechanism of action of topical minoxidil, available in 2% and 5% strengths, is most likely to involve its stimulation of follicular proliferation and vascularization of the follicle. Application of minoxidil must be continued, however, to maintain hair growth. After stopping treatment, the newly grown hairs are lost within 6 months. The most common side-effect of topical minoxidil is irritation, usually from the propylene glycol in the solution. Hypertrichosis has been described on non-scalp sites, possibly from transfer of the solution.[284] Oral finasteride is the only approved systemic medication for androgenetic alopecia, but is not approved for use under the age of 18 years and should be considered only for males. Finasteride inhibits specifically type II 5-α-reductase, leading to reduction in both serum and scalp levels of dihydrotestosterone. The only statistically significant side-effect of finasteride is sexual dysfunction, but it is known to cause feminization of the male fetus.[285] Spironolactone has shown some benefit in girls with androgenetic alopecia at doses of 50–200 mg/day;[286] similarly, cyproterone acetate in doses of 50–100 mg/day in combination with ethinyl estradiol has been successful in inducing hair regrowth and preventing progression, but is not currently available in the USA. Hair prostheses or surgical procedures, such as scalp reduction with or without tissue expansion, scalp flaps, and multiple-punch autografting hair transplantation, may also be considered in patients with advanced androgenetic alopecia.

Traumatic alopecia

Traumatic alopecia results from the forceful extraction of hair or the breaking of hair shafts by friction, pressure, traction, or other physical trauma. The usual causes are cosmetic practices and trichotillomania. Other causes of traumatic alopecia include pressure, such as occurs in neonates who develop caput succedaneum with a scalp ring from birth trauma or use of suction at delivery[205] (Fig. 7.2; see also Ch. 2), and as is seen on the occiput of infants who lie on their backs or are in the habit of 'head-banging'; prolonged bed rest in one position such as may be seen in chronically ill patients; postoperative alopecia (as a result of pressure-induced ischemia during long surgical procedures); thermal or electric burns; repeated vigorous massage; a severe blow to the scalp; occipitoparietal alopecia such as may be induced by spinning on the crown of the head during 'break-dancing'; pressure from orthodontic headgear;[287] or prolonged use of wide-strapped heavy headphones, such as those frequently used by individuals while jogging. Prolonged or forceful trauma may cause scarring alopecia.

Alopecia from cosmetic practices most often results from traction, but has been described from pulling, frequent brushing with nylon bristles, the use of hot combs and oils, and hair-straightening practices such as teasing. *Traction alopecia* is characterized by oval or linear areas of hair loss at the margins of the hair line, along the part, or scattered through the scalp, depending on the type of traction or trauma.[288,289] Peripheral scalp hair loss may occur in individuals who wear their hair in pony-tail style, braids, or use hair extensions[290] or barrettes (Fig. 7.40). In one study, 17.1% of school-aged African girls showed traction alopecia, with the percentage increasing towards the end of high school and with a history of braids on relaxed hair.[291] The hair loss from hair rollers is usually most conspicuous in the frontocentral area or around the margins of the scalp. Hot comb alopecia, seen primarily in African-American individuals who straighten their hair for cosmetic purposes, generally occurs on the vertex or marginal areas of the scalp. In severe chronic forms, however, the entire scalp may be involved. Traction folliculitis may present as perifollicular erythema and pustules at sites of traction.[292]

Trichotillomania is a self-limiting, self-induced form of traction alopecia produced either consciously or habitual plucking, pulling, or cutting the hair in a bizarre manner.[293,294] Trichotillomania-by-proxy has also been described, in which a parent with trichotillomania pulls the hair of a child as part of the overwhelming urge to depilate.[295] Seen in both sexes, it usually occurs in children above 5 years of age and in young adolescents, although the condition may occur in children as young as 18 months of age. The scalp is the most common site of involvement, but the eyebrows and eyelashes may also be affected as the patient plucks, twirls, or rubs hair-bearing areas, resulting in the epilation or breakage of hair shafts (Fig. 7.41).

The habit is usually practiced in bed before the child falls asleep (when the parent does not notice the habit) or when the child is reading, writing, or watching television. In young individuals the

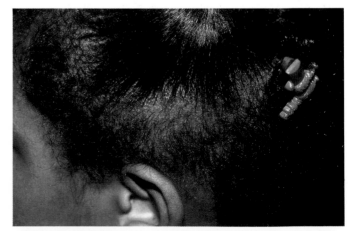

Figure 7.40 Traction alopecia. Hair loss can be seen at the margins where hair is pulled most tightly through use of barrettes.

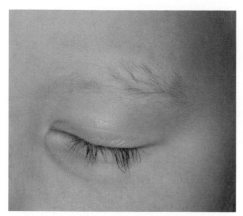

Figure 7.41 Trichotillomania. The eyebrows and eyelashes may be pulled out or broken by repetitive plucking, twirling, or rubbing.

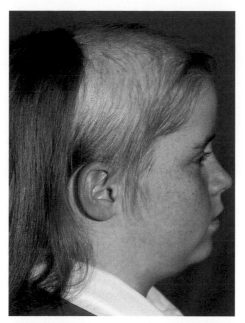

Figure 7.43 Trichotillomania. The affected areas have irregularly-shaped, angular outlines and are never completely bald. They tend to be sites that are easy to reach.

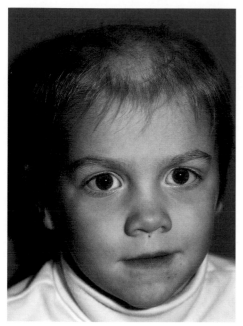

Figure 7.42 Trichotillomania. In younger children trichotillomania is often a habit of twirling or plucking associated with finger or thumb sucking, and does not reflect significant psychological disturbance.

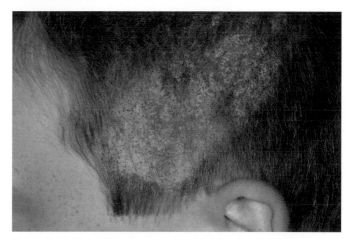

Figure 7.44 Trichotillomania. This boy tried to cover patch of trichotillomania with eyebrow pencil, but continued to pluck hairs.

condition is frequently associated with a habit of finger or thumb sucking (Fig. 7.42). In older children, other compulsive behaviors may be seen as well, such as nail biting (onychophagia), skin picking, picking at acne (acne excoriée), nose picking, lip biting, and cheek chewing. Trichotillomania is classified by the American Psychiatric Association as an impulse-control disorder. The condition is distinguished from obsessive-compulsive disorder in that pulling out the hair is considered pleasurable to affected patients, carried out in response to anxiety, and is performed with minimal awareness. Obsessive-compulsive acts are not pleasurable, are performed in full awareness, and are performed in an effort to avoid anxiety.[294]

Trichotillomania usually begins insidiously as an irregular linear or rectangular area of partial hair loss. Affected areas are generally single, often frontal, fronto-temporal, or frontoparietal, and frequently appear on the contralateral side of right- or left-handed individuals. The affected patches have irregularly shaped angular outlines and are never completely bald (Fig. 7.43). Within the involved regions, the hair is short or stubbly and broken off at varying lengths (Fig. 7.44).

If one maintains a high index of suspicion, trichotillomania can generally be distinguished from other forms of hair loss by its characteristic configuration and distribution. Occasionally, the diagnosis can be confirmed by the finding of wads of hair under the pillow or bed or by observation of the habit by a parent, teacher, or physician. When the diagnosis is suspected, regrowth of hair in a carefully shaved or occluded patch of scalp in the involved area (to prevent manipulation) may confirm the correct diagnosis. Trichotillomania should be distinguished from alopecia areata, although both have been described in the same individuals, often with the alopecia areata as the trigger to the trichotillomania.[296] Clinical differentiation from alopecia areata is usually based on the bizarre configuration, irregular outline, and presence of short stub-like broken hairs. Differentiation from tinea capitis may require microscopic examination of plucked hairs with potassium hydroxide and fungal culture (see Ch. 17). Of particular significance is the fact that the broken hairs of trichotillomania, unlike those of certain forms of tinea capitis, remain firmly rooted in the scalp, and the cutaneous surface is normal and stubbled rather than erythematous or scaly. If the diagnosis remains in doubt, biopsy of the involved area may be helpful.

The management of trichotillomania is often difficult and requires a strong relationship among the doctor, patient, and parents. Although patients occasionally will admit to touching the affected areas, they frequently will deny plucking, rubbing, or excessive manipulation. Blunt accusation is frequently detrimental, but gentle suggestion of the cause may lead to dialogue that is important for reversal. Psychopathologic changes are reported to be present in some 50–75% of affected individuals. These changes are usually mild, but severe psychological disturbance occurs in approximately 5% of patients with trichotillomania, most commonly in older children and teenagers. In general, the disorder is limited in pre-school-age children, and may be more episodic in children than in affected teenagers.

If patients are reassured, given an opportunity to express their emotional needs, and offered a reasonable therapeutic regimen, such as a mild shampoo, mild topical steroid (e.g., hydrocortisone 1%) lotion, and behavioral modification techniques, the habit will frequently disappear. For those individuals with persistent or severe obsessive-compulsive or emotional problems, however, clomipramine or a highly selective serotoninergic reuptake inhibitor (SSRI; e.g., fluvoxamine, fluoxetine, paroxetine, sertraline, or citalopram) and psychiatric intervention should be considered. The possibility of trichophagia and trichobezoar should be also be entertained.[297] Cognitive behavioral therapy with relapse prevention can reduce trichotillomania severity by 64% at 6-month follow-up.[298] For habitual trichotillomania in young children, substitution therapy (such as with a soft tag to stroke or a long-haired doll) and provision of rewards can be helpful.[299]

Eruptive Vellus Hair Cysts

Eruptive vellus hair cysts are characterized by 1–3 mm, skin-colored to hyperpigmented follicular papules, most commonly on the anterior chest (Fig. 7.45). Lesions usually are not grouped and tend to be smooth surfaced with a round or domed shape. Vellus hair cysts have less commonly been described on the upper and lower extremities, face, neck, abdomen, axillae, posterior trunk, and/or buttocks. If darker blue in color and on the face, they have been confused

with nevus of Ota.[300] Although usually seen in children between 4 and 18 years of age, these cysts can occur at any age.

The histologic picture of eruptive vellus hair cysts shows small, mid- to upper dermal keratinizing cysts filled with lamellar keratin and small-diameter non-pigmented or lightly pigmented hair shafts. Vellus hair cysts can be distinguished from steatocystoma multiplex by the inclusion of sebaceous glands in the cyst wall of steatocystoma multiplex.[301] However, lesions with features of both types of cysts have been described; both types of lesions have been seen in the same individuals; and kindreds with the autosomal dominant inheritance of both vellus hair cysts and steatocystoma multiplex have been reported with keratin 17 mutations, suggesting a common causation for the two types of cystic lesions.[302,303] An alternative diagnostic technique to biopsy is to perform a tiny incision at the top after topical anesthesia, and examine the expressed contents microscopically for vellus hairs.[304]

Vellus hair cysts are most commonly confused with milia, molluscum contagiosum, syringomas, folliculitis, keratosis pilaris, steatocystoma multiplex, and other adnexal tumors. The cysts may resolve spontaneously during a few months to years by transepidermal elimination. Patients desiring therapy can be treated by incision of individual cysts and expression of their contents followed by gentle curettage, light electrodesiccation with expression of contents,[305] therapy with topical vitamin A acid (tretinoin), lactic acid (12% lotion), or laser.[306]

Hypertrichosis and Hirsutism

Excessive hairiness may be localized or diffuse, congenital or acquired, and normal or pathologic.[233] Hair in the pubic area of infants may be benign and often resolves spontaneously by 1 year of age, especially if on the scrotum in boys and labia majora or mons in girls without other evidence of virilization or sexual development.[307] The terms *hypertrichosis* and *hirsutism* are frequently and inappropriately used synonymously to describe excessive hair on the body.[308,309] *Hirsutism* implies an excessive growth of body hair in women or children (mostly girls) in an androgen-induced hair pattern (upper lip, chin, sideburn areas, neck, anterior chest, breasts, linea alba, abdomen, upper inner thighs, and legs).[310] Hirsutism most commonly represents a physiologic variant of hair growth, often seen in several family members, which comes to medical attention only because of societal pressure to remove excessive hair. *Hypertrichosis*, conversely, refers to a generalized or localized pattern of *non-androgen-dependent* excessive hair growth in a male or female without evidence of masculinism or menstrual abnormality.

Acquired generalized hypertrichosis

Generalized hypertrichosis may be associated with neurologic disorders (post-encephalitic hypertrichosis, multiple sclerosis), anorexia nervosa, acrodynia, hypothyroidism, porphyria, dermatomyositis, gross malnutrition, and various forms of drug-induced hypertrichosis. Drug-induced hypertrichosis (Fig. 7.46) is most commonly seen in children who are administered phenytoin or cyclosporine, usually after 2 or 3 months of treatment, but other medications have been implicated as well (Table 7.6). In adults, but not in children, acquired forms of hypertrichosis lanuginosa are strongly associated with internal malignancy, especially adenocarcinoma.

Congenital hypertrichosis

The original fine soft unmedullated and usually unpigmented lanugo hairs are shed *in utero* during the 7th or 8th month of gestation. Premature infants, however, frequently display this fine coat

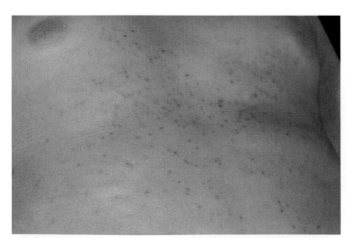

Figure 7.45 Vellus hair cysts. Size 1–3 mm, skin-colored to hyperpigmented follicular papules on the anterior chest.

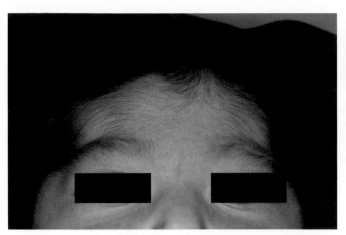

Figure 7.46 Drug-induced hypertrichosis. This infant girl developed hypertrichosis from administration of diazoxide for hyperinsulinemia.

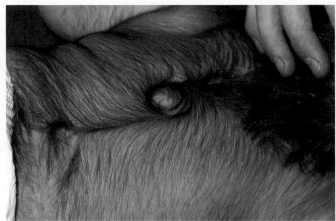

Figure 7.47 Hypertrichosis. Generalized terminal hair growth in this girl with gingival hyperplasia.

Table 7.6 Medications that may cause hypertrichosis
ACTH
Anabolic steroids
Cyclosporine
Danazol
Diazoxide
Glucocorticosteroids
Hexachlorobenzene (drug-induced porphyria cutanea tarda)
Minoxidil
Penicillamine
Phenytoin
Psoralens and ultraviolet light exposure
Streptomycin
Testosterone
Valproic acid

of lanugo hair, particularly on the face, limbs, and trunk. In these infants the fine lanugo hairs are shed during the first months of life and replaced by normal terminal hair growth, generally before the first 6 months.

Hypertrichosis lanuginosa is a rare inherited disorder in which lanugo hairs persist or are overproduced throughout life.[311] Affected infants may be unusually hairy at birth or may develop hypertrichosis during early childhood. In some children, the hair will be spontaneously lost during childhood; in others, it will remain into adulthood. Generalized hypertrichosis can be very disfiguring. Affected children have been called 'monkey-men,' 'dog-face,' and 'human Skye terriers'. Sporadic, autosomal recessive, and autosomal dominant cases have been described. Congenital glaucoma, skeletal abnormalities, and missing teeth have been described in association.

Ambras syndrome is a generalized condition of hypertrichosis in which the hair appears to be vellus, rather than lanugo hair.[312–314] The hypertrichosis is most evident on the face, ears, and shoulders, and persists throughout life. Dysmorphic facial features have been associated. Ambras syndrome has recently been linked to a rearrangement in chromosome 8q that downregulates the expression of TRPS1 (mutated in tricho-rhino-phalangeal syndrome).[315]

Hypertrichosis with gingival hyperplasia is a distinct autosomal dominant disorder in which affected individuals have excessive body and facial hair in an identical distribution to that of hypertrichosis lanuginosa but patients tend to have terminal hair and have associated gingival hyperplasia (Fig. 7.47). Although the hypertrichosis is most commonly present at birth or in infancy, in up to half of reported cases the hypertrichosis begins at puberty. The gingival hyperplasia is usually noted with delayed tooth eruption, and has been described as pink, firm, and pebbly. The disorder is complicated by interference with chewing, respiration, and speech, and periodontal abscesses have been described because of difficulty in dental eruption. Gingival debulking may be required. A large deletion on 17q24.2–q24.3 has been found to be responsible for congenital generalized hypertrichosis, with or without gingival hyperplasia.[316]

X-linked dominant hypertrichosis has been described in a Mexican pedigree. Affected males show excessive generalized terminal hair growth, especially on the face and upper torso; female individuals are less severely affected, and can show asymmetric hairiness thought to represent random inactivation (lyonization) of the affected chromosome. This condition sometimes improves after puberty.[317] In another Mexican kindred, congenital universal hypertrichosis was associated with deafness and dental anomalies as an X-linked recessive disorder.[318]

Generalized hypertrichosis is also a feature of several syndromes (Table 7.7), most commonly, the *Cornelia de Lange syndrome*. This congenital disorder features marked hypertrichosis; cutis marmorata; hypoplastic genitalia, nipples, and umbilicus; growth and skeletal abnormalities; mental retardation; and a characteristic low-pitched and growling cry. The vast majority of cases are sporadic, but rare familial cases appear to be autosomal dominant.[319] The face of afflicted individuals is characterized by overgrowth of the eyebrows, long eyelashes, high upper lip, saddle-nose, and a cyanotic hue about the eyes, nose, and mouth. Children with this disorder often have recurrent respiratory tract infections and gastrointestinal upsets; seizures have been observed in about 20% of reported cases, and most patients die before the age of 6 years. Hypertrichosis is also a feature of congenital erythropoietic porphyria (see Ch. 19).

Localized Forms of Hypertrichosis

Nevoid hypertrichosis

Growth of hair abnormal in length, shaft diameter, or color may occur in association with other nevoid abnormalities or as isolated circumscribed developmental defects.[320] Abnormal tufts of hair in the lumbosacral and, at times, the posterior cervical or thoracic areas (the faun-tail nevus, Fig. 7.48) may be associated with an

Table 7.7 Congenital syndromes associated with generalized hypertrichosis

Barber–Say syndrome
Cantu syndrome (hypertrichosis with osteochondrodysplasia)
Coffin–Siris syndrome
Cornelia de Lange (Brachmann–de Lange) syndrome
Craniofacial dysostosis
Hemi-maxillofacial dysplasia
Lipodystrophies
    Berardinelli–Seip syndrome
    Donohue syndrome (Leprechaunism)
MELAS syndrome
Mucopolysaccharidoses
    Hunter syndrome
    Hurler syndrome
    Sanfilippo syndrome
Rubinstein–Taybi syndrome
Schinzel–Giedion syndrome (Albano 15122424)
Porphyrias (Ch. 19)
    Erythropoietic porphyria (Gunther disease)
    Familial porphyria cutanea tarda
    Hepatoerythropoietic porphyria
Stiff skin syndrome
Toxin exposure
    Fetal alcohol syndrome
    Fetal hydantoin syndrome
Winchester syndrome (Ch. 6)

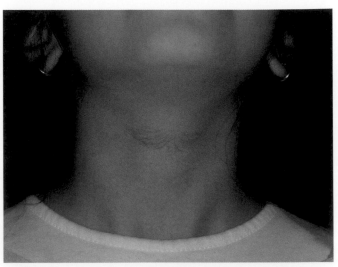

Figure 7.49 Anterior cervical hypertrichosis. A form of nevoid hypertrichosis, this patch of hair at the anterior aspect of the neck is usually not associated with other pathology.

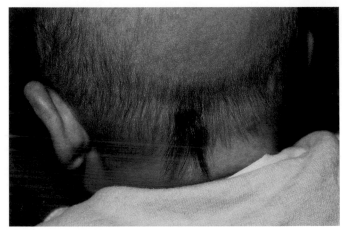

Figure 7.50 Nevoid circumscribed hypertrichosis. This hair follicle hamartoma shows congenital growth of thicker, darker, and longer hairs without associated hyperpigmentation or associated follicular prominence.

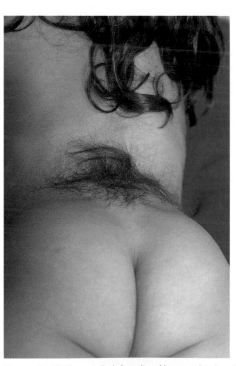

Figure 7.48 Faun-tail deformity. Abnormal tufts of hair in the lumbosacral area suggest an underlying tethered cord or diastematomyelia.

underlying kyphoscoliosis, duplication of a portion of the spinal cord (diastematomyelia), or tethered cord. Although neurologic signs of this disorder generally appear during early childhood, they may be delayed until the affected person's teenage or adult years. Early detection by imaging allows neurosurgical intervention and prevents the potential neurologic sequelae. Symmetrical localized hypertrichosis has also been described at the elbows (hypertrichosis cubiti)[321] and anterior cervical area (anterior cervical hypertrichosis) (Fig. 7.49). Both hypertrichosis cubiti and anterior cervical hypertrichosis are usually an isolated phenomenon. However, anterior cervical hypertrichosis has been described as an autosomal recessive disorder in association with developmental delay and peripheral neuropathy with or without retinal abnormalities,[322] and hypertrichosis cubiti with short stature, facial asymmetry, intrauterine growth retardation, developmental and speech delay, and infantile spasms.[323]

Hypertrichosis is frequently a characteristic of melanocytic nevi, smooth muscle hamartomas and Becker's nevus, plexiform neurofibromas, and linear epidermal nevus. Nevoid circumscribed hypertrichosis (Fig. 7.50), a hair follicle nevus, presents as an isolated patch of hypertrichosis. Increased local hair growth may be seen after wearing a cast, or at sites of thrombophlebitis, stasis dermatitis, X-ray or ultraviolet light irradiation, chemical irritation, or local hormonal stimulation. Extensive congenital smooth muscle hamartomas may show hypertrichotic and skin-colored to lightly hyperpigmented patches in association with excessive skin-folds and follicular dimpling (sometimes called Michelin baby syndrome).[324] Multiple patches of congenital hypertrichosis in association with blaschkoid streaks of hypopigmentation have spontaneously cleared shortly after birth.[325] Symmetrical large hypertrichotic indurated hyperpigmented patches on the middle and lower body first appear during the first or second decade in autosomal recessive *H* syndrome.[326] In addition to *h*yperpigmentation and *h*ypertrichosis, patients show *h*epatosplenomegaly, *h*eart anomalies, *h*earing loss, *h*ypogonadism, *h*allux valgus, low *h*eight, camptodactyly and occasionally *h*yperglycemia. Mutations have been found in the nucleoside transporter hENT3, encoded by SLC29A3.[327]

Idiopathic hirsutism

Idiopathic hirsutism describes the presence in girls of excessive body hair in a male sexual pattern (the face, particularly the upper lip, chest, abdomen, arms, and legs) in the absence of clinical evidence of disturbed endocrine or metabolic function (see Fig. 23.12). Idiopathic hirsutism is assumed to relate to increased stimulation of the hair follicles of genetically predisposed girls by normal levels of androgenic hormones. Hirsutism is quantified by the Ferriman–Gallwey scale, with scores of 6–8 considered mildly hirsute, 8–15 serious, and >15 overt hirsutism. Other signs of hyperandrogenism are acne, oligo- or amenorrhea, and androgenetic alopecia.

The incidence of hirsutism in any population is difficult to assess, since the range of normal is quite wide and subject to individual acceptance, and includes that which is not always socially acceptable in a particular culture. Hispanic, Jewish, and Welsh women in general have more hair than their counterparts of Northern European, Japanese, and Indian heritage. The physician should be cognizant of what is normal and acceptable to some individuals, yet unacceptable and a source of anguish to others. Performing a history and physical examination (including BMI and abdominal circumference) will determine the need for full endocrinologic investigation. When hirsutism is observed in a post-pubertal girl without other signs of masculinity (receding hairline, deepening of the voice, or evidence of menstrual disturbance), endocrine disease is unlikely. When the disorder does not appear to be physiologic and particularly if associated with other signs of androgen excess or premature puberty (sexual hair before 8 years of age in girls), abnormalities of the pituitary, adrenals, and ovaries must be ruled out. These include 'exaggerated adrenarche', late-onset congenital adrenal hyperplasia, virilizing tumors,[328,329] Cushing syndrome, hyperprolactinemia, acromegaly, Achard–Thiers (diabetes, hypertension, and hirsutism) syndrome, and polycystic ovary syndrome (PCOS) (see Ch. 8).[330,331] Of these, PCOS is by far the most common and is increasing in prevalence in parallel to the increasing trend towards obesity in teenagers (3% of unselected adolescents in one study).[332]

In addition to signs of hyperandrogenism,[333] the presence of oligo- or amenorrhea and acanthosis nigricans are a clue to PCOS.[334] Oligomenorrhea is defined as menstrual cycles of >35 days, with fewer than eight menstrual cycles defined as chronic anovulation. It is harder to diagnose oligomenorrhea in adolescents, but persistent irregularity more than 2 years after the onset of menses should be considered abnormal. Obesity is a significant risk factor for PCOS, and 40–60% of women with PCOS are overweight or obese, especially with abdominal adiposity.

If an endocrine abnormality is suspected, minimal laboratory testing for excessive androgen production should include levels of 17-ketosteroids (for mild adrenal hyperplasia), free plasma testosterone, dehydroepiandrosterone sulfate levels, and morning and evening cortisol; luteinizing hormone and follicle-stimulating hormone ratios and transabdominal ultrasound (to rule out small ovarian cysts) may be useful. Hormonal evaluations are best carried out in the morning during the third-fifth day of menstruation. If PCOS is suspected, fasting levels of glucose and insulin should be obtained.[335] A recently proposed definition of PCOS in adolescents includes four of the following criteria: (1) clinical hyperandrogenemia; (2) biochemical hyperandrogenemia (serum testosterone >50 ng/dL and LH:FSH ratio of >2; (3) insulin resistance and hyperinsulinemia (acanthosis nigricans, visceral adiposity, and impaired glucose tolerance); (4) oligomenorrhea persisting 2 years after menarche; and (5) polycystic ovarian morphology on ultrasound.[336]

Treatment of hypertrichosis and hirsutism

The appearance of excessive hair may be modified in several ways. Cutting with scissors or shaving with a razor or electric shaver, although occasionally not psychologically acceptable to the patient, are the simplest methods and least likely to irritate the skin. These techniques do not stimulate faster or thicker growth.[308] Bleaching with hydrogen peroxide may make excessive hair less conspicuous for up to 4 weeks, and works best for light-skinned children, because yellow bleached hair may be emphasized when viewed against darkly pigmented skin. Plucking or wax epilation (essentially a form of widespread plucking) by application of a warm wax preparation to the affected areas, are too painful for children, but may be an option for older adolescents. Chemical depilatories that contain sulfides or thioglycolates, or enzymatic depilatory agents destroy the projecting hair shafts, causing minimal damage to underlying skin. Of these, the sulfide-containing preparations are more effective, but more irritating, and produce a disagreeable hydrogen sulfide odor. The thioglycolate-containing agents are less irritating but slower in action and less effective on coarse hairs. Enzymatic agents are less offensive, but not as effective as other types. Children with extensive hypertrichosis must limit treatment with chemical depilatories to localized sites because of the risk of systemic absorption and toxic reactions.

Electrolysis and laser are more permanent hair removal techniques that have not been studied and are probably too uncomfortable for pre-pubertal children. In electrolysis, an electric current is delivered to the hair follicle, destroying it. Laser and intense pulsed light therapy remove unwanted hair through the selective photothermolysis of melanin-rich structures; light energy is absorbed in hair follicles with minimal absorption by surrounding tissues.[337,338] Long-pulse alexandrite and long-pulse Nd:YAG lasers have been used in lighter skin and darker skin children, respectively, for a variety of indications and with good tolerance.[339] Application of topical anesthesia may be required. Eflornithine cream 15% is prescription medication for twice-daily application that inhibits ornithine decarboxylase, a hair follicle enzyme that participates in hair growth. As a result eflornithine may decrease further growth, although it does not minimize existing hair. Local irritation may occur.

If an adolescent has hirsutism and hyperandrogenemia, therapy should be specific to the underlying trigger, under the guidance of a gynecologist or endocrinologist. For example, dexamethasone 0.25–0.5 mg at night generally reverses the hyperandrogenic signs of adrenal hyperplasia.[340] For PCOS in adolescents, the most important intervention is lifestyle modification with increasing exercise and controlling dietary intake. In PCOS, loss of at least 10% of initial body weight improves menstrual function and metabolic abnormalities.[341] The administration of metformin or other insulin sensitizers is adjunctive to lifestyle changes, but can improve insulin resistance, adiposity and serum androgen levels. Anti-androgens and oral contraceptives are the traditional treatment for management of hirsutism. The combination of ethinyl estradiol and drospirenone, for example, reduces the Ferriman–Gallwey score in adolescents by approximately 50% over a 12-month period.[342] Spironolactone in doses of 50–200 mg/day, cyproterone acetate, 50–100 mg/day (available in Europe), and cimetidine have anti-androgenic activity.

Pigmentary Changes of Hair

Premature graying

Graying of human hair is caused by a reduction in the activity of melanocytes within hair follicles. Premature graying of hair, termed *canities*, refers to a loss of color, especially of scalp hair, at an age earlier than that generally accepted as physiologic (before the age of 20 in Caucasians and 30 in African-Americans). It most commonly occurs in children with vitiligo or alopecia areata. Canities have also been described in children with pernicious anemia, hyperthyroidism and other thyroid disorders, progeria, Werner syndrome, ataxia-telangiectasia, Rothmund–Thomson syndrome, tuberous sclerosis, neurofibromatosis, and the Waardenburg and Vogt–Koyanagi syndromes. Premature graying may be readily masked, if desired, by chemical rinses and dyes. Chloroquine interferes with pheomelanin synthesis and may lead to lightening of hair with a silvery discoloration in blonde and red-haired persons.[343]

Green discoloration

The spontaneous appearance of green discoloration in the hair of light-haired individuals may occur as a result of exposure to copper used as an algae-retardant in swimming pools or household tap water containing excessive amounts of copper.[344] The introduction of fluoride into a town water supply may acidify water and cause copper to be leached from the plumbing system. Sometimes a ground wire connects a faulty electrical apparatus to the copper water pipes, thus diverting sufficient flow of electric current through the water system to dissolve copper.

If resulting from swimming, the use of a copper-based algicide should be discontinued. In cases related to household tap water, electrical grounding of household plumbing and adjustment of the pH of the tap water will help to prevent recurrences. Copper-induced discoloration of the hair can be treated in several ways: bleaching with 3% hydrogen peroxide for 2–3 h; washing with the chelating agent edetic acid (EDTA-Metalex) for 30 min; use of a penicillamine-containing shampoo; or application of 1.5% 1-hydroxyethyl diphosphonic acid.[151]

Nails

The nails are convex horny structures originating from a matrix that develops from a groove formed by epidermal invagination on the dorsum of the distal phalanges at 9 weeks' gestation. At 10 weeks' gestation, a smooth shiny quadrangular area can be recognized on the distal dorsal surface of each digit, and formation is completed by 20 weeks' gestation. The nail apparatus consists of a nail matrix of proliferating epidermal cells (Fig. 7.51), largely located under the proximal nail fold. In the thumbs and in a variable number of digits, a white crescent-shaped lunula is usually seen projecting from under the proximal nail folds, and represents the distal portion of the matrix. The cells of the lunula form the lower surface of the nail plate, whereas the more proximal matrix forms the exposed surface of the nail plate. Although the nail plate is translucent and essentially colorless, most of the exposed nail appears pink as the result of transmission of color from the adherent richly vascular

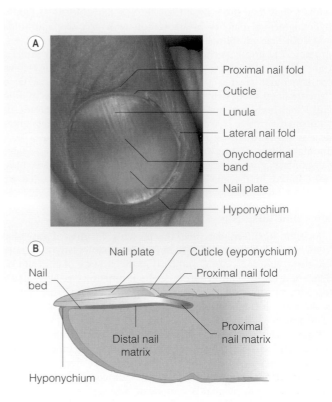

Figure 7.51 (A) Visible structures of the nail. (B) Anatomic structure of the nail apparatus.

underlying nail bed. The lateral borders of the nail plate lie under the edge of the lateral nail folds. The hyponychium is the area of skin where the distal border of the nail plate becomes detached from the nail bed.

Unlike hair, nails grow continuously throughout life and normally are not shed. Although the nails of individual fingers grow at different rates, the normal rate of growth of fingernails varies between 0.5 and 1.2 mm per week; the rate of toenail growth is slower than that of the fingernails. Nails grow more quickly in children than in adults. Many dermatoses that characteristically involve the skin and hair may also affect the nails. Among these are atopic dermatitis, psoriasis, lichen planus, Darier disease, alopecia areata, onychomycosis, dyskeratosis congenita and other ectodermal dysplasias, and certain forms of epidermolysis bullosa. Some nail deformities require surgical correction for cosmetic or functional improvement.[345]

Median Nail Dystrophy

Median nail dystrophy (dystrophia unguium mediana canaliformis) is an uncommon temporary nail disorder in which a split or canal-like dystrophy develops in one or more nails, usually those of the thumb. Often described as having an inverted fir tree or Christmas tree appearance, the condition shows feathery cracks extending laterally from the split toward the nail edge. A temporary defect in the matrix that interferes with nail formation is thought to be the cause. The split occurs at the cuticle, generally slightly off the midline, and proceeds outward as the nail grows. The disorder may at times improve spontaneously after a period of several years and, other than avoidance of trauma, there is no effective treatment. Median nail dystrophy has been described during administration of isotretinoin[346,347] and with habitual use of personal digital assistants.[348]

Habit-tic Dystrophy

Injuries to the base of the nail and nail matrix may result in longitudinal ridging or splitting of the nail (Fig. 7.52); a common form of nail injury. Habit-tic dystrophy is caused by continuous picking of the nail cuticle of the affected digit; it has recently also been described in association with guitar playing.[349] It is usually characterized by a depression toward the center of the nail plate with several irregularly spaced horizontal ridges extending across part of the nail (in contrast to the Christmas tree appearance of median nail dystrophy). The nail changes tend to clear when the habit is stopped.

Onychoschizia

Lamellar splitting of the nail plate at its distal free edge, or onychoschizia, is a common complaint of girls and women. The condition usually results from repeated trauma, frequent exposure to nail polish, or excessive immersion in water with detergents. The defect is aggravated by excessive manicuring and the frequent use of solvents to remove nail polish, which further dehydrates the nail. The regular use of a moisturizer or emollient hand cream to the nail and its cuticles, the avoidance of excessive manipulation, the use of several layers of nail polish in an effort to splint the nail, and avoidance of all but oily polish removers, is beneficial.

Nail Pitting

Pitting of the nails is a common problem of children, and most commonly is associated with the nail involvement of psoriasis,[350] atopic dermatitis, or alopecia areata. The punctate depressions result from alterations in the proximal matrix, and may vary from small to large and deep. One nail or several may be affected. Clustered pits may be seen in children from localized trauma, whereas shallow, randomly distributed pits are usually seen in children with psoriasis (see Fig. 4.14) or atopic dermatitis. Transverse rows of regularly spaced pits have been described in children with alopecia areata (Fig. 7.36). The pathomechanism for nail pits likely involves pinpoint areas of aberrant epidermis and inflammation of the nail matrix.

Nail Matrix Arrest (Beau's Lines and Onychomadesis)

Nail matrix arrest develops as a nonspecific reaction to any stress that temporarily interrupts nail formation and become visible on the surface of the nail plate several weeks or more after onset of the disease that caused the condition. Triggers range from coxsackie infection[351] to chemotherapy[352] to a prolonged intensive care stay.[353] Beau's lines are transverse grooves or furrows that originate under the proximal nail fold (Table 7.8). They first appear at the cuticle and move forward with the growth of the nail. Because normal nails grow at a rate of approximately 1 mm per week, the duration and time of the illness frequently can be estimated by the width of the furrow and its distance from the cuticle. Beau's lines have been described in infants at approximately 4 weeks of age, probably as a result of birth trauma; a normal nail has usually regrown by 4 months of age. Onychomadesis (proximal complete separation of the nail) results from full, but temporary, arrest of growth of the nail matrix (Fig. 7.53).[351] As with Beau's lines, onychomadesis has been described in patients with a wide variety of stressful events (Table 7.8), and the nail grows out normally.

Spoon Nail

Spoon nail (koilonychia) is a common deformity in which the normal contour of the nail is lost. The nail is thin, depressed, and concave from side-to-side, with turned-up distal and lateral edges. Koilonychia of the hallucal nails is common in newborns and young infants, and resolves spontaneously during childhood. The condition may be a secondary feature of several dermatological disorders. It occurs in association with nail thickening in psoriasis, onychomycosis, and pachyonychia congenita, in which subungual thickening from the hyponychium changes the direction of nail growth. Koilonychia can also be seen in disorders with nail thinning or ridging, as in lichen planus, trachyonychia, and focal dermal hypoplasia. Spoon nails have been described in individuals with severe iron deficiency anemia, although the pathomechanism is

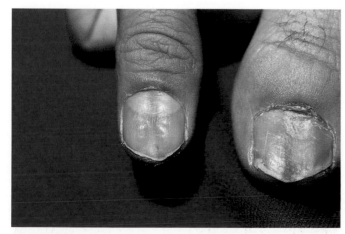

Figure 7.52 Habit-tic deformity. Central depression and irregularly spaced horizontal splits from continuous picking of the nail cuticle of the affected digit.

Table 7.8 Associations with nail matrix arrest		
Insult	**Beau's lines**	**Onychomadesis**
Acrodermatitis enteropathica	+	+
Amelogenesis imperfecta	–	+
Antibiotic usage	–	+
Chemotherapeutic agents	+	+
Coxsackie virus infection	+	+
Epidermolysis bullosa	–	+
Febrile illness	+	+
Hypoparathyroidism	+	+
Kawasaki disease	+	+
Periungual inflammation or trauma	+	+
Radiation therapy	–	+
Retinoid administration	–	+
Stevens–Johnson syndrome	+	+
Syphilis	+	+

Modified from Schachner and Hansen (2003).[182]

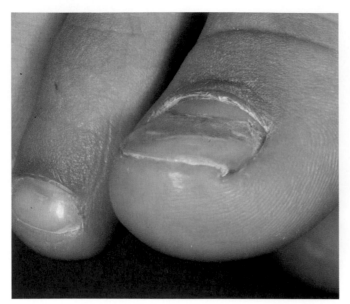

Figure 7.53 Onychomadesis. Nails showed this deep transverse groove and nail separation.

Table 7.9 Clubbing in children		
History	**System**	**Disease**
Acquired		
Generalized	Pulmonary	Cystic fibrosis
		Bronchiectasis
		Tuberculosis, aspergillosis
		Asthma complicated by lung infections
		Sarcoidosis
		Pulmonary fibrosis
		Tumors
	Cardiovascular	Cyanotic congenital heart disease
		Subacute bacterial endocarditis
		Myxomas
	Gastrointestinal	Inflammatory bowel disease
		Gardner's syndrome
		Parasitosis
		Cirrhosis
		Chronic active hepatitis
	Endocrine	Diamond's syndrome (myxedema, exophthalomos and clubbing)
		Hypervitaminosis A
		Malnutrition
Limited to one or more digits		Aortic/subclavian artery aneurism
		Brachial plexus injury
		Trauma
		Maffucci's syndrome
		Gout
		Sarcoidosis
		Severe herpetic whitlow
Hereditary		Pachydermoperiostosis
		Familial, isolated
Pseudoclubbing[a]		Apert's syndrome
		Pfeiffer's syndrome
		Rubinstein–Taybi syndrome

[a]Broad distal phalanges with normally shaped nails.
Reprinted with permission from Schachner and Hansen (2003)[182] (and adapted from Baran R, Dawber PR. Diseases of the nails and their management. London: Blackwell Scientific; 2001.

unclear. Koilonychia may also be inherited as an isolated autosomal dominant trait. Koilonychia can be confused with *platyonychia*, or flattened nails, which have been described primarily in patients with cirrhosis, and with *pincer nails*, characterized by excessive curvature at the lateral aspects of the nail plate, leading to an appearance of ingrown nails. Pincer nails are usually a congenital deformity, but can be acquired in individuals with epidermolysis bullosa, digital epidermoid cysts, and distal phalangeal exostosis. Because they can be quite painful, pincer nails are often corrected surgically.

Racket Nail

Racket nails or brachyonychia are short, wide nails that show loss of curvature. Most commonly found on the thumb and halluces, racket nails are associated with short, stubby phalanges, presumably reflecting an arrest in distal phalangeal formation. This disorder may be inherited in an autosomal dominant mode as an isolated entity, but has been described in association with several pediatric syndromes, such as acrodysostosis, acro-osteolysis, cartilage-hair hypoplasia syndrome, Larsen syndrome, pyknodysostosis, and Rubinstein–Taybi syndrome. Racket nails may be confused with nail *clubbing* or acropachy, which results from overgrowth of the fibrovascular support stroma of the distal phalanx. Increased flexibility of the distal nail plate due to edematous tissue is an early sign of clubbing. Also typical is the angle >180° (Lovibond's angle) formed by the proximal nail fold and nail plate when viewed from a lateral position. Clubbing in children is usually a sign of internal disease (Table 7.9).

Trachyonychia

Trachyonychia is characterized by excessive ridging, longitudinal grooves and striations, opalescent discoloration, a rough sandpaper-like quality of the nails, a tendency towards breakage and fragmentation (onychorrhexis), and splitting at the free margins[354] (Fig. 7.54). When all nails are involved, the condition has been called *twenty-nail dystrophy*. Trachyonychia has been described in association with lichen planus, psoriasis, atopic dermatitis, and alopecia areata, but the trachyonychia may occur months to years before other signs of mucocutaneous disease. The course of trachyonychia is variable, but spontaneous improvement may occur in months to years; in one study 50% showed total resolution or marked improvement in the first 6 years.[355] Application of potent topical corticosteroids to the base of the nail, particularly in the form of flurandrenolide tape, often reverses the changes of trachyonychia after several months of nightly usage. Filing the nails and application of clear nail polish may reduce the tendency toward snagging and tearing of the nail plates.

Onychogryphosis

Onychogryphosis is a hypertrophic nail deformity most commonly seen in the toenails. Some cases of nail hypertrophy are

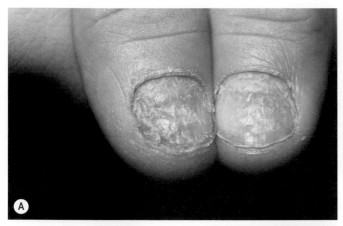

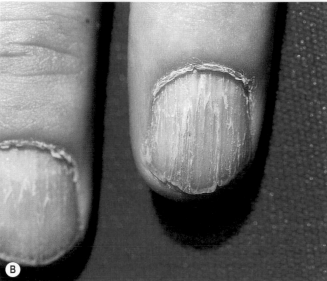

Figure 7.54 Twenty-nail dystrophy (trachyonychia). Opalescent discoloration, excessive ridging, longitudinal striations and a rough texture of all 20 nails in a school-age child (A) and in adolescent (B). Note the rough edges associated with the longitudinal striations in (B).

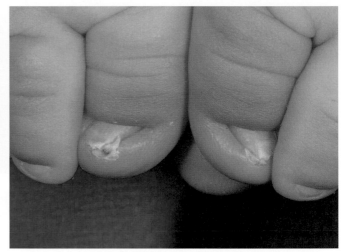

Figure 7.55 Congenital malalignment of the great toenails. Lateral rotation of the nail matrix leads to lateral deviation of the great toenail from the longitudinal axis of the distal phalanx and, at times, thickening, discoloration, and shortening of the nail plate. Note the secondary severely ingrown toenails and overgrowth of the lateral nailfold.

developmental. The nails become thick and circular in cross-section instead of flat (thus resembling a claw). The disorder is most commonly seen in elderly individuals, but may occur in children with poor hygiene. Management requires regular paring or trimming and, when severe, treatment by a podiatrist using files, nail clippers, or mechanical burrs. Onychogryphosis is frequently associated with secondary onychomycosis, but may be seen in a variety of forms of ichthyosis (Ch. 5) and in severe epidermolysis bullosa simplex (Ch. 13).

Congenital Malalignment of the Great Toenails

Congenital malalignment of the great toenails is a disorder in which lateral rotation of the nail matrix leads to lateral deviation of the great toenail from the longitudinal axis of the distal phalanx, and, at times, thickening, discoloration, and shortening of the nail plate (Fig. 7.55).[356] Resultant onychodystrophy may lead to onychogryphosis and chronic ingrown toenails. The disorder may be inherited as an autosomal dominant disorder,[357] and often improves spontaneously.[358] If improvement is not seen during the

first year and the deviation is severe, surgical realignment of the nail with local anesthesia can be performed, preferably before age 2 years.[345]

Ingrown Nails

Ingrown toenails are a common disorder in which the lateral edge of the nail is curved inward and penetrates the underlying tissue, with resulting erythema, edema, pain, and in chronic forms, the formation of granulation tissue. Generally seen on the great toes of affected individuals, the main cause of the deformity is compression of the toe from side-to-side by ill-fitting footwear and improper cutting of the nail (in a half-circle rather than straight across). Pseudo-ingrown toenails, also seen as a transient deformity in newborns, are a common phenomenon (2.4% of infants)[359] and are generally self-corrected by the time the child reaches the age of 12 months. Treatment, if required, consists of the wearing of properly fitting footwear, allowing the nail to grow out beyond the free edge, control of acute infection by compresses, topical and, at times, systemic antibiotics, and in many instances (once the infection has subsided) surgical treatment. In recurring cases, excision of the lateral aspect of the nail with the use of local anesthesia followed by curettage or chemical destruction of the nail matrix will prevent regrowth of the offending portion of the nail.[360]

Nail Atrophy

Atrophic nails range from complete absence of the nail (anonychia) to nails that are poorly or partially developed (micronychia). Anonychia can be associated with junctional epidermolysis bullosa, trauma, infectious paronychia, and inflammation (e.g., Stevens-Johnson syndrome, chronic graft-versus-host disease, and lichen planus). Micronychia has been described in patients with ectodermal dysplasias, teratogen exposure (e.g., fetal hydantoin syndrome), and chromosomal abnormalities (e.g., Turner syndrome, Noonan syndrome, and trisomies of chromosomes 3, 8, 13, and 18). Micronychia is a prominent feature of the nail-patella syndrome and COIF (congenital onychodysplasia of index fingers, see below).

Nail-Patella Syndrome

The nail-patella syndrome, also termed the *nail-patella-elbow syndrome or osteo-onychodysplasia*, is an autosomal dominant disorder characterized by the absence or hypoplasia of the patella and nails and dysplasia of the radial heads and iliac horns. Renal involvement occurs in 30–60% of patients, and presents with (often asymptomatic) proteinuria and/or microscopic hematuria, edema, and hypertension. Progression to nephrotic syndrome occurs in fewer than 20% of patients, and renal failure requiring dialysis or transplantation in 10%.[361] Complete remission of the nephritic syndrome was recently induced by the combination of enalapril and losartan.[362] Affected patients also risk the development of glaucoma.

Nail changes are seen in 98% of affected individuals. They vary from a triangular lunula, especially of the thumbs and index fingers, to severe dysplasia and micronychia to absence of the medial and distal aspects of the index and thumb nails. Occasionally nails of other fingers and sometimes the toes may also be affected. Softening, spooning, discoloration, central grooving, splitting and cracking, narrowing, and less commonly thickening of nails have been described. Nail involvement is symmetrical and often shows progression from index to fifth fingernails.

The disorder results from mutations in *LMX1B*, a transcription factor that regulates nail, bone, and glomerular basement membrane development, as well as continuing renal glomerular podocyte function.[363,364] Deletion of the LMX1B gene on one allele also causes disease, suggesting a role for haploinsufficiency.[365] A support group is available at: www.nailpatella.org.

Congenital Onychodysplasia of the Index Fingers (COIF)

COIF, also known as Iso and Kikuchi syndrome, is characterized by asymmetric, ulnar-deviated micronychia of the index fingers. Involvement may be unilateral of bilateral, and polyonychia may be associated. X-rays of the underlying phalangeal bone show a characteristic Y-shaped bifurcation or a sharp distal phalangeal tip. Deformities of other fingers are rarely present.[366] Usually a sporadic condition, autosomal dominant inheritance and occurrence in twins have been described.[367]

Pachyonychia Congenita

Pachyonychia congenita (PC) is an autosomal dominant group of disorders characterized by dyskeratosis of the fingernails and toenails.[368–373] The historical designations of type 1 (Jadassohn–Lewandowsky) and tpe 2 (Jackson–Lawler) have been abandoned. PC results from mutations in one of four genes, *KRT6a, KRT6b, KRT16*, and *KRT17*, leading to a new designation based on genotyping of PC-6a, PC-6b, PC-16, and PC-17. The Pachyonychia Congenita Project provides genotyping at no cost through its registry (www.pachyonychia.org)..

The nail changes often begin during the first year of life, but may have their onset as late as teenage years.[369] Nails show progressive discoloration, tenting, and thickening, particularly owing to accumulation of a horny, yellowish brown material of the undersurface that causes the nail to project upward from the nail bed at the free margin (Figs 7.56–7.58). Paronychial inflammation and recurrent loss or shedding of nails are common

Progressive painful focal hyperkeratosis of the soles is seen in almost all cases by childhood, with palmar thickening in 60%. Bullae may occur on the toes, heels, sides of the feet, and

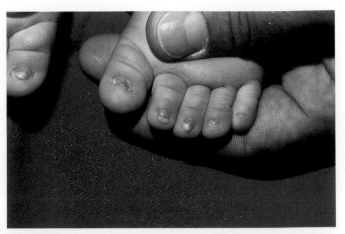

Figure 7.56 Pachyonychia congenita. The nails may be thickened or discolored at birth, but often show changes first on the toenails and during infancy.

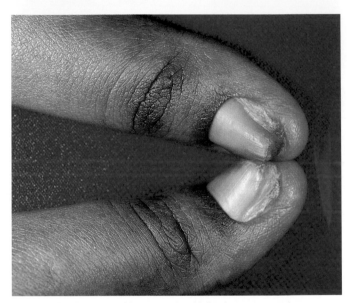

Figure 7.57 Pachyonychia congenita. Nails show progressive discoloration, tenting, and thickening, particularly owing to accumulation of a horny, yellowish brown material of the undersurface that causes the nail to project upward from the nail bed at the free margin. Although unusual, this adolescent's nail changes began during teenage years.

occasionally palms, particularly during warm weather. Hyperhidrosis of the palms and soles may be associated. Pinhead-sized follicular papules may appear in areas of trauma on the extensor surfaces of the extremities, popliteal fossae, lumbar region, buttocks, and, less commonly, on the face and scalp. Early oral lesions are frequently present in the form of opaque white plaques (leukokeratosis) on the dorsum of the tongue or the buccal mucosa at the interdental line, and are often confused with through. Less frequently associated findings include cheilitis, scrotal tongue, corneal dystrophy, and hoarseness, the latter specific for PC-6a.

Steatocysts and pilosebaceous cysts, formerly thought to be specific to PC-6b and PC-17, are now known to be common in PC-6a as well. These cysts usually first manifest at early puberty, particularly on the head, neck, upper chest, and upper arms. Hair defects are not seen in autosomal dominant PC and, in fact, an alternative diagnosis of Clouston ectodermal dysplasia due to connexin 30 mutations should be considered if alopecia is present, as well as PC-like changes and palmoplantar keratoderma. More recently, mutations in keratin K6c have been asociated with focal palmoplantar keratoderma with minor or no nail changes.[374]

The subungual hyperkeratosis persists for life, and treatment is directed towards relief of the painful hyperkeratosis of the soles and nails.[375] Filing and trimming of the nails with professional nail clippers is most commonly performed. Topical keratolytics under occlusion, such as 20% urea in an emollient cream, 60% propylene glycol in water, 6% salicylic acid in a gel containing propylene glycol, or 10% salicylic acid, or 40% urea in petrolatum, can be applied overnight to decrease the thickened skin or nail. Administration of systemic retinoids has been successful for some, but not all, patients, but is rarely appropriate in pediatric patients. As a last resort, surgical avulsion and matrix destruction followed by scarification of the nail bed to prevent regrowth can be performed. Plantar sweating has been shown to increase the painful blistering of at hyperkeratotic sites and can be controlled by oral administration of glycopyrrolate or injections of botulinum toxin.[376] Oral rapamycin decreased painful plantar thromboses and keratoses in patients with K6a mutations (based on suppression of K6a expression), but led to unacceptable gastrointestinal and mucocutaneous adverse events.[377] K16 siRNA injections into the palmoplantar keratoderma have resulted in clearance, but are too painful to sustain.[378]

Dyskeratosis Congenita

Dyskeratosis congenita is characterized in 80–90% of patients by the triad of nail dystrophy, reticular pigmentation and oral leukoplakia, but many additional features have been described (Table 7.10).[379,380] Most cases have been in males, consistent with an X-linked disorder, but carrier females may show mild to complete clinical features. The disorder may also be inherited as autosomal dominant or recessive, and six mutated genes have been described to date, accounting for 50% of studied individuals with dyskeratosis congenita (see Table 7.11, online only).[379,381,382] The median age of diagnosis is 15 years, as many patients first present as teens or young

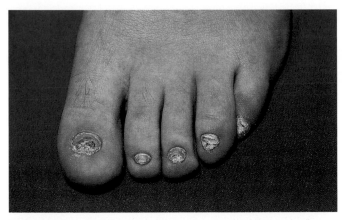

Figure 7.58 Pachyonychia congenita. The nails may be markedly shortened and fragile, but show the tenting and subungual thickening.

Table 7.10 Complications of dyskeratosis congenita and suggested monitoring

System	Findings	Potential complications	Monitoring/treatment
Skin	Nail dystrophy Reticulated pigmentation Hyperhidrosis Early hair graying Palmoplantar keratoderma Absent dermatoglyphics	Cutaneus SCCs	Annual skin examination Sun protection
Oral	Leukoplakia Erythematous patches Dyspigmentation Taurodontism	Oral cancer	Biannual dental examinations
Growth and development	Short stature Developmental delay		
Head and neck		SCC	Annual otolaryngology examinations
Eyes	Epiphora Ectropion, entropion Trichiasis, sparse lashes	Corneal abrasion Infections	Annual eye examinations
Gastrointestinal	Esophageal stenosis Hepatic fibrosis	Dysphagia	Esophageal dilatation Annual liver function tests Liver ultrasounds
Genitourinary	Urethral stenosis Epithelial malignancy		
Lungs	Pulmonary fibrosis	High risk with transplant	Annual PFTs
Bones	Osteoporosis Avascular necrosis hips, shoulder	Fractures	Ca++, Vitamin D$_3$
Hematologic	Low blood counts	Bone marrow failure Myelodysplastic syndrome Leukemia	Biannual blood counts Baseline bone marrow Chemotherapy as appropriate

SCC, squamous cell carcinoma; PFT, pulmonary function test; Ca++, calcium.

adults. Overall, approximately 90% of patients develop life-threatening bone marrow failure, characterized by severe aplastic anemia with neutropenia, splenomegaly, and a hemorrhagic diathesis. Pulmonary fibrosis and hepatic cirrhosis are other life-threatening complications. Epithelial tumors often first develop by the mid-teens, frequently in areas of mucosa with leukoplakia. Squamous cell carcinoma of the tongue is most common, but cutaneous SCC, acute myeloid leukemia and myelodysplastic syndrome are not uncommon.

The thin, dystrophic nails usually appear first, between the ages of 5 and 13 years. Mildly affected nails show ridging and longitudinal grooving; severely affected nails are shortened and show pterygium formation (Fig. 7.59). Cutaneous changes usually develop after the onset of nail changes, most commonly during late childhood to teenage years. A fine reticulated grayish-brown hyperpigmentation, sometimes surrounding hypopigmented, atrophic, telangiectatic patches, on the face, neck, shoulders, upper back, and thighs is characteristic (Fig. 7.60). Other cutaneous changes may include telangiectasia of the trunk; redness and atrophy of the face with irregular macular hyperpigmentation; acrocyanosis; palmoplantar hyperkeratosis; hyperhidrosis and bullae of the palms and soles; wrinkled atrophic skin over the elbows, knees, and penis; and a diffuse atrophic, transparent, and shiny appearance on the dorsal

aspects of the hands and feet. The hair of the scalp, eyebrows, and eyelashes is often sparse and lusterless, and patients with this disorder frequently have atrophic changes of the muscles and bones of the feet and hands, giving a 'cupped' appearance to the palms.

Mucous membrane changes consist of leukoplakia, and rarely blisters and erosions, of the oral (Fig. 7.61) and anal mucosae, esophagus, and urethra. Similar changes of the tarsal conjunctiva may result in atresia of the lacrimal ducts, excessive lacrimation, chronic blepharitis, conjunctivitis, and ectropion. The teeth tend to be defective and subject to early decay. Periodontitis may develop, and affected persons have an increased incidence of cutaneous malignancy, predominantly squamous cell carcinoma in the areas of leukoplakia.

Recommended disease surveillance includes biannual blood counts, bone marrow evaluations annually, hepatic ultrasounds, annual pulmonary functional tests and skin cancer screening. Treatment of bone marrow failure is recommended with a hemoglobin persistently below 8 g/dL, platelets <30 000/mm^3, and neutrophils <1000/mm^3. If a matched donor without genetic and clinical evidence of dyskeratosis congenita is available, stem cell transplant should be considered, but carries substantial risk, including an increased risk of pulmonary fibrosis with graft-versus-host disease. Long-term survival after transplantation has been poor. A trial of androgens, such as oxymetholone, may be considered before transplantation from an unrelated donor, and improved blood counts in 60% of treated patients;[381] however, androgens may cause hepatic tumors, and the combination of androgen and G-CSF has led to splenic rupture. Management of patients otherwise consists of bougienage for esophageal stenosis; fulguration, curettage, and surgical excision of leukokeratosis of the buccal and anal mucosae; and lifelong, regular supervision for early detection of mucosal or cutaneous carcinomas.

Disorders of the Nail Bed

Onycholysis refers to separation of the nail plate from the underlying hyponychium, and can occur for a wide variety of reasons (Table 7.12).[383,384] Vigorous cleaning of the subungual debris that tends to accumulate exacerbates this condition. Onycholysis may result from exposure to sunlight (photo-onycholysis)[385] in individuals administered tetracyclines, especially doxycycline (see Fig. 8.16), or thiazides.

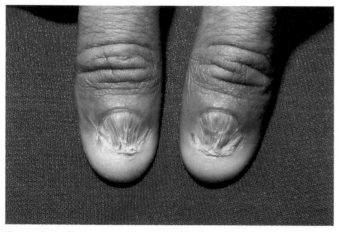

Figure 7.59 Dyskeratosis congenita. Shortened nails with pterygium formation.

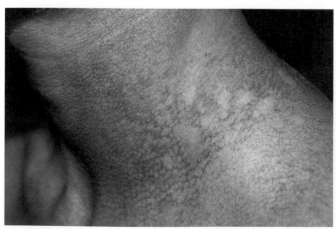

Figure 7.60 Dyskeratosis congenita. Reticulated hyperpigmentation surrounding hypopigmented, atrophic, telangiectatic patches.

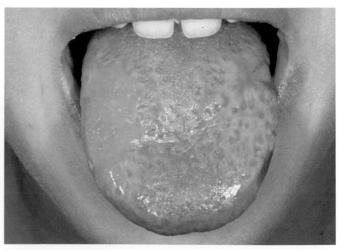

Figure 7.61 Dyskeratosis congenita. Leukoplakia of the oral mucosa.

Table 7.12 Underlying causes of onycholysis
Chemical irritants
Cosmetics, especially with formaldehyde
Depilatories
Detergents
Nail polish removers
Organic solvents
Inflammatory disorders
Alopecia areata
Atopic dermatitis
Contact dermatitis
Lichen planus
Psoriasis
Infectious disorders
Bacterial paronychia
Candidiasis
Herpes simplex (whitlow)
Onychomycosis
Verrucae
Medications
Anticonvulsants (valproic acid)
Chemotherapeutic agents (esp. taxanes)
Retinoids (isotretinoin)
Tetracyclines (photo-onycholysis)
Thiazides (photo-onycholysis)
Systemic disorders
Iron deficiency anemia
Rheumatic disease
Thyroid disease (hyper- or hypo-)
Trauma
Compulsive subungual cleaning
Sportsman's toe

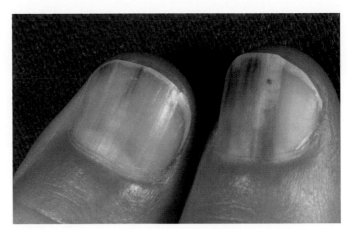

Figure 7.62 Darier disease. Longitudinal reddish-purple and white streaks of the nail.

Abnormalities of the nail bed may be seen through the transparent nail plate. Onycholysis that occurs proximal to the hyponychium may resemble a yellow-brown 'oil spot,' a nail change that is considered pathognomonic of psoriasis, but is rarely seen in children. Notching of the distal nail plate may be seen in Darier disease, in association with longitudinal red and white streaks (Fig. 7.62) (see Ch. 5). Nail bed hemorrhages are usually due to trauma. As the hemorrhage ages, it changes color from red to purple to brown, and moves more distally. Larger hematomas may resemble melanocytic nevi, although more commonly melanocytic nevi of the nail bed manifest as longitudinal pigmented streaks of the nail.

Paronychia

Paronychia refers to inflammation surrounding the nail resulting from infection.[386] At times, the cuticle is obscured, and the nail fold is replaced by granulation tissue. Acute paronychia, characterized by painful, erythematous, indurated swelling of the proximal or lateral nail folds, often with purulent draining, is usually caused by *Staphylococcus aureus* infection; bacterial cultures can be performed to consider a bacterial etiology (see Ch. 14). Chronic paronychia with nail dystrophy, presenting with non-purulent erythema of the periungual areas, nail ridging and cuticle loss, is more commonly owing to candidal infection. Candidal paronychia is often associated with repeated exposure of the fingers to wetness (see Fig. 17.34). Toddlers who suck their fingers or thumb usually have candidal paronychia, but a more acute process with purulence and crusting overlying the erythema and swelling may also reflect a

herpetic whitlow of the finger or toe. Infants with sucking blisters show blisters filled with clear fluid. Potassium hydroxide scrapings to detect the pseudohyphae of *Candida albicans* (Ch. 17) and direct fluorescence assays and cultures to consider *herpes simplex* infection (Ch. 15) should be performed to distinguish these disorders. Treatment of paronychia should be directed toward clearance of the infecting organism. In individuals beyond the age of infancy, efforts to keep the fingers dry, including avoidance of sucking and wet work, are critical for clearance. Periungual inflammation may also be seen in children with psoriasis and acropustulosis (Ch. 4) and rarely with tinea unguium (Ch. 17). Paronychia can result from exposure to medications, particularly from isotretinoin[384] and indinavir,[387] and nail cosmetics.[388]

Disorders of Nail Coloration

Abnormal nail pigmentation may be seen in systemic diseases[389] or in association with the ingestion of various chemicals or medications. Brown pigmentation of nails may be associated with the ingestion of phenolphthalein, as a reaction to antimalarials, minocycline, or gold therapy, or as a manifestation of Addison's disease. In argyria the lunulae show a distinctive slate blue discoloration, and in hepatolenticular degeneration (Wilson's disease) the lunulae may present an azure blue discoloration. Blue discoloration of the nails has also been described from administration of azidothymidine (AZT).[384] Lithium carbonate can cause brownish black transverse bands at the margins of the lunulae, and pigmentation in the form of transverse bands has been reported in patients receiving zidovudine, bleomycin, and doxorubicin. Gray or blue-gray nails can occur in individuals with ochronosis or argyria or as a reaction to quinacrine or phenolphthalein. Brown-black pigmentation of the nail fold and nail matrix can be seen as a sign of melanoma of the nail bed (Hutchinson's sign), Addison's disease, Peutz–Jeghers syndrome, and Laugier–Hunziker syndrome. Most commonly, however, a longitudinal streak of brown pigmentation of the nail ('melanonychia striata') and even including the nail bed represents a benign melanocytic nevus (see Ch. 9). When a green discoloration is seen in association with onycholysis, *Pseudomonas aeruginosa* infection must be considered.

Red lunulae can be seen in patients with alopecia areata, lupus erythematosus, dermatomyositis, congestive heart failure, reticulosarcoma, psoriasis, carbon monoxide poisoning, and lymphogranuloma venereum. When the distal 1–2 mm portion of the nail has a normal pink color and the rest of the nail has a white appearance, the disorder has been termed *Terry's nails* (Fig. 7.63).

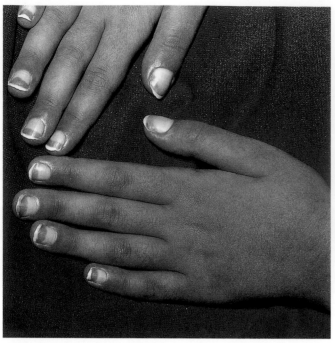

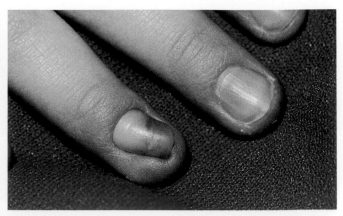

Figure 7.64 Yellow nail syndrome. Yellowish discoloration of the nails is associated with slow growth, thickening, excessive curvature, and an absence of lunulae in some of the nails of this 6-year-old boy who had congenital chylothorax. The toenails were almost all still affected.

Figure 7.63 Terry's nails. The distal 1–2 mm portion of the nail has a normal pink color and the rest of the nail has a white appearance. This girl had hepatic cirrhosis.

Seen in patients with cirrhosis, chronic congestive heart failure, adult-onset diabetes, and POEMS syndrome, Terry's nails may also be seen in normal children younger than 4 years of age, in the very elderly, and at times in normal individuals without evidence of cirrhosis or other systemic disease.

The term *leukonychia* (white nails) is used to describe a disorder in which at least a portion of the nail becomes white. The white color may be seen as punctate, striate (leukonychia striata, usually due to local manipulation), or superficial onychomycosis; as paired narrow white bands (seen in patients with cirrhosis and hypoalbuminemia); as transverse 1–2 mm white bands (Mees' bands), described in arsenic or heavy metal poisoning, septicemia, dissecting aortic aneurysm, and renal failure; as white transverse bands in the nail bed occurring in pairs (Muehrcke's nails) as a sign of hypoalbuminemia; or as the half-and-half nail, a disorder characteristic of renal disease and azotemia in which the proximal nail bed is white and the distal half is red, pink, or brown.

The yellow nail syndrome is a disorder associated with severe long-term lymphedema and, most commonly, respiratory disease, especially chronic bronchitis, bronchiectasis, interstitial pneumonitis, and pleural effusion. Other associations include persistent hypoalbuminemia, thyroid disease, immunologic deficiencies (IgA), lympho-reticular malignancy, rheumatoid arthritis, lupus erythematosus, Hodgkin disease, and the nephrotic syndrome. Most often a phenomenon of middle-aged individuals, but also described

in neonates and young children, the nails show a pale yellow or greenish-yellow to brown discoloration of the nails (Fig. 7.64) associated with slow growth, thickening, and excessive curvature from side to side (on its long axis), increased hardness, onycholysis, or spontaneous shedding of the nails; absence of lunulae; and swelling of the periungual tissues, as might be seen in patients with chronic paronychia. The nail changes are often permanent, but administration of oral and topical vitamin E have been reported to be effective in some individuals.[390,391]

Key References

 The complete list of 391 references for this chapter is available online at **www.expertconsult.com.**
See inside cover for registration details.

Berk DR, Bayliss SJ. Milia: a review and classification. *J Am Acad Dermatol.* 2008;59:1050–1063.

Cantatore-Francis JL, Orlow SJ. Practical guidelines for evaluation of loose anagen hair syndrome. *Arch Dermatol.* 2009;145:1123–1128.

Cheng AS, Bayliss SJ. The genetics of hair shaft disorders. *J Am Acad Dermatol.* 2008;59:1–22.

Faghri S, Tamura D, Kraemer KH, et al. Trichothiodystrophy: a systematic review of 112 published cases characterises a wide spectrum of clinical manifestations. *J Med Genet.* 2008;45:609–621.

Kim BJ, Kim JY, Eun HC, et al. Androgenetic alopecia in adolescents: a report of 43 cases. *J Dermatol.* 2006;33:696–699.

Priolo M. Ectodermal dysplasias: an overview and update of clinical and molecular-functional mechanisms. *Am J Med Genet A.* 2009; 149A:2003–2013.

Savage SA, Alter BP. Dyskeratosis congenita. *Hematol Oncol Clin North Am.* 2009;23:215–231.

Schweizer J, Langbein L, Rogers MA, et al. Hair follicle-specific keratins and their diseases. *Exp Cell Res.* 2007;313:2010–2020.

Wallace MP, de Berker DA. Hair diagnoses and signs: the use of dermatoscopy. *Clin Exp Dermatol.* 2010;35:41–46.

Disorders of the Sebaceous and Sweat Glands

8

Disorders of the sebaceous glands

Acne Vulgaris

Acne vulgaris is the most common skin problem in the USA, affecting nearly 80–85% of individuals at some point between 11 and 30 years of age.[1,2] Although not a serious disease, acne may be the source of permanent scarring and, even more important, psychosocial morbidity and decreased emotional wellbeing. Withdrawal from society, depression, and decreased self-esteem may occur in individuals with more significant disease. In one study, acne severity was directly correlated with extent of embarrassment and lack of enjoyment of/participation in social activities.[3] Patients with even mild to moderate acne have demonstrated high scores on the Carroll Rating Scale for Depression, and an increased prevalence of suicidal ideation.[4] In addition, patients with severe acne may have poorer academic performance[5] and higher unemployment rates.[6] Issues such as these highlight that the potential benefits of acne therapy extend far beyond the simple cosmetics of the disease.

Acne vulgaris is seen routinely by primary care physicians, and so familiarity with the treatment of this condition is vital. The majority of acne patients with mild to moderate disease respond well to traditional therapies; patients with severe or recalcitrant disease may merit treatment with agents most appropriately prescribed by dermatologists. Although the underlying cause of acne vulgaris remains unknown, considerable data concerning its pathogenesis have accumulated in recent decades to allow a rational and therapeutically successful approach to its management. There is no single 'Gold Standard' therapy for acne, and treatment regimens must be individualized and occasionally 'fine-tuned' in order to achieve the optimal response.

The tendency to develop acne is often familial, and is felt by some to be inherited as an autosomal dominant trait. However, because of the high prevalence, the genetics of the disease remain unclear. Adolescent acne usually begins around the time of onset of puberty, occurring earlier in girls (12–13 years) than boys (14–15 years). However, the onset of acne may occur significantly earlier, and it may be the first sign of pubertal maturation in girls, correlating with increasing levels of dehydroepiandrosterone sulfate, an adrenal androgen.[7] Natural history studies show that in 80% of patients, the incidence and severity of acne decline by the early 20s, although as many as 50% of adults older than 25 years are affected and a minority may have persistence into middle-age.[8,9]

An understanding of acne pathogenesis helps the practitioner to conceptualize and formulate the therapeutic plan. Four interrelated processes, including hyper-keratinization, androgen stimulation, bacterial infection, and inflammation, are involved in this multifactorial disease. A pictorial representation of acne pathogenesis is shown in Figure 8.1.[10] Individual acne lesions usually begin with obstruction of the pilosebaceous unit (composed of the hair follicle and the sebaceous gland). These units are localized primarily to the face and trunk, and these 'follicular plugs' (or *microcomedones*) are caused by excessive numbers of desquamated epithelial cells from the wall of the follicle, in combination with excessive amounts of sebum, the oily, lipid-rich substance produced by the sebaceous glands. Sebum production is stimulated by adrenal and gonadal androgens, and rises to maximum levels during late adolescence. These microcomedones enlarge into *comedones*, which may be open (blackheads) or closed (whiteheads). The reason for the black appearance of open comedones is unclear; one hypothesis suggests compaction and oxidation of the keratinous material at the follicular opening results in this finding. Melanin pigment may also play a role.[11,12]

Propagation of acne lesions occurs when *Propionibacterium acnes*, a resident anaerobic organism, proliferates in this environment of sebum and follicular cells, with the production of chemotactic factors and proinflammatory mediators, which contribute to inflammation.[13] Hypersensitivity to this organism may also play a part in the more severe forms of acne.[14] The clinical counterpart to these infectious and inflammatory events are *papules* and *pustules*. With continued inflammation and macrophage recruitment, larger lesions (*cysts* and *nodules*) may result. Finally, sequelae of active acne lesions include *dyspigmentation* (usually hyperpigmentation or, occasionally, hypopigmentation) and *scarring*. Table 8.1 summarizes the various types of acne lesions.

In addition to the established pathogenic factors discussed previously, there may be other triggers or exacerbating conditions that contribute to acne vulgaris. These other factors are less well understood and, in some cases, controversial. Stress appears to be a common trigger for acne, possibly via increased activation of the hypothalamic–pituitary–adrenal axis and the resultant increase in androgen production. Acute worsening of acne has been documented in college students during examination periods, and correlated with an increased perceived stress score.[15] Mechanical factors, such as skin occlusion from sportsgear (i.e., helmets, chin straps, shoulder pads, etc.), may exacerbate the condition. Topically applied preparations, especially pomades and greasy ointments, to hair or skin may contribute to physical obstruction of the pilosebaceous unit and worsen the disease. Several medications may worsen acne, including anabolic steroids, progestins, lithium, isoniazid, hydantoin, and gold.[16] Pathologic androgen excess is often associated with acne (see below), and although endocrinologic evaluation is not indicated for the majority of patients, it should be considered in patients who have additional signs as listed in Table 8.2.[17]

The role of diet in the pathogenesis of acne vulgaris remains controversial, and controlled studies have refuted the value of dietary restrictions. For many years the elimination of various foods such as chocolate, soft drinks, milk, ice cream, fatty foods, shellfish, and iodides was recommended. The misconception that iodine is injurious to patients with acne vulgaris originated with the concept that iodides administered orally as a medication occasionally initiate a papulopustular acneiform eruption. The concept that chocolate exerts an adverse effect on acne has been challenged, and in

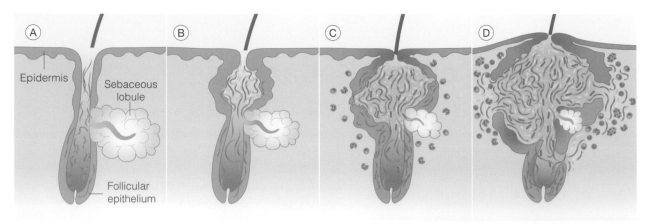

Figure 8.1 Acne pathogenesis. (A) Early comedone, with mild follicular plugging. (B) Later comedone. (C) Inflammatory papule/pustule. (D) Nodule/cyst. (Reprinted with permission from Bolognia et al. 2003.[10])

Table 8.1 Types of acne lesions
Active lesions (increasing severity)
Microcomedone
Open comedone (blackhead)
Closed comedone (whitehead)
Papule
Pustule
Cyst
Nodule
Sequelae
Dyspigmentation (usually hyperpigmentation)
Scarring (sometimes keloidal)

Table 8.2 Potential signs of androgen excess in acne patients
Young children
Body odor
Axillary hair
Pubic hair
Clitoromegaly
Adult women
Recalcitrant/late-onset acne
Menstrual irregularity
Hirsutism
Male- or female-pattern alopecia
Infertility
Acanthosis nigricans
Truncal obesity

Adapted from Strauss et al. (2007).[17]

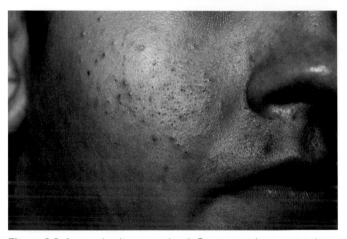

Figure 8.2 Acne vulgaris – comedonal. Open comedones present as 'blackheads'.

one controlled double-blind study, it was found that it failed to affect either the course of the disease or the production and composition of sebum.[18] However, the possibility that diet plays a role in the pathogenesis or exacerbation of acne remains unclear. An interesting review of two non-Westernized populations (one in Papua New Guinea and the other in Paraguay) revealed an astonishing difference in acne prevalence in comparison to individuals in Westernized societies.[19] One potential explanation asserted for these differences is the diets of these populations, which are composed mainly of minimally processed plant and animal foods and are nearly devoid of the carbohydrates typical in Western diets, which

may result in high insulin levels. Hyperinsulinemia, in turn, may promote the development of acne by its ability to increase androgen production.[19] It remains unclear, however, whether adhering to a diet with a low glycemic load can effect a change in acne.[20–22] Recently, the association between milk consumption and development of acne has been explored, with some studies suggesting a positive association, possibly related to a combination of exogenous hormones and growth factors, and stimulation of endogenous hormones.[23–25]

Acne presents with a combination of the various lesion types previously discussed: comedones, papules, pustules, cysts, nodules, scarring, and dyspigmentation. The earliest lesion type is usually the comedone, and mild acne may be limited to these lesions (Figs 8.2, 8.3). With increasing severity, patients develop inflammatory lesions, including papules and pustules (Figs 8.4, 8.5). Nodules and cysts may be present in patients with moderate to severe disease (Figs 8.6, 8.7) and may result in permanent acne scarring (Figs 8.8, 8.9). Dyspigmentation is a common sequela, especially in patients with darker complexions (Figs 8.10, 8.11). The primary sites for acne lesions correlate with the areas most concentrated with sebaceous glands: the face, chest, back, and shoulders. In patients with regressing acne lesions, macular erythema (Fig. 8.12) and hyperpigmentation are frequently seen. Although patients commonly regard these as active lesions and 'scars,' they usually imply effectiveness of the therapy, and their temporary nature should be explained to the

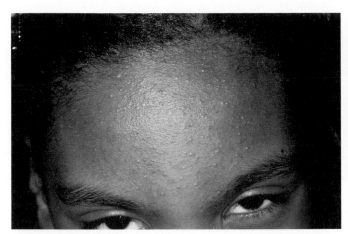

Figure 8.3 Acne vulgaris – comedonal. Closed comedones present as 'whiteheads'.

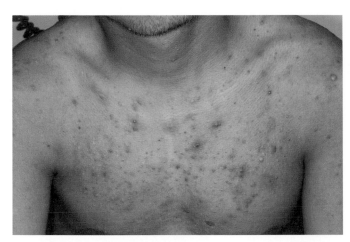

Figure 8.4 Acne vulgaris – inflammatory. Note the erythematous papules and pustules, as well as open and closed comedones.

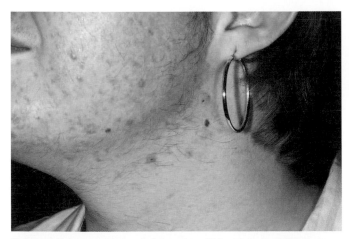

Figure 8.5 Acne vulgaris – inflammatory. This adolescent female has inflammatory papules and papulopustules, and hirsutism.

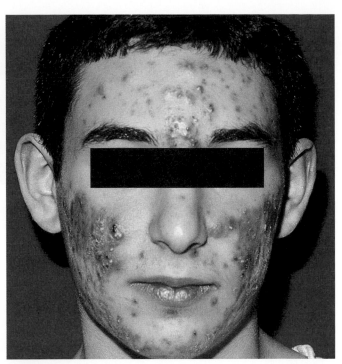

Figure 8.6 Acne vulgaris – nodulocystic.

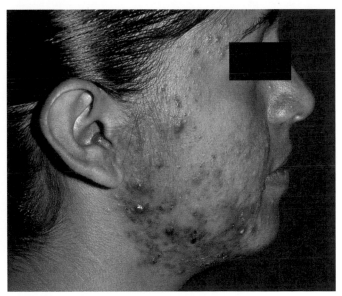

Figure 8.7 Acne vulgaris – nodulocystic.

patient. The scarring that occurs in patients with the more severe papulopustular and nodulocystic forms of acne develops because of fibrous contraction following the inflammatory phase. In addition to sharply punched-out pits and craters, hypertrophic or keloidal scars may also develop. The severity of the scarring depends on the depth and degree of the inflammation and on the patient's individual susceptibility.

Acne fulminans is a rare and severe form of acne vulgaris, occurring almost exclusively in young males. Patients present with an acute onset of painful, nodular, and occasionally ulcerative acne lesions concentrated on the chest (Fig. 8.13), shoulders, back, and face. Fever, leukocytosis, and musculoskeletal pain may also be present, and the skin lesions usually result in permanent scarring. Osteolytic bone lesions may be present, especially in the clavicle, sternum, and long bones.[26] Systemic corticosteroids are the mainstay of therapy, with the addition of isotretinoin after the acute inflammatory stage has subsided.

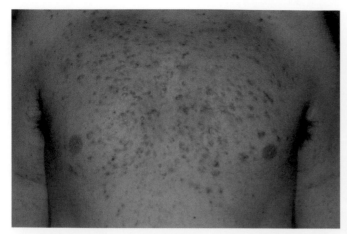

Figure 8.8 Acne scarring. This patient has severe nodular acne vulgaris with scarring involving the trunk.

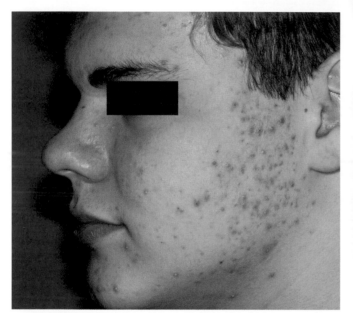

Figure 8.9 Acne scarring.

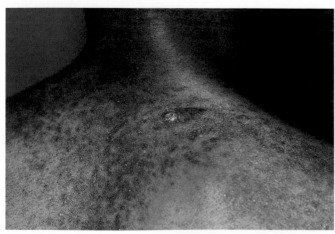

Figure 8.10 Acne-induced dyspigmentation.

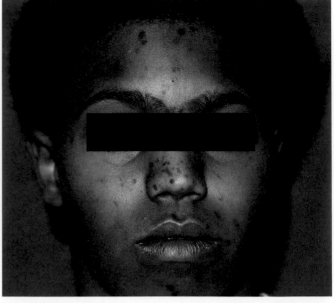

Figure 8.11 Acne-induced dyspigmentation. Note the 'T-zone' distribution corresponding to prior acne lesions.

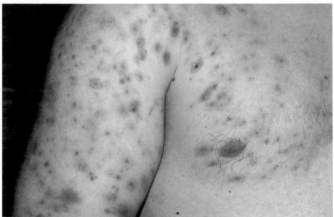

Figure 8.12 Residual post-acne erythema. Note erythematous macules at sites of prior lesions.

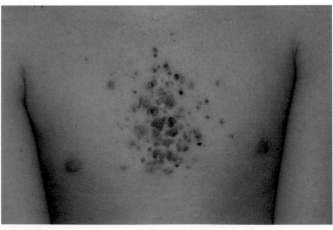

Figure 8.13 Acne fulminans. This patient developed acute worsening of his acne lesions upon starting isotretinoin therapy, and required systemic corticosteroids.

Acne therapy

Before any attempt is made to treat acne, patient education is vital. Important considerations include explaining the nature and natural history of acne vulgaris; dispelling acne myths regarding causes and treatments; highlighting the need for compliance with therapy and appropriate follow-up with the physician; reviewing the correct usage of medications and the potential side-effects; and emphasizing the expected *gradual* improvement in symptoms with therapy. Patient educational materials are very useful to this end and will help to increase compliance with treatment. Such materials can be created and personalized by the physician, or purchased from national organizations such as the American Academy of Dermatology (www.aad.org) or the American Academy of Pediatrics (www.aap.org).

Acne treatment in the past was hindered by mythical concepts regarding its causes, a more limited armamentarium of treatment options, and a lack of appreciation for the dire psychosocial consequences that can result for the acne patient. With our current level of understanding of acne pathogenesis, the ever-expanding array of therapeutic approaches, and a recognition of both the physical and emotional benefits of successful therapy, every acne patient desiring treatment should be able to benefit from physician intervention.

The primary care provider is optimally situated to offer therapy to patients with mild and moderate disease. For those with recalcitrant or severe involvement, referral to a dermatologist is often necessary. Although acne therapy is a combination of art and science, a solid understanding of the various classes of medication and their proper use in both monotherapy and combination therapy provides the foundation for designing treatment plans. A conceptual framework is shown in Figure 8.14, which is an acne treatment algorithm.

Topical therapies are first-line treatment for patients with mild acne, and are very useful as part of a combination therapy regimen for patients with moderate or severe acne. Prescription-strength topical agents are summarized in Table 8.3. Benzoyl peroxide (BP) and topical retinoids (vitamin A acids), although potential irritants, appear to be the most effective topical agents. Based on our current understanding of acne pathogenesis, these two products offer a highly effective therapeutic approach that can be tailored to each patient. Although success in the management of acne vulgaris can be achieved by the use of these agents alone, the therapeutic effect can be increased substantially by their use in combination, although applied at separate times.

BP and salicylic acid are the active ingredients in most over-the-counter (OTC) acne products. The latter helps to reduce sebum and

Severity (lesion type) ⟶	Mild (comedonal)	Mild (inflammatory/mixed)	Moderate (inflammatory/mixed)	Severe (inflammatory/mixed)	Severe (nodular/cystic)
Initial therapy options*	Topical retinoid Salicylic acid cleanser	BP/antibiotic combo BP/retinoid combo Antibiotic/retinoid combo	BP/antibiotic combo ± topical retinoid BP/retinoid combo Antibiotic/retinoid combo ± oral antibiotic	BP/antibiotic combo + topical retinoid + oral antibiotic BP/retinoid combo + oral antibiotic Antibiotic/retinoid combo + oral antibiotic	Isotretinoin
Alternative therapy options*,β	Add BP or BP/antibiotic combo BP/retinoid combo Antibiotic/retinoid combo	Substitute another combo product Add missing component (i.e., topical retinoid, BP, topical antibiotic)	Substitute another combo product Add missing component (i.e., topical retinoid, BP, topical antibiotic, oral antibiotic) Consider hormone therapy for females	Substitute another combo product Add missing component (i.e., topical retinoid, BP, topical antibiotic, oral antibiotic) Consider hormone therapy for females Consider isotretinoin	Consider hormonal therapy for females
Maintenance therapy	Topical retinoid or BP/retinoid combo	Topical retinoid or BP/retinoid combo	Topical retinoid or BP/retinoid combo	Topical retinoid or BP/retinoid combo	Topical retinoid or BP/retinoid combo

*, if combination products not available to patient, consider substitution of individual components as separate prescriptions
β, if needed as determined by physician assessment and patient satisfaction
BP, benzoyl peroxide
Adapted from Zaenglein AL, Thiboutot DM.[46,72–74]

Figure 8.14 Acne treatment algorithm.

Table 8.3 Prescription topical therapies for acne vulgaris

Drug	Brand[a]	Formulation
Antibiotics		
Clindamycin	Cleocin T	1% solution, gel, pledgets, lotion
	Clindets	1% pledgets
	Evoclin	1% foam
Clindamycin/BP[b]	BenzaClin	1% (5% BP) gel
	Duac	1% (5% BP) gel
	Acanya	1.2% (2.5% BP) gel
Dapsone	Aczone	5% gel
Erythromycin	Emgel, Erygel	2% gel
	Eryderm, Erymax, T-Stat	2% solution
	Staticin	1.5% solution
	Akne-mycin	2% ointment
	Theramycin Z	2% solution + ZA
Erythromycin/BP[b]	Benzamycin	3% (5% BP) gel, pak
Sulfacetamide	Klaron, Novacet, Sulfacet-R	10% lotion
	Plexion	10% emulsion
Azelaic acid	Azelex	20% cream
BP	Benzac	5, 10% gel
	Benzac AC (water base)	2.5, 5, 10% gel, wash
	Benzac W (water base)	2.5, 5, 10% gel
	Benzagel	5, 10% wash
	Brevoxyl	5, 10% gel
	Desquam-X	4, 8% gel, wash kit
	NeoBenz Micro	5, 10% gel
		3.5, 5.5% cream
		7% wash
	Panoxyl	5, 10% gel
	Panoxyl AQ (water base)	2.5, 5, 10% gel
	Triaz	3, 6, 10% gel, wash
Retinoids		
Adapalene	Differin	0.1% cream, gel, solution, pledgets
		0.3% gel
Adapalene/BP[b]	Epiduo	0.1% (2.5% BP) gel
Tazarotene	Tazorac	0.05, 0.1% cream
		0.05, 0.1% gel
Tretinoin	Retin-A	0.025, 0.05, 0.1% cream
		0.01, 0.025% gel
	Retin-A Micro	0.04, 0.1% gel
	Avita	0.025% cream, gel
	Atralin	0.05% gel
Tretinoin/Clindamycin[b]	Ziana	0.025% (1.2% Clindamycin) gel

[a]Listed are examples; this list is not exhaustive; many of these preparations have generic alternatives.

[b]Combination therapy product. BP, benzoyl peroxide; ZA, zinc acetate.

decrease comedones, and is found in various concentrations as a gel, lotion, wash, or cream. It may be an alternative comedonal therapy for those who cannot tolerate topical retinoids. Glycolic acid, one of the α-hydroxy acids, is found naturally in fruits and yogurt, and may be useful in decreasing hyperkeratosis associated with acne.

BP is the most frequently used topical preparation for acne vulgaris, and is available both as an OTC and a prescription product. It is a powerful antimicrobial, useful for reducing colonization of *P. acnes*, and also has some comedolytic and antiinflammatory effects. BP is available in a variety of strengths, including 2.5%, 3%, 4%, 5%, 6%, 9%, and 10%, and comes as a gel, wash, lotion, and even shaving cream. It is usually used once to twice daily. BP products may bleach colored clothing or linens, and patients should be warned of this possibility. More recently, combination products of BP with topical antibiotics (erythromycin or clindamycin) have become available, and these agents appear to be more effective than either ingredient used alone.[27–29] A combination BP/topical retinoid product is also available. These agents are discussed in more detail in the paragraphs that follow.

Potential side-effects of BP include an irritant contact dermatitis, and rarely an allergic contact dermatitis.[16,30] Irritant dermatitis is particularly problematic when the product is used excessively or in association with abrasive soaps or astringents or both. Therapy must be individualized and initiated gradually, particularly in fair-skinned or atopic individuals. BP should be applied as a thin film and rubbed in gently, gradually increasing the frequency and strength of the preparation as tolerance is developed (generally over several weeks). As with most topical agents, a small 'pea-sized' portion of the product is generally sufficient for application to the entire face. If irritation or excessive dryness develops, the preparation may be discontinued for several days and then restarted more sparingly, and/or non-comedogenic facial emollients may be used (in small amounts).

Topical retinoids (Table 8.3) are a very effective class of medication used in the treatment of acne. These drugs normalize the keratinization process within the follicles, which reduces obstruction and therefore the formation of microcomedones and comedones. These agents are thus both comedolytic and anticomedogenic and, as such, function to help prevent new acne as well as to treat existing lesions. The prototype drug in this class is tretinoin, an acid of vitamin A. Newer-generation agents include adapalene and tazarotene. Tazarotene is used primarily in the treatment of psoriasis, and subsequently received approval for the treatment of acne vulgaris. Although success in the management of acne can often be achieved by the use of topical retinoids alone, the therapeutic effect can be substantially increased by their use in combination with benzoyl peroxide or a topical antibiotic. A tretinoin/clindamycin combination (Table 8.3) has been found to improve both comedonal and inflammatory acne. More recently, an adapalene/BP combination product has become available and was found to be more effective than either agent alone or placebo.[31]

Topical retinoids are generally applied once nightly, and should be applied sparingly. A useful analogy for the patient is to use a 'pea-sized' amount of product for a full-face application. The traditional recommendation was for retinoids to be applied to a dry face, with 30–45 min of 'air drying' allowed after washing and before applying the product. However, this appears to be unnecessary with the newer 'micro' forms of tretinoin, adapalene, and tazarotene. The primary side-effect of topical retinoids is irritation, which can be minimized by appropriate application and use. In general, the cream forms are less drying than the gels, solutions, or pledgets. In patients with sensitive skin, good initial choices for retinoid therapy would be tretinoin cream (in a lower strength), adapalene cream, or one of the micro preparations. If the product is tolerated well and more effect is desired, the patient can then be advanced to higher strengths, a gel or pledget formulation, or tazarotene. Another useful strategy to decrease the incidence of irritation is to have the patient begin therapy 3 nights weekly, increasing as tolerated over a few weeks to nightly application.[32] Since retinoids may degrade significantly when mixed with benzoyl peroxide, such combination therapy should be used only in the form of pre-formulated combination products (Table 8.3).[33]

Increased sun sensitivity is another potential side-effect of topical retinoids, and patients should be counseled regarding the appropriate use of a sunscreen with a sun protection factor of 15–30, especially if they are also using a photosensitizing oral agent. The risk of teratogenicity with use of the topical retinoids is controversial, but remains a concern given the well-established teratogenic potential of the oral retinoid, isotretinoin. There are sporadic reports of congenital malformations in infants born to women who used topical tretinoin during pregnancy, but controlled human studies are lacking for this drug, which is classified as a pregnancy category C ('studies in animals have revealed adverse effects on the fetus and there are no controlled studies in women or studies in women and animals are not available'). The limited transdermal uptake, lack of alteration of plasma retinoid levels, epidemiologic data, and margin of safety when compared to known teratogens all suggest the unlikelihood of tretinoin being a human developmental toxicant.[34–37] However, until a formal consensus exists, the potential risks of topical retinoids should be discussed in detail with women of child-bearing potential, and their use should probably be avoided during pregnancy.

Topical antibiotics (Table 8.3) exert their effect primarily by decreasing the population of *P. acnes*, and they may also have anti-inflammatory effects. The most commonly utilized topical antibiotics for acne are clindamycin, erythromycin, and sulfacetamide. These agents are most useful for inflammatory acne and, in patients with mixed inflammatory and comedonal disease, should be used in combination with another agent that has comedolytic properties (i.e., benzoyl peroxide or retinoid). These agents are usually well-tolerated, and are applied once to twice daily. As with other topical agents, lotions and creams are less drying than solutions, pledgets, and gels.

Topical erythromycin has been used for decades in the treatment of acne, and is usually well-tolerated. The addition of zinc to erythromycin may increase its therapeutic efficacy.[38] For patients with extremely dry skin, an ointment-based topical erythromycin product (Aknemycin) is available. Topical clindamycin is another well-tolerated antibiotic preparation for acne. Although pseudomembranous colitis is usually associated with oral clindamycin, there are only rare reports of this complication following topical application of this agent.[39,40] Therefore, if a patient using topical clindamycin develops persistent diarrhea, this rare complication should be considered. Topical sulfonamide preparations (mainly sulfacetamide) are also available by prescription, and may be particularly useful in patients who also show evidence of rosacea. These medications are often well-accepted, although some patients may find their odor offensive. Patients with allergies to oral sulfa drugs should not use topical sulfonamides. Topical dapsone, a newer arrival in the acne antibiotic market, may result in clinically-insignificant mild hemolysis in patients with glucose 6-phosphate dehydrogenase deficiency.[41]

With increasing use of topical antibiotics for the treatment of acne vulgaris, the development of resistant strains of *P. acnes* is being observed. Cross-resistance of *P. acnes* to erythromycin and clindamycin is now widespread.[42] In one study, erythromycin-resistant organisms were isolated from 51% of patients treated with oral erythromycin, but also from 42% of patients treated with topical clindamycin.[43] Antibiotic-resistant propionibacteria may be transmissible between acne-prone individuals as well as between patients and their physicians.[44] Data suggest that the concomitant use of benzoyl peroxide with topical (as well as oral) erythromycin or clindamycin diminishes the emergence of resistant bacterial strains.[17,45,46]

Azelaic acid is a naturally occurring dicarboxylic acid produced by the fungal organism *Pityrosporum ovale*. It has antibacterial and anticomedonal properties, and is felt by some to be equal in efficacy to benzoyl peroxide or tretinoin. The effectiveness of azelaic acid may be increased by using it in combination with other topical medications such as retinoids, antibiotics, or benzoyl peroxide.[47] Another benefit of this agent is its ability to decrease hyperpigmentation caused by acne. Azelaic acid is marketed as a 20% cream, and is applied twice daily. Side-effects are rare, but include burning, tingling, mild erythema, and pruritus.

Physicians are frequently consulted regarding the safety of acne treatment in women who are pregnant, may become pregnant, or are breast-feeding an infant. Although there are no long-term studies on the use of topical antibiotics during pregnancy, erythromycin seems to be safe. Since it is estimated that approximately 8% of topically applied clindamycin can be absorbed,[34] this drug is probably best avoided for women who are breast-feeding, are pregnant, or are contemplating pregnancy. Although approximately 5% of topically applied benzoyl peroxide is absorbed through the skin, it is rapidly metabolized to benzoic acid, enters the dermal blood vessels as benzoate, and is then transported to the kidneys and excreted in the urine. Thus, benzoyl peroxide appears to be safe during pregnancy, although controlled studies are lacking. The use of tretinoin is discussed earlier in this section.

Oral antibiotics (Table 8.4) are the most common form of systemic therapy utilized in the treatment of acne vulgaris. These agents are quite effective, and are best reserved for patients with moderate or severe inflammatory acne. They are useful in decreasing *P. acnes*, free fatty acids found in sebum, and inflammation (via their inhibitory effect on neutrophil chemotaxis). Oral antibiotics generally require 4–8 weeks to achieve their maximum effect, and it is usually necessary to continue therapy for several months, with gradual tapering as tolerated once the disease activity has diminished. The most commonly utilized antibiotics for treating acne are the tetracycline-class drugs (tetracycline, minocycline, doxycycline) and erythromycin. Less commonly, clindamycin, trimethoprim-sulfamethoxazole, azithromycin, and cephalexin are used. These medications are usually given on a twice-daily basis.

The safety of long-term antibiotic therapy for acne has been a concern of patients, parents, and physicians. Although the risk-to-benefit ratio of the most commonly used medications is favorable, each agent carries its own inherent potential toxicities, some of greater concern than others. The development of *P. acnes* resistance has been demonstrated for most of the agents utilized in this setting, especially erythromycin and clindamycin, in which case cross-resistance patterns may emerge.[48,49] General guidelines for oral antibiotic usage in acne include avoiding the oral agent if a topical agent will suffice, continuing treatment for no longer than is necessary, reusing the same drug when possible (if restarting oral therapy is required), and avoidance of concomitant oral and topical treatment with dissimilar antibiotics.[49] In patients who do not respond to oral antibiotics, the possibility of resistant strains should be considered. Overall, the commonly used oral antibiotics for acne are well-tolerated, side-effects are uncommon, and routine laboratory testing is unnecessary. Concomitant use of antibiotics and oral contraceptive agents may result in decreased efficacy of the latter, and this possibility should be discussed with female patients.

Table 8.4 Oral antibiotics for acne vulgaris

Drug	Usual dosage[a]	Comments/side-effects
Commonly used		
Tetracycline	250–500 mg	Dental staining <9 years Dairy products decrease absorption GI upset, photosensitivity, teratogenic, PTC, VVC
Minocycline	50–100 mg 45, 90 or 135 mg ER, once daily	Dental staining <9 years Dairy products decrease absorption Vertigo, GI upset, blue-gray skin pigmentation, severe drug/ lupus-like reactions, teratogenic, hepatitis, PTC, VVC
Doxycycline	50–100 mg 75, 100, 150 mg ER, once daily 20 mg ('subantimicrobial dose')	Dental staining <9 years Dairy products decrease absorption Photosensitivity, photo-onycholysis, GI upset (rare), teratogenic, PTC, VVC
Erythromycin	250–500 mg	GI upset (common), VVC
Less commonly used		
Trimethoprim-sulfamethoxazole	80/400 mg, 160/800 mg	Severe drug reactions, bone marrow suppression, hepatitis, GI upset, VVC
Clindamycin	75–150 mg	Pseudomembranous colitis, GI upset, drug reactions, VVC
Cephalexin	250–500 mg	GI upset, drug reactions, VVC

[a]Usually given twice daily for acne, unless otherwise noted in Table. GI, gastrointestinal; PTC, pseudotumor cerebri; VVC, vulvovaginal candidiasis; ER, extended release formulation.

Tetracyclines are the gold standard of oral antibiotic therapy for acne. These agents have a long track record of safety and efficacy, although side-effects are possible. The possibility of dental staining (Fig. 8.15) in children under 9 years of age precludes their use in this population, who only occasionally have moderate to severe acne. Tetracycline-class antibiotics should also not be used in pregnant females, given the deposition of the drug in developing teeth as a result of its chelating properties and the formation of a tetracycline–calcium orthophosphate complex.

The most common side-effects of the tetracyclines are photosensitivity and gastrointestinal upset. The risk of phototoxicity is greatest with tetracycline and doxycycline, and extremely rare with minocycline. Pseudotumor cerebri is a rare side-effect, the risk being greatest when isotretinoin and a tetracycline are taken concomitantly. Tetracyclines cannot be taken with dairy products or antacids, as this results in impaired absorption. In addition, tetracycline (but not doxycycline or minocycline) absorption is impaired in the presence of food, and thus the medication must be taken 1 hour before or 2 hours after a meal. This feature may result in decreased compliance among active teenagers. Tetracyclines should be used with caution in patients with renal disease.

Doxycycline has the benefit of sustained absorption in the presence of food, but may result in severe photosensitivity reactions. One such type of reaction is 'photo-onycholysis,' which presents with erythema and separation of the nail plate from the nail bed (Fig. 8.16). These patients usually also have an associated photosensitivity rash on exposed areas of skin. Off-label use of subantimicrobial-dose doxycycline hyclate (20-mg tablets taken twice daily) has been reported in acne vulgaris, and has been shown to significantly reduce the number of lesions without any detectable antimicrobial effect on skin flora or alteration of resistance patterns.[50] An extended-release formulation of doxycycline is available, and can be administered once daily.

Minocycline is the most widely prescribed systemic antibiotic for the management of acne in the USA, Canada, and the UK, and it is estimated that 65% of prescriptions for this drug are for acne.[51] It is particularly effective against *P. acnes* and also has antiinflamma-

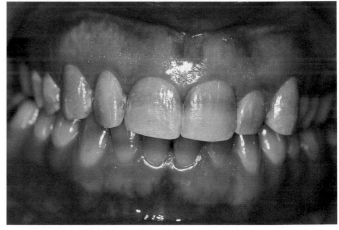

Figure 8.15 Dental staining from tetracycline. (Courtesy of Maria Simon, DDS.)

tory properties. Similar to doxycycline, an extended-release formulation of minocycline is now available, and may improve compliance. Although the side-effect profile is somewhat similar to that of other tetracyclines, minocycline rarely causes photosensitivity. Other side-effects more specific to minocycline are headache, dizziness, vertigo, and a blue-gray pigmentation of mucosae (Fig. 11.57) or at sites of previous inflammation such as acne scars.

Occasional potentially-serious toxicities may be associated with minocycline, including autoimmune hepatitis, drug-induced lupus (DIL), serum sickness-like reaction (SSLR), and a drug hypersensitivity reaction (HSR).[51,52] This HSR is characterized by a diffuse erythematous rash, facial (especially periorbital) edema, lymphadenopathy, fever, and internal organ involvement (most commonly the liver). It tends to occur within 6–8 weeks of starting the drug, and is similar to the hypersensitivity reaction occasionally seen with the aromatic anticonvulsants (phenytoin, carbamazepine, phenobarbital). SSLR presents with fever, urticarial rash, periarticular

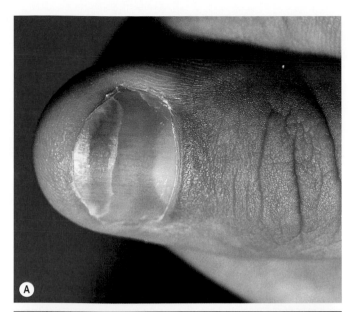

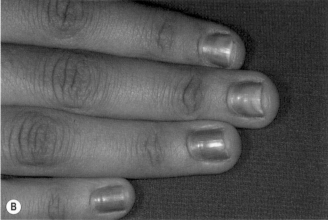

Figure 8.16 Doxycycline-induced photo-onycholysis in two patients. Note distal nail plate separation with new nail growing in proximally (A) and separation of nail plate from underlying nail bed in the index and middle fingers (B).

Erythromycin is a useful antibiotic for acne vulgaris, but its use is frequently limited by the fairly high incidence of gastrointestinal disturbance, even with the enteric-coated preparations. It, otherwise, has few side-effects and carries the distinct benefit of no phototoxicity. Other antibiotics occasionally used for acne include clindamycin, trimethoprim-sulfamethoxazole, and cephalexin. Prolonged use of oral clindamycin is not desirable because of the risk of pseudomembranous colitis due to the toxin liberated by *Clostridium difficile*, which is able to grow in large numbers in the intestinal tract of some patients who receive this drug. Trimethoprim-sulfamethoxazole can be very effective for acne, but is not recommended as a first-line agent given the severe and potentially life-threatening reactions (i.e., HSR or toxic epidermal necrolysis) as well as bone marrow suppression that may occur.

The most frequent complication of antibiotic therapy in adult female patients is vaginal candidiasis, but it rarely occurs in teenagers. This complication is proportionately more common in women who take oral contraceptives (OCPs) concomitantly with their systemic antibiotics. Another concern in patients who are also taking OCPs is the possibility of the oral antibiotic diminishing the effectiveness of the contraceptive. Although this possibility remains controversial, it should be discussed with patients and alternative forms of birth control considered during the period of treatment. Patients on long-term antibiotic therapy may rarely develop a condition termed *Gram-negative folliculitis*, due to superinfection of the pilosebaceous units with Gram-negative organisms. This complication is manifested by a pustular folliculitis or deep nodulocystic lesions recalcitrant to the acne regimen. It may respond to a change in antibiotics to reduce Gram-negative organisms, but responds more consistently to isotretinoin.[55]

Hormonal therapies are another option for the treatment of acne in female patients. The primary goal of these therapies is to oppose the effects of androgens on the sebaceous glands.[56] These medications include androgen receptor blockers, adrenal androgen production blockers, ovarian androgen blockers and enzyme inhibitors, and they may be prescribed in consultation with a gynecologist or endocrinologist. This group of medications may have other beneficial effects on hirsutism, androgenetic alopecia, and menstrual irregularities in some females.[16] OCPs contain both an estrogen and a progestin, and those with a lower intrinsic androgenic activity type of progestin (desogestrel, norgestimate, gestodene and drospirenone) are most desirable for acne therapy. Drospirenone, a novel progestin, has both antiandrogenic and antimineralocorticoid activity, and is reportedly better tolerated in terms of weight gain and mood changes.[57] Currently, Ortho Tri-Cyclen (norgestimate and ethinylestradiol), Estrostep (norethindrone and ethinylestradiol) and Yaz (drospirenone and ethinylestradiol) are FDA-approved for use in the treatment of acne vulgaris. OCPs may be the first-line treatment in females with skin manifestations of hyperandrogenemia.[58]

Antiandrogenic agents include spironolactone, flutamide, cyproterone acetate, gonadotropin-releasing hormone antagonists, and 5-α-reductase inhibitors. Spironolactone, which is used primarily as a diuretic in the treatment of hypertension, competes for androgen receptors on target cells. It is usually started at 25–50 mg/day and maintenance doses, which vary by the individual, are in the range of 25–200 mg/day.[58] Potential side-effects of spironolactone therapy include menstrual irregularities, breast tenderness, hyperkalemia, and fatigue. In a study of 27 women with severe acne who were treated with spironolactone and a combined contraceptive (drospirenone and ethinylestradiol), this combination was demonstrated effective and safe, without hyperkalemia or other serious side-effects.[59]

swelling with arthralgia, and occasional nephritis and lymphadenopathy. A comparative study reviewing tetracycline, minocycline, and doxycycline adverse events revealed that these reaction patterns (DIL, SSLR, HSR) are all more commonly seen with minocycline than with the other two medications.[53] Also of note is the fact that SSLR and HSR usually occur within 2 months of beginning treatment, whereas DIL may be delayed for up to 2 years.[53]

Autoimmune hepatitis, DIL, arthritis, vasculitis, and development of autoantibodies have been unified under the moniker of minocycline induced autoimmunity (MIA). A recent study of 27 children with MIA revealed a mean duration of treatment of 13 months before the diagnosis. The majority of patients had polyarthralgia or polyarthritis, mostly of the hands and feet. Other features included constitutional symptoms, livedo reticularis, Raynaud phenomenon, elevation of liver enzymes, and elevated antinuclear antibody titers. Importantly, 26% of patients had chronic autoimmunity, manifested mostly as persistent arthritis.[54] Although these major types of tetracycline class drug reactions are rare overall, their possibility should be discussed with the patient, especially when minocycline is being considered. Many experts consider doxycycline to be a safe alternative, even in patients who have a history of MIA.

Isotretinoin (13-*cis* retinoic acid, Amnesteem, Claravis, Sotret) is a derivative of vitamin A that is highly effective for recalcitrant nodulocystic acne, and the availability of this agent revolutionized the treatment of severe disease. Although the precise mechanism of action is unknown, its effects appear to be related to marked inhibition of sebum synthesis, lowering of *P. acnes* concentration, inhibition of neutrophil chemotaxis, and comedolytic and antiinflammatory effects. Isotretinoin therapy often results in complete and often, but not always, permanent remission of acne vulgaris.[60] Pre-teens and young teenagers seem to have the highest rate of relapse. In patients who experience a recurrence of disease, however, the flares may be milder and more responsive to therapies utilized prior to isotretinoin therapy. Repeat courses may occasionally be necessary. The availability of isotretinoin was met with much enthusiasm given its potential to prevent permanent scarring. Prescriptions for isotretinoin increased 250% in the 8-year period between 1992 and 2000.[61]

Patients are usually started on 0.5 mg/kg per day of isotretinoin and increased to 1 mg/kg per day, usually for 16–24 weeks. Cumulative dosing goals, ranging from 100 to 150 mg/kg for the entire course of treatment, have been advocated as they may decrease the rate of relapse.[62,63] Early in the course of isotretinoin therapy, there may be a temporary flare of lesions, and patient education regarding this possibility is vital. Although isotretinoin is truly a 'miracle' drug for severe forms of acne, it has many potential side-effects and prescribing should be done only by physicians experienced in its use.

Potential adverse effects of isotretinoin are numerous and are summarized in Table 8.5. A newer risk management program, iPLEDGE (www.ipledgeprogram.com), was approved by the FDA and drug manufacturers and implemented in March of 2006. This program requires prescribers, patients, pharmacies, drug wholesalers, and manufacturers in the USA to register and comply. This mandatory distribution program was created in an effort to prevent the use of isotretinoin during pregnancy, given its teratogenic effects

(see below). Under this system, prescribers must record two negative pregnancy tests before a patient can commence therapy with isotretinoin. The iPLEDGE program represents the most rigorous risk management program in history for such a widely prescribed drug.[64] Overall, the risk of major side-effects (assuming pregnancy is avoided) from isotretinoin, is quite low.

Isotretinoin is a known human teratogen, and is a pregnancy category X drug. Major fetal malformations have been observed in exposed infants, including abnormalities of the skull, ear, eye, central nervous system, and heart. As little as one pill can have devastating consequences on the developing fetus.[16] To qualify for therapy, females of child-bearing potential must have two negative serum or urine pregnancy tests, and commitment to two forms of contraception, one of which must be a primary form (OCPs, intrauterine device, injectable or implantable hormonal birth control product, partner's vasectomy or tubal ligation), for at least 1 month prior to initiation of therapy and for 1 month after discontinuing therapy. Abstinence is most desirable for females on isotretinoin therapy. A signed patient consent form is required. Unfortunately, even with dedicated pregnancy prevention programs and education regarding isotretinoin-associated teratogenicity, inadequate birth control efforts continue to be practiced by some treated females. Ongoing fetal exposure to isotretinoin has been demonstrated to be an international problem, highlighting the need for more effective strategies which incorporate considerations for cultural differences.[65]

The risks of isotretinoin-related depression and suicidal ideation have come to the forefront in recent years. The exact association, if any, remains controversial, and arguments both supporting and refuting the potential for mood disturbance have been made. Epidemiologic data have demonstrated a lower suicide rate of 12- to 18-year-old isotretinoin users when compared with the annual rate of suicide for that population in the USA. Critical literature reviews have failed to confirm an association, and although retinoid receptors are widely distributed in the brain, there is no known pharmacological mechanism to account for isotretinoin-induced psychiatric symptoms.[66–68] In one systematic literature review, it was noted that studies comparing depression before and after treatment did not show a significant increase and that, surprisingly, some revealed a trend toward fewer or less severe depressive symptoms after isotretinoin therapy.[68] Nonetheless, patients and parents must be thoroughly informed of the potential risks of depression and suicidal ideation, and patients on therapy must be monitored closely and referred for psychiatric evaluation if indicated.

There are a variety of miscellaneous treatments for acne vulgaris, and these are listed in Table 8.6.[16,69–71] Table 8.7 lists examples of therapeutic approaches based on acne type and severity.

Neonatal and Infantile Acne

Although acne is usually a disorder of adolescents and young adults, neonates and infants are occasionally affected. Neonatal acne has its onset within the first weeks of life, and may be congenital in up to 20% of newborns.[75] Infantile acne, on the other hand, usually presents between 3 and 6 months of life and tends to be more severe and more persistent.[76] Both types occur more often in boys than in girls, and the clinical presentation is similar to that of acne vulgaris, with involvement usually limited to the face. Open and closed comedones are most common, and inflammatory papules and pustules (Fig. 8.17) occasionally occur. Infants may also develop deep papules, cysts and nodules (Fig. 8.18) with the potential for scarring, even without comedonal lesions.

The causes of neonatal and infantile acne are unclear. A family history of acne may or may not be present.[77] Neonatal disease is

Side-effect	Comment
Dry skin and nasal membranes	Occasional epistaxis
Dry eyes	Most problematic for contact lens-wearers
Cheilitis	May be quite severe
Photosensitivity	
Decreased night vision	
Corneal opacities	
Alopecia	Diffuse thinning
Headache	
Pseudotumor cerebri	Most common with concomitant use of tetracycline-class antibiotic
Musculoskeletal pain	
Hyperostosis	Mainly seen with prolonged use
Elevated triglycerides, cholesterol	Rare pancreatitis
Hepatitis	
Inflammatory bowel disease	
Rhabdomyolysis	
Teratogenicity	See text for discussion
Depression, suicidal ideation	See text for discussion

Table 8.5 Potential isotretinoin-associated adverse effects

Table 8.6 Alternative treatments for acne vulgaris[16,69–71]

Treatment	Comment
Comedone extraction	Performed with comedo extractor
Injections	Intralesional triamcinolone injected into large cysts or nodules
Light therapy	420 nm ultraviolet free blue light; photodestruction of acne bacteria
Resurfacing lasers	Useful for acne scarring
Dermabrasion, dermasanding	Useful for acne scarring
Collagen injection	Useful for acne scarring
Chemical peels	Useful for acne scarring and hyperpigmentation
Punch grafts, tissue augmentation	Useful for acne scarring
Trichloroacetic acid	Useful for atrophic acne scars
Radiation therapy	Outdated modality

Table 8.7 Acne treatment vignettes[a]

Mild comedonal acne
  Topical retinoid once daily, *or*
  Topical salicylic acid cleanser once-twice daily, *or*
  Topical retinoid/BP combination product once daily

Mild–moderate combined acne (inflammatory and comedonal lesions)
  BP cleanser twice daily and topical retinoid once daily, *or*
  BP/topical antibiotic combination product in AM and topical retinoid in PM, *or*
  Topical retinoid/topical antibiotic combination product once daily

Moderate–severe combined acne (inflammatory and comedonal lesions)
  Oral antibiotic and topical retinoid once daily, *or*
  Oral antibiotic and topical retinoid/BP combination product once daily, *or*
  Oral antibiotic and spironolactone (female patient), *or*
  OCP + oral antibiotic and topical retinoid once daily

Severe or scarring acne
  Isotretinoin

[a]The above vignettes are therapeutic examples only, and not intended to be specific recommendations; acne therapy should always be tailored to the specific patient and severity of involvement. BP, benzoyl peroxide; OCP, oral contraceptive pill.

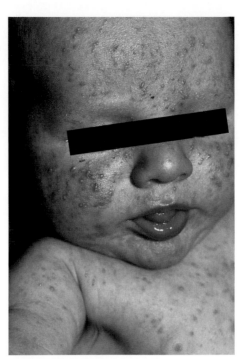

Figure 8.17 Neonatal acne. This newborn had typical papules and pustules, with rapid resolution over 1 month.

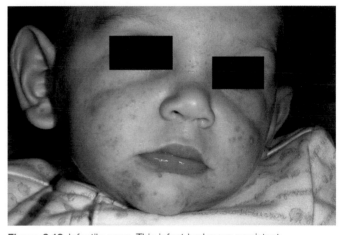

Figure 8.18 Infantile acne. This infant had more persistent involvement with larger lesions, such as the deep papulopustule on the left cheek.

believed to be related to either stimulation of sebaceous glands by maternal androgens or transient adrenal and gonadal androgen production.[75,78] Testicular androgen production serves as a stimulus to primed adrenal glands, which may partially explain the increased incidence of neonatal acne in males.[60] Infantile acne may occasionally be associated with hormonal alterations, namely hyperandrogenism. In any infant with unusually severe or persistent acne, a thorough history and examination should be performed, and diagnostic studies for abnormal androgen production considered. In children between 2 and 7 years of age, acne is unusual and hyperandrogenemia should be ruled out based on thorough examination and laboratory testing. The diagnostic possibilities in this age group include premature adrenarche, mild forms of congenital adrenal hyperplasia, gonadal or adrenal tumors, Cushing's syndrome, and true precocious puberty.[76] Useful screening studies may include serum dehydroepiandrosterone sulfate (DHEA-S), total and free testosterone, 17α-hydroxyprogesterone, gonadotropins (LH and FSH), and prolactin levels, as well as adrenocorticotropin hormone (ACTH) stimulation test and bone age.[75,76,79]

In recent years, a neonatal pustular eruption that presents in a similar fashion to neonatal acne has been described, and is termed 'neonatal cephalic pustulosis'. This disorder presents with multiple facial papules and pustules (see Fig. 2.12) and direct examination of pustule smears shows yeasts of *Malassezia furfur* or *Malassezia sympodialis*.[80,81] These patients respond well to 2% ketoconazole cream. Colonization of neonates with *Malassezia* begins at birth and increases over the first few weeks of life.[82] However, the exact role of *Malassezia* sp. in this setting is poorly understood, and the association between neonatal cephalic pustulosis and neonatal acne remains unclear.[83]

Neonatal acne usually regresses over several months, only occasionally persisting until 9–12 months of age. Infantile acne, however, may be more persistent, lasting as long as several years. Neonatal acne may occasionally evolve into infantile acne. In mild cases of neonatal or infantile acne, therapy is generally unnecessary; daily cleansing with a gentle soap and water may be all that is required. Exogenous oil such as baby oils and lotions may aggravate the condition and should be avoided. When therapy is necessary, it is similar to therapy of acne at any other age, although the use of systemic agents is generally reserved for patients with severe involvement. Mild comedonal acne can be treated with topical tretinoin, although it must be used sparingly and there is a high risk of irritation. Mild inflammatory disease is treated with 2.5% benzoyl peroxide or a topical antibiotic (erythromycin or clindamycin). Treatment should be initiated on an every-other-night basis, and increased as tolerated to nightly. More significant involvement is treated with oral antibiotics, usually erythromycin. Oral isotretinoin is occasionally indicated for infants or young children with cystic involvement and/or scarring.

Androgen Excess and Acne

It is well recognized that androgens may precipitate acne in both men and women. Thus, acne may be produced or aggravated by increased adrenal gland production in response to stress, adrenal tumors, gonadal dysgenesis, Cushing's syndrome, and ovarian androgen excess, such as that which occurs in patients with polycystic ovarian syndrome (PCOS; see Ch. 23). This condition seems to be quite common. In one study of women with acne (but lacking menstrual disorders, obesity, or hirsutism) polycystic ovaries were found in 45%, compared with 17% of age-matched controls.[84] Adolescent females with severe, persistent, or recalcitrant forms of acne, especially in the setting of other signs of androgen excess (i.e., menstrual irregularity and hirsutism) should be screened for this disorder with laboratory examinations and transabdominal ovarian ultrasound. In patients with acne who show rapid development of virilizing signs such as voice deepening, increased muscle mass, or androgenetic alopecia, the evaluation should focus more on a search for a tumor rather than polycystic ovaries.[85] 'Metabolic syndrome' (previously referred to as 'syndrome X') describes the clinical presentation of severe insulin resistance, obesity, hypertension, dyslipidemias, and microvascular angina. Occasionally, ovarian hyperandrogenism and polycystic ovaries may occur in this setting.[86] Treatment for polycystic ovary syndrome typically consists of hormonal agents and antiandrogens such as spironolactone.

Acne Rosacea

Acne rosacea (also known simply as 'rosacea') is a chronic vascular inflammatory disorder usually limited to the face characterized by erythema, telangiectasia, papules and pustules and, occasionally, hyperplasia of the sebaceous glands and the soft tissues of the nose (rhinophyma). Rosacea is primarily a disease of adults between the ages of 30 and 50, but may also appear as early as the second decade of life, at times co-existing with acne vulgaris. Rosacea most often manifests as erythema and telangiectasia of the cheeks. A variety of ocular lesions may occur in the setting of rosacea. This association is termed *ocular rosacea*, is characterized by blepharitis, conjunctivitis, episcleritis, iritis, keratitis, and occasionally corneal ulceration and subsequent opacity. Recently, several aberrant responses have been indentified in rosacea, including altered toll-like receptor 2 (TLR2) expression, enhanced vasodilatation triggered by cathelicidin, and greater lesional skin activity of reactive oxygen species.[87]

There are several potential exacerbating factors in rosacea, including sun exposure, stress, cold weather, hot beverages, alcohol consumption, and certain foods.[88] Avoidance of these factors may help to prevent flares in certain individuals. Although the etiologies of rosacea and ocular rosacea are not well understood, a primary genetic predisposition is suggested since single genes may control mediators involved in rosacea pathways, namely enzymes, neuroendocrine transmitters, and cytokines.[89] Complete clearing of rosacea is rarely achieved, but satisfactory control can usually be accomplished by the use of topical or oral agents. Systemic therapy options include metronidazole, doxycycline, minocycline, tetracycline, or clarithromycin, and the most useful topical therapy is metronidazole.[90] Topical sulfonamide preparations, azelaic acid and sulfabased washes may also be useful. Patients with rosacea tend to tolerate topical retinoids and benzoyl peroxide poorly. Oral isotretinoin has been effective in patients with severe rosacea, predominantly of the granulomatous type. The telangiectasias may improve after pulsed-dye laser therapy. Rhinophyma, if it develops, is a difficult finding to treat, usually requiring aggressive dermatologic surgical procedures with or without laser surgery.

Pomade Acne

A variety of external agents can induce acne-like eruptions upon repeated exposure to the skin of susceptible persons. These include greasy or oily sunscreen preparations, heavy make-up bases, and grooming agents. An acneiform eruption induced by various grooming substances used on the scalp has been termed pomade acne. It is usually seen on the forehead and temples and consists of numerous, closely set closed comedones. The cheek and chin may also be involved if the agent has been applied over the entire face. Pomade acne may in fact represent true acne vulgaris potentiated by the use of occlusive products. It usually responds to standard acne therapy along with discontinuation of the offending comedogenic preparation.

Acne Cosmetica

Acne cosmetica is a variant of acne described in women, usually >20 years, which is attributed to the frequent or heavy use of cosmetics,[91] particularly those containing lanolin, petrolatum, certain vegetable oils, butyl stearate, isopropyl myristate, sodium lauryl sulfate, lauryl alcohol, or oleic acid. The lesions are predominantly small, scattered closed comedones on the face. Although common in women without a history of acne, those with a history of adolescent acne seem to be the most susceptible. A prominent feature is a coarse facial appearance associated with prominent dark follicles that is often more distressing to the patient than the actual acne lesions themselves. The most extensive eruptions are seen in women who attempt to mask the lesions under a heavy coating of cosmetics. Fortunately, most cosmetic companies today are aware of the problem of comedogenicity and many cosmetics are now marketed as 'non-comedogenic'. A variant of acne cosmetica, consisting of deep-seated nodules and closed comedones that heal very slowly with hyperpigmentation, may occur following facial beauty treatments.[92]

Acne Excoriée

Acne excoriée is a form of acne most frequently seen in adolescent girls. It is a self-inflicted skin condition in which the patient feels compelled to pick real or imagined acneiform lesions, which then propagates the disorder.[93] Associated comorbidities may include obsessive-compulsive disorder, body dysmorphic disorder, substance use disorders, eating disorders, trichotillomania, kleptomania, compulsive buying, and borderline personality disorder.[94] Patients usually spontaneously admit the self-inflicted nature of the condition, unlike most artifactual dermatoses[93] (see Ch. 26). Acne excoriée is often precipitated by emotional stress. Excoriation or squeezing of acne lesions may vary from mild to moderate irritation (Fig. 8.19) to severe scarring and occasional gross mutilation. Therapeutic options include behavioral modification or pharmacologic therapies, including selective serotonin reuptake inhibitors, doxepin, clomipramine, pimozide, and olanzapine.[94,95]

Pyoderma Faciale

Pyoderma faciale is a relatively rare condition that presents with he sudden onset of coalescent fluctuant cysts, nodules, and papulonodules with draining sinuses. It is usually confined to the face and occurs exclusively in post-adolescent females. Pyoderma faciale seems to represent a severe form of rosacea, and isotretinoin is the most effective therapy, especially when used in combination with corticosteroids.[96,97] Most patients develop scarring as a sequela.[98]

Acne Conglobata

Acne conglobata is a severe suppurative form of acne vulgaris that is usually chronic and seen in men (especially African-American) between 18 and 30 years of age. It is characterized by cysts, abscesses, and sinus tracts and often heals with cosmetically disfiguring keloidal scars. The SAPHO syndrome is an association of musculoskeletal disorders (synovitis, arthritis, hyperostosis, osteitis) with skin conditions, including palmoplantar pustulosis and acne conglobata.[99,100] Sacroiliitis may also occur, with or without hidradenitis suppurativa (see below) or a peripheral arthropathy.[101,102]

Acne with Facial Edema

Acne may at times be associated with an inflammatory edema of the middle face (cheeks, forehead, periorbital areas, base of the nose, and glabella). Although its pathogenesis is unknown, it is believed to be a manifestation of chronic cutaneous inflammation and edema, analogous to that occurring in the legs of patients with recurrent cellulitis and venous insufficiency. This complication, which tends to be unresponsive to oral antibiotics or topical therapy, may respond to oral corticosteroids and isotretinoin.[103]

Periorificial Dermatitis

Periorificial dermatitis (known traditionally as perioral dermatitis) is a fairly common acneiform condition in children as well as young women, in whom it was originally described. Patients present with erythematous discrete papules and papulopustules distributed in the perioral (Fig. 8.20), nasolabial, and periocular (Fig. 8.21) locations. Occasionally, flesh-colored papules or nodules may be present.[104] As the papules resolve, they may be replaced by a diffuse redness or erythematous scale.

Some consider periorificial dermatitis to be a juvenile form of acne rosacea, in part related to the overlapping histologic features in the two conditions. The etiology of periorificial dermatitis is unknown, but in many patients, use of mid- to high-potency topical corticosteroids seems to be related to the pathogenesis.[105] In one retrospective study of 79 children with the disorder, 72% had a history of previous topical, inhaled or systemic steroid exposure.[106] *Granulomatous periorificial dermatitis* is a less common variant of periorificial dermatitis, and is characterized by discrete

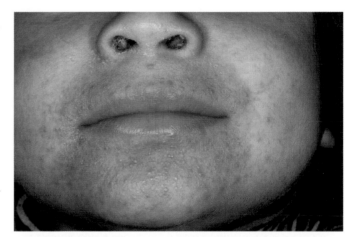

Figure 8.20 Periorificial dermatitis. Numerous erythematous papules in a perioral distribution.

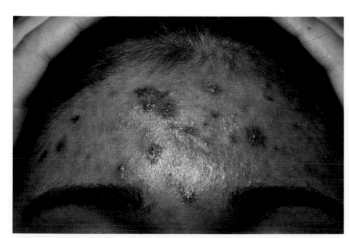

Figure 8.19 Acne excoriée. Note the numerous excoriated and crusted papules of the forehead.

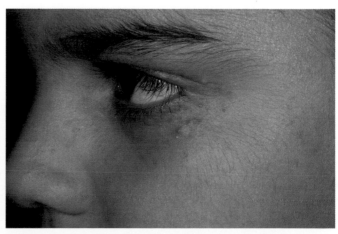

Figure 8.21 Periorificial dermatitis. Erythematous papules, papulopustules and hyperpigmented macules of the inferior eyelid and periorbital region.

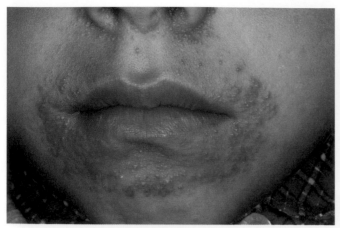

Figure 8.22 Granulomatous periorificial dermatitis. Note the translucent quality of the erythematous papules, and the nasolabial fold involvement.

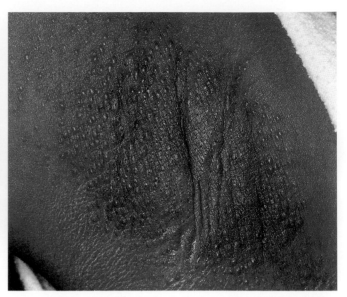

Figure 8.23 Fox–Fordyce disease (apocrine miliaria). Small round follicular papules in the axilla of an adolescent girl.

yellow-brown papules (Fig. 8.22), less prominent erythema, and a granulomatous infiltrate on histologic examination. In addition to facial involvement, these patients may have extrafacial lesions clinically and histologically identical to the facial ones.[107] Blepharitis and conjunctivitis may occasionally occur. Most reported cases of granulomatous periorificial dermatitis have been in prepubertal children, especially in those with a preceding history of topical corticosteroid application to the affected areas. Some patients have been initially misdiagnosed as having sarcoidosis, based primarily on histopathological findings. Nonetheless, sarcoidosis and Blau syndrome (see Ch. 25), an entity which may be difficult to distinguish from sarcoidosis, may be in the differential diagnosis in patients with more extensive periorificial dermatitis (and with more generalized involvement).

Periorificial dermatitis is generally self-limited, although resolution may take months to years, and the lesions may occasionally heal with scarring. Treatment options include topical antibiotics (the most effective being metronidazole, erythromycin or sulfur-based products) and, in more severe cases, oral erythromycin or tetracyclines (in patients >8 years). In patients treated with oral antibiotics, treatment should be continued for a minimum of 6–8 weeks, with gradual tapering, in an effort to avoid the rapid rebounding that is commonly seen with shorter courses of therapy.

Fordyce Spots

Fordyce spots are a relatively common benign condition characterized by minute yellow to yellow-white macules and globoid papules distributed on the vermilion region of the lips and the buccal mucosa. Other less common locations include the glans penis or labia minora. Fordyce spots are composed of 'free' (i.e., not associated with hair follicles) sebaceous glands, and they probably represent a normal anatomic variant. They may present or become more prominent during puberty. Fordyce spots are asymptomatic, and treatment is unnecessary.

Disorders of the apocrine glands

Apocrine sweat glands are found in only a few areas: the axillae, anogenital region, and areolae of the breasts. They are poorly developed in childhood but begin to enlarge with the approach of puberty, triggered by androgen production. Apocrine secretion is

sterile and odorless when it initially appears on the cutaneous surface. Associated odor develops as a result of bacterial decomposition of the secreted substances.

Fox–Fordyce Disease

Fox–Fordyce disease (also known as apocrine miliaria) is a chronic papular eruption of apocrine gland-bearing areas, principally the axillae, the mammary areolae, and the pubic and perineal regions. It is seen primarily in young women, and is a disorder of unknown etiology. It appears to be related to apocrine sweat retention associated with obstruction and rupture of the intraepidermal portions of the affected apocrine glands. Fox–Fordyce disease is usually seen in post-pubescent females, and is quite rare in prepubertal children owing to quiescence of the apocrine glands.

This disorder presents with dome-shaped, flesh-colored to erythematous follicular papules (Fig. 8.23) in the affected areas. Pruritus may be severe, is often paroxysmal, and is aggravated by emotional stress. Treatment is notoriously difficult, and may include topical or intralesional corticosteroids, topical antibiotics, or topical retinoids. Surgical excision of the affected areas is occasionally necessary in severely afflicted patients.

Hidradenitis Suppurativa

Hidradenitis suppurativa (HS) is a chronic suppurative and scarring disease that primarily involves apocrine gland-bearing skin in the axillary, inguinal, and anogenital regions. The breasts and scalp are less commonly involved. HS affects African-Americans and females more often than Caucasians or males, usually develops after puberty, and has traditionally been ascribed to plugging of the apocrine duct and associated bacterial infection. Prepubertal individuals may occasionally be affected.[108] Recent studies have suggested that the primary event may be a folliculitis with secondary involvement of the apocrine glands.[109,110] Some authors have thus suggested the alternative name, *acne inversa*. The etiology of HS is poorly understood. Genetic factors, hormonal influences, obesity, smoking, and tight-fitting clothing have each been hypothesized to play a role.[110,111]

The earliest clinical finding in HS is a painful, inflammatory abscess-like swelling, usually 0.5–1.5 cm in diameter, in the affected apocrine area(s). Within hours to days, the abscess enlarges and may open onto the overlying skin, resulting in purulent drainage. With further development and enlargement of abscesses, sinus tracts form (Fig. 8.24) and eventual scarring ensues with the development of deep fibrosis. Hypertrophic scarring may be seen. HS may be extremely debilitating in severely afflicted patients, with chronic pain, drainage, and secondary infection. Bacteriologic study of early lesions often reveals coagulase-positive staphylococci or streptococci, probably representing secondary infection. Occasionally *Escherichia coli*, *Pseudomonas aeruginosa*, or other Gram-negative organisms contaminate lesions. HS has a significant impact on quality of life, and has been shown to result in more impairment than found with several other dermatologic conditions, including chronic urticaria, psoriasis and atopic dermatitis.[112]

Therapy of HS may be challenging. Management must be individualized based on the severity of disease and symptomatology. Initial measures include antibiotics (especially tetracyclines) and local wound care. Incision and drainage may be useful in certain instances, but for more severe cases, surgical modalities are generally necessary. These include local excision, unroofing of lesions with marsupialization, and wide excision with primary or secondary closure, skin grafting, or flaps.[113,114] Carbon dioxide laser therapy is another option that seems to be quite effective.[115] Low efficacy or a high risk-to-benefit ratio have been suggested as possible limitations for isotretinoin, etanercept and infliximab in this setting,[116–118] although these agents, as well as adalimumab, have been demonstrated helpful in other studies.[119–121]

Disorders of the eccrine glands

The eccrine sweat glands are distributed over the entire skin surface and are found in greatest abundance on the palms and soles and in the axillae. They represent the principal means of maintaining homeostatic balance by evaporation of water. Their secretion depends on their sympathetic nerve supply, which is controlled by various stimuli, including thermal and emotional types. By these mechanisms the quantity and quality of sweat may be varied. Disorders associated with decreased eccrine sweating (i.e., ectodermal dysplasia) are discussed in Chapter 7.

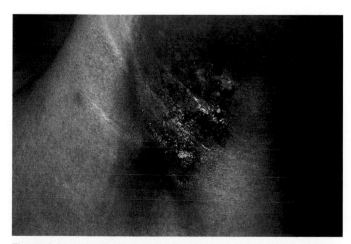

Figure 8.24 Hidradenitis suppurativa. Erythematous papules, cysts, nodules, and sinus tracts are seen in the axilla of this adolescent male.

Hyperhidrosis

Hyperhidrosis (idiopathic hyperhidrosis or primary pediatric hyperhidrosis) is a disorder characterized by the excessive production of sweat in response to heat or emotional stimuli, and not related to an underlying disease or drug toxicity. It is a poorly understood disorder, and the clinical spectrum ranges from a mild increase over the normal level of physiologic sweating to an extreme, debilitating expression of the disease. Such extreme sweating may be socially embarrassing and occupationally disabling, and may negatively affect the patient's psychological wellbeing.[122,123] Hyperhidrosis may be palmoplantar and/or axillary and, in rare instances, generalized. In patients with these forms of idiopathic hyperhidrosis, neurovascular or metabolic abnormalities are absent. *Idiopathic localized unilateral hyperhidrosis* is a rare form of hyperhidrosis localized to a sharply demarcated area on the face or upper extremities of an otherwise healthy individual.[124,125] *Auriculotemporal nerve (Frey) syndrome* is the constellation of facial flushing and hyperhidrosis in response to gustatory stimuli, and is discussed in Chapter 12.

There are a variety of treatment options for idiopathic hyperhidrosis (Table 8.8). The first-line therapies are topical, and consist of both over-the-counter and prescription strength antiperspirant preparations. The active ingredient in many of these is either aluminum chloride or formaldehyde. These products are best applied to dry skin at bedtime, and their effect may be potentiated when they are used along with plastic wrap occlusion overnight (when practical). However, for some patients, occlusion results in more irritation. Systemic anticholinergic agents such as glycopyrrolate or propantheline bromide are often useful, but may be limited by their side-effect profiles, which include dry eyes, dry mouth, and bowel and bladder dysfunction. Sedative agents such as diazepam may be useful before an anxiety-provoking event, but their continual use is not recommended.

Table 8.8 Most common therapies for primary hyperhidrosis	
Treatment	**Comment**
Topical antiperspirants	Aluminum chloride, formaldehyde, others Both over the counter (OTC) and prescription strengths Usually applied at bedtime
Oral anticholinergic agents	Glycopyrrolate, propantheline bromide, others May be limited by side effects (dry eyes, dry mouth, bowel/bladder dysfunction)
Iontophoresis	Safe and well-tolerated Efficacy variable
Botulinum toxin type A	Injected intradermally or intracutaneously Effective, but painful Often requires repeat injections at 3–6 month intervals
Thoracic sympathectomy	Reserved for patients with severe or recalcitrant disease Postoperative compensatory sweating may occur Video-assisted surgery: quicker and fewer complications

Adapted from Stolman LP. Treatment of hyperhidrosis. *Dermatol Clin* 1998;16(4):863–869; and Gelbard CM, Epstein H, Hebert A. Primary pediatric hyperhidrosis: A review of current treatment options. *Pediatr Dermatol* 2008;25(6):591–598. Copyright © 2008 by John Wiley & Sons, Inc. Reprinted by permission of John Wiley & Sons, Inc.

Iontophoresis is a successful therapy for some patients. This therapy utilizes a small device that delivers a direct current utilizing tap water as the conductive medium. Its proposed mechanism of action is the development of keratotic plugs in the eccrine sweat ducts, and its effect may last up to 6 weeks between treatments. This treatment appears to be quite safe, with side-effects limited to dryness and fissuring of treated sites. Iontophoresis units (Drionic, General Medical Co., Los Angeles) are available without a prescription via mail or internet (www.drionic.com) orders.

Botulinum toxin type A, injected either intradermally or 'intracutaneously' (more superficial injections), has been demonstrated to be quite effective in the treatment of axillary or palmoplantar hyperhidrosis.[125-127] Studies have revealed improved quality of life and an excellent safety profile of this modality.[127-129] In patients with severe and recalcitrant idiopathic hyperhidrosis, surgical therapy may be indicated. Thoracoscopic sympathectomy (or endoscopic thoracic sympathectomy) is the traditionally utilized procedure, although postoperative compensatory and gustatory sweating may be a problem.[130-133] Up to 20% of patients may have such severe disabling compensatory sweating that they regret having had the procedure.[134]

Dyshidrosis

Dyshidrosis (dyshidrotic eczema or pompholyx) is the term applied to a condition of recurring vesiculation of the palms, soles, and lateral aspects of the fingers in which hyperhidrosis is often associated. It is not a primary disorder of eccrine glands, but rather a type of eczematous eruption. It is discussed in more detail in Chapter 3.

Anhidrosis

Anhidrosis is the abnormal absence of (or, in the case of hypohidrosis, decrease in) perspiration from the surface of the skin in the presence of appropriate stimuli, which may result in hyperthermia. This condition may be caused by a deficiency or abnormality of the sweat glands (as in hypohidrotic ectodermal dysplasia, see Ch. 7) or of the nervous pathways from the peripheral or central nervous system leading to the sweat glands (as in syringomyelia, leprosy, anticholinergic drug therapy, or sympathectomy). Cool baths, air conditioning, light clothing, and reduction of the causes of normal perspiration help to relieve symptoms.

In *congenital insensitivity to pain with anhidrosis*, patients have recurrent episodes of fever, anhidrosis, absence of reaction to noxious stimuli, self-mutilating behavior, and mental retardation. These patients frequently show evidence of oral self-mutilation, including biting injuries and scarring of soft tissues of the mouth and oral mucosa.[135] This autosomal recessive condition has been ascribed to defects on the *NTRK1* gene, which encodes the receptor tyrosine kinase for nerve growth factor.[136]

Bromhidrosis

Bromhidrosis is an embarrassing malodorous condition in which an excessive, usually offensive, odor emanates from the skin. It may be of two types: (1) apocrine, resulting from bacterial degradation of apocrine sweat, or (2) eccrine, from the microbiologic degradation of stratum corneum softened by excessive eccrine sweat.

The term *apocrine bromhidrosis* refers to an exaggeration of the axillary odor normally noted by all postpubertal individuals. *Eccrine bromhidrosis* refers to the excessive odor produced by bacterial action on the stratum corneum when it becomes macerated by eccrine sweat. This disorder occurs primarily on the plantar surfaces of the feet and intertriginous areas, particular the inguinal region. Eccrine

bromhidrosis may also occur in association with metabolic disorders, including phenylketonuria, maple syrup urine disease, and isovaleric acidemia.

Bromhidrosis is best managed by regular thorough cleansing (preferably with an antibacterial soap), the use of commercial deodorants and antiperspirants, the application of topical antibiotics as necessary, and frequent changes of clothing. Plantar bromhidrosis may be associated with pitted keratolysis (see Ch. 14).

Miliaria

Miliaria (see also Ch. 2) is a common dermatosis caused by sweat retention, and is characterized by a papulovesicular eruption secondary to prolonged sweating with obstruction of the eccrine ducts. The pathophysiologic events that lead to this disorder are keratinous plugging of eccrine ducts followed by disruption of the normal escape of eccrine sweat into the skin. The clinical findings vary depending on the depth of obstruction of the eccrine duct within the skin. The three forms of miliaria are miliaria crystallina (sudamina), miliaria rubra (prickly heat), and miliaria profunda. The incidence of miliaria is greatest in the first few weeks of life, owing to a relative immaturity of the eccrine ducts that favors poral closure and sweat retention. In addition, older infants and children may develop miliaria in any situation predisposing them to increased sweating and/or skin obstruction (i.e., warm summer climates, swaddling with several layers of clothing during winter months, febrile illnesses).

Miliaria crystallina is characterized by clear, thinwalled, noninflammatory vesicles, 1–2 mm in diameter, occurring in crops on otherwise normal-appearing skin. The vesicles are asymptomatic and occur most frequently in intertriginous areas, particularly on the neck and axillae, or on parts of the trunk covered by clothing. Lesions of miliaria crystallina are highly characteristic and easily differentiated from other vesicular diseases. When the diagnosis is in doubt, rupture of vesicles with a fine needle results in release of the clear, entrapped sweat. The obstruction in miliaria crystallina is quite superficial, either within or just beneath the stratum corneum.

Miliaria rubra (prickly heat) is the most common form of miliaria. These lesions have a predilection for occluded areas of skin, especially the upper trunk, back, volar aspects of the arms, and body folds. The face may also be involved. Clinically, there are discrete but closely aggregated, small erythematous papules or papulovesicles (see Ch. 2, Fig. 2.8). The lesions of miliaria rubra are always non-follicular, which helps to differentiate this disorder from folliculitis. Viral exanthems and drug reactions may sometimes be in the clinical differential diagnosis, but the distribution of lesions combined with the history and physical examination usually allow for distinction. *Miliaria pustulosa* is a variant of miliaria rubra consisting of distinct superficial pustules, also not associated with hair follicles. Lesions tend to occur in areas of skin that have had previous inflammation and frequently appear coexistent with lesions of miliaria rubra.

Miliaria profunda is a more pronounced form of miliaria quite uncommon outside of the tropics. This disorder usually follows repeated episodes of miliaria rubra and is characterized by firm, white, 1–3 mm papules. This papular presentation is related to the deep level of obstruction. Lesions are most prominent on the trunk and proximal extremities, and this form of miliaria is extremely rare in infants and children.

The key to the management of miliaria is prevention by avoidance of excessive heat and humidity. In infants, all that is generally required is parental reassurance and advice on proper clothing and temperature regulation. The lesions of miliaria are self-limited, but simple strategies such as cool baths, light clothing, and use of air conditioning can make the patient more comfortable while awaiting resolution. Topical preparations are of little value, and in fact may further propagate the condition by compounding eccrine duct obstruction.

Granulosis Rubra Nasi

Granulosis rubra nasi is a rare chronic disease that occurs on the nose (occasionally the cheeks and chin) of prepubertal children, with the highest reported incidence between the ages of 7 and 15 years. It is characterized by diffuse redness, persistent hyperhidrosis, and discrete red or brown-red macules and soft papules on an erythematous base. Vesicles and small cystic lesions may also occur. The etiology of granulosis rubra nasi is unknown, but it appears to represent an inherited disorder. The role of the sweat glands and cutaneous vasculature is obscure, although occasionally this disease is associated with hyperhidrosis of the palms and soles. The condition may be a complication of hyperhidrosis, and was noted to occur in a patient with pheochromocytoma, with involution of the lesions following surgical excision of the tumor.[137]

No effective local or systemic therapy is available for this disorder, although simple drying lotions, tinted to help obscure the erythema, may provide symptomatic and cosmetic relief. Although granulosis rubra nasi may sometimes persist into later years, it usually disappears by puberty.

Key References

The complete list of 137 references for this chpater is available online at **www.expertconsult.com.**
See inside cover for registration details.

El-Hallak M, Giani T, Yeniay BS, et al. Chronic minocycline-induced autoimmunity in children. *J Pediatr.* 2008;153(3):314–319.

Gelbard CM, Epstein H, Hebert A. Primary pediatric hyperhidrosis: A review of current treatment options. *Pediatr Dermatol.* 2008; 25(6):591–598.

George R, Clarke S, Thiboutot D. Hormonal therapy for acne. *Sem Cutan Med Surg.* 2008;27:188–196.

Nguyen V, Eichenfield LF. Periorificial dermatitis in children and adolescents. *J Am Acad Dermatol.* 2006;55:781–785.

Strauss JS, Krowchuk DP, Leyden JJ, et al. Guidelines of care for acne vulgaris management. *J Am Acad Dermatol.* 2007;56:651–663.

Thiboutot D, Gollnick H, Bettoli V, et al. New insights into the management of acne: An update from the Global Alliance to Improve Outcomes in Acne Group. *J Am Acad Dermatol.* 2009;60:S1–50.

Zaenglein AL, Thiboutot DM. Expert committee recommendations for acne management. *Pediatrics.* 2006;118(3):1188–1199.

9 Cutaneous Tumors and Tumor Syndromes

Because of the increasing public awareness and frequency of skin cancer, physicians are frequently consulted regarding tumors of the skin. In children, the vast majority of cutaneous tumors are benign, and their importance lies predominantly in the cosmetic defect they may create or in their occasional association with systemic disease. Malignant skin lesions, however, despite their relative rarity in children, cannot be completely disregarded or ignored. Each lesion in children, as in adults, must be assessed individually with a consideration of its cosmetic effect, its possible association with systemic manifestations, and its capacity for malignant degeneration.

Cutaneous tumors can be differentiated into those arising from epidermal (or mucosal) cells, from melanocytes, from the epidermal appendages, or from dermal or subcutaneous cells or tissues. The latter category includes tumors of fibrous, neural, vascular, fatty, muscular, and osseous tissues. Skin tumors can also be divided into benign (the vast majority of lesions in children) and malignant. The term *nevus* (plural *nevi*) has a broad meaning in dermatology. Strictly defined, this term refers to a circumscribed congenital abnormality of the skin. When this term is used, therefore, it is appropriate to include a qualifying adjective (i.e., epidermal nevus, melanocytic nevus, or vascular nevus), thus specifying the cell of origin. In commonplace practice, however, the term *nevus* is usually used to imply a benign tumor of pigment cells (melanocytes). Hence, to many practitioners, a nevus is the same as a 'mole'.

In this chapter, we will discuss several cutaneous tumors (and corresponding tumor syndromes, where applicable). Pigmented lesions are discussed as a separate entity apart from the above classification, given their high incidence.

Pigmented lesions

Pigmented lesions, especially melanocytic nevi (moles), are the most common neoplasms found in humans. In this section, we will discuss melanocytic nevi (both congenital and acquired) and several variants, including dysplastic, Spitz, and halo types. Nevus spilus and Becker's nevus, two distinct pigmented lesions, will also be discussed as will malignant melanoma, which, although rare in childhood, does occasionally occur.

Melanocytic Nevi

Melanocytic nevi are extremely common skin neoplasms composed of 'nevocytes' or nevus cells, which are believed to be slightly altered melanocytes. The melanocyte is a dendritic cell that produces melanin and transfers it to keratinocytes (epidermal cells) and hair cells, thus supplying the normal brown pigment to skin and hair. Both melanocytes and nevus cells are of neural origin. Melanocytes originate in the neural crest and early in fetal life migrate from there to the skin. After birth, some melanocytes will occasionally remain in the dermis of certain races (Asians, Native Americans, African-Americans, and individuals from the Mediterranean region), where

they may appear as Mongolian spots (Ch. 11). Blue nevi and the nevi of Ota and Ito (Ch. 11) also represent examples of arrested melanocytic migration in which the melanoblasts remain in the dermis.

Melanocytic nevi can be either congenital (described in more detail below) or acquired. Acquired nevi usually appear after infancy, increase in size and number during early childhood, and peak during the third or fourth decade, with slow involution as aging progresses. The predisposition of an individual to the development of acquired melanocytic nevi seems to be related to several factors, including skin type, race, genetic predisposition, and ultraviolet light exposure. These lesions tend to be few in childhood, increasing in number with age to a peak in the third decade. Sun exposure, sunburns, and fair skin pigmentation seem to be associated with their development in childhood.[1] In one large cross-sectional study, nevus counts were found to steadily increase with age from a median of three at age 2 years to 19 at age 7 years.[1] High numbers of nevi were associated with moderate sun exposure and outdoor activities. In another study, 5- and 6-year-old children with a history of sunburns or an increased number of holidays in foreign countries with a sunny climate had significantly higher nevus counts than controls without these characteristics.[2] Higher numbers of childhood nevi have been demonstrated in areas of skin chronically exposed to the sun, and in children with lighter skin, blond hair, and blue eyes.[3] Higher nevus counts are noted in children who reside in sunny climates (i.e., Australia) when compared with age- and race-matched control children. Melanocytic nevi may also occur in higher numbers in children with a history of leukemia and/or a history of chemotherapy, and in these settings, the lesions may occur with greater frequency on acral areas such as the palms and soles.[4–6]

The primary importance of melanocytic nevi lies in their possible transformation into malignant melanoma. These lesions are felt to be both markers of an increased risk of cutaneous melanoma and, in some cases, direct precursor lesions.[7] The annual transformation rate of a single mole into melanoma seems extremely low, with an estimate of ≤0.0005% for individuals younger than 40 years.[7] Nonetheless, melanocytic nevus cells were seen histologically in proximity to malignant melanoma in 51% of cases in one study.[8] Genetic analyses of nevi and melanoma reveal non-random patterns of genetic alteration (loss of heterozygosity), confirming the notion that the former are precursor lesions for the latter.[9] These findings highlight the relevance of close monitoring of melanocytic nevi for atypical features as well as the importance of sun protection education.

Melanocytic nevi are subdivided and clinically described based on the microscopic location of the nevus cells. Accordingly, they are divided into *junctional*, *intradermal*, or *compound* lesions. Junctional nevi have proliferation of nevocytes at the dermal-epidermal junction, compound nevi reveal cells at the junction and in the dermis, and intradermal nevi reveal loss of the epidermal component with nests of cells limited to the dermis. Interestingly, these histologic

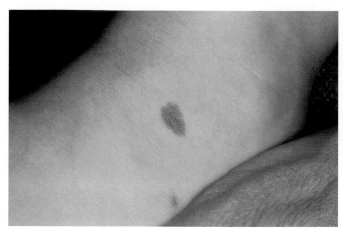

Figure 9.1 Junctional melanocytic nevus. A well-demarcated, tan macule.

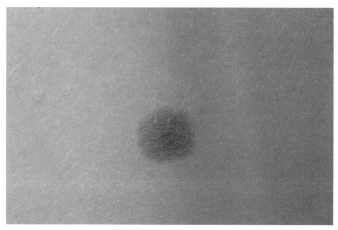

Figure 9.2 Compound melanocytic nevus. A well-demarcated, tan papule with some darker speckling centrally.

subtypes progress in parallel to the natural history of nevus maturation (junctional nevi early in life, then compound nevi, and finally intradermal nevi with eventual atrophy of the dermal component during later adulthood).[10] Melanocytic nevi have a wide range of clinical appearances. They may occur anywhere on the cutaneous or mucocutaneous surface and may be flat, slightly elevated, dome-shaped, nodular, verrucous, polypoid, cerebriform, or papillomatous.

Junctional nevi

Junctional nevi usually occur as hairless, light to dark brown or black macules (Fig. 9.1). They range from 1 mm to 1 cm in diameter, with a smooth and flat (non-palpable) surface and preservation of skin furrows. Although most junctional nevi are round, elliptical, or oval and show a relatively uniform pigmentation, some may be slightly irregular in configuration and color. Most junctional nevi represent a transient phase in the development of compound nevi and are found only in children. An exception to this rule, however, is seen on the palms, soles, and genitalia where the lesions often retain their junctional appearance.

Compound nevi

Compound nevi are more common in older children and adults, but may also be present in younger children. They may appear similar to junctional nevi, but tend to be more elevated and accordingly vary from a slightly raised papule to a larger, papillomatous papule or plaque. They are flesh-colored to brown (Fig. 9.2), may have a smooth or verrucous surface, and may have dark coarse hairs within them (Fig. 9.3), especially when occurring on the face. During later childhood and adolescence, compound nevi tend to increase in thickness and depth of pigmentation. It is at this stage that many children are brought to the physician for evaluation.

Intradermal nevi

Intradermal nevi are seen most frequently in adults. They are usually dome-shaped, soft, 'fleshy' papules (Fig. 9.4). They may be sessile (attached by a broad base) or more pedunculated (attached by a more narrow base) and range from a few millimeters to ≥1 cm in diameter. Intradermal nevi may be clinically indistinguishable from compound nevi, and their color varies from non-pigmented (flesh-colored) lesions to those of varying shades of brown. They may occur anywhere on the skin surface and are frequently found on the head and neck; coarse hairs often are present. After the third decade

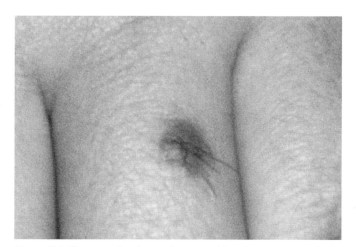

Figure 9.3 Compound melanocytic nevus. Note the coarse, terminal hairs within the nevus.

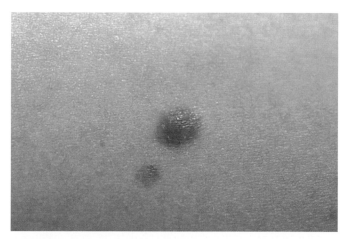

Figure 9.4 Intradermal melanocytic nevus. A tan, fleshy papule with adjacent intradermal nevus.

of life, as nevus maturation continues, there is destruction and replacement of nevus cells by fibrous or fatty tissue, and by 70 years of age most individuals have few remaining nevi. In fact, nevi that persist into old age appear to have an increased risk of malignant degeneration.[7]

Treatment decisions regarding melanocytic nevi are usually related to their cosmetic appearance, repeated irritation of the lesion, or fear of potential malignant transformation. The majority of melanocytic lesions require no treatment; by careful clinical evaluation the patient can frequently be reassured as to their benign nature. Removal of nevi, when indicated, is best achieved by punch biopsy or complete surgical excision. Any nevus being removed because of concern for malignant degeneration should be removed with a full-depth excision, since microscopic tumor depth is the primary prognostic indicator in malignant melanoma. Every excised nevus should be subjected to histopathologic examination.

Many authors advocate for the routine excision of pigmented lesions in certain anatomic locations (i.e., palms, soles, scalp and genitalia), owing to the belief that the likelihood of malignant transformation is greater in these areas. It seems that prophylactic excision of all nevi in these locations is unwarranted. However, lesions in acral sites may reveal atypical clinical and histologic features,[11,12] possibly in relation to repetitive trauma. Recognition of these histologic variations is vital in order to avoid the misdiagnosis of the 'acral lentiginous' subtype of malignant melanoma, which occurs primarily after the seventh decade of life. Additionally, scalp nevi in children (and particularly adolescents) may commonly reveal mild clinical atypia, both clinically and histologically, although the vast majority behave in a biologically benign fashion.[13] Scalp nevi which reveal significant atypia and/or which may be difficult to follow clinically, however, may merit excision.

Occasionally, pigmented nevi will show recurrence after excision, which may be a significant source of anxiety for the patient, parent, and at times, the physician. Recurrent lesions (which have been called 'pseudomelanoma' by some) present as circumscribed pigmentation within the surgical scar (Fig. 9.5). This finding is usually not an indication of malignancy, but instead represents proliferation of nevus cells from the peripheral epidermis, sweat ducts, or hair follicles. Options for management include close clinical follow-up (assuming the original pathologic examination revealed no atypical findings) or repeat excision.

Melanonychia Striata

Melanonychia striata (also known as longitudinal melanonychia) is most commonly seen in individuals with darker skin complexions, especially African-Americans in whom up to 90% may have at least one such streak. It is significantly less common in children with white skin. Melanonychia striata presents as a brown to brown/black linear band of pigmentation on a fingernail (Fig. 9.6) or toenail. The pigmentation extends from the proximal nail fold to the distal margin of the digit, and the width may vary from <1 mm to several millimeters. Drugs, pregnancy, trauma, and HIV infection may all be associated with melanonychia striata, although the majority of patients have no underlying association.

Melanonychia striata may represent benign melanocytic hyperplasia (i.e., melanocytic nevus or lentigo) or a nail matrix melanoma. In children, the majority of cases seem to be related to benign lesions,[14,15] although the possibility of melanoma must always be entertained. The presence of multiple bands, as occasionally seen in darker races, is reassuring and mitigates against malignancy. Worrisome features may include very dark, broad bands and extension of the pigmentation onto the proximal or lateral nailfolds (Hutchinson's sign; Fig. 9.7).[16] In patients with melanonychia striata and any such atypical or concerning features, nail matrix biopsy for histologic evaluation should be highly considered. Although this procedure may result in permanent nail plate dystrophy, this risk is justified when concerns for possible melanoma exist.

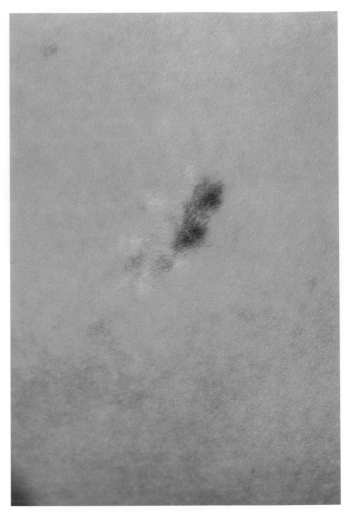

Figure 9.5 Recurrent melanocytic nevus (within a surgical scar). The initial nevus had been incompletely excised.

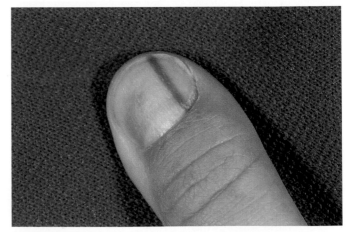

Figure 9.6 Melanonychia striata. A 2 mm, evenly pigmented band. Note the absence of pigmentation of the proximal nail fold (negative Hutchinson's sign).

Congenital Melanocytic Nevi

Congenital melanocytic nevi represent a special group of melanocytic lesions with an increased risk of transformation to malignant melanoma. By strict definition, these lesions are present at birth. However, in some patients with small and medium-sized lesions,

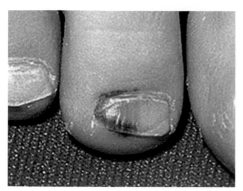

Figure 9.7 Hutchinson's sign. Note pigmentation involving both the proximal nail fold and the distal nail fold regions. This patient underwent nail matrix biopsy; the lesion was a compound nevus without atypia.

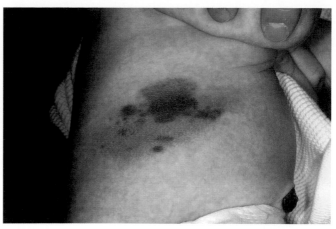

Figure 9.8 Early congenital melanocytic nevus. Note the various shades of brown and red in this 2-week-old infant boy.

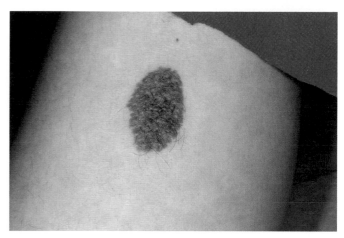

Figure 9.9 Congenital melanocytic nevus. A well-demarcated, brown plaque with some pigment variation and hypertrichosis.

they may be initially noted sometime during the first year of life rather than immediately at birth. Congenital nevi have been classified traditionally according to their greatest diameter in *adulthood*. According to this nomenclature, they are defined as *small* (<1.5 cm in greatest diameter), *medium-sized* (1.5–19.9 cm), or *large* (≥20 cm) congenital nevi. Approximately 1% of newborns have a small congenital nevus, and large lesions occur in around 1 in 20 000 newborns.[17-20] Giant melanocytic nevi occur in 1 in 500 000 newborns.[21] Nevus spilus, or speckled lentiginous nevus (see below), may represent a distinct subtype of congenital melanocytic nevus that presents early in life as a café-au-lait macule, with the development of the more characteristic nevi a bit later in life.[22]

Congenital nevi have some characteristic histopathologic features, including extension of nevus cells into the deeper dermis and subcutis, between the collagen bundles (as single cells), and in association with appendages, nerves, and vessels.[23,24] These features may be useful when histologic confirmation of a congenital lesion is desired, but such findings may not be noted in every congenital nevus. This pattern of deep extension is important to keep in mind when surgical intervention of such a lesion is being considered. While the etiology of congenital nevi is unclear, one series revealed frequent activating mutations in the *NRAS* gene, distinct from nevi developing after birth (acquired nevi), which are more likely to reveal mutations in *BRAF* (see also below).[25,26]

Small and medium-sized congenital melanocytic nevi usually present as flat, light to dark brown or pink macules (Fig. 9.8) or papules or as brown to dark brown, well-circumscribed patches or plaques. They may reveal some pigment variation and the surface may have hair (Fig. 9.9). With time they tend to become more elevated, and coarse dark brown hairs may become more prominent. When an extremity is circumferentially involved with a medium- or large-sized congenital nevus, limb underdevelopment may occur (Fig. 9.10).[10]

Large congenital nevi are uniformly present at birth and present as dark brown to black plaques, often with a verrucous or cobblestoned surface and hypertrichosis (Fig. 9.11). Color variation is common in these lesions, and may make clinical examination for concerning features more challenging. Giant congenital nevi often occur on the posterior trunk, and may occupy a significant portion of the skin surface. They may have a dermatomal distribution, and may involve an entire upper or lower extremity or the scalp. These lesions have been variably named *coat-sleeve, stocking, bathing trunk, or giant hairy* nevi, depending on their site(s) of involvement. As with large congenital nevi, giant nevi present as large, brown to black plaques with varying degrees of nodularity, color variation,

and hypertrichosis (Fig. 9.12). Erosions or ulcerations in these giant lesions may occur (Fig. 9.13), and although once believed to be consistently ominous findings, are often benign and usually not indicative of malignant melanoma.[27] Large and giant congenital nevi may be associated with cosmetic disfigurement, an increased risk of malignant melanoma, and underlying neurocutaneous melanosis (see below). These lesions frequently have associated 'satellite' nevi, which may be disseminated over the entire skin surface. Satellite nevi are usually tan to brown macules or papules, with varying degrees of hypertrichosis (Fig. 9.14). They may be present at birth or continue to develop during infancy.[20]

The congenital nature of nevi is one of several known risk factors for malignant melanoma, but the exact magnitude of risk remains controversial, especially for small and medium-sized lesions. All congenital nevi should be considered as potential precursors to melanoma. The risk in small and medium-sized lesions seems low, and if melanoma occurs, it tends to occur during adulthood.[10,28,29] Factors that might increase the level of concern include atypical clinical features (deeply or irregularly pigmented, rapidly growing, etc.), an abnormal nevus phenotype, or a strong family history of malignant melanoma. The risk of malignant transformation of congenital nevi in African-American patients is extremely small.[30]

The risk of malignant melanoma in large congenital nevi appears to be significantly greater than that for small and medium-sized

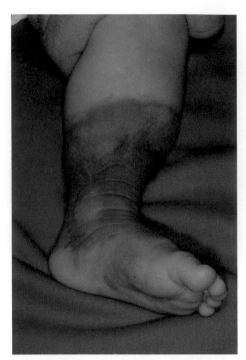

Figure 9.10 Congenital nevus of the lower extremity. Note the limb hypoplasia in the ankle region associated with this circumferential lesion.

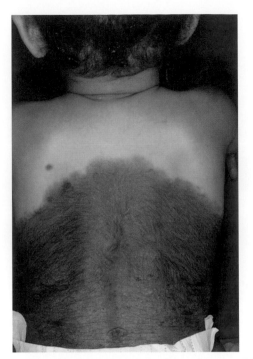

Figure 9.12 Giant congenital melanocytic nevus. Note the marked hypertrichosis and adjacent satellite lesions.

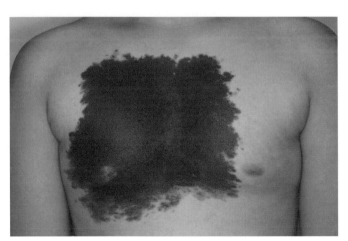

Figure 9.11 Large congenital melanocytic nevus.

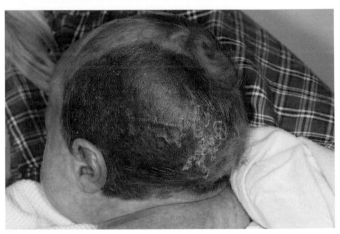

Figure 9.13 Giant congenital melanocytic nevus with erosions. Surface erosion and crusting was present at birth, and healed rapidly over a few weeks with topical care.

lesions, with melanoma often (but not always) occurring before the age of 5 years.[31,32] It is unclear whether axial lesions pose a greater risk than those occurring on the extremities, as traditionally suggested.[33] When melanoma occurs in patients with large congenital nevi, it may occur within the skin or in extracutaneous sites such as the central nervous system.[34,35] Development of melanoma in satellite lesions is exceedingly unlikely.[34] The overall lifetime risk of development of malignant melanoma in patients with large congenital nevi has been reported to range from 0% to 31%, but is best estimated at between 4.5% and 10%.[31,32,36] In addition to melanoma, other malignancies may occur with increased frequencies in these patients, including rhabdomyosarcoma, liposarcoma, malignant peripheral nerve sheath tumor, and other sarcomas.[18,34]

Large and giant congenital nevi, particularly those on the head, neck and back, may be associated with a condition termed *neurocutaneous melanosis* (NCM). NCM, as well as melanoma risk, appears to be more common in patients with greater numbers of satellite nevi.[37,38] Patients with NCM have a proliferation of nevus cells in the central nervous system (leptomeningeal melanocytosis), and are predisposed to seizures, malignant melanoma of the CNS, and neurologic symptoms related to increased intracranial pressure or spinal cord compression. They often present with symptoms during the first 3 years of life, including lethargy, irritability, headache, recurrent vomiting, seizures, increased head circumference, bulging anterior fontanelle, photophobia, papilledema, neck stiffness, and occasionally nerve palsies, particularly of cranial nerves VI and VII. Magnetic resonance (MR) imaging of NCM reveals focal areas of high signal on T1-weighted images in one or multiple areas of the brain, including the temporal lobes, cerebellum, pons, and medulla.[39,40] T2 shortening may also occur.[40] In one study, 45% of

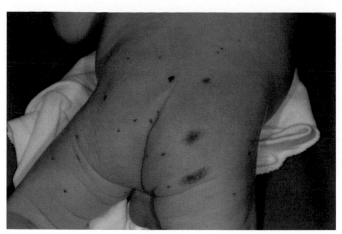

Figure 9.14 Satellite melanocytic nevi. This patient had a giant nevus of the scalp.

Table 9.1 Risk factors for malignant melanoma in children
Familial atypical multiple mole-melanoma (FAMMM) syndrome
Xeroderma pigmentosum
Congenital melanocytic nevi
Atypical ('dysplastic') nevi
Personal history of melanoma
Family history of melanoma
High numbers of melanocytic nevi
Fair complexion
Excessive sun exposures
History of blistering sunburns
History of immunosuppression

neurologically asymptomatic children with giant congenital nevi had these radiologic findings.[39] However, a questionnaire-based study of 186 patients with large congenital nevi who were imaged revealed that only 4.8% of those with positive MR findings for NCM were asymptomatic.[41] Hence, the exact prevalence of asymptomatic NCM remains unclear. Overall, the prognosis for *symptomatic* NCM is poor, with >90% of patients dying of the disease, and around 70% of those dying before 10 years of age.[35,42]

The management of congenital nevi must be individualized for each patient. There are many factors that must be considered in the decision-making process regarding surgical excision of such lesions. These include location of the nevus, size, cosmetic issues (and potential psychosocial ramifications), and the risks of anesthesia, malignant melanoma, and neurocutaneous melanosis.[43] There appears to be less consensus regarding the role of surgical excision of small and medium-sized congenital nevi than that of large lesions. Small congenital nevi with uniform pigmentation, smooth texture, and lack of nodules can be clinically followed, whereas lesions with atypical or deep pigmentation or uneven textures may warrant surgical excision given the heightened difficulty of melanoma detection in this setting.[18] Other risk factors, such as a strong family history of malignant melanoma or the presence of numerous atypical-appearing nevi, may influence the decision regarding surgical removal of small and medium-sized congenital nevi. Lesions located in areas that may be difficult to follow clinically, such as the scalp or groin, may be better served by excision, although in the case of benign-appearing lesions, this decision may be delayed until the child is older and the procedure can be performed under local anesthesia.

Large congenital nevi are often treated with surgical excision. The primary reason for this recommendation is the potentially-decreased risk of malignant transformation, although controlled studies supporting this hypothesis are lacking.[43] Unfortunately, excision of large lesions does not usually result in complete removal of all nevus cells, and melanoma may still develop from this residual tissue. In addition, melanoma may develop with increased frequency at extracutaneous sites in these patients, and the significance of neurocutaneous melanosis (if present) must also be factored into this decision. Nonetheless, most still advocate for surgical excision in an effort to reduce the risk of malignancy.[44,45] Removal of these lesions has been refined with the use of tissue expanders and skin grafting, but multiple procedures are usually required. Partial thickness removal techniques (i.e., dermabrasion, curettage, and laser therapy) have been advocated by some, but the impact of these procedures on malignant transformation or clinical surveillance of the lesion must be further defined.

Close periodic clinical surveillance is important for all patients with congenital melanocytic nevi. Parent education in the importance of sun protection, sunscreen use, and danger signs of atypical nevi or melanoma (see below) is vital. Risks of malignant transformation should be discussed, and parents and patients allowed to reach an informed decision regarding therapy. Educational materials regarding moles, melanoma, and sun protection are useful, and may be obtained from the American Academy of Dermatology (www.aad.org). A multidisciplinary approach must be employed for families of children with large congenital nevi. This includes the primary care physician, dermatologist, plastic surgeon, and diagnostic radiologist. Emotional support should be provided, and the family should be given information on support groups. One such organization is Nevus Outreach, Inc. (www.nevus.org), which was founded by parents of children with large congenital nevi, and offers an annual family conference, newsletters, and a social support network.

Atypical Nevi/Familial Atypical Multiple Mole–Melanoma (FAMMM) Syndrome

Atypical nevi, also known as dysplastic nevi, are defined based on their clinical and/or histologic appearance. These acquired nevi, which often do not present until at or after puberty, are regarded as markers and potential precursors for malignant melanoma. The frequency of histologically confirmed atypical nevi in patients under 18 years of age is very low,[46] although in children who come from melanoma-prone families, their incidence seems much higher.[47] Clinically, these lesions share some or all of the features of malignant melanoma (Table 9.1). These include larger size and irregularities of color, texture, or borders (Fig. 9.15). Atypical nevi are frequently larger than common acquired nevi, usually measuring 6–15 mm in diameter, and display marked lesion-to-lesion variability, often with a cobblestone appearance or a small, dark, central papule surrounded by a lighter brown periphery (the 'fried egg' appearance, Fig. 9.16).

Atypical nevi may occur anywhere, especially on sun-exposed sites, but also frequently occur on covered areas such as the back and in unusual locations such as the buttocks, breasts, and scalp.[48] In fact, a fairly high proportion of nevi removed from the scalp may demonstrate histologic features of atypical nevi.[14,49] Individuals with atypical nevi have been demonstrated to have an increased risk of melanoma, despite the presence or absence of a family history of melanoma.[50,51] A distinct clinical phenotype characterized by numerous (>100), small, darkly pigmented atypical nevi has been described and termed the 'cheetah' phenotype.[52] Longitudinal

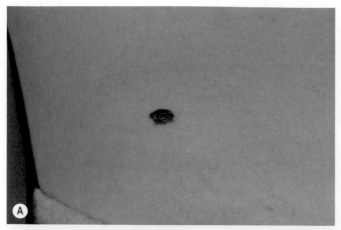

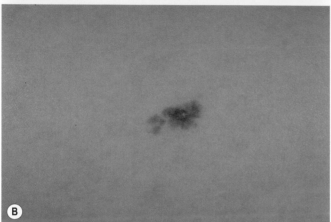

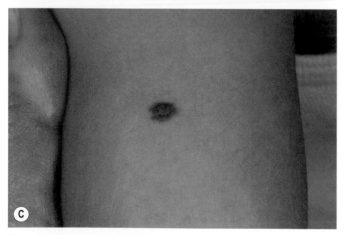

Figure 9.15 (A–C) Atypical melanocytic nevi. These lesions revealed clinically atypical features, including asymmetry and border and color irregularity. All of them were benign histologically.

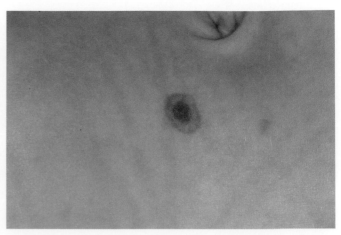

Figure 9.16 'Fried egg' melanocytic nevus. Note the elevated, dark brown papule centrally and surrounding tan macular area.

follow-up of such patients is very challenging given the similar clinical appearance of several histologic patterns, ranging from benign to cytologically atypical.[52]

The familial atypical multiple mole–melanoma (FAMMM) syndrome is a disorder of autosomal dominant inheritance, in which atypical nevi develop during the late second to third decade of life.[53] It was originally described in 1978 by Clark and colleagues, when they noted individuals with increased numbers of melanocytic nevi that displayed atypical clinical and histologic features.[54] Since the original description, FAMMM syndrome has been better

characterized as a hereditary cancer predisposition syndrome, entailing not only an increased risk of malignant melanoma, but also other cancers in some kindreds, especially pancreatic cancer.[55–57] It has been estimated that individuals with a family history of FAMMM and atypical nevi have nearly a 100% lifetime risk of acquiring malignant melanoma. In addition to melanoma of the skin, these individuals may develop intraocular melanoma.

The classic features of FAMMM syndrome are high numbers of melanocytic nevi, often >50, some of which are atypical and often with large variability in size (Fig. 9.17), and in the setting of a family history of malignant melanoma in one or more first- or second-degree relatives.[48] Identification of at-risk children is vital, since melanoma may occur before 20 years of age in up to 10% of individuals.[10] Although most of the atypical nevi develop during or after adolescence, prepubertal children may occasionally show the atypical nevus phenotype, particularly in scalp nevi. In fact, the development of scalp nevi during childhood, as well as large nevus counts early in life, may represent early indicators of increased risk for the atypical mole phenotype later in life.[47,58]

There are several known melanoma susceptibility loci, most notably the *p16/CDKN2A* gene on chromosome 9, which is a tumor suppressor gene responsible for melanoma susceptibility in some kindreds with FAMMM syndrome.[53] Deletion of p16 may play a role in the development of atypical nevi as an early event, as well as in the development of malignant melanoma (see below).

Management of the patient with atypical nevi should include a thorough family history, total body inspection, and regular clinical follow up every 6–12 months, depending on the individual patient. Patients (and parents) should be educated regarding sun protection, regular skin self-examination, and atypical features of nevi, and surgical excision should be performed for lesions with concerning features. A helpful guideline in following children with many nevi is the 'ugly duckling' principle, which dictates that a lesion that stands out from the rest (i.e., markedly darker pigmentation, more irregularity of texture or borders) should be more closely scrutinized and considered for removal. Epiluminescence microscopy (dermatoscopy) is a useful non-invasive instrument that provides magnification of nevi and may be useful in differentiating benign from atypical lesions. It is most often used by dermatologists, and its use requires training and experience in order to provide acceptable sensitivity and reliability. Serial photography of nevi may also be a useful adjunct in the longitudinal follow-up of patients with multiple or atypical nevi.

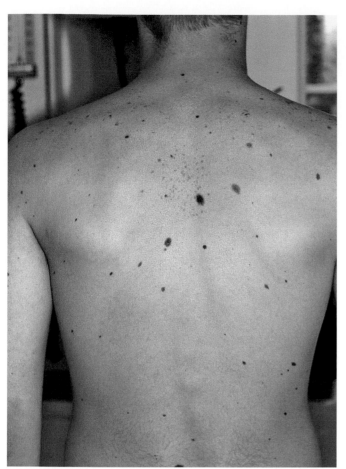

Figure 9.17 Multiple atypical melanocytic nevi (FAMMM type). This adolescent male had a family history of atypical nevi and malignant melanoma.

	Clinical feature	Comment
A	Asymmetry	The two halves of the lesion are not alike
B	Border irregularity	Borders notched, scalloped, irregular
C	Color changes	Especially blue, red, black, white
D	Diameter >6 mm	Size of a pencil eraser; not applicable to congenital nevi which are often >6 mm early in their evolution
E	Enlargement	Evolutionary change in the lesion

Table 9.2 Clinical features (the ABCDE signs) of malignant melanoma

Malignant Melanoma

The incidence of malignant melanoma (MM), the most deadly form of skin cancer, continues to rise and, although childhood MM continues to be rare, the incidence in this population may also be rising.[59,60] The lifetime incidence of melanoma is estimated at around 1 in 58 individuals,[61] which is an alarming increase from the incidence of 1 in 1500 estimated in 1935.[62] The challenges of diagnosing MM in children are multiple, and include lack of recognition, hesitancy to perform skin biopsies in children, and poor reliability in making the histopathologic diagnosis in this population.[63] Melanoma in individuals under 20 years of age accounts for only 1–3% of all MM, and prepubertal cases are even rarer, accounting for 0.3–0.4% of all cases.[64–66] Despite this rarity, the course of melanoma, when it does occur in a child, bears the same prognosis as it does in adults.[65,67,68] Interestingly, many lesions previously thought to be melanomas of childhood are now recognized to be benign Spitz nevi (see below). Congenital MM represents a small subset of all pediatric MM, and is extremely rare, with only 23 cases reported in the English literature between 1925 and 2002.[65] It most commonly arises in a congenital melanocytic nevus, and less commonly is de novo or related to transplacental transmission of MM from the mother.

Malignant melanoma most commonly affects individuals with fair skin, blue eyes, and red or blond hair, particularly those of Celtic origin whose pigment cells have a limited capacity to synthesize melanin. Approximately one-half to 65% of MM arise in a pre-existing nevus. Although melanomas may occur in African-American individuals, the incidence is extremely low when compared with that of Caucasians. In African-Americans, tumors usually arise in areas that are lightly pigmented, especially the mucous membranes, nail beds, or the sides of the palms and soles. Exposure to high levels of sunlight in childhood seems to be a strong determinant of risk for MM, although adult sun exposure also plays a role.[69] Some studies have not supported this 'critical risk period' hypothesis of ultraviolet radiation exposure, suggesting that sun protection education should be directed at the entire population with equal effort, rather than concentrating solely on younger age groups.[70] However, maintaining a stringent focus on childhood sun protection still seems reasonable, as a large proportion of overall lifetime sun exposure is likely to occur during these years.[71]

The genetics of MM have more recently been elucidated, and it is now established that molecular defects in both tumor suppressor genes and oncogenes may be pathogenetically linked to melanoma.[72] Mutations in the *CDKN2A* (*p16*) gene predispose to the FAMMM syndrome and have also been noted in families in which only one or two individuals are affected by MM.[73] A subset of melanoma-prone families with *CDKN2A* mutations also manifests an increased risk of pancreatic cancers.[57,72] Activating mutations in one of two Ras/mitogen-activated protein kinase pathway genes, *BRAF* or *NRAS*, are present in up to 80–90% of melanomas.[74,75] Some of the other genes potentially mutated in melanoma include *PTEN*, *CDK4*, *CCND1*, *c-KIT*, *MITF*, β-*catenin*, and various apoptosis genes.[74,75]

Melanoma is classically categorized according to its clinical and histologic features. The most common forms are superficial spreading, nodular, lentigo maligna (usually confined to adults), and acral lentiginous melanoma. However, pediatric cases of MM often cannot be neatly classified into one of these categories. Pediatric melanoma seems to follow the same distribution patterns as adult melanoma, with head and trunk lesions predominating in boys, and arm and leg lesions predominating in girls. Risk factors for pediatric MM are listed in Table 9.1.

The signs of MM are summarized in Table 9.2. Melanoma usually presents with a rapidly enlarging papule or nodule, most often brown to brown/black in color (Fig. 9.18), although blue, red, or white discoloration may also be noted. Importantly, a significant proportion of pediatric melanomas may present in an amelanotic (i.e., pink, white, red or a combination of these colors) fashion.[76] A halo of hypo- or depigmentation may be present around a primary lesion of MM, although most often these halos occur in the setting of benign nevi (see Halo Nevus, below). Melanomas frequently reveal asymmetry and irregularity of the borders, especially scalloping or notching, and tend to be larger than benign nevi, often (but not always) >10 mm in diameter. Bleeding, itching, ulceration, crusting, and pain may be present. Lymph nodes may be palpable and, if present, are an ominous prognostic

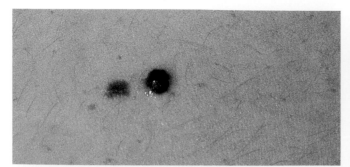

Figure 9.18 Malignant melanoma. This small, black papule was noted on this 10-year-old male with fair skin and red hair; excision confirmed a nodular malignant melanoma.

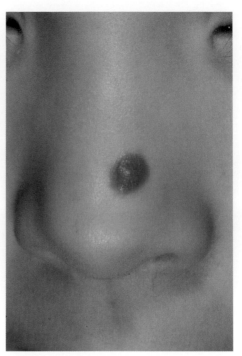

Figure 9.19 Spitz nevus. This patient had the erythematous type of Spitz nevus on her nose.

sign, suggesting metastatic spread. When MM goes undetected and undiagnosed, the lesion proliferates locally, and may spread by satellite lesions or extend through the lymphatics or bloodstream, from which it may eventually invade any organ of the body. Once metastatic disease occurs, the prognosis of MM significantly declines.

Early detection of melanoma is germane to long-term survival. The survival rate for children and adults seems to be similar, and the primary determinants of prognosis have traditionally been tumor thickness and depth of invasion.[62,67] The presence or absence of ulceration has been added to the American Joint Committee on Cancer (AJCC) staging system for MM as another important prognostic criterion (the presence of ulceration correlating with poorer prognosis).[77] The pediatrician (or other primary care provider of children) is in good position to follow pigmented skin lesions over time in their patients. Early referral should be considered for any melanocytic lesion that displays substantial growth changes, especially if asymmetry, ulceration, or other atypical features are present. Melanoma is diagnosed by histopathologic examination of skin tissue from biopsy. When MM is suspected, full-thickness excision of the lesion should be performed, as depth of the lesion must be fully visualized in order to assess this prognostic indicator. Shave biopsies or excisions should be avoided in the removal of concerning pigmented lesions.

Surgical excision is the initial step in melanoma management, along with adequately staging the disease. Once the diagnosis of MM is confirmed, the site is re-excised with appropriate margins (0.5–3 cm), depending on tumor depth in the initial specimen. Clinically suspected lymph nodes are surgically removed and histologically evaluated. Recent developments in tracer techniques have enabled sampling of the first lymph node draining the affected skin site (the 'sentinel' lymph node), which assists in determining whether to proceed with regional lymph node dissection for further staging and therapy. This technique, which is usually performed concurrently with re-excision of the primary lesion, allows for accurate staging of the regional lymph nodes with minimal morbidity.[67]

Treatment of more advanced stages of MM includes chemotherapy, radiotherapy, and immunotherapy, although the results have been somewhat discouraging.[78] Adjuvant interferon α-2b therapy has received much attention in the treatment of high-risk melanoma in adults, with reports of improved disease-free survival and overall survival rates. Recommendations for use of this agent in children have primarily been extrapolated from the adult data, and while potentially effective, its use may be associated with some toxicities at higher doses, which may be limiting when treating the pediatric melanoma patient.[79,80] Immunotherapeutic approaches to MM include melanoma vaccines, cytokine therapy, and passive immunotherapy with monoclonal antibodies, and these and other

approaches continue to be the topics of active investigation.[81] Traditional chemotherapy regimens have shown minimal activity against melanoma.[60] The prognosis for pediatric melanoma is strongly correlated with initial stage. In a review of data from the National Cancer Data Base of 3158 patients aged 1–19 years with melanoma, average 5-year survivals were 98.7% (*in situ* disease), 93.6% (localized invasive disease), 68% (regionally metastatic disease) and 11.8% (distant disease).[82]

Spitz Nevus

Spitz nevus is a distinct subtype of melanocytic nevus that occurs primarily in children. The importance of the Spitz nevus, which was formerly known as 'benign juvenile melanoma', lies in its histologic differentiation from malignant melanoma. This lesion was originally recognized in 1948 when Dr. Sophie Spitz realized that a subset of 'juvenile melanomas' did not behave in the same fashion as adult melanomas.[83] Spitz nevi have subsequently been identified as a distinct nevus variant, occurring most commonly on the face of children and adolescents.

Spitz nevi present usually as a smooth-surfaced, hairless, dome-shaped papule or nodule with a distinctive red-brown color (Fig. 9.19). They are most often solitary, although multiple clustered (agminated, Fig. 9.20) or disseminated lesions have been described.[84] They may vary in size from a few millimeters to several centimeters, although most range from 0.6 to 1 cm in diameter. The lesion may be so red that the differential diagnosis for some includes pyogenic granuloma or early juvenile xanthogranuloma. The presence of brown pigmentation (Fig. 9.21), either with regular clinical examination or when examined through a glass slide compressing the surface ('diascopy'), may be useful in confirming the melanocytic nature of the lesion. Surface telangiectasia may also be a prominent feature. In some lesions, particularly those on the extremities, the red color is replaced by a mottled brown to tan or black appearance, often with verrucous surface changes and irregular borders.

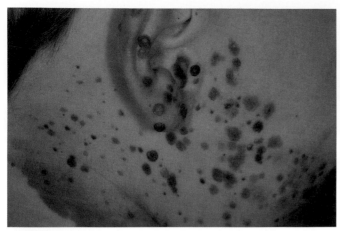

Figure 9.20 Agminated Spitz nevi. This child had multiple lesions of the lateral cheek, ear and neck, several of which were excised, revealing characteristic histologic features of Spitz nevus.

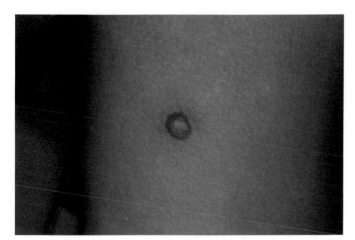

Figure 9.21 Spitz nevus. This pink papule reveals brown speckling, which was easier to see when pressure was applied with a glass slide (diascopy).

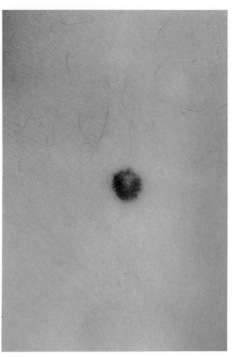

Figure 9.22 Spitz nevus. The dark brown or black type is most often confused clinically with malignant melanoma.

Clinically, it is this type of lesion that is most easily confused with malignant melanoma (Fig. 9.22).

Although most Spitz nevi behave in a benign fashion, local recurrence after excision may occur in as many as 5%.[85] It has been suggested by some that occasional Spitz nevi are 'malignant' in origin, and have the potential for more aggressive biologic behavior. Whether these represent a subtype of Spitz nevus or, on the other hand, a 'Spitzoid' malignant melanoma is unclear. It is obvious that some 'Spitz nevus-like' lesions may pose substantial diagnostic difficulties, especially when atypical features are present, even among dermatopathology experts.[86] A grading system has been proposed for Spitz nevi with atypical features, and application of such a system may be useful in guiding management for patients with atypical Spitz tumors.[87] Recently, *BRAF* mutations were observed in a small subset of Spitz nevi, suggesting that this finding should not be relied upon for distinguishing Spitz nevus from melanoma.[88] The expression of cell cycle and apoptosis regulators in Spitz nevi appears to more closely parallel the findings in benign nevi rather than melanoma.[89]

The management of Spitz nevi is controversial. Many recommend excision of these lesions on the basis of uncertainty in their biologic behavior and occasional reports of aggressive potential. Others advocate for watchful waiting, reserving excision for lesions that demonstrate atypical features or those of psychosocial significance. When these lesions are excised, however, complete removal is advisable. More importantly, surgical specimens should be examined by a dermatopathologist or pathologist experienced in the diagnosis of melanocytic lesions and familiar with Spitz nevi. If an excised lesion is diagnosed unequivocally as a Spitz nevus without atypical features, no further therapy is necessary. However, since incompletely removed lesions may recur and result in a histopathologic appearance that may be more likely to be misinterpreted as malignant melanoma, conservative re-excision is recommended for lesions with positive margins noted on the initial biopsy.

Halo Nevus

A halo nevus is a unique skin lesion in which a centrally placed, usually pigmented nevus becomes surrounded by a 1–5 mm halo of hypo- or depigmentation (Fig. 9.23). These lesions are common in children and young adults. The cause of the spontaneous loss of pigmentation is unknown but appears to be related to an immunologic destruction of melanocytes and nevus cells.[90,91] Adding support to this hypothesis is the fact that several patients with halo nevi have a tendency toward the development of vitiligo (see Ch. 11). Histologic examination of halo nevi reveals reduction or absence of melanin and a dense inflammatory infiltrate around the central nevus. Although compound or intradermal nevi are the tumors most frequently associated with the halo phenomenon, it may also occur around blue nevi, Spitz nevi, neurofibromas, melanomas, and metastatic lesions of melanoma. Giant congenital melanocytic nevi may also reveal the halo phenomenon with pigment regression and, at times, self-destruction.[92,93]

Typical halo nevi are notable for loss of pigmentation in the nevus, with a pink appearance and, frequently, eventual disappearance of the original melanocytic lesion. Occasionally, darkening of the central nevus may occur.[94] Halo nevi may appear on almost any cutaneous surface, but the site of predilection for most lesions is

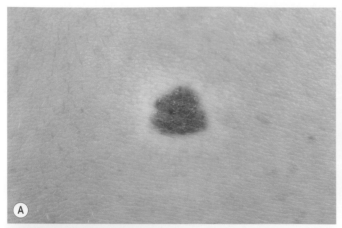

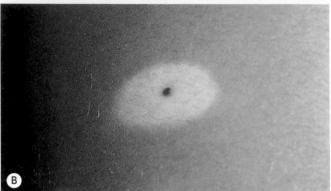

Figure 9.23 Halo nevi. (A) Small halo surrounding a small congenital nevus. (B) Larger halo surrounding an acquired compound nevus.

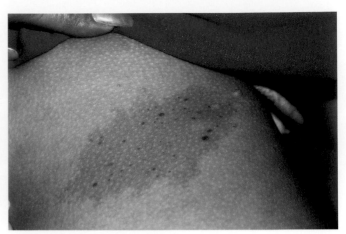

Figure 9.24 Nevus spilus. A tan patch is studded with numerous darker brown macules and papules.

the trunk, particularly the back. In most patients, eventual repigmentation of the halo occurs over a period of months to years.

Halo nevi tend to be benign, although the halo phenomenon may occur around lesions revealing varying degrees of histologic atypia.[95] Potential concern has been raised over reports of malignant melanoma exhibiting the halo phenomenon, and the increased incidence of halo nevi in adults with melanoma.[96] In a survey of pediatric dermatologists, no diagnoses of malignant melanoma in pediatric patients with halo nevi were noted.[96] Clinical features that may suggest an increased probability of an atypical melanocytic lesion within a halo include the 'ABCDE' diagnostic criteria of melanoma (Table 9.2) and asymmetry or irregularity of the surrounding depigmentation. Any patient with a halo nevus, and especially if multiple halo lesions are present, should receive a complete skin and mucous membrane examination to assess for melanocytic lesions revealing atypical features. Patients with the halo nevus phenomenon, concomitant vitiligo and ocular melanoma have been described,[97] but in general, ophthalmologic evaluation is not indicated. If the melanocytic lesion in the central portion of a halo reveals concerning or atypical features, complete excision should be performed. If, on the other hand, the central lesion has benign characteristics, excision is unnecessary and the lesion may be observed at intervals until it has resolved.

Nevus Spilus

Nevus spilus is a solitary, non-hairy flat, brown patch of melanization dotted by smaller dark brown to black macules (Fig. 9.24). This relatively common lesion, although usually present at birth, may

first become noticed during infancy, childhood, or even later. However, clinical and histologic data suggest that these lesions are most likely a subtype of congenital melanocytic nevi.[22] The earliest findings are usually similar to a café-au-lait patch, with eventual development of the secondary superimposed darker melanocytic lesions. Nevi spili may vary in size from 1 to 20 cm in diameter and may appear on any area of the face, trunk, or extremities without relation to sun exposure. Although the darker melanocytic components of these lesions have the potential to develop malignant melanoma, the frequency of this transformation appears to be low.[98,99] Histologic evaluation of a nevus spilus usually reveals components of junctional and congenital nevi.[22,98] Patients with nevus spilus should be followed longitudinally with serial clinical examinations, and if possible, photographic surveillance. Any areas revealing atypical clinical features should be selectively excised and subjected to histologic evaluation, but widespread prophylactic excision seems unwarranted.[20] These lesions (especially when larger) have also been called *speckled lentiginous nevus* (SLN). Although they usually occur in isolation, they may sometimes be associated with other organ abnormalities as part of a syndrome such as phakomatosis pigmentovascularis (Ch. 12), phakomatosis pigmentokeratotica or SLN syndrome (see below).

Becker's Melanosis

Becker's melanosis, also known as Becker's nevus, is an acquired, unilateral hyperpigmentation usually involving the upper trunk of adolescent males. Occasionally, it may present very early in life (as early as birth) and may be distributed in other locations, including the extremities.[100] This pigmentation, which is caused by increased melanization of the epidermis and not by nevocellular proliferation, may be associated with hypertrichosis and, occasionally, proliferation of smooth muscle derived from erector pili muscles. Becker's melanosis is discussed in more detail in Chapter 11.

Tumors of the epidermis

Tumors of the epidermis range in spectrum from benign lesions to those that are malignant. Benign tumors appear much more frequently than malignant lesions in children, and the latter, when they do occur, may be overlooked and/or the diagnosis delayed.

Epidermal Nevi

Epidermal nevi (EN) are benign congenital lesions characterized by hyperplasia of epidermal structures. They are usually apparent at birth or become noticeable during early childhood, affect both sexes equally, and are known by several descriptive names, including nevus verrucosus, nevus unius lateris, and ichthyosis hystrix. In addition, EN can be divided into non-organoid (keratinocytic) nevi and organoid epidermal nevi, such as nevus sebaceous or follicular nevi. Although the exact etiology of EN is unknown, activating fibroblast growth factor receptor 3 (FGFR3) mutations have been demonstrated in some,[101,102] as have mutations in the p110 α-subunit of PI3K (PIK3CA).[103]

Keratinocytic epidermal nevi (frequently referred to simply as 'epidermal nevi') may be slightly or darkly pigmented and unilateral or bilateral in distribution. They often favor the extremities, although they may occur anywhere on the cutaneous surface. Epidermal nevi are usually distributed in a mosaic pattern of alternating stripes of involved and uninvolved skin. This pattern is termed 'Blaschko's lines', and occurs as a result of migration of skin cells during embryogenesis. Disorders that occur along Blaschko's lines usually reveal a linear pattern on the extremities and a wavy or arcuate pattern on the trunk. Although a single EN is most common, multiple lesions may be present, sometimes in association with the 'epidermal nevus syndrome' (see below). The localized form is often present at birth and presents as a tan to brown, velvety or verrucous (warty) papule or plaque. There may be a single lesion (Fig. 9.25) or multiple lesions, and a linear configuration is common (Fig. 9.26). One subtype of epidermal nevus has been termed the *acanthosis nigricans form of EN*, and is characterized by a clinical (Fig. 9.27) and histologic resemblance to acanthosis nigricans.[104]

The term *nevus unius lateris* has been used traditionally to describe extensive unilateral lesions. Nevus unius lateris may present as a single or spiral linear, verrucous lesion or at times as an elaborate, continuous, or interrupted pattern affecting multiple sites (Fig. 9.28), and occasionally involving more than half of the body.

Systematized epidermal nevus has been used to describe extensive lesions that are bilateral and in which truncal involvement predominates.

Epidermal nevi may reveal a variety of histologic features. Importantly, those that reveal 'epidermolytic hyperkeratosis', a distinct pattern of clumping of keratin filaments in the suprabasal cells of the epidermis, imply a mosaic disorder of keratin genes. These patients, especially when skin involvement is extensive, may transmit these mutations to offspring, resulting in a more widespread ichthyosiform condition termed 'epidermolytic ichthyosis' (formerly 'bullous congenital ichthyosiform erythroderma', and epidermolytic hyperkeratosis; see Ch. 5).[105] These epidermal nevi may be clinically indistinguishable from other epidermal nevi (Fig. 9.29).

Epidermal nevi are challenging to treat, given the observation that most superficial destructive therapies are followed by recurrence of

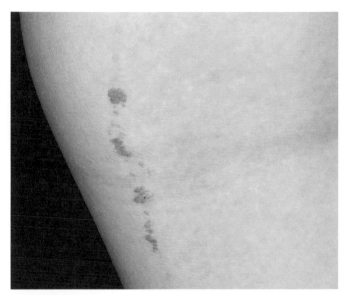

Figure 9.26 Epidermal nevus. Note the warty nature and linear configuration.

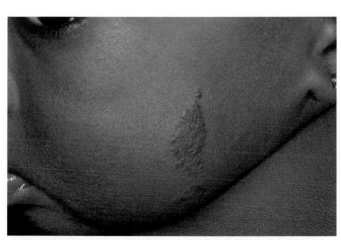

Figure 9.25 Epidermal nevus. This multifocal, verrucous plaque was present since birth.

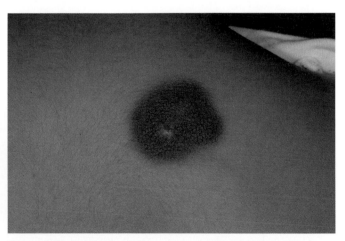

Figure 9.27 Acanthosis nigricans form of epidermal nevus. This form of epidermal nevus reveals a well-demarcated area of velvety thickening, as classically seen with more widespread acanthosis nigricans.

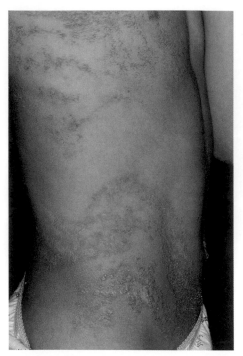

Figure 9.28 Nevus unius lateris. Numerous linear and 'whorled' lesions were present on the right side of this 10-year-old female.

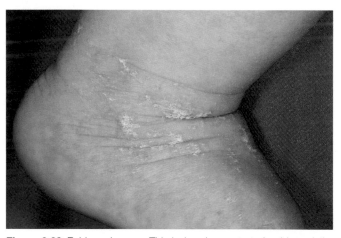

Figure 9.29 Epidermal nevus. This lesion demonstrated epidermolytic hyperkeratosis on histologic evaluation (see text).

the lesion(s). These superficial therapies have included cryotherapy with liquid nitrogen, dermabrasion, electrodesiccation, and laser ablation. CO_2 laser therapy may offer excellent results, but response to therapy is unpredictable.[106] Staged CO_2 laser ablation has been used successfully, both with and without preceding surgical debulking.[107] Topical therapies used with variable success include retinoids, 5-fluorouracil, steroids, and podophyllin, among others. Full-thickness surgical excision or deeper destructive procedures (such as deep dermabrasion) appear effective at removing these hamartomas, but are generally limited to smaller, more localized lesions. Since these lesions may continue to extend during childhood, surgical intervention should be delayed until the full extent of the process is determined.

Epidermal Nevus Syndrome

The epidermal nevus syndrome (ENS) is a sporadic association of epidermal nevi with abnormalities in other organ systems. Some believe that this syndrome is actually a group of several syndromes, each with distinguishing cutaneous and extracutaneous features. Happle suggests that the five well-defined epidermal nevus syndromes are Schimmelpenning syndrome, nevus comedonicus syndrome, pigmented hairy epidermal nevus syndrome, Proteus syndrome (Ch. 12), and CHILD (*c*ongenital *h*emidysplasia with *i*chthyosiform nevus and *l*imb *d*efects) syndrome (Ch. 5).[108] Keratinocytic ENS also merits inclusion on this list.[109] Regardless, patients who fall into the spectrum of having an epidermal nevus syndrome generally present with organoid or nonorganoid epidermal nevi, in conjunction with defects in the central nervous system, eyes, musculoskeletal system, or occasionally other organ systems. The manifestations of ENS are believed to represent genomic mosaicism, with the effects of the genetic defect(s) and timing of the mutation during development determining the spectrum of clinical involvement.[109]

Phakomatosis pigmentokeratotica (PPK) has been used to describe the association of speckled lentiginous nevus with an epidermal nevus that has sebaceous differentiation, and which is accompanied by skeletal and neurologic abnormalities.[110] It has been suggested that PPK patients may have systemic features suggestive of either Schimmelpenning syndrome (extensive sebaceus nevi, mental retardation, seizures, coloboma, lipodermoids of the conjunctiva, skeletal defects and vascular abnormalities) or what has been termed speckled lentiginous nevus syndrome ('SLN syndrome', presenting with SLN, hyperhidrosis, sensory and motor neuropathy, nerve palsy and spinal muscular atrophy).[111,112]

Examples of extracutaneous abnormalities seen in patients with ENS include seizures, mental retardation, hemiparesis, hypotonia, cranial nerve palsies, developmental delay, deafness, kyphosis, scoliosis, limb hypertrophy, hemihypertrophy, facial bone deformity, macrocephaly, ocular lipodermoids, coloboma, corneal changes, cortical blindness, cataracts, and retinal changes.[108,109,113,114] In addition, hypophosphatemic vitamin D-resistant rickets has been observed in patients with ENS, and in some reports, the hypophosphatemia improved following surgical revision of the epidermal nevi.[115–117] It has been suggested that some epidermal nevi may produce a phosphaturic substance that contributes to this association.[115,116] Hyponatremia has also been observed as an early manifestation in a patient with ENS.[118] Cardiac and genitourinary defects may also be associated.

The features of the cutaneous lesions in ENS range from large unilateral nevus unius lateris-like lesions to diffusely distributed, whorled lesions (Fig. 9.30) involving variable degrees of the skin surface or linear, orange-yellow plaques as seen in nevus sebaceous of Jadassohn (see Nevus Sebaceous, below). Plaques of dilated follicular pits filled with keratin may be seen in the 'nevus comedonicus' type ENS, and extensive Becker's nevus is seen in the 'pigmented hairy' type of ENS. In the CHILD syndrome, a unilateral inflammatory epidermal nevus with a sharp midline demarcation and an affinity for body folds is seen in conjunction with the characteristic ipsilateral hypoplasia of limbs and other organ defects. Patients with Proteus syndrome have verrucous epidermal nevi in association with partial gigantism, macrocephaly, and vascular malformations.

Patients with large or extensive epidermal nevi require careful medical, family, and developmental histories and thorough physical evaluation, with particular emphasis on the musculoskeletal, neurologic, ocular, and cardiovascular examinations. Management of ENS should be multidisciplinary, including a dermatologist,

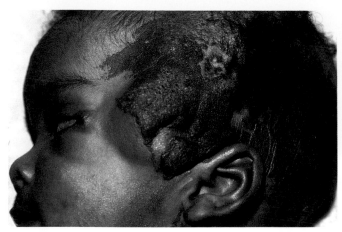

Figure 9.30 Epidermal nevus syndrome. This infant had numerous widespread epidermal nevi in conjunction with multiple congenital anomalies.

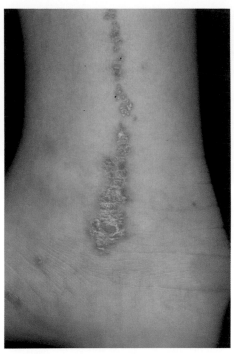

Figure 9.31 Inflammatory linear verrucous epidermal nevus (ILVEN). Multiple red, scaly papules coalescing into a linear plaque on the medial leg, malleolus and foot of a 7-year-old girl.

pediatrician, neurologist, ophthalmologist, and plastic surgeon, with utilization of other subspecialists as necessary. Epidermal nevi can be treated as noted earlier, although treatment is even more challenging given their extensiveness in this setting. Malignant transformation of epidermal nevi is rare but may occur, both in syndromic and non-syndromic lesions, and includes basal cell carcinoma or squamous cell carcinoma, depending on the type of epidermal nevus.

Inflammatory Linear Verrucous Epidermal Nevi

Inflammatory linear verrucous epidermal nevus (ILVEN) appears to be a unique variant of epidermal nevus that presents as a chronic pruritic process with erythematous, scaly, and verrucous papules that coalesce into linear plaques (Fig. 9.31). These lesions are often present at birth or may appear during early childhood, and most often occur on an extremity. They are notable for their chronic and intermittent course and resistance to therapy.[119] Occasionally, lesions may spontaneously improve or resolve, only to eventually reappear. The differential diagnosis of ILVEN includes linear psoriasis, lichen striatus, linear lichen planus, and verrucous epidermal nevus. ILVEN can usually be confirmed by the clinical course, morphologic appearance of lesions, intense pruritus, and resistance to therapy.

Treatment of ILVEN is difficult, as discussed previously for epidermal nevi. Topical or intralesional corticosteroids may reduce inflammation and pruritus and produce a temporary remission, but the lesions generally recur. Topical retinoids, 5-fluorouracil, calcineurin inhibitors (i.e., tacrolimus or pimecrolimus), carbon dioxide laser therapy, and vitamin D derivatives (i.e., calcitriol) have been used with varying results.[120,121] Patients with extensive and symptomatic ILVEN have been treated surgically, with tissue expansion, serial full-thickness excisions, and split-thickness skin grafting, with excellent outcomes.[122]

Basal Cell Carcinoma

Basal cell carcinoma (BCC) is a slow-growing, usually non-metastasizing but invasive malignant skin tumor with varying clinical patterns, which may be triggered by ultraviolet radiation exposure. This disorder arises from the basal cells of the epidermis or its appendages and is most commonly seen in persons of middle-age. BCC is the most common form of skin cancer, and although rarely seen in children, it can occur in childhood and must be considered even in the very young.[123,124] However, misdiagnosis must also be considered in a child, as several benign hamartomas of follicular differentiation (trichoepithelioma, trichoblastoma, trichofolliculoma) may histologically appear similar to BCC to the inexperienced pathologist.

When the diagnosis of BCC is confirmed in a child, one must consider an associated predisposing condition, such as basal cell nevus syndrome (see below), xeroderma pigmentosum (Ch. 19), Bazex syndrome and Rombo syndromes (Ch. 7), albinism (Ch. 11), or an underlying nevus sebaceous of Jadassohn (see Nevus Sebaceous, below). Children treated with irradiation for malignancy or with solid organ transplantation may develop BCC years to decades following the radiation exposure.[123,125] These lesions have occasionally been reported as sporadic cases in children without any underlying predisposition, and appear to be most often located on the head, back and chest.[123,126,127] The diagnosis of BCC in childhood is often delayed because of a low index of suspicion.

The majority of BCC have a predilection for the upper central part of the face. Although they may arise without apparent cause, prolonged exposure to the sun is a predisposing factor, particularly in individuals with a fair skin phenotype. BCC may occur in several clinical forms. *Noduloulcerative* BCC, the most common type, begins as a small elevated translucent papule or nodule with telangiectatic vessels on its surface. It may enlarge, develop central necrosis, and result in an ulceration surrounded by a pearly rolled border. Although this form usually occurs as a single lesion, patients who develop this form of basal cell tumor frequently are likely to develop other such lesions. *Superficial* BCC presents as an erythematous, scaly minimally elevated papule or plaque that may have superficial crusting. Often multiple, these lesions tend to occur on the trunk or extremities, expand slowly, and are easily mistaken for lesions of psoriasis, dermatitis, or tinea. *Pigmented* BCC are similar to noduloulcerative lesions, but also contain irregular brown pigmentation, which may simulate the appearance of a nevus or malignant melanoma. *Sclerosing* or *morpheaform* BCC presents as a firm, yellow-white waxy papule or plaque with an ill-defined border and absence of the translucent rolled edge. Tumors of this type have been known to arise in early childhood and may grow for years before attracting medical attention.

In the pediatric patient who is diagnosed with a BCC, a thorough history and physical examination should be performed, with attention to the regional lymph node examination. An evaluation for an associated predisposing condition should be performed, when indicated. No single method of therapy is applicable to all BCC lesions. The goal, as with any skin tumor, is for permanent cure with the best functional and cosmetic result. Curettage and electrodesiccation is a simple office therapy most frequently used by dermatologists for low-risk, small BCC in areas without a dense hair pattern. Excision (with or without Mohs' micrographic surgery) is the treatment of choice for childhood onset BCC.[123] Radiation therapy can be an effective treatment, but is not desirable in children (and contraindicated in the setting of basal cell nevus syndrome, discussed below, as it may increase the risk for invasive BCC).[124] Other treatment modalities include cryotherapy, CO_2 laser therapy, photodynamic therapy, systemic retinoids, topical chemotherapy (i.e., topical 5-fluorouracil), and biologic response modifiers. The latter include imiquimod, a topical immune-response modifier demonstrated to be effective against superficial BCCs and small nodular BCCs.[128] This agent promotes innate immune responses and exhibits antitumor as well as antiviral effects, having been initially approved for the treatment of anogenital condylomata. Experience with these therapeutic methods in childhood BCC is primarily anecdotal. Sun protection and skin self-examination education is vital.

Basal Cell Nevus Syndrome

The basal cell nevus syndrome (BCNS, also known as Gorlin syndrome or nevoid basal cell carcinoma syndrome) is an autosomal dominant disorder with complete penetrance and variable expressivity, characterized by childhood onset of multiple BCCs associated with other abnormalities, including odontogenic jaw cysts, bifid ribs, and intracranial calcification.[129-132] The most obvious cutaneous feature in patients with BCNS is the appearance of multiple BCC early in life. These basal cell epitheliomas are indistinguishable on histopathologic examination from ordinary BCCs. The diagnostic criteria for BCNS are shown in Table 9.3.

The skin lesions of BCNS may appear as early as the first year of life, but have a mean age of onset of around 20–23 years.[131,132] They involve, in decreasing order of frequency, the face, neck, back, trunk, and upper extremities. The BCCs in BCNS may range in number from one to well over a thousand. In addition, patients with BCNS may develop skin lesions that appear similar to nevi or seborrheic keratoses and tend to follow a more benign course, although after puberty the cutaneous lesions of BCNS tend to be more aggressive. The BCC lesions appear as flesh-colored to pink or tan, dome-shaped papules that measure 1–10 mm (Fig. 9.32A). Secondary changes such as ulceration, crusting, and bleeding rarely occur before puberty, but if left untreated, these lesions can become extremely destructive. Unlike ordinary basal cell carcinomas, BCNS-associated lesions do not appear to be induced by prolonged exposure to sunlight.

In addition to nevoid BCCs, affected individuals have a characteristic facies with coarse features, broad nasal root, hypertelorism, and other cutaneous stigmata. These include multiple small facial milia, comedones, large epidermal cysts, lipomas, fibromas, and

Table 9.3 Diagnostic criteria for basal cell nevus syndrome[a]
Major criteria
Multiple basal cell carcinomas (>5 in a lifetime, or a BCC before 30 years)
Lamellar calcification of the falx (or clear evidence of calcification in an individual younger than 20 years)
Jaw keratocyst (odontogenic keratocyst, confirmed histologically)
Palmar or plantar pits (>2; may be most easily seen following soaking of the hands and feet in warm water)
First-degree relative with BCNS
Minor criteria
Macrocephaly
Childhood medulloblastoma
Cleft lip/palate
Rib/vertebral anomalies: bifid, splayed, missing or extra ribs; bifid, wedged or fused vertebrae
Preaxial or postaxial polydactyly
Cardiac or ovarian fibroma
Lymphomesenteric or pleural cysts
Ocular anomalies (cataract, coloboma, microphthalmia)

Adapted from High and Zedan (2005)[135] and Evans and Farndon (2002).[136]
[a]Diagnosed when an individual has two major criteria and one minor criterion, OR one major criterion and three minor criteria. BCC, basal cell carcinoma; BCNS, basal cell nevus syndrome.

café-au-lait macules. Shallow 2–3 mm palmar and plantar pits (Fig. 9.32B), a characteristic feature of the syndrome, are seen in 70–90% of affected individuals. They may become more prominent after immersion of the hands or feet in water. These defective areas of keratinization usually first appear during the second decade of life or later. Palmar and plantar pits tend to have associated erythema, which on casual observation appears as multiple small red spots on the palms and soles.

Odontogenic jaw cysts occur in around 75% of patients and may present with painless swelling, jaw pain, abnormal taste, or a discharge in the mouth. The first jaw cyst often occurs before the age of 20 years, and symptoms referable to these lesions are often the presenting complaint. Jaw cysts occurring in patients with BCNS present earlier in life than those occurring in patients without BCNS.[133] The cysts may be multiple, and may result in loosening and loss of teeth. Patients with BCNS may become edentulous at an early age.

Musculoskeletal anomalies present in 60–80% of patients include macrocephaly, frontoparietal bossing, high arched palate, and broad nasal bridge.[131] Other abnormalities include splayed or bifid ribs, mandibular and maxillary bone cysts, prognathism, kyphoscoliosis, Sprengel deformity, cervical or thoracic vertebral anomalies, spina bifida, pectus excavatum and carinatum, and shortened fourth metacarpals.

The most common neurologic abnormality is calcification of the falx cerebri, which is seen in up to 90% of patients with BCNS. In addition, mental retardation, electroencephalographic abnormalities, agenesis of the corpus callosum, seizures, hydrocephalus, and deafness may occur. Other associations include anosmia, renal malformations, endocrinopathy, and blindness. Patients with BCNS appear to have a predisposition to malignancy, especially medulloblastoma, which may present early in life.[134] The desmoplastic subtype of medulloblastoma in children younger than 2 years of age is considered by some a major diagnostic criterion for the diagnosis of BCNS.[134,135] This desmoplastic variant has a favorable prognosis.[136] Ovarian and cardiac fibromas and meningiomas also occur with increased frequency in these patients.

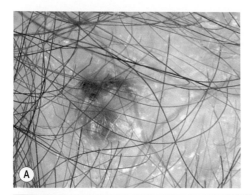

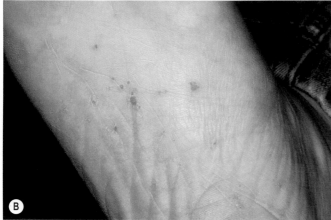

Figure 9.32 Basal cell nevus syndrome (BCNS). (A) Pigmented basal cell carcinoma on the scalp of a 12-year-old girl. (B) Shallow erythematous depressions (pits) on the plantar surface of an adult female with BCNS.

The molecular cause of BCNS has been elucidated. Mutations in the human *patched* (*PTC*) gene have been identified in patients with BCNS as well as in those with sporadic BCCs.[137–139] *Patched* is located on chromosome 9q and encodes a transmembrane receptor that represses growth factor gene transcription. The gene product of *PTC* functions as a tumor suppressor, and *PTC* mutations results in dysregulation of several genes known to play a role in both organogenesis and carcinogenesis.[140] Sequence analysis to detect mutations as well as deletion testing are both clinically available to assist in diagnosis of BCNS.

The management of patients with BCNS must be multidisciplinary and individualized. Genetic counseling is important given the autosomal dominant mode of inheritance. Family members judged to be at-risk may be screened with skeletal surveys, dental radiographs, and neurologic evaluation (both clinical and radiographic). Molecular diagnosis is also possible (GeneDx, Inc., Gaithersburg, MD), with a sensitivity around 60%. Removal of cutaneous BCC may be accomplished with the same techniques as discussed earlier, and general anesthesia may be required for treatment of multiple lesions. Systemic retinoids (i.e., isotretinoin) may be useful in preventing BCCs, but its use must be balanced by potential side-effects and, in females, the known teratogenicity. In addition, if the retinoid is discontinued, the patient may show rapid disease progression. Yearly dental follow-up, with dental radiography, should be performed and jaw cysts removed by an experience oral surgeon. Regular neurologic evaluations should be performed through the early elementary school years, and magnetic resonance imaging considered.

Squamous Cell Carcinoma

Squamous cell carcinoma (SCC) is a malignant tumor of the epidermis rarely seen in children. Occasionally it may arise in normal skin, but generally it is seen in skin that has been injured by sunlight, trauma, thermal burn, or chronic inflammation. Children who develop SCC often have an underlying predisposing condition, including xeroderma pigmentosum (Ch. 19), human papillomavirus infection (especially in the immunocompromised host), or a history of organ transplantation, chemotherapy with immunosuppression, or radiation therapy. In addition, scars related to dystrophic epidermolysis bullosa (Ch. 13) may be predisposed to the development of SCC. Although these tumors generally do not present until the third or fourth decade, they may occasionally occur during childhood.[141] SCC has also been reported to occur within the lesions of pansclerotic morphea of childhood.[142]

The most common sites for SCC are the face (in particular the lower lip and pinna of the ear) and the dorsal aspect of the hands and forearms. Lesions usually present as red, scaly papules or plaques, often with induration. Telangiectasias may be present, as may ulceration or necrosis. Lesions that arise de novo usually appear as solitary, slowly enlarging firm nodules with central crusting, underlying ulceration and an indurated base. The histologic evaluation of SCC offers prognostic information based on the depth of the lesion and the cytologic features and degree of differentiation of the cells.

The prognosis for squamous cell carcinoma of the skin is quite variable. Easily cured small lesions arising in sun-damaged skin have a low propensity to metastasize. Lesions arising in burn scars, prior radiation fields, and chronic wounds (i.e., ulcers or epidermolysis bullosa scars; see Ch. 13) tend to be more aggressive with higher rates of metastases. Complete excision is the treatment of choice for SCC. Other treatment options that may be considered include electro-desiccation and curettage, cryotherapy, photodynamic therapy, and Mohs micrographic surgery. Sun protection and skin self-examination education is again vital.

Keratoacanthoma

Keratoacanthoma (KA) is an epithelial tumor that may be clinically and histologically indistinguishable from SCC. These lesions are considered by many to be benign, and they often involute spontaneously without therapy. However, given rare reports of extensive local destruction and metastases, some consider KAs to be a variant of SCC. Keratoacanthomas are usually seen in older adults, with rare reports of neonatal or childhood involvement.[143,144] Multiple KAs characteristically have their onset in adolescence or early adult life, and may occur in several clinical settings, such as the Ferguson–Smith or Muir–Torre syndromes. Eruptive KA, with the sudden onset of multiple lesions, may also occur (termed the 'Grzybowski' type).

Keratoacanthoma presents as a firm, dome-shaped nodule that generally measures ≥1–3 cm. The center contains a horny plug or is covered by a crust that conceals a central keratin-filled crater. The nodule generally grows rapidly, and reaches its full size within 2–8 weeks. Following a period of quiescence, which may last for 2–8 weeks, most lesions heal spontaneously over several months with only a slightly depressed, somewhat cribriform scar in the previously affected area.

The main problem in the diagnosis of KA is its differentiation from SCC. In most cases, the rapid evolution and typical clinical appearance help to establish the correct diagnosis. Because the architecture of the lesion is as important as the cellular characteristics, full excisional biopsy is recommended to enable appropriate histopathologic evaluation. The treatment of KA is usually approached with a view toward its spontaneous resolution. Its close resemblance to squamous cell carcinoma, however, frequently results in excisional biopsy. Other reported treatment options include intralesional corticosteroids, topical imiquimod, intralesional methotrexate, topical 5-fluorouracil, electrodesiccation and curettage, and radiation therapy.[145–148]

Tumors of the oral mucosa

White Sponge Nevus

White sponge nevus is a rare, autosomal dominant condition that most often affects the oral mucosa, and less commonly the mucosae of other regions. It presents as exuberant, asymptomatic white plaques on the buccal mucosae (Fig. 9.33), palate, gingivae, or sides of the tongue. Other mucosal regions that may be involved include the nasal, vaginal, labial, and anal mucosa. In some instances, the plaques may be quite thickened with fissures and folds, and occasionally a raw, denuded surface may be evident. White sponge nevus may be present at birth, or may have its onset any time from infancy through adolescence. It reaches its maximal severity during adolescence or early adulthood, and the lesions are entirely asymptomatic and often noted incidentally during examination. Both sexes are equally affected. The differential diagnosis of white sponge nevus includes oral leukoplakia, pachyonychia congenita, dyskeratosis congenita, cheek biting, and lichen planus.

Defects in the genes for keratins 4 and 13 have been demonstrated to be responsible for white sponge nevus.[149,150] This disorder is generally benign and asymptomatic, and requires no specific therapy. White sponge nevus should not be confused with focal epithelial hyperplasia (Heck's disease), a rare disorder of the oral mucosa of children believed to be caused by infection with human papillomavirus, especially types 13 and 32. In patients with Heck's disease, the mucosa of the lower lip is most commonly involved and reveals soft papules and plaques, which tend to regress spontaneously over several months.

Leukoplakia

Leukoplakia is a term generally used to describe a white plaque involving the oral mucosa, and which cannot be easily removed by scraping or rubbing with a cotton swab or tongue blade. It is a nonspecific term inconsistently applied to a variety of different etiologic lesions, including white sponge nevus, pachyonychia congenita, dyskeratosis congenita, hereditary benign intraepithelial dyskeratosis, hereditary mucoepithelial dysplasia, and many others. It is also used to describe white changes on the vulva of females, where its use is equally nonspecific.

Oral leukoplakia is the terminology usually used to describe a condition seen most often in adults, and related to a variety of factors, including trauma, poor oral hygiene, chronic irritation, and use of tobacco products. It may occasionally be seen in children, and has been reported in pediatric patients with HIV infection.[151,152] The clinical presentation is notable for either focal or more diffuse involvement with white plaques of the buccal mucosae, hard or soft palate, lateral surfaces of the tongue, and the floor of the mouth. Mucosal biopsy with histopathologic evaluation is usually necessary to confirm the exact diagnosis, and treatment depends on the etiology. Meticulous attention to oral hygiene is useful regardless of the cause. Since oral leukoplakia may have malignant potential (eventuating into squamous cell carcinoma), long-term follow-up is indicated, with repeat tissue biopsy when necessary.

Tumors of the epidermal appendages

Nevus Sebaceous

Nevus sebaceous of Jadassohn is a common congenital lesion that occurs mainly on the face and scalp. These lesions are usually solitary, and present as a well-circumscribed, hairless plaque. A developmental defect, they are generally present at birth, but may first be noted during early childhood and rarely in adult life. Although rare familial forms have been reported, these hamartomas tend to be sporadic. Multiple nevi sebaceous may occur in association with cerebral, ocular, and skeletal abnormalities as part of the epidermal nevus syndrome. This association has been termed Schimmelpenning syndrome.[108]

Classic nevus sebaceous presents as a hairless, yellow to tan plaque on the scalp (Fig. 9.34) or face (Fig. 9.35). The surface may be verrucous or velvety, and the lesions are often oval or linear. In some patients hyperpigmentation may be a prominent feature, making the distinction from a verrucous epidermal nevus difficult.

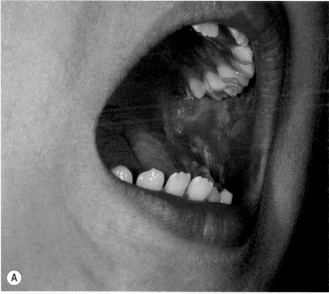

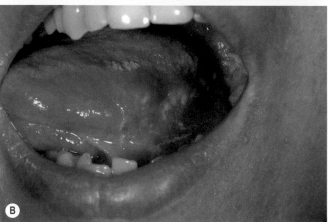

Figure 9.33 Oral white sponge nevus. This 4-year-old boy (A) and his two brothers, father (B), and uncle all had similar white plaques of the oral mucosa.

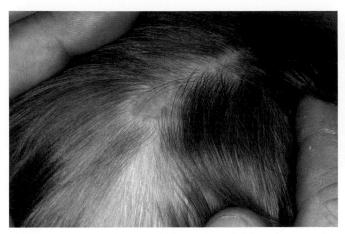

Figure 9.34 Nevus sebaceous. Yellow-orange, hairless plaque on the scalp.

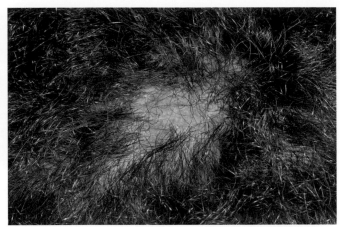

Figure 9.36 Nevus sebaceous. The lesion in this adolescent male demonstrates verrucous (warty) changes that are common with older age.

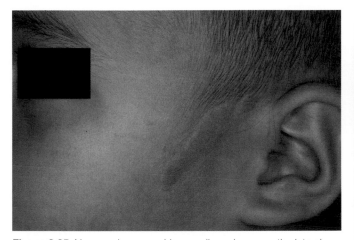

Figure 9.35 Nevus sebaceous. Linear yellow plaque on the lateral cheek.

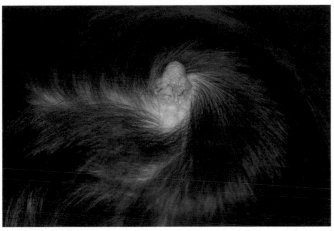

Figure 9.37 Nevus sebaceous with syringocystadenoma papilliferum. This verrucous, exophytic papule developed on the surface of a previously-flat nevus sebaceous.

Nevus sebaceous may vary in size from a few millimeters to several centimeters in length. Their yellow color is related to sebaceous gland secretion, and often this color becomes less prominent after infancy. The lesions tend to enlarge proportionate with growth of the child, until puberty when they may become significantly thicker, more verrucous, and more greasy in appearance (Fig. 9.36), as a result of hormonal stimulation of the sebaceous glands within them. Papillomatous projections may occur, sometimes simulating the appearance of verruca vulgaris.

Surgical excision, the treatment of choice for nevus sebaceous, has traditionally been recommended out of concern for the development of secondary malignant neoplasms within these lesions. Multiple secondary appendageal neoplasms may occur within nevus sebaceous, including syringocystadenoma papilliferum (the most common secondary benign neoplasm, Fig. 9.37), apocrine cystadenoma, spiradenoma, and trichoblastoma.[153–155] The secondary tumor that raises the most concern, however, is BCC, which in the past was estimated to occur in anywhere from 6.5 to 50% of lesions, depending on the source.[156] More recent investigations have documented that the incidence of BCC is actually quite low, and, in fact, trichoblastoma (a benign proliferation that appears to be quite common) may be easily mistaken for BCC.[154,157] Other tumors that have been reported within lesions of nevus sebaceous include keratoacanthoma, leiomyoma, piloleiomyoma, squamous cell car-

cinoma, apocrine carcinoma, and malignant eccrine poroma. Malignant degeneration is usually heralded by the appearance of a discrete nodule with or without ulceration.

The timing of surgery in those patients for whom it is chosen is controversial. Many factors need to be considered, including size and location of the nevus, its cosmetic significance, and the risk-to-benefit ratio of general anesthesia (needed early in life) versus local anesthesia (a possibility when surgery is delayed until later childhood or adolescence). These decisions must be made by the parents (and patient, where appropriate) with input from the involved physician(s). The practitioner should provide parents with the objective data and allow them to make this personal decision, offering support and guidance as necessary.

Nevus Comedonicus

Nevus comedonicus is a rare type of organoid nevus with a hair follicle origin. These lesions are often present at birth, or may become evident over the first decade of life. There is no racial or sexual predisposition. Nevus comedonicus presents as a plaque composed primarily of hyperkeratotic papules and horny plugs (resembling the comedones of acne vulgaris), with varying degrees

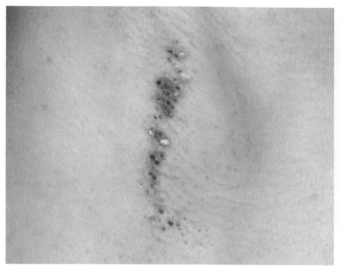

Figure 9.38 Nevus comedonicus. Multiple open (blackheads) and closed (whiteheads) comedones in a linear distribution.

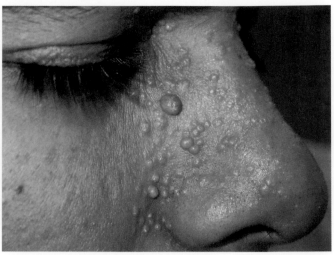

Figure 9.39 Multiple trichoepitheliomas. Multiple flesh-colored papules of the medial cheek and nose. (Courtesy of Keren Horn, MD.)

of erythema (Fig. 9.38). Lesions are most common on the face, neck, trunk, and upper extremities, and are often linear or band-like in distribution. They tend to grow as the child matures, and large lesions extending above the surrounding cutaneous surface may give a grater-like feeling to the skin. There is a spectrum of involvement with nevus comedonicus, from simple comedonal lesions to those with significant inflammation, cysts, and even scarring.[158] Secondary infection and abscess formation rarely occur.

The differential diagnosis of nevus comedonicus includes nevus sebaceous, acne neonatorum, and, in older patients, comedonal acne. Although the lesions usually occur as a sporadic finding, multiple or extensive lesions may be associated with abnormalities in other organ systems as part of the 'nevus comedonicus type' of epidermal nevus syndrome.[108,159] Management of nevus comedonicus is challenging. Topical retinoids, ammonium lactate lotion, or topical antibiotics may each be useful for some patients. Pore strips have been reported useful for removal of the keratin plugs.[160] However, most medical therapies are ineffective, and the definitive therapy for cosmetically significant lesions is surgical excision.

Trichoepithelioma

Trichoepitheliomas may occur as a benign, autosomal dominantly inherited disorder characterized by the presence of multiple small lesions occurring primarily on the face, or as a solitary non-hereditary tumor seen in early adult life or occasionally during childhood. The terminology *Brooke–Spiegler syndrome* (*BSS*) has traditionally been used to describe an autosomal dominant disorder characterized by numerous trichoepitheliomas, cylindromas (see also Cylindroma, below) and spiradenomas, all benign skin appendageal tumors. *Multiple familial trichoepithelioma* (*MFT*) refers to an autosomal dominant disorder characterized by numerous trichoepitheliomas involving the central face, and often starting during childhood. The term *trichoblastoma* has been used to denote benign neoplasms of follicular differentiation. Some now consider these two conditions to be interchangeable, with others considering trichoepithelioma to be one type of trichoblastoma.

Multiple trichoepitheliomas generally begin during early childhood or around puberty as small, firm, flesh-colored papules and nodules on the face (Fig. 9.39), particularly in the nasolabial folds

and over the nose, forehead, upper lip, and eyelids and occasionally the scalp, neck, trunk, scrotum, and perianal area. The lesions measure 2–5 mm in diameter, are firm, and have a translucent sheen. Occasionally, telangiectatic vessels are present over the rounded translucent surface of larger lesions. Trichoepitheliomas may enlarge slowly, reaching up to 5 mm on the face and ears and up to 2–3 cm in other sites; they often coalesce to form nodular aggregates. Mutations in the *CYLD* gene, a tumor-suppressor gene, appear to be the genetic basis for MFT, BSS and familial cylindromatosis (FC, also known as 'turban tumor syndrome'), a disorder characterized by multiple cylindromas as the only tumor type (see also Cylindroma, below).[161–163]

Solitary non-hereditary trichoepitheliomas usually develop during the second or third decade of life and generally appear on the face. They may also be distributed on the scalp, neck, trunk, upper arms, or thighs. Solitary lesions appear as firm, flesh-colored papules and papulonodules and generally reach 5 mm or slightly larger in diameter.

Desmoplastic trichoepithelioma is a variant that presents as an indurated, flesh-colored to red papule or plaque with an elevated annular border and central depression. It occurs most commonly on the face, especially the cheek. Although most commonly seen in early adulthood, desmoplastic trichoepitheliomas may appear during the second decade, are much more common in females, and may occur in a familial fashion.[164]

Although trichoepitheliomas are benign lesions, treatment may be cosmetically desirable, and at times biopsy is indicated to differentiate the lesion from other cutaneous neoplasms. Surgical excision is the treatment of choice, although electrodesiccation, cryotherapy, radiotherapy, dermabrasion and laser therapy have also been utilized.[163]

Trichilemmoma

Trichilemmoma is another benign appendageal neoplasm derived from the hair follicle. These lesions may be solitary or multiple and present as flesh-colored papules or nodules, occasionally with a verrucous (wart-like) surface. The most common location for trichilemmomas is the face, although genitals are another common site and they can occur anywhere on the cutaneous surface. A desmoplastic form (desmoplastic trichilemmoma) may occur, and at times the deeper component of these lesions may histologically simulate invasive carcinoma.[165] Treatment of these benign lesions may be accomplished with surgical excision or ablative procedures, when desired.

Multiple trichilemmomas may be seen in the setting of the multiple hamartoma syndrome, Cowden syndrome (CS). This autosomal dominant disorder is characterized by hamartomas in multiple organ systems, including skin, breast, thyroid, gastrointestinal tract, endometrium, and brain.[166] Mucocutaneous lesions, which are present in nearly all patients, include multiple trichilemmomas, palmoplantar keratoses, oral papillomatosis, and sclerotic fibromas.[166,167] Pigmented macules of the genitalia, café-au-lait macules, acanthosis nigricans, skin tags, lipomas, and vascular malformations may also occur in CS.[167,168] Other benign extracutaneous manifestations include fibrocystic breast disease, breast fibroadenomas, thyroid adenomas, goiter, neuromas, meningiomas, and intestinal polyposis. Patients with CS also have an increased risk of certain malignancies, including those of the breast (up to 30–50% of female patients) and thyroid gland (3–10%).[166,169] The potentially increased risk of other cancers, including renal cell carcinoma, malignant melanoma, and colon cancer is less clear.[169] Skeletal abnormalities may include macrocephaly, scoliosis, and pectus excavatum.

Mutations in the tumor suppressor gene *PTEN*, which encodes a tumor suppressor phosphatase involved in cellular regulation, have been detected in patients with CS as well as in patients with Bannayan–Riley–Ruvalcaba syndrome (BRR, see below), Proteus or Proteus-like syndrome (see Ch. 12), adult Lhermitte–Duclos disease, and autism-like disorders associated with macrocephaly.[169] Cowden syndrome and BRR share many similarities, including the mucocutaneous findings of facial trichilemmomas, acanthosis nigricans, lipomas, palmoplantar keratoses, pigmented macules of the genitalia, and oral papillomatosis.[168] Recently, mucocutaneous neuromas have been highlighted as another overlap finding that may be seen in both CS and BRR.[170] The identification of kindreds with both diseases in the family, as well as identical *PTEN* mutations and overlapping clinical features, suggested that CS and BRR syndrome may represent different phenotypic expressions of the same disease.[166,168,171] Recently, the above disorders thus far attributable to *PTEN* mutations have been collectively referred to as *PTEN hamartoma-tumor syndrome*.[172]

Trichofolliculoma

Trichofolliculoma is an uncommon benign appendageal neoplasm, again of hair follicle derivation, which usually occurs as a solitary lesion. They most often involve the head and neck regions of adults, but may occur during childhood. Trichofolliculomas present as a 2–10 mm, slow-growing, flesh-colored or pearly papule or nodule with a smooth surface. There is often a central pore with a protruding woolly or cotton-like tuft of hair (a highly diagnostic clinical feature). On occasion, the protruding hairs may be so fine that a magnifying lens may be required to detect their presence. Treatment of trichofolliculoma by local surgical excision generally produces a good cosmetic outcome.

Pilomatricoma

Pilomatricoma (also known as calcifying epithelioma of Malherbe) is a benign tumor derived from the hair matrix, which usually develops within the first two decades. Pilomatricomas usually present as a solitary lesion of the face, neck, upper trunk, or upper extremities. The two most common locations in one large study

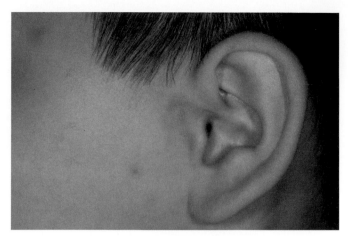

Figure 9.40 Pilomatricoma. This preauricular blue papulonodule was very firm to palpation.

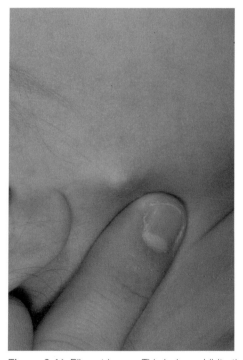

Figure 9.41 Pilomatricoma. This lesion exhibits the 'tent sign' as the adjacent skin is stretched.

were the head (nearly 50%) and the upper extremities (35%).[173] Clinically, pilomatricomas appear as flesh-colored to white, firm papules or papulonodules that may have an overlying pink to blue hue (Fig. 9.40). They are generally very hard, owing to calcification, and may demonstrate a positive 'teeter-totter sign', whereby downward pressure directed at one end of the lesion causes the other end to spring upward in the skin. Another useful sign is the 'tent sign', whereby multiple facets and angles (resembling a tent) are visualized when the skin overlying the lesion is stretched (Fig. 9.41).

Pilomatricomas range in size from 5 mm to over 5 cm. Although pilomatricomas are usually not hereditary, familial cases have been recognized and some familial forms have been associated with myotonic dystrophy, an uncommon autosomal dominant disorder characterized by hypotonia, muscle wasting, cataracts, hypogonadism, progressive mental retardation, and frontal baldness.[174–176] Multiple pilomatricomas have also been noted in patients with Gardner syndrome, Rubinstein–Taybi syndrome, and trisomy 9.[177–180] Other variants include cystic-appearing pilomatricomas, in which hemorrhage may result in blue-red translucent nodules with rapid enlargement; perforating pilomatricomas; pilomatrix carcinoma (extremely rare); and extruding pilomatricomas (draining lesions that spontaneously discharge a chalky material containing calcium). Activating mutations in β-catenin, a participant in the Wnt signaling pathway, have been identified in pilomatricomas in one study.[181]

Pilomatricomas may periodically develop inflammation or swelling, and may be painful when subjected to pressure on the affected region of skin. Definitive therapy is accomplished by surgical excision. Patients with multiple lesions or familial disease should be examined and followed closely for potentially associated disorders, especially myotonic dystrophy and Gardner syndrome. Importantly, the onset of myotonic dystrophy may not occur until adulthood, and molecular diagnosis is possible.[175]

Syringoma

Syringomas represent benign tumors of eccrine (sweat gland) structures and are predominantly seen in females. The lesions may occur at any age but frequently present initially during puberty or adolescence as small, firm, flesh-colored to yellow, translucent 1–3 mm papules (Fig. 9.42). They are usually multiple, and may occasionally be solitary. In more than half of the patients the lesions are located on the lower eyelids. Other common locations include the lateral neck, chest, abdomen, back, upper arms, thighs, and genitalia. Syringomas occur with increased frequency in patients with Down syndrome. They may occasionally occur in an eruptive fashion, and tend to be influenced by hormones, as evidenced by increased size during pregnancy or the premenstrual period, and enlargement in women receiving hormone therapy.

Syringomas gradually enlarge until they attain their full size and then persist, with little tendency for spontaneous resolution. Although they are benign, they may be of significant cosmetic concern. Treatment, however, is difficult. Therapeutic options include electrodesiccation, cryosurgery with liquid nitrogen, or local surgical excision. CO_2 laser ablation and trichloroacetic acid have also been found useful.[182]

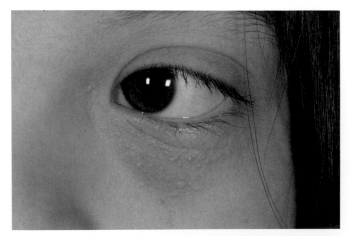

Figure 9.42 Syringomas. These multiple, flesh-colored small papules were present bilaterally in the inferior periorbital regions of this young girl with Down syndrome.

Eccrine Poroma

Eccrine poromas are benign cutaneous tumors that generally arise from the intraepidermal eccrine sweat duct unit. They occur most often during middle age or later, but have been noted to develop as early as 15 years of age. Eccrine poromas present as firm papules, plaques, or nodules, and may be flesh-colored to red. They are usually solitary, and range in size between 2 and 12 mm. They most commonly occur on the plantar surface of the foot and occasionally on the palms, fingers, neck, or trunk. In some lesions, the appearance is quite vascular and may simulate pyogenic granuloma. A striking clinical feature is the presence of a cup-shaped shallow depression from which the tumor grows and protrudes. Malignant eccrine poroma, also known as eccrine porocarcinoma, is a very rare tumor usually occurring in adults, although pediatric cases have been reported.[183] The treatment of choice for eccrine poroma is surgical excision.

Cylindroma

Cylindromas (also known as turban tumors) are benign neoplasms of either eccrine or apocrine origin, characterized by firm, rubbery, pink to bluish plaques and nodules. They may range in size from a few millimeters to several centimeters, and are located primarily on the scalp and occasionally the face, trunk, or extremities. Cylindromas may occur singly or in multiples, and occasionally coalesce to result in large mosaic tumors. Multiple lesions may occur as part of the autosomal dominant Brooke–Spiegler syndrome (with multiple trichoepitheliomas and occasionally other appendageal tumors; see also Trichoepithelioma, above). This disease has been mapped to 16q12–13, and mutations in the *CYLD* gene have been identified in families with this disorder.[184,185] Treatment consists of surgical excision, although CO_2 laser surgery has also been demonstrated useful.[186] Cylindromas are almost invariably benign, although malignant transformation has been rarely reported.

Dermal tumors

Angiofibroma

Angiofibromas are benign dermal neoplasms that may occur as isolated or multiple lesions. The term 'angiofibroma' actually describes the histologic appearance of these lesions (which reveals dermal fibroplasia and dilated blood vessels), but they may present in a variety of clinical fashions. Clinical subtypes include fibrous papule, pearly penile papules, and periungual fibromas. Another presentation pattern is that of multiple facial angiofibromas, which are frequently seen in patients with tuberous sclerosis (Ch. 11), in which setting they have been erroneously referred to as *adenoma sebaceum*, multiple endocrine neoplasia type 1 (see Ch. 23), and Birt–Hogg–Dube syndrome (characterized classically by fibrofolliculomas, trichodiscomas and acrochordons).[187]

Fibrous papule presents as a solitary, flesh-colored shiny papule, most often on the nose of adults. The differential diagnosis may include intradermal nevus, basal cell carcinoma, or other appendageal tumor. These lesions are treated with shave excision or electrocautery. Pearly penile papules present as tiny, flesh-colored to white papules on the glans penis of post-pubertal men. They are most commonly distributed along the corona, and their importance lies in distinguishing them from genital condylomata (often a source of anxiety for the affected individual). This distinction is usually quite simple given their appearance, multiplicity, and localization. Treatment of pearly penile papules is unnecessary. Periungual fibromas present as flesh-colored filiform growths arising from the

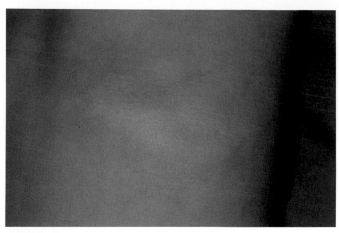

Figure 9.43 Connective tissue nevus. This flesh-colored, dermal plaque on the back of a school-aged boy had been present for several years.

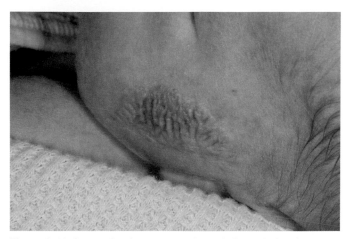

Figure 9.44 Connective tissue nevus. A cerebriform, fleshy plaque on the cheek of a newborn male.

proximal nail fold region. Although they occasionally occur sporadically, multiple lesions are pathognomonic for tuberous sclerosis.

Connective Tissue Nevus

Connective tissue nevus (also known as connective tissue hamartoma) is a localized hamartoma of either dermal collagen or elastic fibers or both. These benign skin lesions may be sporadic or hereditary, and can be seen as a component of several syndromes. For instance, the shagreen patch and fibrous forehead plaque seen in tuberous sclerosis (Ch. 11) are both forms of connective tissue nevi. In addition, the palmoplantar cerebriform hyperplasia that occurs in patients with Proteus syndrome (Ch. 12) represents excess collagen, and thus could also be classified under this umbrella term. This section discusses primarily the sporadic, non-syndromic form of connective tissue nevus.

These lesions usually present as asymptomatic, flesh-colored dermal plaques composed of multiple papules. They may be quite subtle (Fig. 9.43), or may be associated with significant thickening, cobblestoning, or cerebriform changes (Fig. 9.44). Solitary plaques may occur anywhere on the cutaneous surface, and multiple lesions are often distributed symmetrically on the back,

buttocks, and extremities. The differential diagnosis may include smooth muscle hamartoma (see Congenital Smooth Muscle Hamartoma, below).

Another form of connective tissue nevus, dermatofibrosis lenticularis disseminata, has been reported in association with a specific bone dysplasia termed osteopoikilosis. This association is also known as Buschke–Ollendorf syndrome (see Ch. 6). The cutaneous lesions in this setting usually appear in adult life, but their onset has also been reported during the first year or early childhood. They appear as flesh-colored to yellow papules, usually a few millimeters in size, distributed on the trunk, buttocks, and extremities. They often represent hamartomas of elastic tissue (elastomas) histologically. The bony lesions are usually asymptomatic and are often noted incidentally as focal sclerotic areas on bone radiographs. They may occasionally be mistaken for foci of metastatic malignancy, highlighting the importance of familiarity with this disorder and its associated skin lesions.

Connective tissue nevi are generally asymptomatic and not usually of cosmetic significance. If the diagnosis is unclear, incisional biopsy is useful. Surgical excision is otherwise unnecessary.

Mastocytosis

The term mastocytosis refers to a group of clinical disorders characterized by the accumulation of mast cells in the skin and, at times, other organs of the body. It may appear at any time from birth to middle age. In approximately 55% of patients, the onset occurs before the age of 2 years, and for 10%, the onset is between 2 and 15 years of age.[188] Mastocytosis may be congenital in up to 25% of pediatric-onset cases. The growth and regulation of mast cells is dependent on stem cell factor, which is the ligand for the protein product of the c-kit gene. Studies have documented c-kit mutations in adult patients with mastocytosis, and more recently, activating c-kit mutations have also been demonstrated in pediatric mastocytosis, in codon 816 (exon 17) as well as exons 8 and 9.[189] Although mastocytosis is generally a sporadic disorder, familial cases have been reported.[190–192]

The clinical spectrum of cutaneous mastocytosis includes mastocytomas (single or multiple), urticaria pigmentosa, bullous mastocytosis, diffuse cutaneous mastocytosis, and telangiectasia macularis eruptiva perstans (TMEP). The traditional classification of adult disease includes indolent mastocytosis, mastocytosis with an associated hematologic disorder, mast cell leukemia, and lymphadenopathic mastocytosis with eosinophilia.[188] Alternatively, for either pediatric or adults patients, mastocytosis may be divided into cutaneous and systemic forms, with the potential for overlap between these two. Although the disease may be classified by several different schemas, there appear to be some fairly consistent differences between adult and pediatric mastocytosis. These include the following for pediatric disease: early onset, usually within the first year of life; rare occurrence of TMEP; tendency toward spontaneous resolution, often before puberty; rare association with hematologic disorders; and rare infiltration of other organs aside from the skin.[193]

Although the classification of mastocytosis is often confusing, it can be somewhat simplified when considering the typical childhood presentations. Children most commonly present with mastocytomas (either solitary or multiple), urticaria pigmentosa, or occasionally diffuse cutaneous mastocytosis. All three of these childhood forms may display vesicular or bullous variants. Vesiculation is presumably related to histamine- or other chemical mediator-induced transuding leakage in a group susceptible to blister formation by less secure attachments of the epidermis to the underlying dermis.[194]

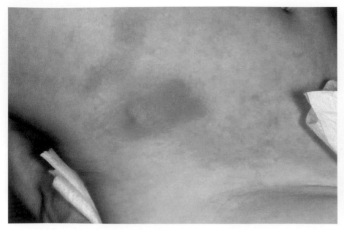

Figure 9.45 Darier's sign in mastocytosis. Edema and surrounding erythema developed within minutes after firmly stroking this lesion.

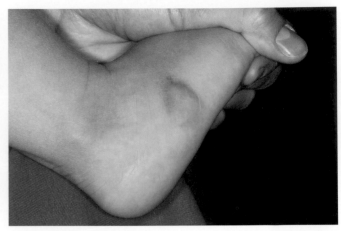

Figure 9.46 Solitary mastocytoma. An edematous plaque with mild surrounding pigmentation.

Table 9.4 Potential triggers of mast cell degranulation

Physical
    Exercise, heat, hot baths, hot beverages, cold exposure,
    sunlight, stress

Medications (systemic)
    Aspirin, alcohol, morphine, codeine, dextromethorphan, NSAIDs,
    opiates, amphotericin B, thiamine

Medications (topical)   Polymyxin B

Medications sometimes used with general anesthesia
    D-tubocurarine, scopolamine, decamethonium, gallamine,
    pancuronium

Local anesthetics   Tetracaine, procaine, methylparaben
X-ray contrast   Iodine-containing contrast media
Venoms   Snakebites, bee stings, jellyfish stings

Foods
    Egg white, crayfish, lobster, chocolate, strawberries, tomatoes,
    citrus, ethanol

NSAID, non-steroidal antiinflammatory drug.

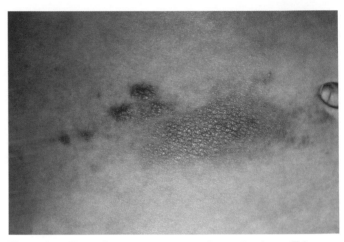

Figure 9.47 Peau d'orange appearance of a mastocytoma. This plaque-like mastocytoma shows the characteristic surface changes.

The diagnosis of all forms of cutaneous mastocytosis is aided by the phenomenon known as Darier's sign. This finding, a hallmark of the disorder, is seen in 90% of patients with skin disease and consists of localized erythema and urticarial wheals (Fig. 9.45) that develop after gentle mechanical irritation, such as might be induced by rubbing with a tongue blade or the blunt end of a pen or pencil. This urtication develops within a few minutes after the stimulus, and may persist as long as 30 min to several hours. Occasionally, blister formation may result. It should be noted, though, that Darier's sign may be negative in mastocytosis, especially in patients with entirely flat lesions at baseline.

Mast cell mediators include histamine, prostaglandin D$_2$, heparin, tryptase, chymase, leukotrienes, and others. Cutaneous symptoms related to release of these mediators in the setting of mastocytosis may include flushing, blistering, and itching. Systemic symptoms may include nausea, abdominal pain, diarrhea, bone pain, hypotension, and, less often, pulmonary signs. Whereas the extent and density of cutaneous lesions may correlate with systemic symptoms

in adults, such a correlation is lacking in children with mastocytosis.[195] There are many potential triggers of mast cell degranulation, including physical stimuli, drugs, and foods, and these are listed in Table 9.4. Most of these triggers are clinically insignificant in children with more mild forms of the disease, but exposures should be minimized in those at the more severe end of the spectrum or with a history of related systemic symptoms.

Mastocytomas are a common type of childhood mastocytosis. They may be either solitary or multiple, and present as flesh-colored to yellow-orange-tan papules (Fig. 9.46) or plaques. Some lesions may have a 'bruise-like' appearance, and others may present in similar fashion to café-au-lait macules.[193] They may range in size from a few millimeters to several centimeters, and are present at birth in around 40% of patients.[196] In the remainder, they generally appear by one year of age. The surface of the lesion often reveals a 'peau d'orange' (orange peel-like) appearance (Fig. 9.47), and Darier's sign is notoriously positive. Occasionally, stroking or rubbing of even a solitary lesion may provoke symptoms of flushing or colic. Mastocytomas may occur on any part of the body but are noted most frequently on the arms, neck, and trunk. A history of intermittent blistering of the affected area may be obtained, and in this setting, misdiagnosis of bullous impetigo or herpes simplex infection is common. The tendency toward vesiculation tends to disappear within 1–3 years. Although the course of mastocytomas is generally benign and the lesions usually involute over several years, there have been reports of solitary mastocytosis eventuating in generalized urticaria pigmentosa.[197]

Urticaria pigmentosa is the most common presentation of mastocytosis. It presents with multiple, well-demarcated, tan to red-brown macules and papules (Fig. 9.48) that may occur anywhere on the cutaneous surface. Mucous membranes may be involved, and palms and soles are usually spared. Some lesions may have a purpuric quality, and occasionally a yellow coloration is noted. There may be tens to hundreds of lesions, ranging in size from a few millimeters to several centimeters. Darier's sign is positive, and dermatographism may be present in 30–50% of patients. The lesions of urticaria pigmentosa may become vesicular or bullous (Fig. 9.49), a presentation termed *bullous mastocytosis*. These blisters may result in pain and secondary infection, but generally heal without scarring. Beyond the age of 2 years, bullous changes are unusual.[188]

Diffuse cutaneous mastocytosis is a less common variant of mastocytosis, especially in children. This presentation is characterized by diffuse infiltration of the skin by mast cells, with skin that may appear grossly normal, thickened, doughy, reddish-brown, or peau d'orange in texture (Fig. 9.50). There may be a yellow, carotenemia-like color present, and occasionally these patients present with extensive bullous eruptions. Patients with the diffuse cutaneous form appear to have the highest frequency of systemic disease, and may experience intense generalized pruritus, flushing, temperature elevation, vomiting, diarrhea, abdominal pain, gastrointestinal ulceration, or respiratory distress. Overt shock may occur in this form of mastocytosis.

Telangiectasia macularis eruptive perstans is a variant of mastocytosis seen usually in adults, and only rarely reported in children. Patients with TMEP have an eruption of small, red-brown, telangiectatic macules on the trunk and extremities with little or no tendency toward urtication.

Systemic mastocytosis is markedly more common in adults than in children with mastocytosis. The most frequently involved systems are gastrointestinal and skeletal, although the lungs, kidneys, lymph nodes, myocardium, pericardium, liver, spleen, and bone marrow may also be affected. Skeletal lesions may consist of radio-opacities, radiolucencies, or a mixture of both. These changes are quite rare in children with the disorder.[198] Hepatomegaly, splenomegaly, and lymph node enlargement may also occur. Gastrointestinal symptoms include abdominal pain, diarrhea, nausea, and vomiting. Gastrointestinal hemorrhage may occasionally occur, and is often

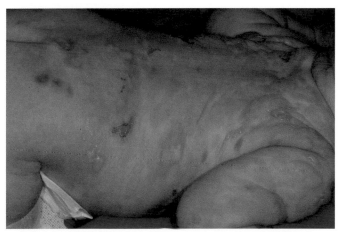

Figure 9.49 Bullous mastocytosis. This 8-month-old female had widespread mastocytosis with blister formation. Note the diffuse distribution of infiltrative plaques, peau d'orange changes, superficial erosions, and intact bullae of the shoulders, upper back and flank.

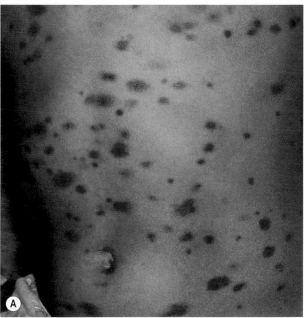

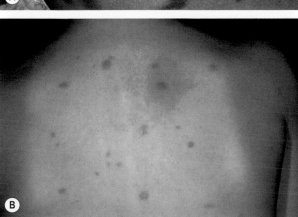

Figure 9.48 Urticaria pigmentosa. (A) Multiple hyperpigmented macules and papules in this 2-year-old girl. (B) Light tan macules and papules in a school-age boy. Note the Darier's sign, which occurred after rubbing the lesion.

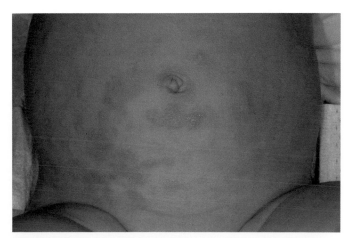

Figure 9.50 Diffuse cutaneous mastocytosis. This child had diffuse erythematous-yellow plaques and peau d'orange surface changes.

secondary to gastritis or peptic ulcer disease. Children with the diffuse cutaneous form of mastocytosis may be at particular risk for this complication.[188] The 'mastocytosis syndrome' results from massive histamine release with symptoms including bronchospasm, headache, flushing, diarrhea, pruritus, and hypotension. It occurs most often in infants or young children with the diffuse cutaneous form of the disease, and death may occasionally result.

The increased risk of development of a hematologic malignancy is a major concern in adults with mastocytosis. The hematopoietic and reticuloendothelial systems in pediatric patients, however, are rarely involved, and the level of increased risk, if any, in childhood mastocytosis remains unclear.

Anesthetic management of pediatric patients with mastocytosis has traditionally been viewed as complex and risky, given the nature of the disease, the degranulation effects of some anesthetic agents, and the reported adult literature. Recent reports, however, suggest that pediatric patients with cutaneous (vs systemic) mastocytosis are at fairly low risk for major anesthesia-related complications.[199,200] Anesthesia considerations for pediatric mastocytosis patients are listed in Table 9.5.

The diagnosis of pediatric mastocytosis is often based on the characteristic cutaneous findings and positive Darier's sign. Although it is usually a straightforward diagnosis, atypical or unusual presentations or those lacking skin involvement may pose a diagnostic challenge. When skin lesions are present, the diagnosis can be confirmed with skin biopsy, which reveals an accumulation of mast cells in the dermis. Special immunohistochemical stains, such as Giemsa, toluidine blue, or tryptase antibodies, maybe useful in confirming the mast cell nature of the infiltrate. Biopsy of the bone marrow or GI tract may be necessary if such organ involvement is suspected and the patient lacks cutaneous lesions.

Indirect methods for diagnosing mastocytosis are also available. Measurement of serum tryptase, a protease produced by mast cells, is helpful in supporting the diagnosis.[201] Two forms (α and β) have been identified, and measuring both of these mediators can be useful for correlation with the extent of mast cell disease. Urinary histamine and its metabolites may also be helpful. High levels of urinary N-methylhistamine may be suggestive of more extensive

involvement.[202] Urinary N-methylimidazoleacetic acid is another histamine metabolite that is useful as a chemical marker for the disease.[203]

Extensive laboratory or radiographic studies, or invasive diagnostic procedures, in pediatric patients with mastocytosis are generally not indicated. However, in patients with extensive disease (i.e., extensive urticaria pigmentosa or diffuse cutaneous mastocytosis), complete blood cell count with peripheral smear and blood chemistry studies should be performed, with occasional follow-up. Other diagnostic studies, such as abdominal ultrasound, endoscopy, bone scan, or bone marrow biopsy, should be reserved for patients in whom specific symptoms suggest systemic disease.[188]

The course and prognosis of mastocytosis depends on the clinical subtype, severity of disease, and age of onset. In general, the prognosis for childhood mastocytosis is favorable in most patients. Symptoms improve by adolescence in up to 50% of patients,[204] but complete resolution may occur less often than previously believed. In one study, 5 of 33 children had complete resolution, and 21 of the 33 had improvement by adolescence.[205] When mastocytosis persists into adulthood, patients have the same risk of systemic disease as do those with adult-onset mastocytosis.[188]

The treatment of mastocytosis is primarily symptomatic, as no specific therapy or cure currently exists for this disorder. Patients (and/or their parents) should be counseled about the disease, its natural history, differences between pediatric and adult mastocytosis, and possible triggers of mast cell degranulation (Table 9.4). Non-sedating histamine type 1 receptor (H1) antagonists are a good initial treatment of choice, and include cetirizine, levocetirizine, loratadine, and fexofenadine. The long half-life and nonsedating nature of these medications offers advantages over traditional antihistamines. In patients with severe involvement or symptoms, a classic H1 antagonist (i.e., hydroxyzine, diphenhydramine, and cyproheptadine) may be useful. The addition of an H2 antagonist (i.e., cimetidine, ranitidine, famotidine) may be considered, especially in patients with flushing or marked gastrointestinal symptoms.

Oral cromolyn sodium has been found useful in treating gastrointestinal symptoms of mastocytosis, although controlled studies in children are lacking. Ketotifen, a mast cell stabilizer unavailable in the oral form in the USA, has shown promise in alleviating symptoms. Psoralen plus UVA (PUVA) therapy has been demonstrated useful in urticaria pigmentosa, diffuse cutaneous mastocytosis, and systemic mastocytosis.[206,207] This therapy is more challenging though, and has a higher risk-to-benefit ratio in children. Aspirin and NSAIDs, although they may induce mast cell degranulation, may paradoxically be used to reduce prostaglandin-dependent flushing in some patients. Mastocytomas have been noted to improve or disappear after therapy with a potent topical corticosteroid under occlusion. A brief course of oral corticosteroids (i.e., 1 mg/kg per day of prednisone or prednisolone for 4–6 weeks) may be quite effective for symptomatic patients, but obviously is not an appropriate long-term therapy. Cyclosporin and interferon-α2b have been used in some adults with more aggressive forms of mastocytosis. Lastly, patients (parents of children) at risk for recurrent hypotensive episodes or mastocytosis syndrome should have a premeasured epinephrine pen kit (EpiPen or EpiPen Jr) with them at all times for emergency use. Lastly, information regarding patient support groups and education for pediatric mastocytosis (www.mastokids.org) should be given.

Granuloma Annulare

Granuloma annulare (GA) is a fairly common skin disorder characterized by papules or nodules grouped in a ring-like or circinate configuration. Although GA may occur on any part of the body, it

---

Table 9.5 Anesthesia considerations in pediatric mastocytosis patients

Ensure adequate familiarity of anesthesiologist with pediatric mastocytosis and preparedness to treat possible adverse events during anesthesia
Review detailed history of past clinical drug reactions prior to anesthesia
Consider baseline serum tryptase, which may be useful to: Suggest systemic mastocytosis (and concomitant higher risk of anesthetic reaction), if extreme elevation   Diagnose possible anesthesia-related adverse events, if significantly elevated from baseline
Avoid preoperative drug skin testing
Continue scheduled maintenance mastocytosis medications
Consider administration of incremental (vs single boluses) of necessary agents known to be mast cell degranulators
Administer NSAIDs with caution and only in the absence of a history of sensitivity
Consider patient positioning to minimize mechanical pressure on skin during anesthesia

Adapted from Carter et al. (2008)[199] and Ahmad et al (2009).[200] NSAID, non-steroidal antiinflammatory drug.

often involves the lateral or dorsal surfaces of the hands, feet, wrists, and ankles. Patients may have solitary lesions or multiple sites of involvement. Granuloma annulare may occur at any age, and is especially common in school-age children.

The cause of GA is unknown. Various studies have suggested a possible association between GA and diabetes mellitus, but this hypothesis remains controversial and some studies refute it.[208] Other purported associations have included tetanus or BCG vaccination, hepatitis B infection, *Borrelia* infection, Hodgkin's disease, leukemia or a hypersensitivity reaction to an unidentified antigen.[209–212] In some individuals GA has been noted following trauma, sun exposure, and insect bites.

Granuloma annulare most classically presents with an annular, smooth, non-scaly plaque with a border composed of numerous small papules (Fig. 9.51). Patients are often misdiagnosed with tinea corporis and have previously failed topical antifungal therapy. Early lesions begin as smooth, flesh-colored to pink papules that slowly enlarge peripherally and undergo central involution to form the classic rings with clear centers and elevated borders. Lesions may range in size from 5 mm to several centimeters.

There are several clinical variants of GA. A *generalized* form may occur, in which patients have multiple, disseminated, small papular lesions. *Perforating GA* presents as grouped papules, some of which have a central umbilication or crusting and scaling. This form is seen mainly on the extremities. *Subcutaneous GA* (Figs 9.52, 9.53) is an important subtype in children, in whom it is most common. This form presents as subcutaneous nodules, distributed mainly on the feet, anterior tibial surfaces, fingers, hands, and scalp.[213,214] Penis lesions have also been rarely reported.[215] These lesions are usually painless and only occasionally slightly tender. The differential diagnosis of these lesions includes rheumatoid nodules, trauma, infection, malignancy, and tumor. Incisional biopsy is often necessary to confirm the diagnosis, unless there are classic cutaneous GA lesions present elsewhere on the skin surface.

Lesions of granuloma annulare usually disappear spontaneously, without sequelae, within several months to years. There is no satisfactory therapy for GA, but since the lesions are nearly always asymptomatic, watchful waiting is often acceptable. Topical corticosteroids, either ointments or creams, or impregnated into tape may be effective, but are limited by their potential in causing skin atrophy. Intralesional corticosteroid injection has also been utilized in some patients. Cryotherapy has been used, as have a variety of systemic agents (including isotretinoin, prednisone, dapsone, and cyclosporine), but the risk-to-benefit ratio is generally not justified for these drugs. Occasionally, the lesions spontaneously regress

following skin biopsy. Until the association with diabetes mellitus is clearly established or refuted, patients with GA should be followed by their primary physician for signs or symptoms, and if there is any concern or a strong family history, testing should be considered.

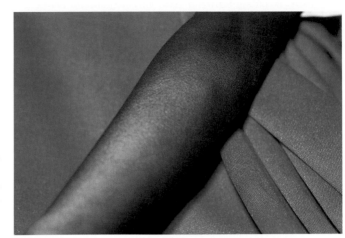

Figure 9.52 Subcutaneous granuloma annulare. Subcutaneous nodules on the forearm.

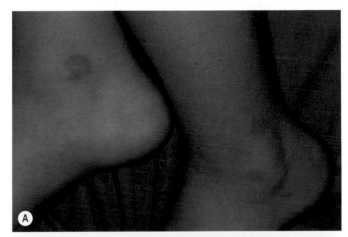

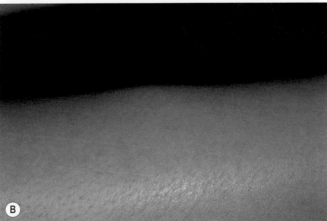

Figure 9.53 Granuloma annulare. This patient had both cutaneous lesions (A) on the malleolar surfaces and subcutaneous lesions (B) on the anterior tibial surfaces.

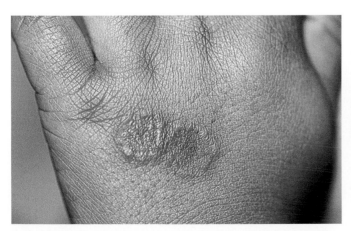

Figure 9.51 Granuloma annulare. Annular, flesh-colored, non-scaly plaques.

Neurofibroma

Neurofibromas may appear as isolated, usually single lesions in a healthy individual or as a cutaneous marker of dominantly inherited type 1 neurofibromatosis (NF1, von Recklinghausen's disease) (see Ch. 11). Lesions not associated with NF1 are discussed here.

Neurofibromas are benign tumors composed of neuromesenchymal tissue, including Schwann cells, endoneurial and perineurial cells, and other cellular components. They often present during young adulthood, and occasionally early in life. Clinically, a neurofibroma presents as a soft, flesh-colored, solitary papule or papulonodule. They may occasionally be red, blue, or brown. They range in size from 2 mm to 2 cm, and with further growth, they become globular, pear-shaped, pedunculated, or pendulous. Neurofibromas exhibit a positive 'buttonhole' sign, felt to be pathognomonic, whereby direct pressure on top of the lesion results in easy invagination into the dermis. This sign may be useful in differentiating neurofibromas from intradermal nevi or dermatofibromas.

When multiple neurofibromas are present, the diagnosis of NF1 must be considered. The presence of café-au-lait macules, axillary or inguinal freckling, or a plexiform neurofibroma lends further support to this diagnosis. *Plexiform neurofibroma* presents as a large, lobulated nodular plaque that may have a 'bag of worms' consistency on palpation. These lesions are considered pathognomonic for NF1 (for further discussion, see Ch. 11). Sporadic neurofibromas are best treated with surgical excision.

Dermatofibroma

Dermatofibroma (fibrous histiocytoma) is a benign neoplasm of connective tissue generally seen in adults; occasionally it is seen in children. It presents as a small, well-defined dermal nodule, firmly fixed to the skin but freely movable over the subcutaneous fat. There is often a tan to brown color of the surface (Fig. 9.54). Dermatofi-

bromas may be found on any part of the body and are common on the extremities, particularly the anterior surface of the leg. They range in size from 1 mm to 2 cm. A useful diagnostic feature is the 'dimple sign', whereby pinching the lesion results in downward displacement.

The differential diagnosis may include melanocytic nevus or cyst. Although treatment of dermatofibromas is unnecessary, surgical excision may be performed for cosmetic purposes or diagnostic confirmation.

Dermatofibrosarcoma Protuberans

Dermatofibrosarcoma protuberans (DFSP) is a slowly growing fibrohistiocytic tumor with intermediate malignant potential, seen primarily in adults between the second and fifth decades. These lesions tend to be locally invasive, have a high recurrence rate after excision, and occasionally result in metastatic disease. Pediatric, and even congenital, cases are occasionally observed, although most lesions present during the second to fifth decades of life.

DFSP usually begins as erythematous to blue papules and nodules that increase in size and may ultimately become multinodular and protuberant. Some lesions present as an atrophic plaque. Ulceration may be present. The majority of lesions occur on the trunk or proximal extremities, and the scalp, neck, and face are occasionally involved. During infancy or early childhood, DFSP may be misdiagnosed as a vascular malformation or tumor given the vascular appearance of many lesions.[216,217] Other initial impressions may include keloid, dermatofibroma, morphea, scar or epidermal cyst.[218] Significant variability in presentation appears to be common with congenital lesions, which are rare but well documented.[217]

Dermatofibrosarcoma protuberans has been linked to a chromosomal translocation, t(17:22), which fuses the collagen type1, alpha 1 (COL1A1) and PDGF-beta genes.[219] The treatment of choice for DFSP is complete surgical excision with adequate margins. In recent years, Mohs micrographic surgery has evolved as the therapeutic standard of care, and it has more recently been demonstrated to offer superior cure rates, smaller surgical margins and fewer surgical sessions when compared to wide local excision in treating congenital DFSP.[220] In patients with DFSP, lifelong clinical follow-up is recommended given the risk of recurrence, however, metastatic spread is fortunately quite rare.[221]

Fibromatoses

The fibromatoses are a group of disorders marked by fibrous and fibrohistiocytic proliferations in the skin. These disorders may represent neoplastic or reactive processes and tend to be benign in nature, although several have the potential for recurrence following excision. In this section, three pediatric fibromatoses are discussed.

Recurring Digital Fibroma of Childhood

Recurring digital fibroma of childhood (RDFC, also known as recurring infantile digital fibromatosis) is a rare, benign childhood fibromatosis. It usually occurs on the dorsal and lateral aspects of the fingers and toes, and presents at birth or, less commonly, during infancy or later childhood. The majority of lesions are present by 12 months of age.[222] Interestingly, the thumbs and great toes are usually spared.

RDFC presents as flesh-colored to slightly erythematous papules and nodules (Fig. 9.55). Lesions are usually multiple and tend to affect multiple digits. They may become as large as 2 cm in size.

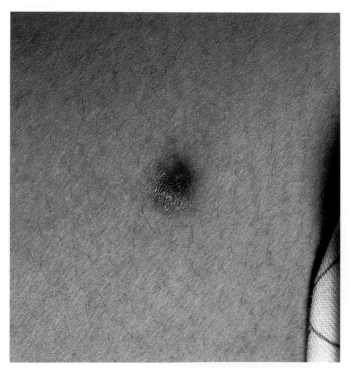

Figure 9.54 Dermatofibroma. This gray-brown papule was firm to palpation.

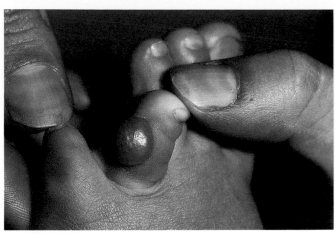

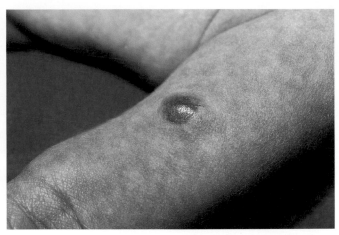

Figure 9.55 Recurring digital fibroma of childhood. A firm, erythematous tumor on the lateral surface of the fourth toe.

Figure 9.56 Solitary myofibroma. This lesion was congenital, and spontaneously resolved by 1 year of age.

Joint deformities and lateral deviation or flexion deformities may occasionally be associated.[222,223]

The etiology of RDFC is unknown, and although a viral etiology was once postulated based on eosinophilic inclusion bodies seen on histologic examination, there appears to be little evidence in support of this hypothesis.[224] Management of RDFC is controversial. Arguments in favor of a conservative 'watchful waiting' approach include the observation that many lesions spontaneously regress over a few years, that excision of the lesions does not alter the natural history of the joint disease (when present), and that excision is often followed by recurrence.[225] However, some assert that surgical excision is indicated to prevent continuous growth and involvement of deeper tissues, and because some lesions do not spontaneously resolve. For smaller lesions without functional impairment, it seems that conservative management of RDFC is most appropriate.

Infantile Myofibromatosis

Infantile myofibromatosis is a term used to describe two fibrous disorders (infantile myofibromatosis and congenital generalized myofibromatosis) that represent two variants of the same process. Patients with these conditions have neoplasms composed of myofibroblasts, a distinct cell type that appears to also be involved in recurring digital fibroma of childhood (see above). Some cases of infantile myofibromatosis may mimic congenital infantile fibrosarcoma, and in these patients, molecular analysis for the ETV6-NTRK3 gene fusion transcript (present in some infantile fibrosarcomas) may be useful.[226]

In infantile myofibromatosis, fibrous nodules may occur in skin, subcutaneous tissue, skeletal muscle, and bone. Most patients have solitary lesions, and the most common sites of involvement are the head and neck regions.[227] The myofibromas, which are often present at birth, appear as flesh-colored to purple, firm or rubbery papules (Fig. 9.56), nodules, or plaques. The differential diagnosis of a solitary myofibroma may include infantile hemangioma, histiocytoma, mastocytoma, and infantile digital fibroma. Visceral involvement is rare when the cutaneous lesion is solitary.

Multiple myofibromas, a condition that has also been termed congenital generalized myofibromatosis, presents with scattered cutaneous and subcutaneous tumors (Fig. 9.57) in addition to lytic bony lesions. Radiography reveals multiple radiolucent areas in the metaphyseal regions.[228] These patients may also have muscle and visceral involvement, with lesions in the gastrointestinal tract,

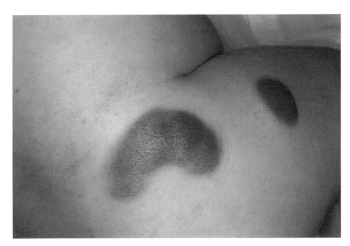

Figure 9.57 Multiple myofibromas. Firm, rubbery nodules and plaques on the thigh of an infant.

lungs, kidneys, spleen, lymph nodes, meninges, nerves, thyroid, adrenal gland, and heart. Spinal canal involvement has also been reported.[229] Although the lesions do not tend to be locally aggressive nor metastasize, their space-occupying nature in some anatomic regions may interfere with vital functions. The differential diagnosis of multiple myofibromas includes hemangiomatosis, juvenile xanthogranulomas, cutaneous metastases (i.e., from neuroblastoma or leukemia), mastocytosis, and sarcomas.

Since the cutaneous and subcutaneous nodules of infantile myofibromatosis tend to regress spontaneously, surgical excision is indicated only for diagnostic confirmation, to alleviate obstruction or potential trauma, or to treat lesions in which the clinical course is prolonged and progressive. Patients with lesions limited to skin and/or bone have a good prognosis. Those with disseminated multiorgan involvement have a higher incidence of morbidity and mortality. Chemotherapy has been utilized for patients with severe involvement.

Fibrous Hamartoma of Infancy

Fibrous hamartoma of infancy is a rare, benign, soft tissue tumor that usually presents during the first two years of life. One in four cases is congenital, and around 90% occur within the first year of

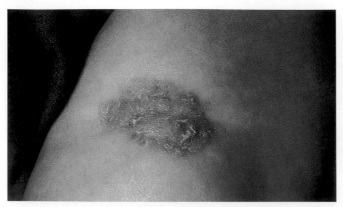

Figure 9.58 Fibrous hamartoma of infancy.

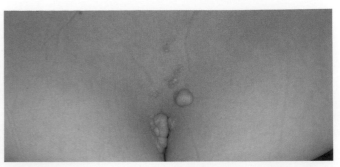

Figure 9.59 Nevus lipomatosus superficialis. This soft, multilobulated plaque was present at birth in the superior gluteal cleft region.

life.[230] It appears to be more common in boys, and has a predilection for the upper trunk, axillae, upper extremities, groin, or genitalia.[231]

Fibrous hamartoma presents as a painless, flesh-colored subcutaneous nodule or nodular plaque (Fig. 9.58). Most cases are solitary, although multiple lesions may occur. They may be mobile or appear to be fixed to underlying tissues. The clinical differential diagnosis may include infantile myofibromatosis (see above) and malignant soft tissue sarcoma. The natural history of fibrous hamartoma is characterized by slow growth, although rapid growth of lesions has been reported.[230] Histologic examination of biopsy tissue reveals the characteristic triad of tissues: adipose, fibrous, and myxoid mesenchymal tissue.

The treatment of choice for fibrous hamartoma of infancy is full surgical excision, although for excessively large lesions this may not be a feasible option. Local recurrence may occur in up to 15% of cases, and is often noted within a few months following the primary surgery.[232] In lesions left untreated, growth continues until around 5 years of age, at which time it plateaus.[233]

Tumors of fat, muscles, and bone

Lipomas

Lipoma, one of the most common benign tumors, is composed of mature fat (adipose) cells. It can be seen at any age but usually occurs at or after puberty. Lesions may be present on any part of the body but predominantly involve the subcutaneous tissues of the neck, shoulders, back, and abdomen. They may be single or multiple and their size is variable, with a characteristic soft, rubbery or putty-like consistency. Microscopic examination reveals encapsulated tumors of adipose tissue with essentially the same appearance as that of normal subcutaneous fat.

A rare nevoid variety, *nevus lipomatosus superficialis* (Fig. 9.59), is characterized by clusters of soft, flesh-colored to yellowish papules, nodules, or plaques often located on the buttocks, lumbosacral region, or thighs. These lesions are often present at birth or develop over the first decade of life. Another lipoma variant, *angiolipoma*, is clinically indistinguishable except that the lesions are often tender or painful and have a greater tendency to be multiple. Angiolipomas occur primarily in teenagers and young adults, and commonly present on the upper extremities or trunk.

Lipomas and the discussed variants are benign lesions. Surgical excision is generally curative, and is indicated for lesions that are painful or of cosmetic significance, or in those lesions for which the diagnosis is uncertain (although incisional biopsy is another option

in this setting). Three syndromes that have lipomas as a component will be briefly discussed: Bannayan–Riley–Ruvalcaba syndrome, encephalocraniocutaneous lipomatosis, and the Michelin tire baby.

Bannayan–Riley–Ruvalcaba syndrome

Bannayan–Riley–Ruvalcaba syndrome (BRR, Bannayan–Zonana syndrome) is an autosomal dominant, multiple hamartoma syndrome, shown to be caused by mutations in the PTEN gene. The hallmark of BRR is macrocephaly. Patients also have multiple subcutaneous or visceral lipomas and vascular malformations. Pigmented macules of the penis are common. Facial trichilemmomas, as described in Cowden syndrome (CS), may also be seen and the same PTEN mutations have similarly been described in this syndrome (see above). Other clinical findings in BRR include oral papillomas, acral (palmoplantar) keratoses, acanthosis nigricans, joint hyperextensibility, scoliosis, pectus excavatum, and downslanting palpebral fissures. Hypotonia, developmental delay, and hamartomatous intestinal polyps may also occur.[166] The latter may result in chronic anemia, diarrhea, failure to thrive or small bowel intussusception.[234] Careful phenotyping has suggested that BRR and CS represent one condition with variable expression and age-related penetrance.[235]

Encephalocraniocutaneous lipomatosis

Encephalocraniocutaneous lipomatosis (ECCL) is a rare neurocutaneous syndrome characterized by mental retardation and unilateral skin and ocular lesions with ipsilateral cerebral malformations. The cutaneous lipomas in ECCL are most often limited to the scalp, and may be accompanied by alopecia. Various ocular abnormalities, including eyelid defects, epibulbar dermoids, scleral desmoid tumors, and corneal clouding, may occur.[236,237] CNS malformations are variable, and include intracranial/spinal lipomas (most common), hemisphere asymmetry, cortical dysplasia, cysts, ventricular dilatation, calcifications, and corpus callosum abnormalities.[238] Seizures are common and tend to start during infancy. The differential diagnosis includes Proteus syndrome, epidermal nevus (nevus sebaceous) syndrome, and oculocerebrocutaneous syndrome.

The Michelin tire baby

Michelin tire baby (Michelin tire syndrome) is a term used to describe a very rare disorder of newborns characterized by numerous, conspicuous cutaneous folds, presumably caused by excessive fat. Elastic fiber abnormalities have also been noted on ultrastructural examination of lesional skin (see Ch. 6).[239] The terminology is derived from the resemblance of affected patients to the mascot for the tire manufacturer, Michelin. Other histologic abnormalities that have been noted in these patients include nevus lipomatosis and smooth muscle hamartoma. A variety of extracutaneous defects, including developmental delay/mental retardation, facial dysmorphism, microcephaly, musculoskeletal anomalies (including rocker-bottom feet, metatarsus abductus and lax joints), hirsutism, hemiplegia, hemihypertrophy, chromosomal abnormalities, abnormal ears, and neurologic abnormalities, may be associated. Michelin tire syndrome may represent a nonspecific clinical presentation related to a variety of different causes.[240]

Congenital Smooth Muscle Hamartoma

Congenital smooth muscle hamartoma is a benign skin disorder characterized by a proliferation of smooth muscle within the reticular dermis. It may be seen within or without an associated Becker's nevus (see Pigmented lesions, above). Smooth muscle hamartoma, when presenting independent of Becker's nevus, appears as a localized, slightly elevated, flesh-colored to faintly hyperpigmented plaque. The lesions may be extremely subtle on examination, but a useful feature is mild overlying hypertrichosis (Fig. 9.60), which may best be visualized with side lighting using a penlight or otoscope head. Rubbing of the plaque may cause a 'pseudo-Darier's' sign, with transient piloerection and the appearance of 'gooseflesh'-like surface changes.

Although most lesions are congenital, they may not be noted until childhood or even early adulthood. Smooth muscle hamartoma is nearly always asymptomatic, and rarely of cosmetic significance. Surgical excision is curative, but rarely necessary.

Leiomyomas

Leiomyomas represent benign tumors principally derived from cutaneous smooth muscle. The majority of these lesions arise from arrector pili muscles, the media of blood vessels, or smooth muscle of the scrotum, labia majora, or nipples. Although found among all age groups, leiomyomas generally occur during the third decade of life and are relatively uncommon in childhood.

Cutaneous leiomyomas may be solitary or multiple and generally present as pink, red, or dusky brown, firm dermal nodules of varying size. They are subject to episodes of paroxysmal spontaneous pain. When multiple, leiomyomas are usually red-brown to blue, firm intradermal nodules with a translucent or waxy appearance. They tend to occur on the back, face, or extensor surfaces of the extremities and are usually arranged in groups. Enlarging lesions may coalesce to form plaques with an arcuate or linear configuration. Multiple leiomyomas may be associated with common uterine fibroids, an association termed *multiple cutaneous and uterine leiomyomatosis syndrome*. This disorder, as well as another hereditary leiomyoma syndrome, *hereditary leiomyomatosis and renal cell cancer*, are both caused by heterozygous mutations in the fumarate hydratase (FH) gene.[241]

Leiomyomas may be classified as hereditary or non-hereditary types and are characterized by unencapsulated tumors of smooth muscle bundles and masses with an irregular arrangement. Cutaneous leiomyomas have been divided into three types:

1. Piloleiomyomas, the most common type
2. Solitary genital or mammary leiomyomas, derived from the smooth muscle of the nipple and genital regions (referred to as the dartoic type)
3. Angioleiomyomas, arising from the tunica media of the blood vessels and embryonic muscle rests, and most often found on the lower leg.

Leiomyosarcoma, a rare soft tissue sarcoma, occurs primarily in older individuals and may have histologic overlap with leiomyoma. Clinically, they are larger than leiomyomas and present as nondescript subcutaneous masses, which may enlarge rapidly and ulcerate. Metastases, when they occur, generally spread through the bloodstream and lymphatics, and lung involvement is common. The histologic features most useful in distinguishing these tumors from benign leiomyomas are high cellularity, cytologic atypia, and obvious mitotic figures.

Leiomyomas are benign but have a high incidence of recurrence following removal. Surgical excision is the treatment of choice, and is curative for smaller, localized tumors. When multiple leiomyomas are present, therapy is challenging and has included CO_2 laser ablation.

Myoblastoma

Myoblastoma (granular cell tumor) is an uncommon tumor that occurs most often as a solitary nodule in the head and neck regions, and especially the tongue. It is rare overall in children. Laryngeal involvement may occur in the posterior or anterior larynx, vocal folds and arytenoids.[242] Patients with multiple tumors have been reported, occasionally in association with neurofibromatosis type 1.[243] *Congenital epulis* represents a granular cell tumor of the gingivae in a newborn, usually marked by spontaneous involution. The origin of granular cell tumors is believed to be neural, with a Schwann cell derivation hypothesized but not proven. Surgical excision is the treatment of choice.

Calcinosis Cutis

Calcinosis cutis is a general term for calcium deposition in the skin. It may be related to abnormal calcium or phosphorus metabolism, damage to the dermal collagen, or idiopathic in origin.[244] It may be focal or widespread. Calcinosis cutis has traditionally been divided into the following subtypes: dystrophic, idiopathic, metastatic, and iatrogenic. Tumoral calcinosis is another distinct subtype.

Dystrophic calcinosis cutis occurs following trauma or inflammation in the skin. This form may also be noted in the setting of diseases that predispose to deposition of calcium in the skin, such as juvenile dermatomyositis (Fig. 9.61 and Ch. 22, Figs 22.9, 22.30) scleroderma, and systemic lupus erythematosus. Calcium deposition in the skin may occur years before other stigmata of dermatomyositis become noticeable,[245] although more typically the calcifications occur years after the disease onset. In dystrophic

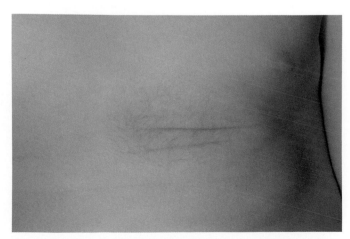

Figure 9.60 Smooth muscle hamartoma. Note the mild hypertrichosis overlying this flesh-colored, dermal plaque.

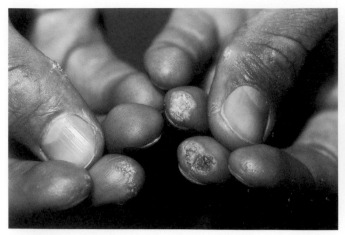

Figure 9.61 Calcinosis cutis in juvenile dermatomyositis. This patient had painful, firm nodules of both knees and both elbows.

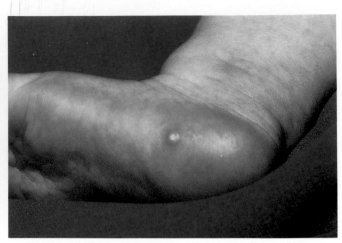

Figure 9.63 Heel stick calcinosis cutis. Firm, white papulonodule at the site of prior heel stick procedures.

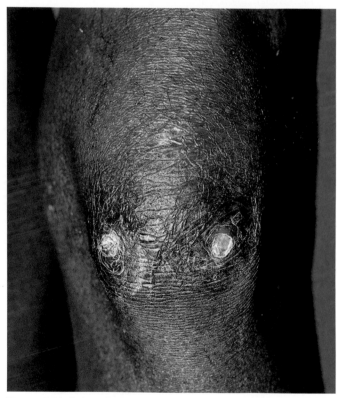

Figure 9.62 Calcinosis cutis in CREST syndrome. Painful, firm deposits with overlying skin breakdown on the distal digits of this teenaged girl with CREST.

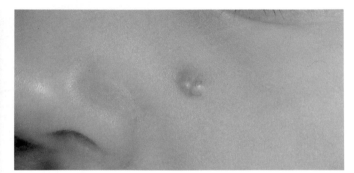

Figure 9.64 Subepidermal calcified nodule. Solitary, firm, white to flesh-colored papulonodule on the cheek.

A common setting for dystrophic calcinosis cutis is in infants following heel stick procedures. These calcifications appear as firm, white to yellow papules on the heels (Fig. 9.63) and are most often seen in high-risk neonates following multiple needle sticks to these locations.[246] They can also occur in healthy neonates after only a single heel stick.[247]

Idiopathic calcinosis cutis occurs in individuals who have normal calcium and phosphorus metabolism, and have no history of trauma or underlying inflammatory diseases. It may occur in various areas of the body, most commonly the scrotum, face, and female genitalia. Labial calcinosis cutis presents as white papules or nodules on the labia majora, and is important to recognize as it may be misdiagnosed as a condition associated with potential sexual abuse (i.e., condylomata or molluscum).[244] *Sub-epidermal calcified nodule* is a solitary, white to flesh-colored, firm papule or papulonodule (Fig. 9.64), most commonly occurring in children. These lesions are often seen on the face. *Milia-like idiopathic calcinosis cutis* presents with small white papules that may discharge a chalk-like substance. These lesions occur most commonly on the hands (Fig. 9.65) and feet, and are usually seen in patients with Down syndrome.[248,249]

Metastatic calcinosis cutis occurs when calcium deposits in the skin and soft tissue of patients who have altered metabolism of calcium and/or phosphorus. One association is chronic renal failure, which results in hypocalcemia with resultant secondary hyperparathyroidism with increased mobilization of both calcium and phosphate. Hypervitaminosis D and milk-alkali syndrome are other potential causes of metastatic calcinosis cutis. *Calciphylaxis*, or

calcinosis cutis, calcium and phosphorus metabolism are normal. Clinically, patients present with firm to rock-hard papules or larger subcutaneous plaques. Elbows, knees, and shoulders are common locations. Secondary ulceration and transepidermal elimination of calcium may occur (presenting as white, chalky material protruding from the affected area). In calcinosis universalis, as may be seen in juvenile dermatomyositis, extensive subcutaneous deposits of calcium occur and patients may present with an exoskeleton. This form has a particularly poor prognosis. Patients with the CREST variant of scleroderma present with painful, calcified papules and nodules over bony prominences and distal digits (Fig. 9.62).

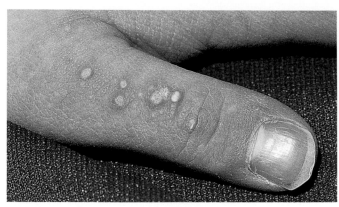

Figure 9.65 Milia-like idiopathic calcinosis cutis in Down syndrome. These firm, white papules were asymptomatic.

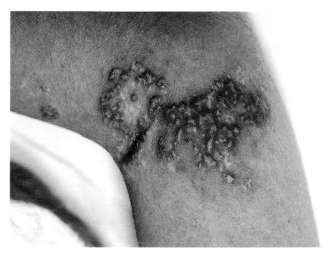

Figure 9.66 Calcinosis cutis following extravasation injury.

calcifying panniculitis, is a severe disorder characterized by vascular calcification with resultant ischemic necrosis of skin and soft tissue. It may result in gangrene and sepsis, and the mortality rate is high. *Tumoral calcinosis* presents with calcifications in juxtaarticular sites, predominantly on extensor surfaces. These grow over months to years and frequently recur following surgical removal.[250] These lesions may attain a fairly large size (up to 20 cm) and may result in disfigurement or impaired function. This disorder may occur sporadically or in an autosomal dominant fashion.

Iatrogenic calcinosis cutis occurs when there is a precipitation of calcium salts in the skin. It most commonly occurs following extravasation of calcium gluconate or calcium chloride. It presents as yellow-white plaques (Fig. 9.66) that frequently reveal secondary inflammation. Lesions are most commonly (but not always) located around sites of prior intravenous line insertions.[251] Central ulceration may occur. These lesions tend to resolve over 4–6 months. Calcinosis cutis has also been reported following application of calcium chloride-containing electrode paste for electroencephalography, electromyography, and auditory-brainstem evoked potentials recordings.[252]

Treatment of calcinosis cutis is challenging, and may include surgical excision, curettage, low calcium and phosphate diet, and administration of aluminum hydroxide, diltiazem, colchicine, or etidronate. The underlying disorder, if present, should obviously be treated.

Osteoma Cutis

Cutaneous ossification (bone formation) is a rare phenomenon, especially in children, that may occur in a variety of settings. It may be primary or secondary. The term *osteoma cutis* is nonspecific, but has traditionally been used to refer to a primary form of spontaneous bone formation in the skin associated with Albright's hereditary osteodystrophy or as an isolated idiopathic occurrence. Secondary cutaneous ossification occurs in areas of inflammation or neoplastic tissue, and may also be seen in any disorder where calcification is present and in benign skin tumors or cysts.

Albright's hereditary osteodystrophy (AHO) (see Ch. 23) is a genetic condition that may present with diffuse cutaneous ossification in conjunction with pseudohypoparathyroidism or pseudo-pseudohypoparathyroidism. These patients tend to be short and obese with a variety of dysmorphic features, including a classic foreshortening of the fourth and fifth metacarpals and metatarsals.

Progressive osseous heteroplasia (POH) is a rare disorder characterized by progressive ossification of skin, muscle, and connective tissue, which may result in significant functional and cosmetic deformity. It usually begins in infancy and tends to be progressive.[253] It can be distinguished from another ossification disorder, *fibro-dysplasia ossificans progressiva* (FOP), by the presence of cutaneous ossification, the absence of congenital malformations of the skeleton, the absence of tumor-like swellings, the asymmetric distribution of lesions, and the predominance of intramembranous rather than endochondral ossification.[254] In both of these disorders, calcium and phosphorus metabolism are normal, in distinction to patients with AHO. The prognosis of FOP is poor, whereas the prognosis of POH is variable. Patients with *plate-like osteoma cutis* (POC) present in infancy with one or a few areas of cutaneous ossification. These lesions tend to remain fairly localized, and these patients do not have abnormalities in calcium or phosphorus metabolism or other associated defects. The prognosis in POC tends to be good.

Miliary osteomas of the face present as small, firm, flesh-colored to white or blue papules on the face. They have been observed in patients both with and without a history of acne vulgaris.

Subungual Exostosis

Subungual exostosis is a solitary hard nodule that occurs on the terminal border of the distal phalanx of a finger or toe. Although the great toe tends to be the most commonly afflicted, this disorder may involve other toes or, occasionally, a finger. However, fifth toe involvement is unusual.[255] Subungual exostosis is a benign osteochondroma that occurs primarily in the second or third decade of life. Patients may report a history of preceding trauma, although for many this history is lacking.

Subungual exostosis presents as a pink or flesh-colored, 5–15 mm exophytic papulonodule that projects from the distal portion of the affected digit (Fig. 9.67). The surface of the lesion may become hyperkeratotic. Pain is common, and the portion of the nail overlying the lesion may be lifted and in some instances become detached. The differential diagnosis includes wart, pyogenic granuloma, glomus tumor, epidermoid carcinoma, and amelanotic melanoma. The bony consistency upon palpation will usually suggest the correct diagnosis, and plain radiography can usually confirm it, revealing an exostotic tumor arising from the dorsal aspect of the tip of the distal phalanx.[255]

Surgical excision, with curettage of the base, is the treatment of choice for subungual exostosis. Recurrences occasionally occur.

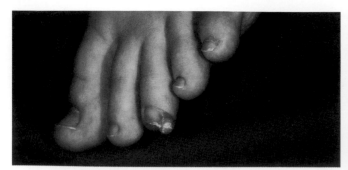

Figure 9.67 Subungual exostosis. This rock-hard papule of the distal digit was painful; excision was curative.

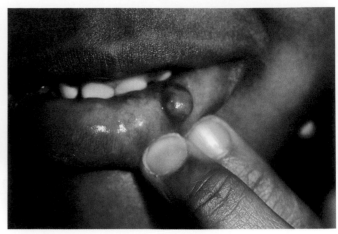

Figure 9.68 Oral mucocele. This lesion was ultimately excised because of continued enlargement.

Miscellaneous

Epidermal Cyst

Epidermal cyst (epidermoid cyst, epidermal inclusion cyst) is a discrete, slow-growing nodule that may appear any time after puberty and most commonly occurs on the face, scalp, neck, trunk, or scrotum. This is a true cyst with an epithelial lining. The term *sebaceous cyst* is an antiquated misnomer for these common tumors.

Epidermal cysts present as well-demarcated, firm to slightly compressible nodules, measuring from a few millimeters to several centimeters. An overlying central punctum, through which keratinous, foul-smelling debris may be extruded, is characteristic. Occasionally the lesions become inflamed, but true secondary infection is quite rare. Such inflammation occurs when rupture of the cyst wall occurs, and this is a frequent scenario prompting a visit to the physician.

Tiny epidermal cysts are termed *milia* (see Ch. 2). These lesions tend to be multiple, 1–2 mm in size, and white in color. In addition to occurring sporadically in healthy newborns, they may occur following abrasion trauma to the skin or in the course of bullous disorders such as epidermolysis bullosa and porphyria. Multiple cysts on the scrotum may occur, and occasionally result in calcinosis cutis (see Calcinosis Cutis, above). *Pilar cysts* (trichilemmal cysts, wens) are epidermal cysts that occur on the scalp, and *chalazions* represent analogous cystic tumors of the eyelids that develop from Meibomian glands.

An important association with multiple epidermal cysts is Gardner syndrome. This autosomal dominant condition is characterized by cutaneous cysts and intestinal polyposis. Gardner syndrome is a form of familial adenomatous polyposis (FAP), an inherited colorectal cancer syndrome characterized by hundreds of adenomas involving the large bowel, with progression (if untreated) to colorectal cancer by the fourth decade.[256,257] The term Gardner syndrome is used to describe the extracolonic manifestations that occur commonly in patients with FAP.[258] The epidermal cysts in Gardner syndrome, which are the most common cutaneous manifestation, are usually multiple, often present during early childhood, and can occur in any location, although they tend to occur most often on the face, scalp and extremities. Multiple pilomatricomas may also be seen in patients with Gardner syndrome.[179] Other findings include desmoid tumors, osteomas, fibromas, lipomas, abnormal dentition, thyroid tumors and congenital hypertrophy of the retinal pigment epithelium (CHRPE).[259] The latter finding is often present at birth and, as such, usually precedes the development of intestinal polyposis.[256] Both FAP and Gardner syndrome have been mapped to the adenomatous polyposis coli (*APC*) gene, a tumor suppressor gene.[256,257,260] Genotype-phenotype correlation studies have led some to suggest that the terminology 'Gardner syndrome' is obsolete.[257]

Malignant degeneration (squamous cell or basal cell carcinoma) of epidermal and pilar cysts is rarely reported. Treatment consists of surgical excision, with an attempt to remove the entire epithelial lining of the cyst in order to minimize the chance of recurrence.

Mucocele (Mucous Cyst)

Mucoceles (mucous cysts of the oral mucosa) present as soft, white to blue, solitary asymptomatic lesions, usually on the mucous surface of the lower lip and occasionally on the gingivae, tongue, or buccal mucosa. They are usually <1 cm in diameter and translucent (Fig. 9.68), containing a clear viscous fluid. Mucoceles are the result of minor trauma, causing rupture of a mucous duct and extravasation of sialomucin into the tissues. Treatment options include surgical excision, incision, and drainage followed by coagulation of the sac, CO_2 laser ablation, or cryosurgery. Occasionally, lesions may rupture spontaneously, although this is usually followed by eventual recurrence.

Digital Mucous Cyst

Digital mucous cyst (myxoid cyst) is a focal accumulation of mucin that presents as a soft, translucent, pink to blue, dome-shaped nodule on the dorsal aspect of the distal interphalangeal joint or proximal nail fold. Occasionally, the overlying nail plate reveals a longitudinal depression distal to the cyst. There is controversy over whether these lesions arise from degenerative changes or as a direct extension from the underlying joint space. Regardless, there appears to be a metabolic derangement of fibroblasts with increased production of hyaluronic acid in sites exposed to friction or minor trauma. In some patients, there may be a communication between the cyst and the underlying joint space.

Surgical excision is frequently effective, but recurrences are common. Other therapeutic options include corticosteroid injection, cryosurgery, repeated incision and drainage, and CO_2 laser ablation.[261–263]

Steatocystoma Multiplex

Steatocystoma multiplex (SM) is a disorder characterized by numerous, 2–4 mm moderately firm, yellow to flesh-colored cutaneous

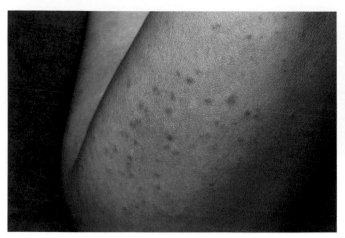

Figure 9.69 Steatocystoma multiplex. Yellow-tan, small papules of the forearm in this patient who also had lesions on the chest.

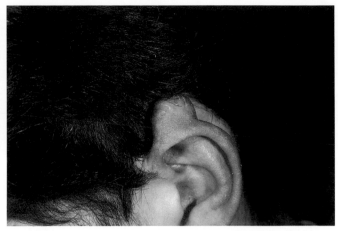

Figure 9.70 Keloid. This early lesion is erythematous and only slightly firm to palpation.

cysts, located primarily on the chest and occasionally the face, genitals, arms (Fig. 9.69), and thighs. The disorder has a high familial tendency and is often inherited in an autosomal dominant fashion. Lesions often appear or become larger around the time of puberty. In some patients, there may be overlap with eruptive vellus hair cysts (see Ch. 7), and both conditions seem to originate from the pilosebaceous duct.[264] SM may also occur in association with pachyonychia congenita (see Ch. 7), and both conditions may be caused by mutations in keratin 17.[265] In addition, persistent infantile milia may at times be associated with both SM and eruptive vellus hair cysts, and may represent a disorder with predisposition to multiple pilosebaceous cystic lesions.[266]

The lesions of SM are rarely symptomatic, but may occasionally be of cosmetic concern to the patient. Treatment can be accomplished with surgical excision or cyst puncture with evacuation of the contents.

Keloid

Keloids, which are benign dermal tumors characterized by invasive growth of fibroblasts and increased synthesis of collagen, represent an exaggerated connective tissue response to skin injury. They are rare in infancy, and their incidence increases throughout childhood, reaching a maximum between puberty and 30 years of age. African-Americans and other darkly pigmented individuals are more susceptible to keloids than individuals with fair skin, and the tendency toward keloid formation often runs in families.

Early lesions are pink, smooth, and rubbery (Fig. 9.70) and may be tender. With increasing age, keloids become less erythematous, more pigmented (Fig. 9.71), and firmer to palpation. Although they may occur anywhere on the skin surface, keloids are most common on the earlobes, upper chest, and back, and in wounds located in areas under tension. As opposed to *hypertrophic scars*, keloids frequently persist at the site of injury, often recur after excision, and always overgrow the original boundaries of the wound.[267]

Treatment of keloids is notoriously difficult and frequently ineffective. In fact, lesions not infrequently become larger following attempts at therapy. Regardless, these lesions are a source of much psychosocial anxiety and suffering for patients, and hence, therapy is often attempted. Intralesional injection of corticosteroid (usually triamcinolone acetonide) is the most frequently utilized treatment, and often requires multiple injections. This therapy is most effective for smaller lesions. Surgery is generally not recommended, given the propensity for lesions to recur or even worsen, but is often used

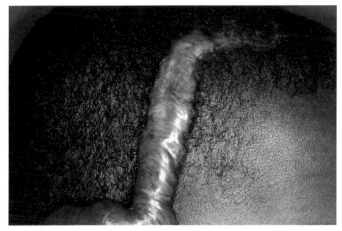

Figure 9.71 Keloid. This older keloid is very firm and hyperpigmented; it had recurred after an initial attempt at surgical removal.

given the lack of other consistently effective therapies. It is often combined with adjunctive therapies such as steroid injections, silicone sheeting, and compression. Keloid core extirpation, a surgical approach involving excision of the inner core followed by a keloid rind flap, may be a more effective approach.[267] Other therapeutic options, each used with varying levels of success, include radiotherapy; pulsed dye, argon or carbon dioxide laser therapy; and intralesional injections of bleomycin, interferon or fluorouracil. Silicone gel and silicone sheeting have been used with variable success to treat both keloids and hypertrophic scars, but their mechanism of action remains unclear. It appears that the increased wound hydration that occurs with occlusive therapies may prompt keratinocytes to alter growth factor secretion and may, hence, affect fibroblast regulation.[268] More recently, intralesional verapamil injections and topical imiquimod cream have been used in combination with surgical excision.[268,269]

Key References

 The complete list of 269 references for this chapter is available online at **www.expertconsult.com.**
See inside cover for registration details.

Briley LD, Phillips CM. Cutaneous mastocytosis: A review focusing on the pediatric population. *Clin Pediatr.* 2008;47(8):757–761.

Efron PA, Chen MK, Glavin FL, et al. Pediatric basal cell carcinoma: case reports and literature review. *J Pediatr Surg.* 2008; 43:2277–2280.

Lange JR, Palis BE, Chang DC, et al. Melanoma in children and teenagers: An analysis of patients from the National Cancer Data Base. *J Clin Oncol.* 2007;25:1363–1368.

Marghoob AA, Agero ALC, Benvenuto-Andrade C, Dusza SW. Large congenital melanocytic nevi, risk of cutaneous melanoma, and prophylactic surgery. *J Am Acad Dermatol.* 2006;54(5):868–870.

Schaffer JV. Pigmented lesions in children: when to worry. *Curr Opin Pediatr.* 2007;19:430–440.

Sugarman JL. Epidermal nevus syndromes. *Semin Cutan Med Surg.* 2007;26:221–230.

Histiocytoses and Malignant Skin Diseases

10

The histiocytoses are a broad group of disorders characterized by an abnormal proliferation of the histiocyte, a type of progenitor cell in the bone marrow (Table 10.1). Some clinically relevant types of histiocytes include the Langerhans cell, the dermal dendrocyte, and cells of mononuclear cell/macrophage lineage. Malignant disorders to be discussed include hematologic malignancies (including leukemia, lymphoma, and Hodgkin's disease), neuroblastoma, and some sarcomas.

Langerhans cell histiocytosis

Langerhans cell histiocytosis (LCH) is the terminology now used to describe a disorder characterized by infiltration of Langerhans cells into various organs of the body. Older synonymous terms, which are now largely obsolete or unnecessary, include histiocytosis X, eosinophilic granuloma, Letterer–Siwe disease, Hand–Schuller–Christian syndrome, and Hashimoto–Pritzker syndrome.[1] The term 'histiocytosis X' was coined by Lichtenstein in 1953 to identify three related clinical entities of unknown etiology, and characterized by histiocyte proliferation.[2] This classification included the triad of Letterer–Siwe disease, Hand–Schüller–Christian disease, and eosinophilic granuloma. The 'X' in this original nomenclature was used to denote the unknown derivation of the histiocyte involved in this disorder. Ultrastructural studies eventually confirmed the relationship of these three different presentations by showing the Langerhans cell to be the proliferative cell in each of them. LCH may occur at any age, from newborn to elderly, although the peak incidence appears to be between 1 and 4 years.[3]

Langerhans cells are derived from the bone marrow and are a type of dendritic cell found primarily in the epidermis (as well as mucosal epithelia, thymus, esophagus, and lung). They are involved in antigen presentation for the skin- and mucosa-associated immune systems, and are identified by strong staining with S100 (a neuronal protein) and CD1a (a cell surface marker). Langerhans cells also have a characteristic organelle, the Birbeck granule, on electron microscopy. The function of this organelle remains unknown. Recently, immunohistochemical demonstration of Langerin (CD207), a mannose-specific lectin found in association with Birbeck granules, has been demonstrated useful for diagnostic confirmation of LCH.[4]

Although numerous etiologies have been proposed for LCH, the pathogenesis remains obscure. Hypothetical causes include somatic mutations, infection (especially viral), immune or cytokine dysregulation, and programmed cell death (apoptosis).[3–6] Whether LCH is a neoplastic disorder also remains unclear. The cells in LCH have been demonstrated to be clonal, and such monoclonality has been demonstrated both in multisystem disease and with solitary organ involvement. While this clonality suggests that LCH may be a neoplastic process with variable biologic behavior, the exact significance and implications remain controversial.[3,4] There are arguments both in favor of and against LCH being a neoplastic process.[7]

LCH may involve multiple organ systems, the most common being the skin and the bones. Table 10.2 lists the spectrum of organ involvement. The older classification system was based on the involved organ systems, such that eosinophilic granuloma referred to localized bone disease; Hand–Schuller–Christian disease the multifocal triad of bone (usually skull) lesions, exophthalmos, and diabetes insipidus; and Letterer–Siwe disease, the acute or subacute disseminated form of the disease. Under the more modern classification, LCH is the umbrella term for the disease, with notation made of the various organ systems involved. Patients may have unifocal, multifocal, or disseminated disease. In general, patients with widespread, multiorgan involvement have the poorest prognosis, and those with isolated bone LCH have the best prognosis.[8]

Cutaneous involvement is very common in LCH, and is often the presenting complaint. The spectrum of skin findings is listed in Table 10.3. The most classic presentation is that of a seborrheic dermatitis-like eruption, with prominent involvement of the scalp, posterior auricular regions (Fig. 10.1), perineum, and axillae. The rash tends to be resistant to standard therapy, which is an important clue that should prompt consideration of the diagnosis. Erythematous, red-brown papules are often seen, especially on the scalp and in flexural areas, and may have secondary erosion, hemorrhage, or crusting (Fig. 10.2). Crusted papules on the palms and/or soles (Fig. 10.3) are another important feature, especially in infants in whom the diagnosis of scabies has been excluded. Although this finding has traditionally been felt to portend a poor prognosis, this observation has not been validated.

In neonates with LCH, vesiculopustular lesions (Fig. 10.4) tend to predominate, and may be misdiagnosed as congenital varicella or herpes.[9] These lesions may become hemorrhagic or crusted. Petechiae and hemorrhage may also be present in association with the dermatitis or the papular lesions of LCH, and may be seen both with and without associated thrombocytopenia. Other less commonly seen cutaneous presentations include nodules and granulomatous, ulcerative lesions.[10] Table 10.4 lists some cutaneous clues to the diagnosis of LCH.

Table 10.1 Histiocytoses
Langerhans cell histiocytosis
Juvenile xanthogranuloma
Xanthoma disseminatum
Benign cephalic histiocytosis
Necrobiotic xanthogranuloma
Generalized eruptive histiocytoma
Progressive nodular histiocytoma
Indeterminate cell histiocytosis
Multicentric reticulohistiocytosis
Sinus histiocytosis with massive lymphadenopathy (Rosai–Dorfman)
Hemophagocytic syndromes
Malignant histiocytic syndromes

Table 10.2 Organ involvement in Langerhans cell histiocytosis

Organ	Comment
Skin	Often the initial presenting sign
Bone	Painful swelling common; frequency: skull > long bones > flat bones (ribs, pelvis, vertebrae)
Lymph nodes	Cervical most common
Liver	
Spleen	
Lungs	Diffuse micronodular pattern on radiography
Gastrointestinal tract	
Thymus	
Bone marrow	Pancytopenia portends a poor prognosis
Gingivae, buccal mucosa	Swelling, erythema, erosions, petechiae
Kidney	
Endocrine glands	Diabetes insipidus most common
Central nervous system	

Table 10.3 Cutaneous manifestations of Langerhans cell histiocytosis

Presentation	Comment
Scaly red-brown papules	Especially in scalp, flexural areas; may have associated crusting; may be umbilicated or lichenoid; palm and sole involvement common
Erythematous, scaly dermatitis	May simulate seborrheic dermatitis
Erosion or ulceration	Common secondary finding, especially in fold areas
Petechiae, hemorrhage	With or without associated thrombocytopenia
Vesiculopustular lesions	Most common in neonates; may simulate congenital varicella or herpes; often have hemorrhagic crusts
Red nodules or plaques	Less common
Granulomatous plaques	Rare

Table 10.4 Cutaneous clues to Langerhans cell histiocytosis

Recalcitrant seborrheic dermatitis-like eruption
Localization of rash to scalp, posterior auricular regions, perineum, axillae
Eroded papules in flexural areas
Petechial or purpuric papules
Crusted papules on palms and/or soles (scabies preparation negative)
Any of the above lesions in combination with lymphadenopathy

Mucosal involvement may occur in patients with LCH, especially those with more disseminated involvement. Gingival erythema, erosions, and hemorrhage may be seen. In some infants, gingival and oral mucosal erosions with premature eruption of teeth may be the initial manifestations of LCH.[11] Loosening of the teeth may occur as a result of severe gingivitis, and especially when there is concomitant bony involvement of the alveolar ridge and jaw. Involvement of the external auditory canals may result in chronic otitis externa.

Bone lesions are very common in patients with LCH. When they occur, painful swelling is the most common presenting complaint, and patients may complain of discomfort both during activity and when at rest.[8] Bony involvement occurs most frequently in the skull, followed by the long bones of the extremities and the flat bones (pelvis, vertebrae, ribs). Radiographic studies usually reveal single or multiple lytic lesions of bone (Fig. 10.5), which often have a 'punched-out' appearance.[11] Proptosis may result from orbital wall involvement, and the radiographic appearance may simulate mastoiditis when there is involvement of the mastoid process.[3] Middle ear extension may cause destructive changes with resultant deafness, and chronic otitis media may also occur as a result of mastoid and temporal bone disease. Vertebral body involvement may result in compression with the radiographic finding of vertebra plana (Fig. 10.6).

The classic triad (historically 'Hand–Schuller–Christian disease') of skull lesions, diabetes insipidus, and exophthalmos is the prototype for 'multifocal' LCH, but many other organs may be involved in this setting. 'Disseminated' LCH (historically 'Letterer–Siwe disease') is the most serious form of the disorder, differing only in extent and severity from multifocal involvement.[11] Lymph node involvement may be seen with localized or widespread LCH, and most often the cervical nodes are involved. Hepatosplenomegaly biliary cirrhosis, and liver dysfunction may occur. Pulmonary LCH may present with cough, hemoptysis, dyspnea, or pain and is most common in the third decade.[3] Pulmonary involvement may also be asymptomatic, especially in younger children. Chest radiography reveals a diffuse micronodular or reticular pattern, and

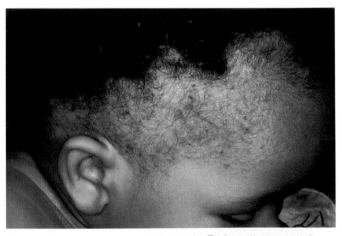

Figure 10.1 Langerhans cell histiocytosis. Erythematous, crusted papules and plaques, with accentuation in the posterior auricular scalp.

pneumothoraces may result. Gastrointestinal tract involvement may present as anorexia, malabsorption, vomiting, diarrhea, and failure to thrive. However, gastrointestinal involvement may be asymptomatic and thus is, at times, overlooked. Thymus abnormalities have been reported, and may present with enlargement of the gland on chest radiography. Bone marrow involvement may result in pancytopenia, and with concomitant hypersplenism may contribute to life-threatening sepsis and hemorrhage.[3,11] Nonspecific

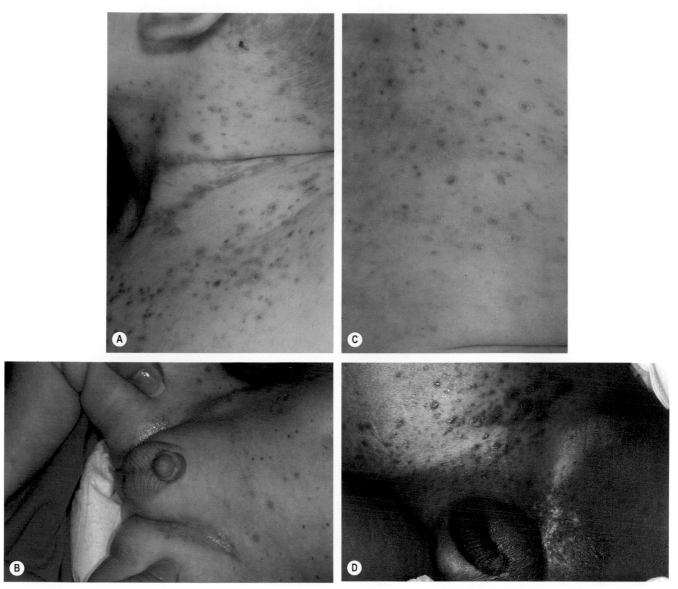

Figure 10.2 Langerhans cell histiocytosis. (A–C) Erythematous and eroded papules in the neck fold, inguinal creases, and over the trunk. Note the associated crusting, purpura, and umbilicated nature of some of the papules. (D) Eroded, erythematous, and hemorrhagic papules in the groin of this infant with disseminated LCH. Note the associated jaundiced appearance, a result of massive liver involvement.

constitutional symptoms, including fever, weight loss, and malaise, are common in patients with multiorgan involvement.

Central nervous system involvement in LCH may include infiltration of the hypothalamic-pituitary regions, which can result in diabetes insipidus (DI), even years after the initial diagnosis. DI seems to develop more often in patients with bony involvement of the skull.[3] Posterior pituitary infiltration may be evident on magnetic resonance imaging as absence of a normally bright signal in the posterior pituitary gland or thickening of the pituitary stalk.[12] Growth retardation may result from anterior pituitary involvement, although growth hormone deficiency is relatively uncommon.[13] Other manifestations of CNS involvement include hyperreflexia, dysarthria, cranial nerve defects, and rarely seizures. Progressive or, rarely, acute ataxia has been observed as a complication.[14] Basilar invagination, which is associated with hydrocephalus and usually occurs as part of the Arnold–Chiari malformation or in patients with diseases that result in bone softening (i.e., osteogenesis imperfecta), has been reported in long-term survivors with LCH.[15]

Magnetic resonance imaging is useful in diagnosing CNS disease. Positron emission tomography (PET) scan has been demonstrated useful in identifying areas with altered metabolism related to CNS LCH, and may provide a tool for longitudinal involvement in some patients.[16] Neuropsychologic deficits that may occur in children with LCH include cognitive deficiencies and deficits in memory, attention and concentration, and perceptual-organizational capabilities.[17] Cognitive defects are noted especially in patients with multisystem LCH with CNS involvement.[18]

Congenital self-healing reticulohistiocytosis deserves special mention. This entity, also known as Hashimoto–Pritzker disease (and more recently as 'congenital self-healing Langerhans cell histiocytosis', or CSHLCH), is marked by the congenital presence of LCH lesions, usually papules and nodules,[19] which may break down in the center and form crater-shaped ulcers. Systemic signs are often absent, and the lesions involute over a few months and are usually gone by 12 months.[19] There may be some distinct histologic features, but not always. It is generally accepted that CSHLCH is a variant of LCH,

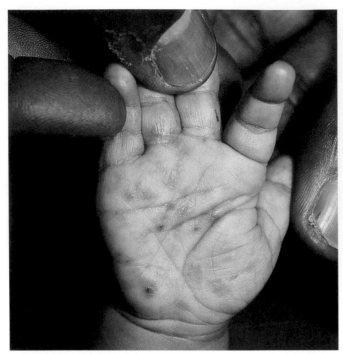

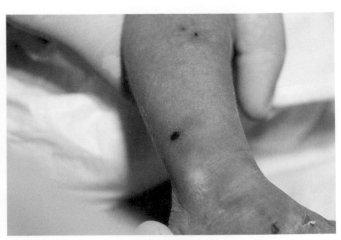

Figure 10.4 Langerhans cell histiocytosis. Hemorrhagic papules and papulovesicles in a neonate with congenital cutaneous LCH.

Figure 10.3 Langerhans cell histiocytosis. Erythematous, crusted papules on the palm in this newborn with congenital multisystem LCH.

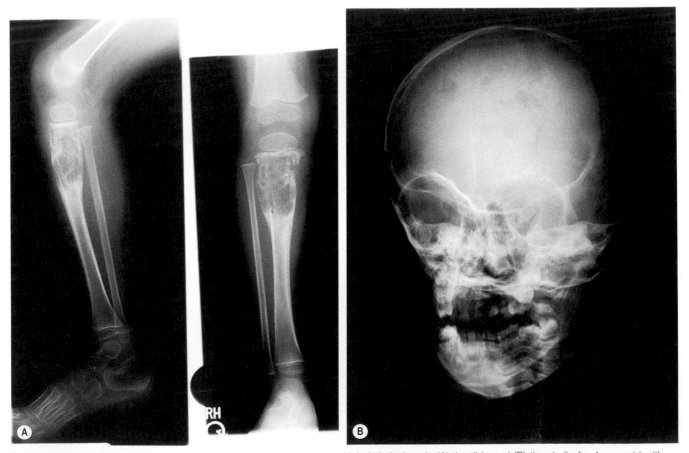

Figure 10.5 Langerhans cell histiocytosis. Plain radiography reveals multiple lytic lesions in (A) the tibia and (B) the skull of a 4-year-old with disseminated disease.

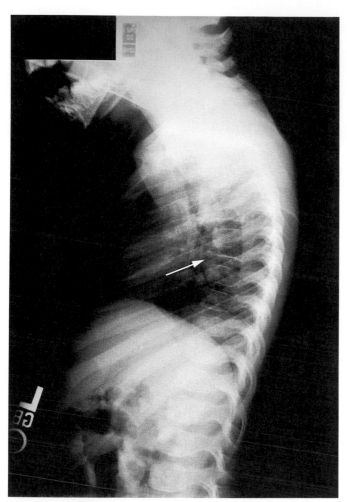

Figure 10.6 Langerhans cell histiocytosis. Plain radiography demonstrates vertebral body compression ('vertebra plana', arrow) in the same patient as that shown in Figure 10.5.

Table 10.5 Recommended evaluation of the patient with suspected Langerhans cell histiocytosis

Physical examination, including growth parameters
Laboratory evaluation:
    Complete blood cell count
    Coagulation studies
    Hepatic function testing
    Urine osmolality
Complete skeletal radiographic survey
Chest radiography
More specific studies as guided by initial results (i.e., bone marrow examination, pulmonary function testing, lung biopsy, liver biopsy, panoramic dental films, CT or MR imaging of the CNS, endocrine evaluation)

Adapted from Satter EK, High WA. Langerhans cell histiocytosis: A review of the current recommendations of the Histiocyte Society. *Pediatr Dermatol* 2008;25(3):291–295. Copyright © 2008 by John Wiley & Sons, Inc. Reprinted by permission of John Wiley & Sons, Inc.[23] CT, computed tomography; MR, magnetic resonance; CNS, central nervous system.

presents with polyuria and polydipsia, occurs in around 15–25% of patients, and may even occur as a late complication in patients who present with 'skin-limited' disease or 'CSHLCH'.[22–25]

The recommended evaluation for the patient suspected of having LCH is shown in Table 10.5. Clinical stratification based extent of disease has been recommended, as follows: single organ system disease (unifocal or multifocal), multiorgan disease (without organ dysfunction), and multiorgan disease (with organ dysfunction). The latter category, multiorgan disease with organ dysfunction, is further stratified as low risk (skin, bone, lymph node, pituitary) or high risk (lung, liver, spleen, hematopoietic cells).[23]

Therapy for LCH depends on the extent of disease. In patients with disease limited to the skin, observation alone is often appropriate, since the lesions may resolve spontaneously. Topical corticosteroids are only occasionally effective. Topical treatment with nitrogen mustard may be used, and in patients with severe skin disease, systemic therapy as is given for multiorgan LCH may be considered. Treatment for disease limited to bone is dictated by the extent of bone involvement and symptomatology. Single bone lesions may resolve spontaneously, and simple observation is appropriate in this setting in patients who are not experiencing pain.[3,11] Painful lesions may be treated with curettage, surgical excision, or intralesional steroid injection. Localized radiation therapy is another treatment option.

In patients with more extensive LCH, there are a variety of therapeutic options. Most patients are treated with systemic chemotherapy, most commonly vinblastine or etoposide. These two agents have been found equally effective in the treatment of multisystem LCH.[26] Prednisone or methylprednisolone is frequently used during the induction phase of therapy for patients with multisystem LCH. Other reported therapies include cyclosporine A, 2-chlorodeoxyadenosine, interferon-α, and allogeneic bone marrow or cord blood transplantation.[27–30]

LCH is a potentially fatal disorder that can be recognized and diagnosed early based on the characteristic cutaneous manifestations. The skin signs may appear alone or in combination with systemic disease, and all patients require a thorough evaluation for extracutaneous involvement before they can be diagnosed as having 'skin limited' disease. Although there is often a delay in the diagnosis of patients with LCH, becoming familiar with the cutaneous clues (Table 10.4) will optimally position the pediatrician or other pediatric health care provider to recognize the disorder. Patients with LCH are usually treated by a pediatric oncologist, and all patients require long-term surveillance for late sequelae or relapse.

and that most patients have a favorable prognosis. However, patients do not always have disease limited to the skin, and thus require an evaluation for systemic involvement. In addition, reports of cutaneous and systemic relapse (including DI) months to years after resolution of the skin lesions highlight the importance of vigilant long-term follow-up as one would do for patients with classic LCH.[4,20,21]

LCH is diagnosed by examination of tissue specimens from affected organs. Skin is a readily accessible organ for biopsy in patients who have cutaneous involvement. Routine histologic sections reveal an infiltrate of typical Langerhans cells, which can be confirmed by positive S100, CD1a or Langerin immunostaining. Electron microscopy, although rarely performed now because of the availability of special stains, reveals the characteristic Birbeck granules within the cytoplasm of the cells. The prognosis for patients with LCH is quite variable and dependent on many factors, including the extent of organ involvement. In general, the younger the age at diagnosis, the shorter the event-free survival and overall survival, although this association does not appear to be as strong as once believed.[22] Interestingly, neonates with isolated cutaneous lesions tend to do very well.[23] Other prognostic factors include the type and number of disease sites, organ dysfunction, and response to therapy.[24] Morbidity and mortality may be related to progressive disease or late sequelae, which include skeletal defects, dental problems, diabetes insipidus, growth failure or other endocrinopathies, hearing loss, and CNS dysfunction.[21] Diabetes insipidus, which

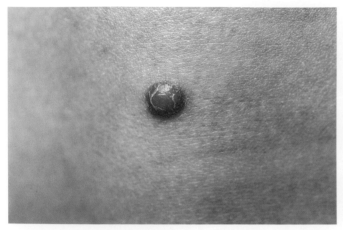

Figure 10.7 Juvenile xanthogranuloma. An early lesion demonstrates erythema and mild surface scaling.

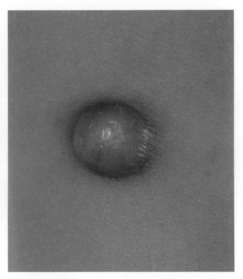

Figure 10.9 Juvenile xanthogranuloma. An established lesion revealing the characteristic yellow to orange-brown appearance.

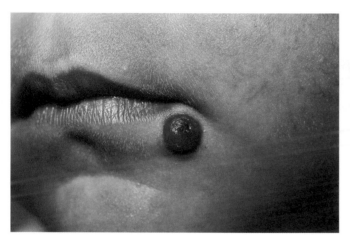

Figure 10.8 Juvenile xanthogranuloma. This early lesion reveals a red to orange color.

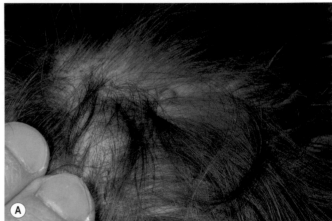

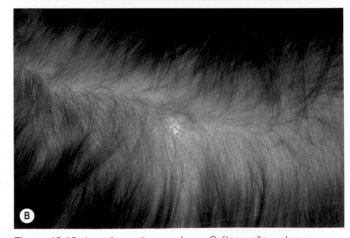

Figure 10.10 Juvenile xanthogranuloma. Solitary yellow, dome-shaped nodular papule (A) and plaque (B), both distributed on the scalp.

Juvenile xanthogranuloma

Juvenile xanthogranuloma (JXG) is a common form of non-Langerhans cell histiocytosis. It is generally a benign, self-limited disease of infants, children, and occasionally adults. Lesions occur most often in skin, although extracutaneous disease may occasionally be present. Most JXGs occur early in life, and the true incidence may be underestimated as many of them may go undiagnosed or misdiagnosed as other common skin tumors, such as nevi. JXG seems to be derived from dermal dendrocytes, and although the term 'xantho-' appears in the name, there is no association of this condition with hyperlipidemia or other metabolic abnormalities.[31]

Juvenile xanthogranuloma presents as a firm, round papule or nodule, varying in size from 5 mm to 2 cm, with giant lesions (i.e., up to 5–10 cm) occasionally seen. Some authors have divided JXG into a 'micronodular' form (lesions <10 mm) and a 'macronodular' form (lesions >10 mm). Early JXGs are erythematous (Fig. 10.7) to orange or tan (Fig. 10.8), but with time they become more yellow in color (Figs 10.9, 10.10). Lesions may be solitary (up to 90% of all patients with JXG[32]) or, less commonly, multiple (Fig. 10.11), and they are usually asymptomatic. Ulceration and crusting may occasionally occur. The head, neck, and trunk are the most common

areas to be involved. Lesions may also occur on mucous membranes or at mucocutaneous junctions (mouth, vaginal orifice, and perineal area). Oral lesions occur on the lateral aspects of the tongue, gingival, buccal mucosa, and midline hard palate, and may ulcerate and bleed. Oral lesions may appear verrucous, pedunculated,

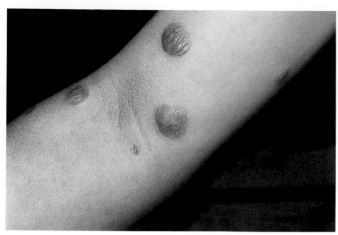

Figure 10.11 Juvenile xanthogranuloma. Multiple lesions were present in this 11-year-old boy, with spontaneous involution evident. Note the fibrofatty tissue residua.

umbilicated, or fibroma-like.[33] Typically, the lesion of JXG present at birth (20%) or during the first 6 to months of life, and may persist or continue to erupt for years.[34]

Histologic evaluation of JXG tissue reveals a dense dermal infiltrate of foamy histiocytes, foreign body cells, and the characteristic Touton giant cells, which are virtually pathognomonic for the condition. The Touton cell is a giant cell with a central wreath of nuclei and a peripheral rim of eosinophilic cytoplasm.[35] Lymphocytes and eosinophils are often seen, and the histiocytes in JXG are S100- and CD1a negative on special staining.

Extracutaneous involvement occasionally occurs with JXG. The eye is the most common organ of involvement second to the skin. The iris is the site most often involved, and potential complications of ocular JXG include hyphema, glaucoma, or blindness.[36] Patients may complain of eye redness, irritation, or photophobia. Children at greatest risk for ocular JXG include those ≤2 years of age and those with multiple skin lesions.[36] Intramuscular JXG presents as a deep, soft tissue lesion that may have imaging features similar to those of malignant tumors of infancy.[37] This form tends to affect exclusively infants and toddlers and occurs as a solitary lesion in skeletal muscles of the trunk.[38] Other sites of extracutaneous involvement include lung, liver, testis, pericardium, spleen, CNS, bone, kidney, adrenal glands, and larynx.[31,35] Solitary as well as multiple intracranial and intracerebral lesions have rarely been reported.[39,40] Systemic JXG generally exhibits a benign clinical course, but may occasionally be fatal, especially when the liver is involved.[32] There are rare reports of JXG in association with LCH, suggesting a possible common progenitor cell and overlap within the histiocytic spectrum of disorders.

An important association is that of JXG and childhood leukemia. The most common association has been with juvenile chronic myelogenous leukemia (JCML), which may be seen with increased frequency in patients with multiple JXG lesions. It has been noted that several such reported patients also had café-au-lait macules and a family history of type 1 neurofibromatosis (NF1).[41] A systematic review of the literature revealed that the frequency of the triple association of JXG, JCML, and NF is 30–40-fold higher than expected, and it is estimated that children with NF and JXG have a 20–32-fold higher risk for JCML than do patients with NF who do not have JXG.[42] However, it should be noted that the vast majority of patients with multiple JXG, even with associated NF, do not develop JCML. The role of surveillance complete blood cell counts

is controversial, and most practitioners follow these patients primarily with regular, thorough physical examinations.

JXGs usually run a fairly benign course, with spontaneous regression occurring over 3–6 years. Pigmentary alteration, atrophy, or 'anetoderma-like' changes may persist in areas of prior skin involvement. Although rare cases lasting until adulthood have been reported, generally those that have their onset early in life manifest complete spontaneous healing. The risk of complications is fairly high when ocular involvement is present. For this reason, once disease has been confirmed in the eye, therapy should be initiated. Intraocular JXGs are treated with intralesional or systemic steroids, radiation therapy, or excision.[43,44] Lesions limited to skin require no therapy, although surgical excision is occasionally performed for diagnostic or cosmetic purposes. Systemic involvement is treated if it interferes with vital functions, and has shown response to chemotherapy regimens similar to those used in LCH.[31,32] Patients with JXG and NF should be followed for the development of leukemia given the increased risk.

Xanthoma disseminatum

Xanthoma disseminatum, a rare disorder of mucocutaneous xanthomatous lesions, is another non-Langerhans cell histiocytosis. This disorder usually occurs in adults, although it may have its onset during childhood.[45,46] Patients present with numerous (sometimes hundreds of) round to oval, yellow-orange or brown papules, nodules, and plaques. They occur primarily on the face and the flexural and intertriginous surfaces, including the neck, antecubital fossae, periumbilical area, perineum, and genitalia. The lips, eyelids, and conjunctivae may be involved, and xanthomatous deposits have also been observed in the mouth and upper respiratory tract (epiglottis, larynx, and trachea), occasionally leading to respiratory difficulty.[47,48] Facial lesions may become exuberant and may cause disfiguration.[49] Osseous lesions, presenting radiographically as well-demarcated areas of osteolysis, may be present.[49] Ocular mucosal lesions may result in blindness. Liver involvement is occasionally present.[50]

As with juvenile xanthogranuloma, there is no perturbation in lipid metabolism in patients with xanthoma disseminatum, although it has been rarely reported in affected children.[50] Diabetes insipidus occurs in many patients with the disorder, and severe laryngeal involvement may necessitate tracheostomy. The lesions of xanthoma disseminatum often persist indefinitely, but have been known to involute spontaneously.[51] Treatment of the cutaneous lesions has been performed with cryotherapy, excision, and carbon dioxide laser.[52] Respiratory tract involvement, when severe, may justify a more aggressive approach with localized radiation therapy or chemotherapy.

Benign cephalic histiocytosis

Benign cephalic histiocytosis (BCH) is a self-healing, cutaneous, non-Langerhans cell histiocytosis that classically involves the face and head. The average age of onset is 15 months, and 45% of cases occur in infants under 6 months of age.[53] Clinically, BCH is characterized by small, 2–6 mm yellow-brown macules and minimally elevated papules (Fig. 10.12). The lesions may occasionally coalesce to give a reticulate pattern.[54] BCH most commonly occurs on the face, and less commonly on the neck and trunk. The extremities, buttocks, and pubic area may be involved later in the course.[53] The differential diagnosis may include flat warts, micronodular JXG, LCH, multiple melanocytic nevi, and urticaria pigmentosa.

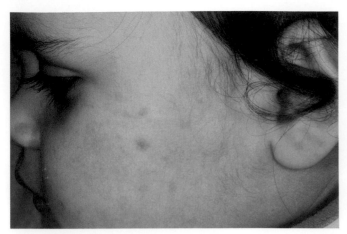

Figure 10.12 Benign cephalic histiocytosis. Faintly tan to erythematous macules and papules on the cheek.

The diagnosis of BCH can be confirmed by skin biopsy, which reveals a histiocytic infiltrate with negative stains for S100 and CD1a. Electron microscopy is useful in confirming the diagnosis, as the cells classically reveal 'intracytoplasmic comma-shaped or worm-like' bodies and the absence of Birbeck granules,[54,55] clearly differentiating it from LCH.

There is significant clinical overlap between some of the non-Langerhans cell histiocytoses. Some authors have considered BCH to be a variant of generalized eruptive histiocytoma (see below). In addition, there are reports of BCH progressing into JXG,[56,57] and although BCH tends to be limited to the skin, there are some reports of associated internal involvement. One patient with BCH developed diabetes insipidus 1 year later, with infiltration of the pituitary stalk on imaging.[58] In another patient with classic lesions of BCH on the face, lytic lesions in the skull, spine, and tibia were demonstrated to be LCH on tissue examination.[59] These clinical observations again highlight the potential overlap among the histiocytic syndromes.

BCH generally runs a benign course with spontaneous healing, often leaving behind flat or atrophic pigmented scars. Treatment is unnecessary, but given the clinical variation in presentation and overlap with other histiocytic syndromes, clinical follow-up for progression or internal involvement is advisable.

Necrobiotic xanthogranuloma

Necrobiotic xanthogranuloma, a rare disorder usually reported in adults, is characterized by sharply demarcated, indurated plaques and nodules that are usually yellow to red-brown or violaceous and have a predilection for periorbital areas, the trunk, and proximal extremities.[60] Lesions vary in size, may at times be as large as ≥10 cm in diameter, and often ulcerate and heal with areas of atrophy and telangiectasia. Ocular involvement is fairly common and includes ectropion, ptosis, keratitis, uveitis, proptosis, and orbital masses. Visceral lesions of necrobiotic xanthogranuloma may involve the heart, skeletal muscles, larynx, spleen, and ovary. A hallmark of this disease is an associated paraproteinemia, IgG monoclonal gammopathy. The course of necrobiotic xanthogranuloma is chronic and progressive and may be associated with proliferation of plasma cells in the bone marrow or multiple myeloma. Treatment options include systemic or intralesional corticosteroids, cytotoxic drugs, radiation therapy, and plasmapheresis. Surgical removal of lesions is associated with a high recurrence rate.[61]

Generalized eruptive histiocytoma

Generalized eruptive histiocytoma is a rare, self-healing histiocytosis characterized by recurrent crops of small, yellow to red-brown papules on the face, trunk, extensor extremities, and, rarely, mucous membranes. The lesions number in the hundreds, and tend to occur in a symmetric distribution. They resolve over months with hyperpigmented macules left in their place. As a result of the continuous development of new lesions, however, the disorder may persist indefinitely. Although generally regarded as a disorder of adults, generalized eruptive histiocytoma has been seen in childhood, even in infants as young as 1 month of age.[62]

The differential diagnosis includes JXG (which may be very difficult to differentiate histologically from early lesions of generalized eruptive histiocytoma), LCH, benign cephalic histiocytosis, and urticaria pigmentosa. Xanthoma disseminatum has developed in a child with the prior diagnosis of generalized eruptive histiocytoma.[45] No treatment is generally necessary for this disorder. However, since there is considerable overlap within the non-Langerhans cell histiocytoses, patients should be followed carefully for the development of signs or symptoms of other organ involvement.

Progressive nodular histiocytoma

Progressive nodular histiocytoma is characterized by a widespread eruption of hundreds of yellow-brown, 2–10 mm papules and deeper, larger subcutaneous nodules. Conjunctival, oral, and laryngeal lesions may occur. The face typically is heavily involved with numerous coalescent lesions, which may result in a leonine appearance. New lesions progressively occur, and ulceration is common. Occasionally, bleeding may occur within the subcutaneous nodules, resulting in marked pain.[63] Lesions of progressive nodular histiocytoma histologically show features typical of xanthogranuloma, and some authors suggest that this entity and JXG may represent a variation of the same process.[64] Treatment for this condition is difficult, and includes excision of large or symptomatic lesions, chemotherapy with vinblastine, and electron beam therapy.

Multicentric reticulohistiocytosis

Multicentric reticulohistiocytosis is a rare systemic disorder of unknown cause. It is characterized by cutaneous lesions and a destructive arthritis, and is seen almost exclusively in adults, with rare reports of pediatric disease.[65,66] The skin lesions present as firm red-brown papules, most often distributed on the hands, fingers, lips, ears, and nose. Facial disfigurement may occur, with cartilaginous destruction and the appearance of a leonine facies. The 'coral bead' sign refers to the presence of a chain of papules along the cuticle.[63] Nodular lesions on the arms, elbows, and knees may occur and at times resemble rheumatoid nodules.[67] Mucous membrane involvement may occur in up to one-half of patients. They most often present on the lips, buccal mucosa, nasal septum, tongue, palate, and gingivae.

Joint involvement is the presenting sign in more than half of the patients, and is highly destructive. It may involve any joint, especially the interphalangeal joints, and co-existing synovitis is common. Shortening of the digits may occur with a 'telescopic' or 'opera-glass' deformity. Rheumatoid arthritis may be mistakenly diagnosed in some patients. Microscopic examination of skin, bone, or synovial tissue reveals a characteristic histiocytic process, with multinucleated giant cells and a 'ground-glass' appearance. Visceral involvement may include pleural effusion, pericarditis, heart failure, salivary gland enlargement, muscle weakness, lymphadenopathy and gastric ulcer.[68] Multicentric reticulohistiocytosis may regress spontaneously over 6–8 years, but for many patients, the articular destruction results in permanent joint deformities. The response of this disorder to therapy is frequently disappointing, with treatments including non-steroidal antiinflammatory agents, corticosteroids, cyclophosphamide, chlorambucil, methotrexate, hydroxychloroquine, and interferon.[63,68–70]

Hemophagocytic syndrome

Hemophagocytic syndrome (HS) refers to a condition characterized by fever, wasting, jaundice, and hepatosplenomegaly resulting from diffuse infiltration of phagocytizing histiocytes in various tissues.[71] This disorder is heterogeneous in its etiologies, which include a familial form ('familial hemophagocytic lymphohistiocytosis') and a secondary/reactive form, which may be associated with a variety of infectious agents (most notably viral, bacterial or parasitic), malignancy and collagen vascular disorders.[72,73] The infection-associated form is seen primarily in immunocompromised patients with evidence of preceding viral (usually Epstein–Barr virus, EBV) infection, in which case it is also known as 'virus-associated hemophagocytic syndrome'. The other viral agents reported in association with HS include cytomegalovirus, enterovirus, and parainfluenza virus.[72,73] The term 'malignant histiocytosis' has also been used to describe this condition, in response to the cytologic atypia and 'malignant' nature of the infiltrating histiocytes. HS has been observed as a complication of allogeneic hematopoietic stem cell transplantation, and in association with hematologic malignancies.[71,74] There also seems to be a relationship between EBV-associated HS and EBV-associated T-cell lymphoma, with HS representing the major cause of death in these patients.[71]

The cutaneous manifestations seen in patients with HS are variable. Most common is a transient, generalized maculopapular eruption. Petechial and purpuric macules, generalized erythroderma, and morbilliform erythema may also occur.[75] Although the skin findings are not specific, their presence in the patient with a supportive history and/or the concomitant findings of fever, lymphadenopathy, hepatosplenomegaly and cytopenias should prompt consideration for this diagnosis. The most common hematologic findings are leukopenia and thrombocytopenia, and coagulopathy is fairly common.[72] The clinical differential diagnosis may include extramedullary hematopoiesis (as may be seen with a variety of infectious or malignant disorders) and metastatic lesions from an underlying malignancy. Langerhans cell histiocytosis and myofibromatosis may also be in the differential.[75] Skin biopsy may be useful in eliminating some diagnoses, but the histologic findings are often nonspecific and the changes of erythrophagocytosis are often absent in skin specimens. Examination of bone marrow or other solid organ (lymph node, spleen, liver) biopsy tissue may be necessary to confirm the diagnosis. HS has a high mortality rate, although chemotherapy, steroids, intravenous immunoglobulin and bone marrow transplantation may offer hope for some patients.

Sinus histiocytosis with massive lymphadenopathy (Rosai–Dorfman)

Sinus histiocytosis with massive lymphadenopathy (SHML, or Rosai–Dorfman disease) is a rare disorder of reactive proliferation of histiocytes in the sinuses of lymph nodes. It occurs primarily in children, who present with massive lymphadenopathy, especially cervical. Extranodal involvement may occur, and when it does, the skin is one of the more common organs to be involved. Papules and nodules are the most common skin lesions, and purely cutaneous SHML may occasionally occur.[76,77] The lesions often involute spontaneously. There are isolated reports of patients with both SHML and lymphoma.[78,79]

Cutaneous pseudolymphoma

Cutaneous pseudolymphoma (CPL, lymphocytoma cutis, lymphadenosis benigna cutis, pseudolymphoma of Spiegler–Fendt, cutaneous lymphoid hyperplasia) refers to a benign process that may clinically and/or histologically mimic lymphoma. CPL may occur at any age, but most characteristically develops during early adult life. The diagnosis of CPL is nonspecific and does not imply the etiology. Some of the various causes of this process are listed in Table 10.6.

One of the most common etiologic categories of CPL is drugs. Many classes have been implicated, including anticonvulsants, antipsychotics, antihypertensives, angiotensin-converting enzyme inhibitors, beta blockers, calcium channel blockers, antibiotics, cytotoxic agents, and even antihistamines.[80] The anticonvulsant hypersensitivity syndrome or DRESS (see Ch. 20) is a prototype for such a reaction, presenting with fever, lymphadenopathy, edema, hepatosplenomegaly with hepatitis, and a diffuse cutaneous eruption that may reveal histologic changes of pseudolymphoma.

Typically, CPL presents as a more localized process, with papules, nodules, and tumors in the skin. The lesions are flesh-colored to red (Fig. 10.13) or violaceous, and may be single or multiple. They are usually not associated with a drug ingestion, and may reach up to 4 or 5 cm in size with continued enlargement. The most common locations are the face, ears, and scalp, with occasional involvement of other body regions. Borrelial lymphocytoma, which follows infection with the Lyme disease agent *Borrelia burgdorferi*, occurs primarily in Europe and usually presents with red nodules involving the ear lobe and areola.[81] CPL resulting from past scabies infestation (scabies nodules) presents as erythematous to red-brown papules and nodules, usually in an infant previously treated for scabies (Fig. 10.14). These lesions may persist for several months following adequate therapy for the infestation. CPL may occasionally be noted in association with molluscum contagiosum (see Ch. 15, Fig. 15.42), a common childhood viral infection.[82]

A more disseminated form of CPL may occur, usually in adults, and presents with firm, red to violaceous papules and nodules with a more diffuse distribution. These lesions may grow rapidly, are prone to recurrence, and tend to persist throughout life. Actinic

Table 10.6 Some causes of cutaneous pseudolymphoma

Idiopathic
Arthropod bite reaction
Drug reaction
Contact dermatitis
Infestation (i.e., scabies nodules)
Lymphomatoid papulosis
Borrelia burgdorferi
Tattoo pigment
Vaccinations
Actinic reticuloid
VZV infection
HIV infection
Molluscum contagiosum

VZV, varicella-zoster virus; HIV, human immunodeficiency virus.

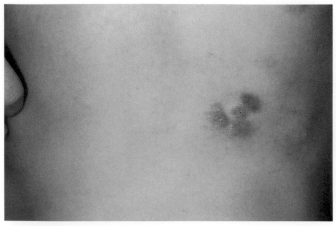

Figure 10.13 Cutaneous pseudolymphoma. Infiltrative, erythematous papules and nodular plaques on the chest of a 7-year-old boy.

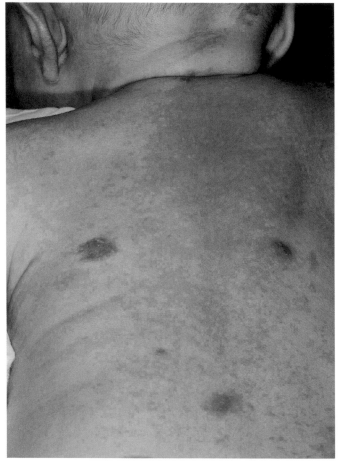

Figure 10.14 Nodular scabies. Erythematous papulonodules with mild scaling in a 10-month-old who was treated for scabies 3 months before.

reticuloid is a severe, chronic photosensitive dermatosis that occurs primarily in older men, and presents with erythematous to violaceous, lichenified papules and plaques on sun-exposed skin. It is categorized as a form of CPL by several authors.

The diagnosis of CPL is based upon the combination of clinical features, histologic evaluation, and often immuno-histochemical and/or gene rearrangement studies.[80] At times, the microscopic

findings of CPL may be very difficult to differentiate from cutaneous lymphoma, and consist of a mixture of B, T or mixed lymphocytes with macrophages and dendritic cells.[83] Treatment of CPL depends on the underlying etiology. Removal of any offending drug or physical stimulus that is identified may be sufficient. In idiopathic cases, lesions may involute spontaneously over months to years. For persistent lesions, treatment options include topical or intralesional corticosteroids, cryosurgery, surgical excision, local radiation therapy, photochemotherapy and antimalarial and cytotoxic agents.[80] Antibiotics appropriate for Lyme disease are indicated for treatment of borrelial lymphocytoma.

Leukemia cutis

Leukemia is the most common malignancy of childhood. Cutaneous findings in leukemia may be primary (i.e., leukemic infiltrates in the skin) and secondary (i.e., Sweet's syndrome, Ch. 20; pyoderma gangrenosum, Ch. 25; opportunistic infections). Cutaneous leukemic infiltrates may be known by a variety of names, including leukemia cutis, granulocytic sarcoma, and chloroma. 'Myelosarcoma' is the modern term for any extramedullary infiltrate with myeloid blasts.[84] Leukemia cutis, hence, is a form of myelosarcoma that results from infiltration of the epidermis, dermis, or subcutaneous tissues by neoplastic leukocytes or their precursors. Although biopsies of lesions of leukemia cutis may suggest the diagnosis, the findings may mimic a variety of inflammatory or neoplastic diseases. Therefore, immunophenotyping and examination of peripheral blood smears and bone marrow aspirates are often required in an effort to confirm the diagnosis.

Cutaneous involvement may be associated with various types of childhood leukemias, including acute lymphoblastic leukemia (ALL), acute myeloid leukemia (AML or ANLL, acute nonlymphocytic leukemia), and chronic leukemias (i.e., CML and CLL). In general, leukemia cutis is associated with a grave prognosis, the exception being in patients with congenital leukemia (see below). Cutaneous leukemic infiltrates are most common with the myeloid leukemias (between 3% and 30% of patients, depending on the subtype), especially acute myelomonocytic and monocytic leukemia.[84–86] Gingival hypertrophy is a notable feature seen with these subtypes of leukemia, less so with other acute leukemias, and rarely with chronic leukemias.[85] Leukemia cutis is less common in patients with ALL (around 1–3%), in which case it seems to be most common on the head and may be an early manifestation in children in both standard risk and high-risk categories.[85,87] Leukemia cutis may also occur in patients with myelodysplastic syndrome, usually before or simultaneously with identifiable leukemic transformation in the peripheral blood or bone marrow.[88]

The clinical appearance of leukemia cutis is variable. Lesion types include macules, papules, plaques, nodules, ecchymoses, erythroderma, palpable purpura, ulcers, bullous lesions, and urticaria-like lesions.[85] A 'seborrheic dermatitis-like' presentation with scaling and papules of the scalp was observed in a 7-month-old with AML in remission.[89] Brown macules and nodules exhibiting a positive Darier's sign and mimicking mastocytosis have been noted.[88] The most characteristic lesions of leukemia cutis are flesh-colored to red-brown to violaceous papules (Fig. 10.15), nodules, and plaques that may become purpuric (especially with co-existing thrombocytopenia). Leukemia cutis lesions may localize to sites of skin trauma, burns, surgical sites, or sites of cutaneous infections.

The clinical features of the skin lesions are not distinct for the different types of leukemias. However, certain subtypes may be more likely to result in cutaneous infiltrates with certain characteristics. For example, granulocytic sarcoma (or chloroma) presents as

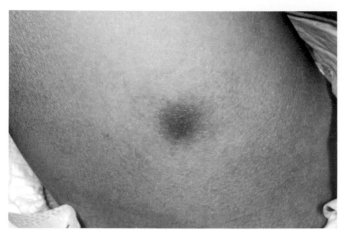

Figure 10.15 Leukemia cutis. Erythematous nodule in a 3-year-old with diagnosed acute lymphocytic leukemia.

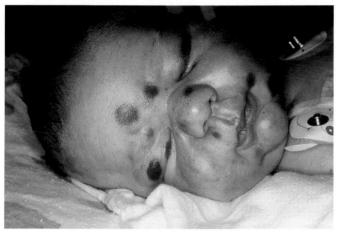

Figure 10.16 Congenital leukemia cutis. Congenital acute lymphocytic leukemia with cutaneous facial lesions. (Courtesy of Anne Lucky, MD.)

Table 10.7 Causes of 'blueberry muffin' cutaneous lesions in a newborn

Neoplastic infiltrates
    Leukemia
    Neuroblastoma
    Histiocytosis

Extramedullary hematopoiesis
    Congenital infection
        Rubella
        Toxoplasmosis
        Cytomegalovirus
        Parvovirus B19
    Anemia
        Hemolytic disease of the newborn
        Hereditary spherocytosis
        ABO incompatibility
        Twin–twin transfusion syndrome

Transient myeloproliferative disorders:
    with Down syndrome
    without Down syndrome

a rapidly growing, firm nodule that at times has a green hue. This tumor is usually associated with acute myeloid leukemia, and the greenish color is related to myeloperoxidase in the granulocytes. Granulocytic sarcoma may occur in patients with known AML, in those with a myeloproliferative disorder with an impending blast crisis, or in patients without any known hematologic disease.[86] At times, leukemia cutis may precede the development of the systemic leukemia. This phenomenon is termed *aleukemic leukemia cutis*, and the cutaneous lesions can sometimes precede the systemic malignancy by years.

Congenital Leukemia Cutis

Congenital leukemia is defined as leukemia presenting at birth or within the first month of life. Congenital leukemia cutis, as compared with later-onset leukemia cutis, is believed to be quite common in the setting of this malignancy, with incidence estimates in the literature ranging between 25% and 30% of patients with congenital AML.[90] The cutaneous lesions range in size from a few millimeters to several centimeters, and are usually red to brown to violaceous papules and nodules (Fig. 10.16). This latter clinical presentation in the neonate (with multiple violaceous papules and nodules) has been termed 'blueberry muffin' baby, and such skin findings may represent malignant cutaneous infiltrates or any of

several possible causes of extramedullary hematopoiesis. Table 10.7 lists the various causes of blueberry muffin skin lesions. As with non-congenital leukemia cutis, cutaneous infiltrates are more common with the myelogenous type of congenital leukemia.[90] Congenital leukemia cutis is felt to portend a poor prognosis, although some reports describe spontaneous remission.[91,92] However, since late relapses have been noted in some of these patients, they deserve close long-term follow-up. Occasionally, infants with congenital leukemia cutis may present with a solitary nodule.[93,94]

Patients with Down syndrome have an increased risk of hematologic aberrations, including leukemia, leukemoid reaction, and transient myeloproliferative disorder. A leukemoid reaction is a temporary overproduction of leukocytes in response to infection, hemolysis, or other stress. Transient myeloproliferative disorder, which is also self-limited, is similar except that there is no identifiable trigger.[95] Down syndrome patients with a leukemoid reaction or transient myeloproliferative disorder have been described with pustular or vesiculopustular skin eruptions, and smears or biopsies of these lesions have revealed immature myeloid forms.[95,96] This vesiculopustular presentation (Fig. 10.17) is quite distinct from the typical papules and nodules that occur with leukemia cutis. The significance of this eruption is unclear, and the findings resolve without therapy as the hematologic disorder subsides. However, true leukemia may develop months to years later, and therefore long-term follow-up is again indicated.

Lymphoma cutis

Lymphoma involving the skin is quite rare in children. The most common form of cutaneous lymphoma is cutaneous T-cell lymphoma (CTCL, mycosis fungoides) (see below). Other forms of lymphoma cutis include subcutaneous panniculitic T-cell lymphoma, anaplastic large cell lymphoma, cutaneous B-cell lymphoma, natural killer cell lymphoma, angiocentric cutaneous T-cell lymphoma, and Hodgkin lymphoma. Some types of lymphoma that can also have skin involvement but will not be discussed include lymphoblastic lymphoma, marginal zone lymphoma, Burkitt lymphoma, and HTLV-1-associated lymphoma. Lymphoma cutis may be a primary cutaneous process, or skin involvement may be associated with a systemic lymphoma. In non-Hodgkin lymphoma patients overall, cutaneous involvement occurs in 1–5% of

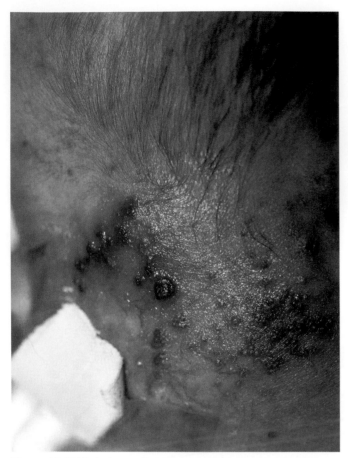

Figure 10.17 Vesiculopustular eruption in Down syndrome patient with transient myeloproliferative disorder. (Courtesy of Beth Drolet, MD.)

cases, and skin as the primary site (primary cutaneous lymphoma) is quite rare.[97-99]

Head and neck involvement is the most common pattern of cutaneous lymphoma in children.[97-99] The second most common site of involvement appears to be the abdomen.[97] Most patients present with solitary nodules in the skin, and less often multiple nodules are present. Papules or plaques are occasionally seen. The lesions are usually 5–10 cm in diameter, erythematous, and firm. *Subcutaneous panniculitic T-cell lymphoma* (SCPTCL) is a rare T-cell lymphoma in children, which presents with subcutaneous nodules or nodular plaques. This tumor involves the subcutaneous fat in a manner mimicking panniculitis.[100] The clinical presentation of SCPTCL may mimic several processes, including lupus panniculitis and erythema nodosum, and hence this disorder may elude diagnosis.[101] SCPTCL has been associated in some patients with hemophagocytic syndrome, and concomitant histiocytic cytophagic panniculitis has been observed.[102,103] Hence, in any child with panniculitis and hemophagocytic syndrome, investigations for T-cell lymphoma should be performed.

Ki-1/CD30-positive (anaplastic large cell) lymphoma is a form of lymphoma that may simulate a metastatic carcinoma or malignant histiocytosis.[104,105] A significant proportion of patients with this neoplasm are children or young adults. Patients present with fever, wasting, lymphadenopathy and often cutaneous lesions. Skin involvement may consist of fleeting eruptions or more specific lesions, usually painful nodules, which occasionally undergo spontaneous involution.[104,106] In 36% of children in one series with peripheral lymph node involvement, lymphomatous infiltration of contiguous skin occurred and presented as erythematous, thickened, desquamating, and ulcerative plaques.[107] Anaplastic large cell lymphoma is a high-grade non-Hodgkin lymphoma with a relatively good prognosis with early multiagent chemotherapy.[105,107] Biopsies of affected skin reveal large, atypical lymphoid infiltrates that stain positive with the activation antigen Ki-1, also known as CD30.

Cutaneous B-cell lymphoma is fairly rare, even though B-cell lymphomas represent the majority of non-Hodgkin lymphomas occurring in lymph nodes. As with T-cell lymphomas, B-cell lymphomas may involve the skin in a primary fashion or be secondary in relation to dissemination of nodal disease. Hence, complete staging and evaluation is indicated for any patient diagnosed with a cutaneous B-cell lymphoma. This form of lymphoma cutis is notoriously rare in the pediatric population. The clinical presentation of B-cell lymphoma cutis includes papules, plaques, and tumors, occasionally with associated ulceration. The head, neck, upper trunk, and extremities seem to be sites of predilection in most patients, although some subtypes favor the lower extremities.

Natural killer cell (CD56+ NK/T cell) lymphoma is classically an aggressive nasal lymphoma, although patients can also present with cutaneous plaques and subcutaneous nodules. This neoplasm may occur in a primary cutaneous or secondary form, and these two variants show considerable clinicopathologic differences with a more favorable prognosis associated with primary skin disease.[108] This neoplasm occurs primarily in older adults, seems to have an association with EBV infection, and usually is associated with a high mortality rate. *Angiocentric cutaneous T-cell lymphoma* is an unusual T-cell lymphoma of childhood that presents with a vesiculopapular eruption that may mimic hydroa vacciniforme (see Ch. 19).[109] It occurs mainly in children from Asia and Latin America, and may be related to EBV infection.

Hodgkin lymphoma is a fairly common childhood lymphoma that often occurs prior to adolescence. It rarely occurs before the age of 5 years, and there is another peak of involvement later in adulthood. In the majority of cases, Hodgkin lymphoma, which is now classified as a B-cell lymphoma, is initially limited to the lymph nodes, with superficial lymph nodes more commonly initially involved than visceral lymph nodes. It presents as painless lymph node enlargement, usually in the neck. Hodgkin lymphoma is histologically characterized as one of several subtypes, and staging depends on the extent of lymph node involvement and the presence or absence of constitutional symptoms. Skin involvement resulting from infiltration of the malignant cells is quite rare (<1%), but nonspecific secondary findings may occur and include pruritus, purpura, ichthyosis, and pigmentary changes. When specific cutaneous lesions are present, they are usually pink to red-brown or violaceous papules or nodules, which may coalesce to form larger plaques or tumors.

The treatment of cutaneous lymphomas can be planned only after thorough evaluation and staging for the extent of extracutaneous disease. Occasionally, patients with low-grade neoplasms with limited involvement may be appropriately managed by 'watchful waiting'. Therapeutic options otherwise include radiotherapy, chemotherapy, surgical excision (i.e., for localized primary cutaneous tumors), and newer cytokine and biologic therapies.

Cutaneous T-cell lymphoma

Cutaneous T-cell lymphoma (CTCL, mycosis fungoides) is a primary cutaneous lymphoma that occurs primarily in adults. Although approximately 75% of patients are diagnosed after the age of 50,[110] onset of the disease during childhood may occur in 0.5–5% of cases.[110,111] It has been diagnosed as young as 22 months,[110] and suspected to have started as young as 10 months of age.[112] Many factors may contribute to the seemingly lower incidence of CTCL in children, including lack of recognition of its occurrence and hesitancy to perform skin biopsies in younger patients. Delay in diagnosis is most common in the youngest age group (0–3 years).[112] The possibility of CTCL should be considered in the setting of chronic dermatoses recalcitrant to therapy, and serial skin biopsies may be necessary.[113] In general, patients who present with CTCL during childhood are more likely to present with limited disease and, as a result, seem to have a better disease-specific survival than older CTCL patients.[110,114] Some studies, however, have found no statistically significant differences in the course between early childhood- and adult-onset disease.[115] Table 10.8 lists the staging and classification for CTCL.

The clinical presentation of CTCL is quite variable. Most pediatric patients present with erythematous, scaly patches, papules, and plaques (Fig. 10.18) with variable degrees of pruritus. Thin, erythematous, atrophic patches on the trunk and buttocks are a classic presentation. At times, central clearing develops and the lesions assume serpiginous, arciform, horseshoe, or other bizarre shapes. The lesions of CTCL may simulate many other skin disorders, including atopic dermatitis, psoriasis, parapsoriasis, hypopigmented diseases (i.e., vitiligo or pityriasis alba; see below), and pityriasis lichenoides. Some patients show changes of poikiloderma, characterized by the combination of hyper- and hypopigmentation, atrophy, and telangiectasia. Although the lesions themselves may not be pathognomonic for CTCL, their chronic nature and history of recalcitrance to therapy often prompt further diagnostic investigations. Skin nodules and tumors, which may grow aggressively and occasionally ulcerate, are an uncommon presentation of pediatric CTCL, and are more often seen in adult and elderly patients. Occasionally, focal skin nodules may intermittently occur superimposed on a background of patch- or plaque-type CTCL, with CD30+ cells and a self-limited clinical course consistent with lymphomatoid papulosis[116] (see Ch. 4) (Fig. 10.19). Occasionally, patients present with skin findings suggestive of pigmented purpuric dermatosis.[117,118] In some patients, the entire cutaneous surface may become infiltrated, producing thickened red skin with or without scaling, and with islands of normal skin often remaining for a time before the universal erythroderma becomes complete.

Hypopigmented CTCL is a variant of the disease that occurs most commonly in children. It tends to present most often in patients with black or darkly pigmented skin, although more fair-skinned individuals may also manifest these findings.[119–121] Patients with this form of CTCL present with hypopigmented macules and patches (Fig. 10.20) that are usually asymptomatic. The clinical appearance most often simulates disseminated pityriasis alba, tinea versicolor, or post-inflammatory hypopigmentation. Lesions may be round, arcuate, or gyrate, and often there is some subtle overlying scale.[111] Histologically, biopsies of hypopigmented lesions show the same features as the inflammatory lesions of CTCL, although on immunophenotyping, the infiltrate may be shown to be composed predominantly of CD8+ T cells rather than CD4+ T cells.[122]

Granulomatous slack skin is an extremely rare form of CTCL characterized by the insidious onset of papules and violet-colored plaques with progression to pendulous skin masses.[123] The lesions appear erythematous and wrinkled, and are most commonly distributed in the axillary and inguinal regions. There is a male

Stage	Skin (T)[a]	Nodes (N)[b]	Viscera (M)[c]	Blood (B)[d]
Ia	1	0	0	0
Ib	2	0	0	0
IIa	1–2	1	0	0
IIb	3	0, 1	0	0
III	4	0, 1	0	0
IVa	1–4	2, 3	0	1
IVb	1–4	0–3	1	1

Table 10.8 TNMB staging/classification of cutaneous T-cell lymphoma (CTCL)

[a]Skin: T0, clinically suspicious lesions; T1, limited papules or plaques (<10% BSA); T2, generalized papules or plaques (>10% BSA); T3, tumors; T4, generalized erythroderma. [b]Nodes: N0, none; N1, clinically abnormal nodes, negative pathology; N2, no clinically abnormal nodes, positive pathology; N3, clinically abnormal nodes and positive pathology. [c]Viscera: M0, no visceral involvement; M1, visceral involvement confirmed by pathology. [d]Blood: B0, atypical circulating cells not present (<5%); B1, atypical circulating cells present (>5%).

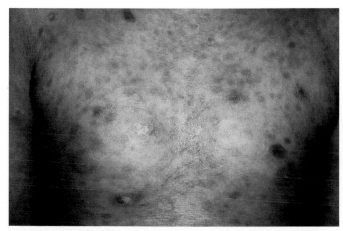

Figure 10.18 Cutaneous T-cell lymphoma. Erythematous macules, papules, plaques, and nodules in this 6-year-old male. Skin biopsy revealed an atypical T-cell infiltrate, with similar circulating cells noted in the blood.

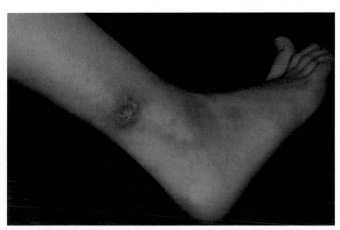

Figure 10.19 Lymphomatoid papulosis in a patient with cutaneous T-cell lymphoma. This 10-year-old male with a long history of patch- and plaque-stage CTCL developed intermittent self-healing ulcerative nodules, noted to be CD30+ on histologic evaluation.

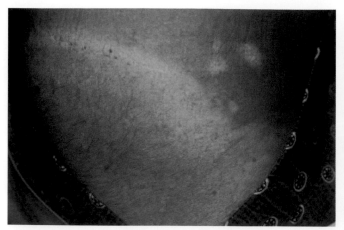

Figure 10.20 Hypopigmented cutaneous T-cell lymphoma. Hypopigmented macules and patches with minimal scaling. (Courtesy of Youn Kim, MD.)

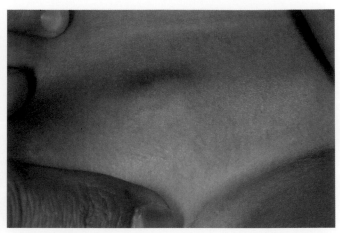

Figure 10.21 Neuroblastoma with cutaneous metastases. This male infant had numerous firm blue subcutaneous nodules which revealed neuroblastoma on histologic examination. He was found to have a large retroperitoneal primary tumor with disseminated metastatic disease.

predominance in the literature.[111] Histologically, a granulomatous T-cell infiltrate is seen along with fragmentation of elastic fibers.[124]

Alopecia mucinosa (follicular mucinosis) (see also Ch. 7) has also been seen as a feature of CTCL, primarily in adults. Although it occasionally occurs as a manifestation of the disorder in children, in the majority of patients (children and adults <40 years), it is generally regarded as a benign condition not associated with CTCL. Alopecia mucinosa presents as grouped follicular papules and boggy erythematous plaques in association with alopecia. Although most cases in childhood represent a benign self-limiting process, when lesions are persistent, evaluation for possible CTCL should be considered. *Pityriasis lichenoides-like CTCL* presents with erythematous papules with scaling and crusting, which simulate pityriasis lichenoides chronica or pityriasis lichenoides et varioliformis acuta (see Ch. 4).[125,126]

Sézary syndrome, which is characterized by erythroderma, lymphadenopathy and circulating atypical lymphocytes ('Sézary cells'), is felt to be a systemic variant of CTCL. It is rare in children. The cutaneous eruption is scaly, pruritic, and resistant to multiple therapies. As with many forms of CTCL, repeat skin biopsies may be necessary to confirm the diagnosis.

The diagnosis of CTCL is established based on the histologic findings of skin biopsy tissue, in conjunction with immunohistochemical studies. Although there are characteristic histologic features in well-developed disease, biopsy findings in patients with early involvement may be difficult to distinguish from other, more benign processes such as inflammatory dermatoses.[111] Immunohistochemical studies usually reveal an infiltrate of CD4+ T cells, with loss of CD7+ (leu-9) cells. Southern blot analysis and polymerase chain reaction (PCR) may be used to evaluate for T-cell receptor gamma gene rearrangement, which is seen in many but not all CTCL specimens.[127] A more specific technique, combining PCR and denaturing gradient gel electrophoresis (PCR/DGGE), demonstrates more sensitivity for detecting clonality but poorer specificity as it may detect rearrangements in a subset of patients with chronic dermatitis.[128]

There are a variety of treatment options for children with CTCL, but no standard protocols exist and the ideal therapy remains unclear. Potent topical corticosteroids are often sufficient for limited patch or plaque stage CTCL, but patients must be monitored for adrenal suppression and cutaneous atrophy.[129] Topical nitrogen mustard has demonstrated efficacy in adults with patch or plaque stage disease, and long-term follow-up studies have confirmed its

safety.[130] Psoralen plus ultraviolet A (PUVA) photochemotherapy is effective, but may be difficult and have limiting side-effects in children. Topical PUVA has been demonstrated useful in children with patch and plaque stage disease.[131] Other therapies used for CTCL include ultraviolet B therapy, carmustine, imiquimod, tazarotene, electron beam therapy, systemic chemotherapy, denileukin diftitox (a fusion toxin), interferon, photopheresis, and bexarotene (a systemic rexinoid, a cousin of the retinoids). Narrowband UVB therapy may offer similar results as those seen in adults, and has the potential advantages of being well tolerated in children, having fewer unpredictable phototoxic reactions, and requiring shorter treatment sessions.[132] However, pediatric experience with many of these treatments is quite limited. Young patients with CTCL may have an increased risk of Hodgkin lymphoma, and hence should be followed up on a long-term basis.

Neuroblastoma

Neuroblastoma, a tumor derived from primitive cells of the sympathetic nervous system, is the most common malignant tumor affecting infants in the first month of life, and accounts for 30–50% of all tumors occurring in the newborn period.[133] It is a tumor with large variability in its clinical presentation and natural history. Neuroblastoma may regress spontaneously (particularly in infants), mature into a benign ganglioneuroma, or result in extensive metastatic disease with a poor prognosis.[134] These tumors typically present as an abdominal mass due to liver infiltration with malignant cells, and may originate in the adrenal medulla, visceral ganglia, or paravertebral sympathetic ganglia.

Cutaneous metastases of neuroblastoma are seen in around 2% of all patients and 32% of those with a neonatal presentation. These skin lesions, which may be the presenting sign of the disease, appear as firm, blue-purple papules and nodules (Fig. 10.21), and when occurring in a neonate, fall into the spectrum of blueberry muffin lesions (Table 10.6). The catecholamines produced by the tumor cells may result in the classic blanching and peripheral halo of erythema noted after firm stroking. When cutaneous lesions are encountered in the newborn period, it confers a favorable prognosis.[133] Very hard subcutaneous nodules arising from the skull and orbital ridges are caused by skeletal metastases. Orbital metastases may result in the classic presentation of periorbital ecchymoses, so-called 'raccoon eyes'. Another ocular finding is that of heterochromia irides, which is related to involvement of the ophthalmic sympathetic nerve.

Staging of neuroblastoma is based on clinical and radiographic extent of disease and surgical resectability. Tumor tissue is usually necessary to confirm the diagnosis, and when cutaneous lesions are present, skin biopsy with histologic evaluation, immunophenotyping, and genetic analysis may be indicated. Measurement of urine and serum catecholamines or metabolites, computed tomography and/or magnetic resonance imaging, bone marrow aspirate and biopsies, and iodine-123 metaiodobenzylguanidine (MIBG) scintigraphy are recommended as part of the staging evaluation.[135]

Rhabdomyosarcoma

Rhabdomyosarcoma is the most common soft tissue sarcoma in children and adolescents, accounting for 50% of all soft tissue sarcomas in those under 15 years of age.[136,137] It is a malignant soft tissue neoplasm of skeletal muscle origin, and is seen primarily in the first and second decades of life. Although rhabdomyosarcoma is not a primary skin tumor, it is included in this section because it may simulate other cutaneous tumors, may extend or metastasize to the cutaneous surface, and may initially present to the pediatrician or other pediatric health care provider.

Rhabdomyosarcoma usually presents as an asymptomatic mass that is occasionally painful.[138] The head and neck, especially the nasal cavity and paranasal sinuses, are the most common sites of involvement in children. The genitourinary tract and extremities are other common sites of predilection. Patients may present with small to large nodules or rapidly expanding swellings. The surface may be flesh-colored to erythematous and, at times, may appear vascular with prominent vessel markings. The differential diagnosis may include infantile hemangioma, vascular malformation, fibrosarcoma (Fig. 10.22), cyst, infection, or other inflammatory or neoplastic process. Perianal rhabdomyosarcoma may mimic perirectal abscess.[139] *Congenital alveolar rhabdomyosarcoma* is a rare subtype, with >50% of patients presenting with multiple cutaneous metastases.[140] Tumor-specific translocations are detected in the majority of cases, and the disorder is invariably fatal.

Treatment of rhabdomyosarcoma consists primarily of surgery, radiotherapy, and chemotherapy. Although challenging, the overall 5-year survival of children and adolescents with both non-metastatic and metastatic tumors approaches 80%.[141]

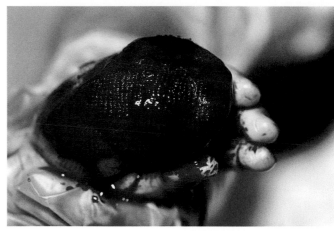

Figure 10.22 Fibrosarcoma. This congenital, vascular, friable mass was initially thought to be an infantile hemangioma; it grew rapidly and ultimately required full excision with amputation.

Key References

The complete list of 141 references for this chapter is available online at **www.expertconsult.com**.
See inside cover for registration details.

Chang MW, Frieden IJ, Good W. The risk of intraocular juvenile xanthogranuloma: Survey of current practices and assessment of risk. *J Am Acad Dermatol.* 1996;34(3):445–449.

Loeb DM, Thornton K, Shokek O. Pediatric soft tissue sarcomas. *Surg Clin N Am.* 2008;88:615–627.

Monclair T, Brodeur GM, Ambros PF, et al. The International Neuroblastoma Risk Group (INRG) staging system: An INRG task force report. *J Clin Oncol.* 2009;27(2):298–303.

Nijhawan A, Baselga E, Gonzalez-Ensenat A, et al. Vesiculopustular eruptions in Down syndrome neonates with myeloproliferative disorders. *Arch Dermatol.* 2001;137:760–763.

Satter EK, High WA. Langerhans cell histiocytosis: A review of the current recommendations of the Histiocyte Society. *Pediatr Dermatol.* 2008;25(3):291–295.

Weitzman S, Egeler RM. Langerhans cell histiocytosis: update for the pediatrician. *Curr Opin Pediatr.* 2008;20:23–29.

11 Disorders of Pigmentation

Although chiefly of cosmetic significance, disorders of pigmentation are among the most conspicuous and thus can have profound psychosocial implications for pediatric patients. The most important pigments in skin are melanin, reduced and oxygenated hemoglobin, and carotene. Melanin is a pigment produced by melanocytes, specialized dendritic cells derived from the neural crest that migrate to the basal layer of the epidermis during embryogenesis. Melanocytes synthesize and package melanin within discrete membrane-bound organelles called melanosomes, which are then transferred via melanocytic dendrites to surrounding keratinocytes of epidermis and hair follicles; on average, there is one melanocyte to every 36 surrounding keratinocytes.[1-4] Variations in skin color among different individuals reflect the number and size of mature melanosomes, not the number of melanocytes.

Four stages of melanosome maturation have been described and can be distinguished by ultrastructural examination:

1. Membrane vesicles that contain no visible pigment (stage I or premelanosomes)
2. More elongated vesicles with an ordered internal membrane, but no pigment (stage II melanosome)
3. The presence of melanin on ordered internal fibers (stage III melanosome)
4. Structures so full of melanin that the luminal structures cannot be seen (mature or stage IV melanosomes).

Darkly pigmented individuals have more numerous, larger, singly dispersed melanosomes, whereas individuals with light pigmentation have fewer, smaller melanosomes that are aggregated into complexes and are more rapidly degraded.[5] The presence of melanin in the epidermis helps protect against ultraviolet radiation and associated cutaneous damage, including pigmented nevi,[6] actinic damage, and cutaneous neoplasia. Red hair color, usually associated with an inability to tan, increases the risk of developing melanoma fourfold and has been associated with polymorphisms in the melanocortin receptor 1 (MCR1).[7]

Melanin exists in two forms in human skin, brown-black eumelanin and yellow-red pheomelanin. Melanin biosynthesis is primarily regulated by tyrosinase, a copper dependent enzyme that allows the initial conversion of tyrosine to dihydroxyphenylalanine (DOPA). Eumelanin synthesis involves increased levels of tyrosinase activity and additional melanogenic enzymes, such as tyrosinase-related protein (TRYP)-1 and TRYP-2/dopachrome tautomerase, both regulators of distal steps in the pathway to melanin and/or stabilizers of tyrosinase. Pheomelanin synthesis, however, involves the addition of a cysteinyl group that accounts for the yellow-red color, and is associated with reduced tyrosinase activity and absence of TRYP-1, TRYP-2, and a protein called P (pink-eyed dilution) protein.

The ratio of eumelanin to pheomelanin, as well as the total content of melanin, is higher in skin types V–VI (the darkest skin colors) than in skin types I and II (the lightest skin colors, most prone to burning with ultraviolet light exposure). Pheomelanin levels tend to be greatest in individuals with bright red hair, whereas eumelanin is the predominant pigment in individuals with brown or black hair.[8]

In all races the dorsal and extensor surfaces are relatively hyperpigmented, and the ventral surfaces are less pigmented. This is most evident in races with darker skin (African-Americans, Hispanics, and Asians). The separation of the dorsal and ventral pigmentation is most conspicuous on the extremities and more or less follows Voight's lines.[9] Termed Futcher's or Ito's line, this differentiation of dorsal and ventral pigmentation is present from infancy and persists throughout adulthood. Approximately 75% of blacks and 10% of whites have at least one line of pigmentary demarcation.

Disorders of abnormal pigmentation

Disorders of decreased pigmentation may be classified as:

1. Genetic or developmentally controlled disorders, in which pigmentation tends to be abnormal from birth or early infancy
2. Disorders associated with depigmentation or loss of previously existing melanin.

Congenital disorders of decreased pigmentation include tuberous sclerosis, piebaldism, Waardenburg syndrome, and albinism. Acquired disorders of decreased pigmentation include vitiligo, post-inflammatory hypopigmentation, pityriasis alba, and tinea versicolor. Hypopigmentary disorders may be further divided into patterned and unpatterned groups. Patterned forms of decreased pigmentation include pityriasis alba, cutaneous T-cell lymphoma, tinea versicolor, post-inflammatory hypopigmentation, leprosy, pinta, tuberous sclerosis, pigmentary mosaicism, vitiligo, piebaldism, and the Waardenburg and Vogt–Koyanagi syndromes. Unpatterned decreases in pigmentation may be seen in albinism, phenylketonuria, and the silvery hair syndromes.

Vitiligo

Vitiligo, an acquired form of patterned loss of pigmentation, results from the cytotoxic activity of autoreactive T cells against melanocytes and the failure of circulating T regulatory cells to home to skin.[10-12] Autoantibodies that can destroy melanocytes have been detected in serum samples of patients with vitiligo, and are directed against several melanocyte-specific antigens, including tyrosinase and TRYP-1. The disorder has a genetic component, with a prevalence of 7–12% among 1st-degree relatives, 6% among siblings, and 23% among monozygotic twins.[13] Generalized vitiligo has recently been linked to markers of autoimmunity, autoinflammation (e.g., NALP1) and to the tyrosinase gene.[13,14] Autoimmune disorders are seen with significantly increased frequency in immediate family members of affected individuals, most commonly vitiligo and leukotrichia,[15] but occur in only about 1% of pediatric patients with vitiligo.[16] The vast majority of patients with vitiligo are otherwise healthy. Thyroid disease and alopecia areata occasionally have been reported in association,[17,18] although the presence of autoimmune antibodies is common.[16]

Vitiligo affects approximately 1% of the population and may begin at any age, although rarely is congenital. Its onset is most common in young adults; in about half of the patients it begins prior to the age of 20 years, and in one-quarter of patients it develops before the age of 8 years. The mean age in pediatric patients is 6.2 years.[15,19,20]

The location, size, and shape of individual lesions vary considerably, yet the overall picture is characteristic. Lesions usually appear as partially or completely depigmented ivory white macules or patches, usually with well-defined, sometimes hyperpigmented, convex borders (Fig. 11.1). They tend to have an oval or linear contour and range in size from several millimeters to large patches (Fig. 11.2). Rarely, extensive or near total depigmentation of the body (universal or total vitiligo) occurs (Fig. 11.3). Although usually considered to be a bilateral disorder, vitiligo may be asymmetrical; segmental vitiligo, in which the depigmentation is confined to a localized, usually unilateral area, occurs more frequently in children than in adults (Fig. 11.4). In 75% of affected individuals the first lesions occur as depigmented spots on exposed areas, such as the dorsal surfaces of the hands, face, and neck. Other sites of predilection include the body folds (the axillae and groin), body orifices (the eyes, nostrils, mouth, navel, areolae, genitalia, and perianal regions (Figs 11.5, 11.6), and areas over bony prominences such as the elbows, knees, knuckles, and shins. Approximately 12% of patients show white hairs (leukotrichia or poliosis) (Fig. 11.7). Vitiligo has been divided into several subtypes based on the distribution of lesions. In descending order of frequency in pediatric patients, these include generalized, focal, segmental, acrofacial, mucosal, and universal. Patients with vitiligo commonly show halo nevi,[21] pigmented nevi surrounded by a zone of depigmentation (Fig. 11.8; see Ch. 9, Fig. 9.23), and the discovery of a halo nevus should prompt the search for vitiligo elsewhere.

The Koebner phenomenon (development of a lesion after trauma) has been described in approximately 15% of affected children with vitiligo, particularly related to sunburn. A recent study showed that skin friction induces melanocyte detachment in persons with vitiligo, but not in individuals with normal skin, further emphasizing the role of trauma in triggering new lesions.[22] Other individuals associate the onset of vitiligo with periods of severe physical or emotional trauma.

Ordinarily the diagnosis of vitiligo is not difficult, especially when there is symmetrical depigmentation about the eyes, nostrils, mouth, nipples, umbilicus, or genitalia. In fair-skinned individuals it may be difficult to differentiate areas of vitiligo from the adjacent normal skin. In such cases examination under Wood's light in a darkened room may help to delineate a contrast between normal

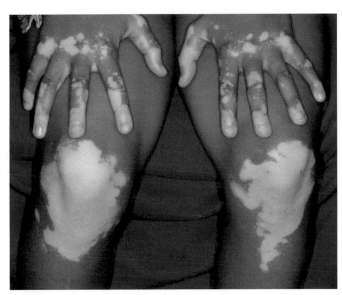

Figure 11.2 Vitiligo. Symmetrical depigmentation of the knees and dorsal aspect of the hands. The distal fingers are particularly hard to repigment.

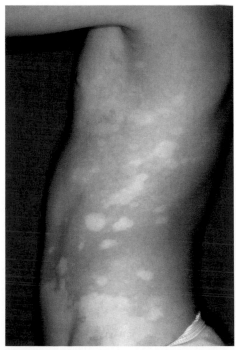

Figure 11.1 Vitiligo. Depigmented, usually well-defined, white macules or patches that tend to have an oval or linear contour.

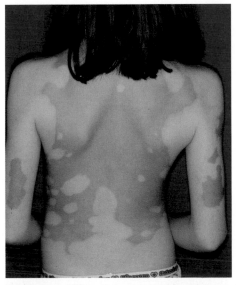

Figure 11.3 Vitiligo. Extensive depigmentation in this 13-year-old girl. Virtually all of her skin was depigmented, except for the pigmented areas on the back. After years of unsuccessfully trying to stimulate repigmentation, at 16 years of age, this girl and her parents elected to initiate 20% monobenzyl ether of hydroquinone.

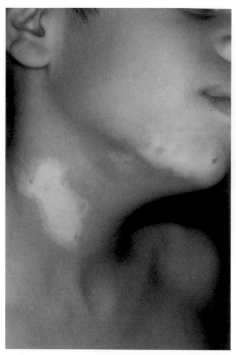

Figure 11.4 Segmental vitiligo. Segmental distribution of depigmentation on the right side of the chin and neck. Note the areas of perifollicular as well as peripheral repigmentation.

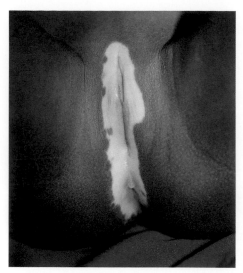

Figure 11.6 Vitiligo. The vitiligo was limited to the vulvar and perianal areas in this African-American girl.

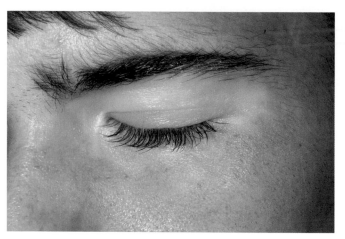

Figure 11.5 Vitiligo. Periorbital depigmentation. The perioral and perinasal areas are also commonly affected on the face.

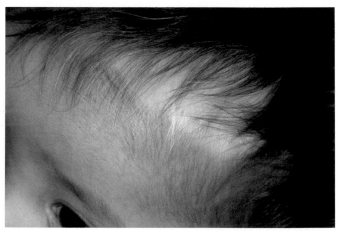

Figure 11.7 Vitiligo with poliosis. When the hair in the affected area is white, there is a decreased likelihood of repigmentation.

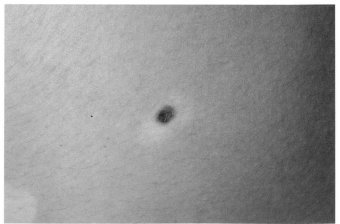

Figure 11.8 Vitiligo. Halo nevi are not uncommonly seen in children with vitiligo, and the pathomechanism of vitiligo and halo nevi is thought to be the same. Although the depigmentation may be limited to the site of the pigmented nevus, a search for other sites of depigmentation should be performed.

and depigmented skin. When the diagnosis is in doubt, the distribution of lesions, the age at onset, the presence of a convex hyperpigmented border, and the characteristic sites of predilection may help establish the correct diagnosis.

Lesions of post-inflammatory hypopigmentation are hypopigmented, not depigmented, and patients usually provide a history of previous localized inflammation. Nevus depigmentosus tends to be a well-defined, usually hypopigmented patch that may be present at birth or appear during infancy as normal pigmentation increases, but is subsequently stable. Pityriasis alba is a hypopigmentary disorder, and may be further differentiated by its frequent distribution on the face, upper arms, neck, and shoulders, and its occasional fine adherent scale (see Ch. 3, Fig. 3.29). Lesions of tinea versicolor may be differentiated by their discrete or confluent small round hypopigmented macules, their fine scales, and their typical distribution

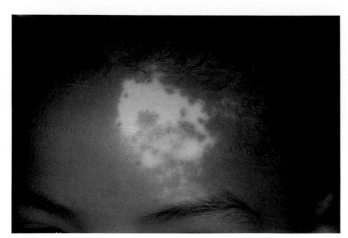

Figure 11.9 Vitiligo. Note the follicular repigmentation on the forehead of this girl.

on the trunk, neck, upper arms, or, particularly in pediatric patients, on the face (see Ch. 17, Figs 17.28, 17.29). The demonstration of hyphae on microscopic examination of epidermal scrapings is confirmatory (Fig. 17.30). The diagnosis of cutaneous T cell lymphoma of the hypopigmented type should be considered in adolescents with more extensive hypopigmented macules resembling pityriasis alba (see Ch. 10, Fig. 10.20).[23]

The presence of a white forelock and the pattern of depigmentation suggest a diagnosis of piebaldism or Waardenburg syndrome (see Piebaldism and Waardenburg syndrome, discussed below). Most individuals with Waardenburg syndrome show characteristic facial features. The diagnosis of albinism (see Oculocutaneous albinism, below) may be established by its presence at birth and by the facts that normal eye color is retained in vitiligo (but not in albinism); in addition, hair on glabrous skin in the vitiliginous patient, in contrast to that in the patient with albinism, often retains most of its pigment.

The hypopigmented macules of tuberous sclerosis (see below) usually lack the characteristic milk-white appearance of lesions of vitiligo, are present at birth or during the first years of life, do not change with age, and have a normal number of melanocytes (with reduction in size of melanosomes and melanin granules within them) in contrast to the absence or decrease in number of melanocytes in patients with vitiligo.

The course of vitiligo is variable. Long periods of quiescence may be interrupted by periods of extension or partial improvement. Complete spontaneous repigmentation is unusual. Some temporary or partial repigmentation, however, may occur, especially in children with lesions of recent onset and during the summer months because of increased exposure to ultraviolet light. Loss of pigmentation in lesions that have at least partially repigmented is common in temperate climates during the winter months. The repigmentation process proceeds slowly, although children tend to respond with more permanent and complete repigmentation than adults. Repigmentation most commonly appears as small, freckle-like spots of repigmentation, reflecting the migration of melanocytes from the hair follicle (Fig. 11.9). As such, the chance of repigmentation in a site is greater if pigmentation of regional hairs is retained. Diffuse repigmentation of lesions or repigmentation from the margins has also been described. The preferential tendency to repigment of the face and neck has been attributed to the high density of hair follicles at these sites, as well as exposure to ultraviolet light. In contrast, sites lacking or poor in hair follicles, such as the dorsal surfaces of the fingers, hands, and feet and the volar aspect of the wrists, do not respond as well as other areas.

Repigmentation can frequently be accomplished, at least partially, by the twice-daily application of potent topical corticosteroids or topical calcineurin inhibitors (tacrolimus ointment, pimecrolimus cream).[24,25] The skin of the head and neck responds best to both of these treatment modalities. Overall, 40–90% of pediatric patients show a response to these treatments, although moderate to high potency steroids can be associated with systemic absorption, especially if applied over large body surface areas or on the head and neck continuously.[18,26,27] Application of a topical calcineurin inhibitor for facial vitiliginous lesions eliminates the risk of cutaneous atrophy and ocular toxicity carried by application of topical corticosteroids. Despite the lack of evidence of photocarcinogenic potential of topically applied calcineurin inhibitors in humans, application of calcineurin inhibitors coupled with phototherapy carries a potential risk until additional experience is accrued. Although topical antiinflammatory therapy has been standard, a recent study described good to excellent repigmentation in 65% of 400 children treated with minipulses of oral methylprednisolone on two consecutive days weekly, and fluticasone ointment twice daily.[28]

The repigmentation of lesional skin can be stimulated most effectively by exposure to ultraviolet light. Most commonly narrow band UVB is utilized, which has been shown to be as effective as topical PUVA therapy.[29,30] In one study, 50% responded to nbUVB and 57% to PUVA.[31] Systemic or topical administration of psoralen compounds or khellin followed by gradually increasing exposure to sunlight or long-wave ultraviolet light (PUVA) is rarely used now in children because of its greater toxicity. Narrow band UVB phototherapy is largely reserved for older pediatric patients who are highly motivated and completely informed about their chances for improvement with these therapies. Treatment is traditionally 2–3 times weekly, beginning at relatively low dose and increasing by about 20% each treatment until slight erythema is reached. The 308 nm monochromatic excimer laser (in the UVB range) is an excellent, painless therapy for more localized lesions. The best responses to excimer laser are at sites that also respond best to narrow band ultraviolet light therapy, with the dorsal aspect of the hands and feet, genital and suprapubic areas the most difficult sites to repigment.[32] In one study of chronic stable vitiligo, >50% showed >75% repigmentation.[33] Responses to the excimer laser may be improved by concurrently using antiinflammatory therapy.[34] Avoidance of burning with phototherapy is important, since cutaneous burning can lead to further depigmentation via the Koebner phenomenon.

Topical therapies can be used jointly with light treatment, although the long-term safety of the combination of topical calcineurin inhibitors and ultraviolet light is unknown. Treatment with the combination of topical tacalcitol (vitamin D derivative) and excimer laser for 12 sessions (over 12 weeks) was significantly more effective than the excimer laser treatments alone.[35] The use of antioxidants, particularly pseudocatalase, has been based on the demonstration of decreased enzymatic and non-enzymatic oxidants in the skin of patients with vitiligo.[36] Pseudocatalase acts as a substitute for the decreased levels of catalase, degrading the increased hydrogen peroxide and recovering enzymatic activity. In one retrospective uncontrolled study of 71 children, twice daily full body application of pseudocatalase coupled with daily low dose (0.15 mJ/cm²) nbUVB stopped the progression of vitiligo in all children and led to >75% repigmentation in 93% of treated children; repigmentation of the hands and feet was most disappointing.[37] Oral antioxidants for vitiligo are under investigation.[36]

Surgical modalities are based on the autologous grafting of nonlesional epidermis or cultured melanocytes from healthy skin sites to depigmented areas that have been deepithelialized by ablative procedures.[38,39] Chinese cupping has recently been shown to be a technique to induce blisters for capturing donor melanocytes.[40]

Grafting has been demonstrated to lead to at least 75% repigmentation in 30–90% of patients, and is most successful for more localized lesions.[41,42] However, these approaches are time-consuming and expensive, and can result in recurrence of vitiligo (including at the donor site), scarring, infection, and keloids in at-risk patients. Grafting should only be considered for stable vitiligo in adolescents at sites that are resistant to medical treatment.

When treatment of vitiligo is unsatisfactory, lesions can be hidden by the use of cosmetic makeup or aniline dye stains, such as Vitadye (Elder), quick-tan preparations,[43] or cosmetic camouflage (Dermablend or Covermark). In those few recalcitrant cases in which vitiligo has progressed to such an extent that >50% of the body is involved (particularly in those persons in whom only a few islands of normal skin remain), an attempt at depigmentation with 20% monobenzyl ether of hydroquinone (Benoquin) may be considered. Such patients should be reminded that the depigmentation is permanent, requiring lifelong vigilant use of sun protection. Owing to the permanence of depigmentation therapy, this treatment is not generally offered to pre-adolescent patients. Quality of life studies have shown that children with vitiligo have impaired social development as young adults, stressing the importance of intervention.[44] Patients with vitiligo and their families can find support through the National Vitiligo Foundation (www.vitiligofoundation.org or www.nvfi.org).

Vogt–Koyanagi Syndrome

The Vogt–Koyanagi syndrome (Vogt–Koyanagi–Harada syndrome) is a rare, possibly autoimmune disorder characterized by bilateral granulomatous uveitis, alopecia, vitiligo, poliosis, dysacousia (in which certain sounds produce discomfort), and deafness. Usually seen in adults in the 3rd and 4th decades of life,[45] the disorder also occurs in children and adolescents.[46,47] Although the etiology is unknown, it has been hypothesized that this syndrome is associated with an abnormal host response to an infective agent, possibly a virus, with an allergic sensitization to uveal melanocyte antigens and destruction of melanin in the hair and skin. The Vogt–Koyanagi–Harada syndrome adds meningeal irritation or encephalitic symptoms in association. In this variant of Vogt–Koyanagi syndrome, a prodromal febrile episode, with lymphocytosis, encephalitic, or meningeal symptoms, and increased pressure of the cerebrospinal fluid, is followed by bilateral uveitis (often with choroiditis and optic neuritis).

The bilateral uveitis occurs in all patients and generally takes a year or more to clear. As the uveitis begins to subside, poliosis (in 80–90%), temporary auditory impairment, usually bilateral vitiligo (in 50–60%), and alopecia (in 50%) develop. The poliosis may be limited to the eyebrows and eyelashes or may also involve the scalp and body hair. The pigmentary changes, which generally appear 3 weeks to 3 months after the onset of the uveitis, tend to be permanent. Although most patients show some recovery of visual acuity, the majority of children and adolescents have a residual visual defect, related to the development of cataracts, glaucoma, choroidal neovascularization, and subretinal fibrosis.[48] Early and aggressive systemic corticosteroid use often leads to response.

Alezzandrini Syndrome

Alezzandrini syndrome is a rare disorder of unknown origin primarily seen in adolescents and young adults. Possibly related to the Vogt–Koyanagi syndrome, it is characterized by unilateral degenerative retinitis with visual impairment, which is followed after an interval of months or years by bilateral deafness and unilateral vitiligo and poliosis, which appear on the side of the retinitis.

Oculocutaneous Albinism

Albinism is a group of inherited disorders of melanin synthesis manifested by a congenital decrease of pigmentation of the skin, hair, and eyes.[49,50] It occurs in two forms: oculocutaneous and ocular. Oculocutaneous albinism (OCA) encompasses at least four major subtypes (Table 11.1) with decreased or absent melanin biosynthesis in the melanocytes of the skin, hair follicles, and eyes. All forms except one (the rare autosomal dominant form of oculocutaneous albinism) are inherited as autosomal recessive traits. In ocular albinism, usually an X-linked recessive form, only the eye pigmentation is consistently abnormal. An oculocerebral syndrome with hypopigmentation (the Cross–McKusick–Breen syndrome) is characterized by oculocutaneous albinism, microphthalmos, spasticity, and mental retardation.[51] The silvery hair syndromes, Chediak–Higashi syndrome, Griscelli syndrome, and Elejalde syndrome, and the Hermansky–Pudlak syndrome are distinct from albinism and will be discussed separately.

Oculocutaneous albinism affects 1 in 17 000 persons in the USA. The highest prevalence (as high as 1% of the population) occurs in the Cuna tribe of Indians on the San Blas Islands off the coast of Panama. Affected Cuna Indian children have been called 'moon children' because they have marked photosensitivity and photophobia and prefer to go outdoors only at night. In some African tribes, the frequency is 1:1500. Oculocutaneous albinism is characterized by varying degrees of unpatterned reduction of pigment

Table 11.1 Forms of oculocutaneous albinism

Type	Mutation	Subtypes or alternate name	Comments
OCA1A	Tyr (absence)	Tyrosinase-negative	1:40000; Most severe cutaneous and ocular defects; highest risk of skin cancer
OCA1B	Tyr (decreased)	Yellow mutant	Yellow hair
		Platinum	Metallic tinge
		Minimal pigment	Only eyes darken
		Temperature-sensitive	Melanin at acral sites
OCA2	P protein	Tyrosinase-positive	1:36000 (whites)
		Brown	1:3900–1:10000; Most common form in patients of African origin; More pigment with advancing age
OCA3	TRYP1	Rufous	Rare; 1:8500 Africans; Reddish-bronze color to skin and hair
OCA4	MATP		Rare (whites); 1:85000 Japanese; Resembles OCA2

Tyr, tyrosinase; P protein, pink-eyed dilution protein; TRYP1, tyrosinase-related protein 1; MATP, membrane-associated transporter protein.

in the skin and hair, translucent irides, hypopigmented ocular fundi, and an associated nystagmus. Melanocytes and melanosomes are present in the affected skin and hair in normal numbers, but fail to produce normal amounts of melanin. Regardless of subtype, affected individuals require vigorous sun protection of the skin and eyes, and are at risk of adverse psychosocial effects because of the cosmetic aspects of albinism, especially in children from darker-skinned backgrounds.

In the past, albinism was divided into tyrosinase-negative and -positive forms, based on the ability (tyrosinase-positive) or inability (tyrosinase-negative) of plucked hair to become pigmented in the presence of tyrosine or DOPA. Tyrosinase-negative albinism, now called type I albinism, results from absence (OCA1A) or partial reduction of the activity (OCA1B) of tyrosinase, the critical enzyme in melanin formation (Table 11.1).[52] The underlying genetic bases for the various forms of tyrosinase-positive albinism are now also known. Type II albinism (OCA2) results from the absence of P ('pink-eyed dilution') protein,[53] which is important for melanosome biogenesis and the normal processing and transport of melanosomal proteins, such as tyrosinase and TRYP1. OCA3 occurs from an absence of TRYP1,[54] an enzyme in the biosynthetic pathway of melanin synthesis that catalyzes the oxidation of 5,6-dihydroxyindole-2-carboxylic acid monomers into melanin and also stabilizes tyrosinase, allowing it to leave the endoplasmic reticulum for incorporation into melanosomes.[55] OCA4 results from mutations in the gene encoding membrane-associated transporter protein (MATP), which is a melanosome membrane transporter.[56]

Individuals with OCA1A are unable to produce melanin at all and show white skin, white hair, and blue irides, regardless of familial skin coloration.[57] Hair may show a slight yellow tint with advancing age because of denaturation of hair keratins. Similarly, ocular abnormalities are most severe with OCA1A. Eye findings include photophobia (with squinting), nystagmus (which typically develops at 6–8 weeks of age), strabismus, and decreased visual acuity; patients with OCA1A are often legally blind. The optic fibers are misrouted, resulting in monocular vision, which is usually not altered by surgical correction of the nystagmus or strabismus.[58,59] Although neurologic development is otherwise generally normal, an increased risk of ADHD has also been described.[60] Actinic damage (cutaneous atrophy, telangiectasia and wrinkling, actinic cheilitis, actinic keratoses) and malignant skin tumors (basal and squamous cell carcinomas, melanomas) are almost always seen in affected young adults and often present during childhood if the skin and eyes are not protected.

Patients with OCA1B have been divided into different phenotypic subgroups (Table 11.1) that occur because of differences in degree of tyrosinase activity and the localization within the *TYR* gene of the mutation. One of these is the 'yellow mutant' form, in which the hair color turns to yellow within the first few years and a golden blond to light brown by the end of the second decade. Patients with platinum OCA develop small amounts of pigment with a metallic tinge in late childhood, while those with minimal pigment OCA show darkening of the eyes with time, but the skin remains without pigmentation. Individuals with temperature-sensitive OCA1B are born with white skin and hair and blue eyes. Usually during the second decade of life, however, areas with lower temperature (esp. hair at acral sites on the upper and lower extremities) are able to produce melanin because the tyrosinase activity is only inactivated above 35°C. This interesting phenotype is shared with that of the Siamese cat, which also results from temperature-sensitive tyrosinase activity.

The OCA2 type of albinism, which includes 'tyrosinase-positive' albinism and Brown OCA, is the most common form, and is usually the type that occurs in African-American individuals (Fig. 11.10).

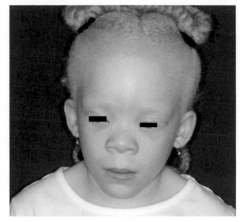

Figure 11.10 Albinism. This African-American girl has type II albinism with light skin and yellow hair.

The phenotype may vary from a slight to moderate decrease in pigmentation of the skin, hair and eyes. With time, however, dark lentigines and pigmented nevi usually develop at sun-exposed sites. These individuals can also have problems with their eyes and an increased risk of cutaneous malignancy, but significantly less than that seen in individuals with tyrosinase-negative albinism. Although the degree of pigment dilution in affected individuals is variable, the diagnosis is usually easily established in those who have striking pigment loss or relative pigment dilution when compared with unaffected siblings or parents. Some patients with OCA2 have red hair, which has been shown to result from concomitant mutations in the melanocortin 1 receptor.[61] OCA2 has also been described in approximately 1% of patients with Angelman syndrome or Prader–Willi syndrome, disorders that result from deletion of the long arm of chromosome 15, the site of the P gene. Prader–Willi syndrome results from deletion of the paternal chromosome at 15q, and is characterized by hyperphagia with obesity, hypogonadism, and mental retardation. In contrast, Angelman syndrome results from deletion of the maternal chromosome at 15q and is characterized by microcephaly, severe mental retardation, ataxia, and inappropriate laughter. Pigment dilution occurs when both copies of the P gene are mutated or deleted. Interestingly, duplication of the 15q chromosomal region has been associated with generalized skin hyperpigmentation.[62]

Rufous OCA or OCA3 presents as 'ginger' red hair, a reddish-bronze color of skin, and blue or sometimes brown irides. This form may be underreported, since the decrease in pigmentation is slight, and may be undetectable in lighter skinned patients. OCA4 is now considered one of the most common forms in Japan,[63] and affected individuals resemble patients with OCA2.[56]

Molecular testing is available commercially for detecting mutations in *TYR* and P protein, while analysis of mutations in TYRP1 and MATP is available on a research basis. Interestingly, only about 50% of patients have mutations in two alleles of any of the known affected genes. Some have one abnormal allele, and a polymorphic variant of *TYR* (R402Q allele) is found in the majority with only one *TYR* mutation, suggesting at least a close association.[64] Patients with albinism should be followed by an ophthalmologist, in addition to the dermatologist. Glasses may help the poor vision, and contact lenses and tinted glasses may ameliorate the photophobia. Nystagmus may be helped by surgery of the eye muscles or contact lenses; eye patching may be needed for the strabismus. High contrast written material, large type textbooks and computers that can enlarge text are all helpful for patients with poor visual acuity. Early actinic changes, keratoses, basal cell tumors, and particularly squamous cell carcinomas are common; the risk of melanoma (often amelanotic)[65] is also increased, even in children and adolescents. Thus, individuals with cutaneous albinism must learn to avoid sunlight exposure, to wear sunglasses, and to use protective clothing and sunscreen preparations on exposed surfaces. NOAH (National Organization for Albinism and Hypopigmentation) is a national support group for patients and their families (www.albinism.org).

Hermansky–Pudlak Syndrome

Hermansky–Pudlak syndrome (HPS) is a group of autosomal recessive disorders (HPS1–8) characterized by pigment dilution, a hemorrhagic diathesis secondary to a platelet storage pool defect and ceroid-lipofuscin depositions within the reticuloendothelial system, oral and intestinal mucosae, lung, and urine.[66–68] HPS is a disorder of biogenesis of melanosomes and other lysosome-related organelles[69–71] including platelet dense granules (Table 11.2). Most commonly seen in Hispanics from Puerto Rico (1:1800–1:400 persons), in persons of Dutch origin, and in East Indians from Madras, the platelet defect in patients with HPS does not produce a severe problem in children. Its expression, however, can be aggravated by ingestion of aspirin and other prostaglandin blockers. Special precautions and sometimes platelet transfusions must be given to avoid excessive bleeding after minor trauma or dental surgery.

The diffuse pigmentary features of the skin and eyes of individuals with HPS include pigmentary dilution of the skin and often the irides with hair that has a peculiar sheen, although not as silvery as in Chediak–Higashi, another syndrome of lysosome-related organelles. The degree of generalized pigment loss is quite variable in intensity, ranging from white skin to brown and light to brown eyes (Fig. 11.11). Ocular pigmentation generally correlates with cutaneous pigmentation. Ocular findings include nystagmus, photophobia, and decreased visual acuity. Extensive ecchymoses are a common clinical manifestation (Fig. 11.12). The bleeding diathesis also commonly manifests as epistaxis and menometrorrhagia. Patients with both HPS and systemic lupus erythematosus have been described.[72] The life-threatening complications of HPS, other than the bleeding diathesis, have been described in certain subtypes and are unusual in most affected children. These include granulomatous colitis,[73] progressive pulmonary fibrosis, and, less commonly, cardiomyopathy and renal failure. The life expectancy is 30–50 years of age. Glasses or contact lenses can help to correct the refractive errors. The bleeding from skin wounds may be stopped

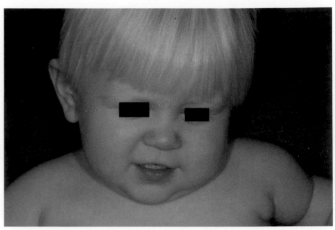

Figure 11.11 Hermansky–Pudlak syndrome. This Puerto-Rican infant shows the white hair and fair skin of Hermansky–Pudlak syndrome.

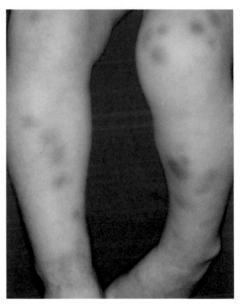

Figure 11.12 Hermansky–Pudlak syndrome. Legs of the baby shown in Figure 11.11, showing extensive ecchymoses.

Table 11.2 Clinical features of Hermansky–Pudlak syndrome (HPS)

Type	Mutation	Underlying cause	Findings associated with the cutaneous pigment dilution
HPS-1 HPS-4	*HPS-1* *HPS-4*	HPS-1 and -4 associate in a complex (BLOC-3) that regulates biogenesis of melanosomes, platelet dense bodies, and the lung lamellar body	Nystagmus, decreased visual acuity; prolonged bleeding; pulmonary fibrosis; granulomatous colitis (up to 1/3 of patients)
HPS-2	*AP3B1*	AP3B1 encodes a subunit of AP-3, which mediates protein trafficking into transport vesicles of the lysosome (and is thus also involved in immune function)	Nystagmus, decreased visual acuity; prolonged bleeding; neutropenia; recurrent infections; conductive hearing loss
HPS-3 HPS-5 HPS-6	*HPS-3* *HPS-5* *HPS-6*	HPS-3, -5, and -6 are associated in a complex (BLOC-2), which localizes tyrosinase and Tryp1, allowing them to function normally	Nystagmus, decreased visual acuity; mild extraocular manifestations: high cholesterol and slightly elevated triglycerides in HPS-5
HPS-7 HPS-8	*DTNBP1* *BLOC1S*	Dysbindin and BLOC1S3 are subunits of BLOC-1, and also involved in skin melanosome biogenesis and platelet function	Nystagmus, decreased visual acuity; prolonged bleeding

BLOC, biogeneses of lysosome-related organelles complex; DTNBP1, dystrobrevin binding protein 1.

with thrombin-soaked gelfoam, while DDAVP has been administered for tooth extraction and other invasive procedures. Transfusions of platelets or erythrocytes are occasionally required. Gene testing is available for mutations of *HPS-1* and *-4*.

Silvery Hair Syndromes

Three syndromes, Chediak–Higashi, Griscelli, and Elejalde (probably a subset of Griscelli), are autosomal recessive disorders characterized by an early silvery sheen to the hair, relative pigmentary dilution of skin with a grayish coloration, and in some patients ocular hypopigmentation.[68]

Chediak–Higashi syndrome

Patients with Chediak–Higashi syndrome (CHS) usually have a characteristic silvery sheen to the hair and skin, with a skin color that may appear lighter than that of other family members.[74,75] In affected individuals of family backgrounds of darker skin, however, the skin of acral, sun-exposed areas (ears, nose) may become intensely hyperpigmented (Fig. 11.13) or show only speckled hypopigmentation.[76,77] Decreased iris pigmentation results in an increased red reflex and photophobia. Strabismus and nystagmus are common, but visual acuity is usually normal. Inflammation and ulceration of the oral mucosa, especially of the gingivae, have been described.

The immunodeficiency of patients with CHS leads to infectious episodes. These episodes are associated with fever and predominantly involve the skin, lungs, and upper respiratory tract. The most common organisms found are *Staphylococcus aureus*, *Streptococcus pyogenes*, and *Pneumococcus*. The skin infections are primarily pyodermas, but infections with these organisms that result in deeper ulcerations resembling pyoderma gangrenosum have been reported.

Approximately 85% of patients with CHS undergo an 'accelerated' lymphohistiocytic phase, characterized by widespread visceral tissue infiltration with lymphoid and histiocytic cells, which are sometimes atypical in appearance.[78] Hepatosplenomegaly, lymphadenopathy, pancytopenia, jaundice, a leukemia-like gingivitis, and pseudomembranous sloughing of the buccal mucosa are associated features. The thrombocytopenia, platelet dysfunction, and depletion of coagulation factors may lead to petechiae, bruising, and gingival bleeding. Granulocytopenia and anemia are found in

90% of patients during the accelerated phase. Viral infection, particularly due to Epstein–Barr virus (EBV) infection, has been implicated in causing the accelerated lymphohistiocytic phase. The accelerated phase must be distinguished from autoimmune hemophagic syndromes and familial hemophagocytic lymphohistiocytosis (genetic defects in perforin or its receptor).

Many patients with CHS develop progressive neurological deterioration, particularly with clumsiness, abnormal gait, paresthesias, and dysesthesias. Peripheral and cranial neuropathies and, occasionally, a form of spinocerebellar degeneration may occur.

Giant abnormal granules or melanosomes are the hallmark of CHS, and result from dysregulated fusion of primary lysosome-like structures. They are found in circulating leukocytes, melanocytes of skin and hair, renal tubular epithelial cells, central nervous system (CNS) neurons, and other tissues. In the hair shaft, these giant melanosomes are smaller than those of Griscelli syndrome (see below) and regularly spaced (Fig. 11.14A). The giant granules within phagocytic cells of affected children cannot discharge their lysosomal and peroxidative enzymes into phagocytic vacuoles. The dysregulated fusion results from mutations in LYST, a lysosomal transport protein. The skin pigmentary disorder has been attributed to the inability of melanosomal fusion and transfer to keratinocytes, leading to giant melanosomes within melanocytes.

Neutropenia is common, and neutrophils are deficient in chemotactic and bactericidal capability. Selective deficiency of natural killer (NK) cells is characteristic. These immune abnormalities have been thought to cause the increased susceptibility to infections and the lymphohistiocytic phase. The mean age of death for patients with CHS without immune reconstitution is 6 years of age. Fatality usually results from overwhelming infection or hemorrhage during the accelerated phase. Approximately 10–15% of affected patients have a milder clinical phenotype and survive into adulthood, but tend to develop the progressive neurologic dysfunction.[79]

Griscelli syndrome

Patients with Griscelli syndrome may be difficult to distinguish clinically from patients with Chediak–Higashi syndrome, as the silver-gray hair and skin color (Fig. 11.15), recurrent episodes of fever with or without infection, increasing hepatosplenomegaly due to lymphohistiocytic infiltration, and progressive neurological deterioration may be part of the clinical spectrum of both disorders.[80] Blood smears show pancytopenia but, in contrast to the patients with Chediak–Higashi syndrome, no leukocyte inclusions. Microscopic examination of the hair shows clumping of pigment in the hair shaft, similar to that of CHS, but with larger, more irregularly spaced macromelanosomes (Fig. 11.14B).

Three subsets of patients with Griscelli syndrome have been described, based on clinical manifestations and underlying gene defects. Two of these subsets are caused by mutations in genes close

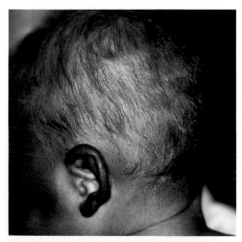

Figure 11.13 Chediak–Higashi syndrome. Note the silvery sheen to the hair and the intense pigmentation of the ear in this affected 8-month-old boy.

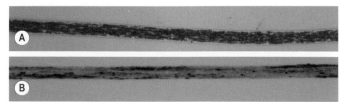

Figure 11.14 Silvery hair syndromes. The giant melanosomes are easily seen in the hair shaft of individuals with Chediak–Higashi syndrome (A) and Griscelli syndrome (B). Note the more regular spacing of the melanosomes in the hair from a patient with Chediak–Higashi syndrome.

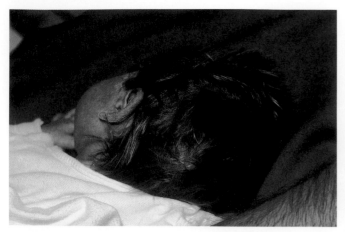

Figure 11.15 Griscelli syndrome. The silvery hair suggests the reason for this child's hepatosplenomegaly and pancytopenia. The child died before bone marrow transplantation could be performed.

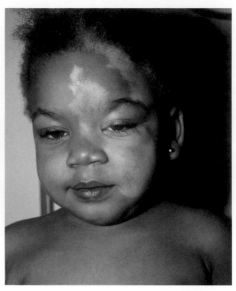

Figure 11.16 Piebaldism. This young girl shows the white forelock with depigmentation on the forehead as two triangular patches. The left cheek is also depigmented.

to each other on chromosome 15q21, *myosin Va* (type 1) and *Rab27A* (type 2). Patients who present with uncontrolled activation of T lymphocytes and macrophages (hemophagocytic syndrome) and immune deficits (especially reduction in T-cell cytotoxicity and cytolytic granule exocytosis) have mutations in *Rab27A*,[81] whereas those patients with neurologic problems and without immune abnormalities or hemophagocytosis tend to have myosin Va mutations.[82] Rare patients with neurologic abnormalities with or without hemophagocytosis have shown a *Rab27A* mutation.[83,84] *Myosin Va* encodes a protein that binds organelles such as melanosomes to actin. *Rab27A* is a GTP binding protein involved in the movement of melanosomes. Melanocytes are unable to transfer melanosomes to epidermal cells, and ultrastructural examination of skin biopsies reveals accumulation of melanosomes in melanocytes.

Elejalde syndrome

Elejalde syndrome (neuroectodermal melanolysosomal disease) is a silvery hair disorder characterized by severe neurologic dysfunction (seizures, severe hypotonia, ocular abnormalities, and mental retardation), but no immunodeficiency or hemophagocytosis.[84,85] The large, irregularly distributed melanosomes in hair resemble those of Griscelli syndrome, and Elejalde syndrome is now thought to be allelic to Griscelli syndrome type, resulting from mutations in myosin Va.[86] Type 3 Griscelli syndrome shows a phenotype restricted to the pigmentary defects and results either from mutation in the gene that encodes melanophilin (Mlph) or from a deletion in the F-exon of myosin Va.[87]

For all of the silvery hair syndromes, early bone marrow or stem cell transplantation is the treatment of choice for patients with an HLA-match. Bone marrow transplantation reverses the immunodeficiency and prevents the often fatal accelerated phase, but has no effect on pigmentation or on neurologic deterioration. Given the lack of success of transplantation in patients with mutations in myosin Va,[88] restriction of transplantation to patients with *Rab27A* mutations has been suggested. Otherwise, management of the disorder is largely supportive. Antibiotics help to control the recurrent infections, and immunoglobulin or immunosuppressive agents have been administered in an attempt to control the lymphohistiocytic or hemophagocytic phases. Splenectomy has been advocated in patients with the accelerated phase unresponsive to other forms of therapy.

Piebaldism

Piebaldism is an autosomal dominant disorder characterized by congenital patterned areas of depigmentation, including a white lock of hair above the forehead (the white forelock) in most affected individuals.[89] The disorder usually results from mutations in the *kit* proto-oncogene, which encodes a cell surface receptor for the stem cell/mast cell growth factor;[90] deletions in *SLUG*, a transcription factor, have also been described.[91] The clinical manifestations of piebaldism may be explained by the resultant defective migration of melanoblasts from the neural crest to the ventral midline and defect in the differentiation of melanoblasts to melanocytes. The distinctive patterns of hypopigmentation or depigmentation usually persist unchanged throughout life, but affected individuals with progressive depigmentation,[92] response to ultraviolet light and partial repigmentation,[93] or forelock regression during infancy[94] have occasionally been described. The white forelock, with a depigmented triangular patch of the scalp and forehead (widest at the forehead, with the apex pointing backward) occurs in 80–90% of piebald individuals (Fig. 11.16). Depigmented areas on the forehead often include the whole or inner portions of the eyebrows and eyelashes and extend to the root of the nose. Hypopigmented or depigmented areas have also been noted commonly on the chin, anterior neck, anterior portion of the trunk and abdomen, and on the anterior and posterior aspects of the mid-arm to the wrist and the mid-thigh to mid-calf. Typical of the lesions of piebaldism are islands of normal and increased pigmentation within the hypomelanotic areas, and sometimes hyperpigmented borders (Fig. 11.17).

The depigmentation of piebaldism can be differentiated from that of vitiligo by the usual presence at birth, lack of convex borders, and predilection for ventral surfaces, in contrast to the predilection on exposed areas, body orifices, areas of trauma, and intertriginous regions in vitiligo. The typical facial characteristics of type I Waardenburg syndrome are not seen in patients with piebaldism, although sensorineural deafness has rarely been described in piebaldism.[95] Treatment consists of cosmetic masking of areas of leukoderma[43] and vigorous sun protection. In the rare patients who show increased pigmentation after ultraviolet exposure,

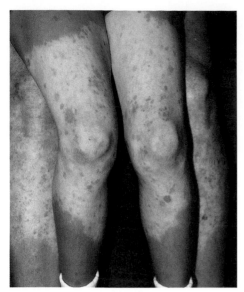

Figure 11.17 Piebaldism. Note the sharply demarcated areas of depigmentation with the islands of normal and hyperpigmentation within both the depigmented and normally pigmented (see top) areas. These are the legs of a mother and her daughter.

Table 11.3 Diagnostic criteria for type I Waardenburg syndrome	
Two major criteria or one major plus two minor criteria allows for the diagnosis of WS type I	
Major criteria	Minor criteria
White forelock, hair depigmentation Pigmentary abnormality of the iris Dystopia canthorum, W index* >1.95 Congenital sensorineural hearing loss Affected 1st-degree relative	Skin depigmentation Synophrys/medial eyebrow flare High/broad nasal root Hypoplastic alae nasi Gray hair before 30 years old

*W index: The measurements necessary to calculate the W index (in mm) are as follows: the inner canthal distance (a), the interpupillary distance (b), and the outer canthal distance (c).

Calculate $X = (2a − 0.2119c + 3.909)/c$

Calculate $Y = (2a − 0.2479b + 3.909)/b$

Calculate $W = X + Y + a/b$.

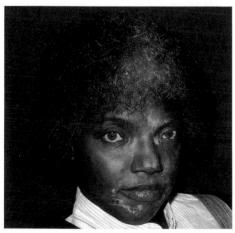

Figure 11.18 Waardenburg syndrome, type 1. Note the white forelock, dappled skin, broad nasal root, and dystopia canthorum. This young woman also had an affected son.

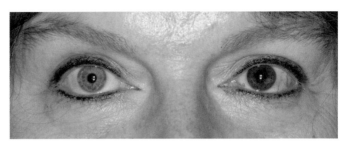

Figure 11.19 Waardenburg syndrome, type II. This affected individual shows iris heterochromia with the 'brilliant blue' iris. She had sensorineural deafness, but none of the facial features seen in type I Waardenburg syndrome.

phototherapy may be considered. Re-epithelialization by grafting with autologous cultured epidermis after laser removal of epidermis has provided permanent repigmentation in patients.[96,97]

Waardenburg Syndrome

Waardenburg syndrome (WS) is a group of autosomal dominant disorders characterized by a white forelock, heterochromia irides, cutaneous depigmentation and, in many patients, congenital sensorineural deafness.[98,99] WS reportedly accounts for 2–5% of cases of congenital deafness.[100] Four subtypes of WS have been described. Individuals with type I WS, the most common form, have characteristic facial features, including a broad nasal root and lateral displacement of the medial canthi and lacrimal puncta of the lower eyelids (dystopia canthorum) (Fig. 11.18). For clinical diagnosis, an individual must have two major criteria or one major plus two minor criteria to be considered affected (Table 11.3). Dystopia canthorum can be confirmed by a W index of >1.95 (Table 11.3).[99]

Congenital, usually non-progressive sensorineural hearing loss occurs in 47–58% of affected individuals, whereas the white forelock and cutaneous depigmentation occur in approximately 45% and 30%, respectively. The white forelock may be present at birth, may appear later (typically during teenage years), or may become pigmented with time. The heterochromic irides and/or hypoplastic (often brilliant) blue eyes (Fig. 11.19) are less common than the hair or skin depigmentation. Type I WS results from loss of function mutations in PAX3, a gene critical for both melanocyte migration and facial embryogenesis.[101,102] Spina bifida has been described in several affected families, leading to the firm recommendation for folate supplementation during pregnancy. Type II WS is a heterogeneous group of disorders that shows no facial characteristics, but more commonly than in WS type I, the iris pigmentary changes and deafness (80%). Approximately 15% of patients with type II WS have mutations in the MITF (microphthalmia-associated transcription factor) gene. Other patients with type II WS have mutations in SNAI2/SLUG or Sox 10, transcription factors critical for the migration and development of neural crest cells. Type III WS is an extreme presentation of type I WS with musculoskeletal abnormalities and rarely associated neural tube defects.[103] Some, but not all, patients with type III WS have homozygous mutations in PAX3. Type IV WS includes the pigmentary defects and sensorineural deafness in association with absence of enteric ganglia in the distal part of the intestine (Hirschsprung disease).[104] Facies are normal. Mutations

Table 11.4 Features of tuberous sclerosis

Two major features or 1 major feature + 2 minor features = Definite tuberous sclerosis
One major feature + 1 minor feature = Probable tuberous sclerosis
One major feature or two or more minor features = Possible tuberous sclerosis

Autosomal dominant disorder
Mutations in tuberin or hamartin
Cutaneous manifestations
   Hypopigmented macules* (≥3)
   Confetti skin lesions†
   Adenoma sebaceum* (angiofibromas)
   Fibrous forehead plaque*
   Shagreen patch* (connective tissue nevus)
   Non-traumatic ungual or periungual fibroma*
   Gingival fibroma†
Systemic manifestations
   Central nervous system involvement, esp. seizures, retardation, tumors
   Cortical tubers*
   Subependymal nodules*
   Subependymal giant cell astrocytoma*
   Cerebral white matter radial migration lines†
   Cardiac rhabdomyomas, single or multiple*
   Renal angiomyolipomas*
   Multiple renal cysts†
   Multiple retinal nodular hamartomas (retinal gliomas; phakomas)*
   Retinal achromic patch†
   Lymphangioleiomyomatosis*
   Cystic lesions in lungs†
   Osseous lytic lesions†
   Dental pits†
   Hamartomatous rectal polyps†

*Major features.

†Minor features.

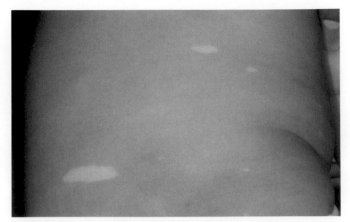

Figure 11.20 Tuberous sclerosis. Several lance-ovate (ash-leaf) and thumbprint white macules are noted on this infant's back.

have been described in three genes: *endothelin 3*;[105] *endothelin B receptor*;[106] and *Sox 10*.[107] Patients with *Sox 10* mutations may also have severe hypotonicity with central nervous system and peripheral nerve abnormalities, because of the important role of Sox 10 in glial cell development.[108] All of the forms of WS show marked variability of clinical characteristics, even within families and in monozygotic twins,[109] and subtle features may be seen, especially in WS1.

Tuberous Sclerosis Complex

Tuberous sclerosis is an autosomal dominant disorder with variable expressivity that occurs in as many as 1 in 6000 persons;[110,111] up to 70% of patients are thought to have new mutation. The disorder results from mutation in one of two different genes, *TSC1* (encoding hamartin; approximately 20% of patients) and *TSC2* (encoding tuberin; approximately 60% of patients); gene mutations have not been discovered in about 20% of affected individuals. Tuberin and hamartin form a complex that suppresses cell growth through regulation of several signaling pathways, most importantly of mammalian-target-of-rapamycin (mTOR) pathway signaling through switching Rheb from an active (GTP-bound) to inactive (GDP-bound) state.[111] In general, patients with mutations in *TSC1* have milder disease.[112] The rate of germline or somatic mosaicism is 10–25%.[113]

The disorder is characterized by the development of hamartomas of the skin, brain, eye, heart, kidneys, lungs, and bone (Table 11.4).[111,114–116] A variety of cutaneous features, including hypopigmented macules, adenoma sebaceum, fibrous tumors, and periungual and gingival fibromas, may be seen.

The hypopigmented macules ('white spots') of tuberous sclerosis are seen in 97% of patients at birth or shortly thereafter, although the appearance of additional lesions as late as 6 years of age has occasionally been described. Once present, the hypopigmented macules tend to be persistent and stable in shape and relative size. Wood's lamp examination in a completely darkened room may be useful in accentuating the macules in fair-skinned children. The white spots most commonly occur on the trunk, but hypopigmented tufts of scalp or eyelash hair have been noted. They range in size from a millimeter to several centimeters, and number from a few to >75. The hypopigmented macules are often round ('thumbprint'), confetti-like (particularly over the pretibial areas), oval or linear, but a lance-ovate shape ('ash leaf spots') is commonly described and easily differentiated from other disorders of localized decreased skin pigmentation, such as nevus depigmentosus and vitiligo (Fig. 11.20).

Lesions of vitiligo tend to be depigmented, and show a bright white coloration with Wood's lamp examination. The hypopigmented white spots of tuberous sclerosis are most difficult to distinguish from nevus depigmentosus (also called nevus achromicus; Fig. 11.21). A single white spot, most commonly nevus depigmentosus, has been described in 0.2–0.3% of all neonates,[117] suggesting that the majority of neonates with a white spot do not have tuberous sclerosis. Nevus depigmentosus may be present at birth or appear during early infancy as normal pigmentation increases. Most individuals will have a solitary lesion of nevus depigmentosus, but multiple lesions and segmental forms of nevus depigmentosus have been described. Nevus depigmentosus tends to persist lifelong, but remains unchanged after onset. Nevus depigmentosus and the hypomelanotic macules of tuberous sclerosis must also be distinguished from nevus anemicus, a developmental anomaly characterized by a circumscribed round or oval patch of pale or mottled skin[118] (see Ch. 12, Fig. 12.56).

Cutaneous angiofibromas (adenoma sebaceum), which are hamartomas composed of fibrous and vascular tissue, appear in 75% of cases. They typically develop between 2 and 6 years of age, but angiofibromas have been described at birth or as late as the mid-20s. These lesions characteristically are 1–4 mm, pink to red, dome-shaped papules with a smooth surface. They occur on the nasolabial folds, cheeks, and chin, and sometimes more extensively on the face. The upper lip is relatively spared, except immediately below the nose (Figs 11.22, 11.23). The angiofibromas in affected

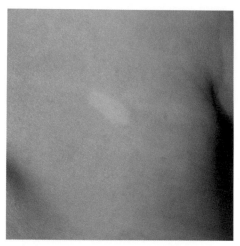

Figure 11.21 Nevus depigmentosus. Well-demarcated patch of hypopigmentation that tends to be round or oval in configuration. Nevus depigmentosus, also known as nevus achromicus, may be noted at birth or may become apparent during infancy.

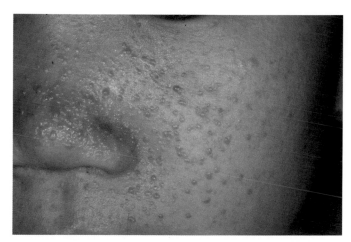

Figure 11.22 Tuberous sclerosis. Facial angiofibromas ('adenoma sebaceum') are typically 1–4 mm, skin-colored to red, dome-shaped papules with a smooth surface.

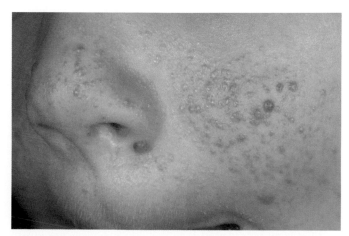

Figure 11.23 Tuberous sclerosis. The cheeks and nose are studded with hundreds of angiofibromas of different sizes. Note the relative sparing of the upper lip. This adolescent girl is concerned about the appearance of these facial lesions and is seeking information about therapy.

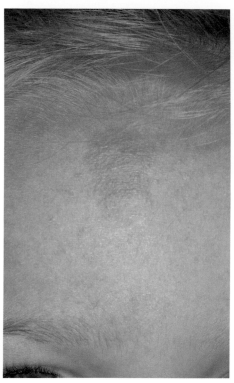

Figure 11.24 Tuberous sclerosis. The fibrous forehead plaque may be present at birth and, together with the hypopigmented macules, may allow a definitive diagnosis of tuberous sclerosis.

adolescents may be masked by or misdiagnosed as acne. Their distribution is usually symmetrical, but may be asymmetrical, especially in patients with a mosaic form of tuberous sclerosis.[119] Multiple angiofibromas, although considered by many to be pathognomonic of tuberous sclerosis, have been described in 43–88% adolescents and adults with multiple endocrine neoplasia (MEN) type 1.[120,121] The facial angiofibromas, however, tend to be fewer in number than in patients with tuberous sclerosis and may involve the upper lip or vermilion border. Collagenomas and confetti-like hypopigmented macules, also hallmarks of tuberous sclerosis, have been observed in 72% and 6% of patients with MEN1, respectively.[121] Patients with MEN1 are at high risk for the development of parathyroid, pituitary, pancreatic, and duodenal tumors.[122] Multiple facial angiofibromas with onset during adulthood have also been described in patients with Birt–Hogg–Dube syndrome,[123] or without signs of any associated disease and negative molecular testing.[124]

Large fibrotic plaques or nodules may occur on the forehead ('fibrous forehead plaque'; Fig. 11.24), cheeks, or scalp in 25% of patients, and are often present at birth. In 14–20% of patients, collagenomas also develop on the trunk, especially in the lumbosacral area, and most commonly during later childhood (shagreen patches or peau de chagrin lesions) (Fig. 11.25). They may be solitary or multiple, and vary from <1 cm to palm-sized. Collagenomas are usually slightly raised with focal depression at follicular openings, leading to comparison with pigskin, elephant skin, orange peel, or gooseflesh. Fibromas under or around the nails of the fingers and especially the toes (periungual and subungual fibromas; Fig. 11.26) and on the gums (gingival fibromas) are also considered pathognomonic. Seen in up to 80% of patients,[125] these fibromas do not tend to appear until after puberty, but may be the only sign of tuberous sclerosis.[126]

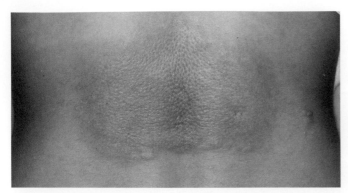

Figure 11.25 Tuberous sclerosis. The shagreen patch is characteristically found at the lumbosacral area and has a peau d'orange texture.

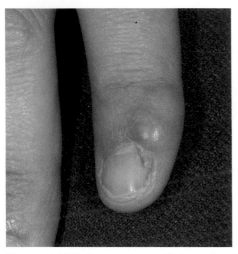

Figure 11.26 Tuberous sclerosis. Periungual and subungual fibromas on the fourth finger of this adolescent boy.

The systemic lesions of tuberous sclerosis may produce severe symptoms and possibly death. Seizures, seen in 80–90% of patients with tuberous sclerosis, may begin as infantile spasms, in which sudden repetitive myoclonic contractions of most of the body musculature are combined with flexion, extension, opisthotonos, and tremors. By 2 or 3 years of age, focal or generalized seizures and mental retardation may become evident. Extensive CNS involvement leads to hypsarrhythmia (salaam seizures), with electroencephalographic findings of multifocal high-voltage spikes and slow chaotic waves. Later in life the seizure pattern may change to a petit mal variety, and in less severe cases generalized or focal motor seizures may develop.

Retardation may be mild or severe and appears in 62% of affected individuals. The severity of mental retardation correlates well with the age of seizure onset. In 50–75% of affected individuals, the brain shows 'tubers,' pale sclerotic patches, which cause elevations or broadening of cerebral gyri. These tubers become calcified and are visible on skull radiographs as curvilinear opacities. Before calcification, these lesions are visible as periventricular or subependymal nodules by CT or MRI scanning.[127,128] Subependymal nodules are not malignant, but may enlarge to cause obstructive hydrocephalus.

By the end of the first decade of life, 80% of patients show renal involvement. Renal hamartomas (angiomyolipomas) occur in about 70% of patients, and larger ones may lead to hemorrhage. With advancing age, 20–30% of patients develop multiple, bilateral renal cysts, resembling those of polycystic kidney disease. These cysts tend to occur in individuals with deletions involving both TSC2 and the contiguous PKD1 (polycystic kidney disease) genes.[129] Abdominal ultrasound or scans are able to detect renal hamartomas or cysts in asymptomatic patients. Cardiac rhabdomyomas are most commonly present in infants and tend to regress spontaneously.[130] Although usually asymptomatic, rhabdomyomas may be associated with congestive heart failure, murmurs, cyanosis, arrhythmias, and sudden death, particularly during the first year of life. Two-dimensional echocardiography is a noninvasive technique that allows detection of asymptomatic cardiac rhabdomyomas.

The eyes may have characteristic retinal lesions (gliomas) referred to as phakomas. These retinal hamartomas have been described in about 50% of patients. Funduscopy may show one of two types of lesions: multiple, raised, mulberry-like lesions on or adjacent to the optic nerve head; or flat, disk-like lesions in the periphery of the retina. Pulmonary lymphangioleiomyomatosis occurs overall in 2.3% of individuals with tuberous sclerosis, particularly in women between the ages of 20 and 40 years.[131] Affected individuals present with shortness of breath, hemoptysis or pneumothorax, and show diffuse interstitial infiltrates with cystic changes by CT examination. About 85% of patients with tuberous sclerosis have osseous manifestations with the bones, particularly those of the hands and feet, demonstrating cysts and periosteal thickenings. Tooth pits (seen as punctate, round or oval, 1–2 mm randomly arranged enamel defects), particularly in the permanent teeth, appear to be another marker of tuberous sclerosis.

The diagnosis of tuberous sclerosis may be difficult, as many affected individuals have subtle manifestations. However, the appearance of characteristic skin lesions in children with seizures, retardation, or both should establish a diagnosis of tuberous sclerosis (see Table 11.4). Diagnosis depends on the cutaneous manifestations, family history (with careful clinical and sometimes imaging examination of family members), magnetic resonance imaging or computed tomography of the brain, renal ultrasound, cardiac echocardiography in infants and young children, and in some cases, ophthalmologic examination, bone survey for cortical thickening and phalangeal cysts, and chest radiography for honeycombing of the lungs.

The prognosis of tuberous sclerosis depends on the severity of the disorder and the presence of neurologic involvement.[132] The leading causes of premature death, status epilepticus and bronchopneumonia, are related to the associated neurologic issues. Seizures can be controlled by anticonvulsant therapy in many patients, and prevention of seizures early in life has been shown to lower the risk of developmental delay and retardation. With routine MRI evaluations and the availability of microscopic surgery for neoplastic brain lesions, patients are surviving longer and have a better quality of life. Neurosurgical intervention may be required in patients with signs of increased intracranial pressure, such as visual disturbances, papilledema, vomiting, or headaches. The facial angiofibromas (adenoma sebaceum) may be a cosmetic problem that responds to cryosurgical, surgical or laser therapy.[133] Recent trials of oral rapamycin, an inhibitor of mTOR signaling, have demonstrated regression of astrocytomas, renal angiomyolipomas, pulmonary lymphangioleiomyomas, and facial angiofibromas,[134,135] leading to studies showing improvement with topical administration of rapamycin for facial angiofibromas.[136] The Tuberous Sclerosis Alliance (at: www.tsalliance.org) and the Tuberous Sclerosis Association, UK (at: www.tuberous-sclerosis.org), are among the groups that offer support for patients with tuberous sclerosis.

Chemically Induced Depigmentation

A number of chemical agents are known to cause depigmentation after topical exposure. Among these compounds are the rubber antioxidant monobenzyl ether of hydroquinone, hydroquinone photographic developer, sulfhydryl compounds, azo dyes, diphenyl-cyclopropenone, phenolic germicidal agents (para-tertiary butylphenol and amylphenol), hydroxyanisole, and 4-tertiary butyl catechol (an additive to polyethylene film). The biochemical mechanism by which phenolic chemicals induce such hypopigmentation appears to be the competitive inhibition of tyrosinase or the release of toxic metabolites that produce injury to the melanocytes. Depigmentation has also occurred after injections of triamcinolone, and in the periorbital area after injection of botulinum A toxin.[137] Oral ingestion of chloroquine,[138] arsenic, and STI-571[139] have also led to depigmentation. A progressive generalized decrease in pigmentation has been reported after drug reaction to sulfonamide.[140]

Idiopathic Guttate Hypomelanosis

Idiopathic guttate hypomelanosis is a common disorder of adults, and its incidence increases with increasing age. It occasionally occurs in children, and is more common in female individuals, although the latter may represent reporting bias. More striking in individuals with darker pigmentation, the lesions of idiopathic guttate hypomelanosis are characteristically 0.5–6 mm sharply defined, porcelain white macules. They are asymptomatic and, once present, do not tend to change. The macules most commonly occur on the extensor forearms and on the shins. The diagnosis is usually made clinically, and no treatment is effective. The underlying cause is unknown, although sun exposure is thought to be a trigger.

Post-inflammatory Hypopigmentation

Post-inflammatory hypopigmentation (or leukoderma) may be associated with a wide variety of inflammatory dermatoses or infections. This relative pigmentary deficiency may be noted following involution of certain inflammatory skin disorders, particularly burns, bullous disorders, infections, eczematous or psoriatic lesions, and pityriasis rosea (see Figs 3.15, 11.27). In the inflammatory dermatoses the intensity of the inflammatory reaction may bear little relationship to the development of post-inflammatory leukoderma. Post-inflammatory hypopigmentation is generally self-limiting, clearing after months to years. It often becomes cosmetically obvious in individuals with darker skin, particularly during summer months, because the preferential darkening with ultraviolet light exposure of surrounding skin accentuates the hypopigmentation.

Although the pathophysiology of post-inflammatory hypopigmentation is unclear, it is postulated that the hypopigmentation is caused when keratinocytes injured by the inflammatory process are temporarily unable to accept melanosomes from the melanocyte dendrites. No therapy is effective, but the condition tends to improve with time.

Pityriasis alba (see Ch. 3) is a common cutaneous disorder characterized by asymptomatic, sometimes scaly hypopigmented patches on the face, neck, upper trunk, arms, shoulders, and at times the lower aspect of the trunk and extremities of children and young adults (see Fig. 3.29). Seen predominantly in children 3–16 years of age, individual lesions vary from 1 to several centimeters in diameter and have sharply delineated margins and a fine branny scale. Although the cause is unknown, this disorder appears to represent a nonspecific dermatitis.

Phenylketonuria is an inborn error of phenylalanine metabolism. Treatment is by avoidance of dietary phenylalanine. Untreated

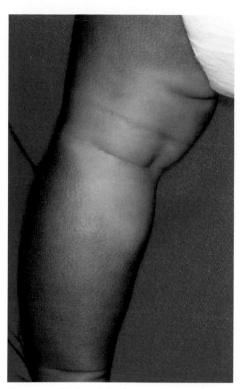

Figure 11.27 Post-inflammatory hypopigmentation. Patches are hypopigmentation are commonly seen at sites of atopic dermatitis after clearance, especially in individuals with darker skin.

patients with this disorder typically show blonde hair, fair skin, and blue eyes (related to the deficiency of tyrosine, the substrate for melanin), mental retardation, seizures, hyperreflexia, dermatitis, and, in rare instances, focal morphea-like skin lesions (see Ch. 22).

Tinea versicolor (pityriasis versicolor; see Ch. 17) is a common condition frequently found on the upper part of the trunk and neck of young adults. Caused by overgrowth of a yeast that normally inhabits skin, *Pityrosporum orbiculare* (*Malassezia furfur*), the condition is characterized by small, either hypopigmented or occasionally hyperpigmented macules, particularly on the trunk and upper arms. The round, individual lesions often coalesce. Facial involvement is more common in affected children than in older individuals. The hypopigmentation results from the production of azelaic acid, which inhibits tyrosinase; the hyperpigmentation is post-inflammatory (Figs 17.28–17.30).

Sarcoidosis (see Ch. 25) is a granulomatous disorder of unknown origin with widespread manifestations involving the skin and many of the internal organs. In addition to the characteristic yellowish brown, flesh-colored, pink, red, and reddish brown to black or blue lesions, subcutaneous nodules, and infiltrated plaques, the spectrum of sarcoidal skin lesions includes hypomelanotic macules and papules. Measuring up to 1.5 cm in diameter, these hypopigmented lesions reveal sarcoid-type granulomas on cutaneous biopsy.

Leprosy (Hansen's disease; see Ch. 14), a chronic infection in which the acid-fast bacillus *Mycobacterium leprae* has a special predilection for the skin and nervous system, can be divided into several types depending on the patient's cellular immune response to *M. leprae*. Tuberculoid leprosy shows characteristic well-defined anesthetic hypopigmented lesions and thickened and palpable peripheral nerves. Lepromatous leprosy, in contrast, more commonly shows nodules or diffuse infiltrates, especially on the eyebrows and ears resulting in a leonine facies. A granulomatous infiltrate on microscopic examination of cutaneous lesions and, particularly in the lepromatous lesions, demonstration of *M. leprae* on cutaneous smear or biopsy specimen generally confirm the diagnosis.

Pinta (see Ch. 14) is a treponemal infection caused by *Treponema carateum*. Seen almost exclusively among the dark-skinned population of Cuba and Central and South America, the disorder is frequently found in children of parents afflicted with this disorder. The cutaneous manifestations may be divided into primary, secondary, and tertiary stages. The late dyschromic stage takes several more years to develop. These lesions have an insidious onset and usually appear during adolescence or young adulthood. They consist of slate-blue hyperpigmented lesions, which, after a period of years, become widespread and are replaced by depigmented macules resembling those seen in patients with vitiligo. Located chiefly on the face, waist, and areas close to bony prominences (elbows, knees, ankles, wrists, and the dorsal aspect of the hands), these depigmented lesions of pinta can be differentiated from those of other depigmented disorders by the presence of pigmented lesions, histologic examination of lesional specimens, identification of antibodies directed against *T. carateum* by serologic testing, and darkfield examination.

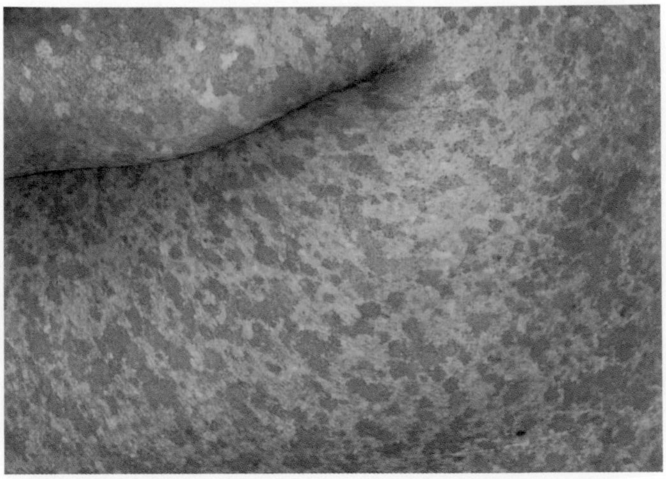

Figure 11.28 Dyschromatosis universalis hereditaria. Reticulated hyperpigmented and hypopigmented macules of various shapes and sizes on the trunk. (Courtesy of Drs S. Worobec and S. Reddy.)

Disorders of both hypopigmentation and hyperpigmentation

Dyschromatoses

Two major forms of dyschromatoses have been described: dyschromatosis symmetrica hereditaria (DSH or reticulate acropigmentation of Dohi) and dyschromatosis universalis hereditaria (DUH), both of which are seen most commonly in Japanese and Chinese individuals (in about 2 per 100 000 individuals). These disorders show only pigmentary manifestations and affected individuals are almost always otherwise healthy. The differential diagnosis of these dyschromatoses includes xeroderma pigmentosum, Dowling–Degos disease,[141] and dyschromic amyloidosis.[142]

DSH is an autosomal dominant disorder characterized by pinpoint to pea-sized hyperpigmented and hypopigmented macules on the dorsal aspects of the distal extremities and face.[143] Lesions first appear during infancy or early childhood, commonly spread until adolescence, and persist lifelong. Neurologic disease has been described in the minority of patients.[144,145] Molecular studies have uncovered mutations in RNA-specific adenosine deaminase (DSRAD or ADAH)[146–148] on chromosome 1q21–22.[149] Infants with hyper- and hypopigmented macules of the palms and soles with limited acral involvement have also been described,[150] but the relation of this presentation to DSH and underlying gene mutations are unclear.

DUH is usually an autosomal dominant disorder in which patients show hyper- and hypopigmented macules of various shapes and sizes with a mottled appearance (Fig. 11.28); some families have shown a pedigree suggestive of recessive inheritance. In DUH skin lesions appear within the first months of life, predominantly on the trunk, and subsequently generalize, including the palms and soles in some cases. The oral mucosa may be involved and nails may show dystrophy with pterygium formation. The numbers of melanosomes is normal, and the disorder presumably reflects increased melanocyte activity. The underlying gene defect has been linked to chromosomes 6q24.2-q25.2[151] and 12q21–23.[152]

Incontinentia Pigmenti

Incontinentia pigmenti (Bloch–Sulzberger syndrome) is an X-linked disorder that predominantly affects the skin, teeth, central nervous system, and eyes.[153–155] The disorder results from mutations in nuclear factor-κB (NF-κB) essential modulator (*NEMO*; *IKBKG*), a gene localized to the X chromosome. In approximately 80% of patients, the mutation is a rearrangement in the *NEMO* gene that eliminates its activity.[156,157] Less commonly, affected girls (often with milder disease) have a missense mutation in exon 10 of the *NEMO* gene; these girls are at risk of having a son with hypohidrotic ectodermal dysplasia with immunodeficiency (see Ch. 7). The mutation in NEMO prevents the activation of NF-κB, which is a regulator of cell proliferation, inflammation and TNF-α induced apoptosis. Some 97% of patients are female, suggesting that the disorder is lethal to affected hemizygous male individuals.[158] Male patients with Klinefelter syndrome (XXY genotype) or with incontinentia pigmenti as a mosaic condition have been described.[159–163] Affected girls show functional mosaicism because of the random inactivation early in embryologic development of one of the X chromosomes (lyonization). As such, the cutaneous lesions of incontinentia pigmenti tend to follow lines of Blaschko, representing the clonal outgrowth of cells that express the affected allele. The variable severity and expression of clinical involvement in the eyes and brain reflect the random activation of the affected X allele in these tissues.

The disorder generally appears at birth or shortly thereafter (90% of patients have cutaneous lesions within the first 2 weeks of life; 96% have their onset before the age of 6 weeks). Although the cutaneous lesions have four distinct phases, their sequence is irregular and overlapping of stages is common (Table 11.5).

The first phase of incontinentia pigmenti begins with inflammatory vesicles or pustules that develop in crops over the trunk and extremities, often persisting for months. These may range from largely papular with scattered vesicles to pustules (Fig. 11.29). Biopsy of a blister during this vesicular stage reveals epidermal vesicles filled with eosinophils, and 74% of affected neonates show eosinophilia (from 18–89%). The vesicles clear spontaneously through cellular apoptosis and repopulation by continuous normal keratinocytes. However, the vesicular phase may be reactivated focally, especially in infants after infection, immunization, or physical trauma; less commonly erythematous whorls without vesiculation may occur in older individuals.[164,165]

Table 11.5 Manifestations of incontinentia pigmenti

X-linked dominant disorder; random X chromosome inactivation dictates extent of disease
Mutations in NEMO (NF-κB essential modulator)
97% of patients are females; probably lethal in males; living males usually represent somatic mosaicism
Four cutaneous phases that may overlap
  Inflammatory vesicles or bullae
  Verrucous lesions
  Streaks of hyperpigmentation
  Streaks of atrophy/hypopigmentation
May have cicatricial alopecia and nail dystrophy
Eosinophilia in >70% of patients (often lasts for 4–5 months)
Systemic manifestations
  Dental
  Ocular
  Central nervous system

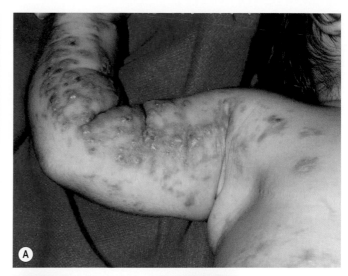

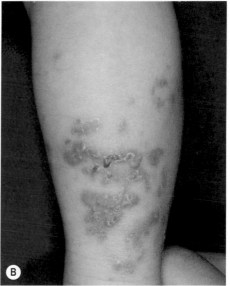

Figure 11.29 Incontinentia pigmenti. (A) The lesions of incontinentia pigmenti tend to follow a curvilinear pattern along lines of Blaschko, lines of the embryological development of ectoderm, as a manifestation of functional mosaicism (i.e., the X chromosome with the mutation in the NEMO gene is the activated X chromosome in the skin at these sites). The lesions of the vesicular phase may range from largely papular with a minor vesicular component to vesiculopustular as shown here and occasionally to bullous. (B) Sometimes the lesions of incontinentia pigmenti do not show a linear pattern. Note the residual inflammation and scaling as the vesicular lesions clear.

In 70% of patients, the vesicular stage is followed by a verrucous phase characterized by irregular, linearly arrayed warty papules on one or more extremities, and often on the hands and feet (Fig. 11.30). This stage resolves spontaneously, usually within a period of up to 2 years.

During or shortly after this verrucous stage, the highly characteristic pigmentary phase occurs in approximately 80% of patients. Lesions typically are thin bands of slate-brown to blue-gray coloration arranged in lines and swirls on the extremities and trunk (Fig. 11.31). These pigmentary bands may coalesce in areas and more closely resemble 'Chinese writing figures' than linear streaks or whorls. When more linear, they must be distinguished from macular amyloidosis in carrier females.[166] Occasionally, these bands appear purpuric at onset (Fig. 11.32), and this appearance has raised the question of child abuse.[167] These pigmentary lesions progress until the patient's second year of life, then stabilize and persist for years. By adolescence, they gradually fade and disappear in two-thirds of affected individuals. Biopsy sections from lesional skin show incontinence of pigment during this phase, leading to the name 'incontinentia pigmenti'. Although the pigmentary changes were originally considered to be a post-inflammatory phenomenon secondary to the vesiculobullous or verrucous stages, the pigment fails to follow the pattern, shape, or location of the vesicular or verrucous lesions.

A fourth phase is characterized by persistent atrophic streaks that are often hypopigmented (Fig. 11.33). Most commonly noted on the arms, thighs, trunk, and particularly the calves of affected individuals, these affected areas show diminished hair, eccrine glands, and sweat pores. These streaks are often subtle and may be accentuated by viewing with side lighting or by Wood's lamp examination. Skin biopsy shows characteristic changes with scattered apoptotic cells, thickened dermis, and absence of hair follicles and sweat glands, allowing diagnosis in older individuals.[168]

Cicatricial alopecia is seen in 38–66% of patients (Fig. 11.34). It occurs most often near the vertex, and does not necessarily relate to the previous presence of lesions at the site. Nail dystrophy is present in 7–51% of affected individuals. In addition, painful grayish-white verrucous or keratotic subungual tumors are seen in up to 10%, usually during the 2nd or 3rd decades of life.[169] Lytic defects on roentgenographic examination of the distal phalanges may be seen as well.

Non-cutaneous manifestations occur in a high percentage of patients with incontinentia pigmenti. Some 70–95% of patients show dental anomalies (delayed dentition, partial anodontia, pegged or conical teeth)[170] (Fig. 11.35), reminiscent of those in boys

with hypohidrotic ectodermal dysplasia (see Ch. 7). Ectodysplasin (which is usually mutated in boys with hypohidrotic ectodermal dysplasia), the ectodysplasin receptor, and NEMO all participate in NF-κB signaling, providing an explanation for these shared phenotypic features. In fact, boys with a form of ectodermal dysplasia with immunodeficiency (Ch. 7) have mutations in NEMO that decrease its function but do not eliminate it.

Up to 30% of patients with incontinentia pigmenti demonstrate involvement of the central nervous system, most commonly seizures. These seizures have been attributed to acute microvascular hemorrhagic infarcts,[171] although recurrent stroke has also been described.[172] Many such neonates are mistakenly thought to have neonatal herpes simplex infection, because of the presence of vesiculopustular lesions and seizures. Overall, 7.5% have severe

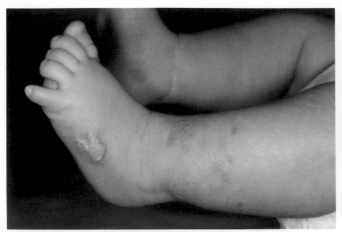

Figure 11.30 Incontinentia pigmenti. The warty papules of the verrucous phase are most commonly found on the hands and feet.

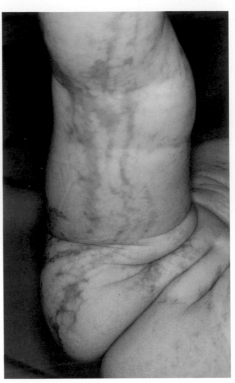

Figure 11.32 Incontinentia pigmenti. The bands of brownish-gray pigmentation may initially appear purpuric, raising the question of child abuse.

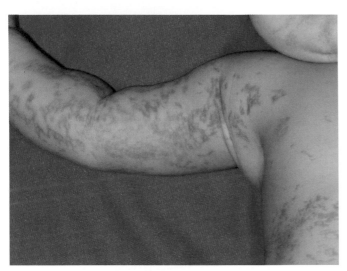

Figure 11.31 Incontinentia pigmenti. The characteristic pigmented lines and swirls tend to be slate-brown to blue-gray in color, and are usually localized to the trunk and extremities. These pigmentary bands may coalesce in areas and more closely resemble 'Chinese writing figures' or a reticulated pattern than linear streaks or whorls. The previous vesicular lesions on this arm are shown in Figure 11.29A. The hyperpigmentation usually fades by late in childhood.

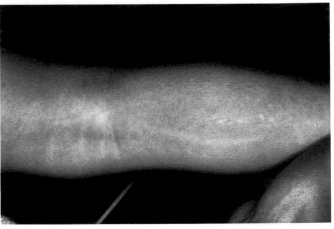

Figure 11.33 Incontinentia pigmenti. Atrophic streaks that are often hypopigmented can be found in the minority of affected individuals. Most commonly noted on the arms and legs, these affected areas show diminished hair, eccrine glands, and sweat pores. The atrophic, hypopigmented streaks are often subtle, and may be accentuated by viewing with side lighting or by Wood's lamp examination.

neurologic abnormalities, including continuing seizures, retardation, and/or spastic abnormalities.[155] Seizures during the 1st week of life have been associated with the worst prognosis for normal development. Ophthalmic changes are present in 35% of patients; 18% have strabismus; and an equal number demonstrate more serious eye involvement (cataracts, optic atrophy, or retinal neovascularization or detachment). Bilateral blindness has been described in 4–8% of individuals with incontinentia pigmenti. Ocular examinations in affected babies are suggested monthly during the first 4 months, every 3 months through the first year, twice yearly to age 3, and then annually.[172] Occasionally, cardiac anomalies and skeletal malformations (such as microcephaly, syndactyly, supernumerary ribs, hemiatrophy, or shortening of the arms or legs) may occur.

The characteristic cutaneous lesions of incontinentia pigmenti allow early diagnosis and investigation for associated ocular and neurologic abnormalities. No special therapy is required for the skin lesions of incontinentia pigmenti, as they tend to clear spontaneously. Early and serial ophthalmologic examination is critical to consider retinal involvement[173] and initiate early intervention with laser or cryotherapy, as needed. If seizures or evidence of developmental delay appear, neurologic consultation is appropriate. Dental evaluation by 2 years of age will allow investigation of missing or misshapen secondary teeth; prostheses can be made in patients with significant dental abnormalities.

Obtaining a history of cutaneous disorders during the neonatal and infantile periods and careful physical examination of mothers who may be carriers is important for genetic counseling; a mother of an affected individual who shows subtle manifestations is at

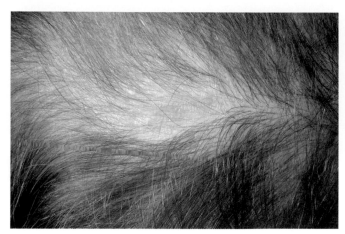

Figure 11.34 Incontinentia pigmenti. Cicatricial alopecia most commonly appears near the vertex, and does not necessarily relate to the previous presence of lesions at the site.

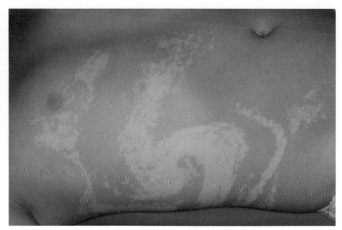

Figure 11.36 Pigmentary mosaicism. Broad linear streaks of hypopigmentation following lines of Blaschko in a patient with developmental delay. This condition used to be called incontinentia pigmenti achromians, but is now known to be a heterogeneous group of disorders of different underlying molecular bases. Most patients with pigmentary mosaicism are otherwise normal, but evidence of neurologic, ocular, and bony defects should be sought, especially with more extensive pigmentary changes.

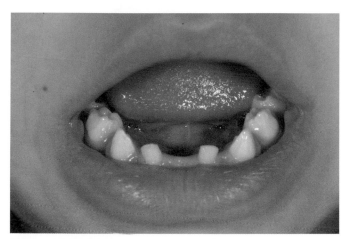

Figure 11.35 Incontinentia pigmenti. Dental anomalies (delayed dentition, partial anodontia, pegged or conical teeth) occur in the majority of affected individuals. Interestingly, these dental changes mirror those of boys with hypohidrotic ectodermal dysplasia, a disorder that shares the NF-κB signaling pathway.

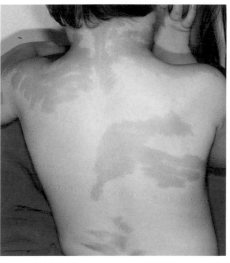

Figure 11.37 Pigmentary mosaicism. Patterned hyperpigmented patches on the neck and trunk. This child was otherwise normal.

increased risk for having another affected daughter (50% probability in daughters) and aborting a male fetus (50% probability in sons). Affected mothers may show subtle signs, such as a patch of cicatricial alopecia,[174] a conical incisor, nail dystrophy[175] or an atrophic streak seen by side lighting examination, or may show no signs at all as an adult, despite a history of a previous blistering disorder in the neonatal period. Prenatal diagnosis is possible and preimplantation genetic diagnosis has been performed.[176] Treatment with topical corticosteroids[177] or tacrolimus[178] may halt the progression of the vesicular phase, although lesions ultimately clear spontaneously. The retinal neovascularization may regress with laser photocoagulation[179] and preliminary studies of VEGF inhibitors appear promising.[180] The Incontinentia Pigmenti International Foundation provides education and support (www.imgen.bcm.tmc.edu/IPIF).

Pigment Mosaicism

The term 'pigment mosaicism' is now preferred for this heterogeneous group of disorders, which includes hypomelanosis of Ito ('incontinentia pigmenti achromians'), linear and whorled nevoid hypermelanosis[181] and the segmental form of nevus depigmentosus,[182] characterized by patterned streaks of hypopigmentation and/or hyperpigmentation (Figs 11.36, 11.37). The linear streaks and whorls tend to follow lines of mosaicism,[183] particularly following the lines of Blaschko (lines of ectodermal embryologic development) or a phylloid pattern of mosaic distribution.[184,185] Both hypopigmented and hyperpigmented streaks may be seen in the same individual.

The pigmentary mosaicism reflects gene mosaicism of affected areas. A large number of gross chromosomal abnormalities have been described in 60% of affected pediatric patients with more extensive pigmentary mosaicism and/or associated noncutaneous abnormalities when peripheral blood leukocytes and cultured fibroblasts or keratinocytes are evaluated.[186–188] These mosaic conditions do not tend to be hereditary, although familial cases have rarely been reported.[189] Study of an unselected patient population with pigment mosaicism showed an incidence of associated abnormalities (particularly of the bones, eyes, and/or central nervous system) in 30% of patients.[190]

The streaks of hypo or hyperpigmentation along Blaschko's lines of embryologic development must be distinguished from the hypopigmented or hyperpigmented streaks of incontinentia pigmenti. The term 'incontinentia pigmenti achromians' for the streaks of hypopigmentation has been abandoned to avoid confusion, since incontinentia pigmenti is unrelated. The lack of preceding vesicular or verrucous lesions of incontinentia pigmenti and the finding of increased melanin deposition at the basal cell layer in hyperpigmented streaks of pigment mosaicism ('linear and whorled hypermelanosis'), rather than the pigment incontinence of incontinentia pigmenti, help to distinguish these disorders.[191] Epidermal nevi may present as flat brown streaks, but more commonly are hyperkeratotic (see Ch. 9).

Disorders of hyperpigmentation

Pigmented nevi are among the most common hyperpigmented lesions and are reviewed in Chapter 9, as are streaks of pigmentation involving the nails (longitudinal melanonychia). Treatment of hyperpigmented lesions with topical agents has generally been unsuccessful. Sun protection is a critical aspect of management in preventing darkening. Lasers have been used to treat a variety of hyperpigmented disorders in children,[192] in particular café-au-lait macules, nevus of Ota and other forms of dermal melanocytosis, Becker nevi, and tattoos. Several therapeutic sessions are required and results are rarely permanent.

Epidermal Melanocyte Lesions

Freckles

Freckles (ephelides) are light brown well-circumscribed macules, usually <3 mm in diameter, which appear in childhood and tend to fade during the winter and adult life (Fig. 11.38). They commonly arise in early childhood, especially between 2 and 4 years of age, and their presence correlates with fair skin, red hair, and an increased risk of developing melanoma.[193] Freckles are most common on the sun-exposed areas of the face (especially the nose and cheeks), shoulders, and upper back.

Freckles become darker and more confluent after ultraviolet light exposure in the sunburn spectrum (290–320 nm) as well as in the long-wave ultraviolet (UVA) range (320–400 nm). UVA light is not blocked by window glass and sunscreen agents that filter out only the sunburn spectrum 290–320 nm. They often become smaller, lighter, and fewer during the winter months. Histopathologic features of ephelides include increased melanin pigmentation of the basal layer without an increase in the number of melanocytes or elongation of the epidermal rete ridges.

Freckles bear cosmetic but no systemic significance. Treatment includes avoidance of sun exposure and appropriate covering makeup. Use of 'full-spectrum' sunscreens that provide protection against both UVA and UVB light (e.g., with avobenzone or titanium dioxide) are more protective than sunscreens that only provide UVB protection. When desired, although seldom necessary, gentle chemical peels or laser may remove the superficial pigmentation and make many of the freckles less conspicuous.

Becker nevus

Becker nevus (Becker melanosis), an irregular macular hyperpigmentation with hypertrichosis, is sometimes congenital, but more commonly starts during early adolescence. It occurs much more commonly in males than females, and affected individuals tend to

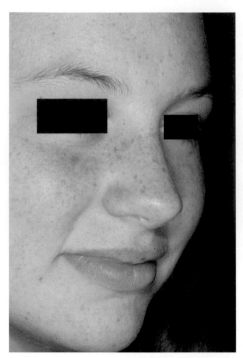

Figure 11.38 Ephelides. Ephelides or freckles are light brown well-circumscribed macules, usually <3 mm in diameter, which most commonly appear during preschool years, especially after exposure to the sun.

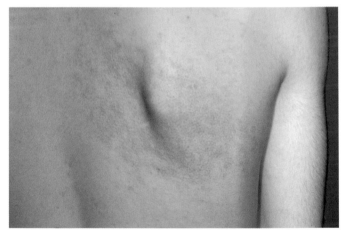

Figure 11.39 Becker nevus. This light brown irregularly-bordered patch without hypertrichosis was recently noticed on the back of this 12-year-old boy.

be otherwise healthy. The first change generally appears as a brown pigmentation on the chest, back, or upper arm that spreads until it reaches an area 10–15 cm in diameter (about the size of a hand or larger) (Fig. 11.39). The outline is irregular, and sometimes surrounded by islands of blotchy pigmentation. Although characteristically seen unilaterally on the upper half of the trunk, especially around the shoulder, it has also been reported in other areas on the trunk, forehead, cheeks, supraclavicular region, abdomen, forearm, wrist, buttocks, and shins, and may be bilateral.[194,195] After a period of time (often 1 or 2 years), coarse terminal hairs appear in the region of, but not necessarily coinciding with, the pigmented area (Fig. 11.40). The intensity of pigmentation may fade somewhat as the patient becomes older, but the hyperpigmentation and hypertrichosis tend to persist for life.

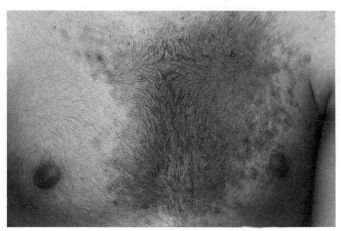

Figure 11.40 Becker nevus. Large patch of grayish brown pigmentation on the chest with associated coarse terminal hairs. These lesions usually appear during late childhood or early adolescence on the upper trunk.

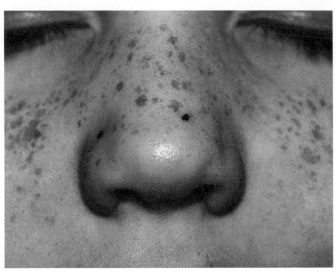

Figure 11.41 Lentigines. These sharply demarcated macules tend to be larger than a freckle but smaller than a café-au-lait spot and range in color from tan to black. This boy shows two black lentigines on the nose.

The etiology of Becker nevus is unknown, but a localized increase in androgen receptor sensitivity may explain the time of onset and clinical features seen in most individuals with this disorder.[196] Reports of familial cases[197] raise the question of a genetic influence in some patients, and the occasional association of significantly increased smooth muscle suggests that Becker nevus and smooth muscle hamartoma may perhaps represent two poles of the same hamartomatous change. Although most Becker nevi occur without other pathologic findings, association with a variety of other abnormalities (such as unilateral breast and areolar hypoplasia, focal acne, pectus carinatum, limb asymmetry, and spina bifida)[198,199] has been called Becker nevus syndrome.[197,200]

Histopathologic features reveal epidermal thickening, elongation of the rete ridges, and hyperpigmentation of the basal layer with increased melanocytes.[196] Malignant transformation does not occur. Treatment of this disorder is purely cosmetic and is generally discouraged. Laser therapy or excision usually does not improve the appearance. The hypertrichosis may be treated with depilation (see Ch. 7).

Lentigines

Lentigines are small, tan, dark brown, or black flat, oval, or circular, sharply circumscribed lesions that usually appear in childhood and may increase in number until adult life. Each lesion ('lentigo simplex') usually measures 3–15 mm in diameter and may occur on any cutaneous surface (Fig. 11.41). Occasionally, lentigines are seen on the mucous membrane or conjunctiva of the eyes. The pigmentation is uniform and darker than that seen in ephelides (freckles) and café-au-lait macules, and the color is unaffected by exposure to sunlight. Lentigines are typically larger than freckles and smaller than a typical café-au-lait macule. Lentigines can also be distinguished from freckles and café-au-lait macules histologically.[201]

Adult forms of this disorder, termed senile lentigines, or 'liver spots' (due to their color and not their origin), are distinguished by their onset with advanced age and localization to the forearms, face, neck, and dorsal aspect of the hands. Lentigines that appear early in life may fade or disappear; those appearing later in life tend to be permanent. Treatment other than for cosmetic purposes is ordinarily not indicated. When desired, however, excision by a small punch biopsy, cryosurgery, or laser may be beneficial. Interestingly, a patient with multiple lentigines shows marked lightening when

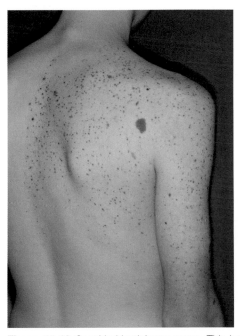

Figure 11.42 Speckled lentiginous nevus. This large patch of lentigines of different sizes overlying an increase in cutaneous pigmentation may represent a mosaic form of multiple lentiginosis syndrome.

treated with imatinib mesylate for familial gastrointestinal stromal tumor syndrome.[202]

Patients with speckled lentiginous nevus or segmental lentiginosis show patches of lentigines, usually overlying a slight increase in cutaneous pigmentation (Fig. 11.42). Eruptive, agminated Spitz nevi may be seen within a segmental lentiginosis.[203] Eruptive lentiginosis is a disorder characterized by a widespread eruption of several hundred lentigines that may develop over a few months or years, usually in adolescents or young adults, without systemic manifestations. Inherited patterned lentiginosis is an autosomal dominant disorder of dark skinned individuals with the onset of lentiginosis during early childhood. Lentigines occur on the centro-facial area, lips, oral mucosae, buttocks, elbows, palms, and soles, and affected individuals are otherwise healthy.

Localized or extensive lentiginosis may also be a component of a multisystem disorder. Although they may occur in children without medical problems, lentigines of the penis are characteristic of Bannayan–Zonana (Bannayan–Zonana–Ruvalcaba) syndrome, an autosomal dominant disorder that results from mutations in the *PTEN* gene and is allelic with Cowden syndrome (see Ch. 9 and Fig. 11.43). Other major features are macrocephaly and lipomas. Lentigines of the hands, feet, and buccal mucosa may also be a feature of Cronkhite–Canada syndrome, in which nail dystrophy, hair loss, and intestinal polyposis are other characteristics. Centrofacial lentiginosis (also called centrofacial neurodysraphic lentiginosis or Touraine's syndrome) is an autosomal dominant process in which lentigines are first noted in the 1st year of life, particularly on the nose and cheeks. Patients with centrofacial lentiginosis may have associated mental retardation, congenital mitral valve stenosis, seizures, sacral hypertrichosis, coalescence of the eyebrows, high-arched palate, absent upper middle incisors, bony abnormalities, defective fusion of the neural tube (dysraphia), psychiatric disorders, dwarfism, and endocrine dysfunction.

The major lentiginous syndromes are Peutz–Jeghers, multiple lentiginosis/LEOPARD syndrome, and Carney complex.

Peutz–Jeghers syndrome

The prevalence of this autosomal dominant disorder of mucocutaneous lentiginous macules and multiple hamartomatous intestinal polyps is approximately 1 in 100 000 individuals.[204] Characteristic bluish brown to black spots, often apparent at birth or in early infancy, represent the cutaneous marker of this syndrome. These discrete, flat pigmented lesions are irregularly oval and usually measure <5 mm in diameter. They are most commonly seen on the lips (Fig. 11.44), buccal mucosa, nasal and periorbital regions, elbows, dorsal aspects of the fingers and toes, palms, soles, and periumbilical, perianal, and labial regions; occasionally the gums and hard palate and, on rare occasions, even the tongue may be involved. The pigmented lesions on the skin and lips frequently fade after puberty; those on the buccal mucosa, palate, and tongue, however, persist.

The hamartomatous gastrointestinal polyps seen in this disorder may be found from the stomach to the anal canal, although the small bowel represents the most frequently involved portion of the intestinal tract (96% of cases). Polyps vary from minute pinhead lesions to those measuring several centimeters in diameter. They may occur in early childhood but the median age of presentation is 12 years, with 50% having symptoms in the first 2 decades. Symptoms in the pediatric patient frequently consist of abdominal pain, melena, or intussusception.[205] The most common symptom, recurrent attacks of colicky abdominal pain, is thought to result from recurring transient episodes of incomplete intussusception. Hematemesis, although less common, may occur owing to involvement of the stomach, duodenum, or upper jejunum. Polyps of the nasal mucosae and gallbladder have occasionally been described, and rarely polyps involve the respiratory and urogenital tracts.[206]

Although the polyps of Peutz–Jeghers syndrome are generally benign, adenocarcinomas of the gastrointestinal tract (stomach, small intestine, colorectum, pancreas, and biliary tract), breast and uterine cervical carcinomas, and gonadal sex tumors (Sertoli cell tumors of the testis and sex cord tumors of the ovary) have been described.[207,208] Overall, the risk of developing malignancy is 18 times that of the general population.[209] Mutations in the serine-threonine kinase *STK11/LKB1* gene have been found in 70% of familial cases and up to 67% of sporadic cases.[204,208]

In the past, therapeutic management focused on relief of symptoms and recurrent resections with the risk of malabsorption. The recommendation now is to remove polyps if technically feasible (especially if >5 mm).[210,211] Endoscopic evaluations by double-balloon endoscopy or videocapsule endoscopy are recommended every 3 years beginning when symptoms occur and every 2 years beginning at 15 years of age if asymptomatic. Yearly evaluation of organs at risk of malignancy (breast, thyroid gland, pancreas, uterus and ovaries, and testes) should begin at adulthood. The lentigines of Peutz–Jeghers syndrome have responded to laser[212] and intense pulsed light[213] therapies, although the lentigines not infrequently recur.[214]

Laugier–Hunziker syndrome is a benign pigmentary disorder that manifests as macular hyperpigmentation of the lips and buccal mucosa. Many patients also show long pigmented bands of the

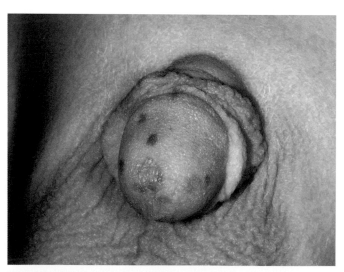

Figure 11.43 Bannayan–Zonana–Ruvalcaba syndrome. Lentigines of the penis are characteristic of Bannayan–Zonana–Ruvalcaba syndrome, an autosomal dominant disorder that also commonly features macrocephaly and lipomas.

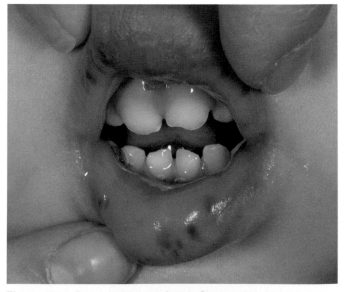

Figure 11.44 Peutz–Jeghers syndrome. Characteristic bluish brown to black spots were first noted in early childhood on the lips of this boy who later developed hamartomatous gastrointestinal polyps.

nails (melanonychia striata), but the visceral manifestations of Peutz–Jeghers syndrome are absent.[214,215]

Multiple lentigines/LEOPARD syndrome

Multiple lentiginoses/LEOPARD syndrome comprises a spectrum of patients who show manifestations ranging from generalized lentigines alone to the complete syndrome that characteristically shows lentigines, electrocardiographic abnormalities, ocular hypertelorism, pulmonic stenosis, abnormal genitalia, retardation of growth, and sensorineural deafness.[216,217] Affected individuals typically show an elongated, marfanoid facies, and several café-au-lait macules admixed within the myriad of lentigines (Fig. 11.45). Mutations in *PTPN11* (chromosome 12q24.1) have been found in 90% patients, while 3% of patients show mutations in *RAF1* (chromosome 3p25).[218-220] Variable expressivity is seen within families, so that some affected individuals show only the multiple lentigines, whereas others show a variety of the visceral manifestations. Nevertheless, a the underlying mutation of a family with multiple lentigines without other features maps to chromosome 6q, a site that is distinct from *PTPN11* and *RAF1*.[221]

The cutaneous markers are the dark, 1–5 mm lentigines, which often do not appear until 4–5 years of age, but then increase dramatically (to thousands of lentigines) by puberty. The cutaneous lesions tend to be concentrated on the neck and upper trunk, but they may also appear on the skin of the face and scalp, arms, palms, soles, and genitalia. The lentigines characteristically spare the mucosa. Occasionally, formes frustes of this disorder occur in which the characteristic lentigines are absent. In most patients, the café-au-lait macules are present before the onset of the lentigines, leading to consideration of the alternative diagnosis of neurofibromatosis type 1 or its allelic variant with café-au-lait spots and pulmonary valve stenosis, Watson syndrome.

Cardiac abnormalities occur in about 85% of affected individuals, mostly hypertrophic cardiomyopathy (up to 75%), which usually appears during infancy and subsequently progresses. Pulmonary valve stenosis and conduction defects have been described

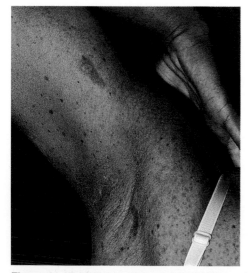

Figure 11.45 Multiple lentiginosis/LEOPARD syndrome. Myriad of lentigines with scattered café-au-lait macules overlying generalized hyperpigmentation in this adolescent with only cutaneous changes. In some individuals, the pigmentary changes are associated with a spectrum of visceral abnormalities, including lentigines, electrocardiographic abnormalities, ocular hypertelorism, pulmonic stenosis, abnormal genitalia, retardation of growth, and sensorineural deafness, leading to the term LEOPARD syndrome.

in 25% and 23% of patients, respectively. Skeletal aberrations may include retardation of growth (below the 25th percentile), hypertelorism, an elongated facies, pectus deformities (carinatum or excavatum), dorsal kyphosis, winged scapulae, and prognathism. Endocrine disorders include gonadal hypoplasia, hypospadias, undescended testes, hypoplastic ovaries, and delayed puberty. The hearing loss of LEOPARD syndrome is congenital and neurosensory, and can be detected by early auditory evoked potentials.

The pigmented lesions (lentigines and café-au-lait macules), facial anomalies, and cardiac defects may resemble those of Noonan syndrome, but the number of pigmented lesions is far fewer in Noonan syndrome, and only 25% show the hypertrophic cardiomyopathy. Mutations in *PTPN11* also cause Noonan syndrome.

Carney complex

Carney complex comprises an autosomal dominant disorder that features the pigmentary abnormalities of lentigines, epithelioid blue nevi, and pigmented schwannomas. The NAME[222] and LAMB[223] syndromes are now included in Carney complex.[224-227] The group of disorders is considered a form of multiple endocrine neoplasia (MEN), in that endocrine abnormalities and tumors are common features, especially pituitary adenomas, ovarian tumors,[228] testicular (Sertoli cell) tumors, and pigmented nodular adrenocortical disease.[229]

Skin manifestations are seen in 80% of patients, most commonly lentigines in 70–75% of patients. The lentigines tend to appear during the peripubertal period, most commonly involving the center of the face, especially the vermilion border of the lips, the conjunctivae, and occasionally the intraoral area. They most commonly fade during adulthood. The blue nevi, including epithelioid blue nevi, tend to be multiple, most commonly on the face, trunk and extremities, and characteristically are dome-shaped dark blue papules (see below). The majority of epithelioid blue nevi in children are associated with Carney complex, but this form of blue nevus has also been described in children without evidence of other features of the syndrome.[230] The lentigines and blue nevi are often accompanied by café-au-lait spots, which do not tend to occur without the other skin features and resemble those of neurofibromatosis. Cutaneous myxomas occur in 30–55% of studied patients, and are most commonly seen on the eyelids, ears, nipples, and external genitalia. They are usually diagnosed during the late teen years. The myxomas are usually multiple and tend to recur. Patients often show myxomas of the oropharynx, heart and breast, and may develop other neoplasia of mesenchymal and neural crest origin. The typical psammomatous melanotic schwannomas occurs in 10% of affected individuals and may involve the skin, posterior spinal nerve roots, gastrointestinal tract, and bone. Biopsies of the blue nevi and schwannomas show characteristic histologic features.[231] Patients have been described both with predominantly cutaneous features[232] and without cutaneous lentigines. The most common endocrine tumors or overactivity include primary pigmented nodular adrenocortical disease (25% of patients), growth hormone-producing pituitary adenoma (10% of patients), large-cell calcifying Sertoli cell tumor, and thyroid adenoma (up to 75% of patients) or carcinoma.

Mutations in the protein kinase A type I-α regulatory sub-unit (*PRKAR1A*)[233] at chromosome 17q22–24 occur in approximately 57% of patients, while an additional 20% of families with Carney complex show linkage to 2p16 (gene not yet identified).

Café-au-lait spots

Café-au-lait spots are large, round or oval, flat lesions of light brown pigmentation found in up to 33% of normal children; having a greater number of café-au-lait spots is more common in children with darker skin color, but having >5 is rare other than in neurofibromatosis or Legius syndrome (see below).[234–237] Frequently present at birth, or developing soon thereafter, they vary from ≤1.5 cm in their smallest diameter to much larger lesions that may measure up to ≥15–20 cm in diameter (Fig. 11.46). Café-au-lait spots may rarely occur anywhere on the body.

The café-au-lait spot(s) of McCune–Albright syndrome are seen in approximately 50% of patients. They tend to be present during infancy or early childhood, with a predilection for areas with particularly bony prominence (the forehead, nuchal area, thorax, sacral areas, and buttocks). They are frequently unilateral, stopping abruptly at the midline and following a dermatomal distribution. They tend to have irregularly jagged or serrated borders (described as resembling the 'coast of Maine,' in contrast to the smooth-bordered café-au-lait spots of neurofibromatosis, which have been compared to the 'coast of California'). The McCune-Albright syndrome in its complete form is a triad characterized by café-au-lait spots, polyostotic fibrous dysplasia, and endocrine dysfunction, often manifesting as precocious puberty (see Ch. 23, Fig. 23.20).

Café-au-lait macules are increased in number in Russell–Silver syndrome,[238] a disorder that also features short stature, musculoskeletal abnormalities, craniofacial dysmorphism, and genitourinary malformations, as well as in multiple lentigines/LEOPARD syndrome (see above and Fig. 11.45). Johnson–McMillin syndrome is an autosomal dominant disorder in which families show truncal café-au-lait macules in association with facial nerve palsy and mild developmental delay.[239]

Not uncommonly, infants may show what appears to be a café-au-lait macule, but sometimes years later the café-au-lait macule develops tiny more darkly hyperpigmented macules or papules. This lesion is called *nevus spilus* (see Ch. 9), and biopsy of the more

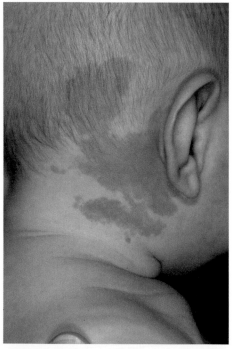

Figure 11.46 Café-au-lait spot. Round or oval patches of light brown pigmentation are common in children, but usually are up to a few centimeters in diameter, in contrast to larger café-au-lait spot of the scalp, neck and retroauricular areas. The segmental distribution of the cafe-au-lait spot should alert one to the unlikely possibility of McCune–Albright syndrome.

darkly pigmented lesions will show typical features of pigmented nevi (see Fig. 9.24). Individuals with red hair or with parents of markedly different skin pigmentation may show hyper-pigmented macules that resemble café-au-lait macules. They can be differentiated by their often irregular shape, tendency to be less well defined than the café-au-lait macules of neurofibromatosis, and the paler coloration of the hyperpigmentation. Observation of these café-au-lait-like macules during the first 5–6 years of life should be performed and annual ophthalmologic evaluations should be considered to be convinced that the macules merely represent a pigment variation. Pigmented purpuric eruptions can also be confused with café-au-lait macules in young children. These benign hyperpigmented macules are often poorly circumscribed and are characterized by pinpoint petechiae and purpura on a hyperpigmented base[240] (see Ch. 12, Fig. 12.86).

Neurofibromatosis

Neurofibromatosis is an autosomal dominant disorder characterized by an increased propensity towards the development of tumors, particularly of the nerve sheath.[241–243] Neurofibromatosis encompasses three distinct disorders: neurofibromatosis type 1 (NF1; von Recklinghausen's disease), neurofibromatosis type 2 (NF2; bilateral acoustic or central neurofibromatosis),[244] and schwannomatosis. The latter is characterized by painful peripheral (non-vestibular, non-dermal) schwannomas and is largely diagnosed in adults.[245] More than 90% of cases of neurofibromatosis are NF1, which occurs in approximately 1 in 3500 births.[246–249] NF2 occurs in 1 in 40 000 individuals and its diagnosis during childhood is unusual. Both disorders show variable expressivity; NF1 shows an approximately 50% rate of new mutations, whereas two-thirds of children with NF2 have an affected parent. Patients with NF1 have mutations in neurofibromin, a large gene localized to chromosome 17q. More than 500 different mutations have been described in this gene,[243] which encodes a large GTPase-activating cytoplasmic protein that negatively regulates Ras activation. The gene mutated in NF2, merlin or schwannomin, localizes to chromosome 22q. Merlin/schwannomin protein is a cytoskeletal protein that inhibits a serine/threonine kinase PAK1, which is essential for Ras transformation.[250]

The cutaneous manifestations of NF1 are of major importance and thus most discussion of neurofibromatosis in this chapter will focus on NF1. However, skin tumors are an important diagnostic clue for patients with NF2, and are frequently present months to years before other features. These tumors, predominantly schwannomas or neurofibromas, are the presenting sign in 27% of individuals with NF2 and eventually occur in 59% of patients.[251,252] A higher number of skin tumors has been correlated with a worse prognosis. Café-au-lait macules are found in 33% of individuals with NF2, but only 2% have six or more café-au-lait spots. Although NF2 is commonly considered a disorder of adults, approximately 15% of patients with NF2 present before 18 years of age,[253] and onset during childhood predicts a worse prognosis. The major criteria for NF2 are shown in Table 11.6. NF2 in children most commonly presents with hearing impairment (one-third of children) or cranial nerve dysfunction (one-third of children). Tumor load is often extensive in pediatric patients (especially vestibular and cranial schwannomas, cranial meningiomas, and spinal cord tumors). Overall, 75% of affected children develop hearing loss. Removal of vestibular schwannomas does not preserve hearing, although early detection and smaller tumors are associated with a better prognosis. Visual impairment occurs in 83% of affected children owing to cataracts and amblyopia. Treatment is primarily surgical. Auditory brainstem implants may partially restore hearing.[254]

Table 11.6 Diagnostic criteria for neurofibromatosis type 2 (NF2)[244,253]

Bilateral vestibular schwannomas seen by MRI scan
or
A 1st-degree relative with NF2
AND
Unilateral vestibular schwannoma
or
Two of the following criteria:
   Meningioma
   Glioma
   Schwannoma
   Juvenile posterior subcapsular cataract

Table 11.7 Diagnostic criteria for neurofibromatosis type 1 (NF1)

Must have two or more of the following:
   Six café-au-lait macules that measure ≥0.5 cm before puberty and ≥1.5 cm in diameter in adults[a]
   Freckling of the axillary and/or inguinal areas[a]
   A plexiform neurofibroma *or* two or more dermal neurofibromas
   Two or more Lisch nodules
   Optic nerve glioma
   Pathognomonic skeletal dysplasia, i.e., tibial or sphenoid wing dysplasia
   An affected 1st-degree relative

[a]Given the recognition that Legius syndrome is distinct from NF1 clinically and genetically, but shares two of the major features, experts on NF1 have recently suggested that having the cutaneous pigmentary lesions alone (café-au-lait spots and freckling) is insufficent for a definitive diagnosis of NF1.

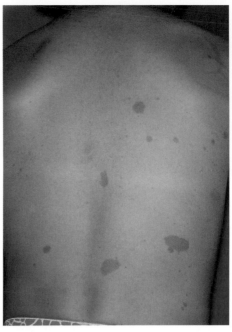

Figure 11.47 Neurofibromatosis type 1. The presence of six or more café-au-lait spots >0.5 cm in diameter in children and 1.5 cm in adolescents suggests the possibility of NF1, although having café-au-lait spots alone does not allow for definitive diagnosis.

NF1 is best known because of Joseph Merrick, the famed 'Elephant Man' of the 1800s. In fact, Mr Merrick had no café-au-lait spots, no family history of neurofibromatosis, and no histologic evidence of neurofibromas. He is now thought to have had Proteus syndrome, a disorder characterized by segmental overgrowth with asymmetry, macrocephaly, lipomas, linear verrucous epidermal nevi, and vascular malformations (see Ch. 12, Figs 12.62, 12.63). The diagnostic criteria for NF1 are shown in Table 11.7. Most children show only multiple café-au-lait macules, and thus the diagnosis cannot be made with certainty until other criteria develop or unless a 1st-degree family member is affected. There is marked variability in the overall severity and progression of neurofibromatosis. It can cause serious problems, and even death in the newborn, or may produce only mild or insignificant problems during the lifetime of the affected individual.

Cutaneous manifestations of NF1

Café-au-lait spots and dermal and plexiform neurofibromas are the characteristic cutaneous findings of NF1. The severity of cutaneous involvement is not indicative of the extent of disease in other organs.

Café-au-lait spots, a hallmark of neurofibromatosis, may occur anywhere on the body. Although they may be present at birth, café-au-lait spots often first make their appearance during the first few months. They continue to increase in size and number during the first decade, especially the first 2 years of life. The diagnostic criterion of 6 or more café-au-lait spots >1.5 cm (15 mm) in diameter probably indicates the presence of NF1 (Fig. 11.47),[255] although having café-au-lait spots alone does not allow for definitive diagnosis. Café-au-lait spots in NF1 tend to have a greater melanocyte density and increased fibroblast secretion of stem cell factor than café-au-lait spots without associated NF1.[256] The number and localization of café-au-lait spots in NF1 does not correlate with the severity of the disorder, except that large café-au-lait spots may be a sign of an underlying plexiform neurofibroma (see below).

Another form of pigmentation, termed axillary freckling (Crowe's sign), also serves as a valuable diagnostic aid in the early recognition of neurofibromatosis (Fig. 11.48).[257] Axillary freckling appears as multiple 1–4 mm café-au-lait spots in the axillary vault. These most commonly appear between 3 and 5 years of age. Lack of sun exposure in this area prevents confusion with true freckles. These freckles are also frequently seen in the inguinal region, and may be more generalized. Overall, almost 90% of affected children have intertriginous freckling by 7 years of age.

Café-au-lait spots without other evidence of NF1 have been inherited as an autosomal dominant trait in some families, although at least two generations of adults with just the café-au-lait spots without neurofibromas or other signs of NF1 are required to confirm the diagnosis of familial multiple café-au-lait spots.[258] Multiple café-au-lait spots and axillary and/or inguinal freckling are features of Legius syndrome (sometimes called neurofibromatosis type 1-like syndrome), which results from mutations in *SPRED1*. *SPRED1* interacts directly with Ras and is involved in its function. Although the clinical features during childhood generally do not allow Legius syndrome to be distinguished from NF1, distinction is important prognostically since, to date, Legius syndrome has been associated with learning disabilities but not with the cutaneous or plexiform neurofibromas, NF1 osseous lesions or symptomatic optic pathway gliomas.[259] Almost 2% of individuals with a previous diagnosis of NF1 are now thought to have Legius syndrome. Although café-au-lait spots and freckling have been distinct criteria that, if both present, allow the definitive diagnosis of NF1, the discovery that Legius syndrome presents with these two criteria has led to the suggestion that multiple café-au-lait spots and freckling be combined into a single criterion for diagnosis.[260]

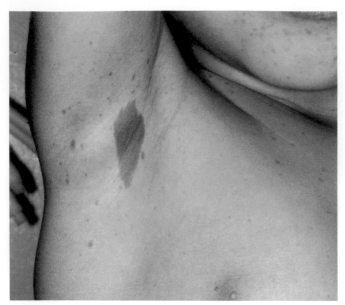

Figure 11.48 Neurofibromatosis type 1. Axillary freckling (Crowe's sign) is present in 20–50% of individuals with NF1 and commonly appears between 3 and 5 years of age. The presence of both axillary freckling and multiple café-au-lait spots allows a definitive diagnosis of NF1 or Legius syndrome.

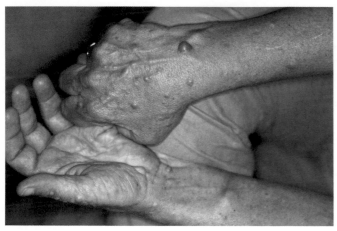

Figure 11.49 Neurofibromatosis type 1. Dermal and subcutaneous neurofibromas are rarely found before adolescence. These tumors, which originate from Schwann cells, increase in number progressively thereafter.

NF1 is also characterized by dermal or subcutaneous neurofibromas, which represent tumors primarily comprised of Schwann cells, mast cells, and fibroblasts. The Schwann cell has been shown to be the cell of origin, in which loss of the normal neurofibromin allele leads to uncontrolled growth in the setting of NF1 ('loss of heterozygosity').[261,262] The dermal and subcutaneous neurofibromas usually occur in late childhood or adolescence; thus, they are generally not found in affected children. Their appearance is frequently associated with puberty and pregnancy, and they have been noted in 84% of affected adults.[263] They are soft in consistency, may range in size from a millimeter to several centimeters in diameter, and often have an overlying violaceous, pink, or blue hue (Fig. 11.49). They may be sessile or pedunculated. With pressure from a finger, dermal neurofibromas may be invaginated, a sign called 'buttonholing'. 'Pseudoatrophic macules' and 'red-blue macules' are unusual

variants of dermal neurofibromas that show replacement of dermal collagen with neural tissue and thick-walled blood vessels in the superficial dermis overlying the neurofibroma, respectively. By adulthood, dermal neurofibromas may number from a few to hundreds, with a progressive increase in size and number as the patient becomes older. Neurofibromas may occur anywhere on the body, with no specific site of predilection. Not uncommonly, patients complain of itchiness at the site of a dermal neurofibroma, perhaps related to the presence of mast cells.

Plexiform neurofibromas may be superficial or deep.[264] They often are oriented along the length of a nerve and involve several fascicles. They may be barely palpable, may be quite firm, or may become huge with a 'bag of worms' consistency. Plexiform neurofibromas not uncommonly are present at birth and have a predilection to involve the extremities. Frequently, a large café-au-lait spot, often with irregular borders, overlies the plexiform neurofibroma (Fig. 11.50); hypertrichosis maybe associated as well (Fig. 11.51). Underlying soft tissue and bone hypertrophy (Fig. 11.52) or bone erosion may be seen. Plexiform neurofibromas may at times cause pain, muscle weakness, atrophy, or slight sensory loss. Given the hyperpigmentation and associated hypertrichosis, a plexiform neurofibroma may be confused with a congenital nevus, Becker nevus, or smooth muscle hamartoma. Isolated plexiform neurofibromas have been described in patients without NF1, although the possibility of mosaicism should be considered (Fig. 11.53).

Although a benign course for neurofibromas is usual, up to 10% of neurofibromas undergo malignant change, virtually always in adults. These 'malignant peripheral nerve sheath tumors' have been attributed to the occurrence of a second mutation within tumor cells, commonly a p53 mutation.[265] Malignant degeneration may be heralded by rapid enlargement or pain, but malignant growth, once it develops, is often slow with few metastases. Malignant peripheral nerve sheath tumors peak in their occurrence during the second and third decades of life.

Systemic manifestations of neurofibromatosis

The ocular manifestations of NF1 include plexiform neurofibromas, Lisch nodules, and optic gliomas. Lisch nodules are asymptomatic yellowish brown melanocytic hamartomas on the iris that cause no problem with vision. These Lisch nodules are found in >90% of affected adults, but are uncommonly found in prepubertal children; the number of Lisch nodules increases with increasing age. They are best detected by slit-lamp examination, although larger ones may be seen without magnification as beige spots on a dark iris or darker spots on a light iris. Their presence virtually ensures the diagnosis of NF1. Since many children with neurofibromatosis do not have Lisch nodules, their absence does not discount the diagnosis. All unaffected parents and children whose status is in question should have a thorough ophthalmologic examination as a part of their evaluation so that appropriate genetic counseling can be provided.

Optic gliomas occur in approximately 15% of children with NF1, and are more indolent than optic gliomas in individuals without NF1. Precocious puberty has been described in up to 40% of patients with gliomas of the posterior chiasm and hypothalamic areas (Fig. 11.54).[266] Overall, only 33% of patients with optic gliomas develop symptoms or signs, such as decreased visual acuity or visual field defects, proptosis, strabismus, and/or optic nerve pallor. A total of 35% of those with symptomatic optic gliomas eventually require treatment, specifically for their progressive loss of vision, gross disfigurement (e.g., from proptosis), or poor weight gain with diencephalic syndrome. Currently, chemotherapy with carboplatin and vincristine is the treatment of choice. Surgical resection is used for cosmetic palliation and radiation therapy is avoided

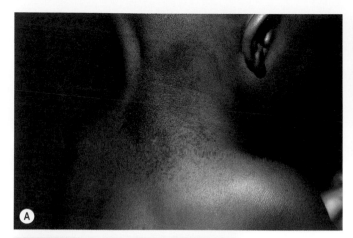

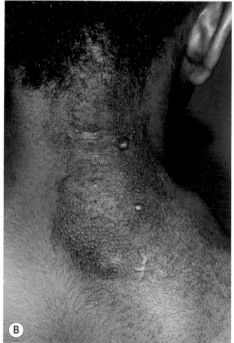

Figure 11.50 Neurofibromatosis type 1. Plexiform neurofibromas are commonly present at birth and can resemble giant café-au-lait spots, although borders are often more irregular (A). With advancing age, plexiform neurofibromas may enlarge and become more elevated with a firm or 'bag of worms' consistency (B). (A) shows a plexiform neurofibroma in a 3-year-old boy, and (B) shows the same plexiform neurofibroma when the child is 11 years of age.

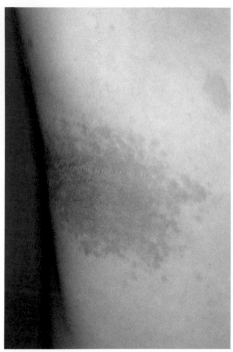

Figure 11.51 Neurofibromatosis type 1. This plexiform neurofibroma is hypertrichotic and was misdiagnosed as a congenital nevus. Café-au-lait macules are unusual on the face and the possibility of an underlying plexiform neurofibroma should be considered.

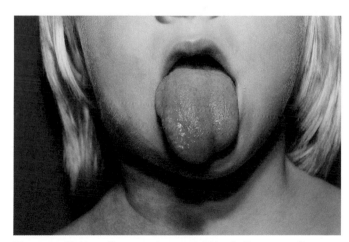

Figure 11.52 Neurofibromatosis type 1. This plexiform neurofibroma of the tongue led to discomfort and difficulty with both speech and mastication. Note the cheek and neck involvement.

because of the risk of second malignancy treatment.[267,268] Progression in optic gliomas occurs by 10 years of age in 90% of patients, suggesting that annual eye examinations until 10 years of age, is appropriate. Although routine baseline MRIs are not necessary, imaging should be performed if abnormalities are found on ophthalmologic evaluation or in the face of signs of a problematic optic glioma.[268] Spontaneous regression of optic gliomas may occur.[269]

Other than the café-au-lait spots, learning disability is the most common manifestation of NF1 in children.[270,271] Learning disability, which occurs in approximately 50% of affected children, includes nonverbal and verbal disability as well as attention deficit disorder. The occurrence of attention deficit disorder in children with NF1 has been linked to the poor development of social skills.[272] The learning disabilities in NF1 appear to be a defect inherently associated with the Nf1± genotype,[273] as well as to the occurrence of

enhanced intensity of T2 signals in brain MRI examinations in the basal ganglia, brainstem, internal capsule, and cerebellum (unidentified bright objects).[274] Brain tumors may lead to neurologic abnormalities. Other than optic pathway gliomas, brainstem gliomas (pilocytic astrocytomas) are the most common intracranial neoplasms,[275] but usually behave less aggressively than histologically identical tumors in non-neurofibromatosis-1 patients. Owing to the indolent nature of these tumors, conservative management with close follow-up is recommended. A total of 23% of meningiomas have been noted in individuals with NF1.[276] More severe developmental delay occurs in only 5% of patients, and has been associated with total deletion of the neurofibromin gene;[277] these patients also have facial dysmorphism and large numbers of neurofibromas.

259

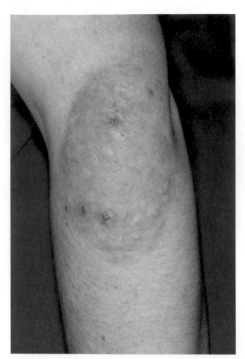

Figure 11.53 Plexiform neurofibroma without NF1. Occasionally typical plexiform neurofibromas occur in individuals without evidence of NF1; mosaicism should be considered.

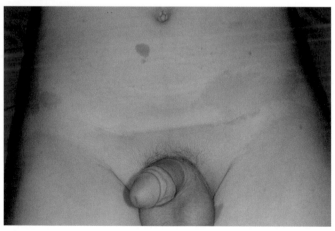

Figure 11.54 Neurofibromatosis type 1. Precocious puberty in a 5-year-old boy with an optic chiasm/hypothalamic glioma.

Skeletal manifestations are most commonly bone dysplasias, pectus deformity, and scoliosis. Even without osseous abnormalities, children and adolescents with NF1 have decreased bone mineral density.[278] Spinal deformities, particularly scoliosis or kyphosis, may occur in at least 10% of patients, and pectus deformities in approximately 24% of patients.[279,280] The dystrophic form of scoliosis almost always develops before 10 years of age and then progresses, usually involves the lower cervical and upper thoracic spine, and is associated with dysplastic changes of the vertebral bodies. Tibial dysplasia ('congenital bowing'), pathognomonic for NF1, presents as anteromedial bowing of the tibia (Fig. 11.55), usually during the first year of life and has been described in about 1–4% of affected children. The cortex of the bone is thinned and the medulla is sclerotic.[281] Fractures may occur at the site, leading to 'pseudoarthrosis.' Sphenoid wing dysplasia is also an uncommon manifestation of NF1 and may manifest as pulsating exophthalmos.

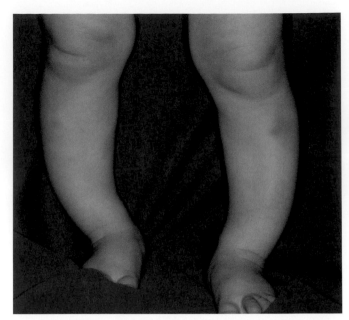

Figure 11.55 Neurofibromatosis type 1. Bilateral tibial bowing without evidence of pseudoarthrosis in an affected infant.

Non-ossifying fibromas have also been described in association with multiple café-au-lait spots (Jaffe–Campanacci syndrome); this group of patients has a high risk of recurrent fractures and significant resultant deformity and disability.[282]

Other features of NF1 that may be seen during childhood are short stature, frequent headaches, macrocephaly, hypertension and rarely seizures. Short stature most often occurs without evidence of neuroendocrine problems.[283,284] The macrocephaly is usually not associated with hydrocephalus, although aqueductal stenosis has rarely been reported. In children, hypertension usually relates to renal artery stenosis and is quite rare;[285] in adults with hypertension and NF1, pheochromocytoma should be suspected. Stenosis or occlusion of several other arteries may occur, leading to cerebral vascular accidents, aneurysms, and even sudden cardiac death.[286,287] Small telangiectatic vessels often form around the stenotic area of the cerebral arteries, leading to a 'puff of smoke' (moyamoya) on cerebral angiography. Watson syndrome is an allelic variant of neurofibromatosis type 1 with associated pulmonic stenosis, and NF1-Noonan syndrome combines the features of Noonan syndrome (ocular hypertelorism, low-set ears, downslanting palpebral fissures, webbed neck and pulmonic stenosis) with NF1, usually with mutations in neurofibromin but not *PTPN11*, the gene usually associated with Noonan syndrome.

NF1 is associated with a 5% lifetime risk of developing malignancy. In addition to the development of malignant peripheral nerve sheath tumors, non-lymphocytic leukemias, carcinoids, and pheochromocytomas are described with increased frequency. Multiple small juvenile xanthogranulomas have been noted with increased frequency in children with multiple café-au-lait spots; a minority of these children have juvenile chronic myelogenous leukemia, but complete blood counts and careful monitoring should be considered.[288]

Therapy of NF1

The current management for most children with NF1 is anticipatory guidance, genetic counseling, and surveillance for potential complications. If available, referral to a multidisciplinary clinic that specializes in seeing individuals with NF1 is optimal. Baseline screening tests, except for annual ophthalmologic examinations until 10 years of age, are not recommended. Monitoring and early intervention for learning disabilities is important. Complete physical examinations should be performed at least twice yearly, including measurements of height, weight, head circumference, and blood pressure; careful palpation for tumors; and assessment for scoliosis or other bony deformities.

Dermal neurofibromas may be excised, but plexiform neurofibromas usually cannot be removed in their entirety.[289] Surgical debulking may be undertaken for tumors that are disfiguring, interfere with function, or are subject to irritation, trauma, or infection. Mast cells appear to play a critical rose in the initiation and progression of plexiform neurofibromas;[290] in one child with an unresectable plexiform neurofibroma that caused airway compression, treatment for 3 months with imatinib mesylate led to 70% diminution in tumor volume without adverse effects. Antiangiogenic agents and farnesyltransferase inhibitors (that block Ras) are currently being tested as new therapies.

Genetic counseling is another important aspect of treatment, since there is a 50% chance of transmitting neurofibromatosis with each pregnancy. Mutations can be found by multistep mutation detection in >95% of individuals with NF1.[243] Mosaicism with postzygotic mutation in neurofibromin, however, is not uncommon.[291,292] Affected patients may show mosaic-generalized NF1, which is indistinguishable clinically from germ-line mutations with generalized manifestations, or mosaic-localized NF1. Patients with mosaic-localized or 'segmental NF1' show typical features of NF1 limited to a specific body segment. Although café-au-lait macules are the most common manifestation of segmental NF1 in children, other cutaneous manifestations (freckling, dermal and plexiform neurofibromas) or non-cutaneous manifestations (pseudoarthrosis, sphenoid wing dysplasia, optic glioma, Lisch nodules) in the localized area may also occur.[293] Individuals with mosaic forms of NF1 who also have germ-line involvement (more common with mosaic-generalized NF1) may have offspring with full NF1 with an up to 50% probability with each pregnancy. A national support group, the National Neurofibromatosis Foundation, Inc (www.nf.org), offers patient information and support.

Reticulated Forms of Hyperpigmentation

The term poikiloderma (poikiloderma atrophicans vasculare) is used to describe a triad of telangiectasia, atrophy, and reticulated dyschromia (hyperpigmentation and hypopigmentation). The disorder may be seen in patients with poikiloderma congenitale (Rothmund–Thomson syndrome), xeroderma pigmentosum, Bloom syndrome, dyskeratosis congenita, juvenile dermatomyositis, and cutaneous T-cell lymphoma. Actinic, thermal, and radiation damage can also leave poikilodermatous changes.

Histopathologic examination of areas of poikiloderma reveals varying degrees of epidermal hyperkeratosis and atrophy, hydropic degeneration of the basal layer, varying numbers of pigment-laden melanophages, and a lymphocytic band-like or perivascular infiltration in the dermis. Management consists of early recognition, avoidance of sun exposure, and the use of protective clothing and topical sunscreen preparations in an attempt to arrest progression of the dermatosis.

Reticulate acropigmentation of Kitamura is an autosomal dominant pigmentary disorder characterized by atrophic, reticulated, or lentiginous hyperpigmentation localized primarily to the dorsal areas of the hands and feet. Its onset is during childhood, and pits on the palms, soles, and dorsal surface of the phalanges are associated.[294] Dowling–Degos disease, which is also an autosomal dominant keratin disorder, typically occurs in adults. Reticulated hyperpigmentation is localized to the intertriginous areas,

primarily the axillae and the inguinal folds. Comedonal lesions and pitted acneiform facial scars are associated.[295] Reticulated hyperpigmentation is also seen in X-linked reticulate pigmentary disorder (also called Partington syndrome or familial cutaneous amyloidosis).[296] Brown pigmentation is distributed along the lines of Blaschko in affected carrier females, and resembles the pigmented streaks and whorls of incontinentia pigmenti. Affected boys may show a more generalized distribution of reticulated hyperpigmentation in association with xerosis, failure to thrive, developmental delay, seizures, hemiplegia, colitis, gastroesophageal reflux, inguinal hernia, and urethral stricture. Dental anomalies, hypohidrosis, photophobia, and corneal clouding are also seen. Skeletal changes may include delayed bone age and shortened metacarpals. The amyloid that has been found in skin biopsies of some affected adults has not been demonstrated in the skin of affected children.

Naegeli–Franceschetti–Jadassohn syndrome and dermatopathia pigmentosa reticularis are autosomal dominant disorders with reticulate hyperpigmentation, palmoplantar keratoderma, absence of dermatoglyphics, onychodystrophy, and decreased sweating with life-long heat intolerance. Both disorders result from nonsense or frameshift mutations in keratin 14 that lead to haploinsufficiency and increased susceptibility of keratinocytes to apoptosis.[297,298] In Naegeli–Franceschetti–Jadassohn syndrome, the reticulated hyperpigmentation is present during the first 2 years of life, primarily involving the abdomen, perioral, and periocular areas.[299] The pigmentation commonly fades during adolescence and may disappear altogether. Dental abnormalities are associated. The pigmentation in dermatopathia pigmentosa reticularis is primarily in a truncal distribution and is associated with non-scarring alopecia.[300] These forms of reticulated hyperpigmentation should be distinguished from the dyschromatoses (see above), which show hyperpigmented and hypopigmented macules, and the reticulated hyperpigmentation that develops in male individuals with dyskeratosis congenita (see Ch. 7). The hyperpigmentation in all of these disorders is nonpalpable, in contrast to the hyperpigmented papules and plaques of confluent and reticulated papillomatosis of Gougerot and Carteaud, an asymptomatic disorder of hyperkeratotic hyperpigmented papules in a reticulated pattern.[301] Seen primarily in adolescents and young adults, this disorder usually occurs on the upper anterior trunk, often in individuals with acanthosis nigricans (see Ch. 23, Figs 23.26, 23.27).

Erythema Dyschromicum Perstans

Erythema dyschromicum perstans (ashy dermatosis) is an acquired chronic, progressive bluish to ash-gray hyperpigmentation that can affect individuals of both sexes from childhood through adulthood. Although more common in darker-skinned individuals, several light-skinned affected children have been described.[302,303] The cause of erythema dyschromicum perstans remains unknown. Lesions usually begin as slate-gray macules (Fig. 11.56), but occasionally show a transient, slightly raised erythematous border. Generally seen on the trunk and upper limbs, lesions may also occur on other areas, with the exception of the scalp, mucous membranes, palms, and soles. Lesions vary from a few millimeters to many centimeters in diameter, and often cover extensive areas. Lesions are usually distinct, but can be confluent. Multiple linear lesions of erythema dyschromicum perstans have been described that follow the lines of Blaschko.[304]

This disorder must be differentiated from the post-inflammatory hyperpigmented lesions of tinea versicolor, pityriasis rosea, and fixed drug eruption,[295] which usually show brown rather than grayish pigmentation.[296] Idiopathic eruptive macular pigmentation is differentiated by the development of brown (rather than grayish)

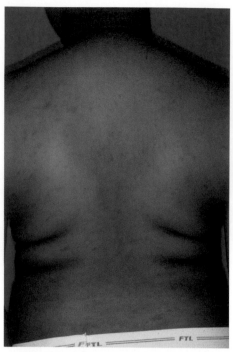

Figure 11.56 Erythema dyschromicum perstans. Oval slate-gray macules, all oriented along the same axis, on the trunk of this otherwise healthy boy. In children with erythema dyschromicum perstans, the hyperpigmented macules often clear spontaneously after years.

non-confluent macules of the trunk, neck and proximal extremities; the absence of preceding inflammation; the lack of exposure to a medication; and basal cell hyperpigmentation without damage to the keratinocytes and without dermal mast cells in biopsy sections.[297] Histologic features of erythema dyschromicum perstans depend on the stage of the lesion. Older lesions show pigment incontinence, but early lesions may show hydropic degeneration of epidermal cells and a lichenoid infiltrate of lymphocytes.[298]

The dermatosis is asymptomatic but chronic. There are frequent exacerbations, with extension into previously uninvolved areas. There is no known effective therapy, but most cases in children clear spontaneously within a few years.[302,305]

Post-inflammatory Hyperpigmentation

Post-inflammatory hyperpigmentation is one of the most common causes of hyperpigmentation, and is characterized by an increase in melanin formation following cutaneous inflammation.[306] Ordinary post-inflammatory hyperpigmentation is of relatively short duration and tends to persist for several weeks or months after the original cause has subsided. Examples include the pigmentation following physical trauma, friction, primary irritants, eczematous eruptions, lichen simplex chronicus, acne vulgaris and dermatoses such as pityriasis rosea, psoriasis, fixed drug eruptions, photodermatitis, and pyoderma. Individuals with dark complexions and those who tan easily following ultraviolet light exposure show the greatest degree and longest persistence of this form of post-inflammatory hyperpigmentation. In cases in which the dermal-epidermal junction and basal layer become disrupted (lupus erythematosus, lichen planus, lichenoid drug eruptions) melanin incontinence occurs (e.g., see Figs 4.37, 4.38). The melanin tends to drop from its normal epidermal position and passes into melanophages of the dermis, leading to more pronounced and persistent discoloration. If areas of post-inflammatory hyperpigmentation can

be protected from further ultraviolet light exposure, fading gradually occurs over a period of months to years. Most patients do not respond to topical agents or resurfacing procedures as well as patients with melasma (see below).[307,308] Topical antiinflammatory medications are appropriate if inflammation is ongoing.

Melasma

Melasma is a term applied to a patchy dark-brown to black hyperpigmentation located primarily on the cheeks, the forehead, and occasionally the temples, upper lip, and neck. Seen in up to 20% of women who take anovulatory drugs or who are pregnant, this disorder has been termed the mask of pregnancy. Typical melasma also can occur in males and in females who are neither pregnant nor taking oral contraceptives. Occasionally it may also appear in patients of both sexes taking phenytoin (Dilantin) or its derivatives. Overall, 10% of affected individuals are male. Since sun exposure tends to trigger and intensify this hyperpigmentation, the disorder characteristically becomes more prominent in the summer months.[309]

Once melasma has developed, it tends to persist for long periods of time, and treatment is generally not very satisfactory. Melasma of pregnancy usually clears within a few months after delivery, only to recur with subsequent pregnancies. Oral contraceptive-induced melasma may persist for up to 5 years after discontinuation of the medication. The treatment of melasma consists of discontinuation of potentially responsible medications, protection from ultraviolet light exposure by the use of appropriate clothing and sunscreen preparations, and the once-daily topical application of hydroquinone bleaching agents (2–4%).[307,308] Hydroquinones act by the inhibition of tyrosinase, and are most effective in combination with tretinoin (0.05–0.1%). A formulation that also includes a mild topical steroid seems to be more effective than the combination of hydroquinone and tretinoin alone, but cannot be used on the face for long periods of time because of the risk of topical corticosteroid application. Twice-daily application of azelaic acid 15–20% can also be efficacious, and tends to be associated with less irritation.[310] Other topical agents that have been used are kojic acid, licorice extract, arbutin, ascorbic acid, soy, N-acetylglucosamine, and niacinamide.[308] Chemical peels may also be helpful in lighter-skinned individuals with melasma. Laser therapy has proved less effective.[311] These preparations often require 3–4 months before a therapeutic effect is achieved. Concurrent sun protection is critical to prevent further hyperpigmentation in patients using hydroquinones. Since continuous use of hydroquinone bleaching creams or lotions can result in excessive pigmentary loss or ochronosis-like hyperpigmentation, once the desired degree of depigmentation is achieved, hydroquinone therapy should be discontinued.

Metabolic Causes of Hyperpigmentation

Cutaneous changes frequently are helpful in the diagnosis of several endocrine disorders, including Addison disease (Figs 23.6, 23.7), hyperthyroidism (Fig. 23.2), hypothyroidism, acromegaly, and Cushing syndrome (see Ch. 23). More than two-thirds of patients with chronic hepatic disease (cirrhosis or prolonged bile duct obstruction) also have some degree of cutaneous hyperpigmentation. Of these, diffuse darkening of the skin is perhaps the most common. Blotchy areas of brown hyperpigmentation occasionally may be seen, and accentuation of normal freckling and areolar hyperpigmentation may appear.

Polycystic kidney disease and other forms of chronic renal disease with nitrogen retention may also be accompanied by pruritus and, at times, a diffuse yellowish brown discoloration of the skin most pronounced on the face and hands. Although urinary chromogens and carotenemia may be present, melanin pigmentation also has been implicated as a cause of this discoloration.

Hemochromatosis

Hemochromatosis is a familial iron storage disorder characterized by cutaneous hyperpigmentation that usually manifests between 40 and 60 years of age. However, type 2 or the juvenile form of hemochromatosis presents during childhood. An autosomal recessive disorder, this type of hemochromatosis maps to chromosome 1q21.[312] Hyperpigmentation is seen in almost every patient with hemochromatosis and is the presenting sign in 25–40% of affected individuals. The increased pigmentation is produced by melanin and not by the deposition of iron in the skin. It appears initially in the exposed areas before it becomes diffuse and is most intense in the skin of the face, arms, body folds, and genitalia. Mucous membranes (the gums, palate, and buccal mucosa), and sometimes the conjunctivae, are involved in 15–20% of affected persons. The skin is soft, dry, thin, shiny, and of fine texture. Spider angiomas are present in 60–80% of affected individuals, and palmar erythema is common. Facial, axillary, thoracic, and pubic hairs are scant or absent. Cardiomyopathy, evidence of hypogonadism, and reduced glucose tolerance are seen by young adulthood. The hepatic cirrhosis characteristic of adult-onset hemochromatosis, however, is less clinically relevant in type 2 hemochromatosis, and icterus is unusual.[313]

Secondary hemochromatosis (hemosiderosis) with associated hyperpigmentation may be seen in patients with anemia who receive numerous blood transfusions. In such instances, visceral fibrosis is unusual, diabetes mellitus is uncommon, and hypogonadism is not present.

The diagnosis of metabolic hemochromatosis is suggested by the presence of cutaneous hyperpigmentation in patients with hepatic cirrhosis and a history of diabetes mellitus. Elevated serum iron and saturation of serum iron-binding globulin confirm the diagnosis. The demonstration of parenchymal iron distribution by skin, liver, and gastric biopsies, and the presence of hemosiderin in urinary sediment are particularly helpful. Histopathologic examination of involved skin shows increased melanin in the basal layer and deposition of iron in the upper cutis (especially in macrophages, endothelial cells of capillaries, and the propria of eccrine glands).

The clinical course of untreated hemochromatosis is characterized by tissue destruction, malfunction of involved organs, and eventual death. Symptomatic treatment of the diabetes, liver dysfunction, and cardiac symptoms and quarterly phlebotomies, when initiated early, frequently result in clinical and pathologic improvement. Dietary restriction of iron is impractical, and chelating agents to date have been of little value.

Ochronosis

Alkaptonuria (ochronosis) is an inborn error of tyrosine metabolism in which homogentisic acid, an intermediate product in the metabolism of phenylalanine and tyrosine, accumulates in the tissues and is excreted in the urine because of a lack of homogentisic acid oxidase. This autosomal recessive disorder usually first becomes manifest in the third decade with scleral blue-black pigmentation (Osler's sign). Affected children rarely show Osler's sign and the characteristic dark urine is usually not noted because the color change only occurs with sitting for 1–2 h, especially in an alkaline environment.[314,315] Dark urine in the diaper may be the first sign in infants. Skin pigmentation first becomes visible around the 4th decade, especially on ear cartilage, eyelids and other facial areas, intertriginous areas and over tendons. Nails may be stained brown. Around this time, the ochronotic arthropathy from pigment deposition also starts to develop, and involves the weight-bearing joints

(spine, knees) most commonly. The mean age of joint replacement is 55 years, of development of renal stones 64 years, of cardiac valve involvement 54 years, and of coronary artery calcification 59 years. The diagnosis can be confirmed by alkalinizing the urine (e.g., with sodium hydroxide), which leads to the typical black color; the homogentisic acid is detected by enzymatic spectrophotometry or gas liquid chromatography. Treatment with ascorbic acid twice daily may reduce the connective tissue damage, and affected children have also been placed on a low protein diet. Nitisinone therapy may decrease homogentisic acid production.[316]

Exogenous ochronosis is clinically and histologically similar to its endogenous counterpart, but is not hereditary and has no internal manifestations. The condition usually occurs in African-American patients from exposure to hydroquinones, and is characterized by asymptomatic hyperpigmentation of the face, neck, back, and extensor surfaces of the extremities. Less commonly, exogenous ochronosis has been described after exposure to antimalarials or products containing resorcinol, phenol, mercury, or picric acid.[317]

Hyperpigmentation due to Heavy Metals

The systemic absorption of chemicals can also cause discoloration of the skin. Although the incidence of hyperpigmentation due to exogenous heavy metals has decreased in recent years, limited exposure to such preparations still occurs, and metallic hyperpigmentation may still be seen in children as well as adults.

Argyria occurs after long-term ingestion or excessive application of silver preparations and presents as localized or widespread bluish-gray or slate-colored discoloration of the skin produced by the deposition of silver within the dermis. The condition is more pronounced on exposed parts of the body, namely the face, forearms, and hands, but may also occur in the sclerae, oral mucous membranes, and lunulae of the nails. Argyria has been increasingly described because of the promotion of colloidal silver-based products for their immunostimulant, antimicrobials, and antiinflammatory properties. The antimicrobial properties are proportional to the bioactive silver ion released and its availability to interact with bacterial or fungal cell membranes.[318] These 'health food' products delivery primarily inactive metallic silver, not the antimicrobial ionized form. Colloidal silver and silver sulfadiazine cream, for example, have high levels of silver release with relatively low levels of ionized silver.[319] Ionized silver dressings have more recently been introduced for wound care;[318] they occasionally cause local dermal argyria[320] but show very low local silver levels. On the other hand, temporary superficial silver staining of the stratum corneum is a common side-effect of these dressings.

Cases with more extensive hyperpigmentation have been described after chronic ingestion of silver-containing water[321] or colloidal silver,[322] or widespread topical application of silver sulfadiazine[323,324] or colloidal silver. Localized staining can be seen periorbitally and on the eyes from ophthalmic preparations containing silver at acupuncture sites[325,326] or after exposure to silver earrings,[327,328] but most commonly is now reported at burn or wound sites after use of silver sulfadiazine or colloidal silver when used as antibacterial agents, for example, for patients with burns or epidermolysis bullosa.[324,329]

The diagnosis of argyria is based on clinical examination and history of exposure and may be confirmed by cutaneous biopsy of affected areas, which shows fine, small round refractive silver granules throughout the dermis, especially around eccrine glands. Increased amounts of melanin may be seen in the basal layer of the epidermis and also within macrophages in the upper dermis. Treatment of argyria depends on recognition of the disorder, discontinuation of the use of the silver-containing preparation, and avoidance of sunlight exposure. The dermal hyperpigmentation is usually irreversible.

Chrysiasis (gold-induced hyperpigmentation) is a rare cutaneous disorder induced by the administration of gold salts followed by exposure to ultraviolet light.[330,331] The pigmentation is bluish gray or purplish and is similar to that seen in argyria except that the hyperpigmentation is more prominent around the eyes, is limited to areas of sunlight exposure, and does not affect the sclerae and oral mucous membranes. Hyperpigmentation may develop after treatment with a Q-switched laser after systemic gold treatment.[332] Other cutaneous manifestations are seen in up to 20% of individuals on gold therapy, which is most commonly administered for rheumatoid arthritis. These include morbilliform, eczematous, urticarial, bullous, purpuric, lichen planus-like, and pityriasis rosea-like eruptions. The histopathologic features of gold-induced hyperpigmentation consist of small, black, round or oval, irregularly shaped gold particles located in a perivascular distribution and in dermal histiocytes.

Chronic exposure to mercury systemically may result in acrodynia (pink disease), a disorder of infants and young children characterized by leg cramps, headaches, hypertension, excessive perspiration, itching, swelling, redness and peeling of the hands, feet, and nose, weakness of the pectoral and pelvic girdles, and nerve dysfunction in the lower extremities. However, exposure to topically applied mercury may lead to slate-gray pigmentation in areas of topical application. The discoloration is exaggerated in the areas of skin folds, and is permanent.[333]

Drug-induced Hyperpigmentation

Hyperpigmentation may be induced by chronic exposure to medication, and tends to be worsened by sun exposure. The diagnosis of a drug eruption is based almost entirely on history and physical examination. The main drugs implicated in causing skin pigmentation are non-steroidal antiinflammatory drugs, minocycline, antimalarials,[334] amiodarone, diltiazem,[335] cytotoxic drugs, heavy metals (see above), clofazimine, imipramine[336,337] and chlorpromazine. Clinical features are variable according to the triggering molecule, with a large range of patterns and shades. Bluish-gray discoloration is most common and especially prominent at sites of exposure to ultraviolet light. The condition is most frequently seen in the pediatric population in adolescents who have been taking minocycline for acne, with the blue discoloration usually notable at sites of acne scarring and on the oral mucosae and shins (Fig. 11.57; see also Fig. 8.15). Three subgroups have been described based on clinical appearance and histopathologic correlates: type I (blue-gray pigmentation in scars); type II (blue-gray pigmentation in previously normal skin, especially of the shins); and type III (brown discoloration at sun-exposed sites).[338] Biopsy specimens tend to show pigmentation within dermal macrophages, often localized to vessels and adnexal structures. Treatment involves interruption of therapy and sun avoidance, although laser may be useful in some cases.[339] These measures are often followed by fading of lesions, but pigmentation may persist for a long time or even be permanent.[340]

The plaques of fixed drug eruptions are circumscribed, usually round or oval, often edematous and sometimes bullous, usually pruritic, and reddish-purple. Drug-induced hyperpigmentation tends to recur in the same location following the readministration of certain drugs, particularly sulfonamides, tetracyclines, acetaminophen, phenolphthalein, barbiturate derivatives, and antineoplastic agents such as cyclophosphamide. Histopathologic examination of lesions of the hyperpigmented phase of fixed drug eruptions

reveals an increase in the amount of melanin in the basal layer of the epidermis and within macrophages of the upper dermis, and is helpful in confirming the diagnosis.

Carotenemia

Carotenemia is a yellowish orange discoloration of skin due to the ingestion of excessive quantities of carotene-containing foods, particularly carrots, squash, pumpkin, yellow turnips, sweet potatoes, peaches, apricots, papayas, mangos, egg yolk, and even green beans.[341-343] The condition is seen primarily in infants and occasionally in older children and adults.[344] The color is most prominent on the palms and soles, in the nasolabial grooves, on the forehead, chin, upper eyelids, postauricular areas, and anterior axillary folds, and over areas of pressure such as the elbows, knees, knuckles, and ankles (Fig. 23.3). Lack of involvement of the sclerae and mucous membranes, coupled with the absence of pruritus and lack of color change in the urine or stool, helps rule out the presence of hepatic or biliary jaundice. Lycopene, a red-colored carotenoid pigment found in fruits and vegetables, especially ripened tomatoes, beets, chili beans, and various fruits and berries, may cause a reddish yellow discoloration of the skin (lycopenemia).

Carotenemia is a benign disorder in infants, and no intervention is required. Rarely, carotenemia may be a sign of systemic disease, especially hypothyroidism, weight loss diets or anorexia, or diabetes. The diagnosis of carotenemia is confirmed by the presence of high carotene levels in the presence of normal serum bilirubin. If the coloration is problematic, reduction of dietary intake of carotene-containing foods to normal levels or correction of the underlying disorder usually results in gradual improvement within 4–6 weeks. Rarely, children will show a genetic defect in the metabolism of carotenoids that is more recalcitrant to dietary intervention.[345,346]

Dermal Melanocytoses

Mongolian spots

Mongolian spots are flat, deep brown to slate gray or blue-black, often poorly circumscribed, large macular lesions generally located over the lumbosacral areas, buttocks (Fig. 11.58), and occasionally the lower limbs, back, flanks, and shoulders of normal infants. They are seen in more than 90% of African-American and Native-American babies; 62–86% of Asians;[347,348] 70% of Hispanic, and 9.6% of Caucasian infants. Mongolian spots are present at birth and tend to fade during the first 2–3 years of life. Mongolian spots were found in 75% of Nigerian neonates; 14% were still present by preschool years, and none were found by 6 years of age.[349] Occasionally, Mongolian spots persist into adulthood.

Mongolian spots may be single or multiple and vary from a few millimeters to 10 cm or more in diameter. They represent collections of spindle-shaped melanocytes located deep in the dermis, probably as the result of arrest during their embryonal migration from the neural crest to the epidermis. The slate blue to blue-black color depends on the Tyndall effect (a phenomenon in which light passing through a turbid medium, such as the skin, is scattered as it strikes particles of melanin). Long-wavelength light rays (red, orange, and yellow) tend to be less scattered and therefore continue to pass downward into the lower levels of the skin; colors of shorter wavelengths (blue, indigo, and violet) are scattered to the side and backward to the skin surface, thus creating the blue-black or slate gray discoloration.

Since Mongolian spots are benign, therapy is unnecessary. However, large and numerous Mongolian spots may be seen in lysosomal storage disorders, among them GM1 gangliosidosis type

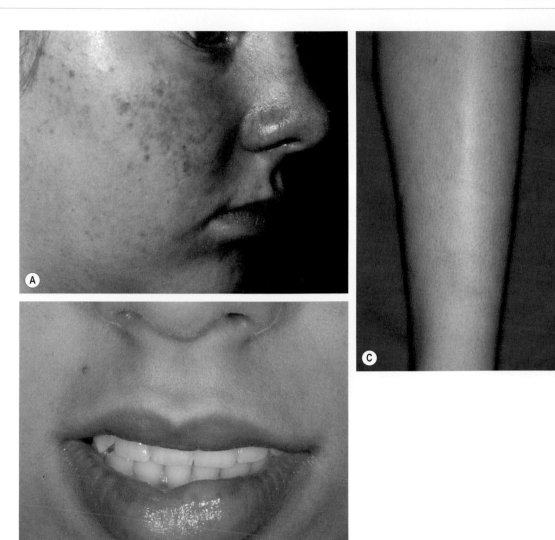

Figure 11.57 Drug-induced hyperpigmentation. Bluish-gray discoloration on the cheeks at sites of acne scarring (A), on the oral mucosae (B) and the shin (C) of adolescents administered minocycline for acne.

1, Hunter syndrome, and Hurler syndrome.[350-354] In these children, the Mongolian spots often fade, but not until at least the 2nd decade of life.[354] Large and extensive Mongolian spots can be seen with phakomatosis pigmentovascularis and phakomatosis pigmentopigmentalis, on association with vascular malformations and other pigmented lesions, respectively.[355]

Nevus of Ota and nevus of Ito

The nevus of Ota (nevus fuscoceruleus ophthalmomaxillaris) represents a usually unilateral, irregularly patchy, blue to bluish-gray to brown discoloration of the skin of the face supplied by the first and second divisions of the trigeminal nerve.[356,357] It typically involves the periorbital region, the temple, the forehead, the malar area, and the nose (Fig. 11.59). About two-thirds of patients with this disorder have a patchy bluish discoloration of the sclera of the ipsilateral eye (Fig. 11.60) and, occasionally, the conjunctiva, cornea, and retina. Palatal involvement has been described in up to 18% of affected individuals.[358] In about 5% of cases the nevus of Ota is bilateral rather than unilateral, and in rare instances, the lips, pharynx, and nasal mucosa are similarly affected.

Although most commonly seen in Asians, nevus of Ota is not infrequently seen in blacks. Unlike Mongolian spots, which tend to disappear with time, the cutaneous coloration of nevus of Ota generally persists and often shows a speckled rather than a uniform discoloration. Approximately 50% of lesions are congenital; the remainder usually appear during the second decade of life. Scleral melanocytosis alone is a much more common finding, which can progress and then recede with advancing age. In a study of Chinese children, only 4–5% were found to have scleral melanocytosis during the first year of life, but that number increased to 45% by 6 years of age with 78% of cases bilateral;[359] only 12% of the children continued to show evidence of scleral melanocytosis by 18 years of age.

The nevus of Ito (nevus fuscoceruleus acromiodeltoideus) has the same features as the nevus of Ota except that the pigmentary changes tend to involve the shoulder, supraclavicular areas, sides of the neck, and upper arm, scapulae, and deltoid regions. It may occur alone or may be seen in conjunction with the nevus of Ota.

Similar to Mongolian spots, biopsy sections of the nevus of Ota and nevus of Ito show elongated dendritic melanocytes scattered

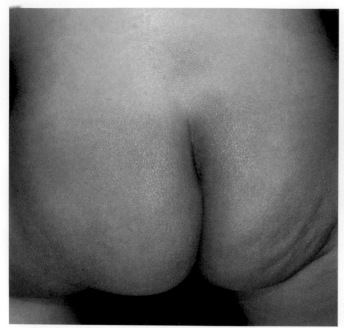

Figure 11.58 Mongolian spots. Large blue-gray patches over the lumbosacral area and buttocks of an African-American baby. These spots often fade or clear within the first few years of life.

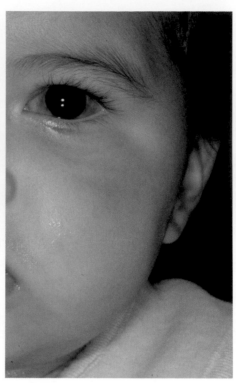

Figure 11.60 Nevus of Ota. About two-thirds of patients with nevus of Ota show a patchy bluish discoloration of the sclera of the ipsilateral eye.

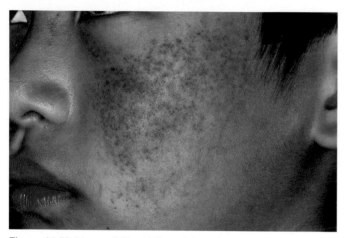

Figure 11.59 Nevus of Ota. Unilateral, irregularly patchy, brownish-gray discoloration of the malar region in an Asian boy.

among the collagen bundles. The melanocytes, however, frequently appear to be situated somewhat higher in the dermis than those seen in ordinary Mongolian spots.

Although these lesions do not disappear spontaneously, changes in color may occur. Darkening of lesions has been noted during and after puberty. These disorders are generally benign. The development of glaucoma and malignant melanoma, however, have been reported in association with the nevus of Ota, and long-term dermatologic and ophthalmologic follow-up is needed. Melanoma arising in a nevus of Ota has been reported to involve the skin, choroid, brain, meninges, orbit, iris, ciliary body, and/or optic nerve.[360–363]

Laser therapy may improve the appearance of nevus of Ota, especially the Q-switched Alexandrite laser.[364] Multiple sessions are required, but resultant scarring is rare. In general, the periorbital pigmentation of nevus of Ota responds relatively poorly to laser treatment, relative to areas of involvement on the zygomatic arch or frontal forehead regions.[365–367] Cosmetic cover-up may also be used.

Nevus of Ota and nevus of Ito may be seen in association with vascular malformations (nevus flammeus or cutis marmorata telangiectatica congenita most commonly) in a disorder called phakomatosis pigmentovascularis (see Ch. 12).[368] The condition may be associated with Sturge–Weber syndrome or Klippel–Trenaunay when the nevus flammeus is on the forehead or limbs, respectively. Occasionally, a nevus spilus is seen in association as well.[369]

Blue Nevi

Blue nevi are a heterogeneous group of congenital and more often acquired melanocytic tumors. Most frequent are common blue nevi and cellular blue nevi, although there may be histological overlap between these types.[370] The nevi appear blue-gray clinically because of the deep (dermal) location of the melanin pigment and the Tyndall effect (selective absorption of longer wavelength components of light by melanin with reflection of the shorter blue components). Blue nevi are thought to result from the arrested embryonal migration of melanocytes bound for the dermal-epidermal junction. It is thus possible that the blue nevus, Mongolian spots, and the nevi of Ota and Ito are closely related and possibly represent different stages of the same physiologic process.

The common blue nevus (also called the classic or dendritic blue nevus) presents as a small, round or oval, dark blue or bluish black, smooth-surfaced, sharply circumscribed, slightly elevated dome-shaped papule, nodule or plaque (Fig. 11.61). Most common blue nevi range from 2 or 3 mm to 10 mm (<1 cm) in diameter. Although usually single, they may be multiple. Lesions may be present at birth but may appear at any age. Although common blue nevi may occur on any part of the body, areas of predilection include the buttocks,

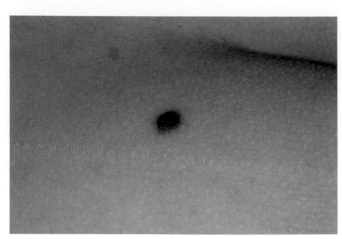

Figure 11.61 Blue nevus. This congenital lesion on the buttocks shows the well-circumscribed bluish-black smooth-surfaced papule of a typical blue nevus.

dorsal aspect of the hands and feet, scalp, and the extensor surfaces of the forearms. They also may occur on the face, bulbar conjunctiva, mucous membranes, and the hard and soft palates.

Once a common blue nevus appears, it usually remains static and persists throughout life. Although fading of color and some degree of flattening may occur with time, malignant degeneration of this form of blue nevus is rare. When a diagnosis of malignant melanoma is considered, the common blue nevus can be differentiated from it by the presence of normal skin markings over the lesion, in contrast to the loss of such markings in lesions of malignant melanoma, the homogeneity of coloration and the smooth borders on routine examination, and the presence of a bluish-gray homogeneous lesion by dermoscopic evaluation.[371]

Cellular blue nevi tend to be larger and generally measure more than 1 cm in diameter. They are usually located on the scalp, buttocks, sacrococcygeal areas, and occasionally the dorsal aspect of the hands and feet. The plaque-type variant of blue nevus is a subset that is present at birth or develops during early childhood, occurs most commonly on the scalp, and may enlarge during puberty. The cellular blue nevus carries a higher risk of malignant transformation than the common blue nevus, but malignant transformation is still rare. Malignant blue nevi are locally aggressive but spread to regional lymph nodes in about 5% of individuals.

The classification of other forms of blue nevi is controversial.[372] Many show clinical and histologic features of more than one form, particularly combinations of variants of blue nevi with common and/or Spitz nevi (see Ch. 9). Among the other forms are the deep penetrating nevus, which often occurs as part of a combined nevus and usually has its onset after the first decade of life, epithelioid blue nevus, which is most commonly seen in individuals with Carney complex (see above), and pigmented epithelioid melanocytoma.[373] Blue nevi may be 'hypochromic' (sclerotic, hypomelanotic and amelanotic forms), eruptive (particularly after sunburn on the upper central chest, shoulders, and 'V' of the neck), or targetoid (preferentially on the back of the hands or feet, leading to a misdiagnosis of melanoma).

Benign-appearing blue nevi do not require excision. If the diagnosis is in question, biopsy can be performed. Histopathologic examination of common blue nevi reveals greatly elongated spindle-shaped melanocytes, mainly in the middle and lower thirds of the dermis, which results in the blue coloration. In addition to spindle-shaped melanocytes, cellular blue nevi also have nodular islands of melanocytes.

Key References

 The complete list of 373 references for this chapter is available online at **www.expertconsult.com.**
See inside cover for registration details.

Barnhill RL, Cerroni L, Cook M, et al. State of the art, nomenclature, and points of consensus and controversy concerning benign melanocytic lesions: outcome of an international workshop. *Adv Anat Pathol.* 2010;17:73–90.

Dessinioti C, Stratigos AJ, Rigopoulos D, et al. A review of genetic disorders of hypopigmentation: lessons learned from the biology of melanocytes. *Exp Dermatol.* 2009;18:741–749.

Halder RM, Chappell JL. Vitiligo update. *Semin Cutan Med Surg.* 2009;28:86–92.

Kaplan J, De Domenico I, Ward DM. Chediak-Higashi syndrome. *Curr Opin Hematol.* 2008;15:22–29.

Kopacova M, Tacheci I, Rejchrt S, et al. Peutz-Jeghers syndrome: diagnostic and therapeutic approach. *World J Gastroenterol.* 2009;15:5397–5408.

Northrup H, Au KS. Tuberous sclerosis complex. In: Pagon RA, Bird TC, Dolan CR, et al, eds. *GeneReviews [Internet].* Seattle: University of Washington; 1993–1999: July 13 [updated May 7, 2009].

Scheuerle A, Nelson DL. Incontinentia pigmenti. In: Pagon RA, Bird TC, Dolan CR, et al, eds. *GeneReviews [Internet].* Seattle: University of Washington; 1993–1999: June 8 [updated January 28, 2008].

Su F, Li F, Jin HZ. Extensive Mongolian spots in a child with mucolipidosis II. *Int J Dermatol.* 2010;49:438–440.

Summers CG. Albinism: classification, clinical characteristics, and recent findings. *Optom Vis Sci.* 2009;86:659–662.

Williams VC, Lucas J, Babcock MA, et al. Neurofibromatosis type 1 revisited. *Pediatrics.* 2009;123:124–133.

Vascular Disorders of Infancy and Childhood

Classification of vascular lesions

Vascular birthmarks, or congenital vascular anomalies, are common lesions that may present in a variety of fashions. There has traditionally been a significant amount of confusion regarding the nomenclature of these lesions, and the term 'hemangioma' has been widely used in the medical literature in reference to a variety of different vascular anomalies.[1,2] In 1982, Mulliken and Glowacki proposed a classification system for vascular birthmarks based on clinical and cellular features.[3] This classification was further refined 6 years later in a book,[4] and in 1996, it was adopted as the official classification system for vascular anomalies by the International Society for the Study of Vascular Anomalies (ISSVA). This nomenclature revolutionized the classification of vascular lesions, and is the basis for continued study into the causes of these lesions and their therapy.

According to this classification system (Table 12.1), vascular birthmarks are divided into *tumors* and *malformations*. Vascular tumors are neoplasms of the vasculature. This category includes hemangioma of infancy (the most common vascular tumor), kaposiform hemangioendothelioma, tufted angioma, and pyogenic granuloma. Vascular malformations represent anomalous blood vessels without any endothelial proliferation or cellular turnover. In distinction to infantile hemangioma, these lesions tend to be present immediately at birth and persist for a lifetime. Vascular malformations are further classified according to their predominant components, i.e., capillary malformation (port-wine stain, salmon patch), venous malformation, lymphatic malformation, and arteriovenous malformation. Figure 12.1 pictorially demonstrates the different natural histories of infantile hemangiomas and vascular malformations.

This chapter will include discussion of vascular tumors and tumor syndromes, vascular malformations and malformation syndromes, disorders associated with vascular dilatation, and a few miscellaneous disorders of the cutaneous vasculature.

Vascular tumors and tumor syndromes

Infantile Hemangioma

Infantile hemangioma (hemangioma of infancy) is the most common benign soft tissue tumor of childhood. It occurs in 1–2% of newborns, and at 1 year of age, 10–12% infants of white skin have one.[5,6] Female infants are three times more likely to have hemangiomas than male infants, and the incidence is increased in premature neonates. Although they occur in all races, infantile hemangiomas appear to be less common in those of African or Asian descent.[7] Multiple gestation pregnancy, advanced maternal age, placenta previa and pre-eclampsia also appear to be risk factors for infantile hemangiomas.[8] Although they are traditionally considered to be sporadic lesions, autosomal dominant segregation within families has been described.[9] These lesions vary considerably in their appearance and significance, relating to their size, depth, location, growth pattern, and stage of evolution. Older descriptive terms for infantile hemangiomas include *strawberry, cavernous,* and *capillary.* These terms are no longer useful and should not be used in the era of more specific vascular lesion nomenclature, as discussed earlier and shown in Table 12.1. Although infantile hemangiomas may occur on any part of the body, they most commonly involve the head and neck regions. Facial hemangiomas have been noted to have a non-random distribution, with the majority of lesions occurring on the central face at sites of development fusion.[10] Four primary segments of facial hemangioma distribution have been identified, as shown in Table 12.2.[11]

The pathogenesis of infantile hemangioma is unknown. Positive endothelial cell staining with GLUT1, the erythrocyte-type glucose transporter protein, has been noted in lesions during all of the growth phases.[12] It is absent in other vascular lesions such as vascular malformations and hemangioendotheliomas. This protein is normally expressed in the microvascular endothelia of blood–tissue barriers, such as the brain, retina, placenta, and endoneurium.[7] As such, it has been suggested that infantile hemangioma may originate from invading angioblasts that have differentiated toward a placental cell type or from embolized placental cells, although some data refute a placental trophoblastic origin for these lesions.[13] Further evidence of a potential relationship between human placenta and infantile hemangioma includes the high level of transcriptome similarity between these tissues,[14] and the higher incidence of pathologic placental findings observed from pregnancies resulting in a child with infantile hemangioma compared with those resulting in healthy infants without infantile hemangioma.[15]

Hemangiomas may occur as *superficial, deep,* or *mixed* lesions. The clinical appearance of the lesion depends on the type of hemangioma present. Superficial hemangiomas, when well formed, present as bright red to scarlet, dome-shaped to plaque-like to lobulated papules, plaques, and nodules (Figs 12.2–12.6). They may partially blanch with pressure and are rubbery or non-compressible on palpation. Deep hemangiomas usually present as subcutaneous, partially compressible nodules and tumors, often with an overlying blue hue, prominent venous network, or telangiectasias (Figs 12.7–12.9). These lesions may be warm to palpation. Combined hemangiomas have both a superficial component and a deep component, and occur in up to 25–30% of patients.[16] They present with both the superficial, bright red component and a deeper, blue nodular component (Figs 12.10, 12.11).

Hemangiomas may present with a variety of precursor lesions, and in up to 50% of affected infants, these premonitory marks may be evident at birth.[7] They include areas of telangiectasias (Fig. 12.12), pallor, ecchymotic macules (Fig. 12.13), and even ulceration (Figs 12.14, 12.15).[17] Fully formed hemangiomas may occasionally present at birth, and are termed *congenital hemangiomas*. These lesions are discussed in more detail later.

The natural history of infantile hemangiomas is characteristic. It is notable for a period of growth (the proliferative phase), a period of stability (the plateau phase), and a period of spontaneous regression (the involutional phase). The majority of infantile hemangiomas first become evident at 2–3 weeks of life, with potential continued growth until around 9–12 months of age. The majority of growth, however, occurs during the first 5 months of age, and in those that continue to grow beyond this age, the growth rate is markedly slower.[18] Occasional lesions have a proliferative phase that lasts for >1 year, sometimes as long as 18–24 months. Deep hemangiomas tend to exhibit both a delayed onset of growth, as well as a sustained, longer growth phase.[18] The onset of the involutional phase, which is difficult to predict in any given patient, is marked by a color change from bright red to dull red, purple, or gray (for superficial lesions) (Figs 12.16, 12.17). It may be more difficult to appreciate early involution in deep hemangiomas, but with time these lesions become smaller, more compressible, and less warm. It is estimated that completed involution of infantile hemangiomas occurs at a rate of 10% per year, such that 30% have involuted by 3 years of age; 50% by 5 years of age; 70% by 7 years of age, and >90% by 9–10 years of age.[7,16,19,20] However, it should be remembered that involution does not necessarily imply totally normal skin. Possible residual changes following hemangioma involution include telangiectasias (Fig. 12.18), atrophy (Fig. 12.19), scarring (Fig. 12.20), or fibrofatty masses (Figs 12.21, 12.22). These possibilities must be explained thoroughly to the parents of patients with infantile hemangioma.

Treatment decisions regarding an infantile hemangioma must incorporate many factors. These include the size and location of the lesion or lesions (see below), the age of the patient and growth phase of the hemangioma, associated findings, and the perceived potential for psychosocial distress both for parents and for the patient later in life. The latter is quite difficult to predict, but must be seriously considered in the patient with a conspicuous hemangioma, especially facial. These lesions may be associated with parental disbelief, fear, mourning, and social stigmatization.[21] The major goals of management should be to: prevent or reverse life- or function-threatening complications; prevent disfigurement; minimize psychosocial stress; avoid overly aggressive procedures; and adequately prevent or treat ulceration in order to minimize infection, pain, and scarring.[22] Treatment decisions can be challenging and must include parental input and a thorough risk-to-benefit analysis. Hemangiomas for which further evaluation, referral to a specialist, and/or therapy should be considered are listed in

Table 12.1 Contemporary classification of vascular birthmarks
Vascular tumors
Hemangioma of infancy
Tufted angioma
Kaposiform hemangioendothelioma
Pyogenic granuloma
Hemangiopericytoma
Vascular malformations
Capillary (CM) (i.e., port-wine stain, salmon patch)
Venous (VM)
Lymphatic (LM)
Arterial (AM)
Arteriovenous (AVM)
Complex/combined (i.e., capillary-lymphatic-venous or capillary-venous)

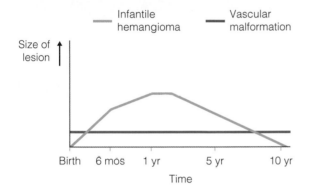

Figure 12.1 Natural history of infantile hemangioma and vascular malformation.

Table 12.2 Distribution patterns of facial infantile hemangiomas			
Segment number/name		**Distribution**	**Comment**
1	Frontotemporal segment	Lateral forehead Anterior temporal scalp Lateral frontal scalp Upper eyelid	Potentially greater risk of associated brain anomalies when PHACES syndrome present
2	Maxillary segment	Lateral cheek Upper lip Spares philtrum, pre-auricular area	
3	Mandibular segment	Pre-auricular area Mandible Chin Lower lip	Potentially greater risk of cardiac defects when PHACES syndrome present
4	Frontonasal segment	Medial frontal scalp/forehead Nasal bridge Nasal tip/ala Philtrum	

Adapted from Haggstrom et al. (2006).[11] PHACES, posterior fossa malformation, hemangioma, arterial anomalies, cardiac anomalies/aortic coarctation, eye abnormalities, sternal clefting/supraumbilical abdominal raphe.

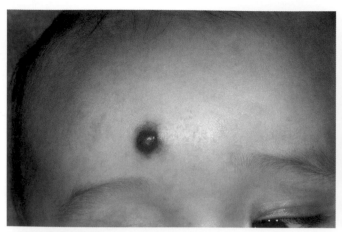

Figure 12.2 Hemangioma, superficial – forehead.

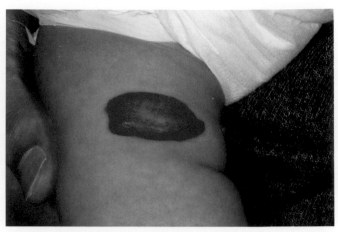

Figure 12.5 Hemangioma, superficial – leg.

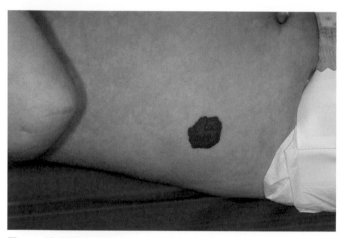

Figure 12.3 Hemangioma, superficial – trunk.

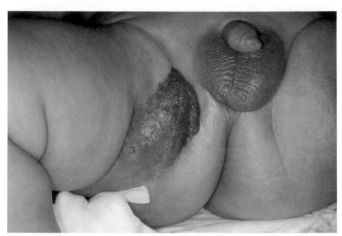

Figure 12.6 Hemangioma, superficial. Note the early ulceration of the lateral inferior portion.

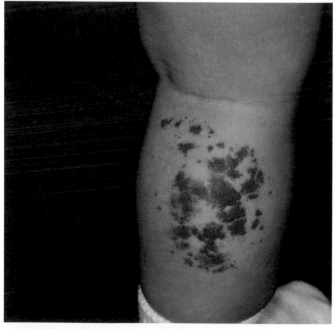

Figure 12.4 Hemangioma, superficial. Note the patchy nature of this lesion, which eventually became confluent.

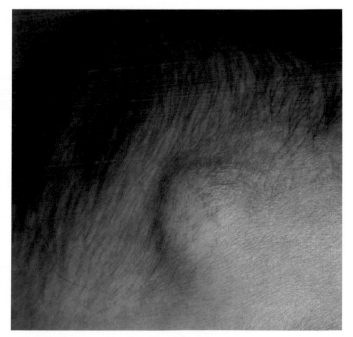

Figure 12.7 Hemangioma, deep. Note the subtle blue hue and surface telangiectasias.

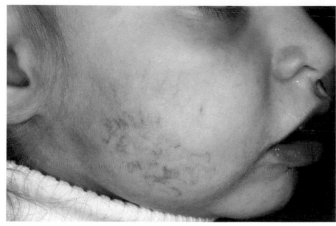

Figure 12.8 Hemangioma, deep. This larger lesion shows the characteristic deep blue hue and surface telangiectasia.

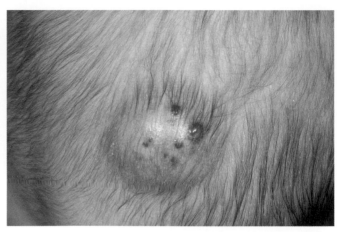

Figure 12.11 Combined hemangioma. This lesion is predominantly deep, with studding of the surface with small, superficial components.

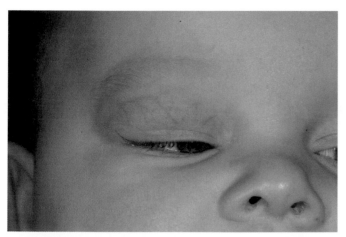

Figure 12.9 Hemangioma, deep. This small, deep lesion resulted in mechanical ptosis, necessitating therapy out of concern for light-deprivation amblyopia. Note the overlying surface telangiectasias.

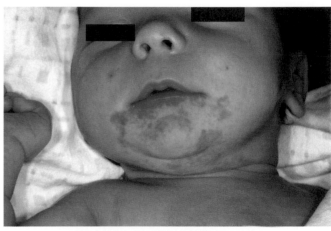

Figure 12.12 Hemangioma precursor, telangiectasias. This lesion might initially be diagnosed as a port-wine stain; within 4 weeks it was thickening, with eventual ulceration of the lip.

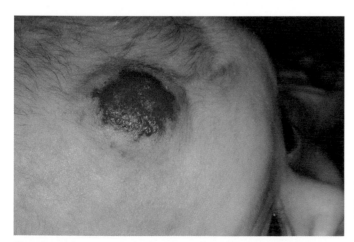

Figure 12.10 Combined hemangioma. Note the larger, deep component and the bright red, superficial component of this combined lesion.

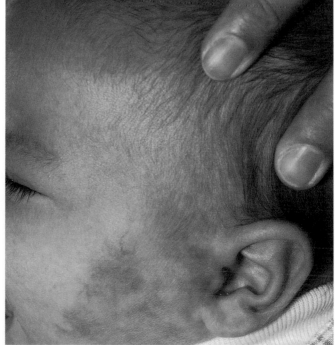

Figure 12.13 Hemangioma precursor, ecchymosis. This 'bruise-like' appearance may be seen before hemangioma proliferation occurs.

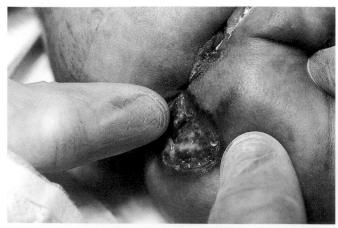

Figure 12.14 Hemangioma precursor, ulceration. This 2-day-old newborn presented with this perianal ulceration; at 3 weeks of age, the ulceration was healing and the lesion had the classic appearance of a superficial hemangioma.

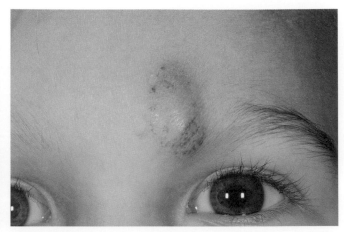

Figure 12.17 Hemangioma, involution phase. The redness has largely resolved and the lesion flattened in this 3-year-old female.

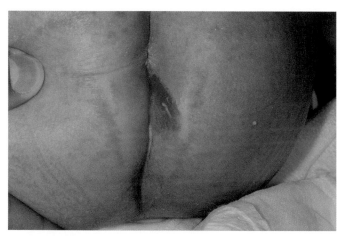

Figure 12.15 Hemangioma precursor, ulceration. This perianal lesion presented at 1 week of age as a vascular plaque with ulceration.

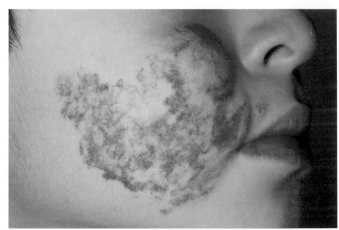

Figure 12.18 Hemangioma, involuted. This lesion demonstrates the residual telangiectasias that may persist after involution of the hemangioma.

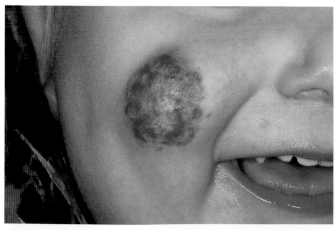

Figure 12.16 Hemangioma, involution phase. Note the patchy vascular appearance in this involuting lesion in a 2-year-old boy.

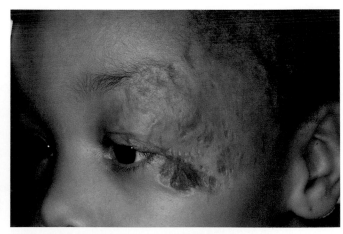

Figure 12.19 Hemangioma, involuted. This hemangioma was very large, with complete obstruction of the visual axis and secondary ulceration. Following involution, atrophy and scarring are both evident.

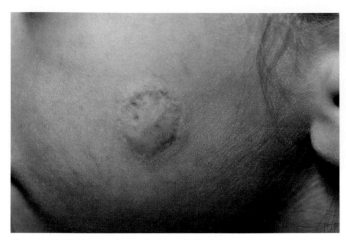

Figure 12.20 Hemangioma, involuted. Residual scarring and atrophy are evident in this fully involuted lesion.

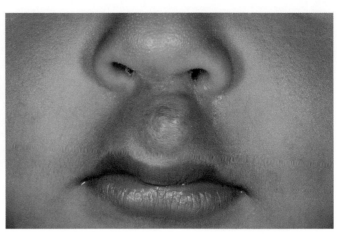

Figure 12.22 Hemangioma, involuted. This philtrum lesion has involuted, but fibrofatty residua remain.

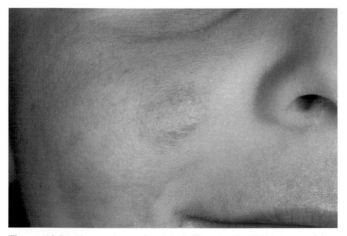

Figure 12.21 Hemangioma, involuted. The cheek of this 4-year-old boy shows the residual fibrofatty tissue that may remain following involution.

Table 12.3 Hemangiomas: Considerations for evaluation, referral, and/or therapy

Life threatening
Function threatening
Periocular
Nasal tip
Ear (extensive)
Lips
Genitalia, perineum
Airway
Hepatic
Large facial
'Beard' distribution[a]
Ulcerating
Lumbosacral
Multiple

[a]See text for discussion.

Table 12.3. (These are discussed in more detail under 'Clinical Variants and Associated Syndromes', below.)

Treatment options for infantile hemangioma are listed in Table 12.4. Probably the most useful principle in the treatment of these lesions is that of *active non-intervention*. This term implies that the physician inquires about the parents' knowledge of the condition, offers education regarding natural history and therapeutic indications, and offers anticipatory guidance and support. Active non-intervention is an appropriate 'therapy' for the majority of infantile hemangiomas, and can be offered by the pediatrician or primary care physician in most instances. Serial photography may be useful for parents of children with hemangiomas, in order to document the gradual spontaneous involution, which may be subtle and underappreciated by them.[16] Referral to support groups and informational resources, like the Hemangioma Investigator Group (www.hemangiomaeducation.org), Vascular Birthmarks Foundation (www.birthmark.org) or the National Organization of Vascular Anomalies (www.novanews.org) is useful for parents of these children.

Corticosteroids are the traditional mainstay of therapy for hemangiomas requiring treatment. They are most often used in the oral form, although both intralesional and topical preparations may be useful. Intralesional corticosteroids are useful for localized lesions. Several injections may be necessary, and periocular lesions should be treated only by a physician experienced in their administration,

given the possibility of embolization of corticosteroid particles and permanent vision loss.[23,24] Topical corticosteroid therapy with clobetasol propionate (a potent, class 1 topical steroid) may be useful for localized hemangiomas.[25,26] In the authors' experience, this therapy is most useful for macular or very thin plaque hemangiomas in the early proliferative stage. This medication should be used cautiously with attention to the risks of atrophy, ocular toxicity, and adrenal suppression.

Oral corticosteroids are the traditional 'gold standard' for complicated infantile hemangioma treatment, although their mechanism of action is poorly understood.[6,24] They are most useful during the proliferative phase, and are generally administered in dosages ranging from 2 to 4 mg/kg per day of prednisolone or prednisone. Some authors advocate doses up to 5 mg/kg per day.[16,27] This therapy is usually continued for several months, with gradual tapering as tolerated. If corticosteroids are tapered too quickly, rebound growth and adrenal suppression may occur. The goals of decreased hemangioma growth or partial shrinkage must be balanced by the risks of long-term therapy. Common side-effects include irritability, weight gain, hypertension, and gastrointestinal upset. Because the immune response is suppressed in patients receiving systemic corticosteroids, live virus vaccinations should not be given during (or within 1 month after discontinuation of) therapy. Although decreased linear growth velocity may occur in treated patients, catch-up growth usually occurs following their discontinuation.[6,7,28]

Table 12.4 Treatments for infantile hemangioma

Treatment	Comment
Active non-intervention	Active emotional support and guidance
Local wound care	When ulcerated: topical antibiotic, non-stick wound dressings, compresses, becaplermin gel
Oral antibiotics	When secondary infection present
Pain control	When ulcerated: may require temporary use of narcotic analgesics
Topical corticosteroids	Potent formulations: may be useful for localized, superficial lesions
Intralesional corticosteroids	Usually triamcinolone; localized lesions; caution with periocular lesions
Oral corticosteroids	Traditional 'gold standard' for systemic therapy; prednisone or prednisolone, 2–4 mg/kg per day
Oral propranolol	Evolving therapy; 2 mg/kg per day; risks include bradycardia, hypotension, hypoglycemia, bronchospasm, hypothermia
Interferon-α	Subcutaneous injection; severe or life-threatening lesions; risk of spastic diplegia
Laser therapy	Usually PDL; mainly useful for ulcerated lesions or residual surface vascularity (i.e., telangiectasias) persisting after involution
Vincristine	Severe or life-threatening lesions; requires venous access; risks include myelosuppression, peripheral neuropathy, extravasation necrosis
Surgical excision	Useful in select situations, i.e., incomplete resolution, disfiguring facial lesions, smaller complicated hemangioma refractory to medical therapy

PDL, pulsed-dye laser.

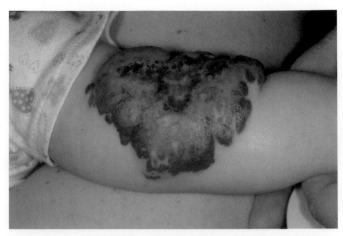

Figure 12.23 Hemangioma, ulcerated. This arm lesion, which was in the proliferative phase, reveals superficial ulceration with crusting.

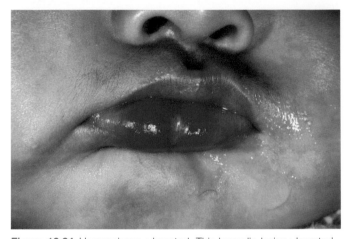

Figure 12.24 Hemangioma, ulcerated. This lower lip lesion ulcerated, with permanent scarring the result.

Adrenal axis suppression is rare, and when it occurs, tends to be reversible.[28,29] Many experts treat concomitantly with H2 blockers (i.e., ranitidine) to diminish the potential for symptomatic steroid-associated gastritis or worsening of gastroesophageal reflux. *Pneumocystis carinii* pneumonia has been rarely reported, which has prompted some experts to recommend trimethoprim-sulfamethoxazole prophylaxis during systemic steroid therapy.[30,31]

Interferon-α2a or 2b, a potent inhibitor of angiogenesis, has been used successfully in patients with hemangiomas refractory to corticosteroid therapy.[32] This medication is administered as a daily subcutaneous injection, in a dose of 1–3 million units/m². Common side-effects include fever, irritability, and malaise. Neutropenia, anemia, and elevation of hepatic transaminases may also occur. However, the most concerning toxicity of this therapy is neurologic in origin, most notably spastic diplegia, which may occur in up to 20% of treated patients.[33,34] Because of this risk, interferon therapy should be reserved for patients with severe life- or function-threatening lesions, and neurologic evaluation before and during therapy should be performed.[35] The chemotherapeutic agent vincristine is also occasionally used for steroid-resistant, life-threatening hemangiomas of infancy.[36–38]

An evolving therapy for infantile hemangioma is propranolol. This non-selective beta blocker, which is traditionally used for cardiac indications such as hypertension or arrhythmia, was incidentally noted to result in marked shrinkage of hemangiomas when administered in two children who had a cardiac indication and who also happened to have hemangiomas.[39] Subsequently, these effects were confirmed in several more patients reported by the same authors. The mechanism of action of propranolol in this setting is unclear. It is most often started at around 0.5 mg/kg per day, with the dose gradually titrated up to 2 mg/kg per day, divided into two to three doses daily. Potential side-effects include hypotension, bradycardia, bronchospasm, hypoglycemia and hypothermia, and this agent should be administered under close supervision with attention to these possible toxicities.[40] Ongoing prospective studies of propranolol for infantile hemangiomas are in progress.

Ulcerated hemangiomas deserve special mention, as this is the most common complication in these lesions, occurring in up to 16% of patients.[41,42] Ulceration usually occurs during the proliferative phase (Fig. 12.23), and is especially common in areas of recurrent trauma such as the lips (Fig. 12.24), genitals (Fig. 12.25), perineum/perianal region, or in moist intertriginous sites, such as

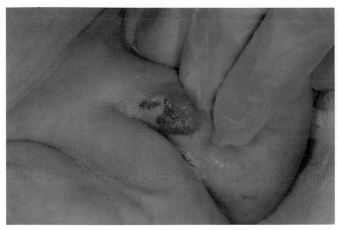

Figure 12.25 Hemangioma, ulcerated. This ulcerated labial hemangioma was very painful, and responded to topical wound care and laser therapy.

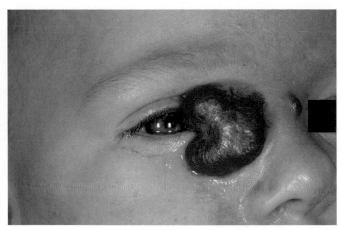

Figure 12.27 Hemangioma, periocular. This large hemangioma was obstructing the visual axis secondary to its size and location.

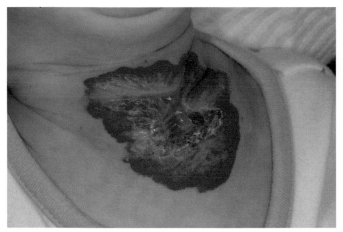

Figure 12.26 Hemangioma, ulcerated. This anterior neck hemangioma ulcerated and healed with marked cribriform scarring.

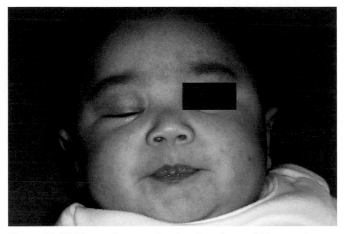

Figure 12.28 Hemangioma, periocular. Superior eyelid hemangiomas may result in ptosis, with a risk for light deprivation amblyopia.

the neck (Fig. 12.26).[42] Tissue breakdown results in bleeding, secondary infection, and pain, and results in permanent scarring. Local wound care with compresses, topical antibiotics (i.e., bacitracin, mupirocin, or metronidazole), and non-stick wound dressings (i.e., petrolatum–impregnated gauze) are useful. Oral antibiotics should be considered if persistent or deep ulceration, drainage, or exudate is present, and should be guided by the results of culture and sensitivity testing. Pain management with acetaminophen or acetaminophen with codeine may be indicated. Topical lidocaine may be helpful for pain control, but should be used with extreme caution given the risks of absorption and possible systemic toxicity. Becaplermin gel, a recombinant human platelet-derived growth factor approved for topical therapy of lower extremity diabetic neuropathic ulcers in patients ≥16 years of age, has been used off-label for the treatment of ulcerated hemangiomas with good success.[43,44]

Pulsed-dye laser (PDL) therapy may be useful in the treatment of ulcerated hemangiomas. This laser emits a wavelength of light specific for oxyhemoglobin, thus imparting specificity for vascular structures ('selective photothermolysis'). Since the light penetrates only 1 mm of depth in the skin, this modality is generally not helpful for non-ulcerated, elevated, or nodular lesions. With ulcerated lesions, though, it is useful in accentuating reepithelialization and decreasing pain.[6,7,45] The choice of PDL therapy must be

individualized to the patient, and occasional patients may show no response or even worsening with this modality.[46] PDL therapy may also be useful for residual surface vascularity following hemangioma involution.

Clinical Variants and Associated Syndromes

Hemangiomas in certain locations may suggest a higher probability of complications or associated findings. Hemangiomas involving various portions of the face may be quite problematic. *Periorbital* hemangiomas may be relatively insignificant when small, but larger lesions (Fig. 12.27) may result in a variety of ocular complications. In addition, any periorbital hemangioma may be indicative of deeper, retrobulbar involvement, which may or may not present with unilateral proptosis. Light deprivation amblyopia may result from visual axis obstruction, most commonly in the setting of significant upper eyelid lesions that result in mechanical ptosis (Fig. 12.28). Astigmatism may occur if the hemangioma compresses the globe, and may result in permanent amblyopia.[7] Rarely, hemangiomas situated near a tear duct may block the drainage system and result in matting and conjunctivitis.[24] Because of these concerns, any child with a periorbital hemangioma should undergo ophthalmologic examination.

Nasal tip/bridge hemangiomas (Fig. 12.29) often require specialist consultation because of their propensity to distort the nasal anatomy (Fig. 12.30), resulting in permanent disfigurement. Slow involution of these lesions may pose significant psychosocial distress to the older child, and the splaying of nasal cartilage combined with redundant fibrofatty tissue following involution may result in the 'Cyrano' nasal deformity (Fig. 12.31). The 'nasal crease sign' refers to a linear, gray atrophic crease in the inferior columella which may occur with segmental facial hemangiomas involving the nose (Fig. 12.32), and which may portend imminent cartilage destruction and nasal collapse.[47] It is for reasons such as these that therapy is frequently indicated for nasal hemangiomas.

Hemangiomas located on the *lips* tend to involute slowly and are more prone to ulceration and bleeding. These changes may in turn contribute to increased pain, feeding difficulties, and permanent scarring. *Ear* hemangiomas may also be cosmetically disfiguring, and when large, may obstruct the auditory canal and result in conductive hearing loss.

Hemangiomas that involve the neck, lower lip, chin, preauricular, and mandibular areas (*beard lesions*) (Fig. 12.33) are clinically important because of the increased risk of associated airway lesions in these patients. In one study, patients with more extensive hemangiomas in this location had up to a 63% incidence of subglottic or upper airway hemangiomatosis.[48] Airway hemangiomas may also occur in the absence of cutaneous hemangiomas. Symptomatic infants usually present within the first few months of life with

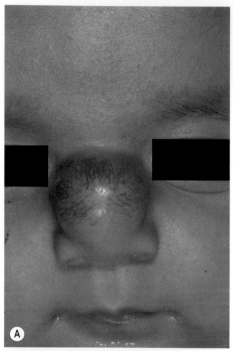

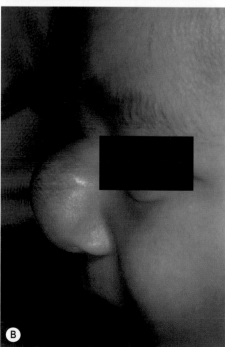

Figure 12.29 Hemangioma, nasal bridge. This large lesion of the nasal bridge (A) results in significant bulbous distortion of the nose (B) and is likely to leave residual deformity.

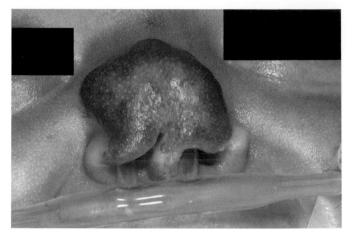

Figure 12.30 Hemangioma, nose. This large nasal lesion resulted in destruction of nasal cartilage and erosion of the columella in this extremely premature infant female.

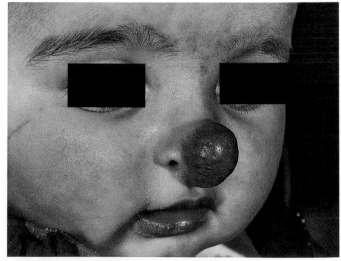

Figure 12.31 Hemangioma, nasal tip. Large nasal tip lesions like this one may leave significant fibrofatty residua, resulting in a 'Cyrano' deformity.

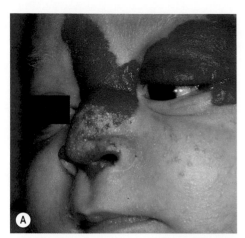

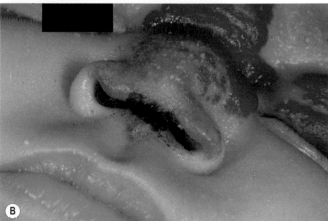

Figure 12.32 Hemangioma, nasal crease sign. This infant girl had a segmental facial hemangioma involving the left forehead, periorbital region, glabella, nasal bridge and nose. At 11 days after noting this linear gray atrophic crease (A), she returned to clinic with complete destruction of the nasal septum and columella, and nasal collapse (B).

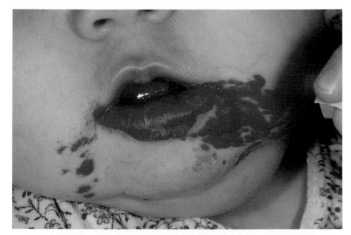

Figure 12.33 Hemangioma, beard distribution. Lesions involving the lower lip, chin, neck, or mandibular regions have a greater risk of airway involvement, as was seen in this female infant.

croup-like cough, hoarseness, and biphasic stridor. Any infant with extensive hemangiomas in this distribution and/or symptoms of upper airway obstruction should be immediately referred for direct visualization of the airway with laryngoscopy. Treatment options in this setting may include tracheotomy, corticosteroids, propranolol, interferon-α, surgical excision, and laser therapy.

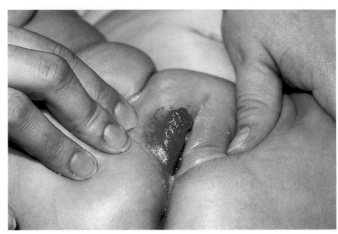

Figure 12.34 Hemangioma, genital. This labial lesion is at increased risk for surface breakdown given its location.

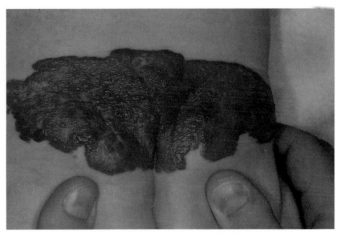

Figure 12.35 Hemangioma, lumbosacral. This large segmental lesion would have an increased risk of association with underlying spinal dysraphism or spinal cord defects. Magnetic resonance imaging in this child was normal.

Parotid hemangiomas often present as mixed superficial and deep lesions, with a prominent deep component of swelling with an overlying blue hue. These lesions may involute more slowly than infantile hemangiomas in other locations and seem to have a poorer response to pharmacologic therapy. *Genital* (Fig. 12.34) and perineal hemangiomas are problematic because of frequent ulceration, with the concomitant risks of bleeding, infection, permanent scarring, and pain. *Hepatic* hemangiomas may be associated with significant morbidity and mortality, and are discussed further in the section 'Diffuse Neonatal Hemangiomatosis', below.

Lumbosacral hemangiomas (Fig. 12.35) are important as they may signal underlying occult spinal dysraphism or spinal cord defects. Tethering of the spinal cord is one of the more common associations,[49] and this anomaly may result in permanent neurological sequelae without release. In addition, sacral hemangioma may be associated with various congenital anorectal or urogenital anomalies, including imperforate anus, renal anomalies, abnormal genitalia, skin tags, and bony sacral anomalies.[50] Any infant with a lumbosacral hemangioma, especially large or segmental types, should be considered for magnetic resonance imaging to assess for such abnormalities.

Segmental hemangiomas are lesions that involve a broad anatomic region (Figs 12.35, 12.36) or a recognized developmental unit.[51] They are often unilateral and sharply demarcated at the midline, although exceptions occur. Segmental hemangiomas are most commonly located on the face. They seem to have a higher frequency of complications and associated abnormalities, such as urogenital anomalies or the PHACES syndrome (see below).[51] In addition, they are more often complicated by ulceration.[10]

The *PHACES syndrome* or *PHACES association* (Online Mendelian Inheritance in Man, 606519) is a constellation of clinical findings associated with extensive facial hemangiomas. Table 12.5 outlines the various features seen in this syndrome. The majority of patients with PHACES syndrome are female.[52,53] Although the pathogenesis of this syndrome is unclear, it appears to be a developmental 'field

defect' that arises around the seventh to tenth week of gestation.[54] The facial hemangiomas in patients with PHACES syndrome are usually large and segmental (Fig. 12.37), and may be unilateral or bilateral. They usually follow an aggressive growth pattern, and ulceration is common.[52] There may be a dermatomal distribution, although these dynamic lesions should not be confused with the static vascular malformations (port-wine stains) associated with Sturge–Weber syndrome (see below). When there is 'beard' area involvement, airway hemangiomatosis should be considered. Hemangiomas may also occur in other nonfacial locations in the setting of PHACES syndrome. Patients presenting with large facial hemangiomas, especially in the presence of ventral developmental defects such as sternal clefting or abdominal raphe, should be screened for this syndrome with magnetic resonance imaging of the brain, echocardiography, ophthalmologic examination, and close neurologic and head circumference examinations. Direct airway visualization should be considered if the infant has extensive involvement in the beard area or symptoms of upper airway obstruction.

Anomalies of the cervical and cerebral vasculature are frequently noted in PHACES syndrome, and these patients appear to have a progressive arterial vasculopathy with risk of arterial ischemic stroke (AIS).[55] Regressive changes in the vascular anomalies have also been noted in some patients.[56] Common CNS structural abnormalities include Dandy–Walker complex, cerebellar hemisphere hypoplasia (ipsilateral to the hemangioma) and arachnoid cysts.[57,58] Aortic arch anomalies, especially aortic coarctation, are the most commonly noted cardiac abnormalities in PHACES syndrome, and tend to be complex and anatomically atypical. These anomalies may remain asymptomatic in the first days of life, until the ductus arteriosus closes, at which time they may result in severe hemodynamic consequences.[59] Table 12.6 lists the recommended evaluation for the infant deemed to be at risk for PHACES syndrome. Diagnostic criteria for PHACE syndrome have been published.[60]

Congenital hemangiomas are lesions that are fully formed at birth. These lesions may follow the typical time course of infantile hemangiomas, may have a more accelerated involution phase, or may persist unchanged. *Non-involuting congenital hemangioma (NICH)* is a specific subtype of infantile hemangioma also known as 'congenital nonprogressive hemangioma.' These lesions may be diagnosed *in utero*, are fully formed at birth, and do not show the postnatal proliferation characteristic of infantile hemangioma.[61] Clinically, NICH lesions are round to ovoid, pink to purple tumors

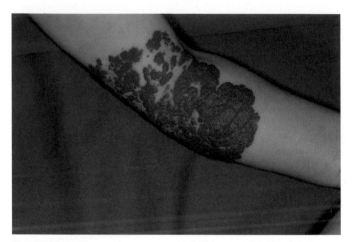

Figure 12.36 Hemangioma, segmental. This superficial hemangioma occupied a large surface area of the distal arm and proximal forearm.

Table 12.5 PHACES syndrome		
Manifestation(s)		**Comment**
P	Posterior fossa malformations	Dandy–Walker malformation; cerebellar atrophy; hypoplasia or agenesis of various CNS structures
H	Hemangioma	Extensive facial; plaque-like; segmental; occasional airway involvement
A	Arterial anomalies	Mainly head and neck; aneurysms, anomalous branches, aberrancy, hypoplasia, stenosis, tortuosity; increased risk of AIS
C	Cardiac anomalies and aortic coarctation	PDA, VSD, ASD, PS, TF, others
E	Eye abnormalities	Horner syndrome, increased retinal vascularity, microphthalmia, optic atrophy, cataracts, coloboma, others
S	Sternal clefting and supraumbilical abdominal raphe	Ventral midline developmental defects

CNS, central nervous system; AIS, arterial ischemic stroke; PDA, patent ductus arteriosus; VSD, ventricular septal defect; ASD, atrial septal defect; PS, pulmonary stenosis; TF, tetralogy of Fallot.

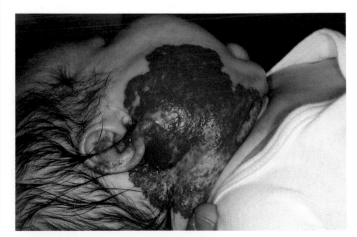

Figure 12.37 Hemangioma, facial. Giant lesions like this one may be associated with the PHACES syndrome.

Table 12.6 Recommended evaluation of the infant at risk for PHACES syndrome

Baseline
Thorough physical examination, including:
   Cutaneous (including assessment for ventral developmental
      defects)
   Cardiac (including pressure measurements in all four
      extremities)
   Respiratory (i.e., for stridor, hoarseness of cry, tachypnea)
   Neurologic (i.e., for hypotonia, developmental delay)
   Abdominal (i.e., for hepatomegaly, abdominal bruit)
MRI/MRA of the brain and neck
Echocardiography
Ophthalmologic evaluation

If indicated
MRI/MRA of the chest
Thyroid function testing (if extensive liver hemangiomatosis)
Other endocrine evaluations (i.e., growth hormone deficiency,
   hypopituitarism, diabetes insipidus)
Airway evaluation/direct laryngoscopy

MRI, magnetic resonance imaging; MRA, magnetic resonance angiography.

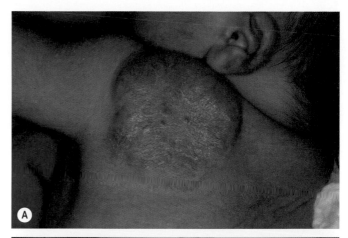

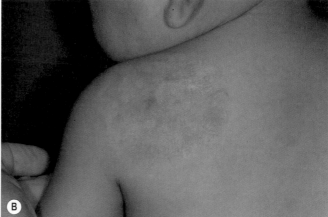

Figure 12.39 Hemangioma, rapidly involuting congenital (RICH). This hemangioma was fully formed at birth (A) and involuted completely by 1 year of age (B).

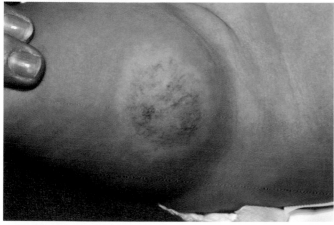

Figure 12.38 Hemangioma, non-involuting congenital (NICH). Characteristic features include prominent surface telangiectasias, and a peripheral rim of pallor.

with overlying prominent telangiectasias and peripheral pallor (Fig. 12.38).[62] Importantly, these lesions also do not undergo the spontaneous involution typical of infantile hemangioma, and hence appear to be a distinctive type of vascular lesion. Interestingly, NICH lesions also have a different histologic appearance and are not immunoreactive for GLUT1.[61]

Rapidly involuting congenital hemangioma (RICH) is the terminology used to describe a congenital hemangioma that undergoes rapid involution early in life. These tumors may present similar to a NICH, or may have the appearance of a typical infantile hemangioma. They often involute completely by 12–15 months of age (Fig. 12.39), and may leave behind dermal and subcutaneous atrophy.[63]

Diffuse neonatal hemangiomatosis

Diffuse neonatal hemangiomatosis (disseminated neonatal hemangiomatosis) describes patients with multiple cutaneous lesions in conjunction with extracutaneous organ involvement. It must be differentiated from *benign neonatal hemangiomatosis*, in which the infant has multiple cutaneous lesions without any symptomatic

visceral lesions or complications.[64,65] Patients with either type of hemangiomatosis may present with only a few or up to hundreds of cutaneous hemangiomas (Figs 12.40, 12.41). Although past data suggested that the risk of internal involvement could be predicted by the number of cutaneous hemangiomas, it appears that there is considerable phenotypic variability, and there is no standard 'cutoff' for number of cutaneous lesions. It is important to remember, in fact, that visceral involvement may occur with few or no cutaneous hemangiomas, although it is more common in the presence of multiple skin lesions. Recent data from a prospective study comparing 151 infants with ≥5 hemangiomas to 50 infants with 1–4 hemangiomas revealed pre-term (<37 weeks' gestational age) delivery and multiple gestation as being associated with a greater risk of having ≥5 hemangiomas. Additionally, 16% of infants with ≥5 skin hemangiomas had hepatic hemangiomas, and those with ≥8 skin hemangiomas had a 2.8 greater probability of having hepatic hemangiomas (ISSVA abstract 2008 and AJM pers comm). Any patient with multiple cutaneous hemangiomas (especially those with ≥5) should receive a thorough physical examination, abdominal ultrasound, and other diagnostic evaluations, as clinically indicated.

The most common extracutaneous site for hemangiomas in patients with diffuse hemangiomatosis is the liver, but multiple other organs can be involved, including the intestine, brain, eyes, spleen, oral mucosa, kidney, and lungs.[66,67] The diagnosis of hepatic hemangiomatosis is usually made clinically, as liver biopsy is undesirable because of the risk of bleeding. Liver lesions may be

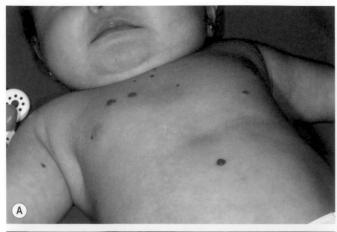

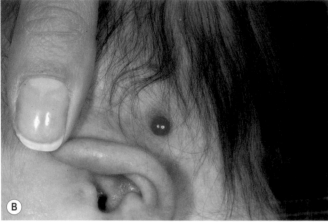

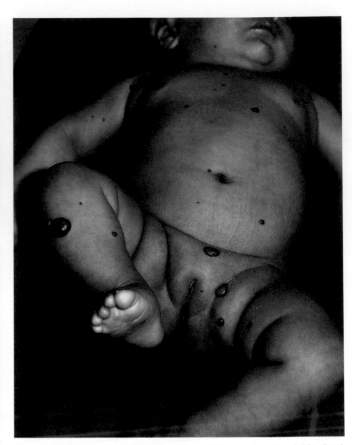

Figure 12.41 Hemangiomatosis, diffuse. This infant had variably sized lesions, and had liver hemangiomatosis.

Figure 12.40 Hemangiomatosis, diffuse. This infant had multiple, small lesions as shown on the trunk (A) and scalp (B), and no internal involvement.

asymptomatic or present with hepatomegaly and congestive heart failure, the latter of which is believed to be due to arteriovenous shunting, which leads to increased venous return and increased cardiac output. Occasionally, anemia or thrombocytopenia is present.

Three patterns of liver hemangiomatosis have been proposed: focal, multifocal, and diffuse.[68] *Focal* lesions are well-defined and solitary on imaging, and are most often clinically asymptomatic. They usually are not accompanied by cutaneous lesions, and tend to involute rapidly. *Multifocal* liver hemangiomas present as multiple spherical tumors, which may be asymptomatic or can result in high-output cardiac failure secondary to arteriovenous shunting. These lesions involute following the same course as seen with cutaneous hemangiomas. *Diffuse* lesions are extensive, may result in near-total replacement of hepatic parenchyma, and may be associated with serious complications including vessel compression, respiratory decompensation, abdominal compartment syndrome, and multiorgan system failure.[68] These lesions may also be associated with severe hypothyroidism.

Abdominal ultrasonography with Doppler studies is the diagnostic modality of choice, although magnetic resonance or computed tomographic imaging may occasionally be necessary. Treatment options may include optimization of cardiac function, corticosteroids, propranolol, interferon-α, vincristine, cyclophosphamide, embolization, hepatic artery ligation, hepatic resection, and liver transplantation.[7,68] Infants with diffuse liver hemangiomas should undergo thyroid hormone monitoring and replacement, as

necessary. Most visceral hemangiomas, like the cutaneous lesions, grow during infancy and, in surviving children, regress during early childhood. Other evaluations that may be useful in the investigation for diffuse hemangiomatosis include complete blood cell counts, stool examinations for occult blood, liver function studies, coagulation studies, urinalysis, echocardiography, electrocardiography, and CNS imaging.

Kasabach–Merritt Phenomenon

Kasabach–Merritt phenomenon (KMP, also known as Kasabach–Merritt syndrome) is characterized by thrombocytopenia (due to platelet trapping), coagulopathy, and microangiopathic hemolytic anemia in association with a rapidly enlarging vascular lesion. It was traditionally felt to be a complication of infantile hemangiomas, but is now known to be associated with vascular tumors other than infantile hemangiomas, namely kaposiform hemangioendothelioma and tufted angioma.[69] These lesions have characteristics that clinically distinguish them from hemangiomas that are discussed below. KMP occurs most often within the first few weeks of life, and presents with sudden enlargement of the vascular lesion, ecchymosis, prolonged bleeding, epistaxis, hematuria, or hematochezia.[70] The cutaneous lesions show purpura, edema, induration, and an advancing ecchymotic margin (Fig. 12.42).[71] In addition to thrombocytopenia, other laboratory findings include anemia, hypofibrinogenemia, elevated D-dimers, fragmentation of erythrocytes on manual smear, and prolonged coagulation studies. The mortality rate is high, from 10% to 30%.

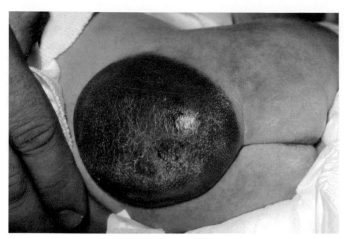

Figure 12.42 Kasabach–Merritt phenomenon. Note the deep purple color of this vascular tumor, which suddenly enlarged and became firm, with accompanying thrombocytopenia.

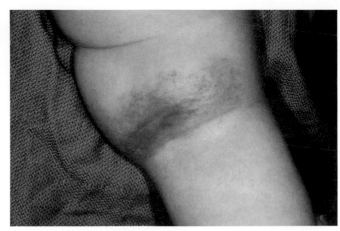

Figure 12.44 Tufted angioma. This vascular plaque was mildly indurated to palpation. (Courtesy of Annette Wagner MD.)

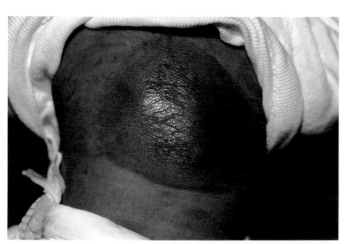

Figure 12.43 Kaposiform hemangioendothelioma. These tumors are characteristically deep purple in color, and may be associated with Kasabach–Merritt phenomenon.

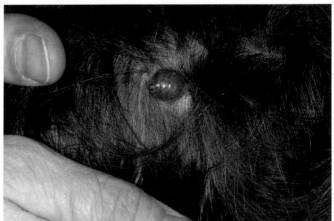

Figure 12.45 Pyogenic granuloma. An acquired, vascular papule.

Kaposiform hemangioendothelioma (KHE)

Kaposiform hemangioendothelioma (KHE) is a locally aggressive vascular tumor, so-named because of the histologic resemblance to Kaposi sarcoma. It presents as a firm, subcutaneous nodule or plaque that expands rapidly and often has a violaceous discoloration (Fig. 12.43).[16,72] Although KHE usually presents in infancy, it may appear months to years later.[73] In addition to involvement of the skin, KHE may involve the deep soft tissues and the bone.[74]

Tufted angioma

Tufted angioma is actually named after its histologic appearance, which reveals groups of dermal capillary tufts. These lesions present clinically as erythematous, annular nodules, or plaques, often with induration (Fig. 12.44).[75,76] Although these lesions may spontaneously involute over years, they tend to persist or gradually progress in most patients. Both KHE and tufted angioma are usually easily distinguished clinically from infantile hemangioma, although in some patients either of the former two may mimic the latter.

Treatment for KMP is challenging. Multiple different regimens have been reported, without randomized studies to support or refute their efficacy. It seems clear that a multidisciplinary approach is optimal, including medical and surgical components of diagnosis and therapy.[71] Hematologic therapies include red blood cell transfusions and administration of fresh frozen plasma and cryoprecipitate. Many experts recommend minimization of platelet transfusions given the risks of further platelet trapping and further expansion of the tumor. High-dose corticosteroids, antifibrinolytics, interferon alpha, vincristine and antithrombotics have been advocated.[77,78] Vincristine was demonstrated useful in a retrospective study of 15 patients with KMP, based on increased platelet count and fibrinogen level, and decreased size of the tumor.[79] Four of these patients had a relapse and were again treated successfully with the agent.[79] Early surgical intervention with full resection has been advocated for smaller lesions where this modality is feasible.[70] Other reported treatments include embolization, compression, and radiation therapy.[80,81]

Pyogenic Granuloma

Pyogenic granuloma (PG) is a common acquired vascular lesion of the skin and mucous membranes in infants and children. It presents as a bright red to red-brown, raised, slightly pedunculated or sessile papulonodule (Figs 12.45, 12.46). The base of sessile lesions may reveal a peripheral collarette of scale (Fig. 12.47). Although they are usually solitary, PG may occasionally present as several lesions. In addition, secondary PG-like proliferations may occasionally occur on the surface of an existing port-wine stain (Fig. 12.48), usually in

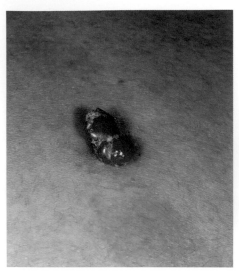

Figure 12.46 Pyogenic granuloma. This lesion is multilobulated.

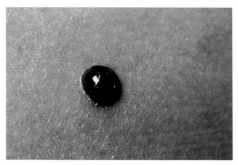

Figure 12.47 Pyogenic granuloma. This lesion demonstrates the collarette of skin around the base of the lesion.

the older child or young adult. PG is prone to superficial ulceration and bleeding, which usually brings the patient to medical attention. The pathogenesis of PG is unknown. Despite the name, the lesions are not considered infectious. Although they may occur on any skin surface, they most commonly appear in areas subject to trauma, especially the hands, fingers, forearms, face, and occasionally the mucosal surfaces of the mouth. They have been described on the penile shaft following circumcision.[82] Although histologic evaluation is usually not necessary for diagnosis, pathologic examination reveals changes similar to those of a well-circumscribed infantile hemangioma.

The traditional therapy for PG is simple shave excision, followed by treatment of the base with electrodesiccation, which achieves hemostasis and seems to help prevent recurrence. Pulsed-dye laser therapy may be useful for the treatment of smaller lesions,[83] and the continuous wave/pulsed carbon dioxide laser has also been demonstrated effective.[84]

Bacillary Angiomatosis

Bacillary angiomatosis (BA) is an exanthem characterized by cutaneous vascular lesions in association with *Bartonella* (previously *Rochalimaea*) infections. *Bartonella* species also cause cat scratch disease, prolonged fever, hepatosplenic disease, ocular manifestations (including Parinaud oculoglandular syndrome), encephalopathy, hemolytic anemia, osteomyelitis, endocarditis, glomerulonephritis and pulmonary disease.[85] BA occurs primarily

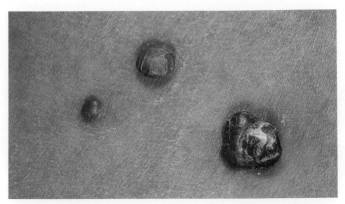

Figure 12.48 This young girl with Klippel–Trenaunay syndrome has multiple, pyogenic granuloma–like papules overlying a port-wine stain of her lower extremity.

in immunocompromised individuals, and was originally described (and once seen quite commonly) in AIDS patients.[86] It has been rarely documented in immunocompetent children.[87,88] BA is caused by *Bartonella henselae* and *Bartonella quintana*, and transmission is via the body louse, a cat scratch, or cat fleas. The lesions may involve various tissues, including brain, bone, lymph nodes, gastrointestinal tract, respiratory tract, and bone marrow. However, skin lesions are the most frequent manifestation, and present as disseminated red to purple papules generally no larger than 1–2 cm in diameter. The clinical differential diagnosis may include pyogenic granuloma and Kaposi sarcoma. Occasionally, BA may present with ulcerative lesions.[89] Liver peliosis is a similar condition affecting the liver and lymph nodes and usually caused by *B. quintana*.

The diagnosis of BA is confirmed by tissue biopsy with histologic examination, which reveals vascular proliferation and plump endothelial cells with the infecting bacilli identified on Warthin–Starry stain. The possibility of HIV infection should be considered if BA is diagnosed. The disorder usually responds to antibiotic therapy with erythromycin, doxycycline, trimethoprim-sulfamethoxazole, or rifampin.

Glomus Tumor

Glomus tumor (glomangioma, glomuvenous malformation) is a benign vascular lesion that usually presents as a blue papule or nodule. It represents a relatively uncommon hamartoma of the glomus body, which is a temperature-regulating arteriovenous shunt that bypasses the usual capillary bed of the dermis. The 'glomus cell', which proliferates in this disorder, is a modified smooth muscle cell. Rarely seen in infants, these lesions may be solitary or multiple and occur in children as well as adults. Occasionally, nodular or plaque-like lesions may also occur.

Solitary glomus tumors, which represent 90% of all lesions,[90] do not appear to have a familial tendency. They are characterized by the clinical triad of paroxysmal pain, local tenderness, and cold sensitivity. Solitary lesions present as a blue-red nodule (Fig. 12.49) from 1 mm to several centimeters in size. They most often appear on the upper extremities, particularly the nail beds, and occasionally on the lower extremities, head, neck, or penis. Although the etiology is unknown, some lesions appear to be associated with previous trauma. The differential diagnosis of a solitary glomus tumor includes venous malformation, blue nevus, melanoma, dermatofibroma, and leiomyoma. If occurring in an infant, hemangioma of infancy may also be in the differential.

In contrast to the solitary type, multiple glomus tumors (often referred to as glomuvenous malformations) are often dominantly

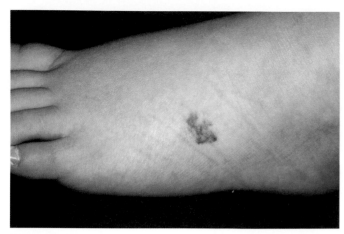

Figure 12.49 Solitary glomus tumor. (Courtesy of Sarah Chamlin MD.)

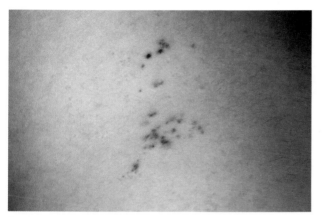

Figure 12.50 Multiple glomus tumors. This patient had multiple, blue papules and papulonodules.

transmitted, may be painful or painless, and vary from a few lesions to several hundred. They are relatively more common in children than adults, and although they can occur anywhere on the cutaneous surface, the majority involve the lower extremities. They may be regionally distributed or generalized, and segmental patterns of presentation have been reported.[91,92] Affected individuals usually have truncating mutations in the glomulin gene.[93] Multiple glomus tumors appear as blue-purple, flat to dome-shaped papules, plaques and nodules (Fig. 12.50) that vary from a few millimeters to several centimeters in size. The differential diagnosis of multiple glomus tumors includes leiomyomas, diffuse hemangiomatosis, and blue rubber bleb nevi.

A congenital variant of glomus tumor has been described and is characterized by a blue-red, nodular plaque that may be painful and tends to grow proportionate with the child's growth.[90] Congenital facial plaquelike glomus tumors may mimic venous malformations and can be quite disfiguring.[94]

Treatment of glomus tumors consists primarily of surgical excision, although this is not a feasible option for patients with multiple lesions, and recurrence tends to be common. Sclerotherapy has been used with some success, as have carbon dioxide lasers.[95] Subungual glomus tumors are usually treated successfully with periungual or transungual surgical excision, although residual nail deformities may result.[96]

Hemangiopericytoma

Hemangiopericytoma is a rare tumor that occurs in both an adult and a childhood form, although children account for <10% of all cases.[97] Congenital lesions are occasionally observed.[98,99] This tumor arises from pericytes, which are smooth muscle cells that surround capillaries. Skin, subcutaneous, and muscular tissues maybe involved, and any part of the body can be affected, the most common location being the lower extremities. Some experts now question whether a majority of lesions previously called hemangiopericytomas actually represent solitary fibrous tumors (originating from fibroblasts).[100]

Hemangiopericytoma may present in a variety of fashions, without a distinctive or pathognomonic appearance. It often presents as a deep soft tissue mass with slow growth. It may be flesh-colored or have a blue-red hue. The diagnosis of hemangiopericytoma is based on the cellular and architectural features on tissue histology.

The prognosis of this tumor in childhood is variable. It appears that children <1 year of age (in which case, it is termed 'infantile hemangiopericytoma') have a better prognosis, with a high response to chemotherapy. In children >1 year of age, the tumor behaves more similar to those in adults and may be more aggressive.[97] Treatment consists of complete surgical resection, when feasible, as well as radiotherapy and rarely chemotherapy.[100]

Angiolymphoid Hyperplasia with Eosinophilia

Angiolymphoid hyperplasia with eosinophilia (ALHE) is an uncommon vascular proliferation disorder occurring most commonly in young adult women, and only rarely in children. It presents as a subcutaneous mass of the head and neck region, especially around the ears or on the scalp. Regional lymph node enlargement and eosinophilia may be present, and treatment is by surgical excision.

Kimura disease is a closely related, yet distinct, chronic inflammatory disorder that occurs primarily in young Asian males. It is characterized by the triad of painless subcutaneous nodules in the head or neck region, blood and tissue eosinophilia, and elevated serum immunoglobulin E levels.[101] Clinically, the lesions of Kimura disease present as solitary or multiple, purple-red papules, nodules, or deep swellings. The parotid and submandibular glands may be involved,[102] as may the oral mucosa, scalp, ears, or orbit. Unilateral cervical lymphadenopathy is commonly present. Laboratory evaluation consistently reveals eosinophilia and increased IgE.[103]

ALHE and Kimura disease may be confused with a variety of other entities, most commonly malignancies such as lymphoma or salivary gland tumors, or histiocytosis. These disorders histologically reveal vascular proliferation with eosinophils and mast cells, and their etiology remains unclear. Treatment options for Kimura disease include surgical excision (although recurrence is common), steroids, chemotherapy, and radiation.

Vascular malformations and malformation syndromes

Salmon Patch

The salmon patch (nevus simplex) is the most common vascular lesion of infancy. It occurs in 30–40% of all newborns and appears as a flat, dull pink, macular lesion on the posterior neck and scalp (Fig. 12.51), glabella (Fig. 12.52), forehead, upper eyelids, and

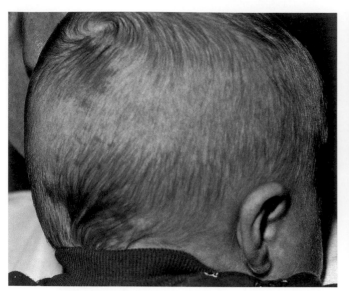

Figure 12.51 Salmon patch. Faint, vascular macules of the occipital scalp.

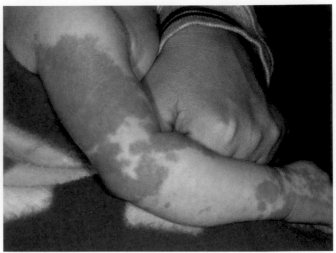

Figure 12.53 Port-wine stain – arm/hand.

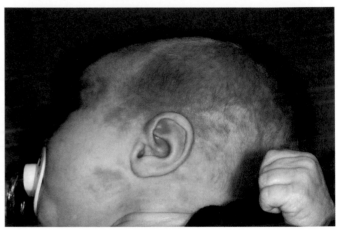

Figure 12.54 Port-wine stain – face/scalp.

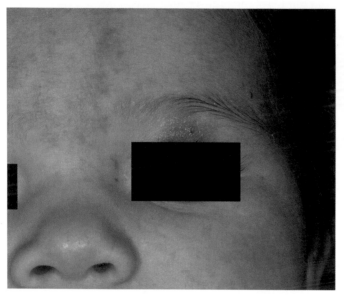

Figure 12.52 Salmon patch. This blanchable vascular patch of the glabella and forehead becomes more prominent with crying or increased body temperature. Note the associated stain over the left superior eyelid.

occasionally the nose or nasolabial regions. When seen on the nape of the neck, it is frequently referred to as a 'stork bite' and, when on the forehead/glabella, as the 'angel kiss'. Although the salmon patch represents the most common form of capillary malformation, it is felt by many to be a form of persistent fetal circulation rather than a true malformation. Although older nomenclature may include salmon patch under the category of 'port-wine stain', this terminology should not be used since these lesions have distinct natural histories and differing significance in terms of potential syndrome associations. Salmon patches are usually isolated lesions without other associated findings.

No treatment is necessary, since 95% of facial salmon patches fade within the first 1–2 years of life. Lesions on the posterior neck or scalp (also known as Unna nevus) may fade, although some of these persist indefinitely. Since they are usually covered by hair,

these lesions do not pose a cosmetic problem. Parents should be educated regarding the common finding of 'reappearance' or accentuation of facial lesions during episodes of crying, breath-holding, straining with defecation, or physical exertion.

Nevus Flammeus/Port-wine Stain

Nevus flammeus, or port-wine stain (PWS), is a congenital capillary malformation that may occur as an isolated lesion or in association with a variety of syndromes. These lesions present as macular (non-palpable) stains with a pink (Fig. 12.53) to dark red (Fig. 12.54) color. Although an early PWS may be indistinguishable from an infantile hemangioma, these lesions are usually distinguished by their congenital presence and their static nature, without the rapid proliferation and thickening that characterizes hemangiomas during the first months of life. PWS may darken progressively over many years, and occasional lesions develop secondary proliferative (pyogenic granuloma-like) vascular blebs on their surface (Fig. 12.48). They may also become somewhat thickened and raised later in life. Port-wine stains are often, but not always, unilateral and the most common site of involvement is the face, although they may occur on any cutaneous surface.

The significance of PWS is two-fold: the potential cosmetic impact of the lesion (especially facial PWS) on the developing child, and the potential for syndrome associations. Table 12.7 lists the various

Table 12.7 Port-wine stain associated syndromes
Sturge–Weber syndrome
Klippel–Trenaunay syndrome
Parkes–Weber syndrome
Phakomatosis pigmentovascularis
Proteus syndrome
Cobb syndrome
Bannayan–Riley–Ruvalcaba syndrome
Beckwith–Wiedemann syndrome
Von Hippel–Lindau disease
Rubinstein–Taybi syndrome
Wyburn–Mason syndrome
Roberts syndrome
Coat disease

Adapted from Requena and Sangueza (1997).[104]

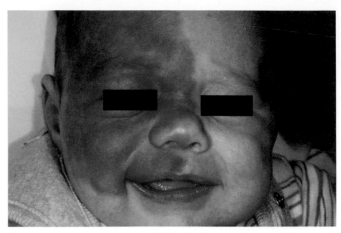

Figure 12.55 Port-wine stain. This lesion involves both the V1 and V2 trigeminal dermatomes in this infant with Sturge–Weber syndrome. (Courtesy of Annette Wagner MD.)

congenital syndromes that may have PWS as a component. Several of these will be discussed later.

PWS lesions show little tendency toward spontaneous improvement or involution, and traditional therapy was limited to the use of tinted 'cover-up' cosmetics (such as Covermark or Dermablend). Laser therapy (the word 'laser' is an acronym for *l*ight *a*mplification by *s*timulated *e*mission of *r*adiation) has revolutionized the treatment of these lesions, and the flashlamp-pumped tunable pulsed-dye laser (PDL) is the most accepted laser for PWS treatment.[105] PDL allows the targeting of short bursts of energy at intravascular hemoglobin (because of the specific wavelength of the emitted light) within the lesional vessels, while sparing other tissue components and thus allowing for precise therapy. Treatment of PWS with PDL is usually performed in conjunction with local or general anesthesia, depending on the size and location of the lesion and the age of the patient. Some smaller lesions can be treated without the need for anesthesia. PDL therapy is usually performed over several sessions, separated in time by 6–8 weeks, and can be quite effective in lightening these lesions, thereby minimizing their cosmetic and psychosocial significance. Although there may be psychological benefits of PDL therapy of facial PWS early in life,[106] studies evaluating efficacy as a function of patient age have yielded mixed results. Some authors have reported optimal treatment response in patients <1 year of age, whereas others have found no evidence that treatment during early childhood is more effective than treatment at a later age.[107,108] In general, lesions over bony areas of the face (i.e., the forehead), lateral cheeks, chest and proximal arms seem to respond best to PDL therapy, while those over the mid-face and distal extremities respond less.[105] PWS of the central face may not respond as well, given the deeper vessels which may escape the effect of the PDL.[109]

Sturge–Weber syndrome

Sturge–Weber syndrome (SWS, encephalofacial or encephalotrigeminal angiomatosis) is a neuroectodermal syndrome characterized by a PWS in the distribution of the first (ophthalmic) branch of the trigeminal nerve (V1) in association with leptomeningeal angiomatosis (presenting usually with seizures) and glaucoma. There are rare reports of patients with classic brain and ophthalmic findings of SWS in the absence of facial PWS.[110–113] The etiology of SWS remains unclear.

Patients with SWS have a PWS in a V1 distribution (Fig. 12.55), and may also have multidermatomal or more extensive cutaneous involvement. Overall, it appears that around 8% of patients with a trigeminal PWS have associated glaucoma and/or seizures.[114] Involvement of the V1 dermatome seems to be consistent in all

patients.[113] Involvement of the other trigeminal dermatomes may be useful in predicting the risk of SWS. In one study, involvement of V1, V2, and V3 was associated with an increased incidence of SWS, as was bilateral trigeminal involvement.[113,114] Another study comparing unilateral to bilateral facial PWS found a higher frequency of glaucoma and leptomeningeal angiomatosis with bilateral involvement, and greater risk of CNS involvement when there was complete (vs incomplete) involvement of V1.[115] Although the exact innervation of the lower eyelid is controversial (V1 vs V2), it seems that involvement of both upper and lower eyelids portends a significantly higher risk of SWS.[113,114] When PWS lesions are unilateral, there is usually a sharp demarcation at the midline.

Central nervous system disease is another component of SWS. Seizures are the most common CNS feature, and often have their onset during the first year of life. The seizures of SWS may be difficult to control, and both early onset and increased seizure intensity are associated with future developmental and cognitive delay.[113,116] Headaches (including migraines), stroke-like episodes, focal neurologic impairments, cognitive deficits and emotional and behavioral problems, including depression, violent behavior, and self-inflicted injury, are also more common in SWS.[113,117] Low self-esteem is common in relation to the facial PWS.

Leptomeningeal angiomatosis is a classic component of the syndrome, and lesions are frequently ipsilateral to the cutaneous vascular stain. Cerebral atrophy is a frequent radiologic finding, as is enlargement of the choroid plexus and venous abnormalities. Magnetic resonance imaging is the modality of choice for identifying these changes, although computed tomography scans are better at detecting the classic cortical calcifications, which are also seen.[118] These calcifications follow the convolutions of the cerebral cortex and are characterized by double-contoured parallel streaks of calcification ('tram lines'). Intracerebral calcifications may be visible during early infancy, and can frequently help confirm the diagnosis before other characteristic features are present. Diffusion MRI, postcontrast fluid-attenuated inversion recovery (FLAIR) imaging, and high-resolution blood oxygen level dependent (BOLD) magnetic resonance venography may be useful in the imaging of suspected SWS.[117]

Ocular involvement occurs in around 60% of patients with SWS.[113,104] Glaucoma is the most frequent ocular finding, and it may present at any time between birth and the fourth decade. It may be unilateral or bilateral, with the latter being more common in patients with bilateral facial PWS. Vascular malformations of the eye in patients with SWS may involve the conjunctiva, episclera, choroid, and retina.[119] Other eye findings include nevus of Ota, buphthalmos, and blindness.[104,120]

Care of the child with SWS should be multidisciplinary. Dermatologic, neurologic, and ophthalmologic follow-up is indicated and the primary care provider must provide anticipatory guidance and support. Other specialty services may become necessary, including plastic surgery, neurosurgery, interventional radiology, and physical and occupational therapy. Referral to support organizations is useful. The Sturge–Weber Foundation (www.sturge-weber.com) provides education and support to individuals with this condition and other disorders associated with PWS.

Although the primary management for seizures is with pharmacologic agents, surgical therapy may become necessary. Visually guided lobectomy with excision of the angiomatous cortex is considered the primary surgical approach in patient with focal lesions.[121] Hemispherectomy is often advised for patients with intractable seizures and unihemispheric involvement. This radical therapy is often successful, with decreased seizure activity and, in some patients, cognitive and behavioral improvement.[122,123]

Phakomatosis pigmentovascularis

Phakomatosis pigmentovascularis (PPV) is a term used to describe the association of a nevus flammeus (PWS) with a pigmented nevus or, in some cases, a nevus anemicus. PPV has traditionally been classified into four types. More recently, a fifth type of PPV has been proposed as the concomitant findings of cutis marmorata telangiectatica congenita and mongolian spots.[124] The classification of PPV is shown in Table 12.8. Nevus anemicus is a distinct vascular birthmark characterized by blanching of cutaneous blood vessels, hence presenting as a 'white' (actually vasoconstricted) patch of skin (Fig. 12.56) that becomes unnoticeable when the surrounding skin is blanched with a glass slide ('diascopy'). The cause of PPV is unclear, but 'twin spotting' has been hypothesized as the genetic explanation.

The most common form of PPV is type II, consisting of nevus flammeus and dermal melanocytosis (i.e., mongolian spots, nevus of Ota) (Fig. 12.57). Without extracutaneous involvement, the subtype designation 'a' is used (i.e., PPV type IIa). When systemic involvement is present, the subtype designation 'b' is used (i.e., PPV type IIb). Systemic involvement usually consists of similar changes to those seen in Sturge–Weber syndrome or Klippel–Trenaunay syndrome.[125] This involvement is usually related to the body surface area affected by the vascular lesion.[126] In one series, nevus of Ota was a common associated finding.[127]

Therapy for the cutaneous lesions of PPV is generally not necessary, although PDL treatment may be useful for the nevus

flammeus. Lesions of dermal melanocytosis may or may not fade spontaneously with time.

Klippel–Trenaunay and Parkes–Weber syndromes

Klippel–Trenaunay (KT) syndrome is a sporadic disorder characterized by the triad of vascular malformation, venous varicosity, and hyperplasia of soft tissue and bone. The vascular malformation is most often a capillary malformation of the PWS type. The various lesions of KT syndrome are usually distributed on the same extremity, although other areas may be involved. The lower extremity is the most common location affected. When arteriovenous malformations are also present, patients have been invariably referred to as having Klippel–Trenaunay–Weber (KTW) syndrome or Parkes–Weber syndrome.[104,128]

Patients with KT syndrome present with a capillary malformation, which may vary from fairly localized, faint lesions to extensive, bright red or purple stains (Figs 12.58, 12.59). These lesions are usually present at birth or become evident during early infancy. Prominent superficial veins may be present, and venous varicosities frequently develop with aging, being present in nearly all patients over 12 years of age.[128] These lesions may become quite large and

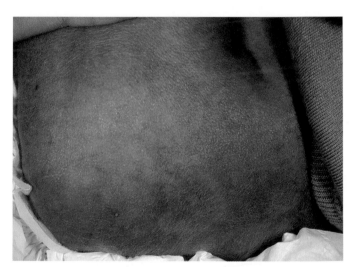

Figure 12.56 Nevus anemicus. Note the subtle area of hypovascular blanching on this toddler's abdomen.

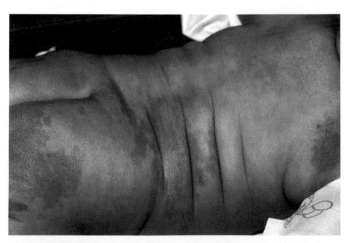

Figure 12.57 Phakomatosis pigmentovascularis type II. This infant has port-wine stains in combination with dermal melanocytosis (mongolian spot, nevus of Ito).

Type[a]	Findings
I	Nevus flammeus + epidermal nevus
II	Nevus flammeus + dermal melanocytosis ± nevus anemicus
III	Nevus flammeus + nevus spilus ± nevus anemicus
IV	Nevus flammeus + dermal melanocytosis + nevus spilus ± nevus anemicus
V	Cutis marmorata telangiectatica congenita + dermal melanocytosis

Table 12.8 Classification of phakomatosis pigmentovascularis

[a]Further subdivided into: A, skin abnormalities only; B, skin abnormalities and systemic abnormalities.

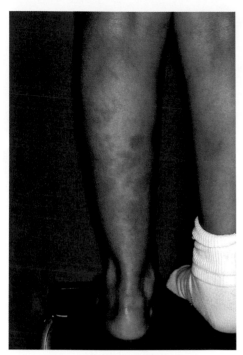

Figure 12.58 Klippel–Trenaunay syndrome. Lower extremity port-wine stain with mild hemihypertrophy.

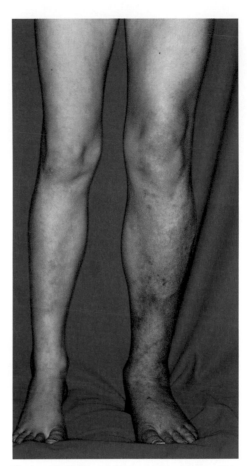

Figure 12.59 Klippel–Trenaunay syndrome. This patient has the characteristic triad, including port-wine stain, hemihypertrophy, and venous varicosities. (Courtesy of Sarah Chamlin MD.)

tortuous, and may predispose patients to episodes of thrombophlebitis. Hypertrophy of the affected body part is another component of the syndrome, and usually presents with increased limb girth and length (Fig. 12.60). The majority of this hypertrophy is related to soft tissue and fat overgrowth, although bony hypertrophy is also observed.[128] Although the cause of this overgrowth is unknown, local hyperemia and augmented arterial flow related to the vascular abnormalities are hypothesized etiologic factors.

Lymphatic disease seems to be more common than originally thought in patients with KT syndrome. This component may be manifested as lymphangiectasia, large lymphatic malformations, lymphedema, vascular blebs (Fig. 12.61), and pseudoverrucous papules. Patients with sharply demarcated and 'geographic' vascular stains may have an increased likelihood of lymphatic involvement.[129]

Complications of KT syndrome, in addition to occasional thrombophlebitis as mentioned previously, include coagulopathy, congestive heart failure (in the presence of hemodynamically significant AV malformation), pulmonary embolism, stasis dermatitis, cutaneous ulcerations, and bleeding. Orthopedic difficulties related to the overgrowth include compensatory scoliosis and hip dislocation. Facial involvement may result in premature dental eruption, facial asymmetry, and malocclusion.[130] Pain is a potentially debilitating problem for KT syndrome patients, and may be related to multiple causes, including superficial or deep thrombosis, cellulitis, calcifications, arthritis and neuropathic origins.[131] Treatments for KT syndrome are primarily supportive, and may include compression garments, chronic pain therapy, laser therapy for the cutaneous stain, and vascular/orthopedic surgical procedures as needed. The clearest indication for surgical therapy is leg length discrepancy, which is projected to exceed 2 cm at skeletal maturity and which can be treated with epiphysiodesis in the growing child.[132] Physical and occupational therapy should be considered, and referral to the Klippel–Trenaunay Support Group (www.k-t.org) is strongly encouraged.

Proteus syndrome is a rare and sporadic disorder characterized by postnatal overgrowth of multiple tissues. This overgrowth may involve the skin and subcutis, connective tissues, central nervous system, and viscera.[133] The involvement characteristically occurs in a patchy (mosaic) and asymmetric pattern. Proteus syndrome was named after the Greek god Proteus, who had the ability to assume various forms to avoid capture.[134] Joseph Merrick, whose life was characterized in the story of *The Elephant Man*, is believed to have had Proteus syndrome, although he was originally thought to have had neurofibromatosis type 1. The etiology of Proteus syndrome remains unclear, although there are some reports of a potential association with mutations in the tumor suppressor gene *PTEN* (see also Ch. 9).

Cutaneous manifestations of Proteus syndrome include connective tissue hamartomas, which primarily involve the palms and soles, resulting in cerebriform hyperplasia (Fig. 12.62). Lipomas and extensive fatty hyperplasia may be found in the subcutaneous tissues as well as more diffusely, at times involving body cavities, muscles, and limbs, and regional absence of fat may also occur. Epidermal nevi are common. A variety of cutaneous and subcutaneous vascular malformations may occur, including capillary, venous, and lymphatic malformations. Patchy hypoplasia of the dermis may occur, resulting in prominent cutaneous venous structures.[135]

Other features of Proteus syndrome include disproportionate overgrowth, which may involve the extremities, hands, feet, digits (macrodactyly, Fig. 12.63), skull (macrocephaly exostoses), vertebrae, external auditory meatus, and viscera.[136] Dysmorphic facial features are occasionally present, and include dolichocephaly,

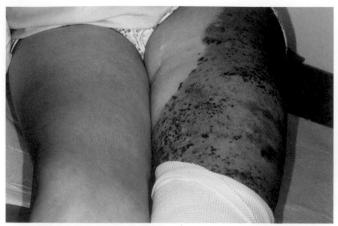

Figure 12.60 Klippel-Trenaunay syndrome. This young girl has massive hemihypertrophy, and her vascular malformation reveals multiple small thromboses, which are often quite painful. (Courtesy of Annette Wagner MD.)

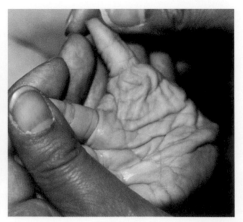

Figure 12.62 Proteus syndrome, cerebriform palmar hyperplasia.

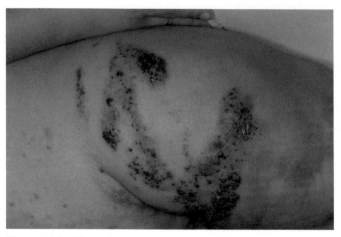

Figure 12.61 Klippel-Trenaunay syndrome with vascular blebs. Note the purple, translucent papules overlying the vascular stain on the lower extremity of this young boy.

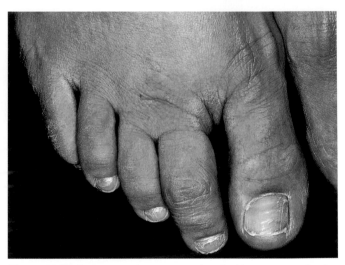

Figure 12.63 Proteus syndrome, macrodactyly. Note overgrowth of the second toe.

elongated facies, low nasal bridge, downslanting palpebral fissures, and wide or anteverted nares. Adenomas of the ovaries or parotid glands may occur with increased frequency in patients with Proteus syndrome. Hemimegalencephaly is the most frequent CNS finding, and ocular manifestations may include strabismus, nystagmus, high myopia, cataracts, and retinal pigmentary abnormalities.[137,138]

Diagnostic criteria for Proteus syndrome, which include general/nonspecific criteria (mosaic distribution of lesions, sporadic occurrence, and progressive course) as well as multiple specific criteria, may be useful both clinically and in the research arena.[139] Evaluation and management of the patient with Proteus syndrome may include skeletal survey, magnetic resonance imaging of clinically affected areas, and consultation with dermatology, genetics and orthopedics when necessary. Both the medical and emotional aspects of the disorder must be considered. Supportive counseling and referral to the Proteus Syndrome Foundation (www.proteus-syndrome.org) are useful.

Bannayan–Riley–Ruvalcaba syndrome

Bannayan–Riley–Ruvalcaba (BRR) syndrome (see Ch. 9) is an autosomal dominant, multiple hamartoma syndrome caused by mutations in the *PTEN* gene. The hallmarks of BRR syndrome are macrocephaly, lipomas, penile lentigines, and vascular malformations. The latter have been inconsistently described in the literature as 'hemangiomas' or 'angiomas' but are actually vascular malformations, usually of the capillary type. Arteriovenous malformation has also been described in patients with BRR syndrome.[140]

Cobb syndrome

Cobb syndrome (cutaneomeningospinal angiomatosis) consists of the association of a cutaneous vascular malformation with a vascular malformation involving the same metamere of the spinal cord. The cutaneous and spinal cord lesions usually correspond within a segment or two of the involved dermatome.[141] The skin lesions present as a dermatomal capillary malformation, with or without a deeper vascular component and occasionally with hyperkeratosis of the surface suggestive of an angiokeratoma. The importance of recognizing this cutaneous lesion lies in the resultant ability to image the spine and refer for neurosurgical therapy before symptoms ensue. Neurological symptoms related to the spinal cord vascular malformation may include root pain, motor dysfunction, paresthesias, and spastic paralysis.[141,142]

Evaluation of the patient with a dermatomal capillary malformation should include magnetic resonance imaging of the corresponding region of the spinal cord, with consideration for spinal angiography. Treatment options may include surgery (when feasible), endovascular embolization, radiation and steroid therapy.

Beckwith–Wiedemann syndrome

Beckwith–Wiedemann syndrome (BWS) is a genetic overgrowth syndrome characterized most classically by visceromegaly, macroglossia, various developmental defects, and neonatal hypoglycemia. It is the most common of the overgrowth syndromes.[143] BWS is a multigenic disorder with dysregulation of the expression of imprinted genes residing in the 11p15.5 region.[144] The inclusion of BWS in this section relates to the common occurrence of a facial capillary malformation involving the mid-forehead, glabella, and upper eyelids. This malformation may extend to involve the nose and upper lip in some patients.

Clinical features of BWS, which are variable, include omphalocele, macrosomia, and macroglossia. Overgrowth may be generalized or limited to specific body regions, and may be associated with an advanced bone age. In addition to omphalocele, other abdominal wall defects include umbilical hernia, prune belly sequence, and inguinal hernia. Visceromegaly may involve the kidneys, liver, spleen, and pancreas. Hypoglycemia is the most common laboratory finding, and tends to regress during early infancy. Patients with BWS have an increased risk of malignant tumors, including Wilms' tumor, adrenocortical carcinoma, and hepatoblastoma.[145] Perinatal features include prematurity, polyhydramnios, enlarged placenta, distended abdomen, and large fetal size.[143] Prenatal ultrasound may be useful in detecting the latter four features, enabling an early diagnosis of the syndrome.[143]

Venous Malformation

Venous malformation (VM) is a fairly common slow-flow type of vascular malformation present at birth. Various inaccurate names have been used to describe these lesions in the literature, including venous angioma, cavernous angioma, and cavernous hemangioma. It should be remembered that VM, like all vascular malformations, is a non-proliferative collection of abnormal vessels distinct from infantile hemangioma and other proliferative vascular tumors. They usually grow with the child. Although these lesions are present at birth, they occasionally may not become obvious until later in life. In addition, VM may rapidly enlarge following trauma, and occasionally this may be the initial presentation.

VM tends to present as blue to purple nodules in the skin (Fig. 12.64). Surrounding veins maybe prominent, and calcified phleboliths may be present within the lesion.[104] These are the result of spontaneous local venous thrombosis within the malformation. Most VM are asymptomatic, although they may occasionally become painful in association with their gradual enlargement and pressure on surrounding structures. Although most VM are isolated, they may occur in association with other syndromic features, such as in Maffucci syndrome and blue rubber bleb nevus syndrome (see below). VM can occur in any body location, although head and neck lesions tend to be the most extensive.[146]

The diagnosis of VM can be confirmed with CT or MR imaging (with or without venography) or Doppler ultrasonography. Plain radiographs may reveal the calcifications associated with phleboliths (which present as painful, firm nodules). Other complications of VM (in addition to thromboses) include disfigurement with psychosocial distress (Fig. 12.65), pain, limitation of motion, bleeding coagulopathy (usually localized intravascular), and functional compromise related to location of the lesion. Treatment is difficult, and may include compression with elastic stockings (which helps to limit swelling, decrease pain, and decrease the risk

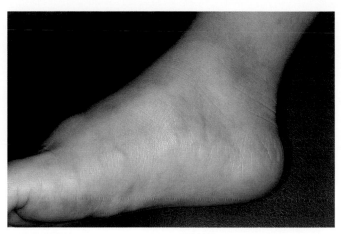

Figure 12.64 Venous malformation. Note venous prominence of the medial and plantar surfaces, and swelling of the dorsal foot.

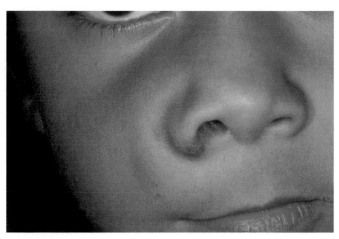

Figure 12.65 Venous malformation. This blue nodular plaque involved the right medial cheek and lateral naris, and became more disfiguring as this young boy grew older, posing a psychosocial concern.

of coagulopathy in extremity lesions), surgery, physical therapy, and percutaneous sclerotherapy. Low-dose aspirin therapy may be useful in patients prone to thrombotic changes within the lesions. A multidisciplinary approach to therapy is desirable, with the goals of improving cosmesis, decreasing pain, limiting bony deformities, and maintaining function.

Maffucci syndrome

Maffucci syndrome is a rare, congenital non-hereditary disorder characterized by the combination of dyschondroplasia and vascular malformations. The cutaneous lesions in this disorder are compressible, red-blue papules and nodules most consistent with venous malformations. They may develop thrombi and phleboliths, with the associated calcifications visible on plain radiography.[147] These vascular malformations may occur anywhere on the skin surface, but are often more extensive on one side of the body and have a preference for the hands and feet.[148] In addition to these lesions, lymphatic malformation[149] and spindle cell hemangioendothelioma[150] (a proliferative vascular tumor) are occasionally present. The vascular malformations of Maffucci syndrome may involve extracutaneous sites in some patients, including mucosal regions, bones, the respiratory tract, and the gastrointestinal tract.

In addition to the vascular malformations, patients with Maffucci syndrome have enchondromas, which are the result of a developmental abnormality in cartilage formation (dyschondroplasia). These lesions start to develop during early infancy, in conjunction with the vascular anomalies. They present as hard nodules over areas of long bones, hands, fingers, and feet. Occasionally they may enlarge and become so numerous as to result in grotesque deformity. Radiographically, enchondromas appear as irregular cystic lucencies. Other progressive skeletal abnormalities (marked bony deformities, pathologic fractures) may occur, as may neurologic deficits related to cerebral encroachment of skull enchondromas.

A significant risk in patients with Maffucci syndrome is that of malignancy, especially chondrosarcoma, which tends to arise from preexisting enchondroma lesions (up to 40% of which may transform into chondrosarcomas).[151] Other malignancies may also occur with increased frequency in these patients. Intracranial chondrosarcoma may rarely occur.[152]

Blue rubber bleb nevus syndrome

Blue rubber bleb nevus syndrome (BRBNS) is a rare disorder characterized by the presence of cutaneous and gastrointestinal venous malformations. Other visceral organs may occasionally be involved. Although usually a sporadic disorder, autosomal dominant inheritance has been reported.[104,153]

Patients with BRBNS present at birth or during early childhood with numerous blue to purple, soft, compressible nodules (Fig. 12.66). The lesions range in size from a few millimeters to 4 cm. Any area of the skin may be involved, as well as mucosal surfaces of the mouth and genitalia. With time, the lesions increase in both size and number. One of the diagnostic features is the ability to compress the nodules, leaving an empty wrinkled sac that then refills rapidly upon withdrawal of the pressure. Gastrointestinal involvement is characterized by hematemesis or melena with chronic anemia. The small bowel is the most common site of GI tract involvement, but lesions can occur anywhere from the mouth to the anus.[153] Blood loss may at times be severe, necessitating transfusion. Various orthopedic complications owing to adjacent venous malformations may occur, and include bowing and pathologic fractures. Central nervous system involvement with vascular malformations may also be a component of the syndrome.[154,155]

BRBNS may be diagnosed based on the clinical presentation, although other diagnostic studies may be necessary, and may include CT, MR, barium studies, skin biopsy, and upper and lower gastrointestinal tract endoscopy. Capsule endoscopy and intraoperative enteroscopy have been reported as useful for thorough investigation of the small bowel.[156] Treatment of the condition is primarily supportive, and may include iron replacement, transfusions, endoscopic sclerotherapy or band ligation, and resection of severely involved portions of the GI tract. The response to pharmacologic agents is variable. Subcutaneous octreotide, a somatostatin analog used to decrease splanchnic blood flow in patients with GI bleeding, may be useful in decreasing the need for blood transfusion.[157]

Arteriovenous Malformation

Arteriovenous (AV) malformations are rare vascular malformations consisting of both arterial and venous components with AV shunting. These lesions may vary in their clinical presentation, from macular erythema to thin vascular plaques to larger pulsating nodules or masses with an audible bruit. A murmur may be appreciated upon auscultation. AV malformations may display aggressive growth patterns and result in functional or cosmetic deformity and, in some patients, cardiovascular compromise. They are the most

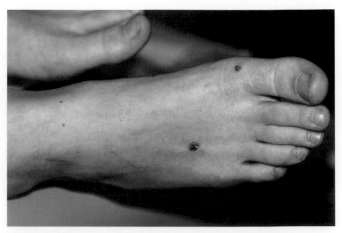

Figure 12.66 Blue rubber bleb nevus syndrome. This patient has multiple blue-purple, compressible papules and papulonodules.

endangering type of vascular anomaly. Diagnostic confirmation of an AV malformation may involve ultrasound with color Doppler study, CT or MR evaluation, or arteriography. Treatment is notoriously difficult and includes surgical excision, embolization, and amputation.

Disorders of lymphatic vessels

The lymphatic system is a complex network of thin-walled vessels responsible for carrying tissue fluid to the venous system.[158] Anomalies of the lymphatic system may include lymphedema and lymphatic malformations. Lymphedema occurs as a result of aplasia or hypoplasia of lymphatic channels or obstruction of lymphatic pathways. Lymphatic malformations occur as a result of hyperplasia of the lymphatic network. Older terminologies for lymphatic malformations are common in the literature, including lymphangioma, cavernous lymphangioma, lymphangioma circumscriptum, and cystic hygroma. These malformations are probably best described, in accordance with the modern classification, as lymphatic malformations, and further classified as macrocystic, microcystic, or combined.

Lymphatic malformations (LM) are composed of interconnected lymphatic channels, and present differently depending on the size of these aberrant vessels.

Macrocystic LM are composed of large interconnected lymphatic channels and cysts. They have been most commonly referred to as cystic hygroma or cavernous lymphangioma in the literature. They may occur in any location, although the head, neck, axilla, and chest are the most common sites. Although macrocystic LM was once considered a diagnostic sign of Turner syndrome, it is now known that these lesions may be associated with other karyotypic abnormalities and malformation syndromes.[158] Other potential associations include Down syndrome, trisomy 18, trisomy 13, and Noonan syndrome. Teratogens may also be associated with macrocystic LM.

Macrocystic LM presents as a large, somewhat translucent mass lying under normal-appearing skin (Fig. 12.67). It enhances with transillumination. Acute hemorrhage within a LM may result in swelling, tenderness, and purple discoloration. Diagnostic confirmation can be made with ultrasound, CT, or MR examination, and prenatal diagnosis is possible with ultrasonography. Prenatal and neonatal complications include lymphedema, facial deformity, and effusions (pleural, pericardial, abdominal). Hydrops fetalis, heart

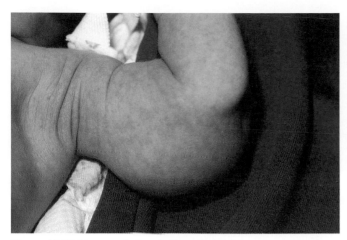

Figure 12.67 Macrocystic lymphatic malformation.

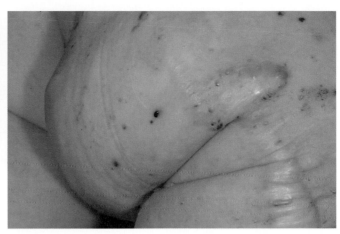

Figure 12.69 Combined microcystic/macrocystic lymphatic malformation with hemorrhage. There are numerous surface blebs (microcystic component), many of which reveal hemorrhage. This young boy also had a large underlying macrocystic lymphatic malformation. Note the surgical scars from past excisions.

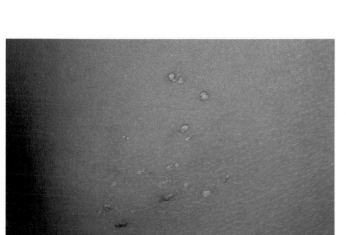

Figure 12.68 Microcystic lymphatic malformation. Note the multiple flesh-colored, translucent papules, with hemorrhagic changes in some of the lesions.

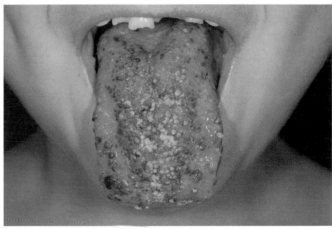

Figure 12.70 Microcystic lymphatic malformation of the tongue. This boy has extensive involvement of his tongue with translucent papules, several of which reveal hemorrhage. The white color of some lesions relates to maceration from the moist environment of the mouth.

failure, respiratory compromise, and intrauterine demise may occasionally occur. Treatment options for macrocystic LM include surgical excision, serial aspirations, and sclerosing therapy with bleomycin, OK-432 (picibanil), or doxycycline.[159–161]

Microcystic LM are a more common form of lymphatic malformation, representing microscopic aggregations of small lymphatic channels. These lesions usually present as cutaneous plaques or nodules with superimposed changes in the overlying skin. These surface changes consist of erythematous to flesh-colored papules, which may be somewhat translucent (Fig. 12.68), accounting for the traditional analogy with frog spawn. The differential diagnosis of the superficial component of microcystic LM may include warts, molluscum contagiosum, herpes simplex, herpes zoster, and epidermal nevus. Perianal lesions may be misdiagnosed as anogenital condylomata.[162] Hemorrhage may occur within the superficial component (Fig. 12.69), and intermittent swelling or bruising may be a feature. Other complications include intermittent leakage of lymph fluid, inflammation, and secondary infection.

Microcystic LM often present during infancy, and may involve any area of the skin or mucosa. Oral lesions are quite common, most often involving the tongue (Fig. 12.70) or cheek. Microcystic LM is often (but not always) treatable by surgical excision.

Lymphedema

Lymphedema refers to a set of conditions characterized by interstitial accumulation of lymphatic fluid, and may be primary or secondary (Table 12.9). Primary lymphedema is related to anatomic abnormalities in the lymphatic system, which may include hypoplasia of vessels, absence of lymphatic valves, and/or impaired contractility of the structures. Secondary lymphedema, which results in disruption or obstruction of lymphatic pathways, arises as a consequence of disease, surgery, or radiotherapy.[163,164] Primary lymphedema most often involves the lower extremity, whereas upper extremity involvement is more common in secondary lymphedema.

Lymphedema presents as edema of the affected extremity. Early in the course the involved region is puffy (Fig. 12.71), whereas later in the course the area becomes more fibrotic and indurated. Secondary cutaneous changes may be present, including a 'peau d'orange' appearance of the overlying skin, pigmentary changes, and recurrent episodes of cellulitis. When a lower extremity is involved, swelling

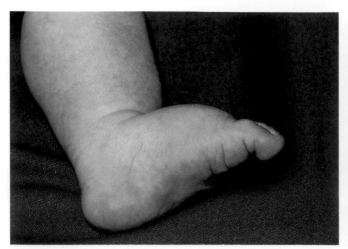

Figure 12.71 Congenital lymphedema. Note the fullness of the dorsal aspect of the foot in this infant male.

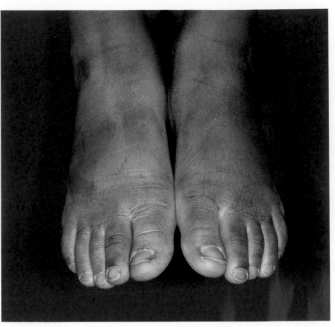

Figure 12.72 Lymphedema. This 10-year-old girl had long-standing, non-pitting edema of her feet bilaterally.

Table 12.9 Classification of lymphedema (L)

Type	Comment
Primary	
Congenital L	Single extremity or multiple limbs
L praecox	Pubertal or post-pubertal females
L tarda	Usually after 35 years
Milroy disease	AD form of congenital familial L; linked to mutation in flt4 locus of VEGFR-3 gene
Lymphedema–distichiasis	AD; L in association with distichiasis (supplementary row of eyelashes); linked to mutations in FOXC2 gene
Hypotrichosis-lymphedema-telangiectasia	AD; linked to mutation in SOX18 gene
Secondary	
L occurring after disruption of lymphatic pathways by:	
Disease Surgery Radiation therapy Burns Pregnancy	i.e., filariasis i.e., lymph node dissection
Large/circumferential wounds to the extremity	

Adapted from Rockson (2001)[163] and (2008).[164] L, lymphedema; AD, autosomal dominant.

of the dorsal aspect of the foot (Fig. 12.72) is common, with a characteristic blunt, 'squared off' appearance of the digits.[163]

Congenital lymphedema may involve a single extremity (upper or lower) or multiple limbs, and the changes are present at birth. Lymphedema praecox, which usually occurs in females around the time of puberty, presents as edema of the foot or ankle, or rarely with upper extremity involvement.[165] Milroy disease is an inherited form of lymphedema, usually occurring with an autosomal dominant pattern of transmission.

The diagnosis of lymphedema is usually a clinical one. Useful findings include edema, fibrosis, *peau d'orange* appearance of the skin, and a positive 'Stemmer sign' (inability of the examiner to tent the skin at the base of the digits in the involved extremity).[164] In cases where further diagnostic confirmation is necessary, available options include indirect radionuclide lymphoscintigraphy, lymphangiography, MR or CT imaging, and Doppler ultrasonography. Therapy for lymphedema includes massage (manual lymphatic drainage), elevation, compression garments, exercise, and meticulous skin care in an effort to prevent skin breakdown and infection. Intermittent pneumatic compression may be useful. Surgical approaches are reserved for patients with severe disease who have failed conservative measures, and include excision of lymphedematous tissues or lymphaticovenous anastomoses.

Gorham Syndrome

Gorham syndrome (Gorham–Stout disease, disappearing bones, vanishing bone disease, massive osteolysis) is a rare condition of unknown origin characterized by progressive bony destruction with intramedullary proliferation of thin-walled vascular structures. Many affected patients have cutaneous vascular lesions as well. Although there is no consensus on the nature of these vascular elements, several authors have proposed that they represent lymphatic vessels.

Patients with Gorham syndrome are usually children or young adults, and they present with pathologic fractures and/or bone pain. Nearly any bone may be involved, but most common are the ribs, scapula, clavicle, humerus, pelvis, spine, femur, and mandible.[166] It may occur in a focal fashion, with spread to contiguous bony structures, and occasionally with multicentric, widespread involvement. Non-skeletal manifestations include respiratory distress, pleural effusions, ascites, and chylothorax. Chylothorax is an uncommon, but often fatal, complication of Gorham syndrome, and may be associated with malnutrition, lymphocytopenia, and infection.[166] The diagnosis of Gorham syndrome is confirmed by the finding of osteolytic changes on radiography without reparative bone formation and in the absence of soft tissue mass, and histologic evaluation of biopsied material.[167]

The natural history of Gorham syndrome is variable, and therapy is difficult. Surgical resection, bone grafting, fractionated radiation therapy, and chemotherapy have all been used with variable results.

Angiokeratomas

Angiokeratomas are skin lesions characterized by ectasia (dilatation) of the superficial vessels of the dermis and hyperkeratosis of the overlying epidermis. They present as hyperkeratotic, dark red to purple or black papules (Fig. 12.73) measuring between 1 mm and 10 mm in diameter. Several types of angiokeratoma are recognized, and although these lesions usually occur sporadically, they may occasionally be associated with potentially serious metabolic disease.

Solitary or multiple angiokeratomas

These usually occur on the lower extremities of young adults. They are blue to black in color, and may sometimes be confused with malignant melanoma. These lesions may be related to preceding trauma or injury.

Angiokeratoma circumscriptum

This presents as a plaque composed of multiple, clustered red to purple papules. These lesions may be present at birth or develop during childhood.

Angiokeratoma of Mibelli

This occurs on the dorsal fingers or toes or in interdigital spaces. These lesions appear during childhood or adolescence, are more common in females, and are inherited in an autosomal dominant fashion.

Angiokeratoma of Fordyce

This is a condition that presents with numerous red to purple papules on the scrotum or vulva of adults. Scrotal lesions may be seen in association with varicocele or inguinal hernia.

Although the above forms of angiokeratoma occur in the absence of associated serious abnormalities, the lesions may occasionally be seen in the setting of potentially serious metabolic disorders.

Angiokeratoma corporis diffusum (ACD)

ACD is the name used to describe these lesions which present as numerous dark red to black papules distributed primarily on the abdomen (Fig. 12.74), genitals, buttocks, and thighs ('bathing-trunk' distribution). The most common disorder associated with ACD is Fabry disease, a rare X-linked recessive disorder due to deficient α-galactosidase A. The genetic cause is a mutation in the *GLA* gene (encoding α-galactosidase A), most often point mutations but occasionally small and large deletions or insertions.[168] Males with Fabry disease have an accumulation of glycosphingolipids, which results in dysfunction of the heart, kidneys, and nervous system. Acral paresthesias and acral and/or abdominal pain occur, often within the first decade of life. Other findings in Fabry disease include corneal and lenticular opacities, hypohidrosis, progressive neuropathy, progressive renal and heart failure, and cerebral artery thrombosis.[169] The angiokeratomas of Fabry disease may number in the thousands and tend to cluster in the iliosacral areas, on the scrotum, and around the umbilicus. The first lesions frequently appear on the scrotum and must be differentiated from angiokeratoma of Fordyce. A majority of patients have pinpoint macular purplish spots on the lips, particularly near the vermilion border of the lower lip. These lesions are smaller than those on the skin. The tongue is generally not affected, but hemoptysis and epistaxis have been reported with involvement of the buccal and nasal mucosae. In addition to the typical cutaneous lesions, fine telangiectasias have been described in the axillae and on the upper chest. Enzyme replacement therapy with recombinant α-galactosidase A is available for treatment of Fabry disease, although it may not lead to complete resolution of symptoms in all patients.

There are other inherited lysosomal storage diseases that may have associated angiokeratomas of the skin. Fucosidosis is an autosomal recessive lysosomal storage disease in which deficiency of α-fucosidase results in multisystem accumulation of oligosaccharides and glycosphingolipids.[170] This disorder is characterized by progressive neuromotor deterioration, seizures, coarse facial features, dysostosis multiplex, visceromegaly, and growth retardation. Recurrent respiratory infections may also occur. The predominant cutaneous feature of fucosidosis is ACD, which may resemble that seen in Fabry disease. In distinction to the lesions of Fabry disease, however, the angiokeratomas associated with fucosidosis tend to occur earlier in life, usually around 5 years, and display a more generalized distribution. Other dermatologic features reported in fucosidosis include hypo- or hyperhidrosis, cutaneous vascular abnormalities, and transverse nail bands.[170]

Other metabolic disorders that may be associated with ACD include GM1 gangliosidosis, galactosialidosis, β-mannosidosis,

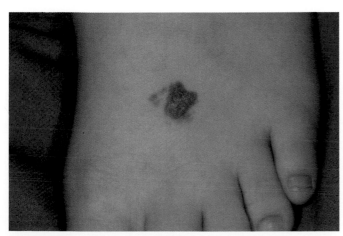

Figure 12.73 Angiokeratoma. This was an isolated lesion in an otherwise-healthy 14-year-old female.

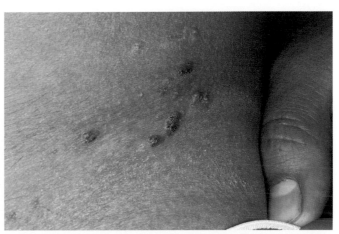

Figure 12.74 Angiokeratoma corporis diffusum in Fabry disease. This 19-year-old male had multiple lesions, involving the trunk, groin, and thighs.

sialidosis, and aspartylglycosaminuria. All of these conditions are inherited in an autosomal recessive fashion, and the diagnosis is made by urine oligosaccharide analysis or enzyme assay.

Disorders associated with vascular dilatation

Livedo Reticularis

Livedo reticularis is a mottled or reticulated, blue-red discoloration of the skin that occurs predominantly on the lower extremities (Fig. 12.75), and less commonly on the trunk or upper extremities. Ulceration may occasionally occur. Although the pathogenesis of livedo reticularis is unclear, the changes seem to be related to slow blood flow and decreased oxygen tension. Exposure to cold environments usually intensifies this vascular pattern. The distinction between livedo reticularis and cutis marmorata may be clinically difficult, although cutis marmorata tends to disappear with rewarming and may be seen as a normal finding in up to 50% of infants.

The significance of livedo reticularis lies in its possible association with a variety of systemic disorders (Table 12.10; see also Ch. 22). Associated disorders may include coagulopathies, autoimmune diseases (including systemic lupus erythematosus, dermatomyositis, rheumatoid arthritis, and scleroderma), systemic vasculitides (including polyarteritis nodosa, Wegener's granulomatosis, and Churg–Strauss syndrome), arterial occlusive disease, and antiphospholipid antibody syndrome. Sneddon syndrome is characterized by the association of livedo reticularis and cerebral ischemic arterial events, such as stroke or transient ischemic attack.[171,172] These patients may have associated antiphospholipid antibodies.

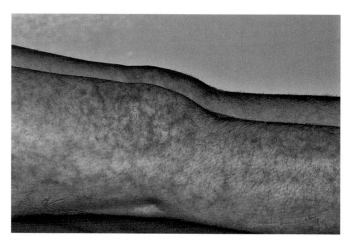

Figure 12.75 Livedo reticularis.

Table 12.10 Associations with livedo reticularis
Autoimmune diseases
Coagulation disorders
Hematologic aberration or malignancy
Hormone-secreting tumors
Arterial occlusive diseases
Sneddon syndrome (cerebral ischemic arterial disease)
Antiphospholipid antibody syndrome
Systemic vasculitis
Paraproteinemia
Drugs

Moyamoya disease, a rare chronic cerebrovascular occlusive disease involving the circle of Willis, has also been reported in conjunction with cutaneous livedo reticularis in a child.[173] In rare instances, recurrent small ulcerations may develop on the lower legs and feet in adults with idiopathic livedo reticularis, and has been termed *livedo vasculitis or livedoid vasculitis*. Mild hypertension and edema of the legs, ankles, and feet may occur in this setting. A variant of this disorder (*atrophie blanche*) is characterized by white atrophic areas, hyperpigmentation, and ulceration with telangiectatic vessels at their periphery. Atrophie blanche usually occurs on the ankles and dorsal feet in young to middle-aged women, but may also occasionally occur in children.

Although there is no specific treatment for livedo reticularis, therapeutic options include avoidance of cold, anticoagulant therapy (especially for patients with ulceration), and treatment of the underlying associated condition.

Flushing and the Auriculotemporal Nerve Syndrome

Flushing, a transient diffuse erythema of the blush areas (the face, neck, and/or adjacent trunk), is caused by dilatation of superficial cutaneous blood vessels mediated by neural mechanisms or the direct action of a vasodilator substance on vascular smooth muscles. Flushing can be caused by emotion; the ingestion of alcoholic or hot beverages; food additives, such as sulfites, nitrites, and monosodium glutamate (MSG) in what has been termed the 'Chinese restaurant syndrome'; calcium channel blockers such as nifedipine; disulfiram (Antabuse); carcinoid syndrome (a disorder caused by a neoplasm that produces large amounts of serotonin and bradykinin); and other tumors that produce catecholamines such as neuroblastoma, renal cell carcinoma, or ganglioneuroma.

The *auriculotemporal nerve (Frey) syndrome* is a phenomenon characterized by unilateral (rarely bilateral) flushing, sweating, or both in the distribution of the auriculotemporal nerve. These changes usually occur in response to gustatory or olfactory stimuli. Frey syndrome is believed to be related to increased irritability of the cholinergic fibers, and possibly to misdirected regeneration of fibers during the healing that follows trauma. It may result following parotid surgery, central nervous system disease (cerebellopontine angle tumors), cervical sympathectomy, and radical neck dissection.[174] When it occurs in one of these settings, it is usually in an adult.

Frey syndrome in infants and children is less common, and is most often noted after the introduction of solid food.[175] It may occasionally be misdiagnosed as a food allergy reaction,[175,176] although the unilaterality of the eruption in most cases should distinguish it from an allergic process. In children, the presentation of Frey syndrome is often limited to facial flushing (without sweating), and these changes occur most often following ingestion of fruits (especially citrus fruits and apple), candy or a favorite food. Perinatal birth trauma from assisted forceps delivery, with subsequent damage to the auriculotemporal nerve, may be responsible in many pediatric cases. In those with no history of trauma to the parotid area, congenital aberration of the auriculotemporal nerve pathway between parasympathetic and sympathetic fibers is suspected. The clinical presentation is that of bright erythema extending in a patch from the corner of the mouth towards the preauricular cheek and as far as the frontotemporal scalp (Fig. 12.76), which occurs within a few seconds after ingestion of the responsible food. The changes resolve spontaneously over 30–60 minutes, and therapy is unnecessary. Spontaneous resolution may occur after a period of time.

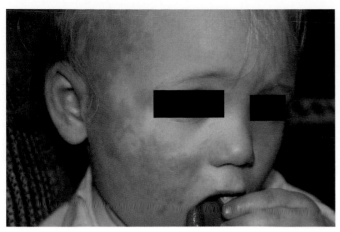

Figure 12.76 Auriculotemporal nerve (Frey) syndrome. Facial flushing extended from the mouth angle to the frontotemporal scalp in this young girl, just seconds following ingestion of solid foods (in this instance, fruit snacks).

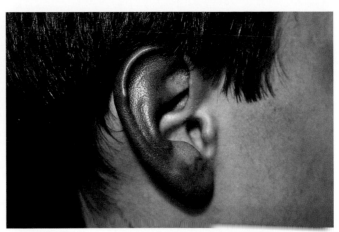

Figure 12.77 Red ear syndrome. This young boy had recurrent episodes of painful burning and redness of the ear.

Erythromelalgia

Erythromelalgia is a rare condition characterized by paroxysmal intense burning pain, erythema, and warmth of the skin. It most often involves the distal limbs, especially the feet, but also the hands. It may occur in primary or secondary forms, and is quite uncommon in childhood. When it does occur in children, it is usually idiopathic.[177,178] Secondary erythromelalgia has been reported in association with various disorders, including hematologic diseases (i.e., polycythemia, malignancy, spherocytosis, and thrombotic thrombocytopenic purpura), embolic disease, cardiovascular disease, connective tissue disorders (including lupus erythematosus, rheumatoid arthritis, and vasculitis), infectious diseases, neurologic disease, and musculoskeletal disease, and as a drug-induced condition.[179] In patients with an associated myeloproliferative disorder, the findings of erythromelalgia may precede the diagnosis by months to years.[180]

Erythromelalgia presents with striking erythema and warmth of the affected distal extremity, which is worsened by heat and relieved by cooling and elevation. It is most often bilateral, although it may occasionally be unilateral. Occasionally, proximal extension of the warmth and redness up the extremity are noted. When severe, erythromelalgia may have a profound effect on quality of life and sleep quality, and may disrupt work and social functioning.[179] Multiple therapies have been utilized for erythromelalgia, with variable success. These include cooling, topical anesthetic agents, aspirin, serotonin-reuptake inhibitors, tricyclic antidepressants, anticonvulsants, calcium channel blockers, sympathetic blocks, sympathectomies, and psychotherapy.[178,179,181]

Red ear syndrome (*erythromelalgia of the ears*) deserves mention here. This entity presents with a painful, burning, bright red ear (Fig. 12.77), which occurs paroxysmally and is usually unilateral. Both ears may be involved. Some have termed this presentation 'otomelalgia' given its similarity in presentation to erythromelalgia. Red ear syndrome may represent a migraine variant, and in fact may be associated with classic symptoms of migraine headache.[182] Other potential associations include irritation of the third cervical root, temporomandibular joint dysfunction, or thalamic syndrome.[183] Patients with this presentation may respond to therapies directed at migraine headache or a tricyclic antidepressant.[184] Cool compresses of the ears often relieves discomfort acutely.

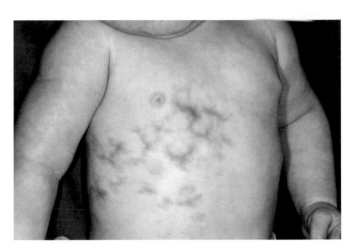

Figure 12.78 Cutis marmorata telangiectatica congenita. The reticulate mottling was limited to the chest in this newborn male.

Cutis Marmorata Telangiectatica Congenita

Cutis marmorata telangiectatica congenita (CMTC, congenital generalized phlebectasia) is a condition characterized by either localized or generalized reticulate erythema. Although the clinical findings may resemble physiologic cutis marmorata, the changes of CMTC do not disappear with rewarming and may be associated with other abnormalities.

Patients with CMTC present with the skin changes either at or shortly after birth. Clinical examination reveals red to violaceous, reticulate, marbled, or mottled patches (Figs 12.78, 12.79). The changes may be limited to a localized region of the body or an extremity, or may show a diffuse pattern of involvement. When localized, the distribution tends to be segmental with a sharp demarcation at the midline.[185] The skin changes are accentuated by a decrease in the ambient temperature. CMTC lesions may resemble livedo reticularis as well as cutis marmorata, and occasionally atrophy or ulceration may be present. The color of the skin lesions may vary from light pink to dark purple.

Additional anomalies may be present in patients with CMTC. A common finding is body asymmetry, especially limb hypoplasia on the affected side.[186,187] Limb hyperplasia may also occasionally occur.[188] Other vascular anomalies may be present in patients with

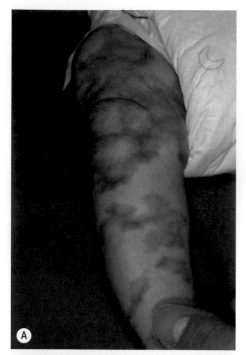

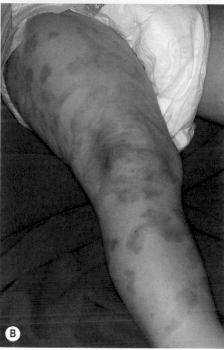

Figure 12.79 Cutis marmorata telangiectatica congenita. This blue-purple, reticulate mottling on the leg of this 2-month-old male (A) does not disappear with rewarming, which distinguishes it from typical cutis marmorata. Marked fading was noted at 2 years of life (B).

associations, most patients with CMTC present with only minor associated anomalies or disease limited to the skin. The incidence of associated findings is unclear, and varies in the literature from 18% to 89%.[186,188,191] In the authors' experience, the majority of patients do not have associated major anomalies.

The combination of CMTC with macrocephaly, abnormal somatic growth, craniofacial and skeletal anomalies, developmental delay, neurologic abnormalities, mental retardation, and connective tissue abnormalities has traditionally been termed *macrocephaly-CMTC*, and is felt by some to be a distinct phenotype within this spectrum of disorders.[190,192] More recently, it has been suggested that the vascular lesions seen in this setting are more consistent with reticulate port-wine stains and that this constellation is more appropriately termed *macrocephaly-capillary malformations (M-CM)*.[193,194] Centrofacial capillary malformations seem to be common in these patients, most notably involving the nose and philtrum.[193,194]

The pathogenesis of CMTC is unclear. Histologic examination, when skin biopsy has been performed, reveals dilated capillaries and veins in the dermis. Vascular proliferation analogous to that seen with infantile hemangioma has been reported.[195] The clinical diagnosis of CMTC is usually straightforward. The differential diagnosis may include reticulate port-wine stain, Klippel–Trenaunay syndrome, and disorders with pronounced cutis marmorata, such as homocystinuria, Down syndrome, and de Lange syndrome.[185] *Diffuse genuine phlebectasia* (Bockenheimer syndrome) is a rare disorder characterized by large venous ectasias usually limited to an extremity. This disorder is unlikely to be confused clinically with CMTC.

The natural history of CMTC is notable for gradual fading of the cutaneous lesions in most patients. When improvement occurs, it tends to be within the first several years of life.[189] Treatment is unnecessary, and in fact, pulsed dye laser seems less effective for these lesions than it is for capillary malformations (i.e., port-wine stains). Ophthalmologic evaluation is probably unnecessary in most patients, but should be considered when there is facial involvement with the vascular process. Referral to a neurologist should be made if neurological symptoms or features of a complex, multiorgan syndrome are present.

Telangiectases

Telangiectases are permanent dilatations of capillaries, venules, or arterioles in the skin that may disappear on diascopy (gentle pressure with a microscope slide). Many processes affecting the blood vessel endothelium and its supporting structure can lead to the development of this common vascular lesion. Some of these are primary disorders of the blood vessels themselves for which the cause is unknown. Others are secondary and are related to a known disturbance, such as aging, sun exposure, radiation, or a systemic disorder, in which they may serve as a useful diagnostic clue. Although telangiectases are usually a sporadic finding without associated underlying abnormalities, a benign hereditary form has also been described. Medical intervention is usually unnecessary, but pulsed dye laser therapy may be considered for cosmetic purposes.

Spider angioma

The spider angioma (nevus araneus) is the best-known type of telangiectasia. It is characterized by a central vascular papule with symmetrically radiating thin branches ('legs') (Fig. 12.80). Spider angiomas appear most commonly on exposed areas of the face, upper trunk, arms, hands, and fingers, and occasionally on the mucous membranes of the lip and nose. They usually blanch with diascopy, only to refill and reappear once the glass slide is removed.

CMTC, most commonly port-wine stain and less often infantile hemangioma.[185,186,189] Sturge–Weber syndrome has been reported in some patients. Ophthalmologic abnormalities include glaucoma, retinal pigmentation, and retinal detachment. Neurologic abnormalities may include macrocephaly seizures, hydrocephalus, and psychomotor retardation.[186,187,190] *Adams–Oliver syndrome* is characterized by CMTC in association with distal transverse limb defects and aplasia cutis congenita of the scalp. Despite the potential

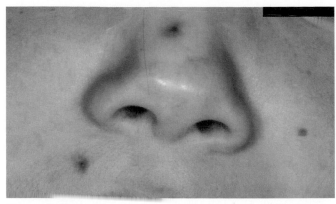

Figure 12.80 Spider angioma. Note lesions on the nasal bridge and the right upper lip.

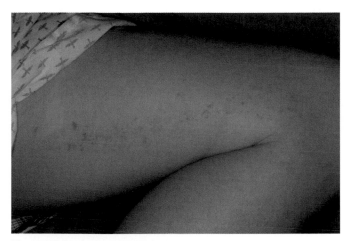

Figure 12.81 Angioma serpiginosum.

The central body is an arteriole, which at times may reveal pulsations with diascopy.

Although spider angiomas can be associated with liver disease, pregnancy, and estrogen therapy, they are frequently idiopathic and may occur in up to 15% of normal children and young adults. The etiology of spider angiomas in patients with liver disease is unclear, but they seem to be related to alcoholism and impaired liver function.[196]

Whereas some spider angiomas may regress spontaneously, in many individuals they tend to persist indefinitely. Treatment options, when desired, include electrocoagulation or pulsed-dye laser therapy.

Angioma serpiginosum

Angioma serpiginosum is a rare condition that manifests as multiple punctate erythematous lesions. It seems to represent a vascular malformation, although vascular proliferation has been reported. The condition is reported most often in young females.

Angioma serpiginosum presents as pinpoint red to violaceous macules that often extend in a serpiginous pattern (Fig. 12.81).[197] There is often some background erythema. The lesions may occasionally appear purpuric, and may be confused with various purpuric dermatoses.[198] The disorder is usually localized, and the most common distribution is on the lower extremities, although more extensive involvement may be seen.[197] Angioma serpiginosum tends to be asymptomatic.

Individual puncta of angioma serpiginosum may disappear, but complete spontaneous clearing of lesions is rare. Treatment

with the pulsed dye laser often leads to improvement or resolution.[199,200]

Hereditary hemorrhagic telangiectasia

Hereditary hemorrhagic telangiectasia (HHT, Osler–Weber–Rendu syndrome) is an autosomal dominant vascular disorder characterized by mucocutaneous telangiectases and a bleeding diathesis, as well as vascular malformations in the lungs, liver, gastrointestinal tract, and central nervous system. It affects approximately 1 in 5000–8000 individuals, and hence is more common than generally appreciated.[201,202] Two molecular subtypes of HHT are recognized: HHT1 and HHT2. HHT1 is known to be caused by mutations in the *endoglin* gene, and HHT2 by mutations in the *activin receptor-like kinase 1 (ALK-1)* gene.[203,204] Mutations in *Smad4* give rise to HHT in association with juvenile polyposis (JPHT).[202] Although there is significant overlap between the clinical findings in HHT1 and HHT2, there appears to be a difference in the frequencies of underlying vascular anomalies.

Patients with HHT most commonly present with epistaxis and anemia, the latter usually being due to gastrointestinal blood loss. The epistaxis may begin in early childhood, but the characteristic mucocutaneous telangiectases often do not appear until adolescence or even later.[104] These vascular lesions have a predisposition for certain anatomic sites, including the lips, ears, oral cavity (especially tongue and palate), palms, fingers, soles, and nasal mucous membranes. Lesions may be present under the nails. Epistaxis occurs spontaneously on more than one occasion, and nighttime bleeds are particularly suspicious for HHT.[205] Other mucous membranes may also be involved, and hemorrhage may occur from any involved mucosal site. Although the distribution of lesions and associated bleeding diathesis are clinically suggestive of HHT, it may occasionally be difficult to distinguish the cutaneous lesions from those seen in benign disorders such as generalized essential telangiectasia. In addition, the classic distribution of HHT-associated telangiectases may not be observable until the third or fourth decade of life,[201] further compounding the challenge of rendering an early diagnosis.

Arteriovenous malformations (AVMs) may occur in HHT patients, and may be responsible for significant morbidity and even death. Pulmonary and cerebral AVMs are the most classically recognized lesions, although hepatic and spinal AVMs may also occur. Previously 'silent' lesions in the lung or brain may hemorrhage, and pulmonary lesions are particularly worrisome because of the risks of hypoxemia or embolism of particulate matter through right-to-left shunts, with neurologic sequelae.[205] Pulmonary AVMs appear less common in HHT2 than in HHT1.[201] Catastrophic intracranial hemorrhage has been reported in infants and children with HHT who were not suspected of having the disease, despite family histories of the syndrome.[206] Screening for pulmonary and cerebral AVMs, when clinically indicated, may include chest radiography, pulse oximetry, blood oxygen determination, and head MRI and MRA (magnetic resonance angiography). Hepatic AVMs in patients with HHT do not appear to pose the same risk for catastrophic events as compared to pulmonary or cerebral lesions.[201]

The diagnosis of HHT generally relies on history, clinical examination, and review of family history. DNA diagnostic testing is technically difficult and costly, but testing is available for diagnosis of an affected individual and for prenatal diagnosis. Newborn screening by endoglin protein expression and mutation analysis of umbilical vein endothelial cells may allow early identification of affected newborns.[207] Treatment of HHT is dictated by the extent of mucocutaneous and organ involvement. Therapies for epistaxis include embolization and septal dermoplasty as well as some pharmacologic alternatives such as estrogens, DDAVP, and antifibrinolytic agents. GI tract bleeding is treated with surgical or medical therapies, including hormones, danazol, and octreotide. Treatments for lung, cerebral, and hepatic AVMs depends on the extent of involvement and may include medical therapies, surgery, embolization, and transplantation.

Unilateral nevoid telangiectasia

Unilateral nevoid telangiectasia is a condition characterized by multiple telangiectases in a dermatomal distribution. The condition may be congenital or acquired, and may be sporadic or associated with medical conditions (such as chronic liver disease), physiologic states (i.e., puberty, pregnancy), or medications (usually estrogen hormonal therapy).[208,209] Although the etiology is controversial, it may be related to an increased level of estrogen receptors in involved skin.[209]

The condition presents with numerous skin telangiectases in a unilateral distribution, especially involving the upper body or extremities (Fig. 12.82). A dermatomal distribution may or may not be evident. Unilateral nevoid telangiectasia occurs most often in females during pregnancy or puberty. When it occurs in adult males, it is often in association with alcoholic cirrhosis. It has also been reported in association with hepatitis C.[209] Treatment is unnecessary, although pulsed-dye laser therapy has been demonstrated to be useful.[210]

Ataxia-telangiectasia

Ataxia-telangiectasia (A-T, Louis–Bar syndrome) is a multisystem autosomal recessive disorder characterized by oculocutaneous telangiectases, cerebellar ataxia, a profound humoral and cellular immunodeficiency, and a predisposition toward hematologic malignancy. A-T is caused by a mutation in the ATM *(ataxia-telangiectasia mutated)* gene, which maps to chromosome 11q.

There is considerable phenotypic variability in patients with A-T, and patients may differ significantly in their rate of progression or appearance of features.[211] The initial clinical manifestation is often truncal ataxia, which may present as early as infancy.[212] Other neurologic features include choreoathetosis, dysarthria, myoclonic jerks, and oculomotor abnormalities. Affected patients may display drooling, peculiar eye movements, a sad mask-like facies, and a stooped posture with drooping shoulders and the head tilted forward and to the side. Confinement to a wheelchair by the second decade is not unusual.

The mucocutaneous telangiectases are a variable feature of A-T, but not infrequently help lead to the correct clinical diagnosis. They usually appear around 3–5 years of age, most often on the medial and lateral bulbar conjunctivae. Skin telangiectases develop primarily on sun-exposed sites, including the ears, cheeks, neck (Fig. 12.83), arms, and upper chest. Other body regions may be affected, and occasionally the cutaneous telangiectases are quite subtle. Other cutaneous findings may include subcutaneous fat loss, progeroid (premature aging) changes of skin and hair, and diffuse hair graying. Segmental, patchy hypo- and hyperpigmentation have been observed,[213] and patients without the telangiectases have been reported.[214] Non-infectious cutaneous granulomas (Fig. 12.84), which present as erythematous plaques, nodules, and ulcers, are a fairly common cutaneous feature in A-T patients.[215,216] These lesions tend to be persistent but are often improved by intralesional injections of triamcinolone.

Chronic sinopulmonary infections occur in the majority of A-T patients. Bronchiectasis with respiratory failure may occur, and is the most common cause of death. Growth failure and mental retardation may also occur. Several immunologic defects have been reported in A-T patients, including decreased IgA, IgE, and IgG, and multiple defects in cell-mediated immune responses. Decreased thymic output and skewed T- and B-cell receptor repertoires have been observed.[217]

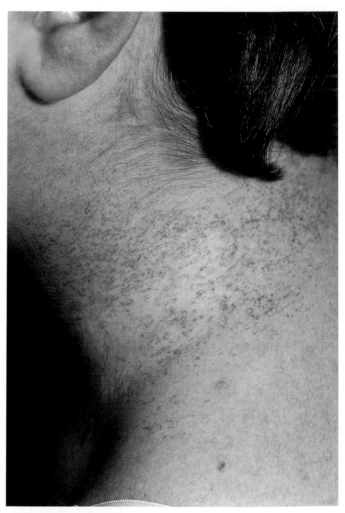

Figure 12.83 Ataxia-telangiectasia, telangiectasias. (Reproduced with permission from Bolognia JL, Jorizzo JL, Rapini RR. Dermatology. Philadelphia: Mosby; 2003.)

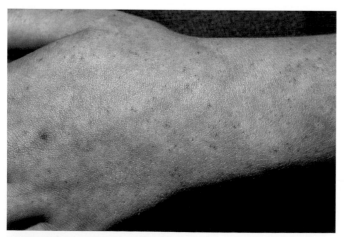

Figure 12.82 Unilateral nevoid telangiectasia. These telangiectatic macules were limited to the hand, forearm, and upper arm.

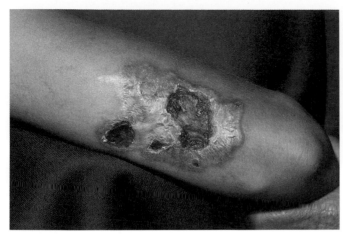

Figure 12.84 Ataxia-telangiectasia, granulomas. These granulomatous skin lesions are very resistant to therapy.

Lymphoid malignancies occur with markedly increased frequency in A-T patients. These include Hodgkin disease, non-Hodgkin lymphoma, and leukemia. There appears to be a four- to five-fold increased frequency of T-cell tumors compared to B-cell tumors in A-T patients.[218] In those with Hodgkin disease, there is a reduced survival compared to Hodgkin disease in the general population.[219] Of the non-Hodgkin lymphomas, diffuse large B-cell lymphomas account for the majority, and T-cell acute lymphoblastic leukemia is the most common form of leukemia.[218,220]

The diagnosis of A-T usually rests on the clinical findings. Elevated levels of α-fetoprotein and carcinoembryonic antigen support the diagnosis. Molecular diagnosis and prenatal diagnosis are possible but not readily available, and the familial mutation must be known. Treatment for A-T is largely supportive, including antimicrobial therapy for infection, early therapy for bronchiectasis, neurodevelopmental follow-up and therapy, and aggressive surveillance for malignancy. Vigorous photoprotection is vital, since A-T patients have a lowered threshold for the development of skin malignancies, and radiation use for treatment of hematopoietic malignancy should be minimized, when feasible. Death is usually the result of chronic bronchiectasis with pulmonary insufficiency and/or pneumonia (55%) or malignancy (15%).

Generalized essential telangiectasia

Generalized essential telangiectasia is a disorder of multiple cutaneous telangiectases without a bleeding diathesis. The condition is notable for a widespread distribution of lesions (Fig. 12.85), progression and/or permanence of the telangiectases, accentuation by dependent positioning, and absence of other epidermal or dermal skin changes (i.e., atrophy, purpura, or dyspigmentation).[221] The most common site of involvement is the lower extremities, and the disorder is more common in females. Oral mucosal and conjunctival telangiectases have occasionally been reported.[104] Although the etiology of generalized essential telangiectasia is unknown, some have suggested a possible autoimmune diathesis.[222] Treatment for this condition is unnecessary. In patients who desire therapy for cosmesis, pulsed dye or Nd:YAG laser treatments appear effective.

Pigmented purpuric eruptions

Pigmented purpuric eruptions (PPE, pigmented purpura, pigmented purpuric dermatosis, progressive pigmented purpura) comprise a group of dermatoses characterized by cutaneous petechiae,

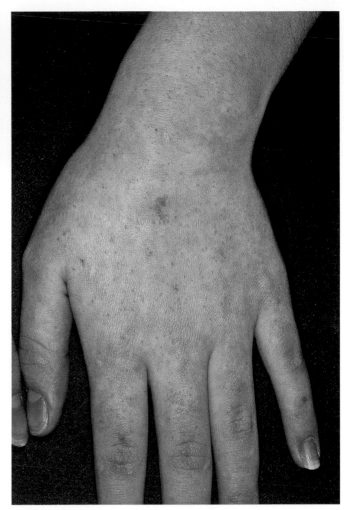

Figure 12.85 Generalized essential telangiectasia. This patient had a widespread distribution of telangiectasias, without any bleeding diathesis.

purpura, and often a yellow-brown pigmentation. Histologically, these disorders all reveal inflammation of the superficial dermal capillaries (capillaritis), without frank vasculitis. Table 12.11 lists the five different subtypes of PPE. The etiology of PPE is unknown, and although they occur primarily in adults, they may also occur in children. Proposed associations with PPE include capillary fragility, cell-mediated immune responses, hepatitis B and C infection, and medication reactions.[223–225] The vast majority of children with PPE are healthy and have no associated medical condition.

Schamberg disease is the prototype for PPE, being the most common type and the most common to present in children. Although rare, it may even occur in infants.[226] The primary lesion is a red-brown punctuate macule, and multiple such lesions ('cayenne pepper spots') occur at the border of red-brown patches (Fig. 12.86).[224,227] The most common location is the lower extremities, although more widespread involvement may occur. Schamberg disease has been associated with the ingestion of several medications, including aspirin and acetaminophen. In addition, there are rare reports of an association between pigmented purpura-like eruptions and progression to cutaneous T-cell lymphoma (mycosis fungoides).[228,229] Although seemingly rare, these reports highlight the need to consider this diagnosis in patients (especially adults) with unusually persistent PPE.

Table 12.11 Subtypes of pigmented purpuric eruptions

Type	Comment
Schamberg disease	Red-brown patches with petechiae ('cayenne pepper spots'); mainly lower extremities
Majocchi disease	Also called 'purpura annularis telangiectodes'; punctate, perifollicular, telangiectases present; tend to become annular and hyperpigmented
Lichen aureus	Rust-yellow lichenoid papules and papules; often linear or along Blaschko's lines; fairly common in children
Doucas and Kapetanakis	Generalized; eczematous, with lichenification and pruritus present
Gougerot and Blum	Red-brown, lichenoid papules and plaques; very rare in children

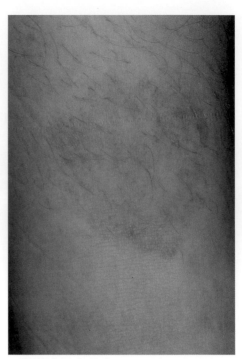

Figure 12.87 Pigmented purpuric eruption, Majocchi disease. Pink-tan patches with petechiae and mild central clearing were present on the lower legs of this adolescent boy.

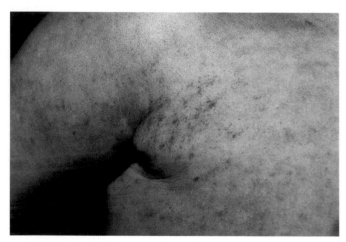

Figure 12.86 Pigmented purpuric eruption, Schamberg disease. Pinpoint, petechial macules coalesce and are superimposed on faint, red-brown patches.

Majocchi disease is an annular variant of PPE, presenting with punctuate, perifollicular petechiae, telangiectases, and hyperpigmented annular patches (Fig. 12.87). It occurs primarily in adolescents and younger adults, and occurs on the lower extremities as well as the trunk and upper extremities.

Lichen aureus is a unique type of PPE in its presentation. Patients present with lichenoid papules that coalesce to form plaques, often with a linear distribution or, in some cases, distribution along the lines of Blaschko. The color of the lesions varies from pink to rust-yellow (Fig. 12.88) to purple, and again the lower extremities are the favored site of involvement.

Eczematoid purpura of Doucas and Kapetanakis is usually a generalized form, with eczematous changes and pruritus. Lichenification (skin thickening with accentuated skin markings) occurs as a result of frequent scratching. *Pigmented purpuric lichenoid dermatosis of Gougerot and Blum* presents with red-brown, polygonal lichenoid papules with telangiectases.

There are no satisfactory treatments for PPE. In cases where a drug reaction is possible, withdrawal of the offending agent may induce regression. Treatments utilized with variable success have included topical and systemic corticosteroids, antihistamines, and PUVA therapy. Therapy with ascorbic acid and bioflavonoids (specifically rutoside), as well as narrowband UVB phototherapy, has also been reported as useful in open-label studies[230-232]

Purpura fulminans

Purpura fulminans is a rare condition characterized by acute, rapidly progressive hemorrhagic necrosis of the skin and disseminated intravascular coagulation. It occurs most often in association with severe bacterial (especially meningococcal meningitis and *S. aureus* sepsis) or viral infection or as a postinfectious syndrome following infections such as varicella or scarlet fever.[233,234] In the latter instance, it usually occurs 10 days to 1 month following the infection. Purpura fulminans has also been described in association with invasive pneumococcal infection.[235] It may also be associated with congenital deficiencies of protein C or S, which are vitamin K-dependent glycoproteins with antithrombotic properties. In fact, infection-associated purpura fulminans may be partly due to acquired deficiencies in these proteins.[236,237] Factor V Leiden, which is a mutated version of factor V, has been shown to be associated with activated protein C resistance, an increased risk of thrombotic events, and exacerbated purpura fulminans in patients with meningococcal disease.[233,238] Purpura fulminans is associated with significant morbidity and is occasionally fatal, especially in the presence of concomitant meningococcal disease.

Purpura fulminans presents with purpura and ecchymoses, often with sharp irregular borders. The lesions are tender, enlarge rapidly, and coalesce with the development of central necrosis, hemorrhagic blebs (Fig. 12.89), and a raised edge with surrounding erythema. The ecchymotic lesions are most commonly distributed on the lower extremities and buttocks, with occasional involvement of the trunk and upper extremities. Deep extension with muscle necrosis and bone involvement may occur. Mucous membranes are usually

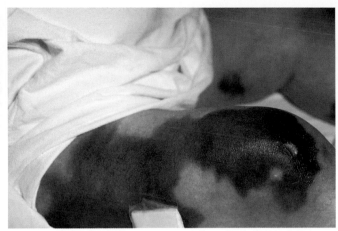

Figure 12.89 Purpura fulminans. Ecchymotic patches and plaques with necrosis and a hemorrhagic bulla over the knee.

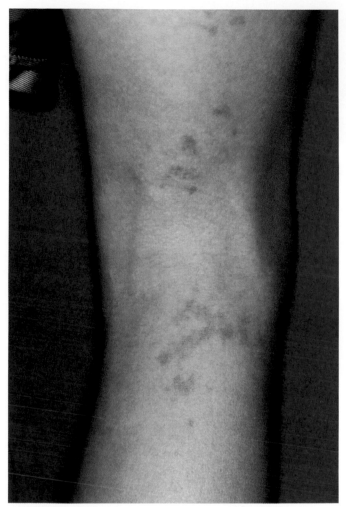

Figure 12.88 Pigmented purpuric eruption, lichen aureus. These golden-tan macules and patches, distributed in a linear fashion, revealed pinpoint petechial macules with diascopy (viewing through a glass slide while applying pressure).

spared. Chills, fever, tachycardia, anemia, and prostration are common. Visceral involvement is less common, but may include central nervous system and retinal vessel thrombosis, hematuria, and gastrointestinal hemorrhage. Adrenal gland thrombosis may result in Waterhouse–Friderichsen syndrome. Skin and muscle necrosis may be severe enough to require grafting, and digital or limb ischemia may necessitate amputation. Epiphyseal growth plate necrosis in a growing child may result in limb foreshortening.[239] Newborn infants with protein C or S deficiency or factor V Leiden present with clinical features of purpura fulminans within 24 hours after birth, and are at high risk for widespread thrombosis of capillaries and venules.[240] Children under 4 years of age, and those with the factor V Leiden mutation, appear to be at increased risk for severe disease and amputation.[234]

Laboratory evaluation in the patient with purpura fulminans reveals decreased fibrinogen and thrombocytopenia. The prothrombin time and partial thromboplastin time are prolonged, and fibrin degradation products are increased. Protein C, protein S, and antithrombin III levels are decreased. Histologic evaluation of the skin lesions reveals dermal vascular thrombosis and hemorrhagic necrosis.[239]

The treatment for purpura fulminans depends upon the underlying disorder and/or associated infection. Initial management consists of fluid resuscitation, ventilatory and inotropic support, and antibiotic administration, when indicated.[241] Administration of protein C and S (i.e., in the form of fresh-frozen plasma or protein C concentrate) may prevent progression of lesions that are not yet necrotic.[236,242] Repeated infusions may be necessary because of the short half-life of protein C.[236] Antithrombin III concentrate has been administered to some patients. Concomitant heparin has been advocated by some (but not by others), and long-term administration of oral anticoagulants is often necessary in patients with congenital protein C or S deficiency. Packed red blood cell transfusion, platelet transfusion, and cryoprecipitate may each need to be considered in certain patients. Surgical modalities include debridement, autologous skin grafting, tissue and muscle flaps, amputation, skin allografts, and tissue-engineered skin.[243,244]

Gardner–Diamond syndrome

Gardner–Diamond syndrome (autoerythrocyte sensitization syndrome, painful bruising syndrome, psychogenic purpura) is a rare disorder characterized by painful bruising and usually seen in patients with emotional or psychiatric disturbance. Historically, the disorder was ascribed to a sensitization reaction to the patient's own erythrocytes, hence the alternative nomenclature 'autoerythrocyte sensitization syndrome'.[245] The majority of patients with Gardner–Diamond syndrome are adolescent or adult females, with only occasional reports of involved males.

The disorder is characterized by recurrent episodes of spontaneous, painful ecchymoses that are often precipitated by emotional stress. The lesions may vary in size, and may involve any part of the cutaneous surface. They tend to resolve over weeks, only to recur again with time. The etiology of Gardner–Diamond syndrome remains unclear. In the original reports, patients were noted to have a positive reaction to intradermal injection of their own erythrocytes, which resulted in an ecchymosis.[246] The significance of this finding has been questioned in subsequent reports, and the immune nature of the condition remains speculative. A number of psychiatric disorders have been observed in association with the cutaneous findings, including depression, anxiety, impulse-control issues, hypochondriasis, hysterical and borderline personality disorders, and obsessive-compulsive behavior.[245] There is no effective treatment for Gardner–Diamond syndrome, although psychotropic medications, hypnotherapy and psychotherapy have been successfully used in some patients.[247]

Scurvy

Scurvy, which is due to vitamin C deficiency, is relatively rare in developed countries, although there are several cases described in the literature in children with an inadequate dietary intake of this vitamin.[248] Clinicians caring for children and adolescents must therefore be aware of this disease and its clinical presentation.

Vitamin C (ascorbic acid) is a vital component of the human diet, due to the inability of humans to derive it from glucose via gluconolactone oxidase.[249] Ascorbic acid is found primarily in fresh fruits, vegetables, and vitamin supplements. When deficiency of this vitamin occurs in a developed country, it is usually in the elderly, indigent, drug- or alcohol-abusing or food faddism populations or those with gastrointestinal disorders or poor dentition.[249,250] Children at risk include those in neglectful social situations, those with neurodevelopmental disabilities or psychiatric illnesses, those with severe food allergies or gastrointestinal disease, and those with unusual dietary habits or with parents who are food faddists.[248-253] Since ascorbic acid is a cofactor in the synthesis of collagen, and collagen is a vital component of the pericapillary network in the skin, capillary fragility results from deficiency of this nutrient.

Clinical manifestations of scurvy include fatigue, petechiae, ecchymoses, purpura, and perifollicular hemorrhages. The latter finding is considered pathognomonic for the condition. In addition, follicular hyperkeratosis and 'corkscrew hairs' may be noted. Purpura often occurs on the lower extremities, but may also involve other body regions. Gingival findings include swelling, bleeding, and loosening of teeth. Bony fractures appear to be more common in pediatric patients when compared to adults, and arthralgias, joint swelling and hemarthrosis may occur. Other findings include gastrointestinal bleeding, conjunctival and intraocular hemorrhage, alopecia, and epistaxis. In some patients, musculoskeletal pain and weakness may be presenting features.[249,252,253] Cardiovascular manifestations of scurvy may include cardiac hypertrophy, postural hypotension, syncope, and possibly, hypertension.[249]

Scurvy is usually diagnosed clinically, with the differential diagnosis including hematologic malignancy, vasculitis, infection, coagulopathy, child abuse, and factitial disorder.[248] A serum ascorbic acid level is usually confirmatory (when <11 µmol/L), although this value may be normal if the patient has had recent intake of vitamin C. Concomitant vitamin deficiencies (especially calcium, vitamin B₁₂, or iron) may also be present.[250] The clinical symptoms usually respond promptly to vitamin C replacement, with dosages for infants and children ranging from 100 to 300 mg/day.

Key References

 The complete list of 253 references for this chapter is available online at **www.expertconsult.com.**
See inside cover for registration details.

Chang LC, Haggstrom AN, Drolet BA, et al. Growth characteristics of infantile hemangiomas: implications for management. *Pediatrics.* 2008;122:360–367.

Garzon MC, Huang JT, Enjolras O, Frieden IJ. Vascular malformations. Part I. *J Am Acad Dermatol.* 2007;56:353–370.

Garzon MC, Huang JT, Enjolras O, Frieden IJ. Vascular malformations. Part II: Associated syndromes. *J Am Acad Dermatol.* 2007;56:541–564.

Govani FS, Shovlin CL. Hereditary haemorrhagic telangiectasia: a clinical and scientific review. *Eur J Hum Genet.* 2009;1–12.

Haggstrom AN, Drolet BA, Baselga E, et al. Prospective study of infantile hemangiomas: Demographic, prenatal, and perinatal characteristics. *J Pediatr.* 2007;150(3):291–294.

Haggstrom AN, Lammer EJ, Schneider RA, et al. Patterns of infantile hemangiomas: New clues to hemangioma pathogenesis and embryonic facial development. *Pediatrics.* 2006;117(3):698–703.

Haggstrom AN, Drolet BA, Baselga E, et al. Prospective study of infantile hemangiomas: clinical characteristics predicting complications and treatment. *Pediatrics.* 2006;118(3):882–887.

Kienast AK, Hoeger PH. Cutis marmorata telangiectatica congenita: a prospective study of 27 cases and review of the literature with proposal of diagnostic criteria. *Clin Exp Dermatol.* 2009;34:319–323.

Leaute-Labreze C, Roque ED, Hubiche T, et al. Propranolol for severe hemangiomas of infancy. *N Engl J Med.* 2008;358(24):2649–2651.

Metry D, Heyer G, Hess C, et al. Consensus statement on diagnostic criteria for PHACE syndrome. *Pediatrics.* 2009;124(5):1447–1456.

Stier MF, Glick SA, Hirsch RJ. Laser treatment of pediatric vascular lesions: port-wine stains and hemangiomas. *J Am Acad Dermatol.* 2008;58:261–285.

Bullous Disorders of Childhood

13

Blisters or bullae are rounded or irregularly shaped lesions of the skin or mucous membranes that result from the accumulation of fluid between the cells of the epidermis, the epidermis and stratum corneum, or the epidermis and dermis. The term *bullae* refers to blistering lesions ≥0.5–1 cm in diameter; those <0.5 cm in diameter are called *vesicles*. The classification of bullous or vesiculobullous disorders is based on clinical morphology and examination of biopsied specimens of lesional or perilesional skin by light microscopy, immunofluorescence analysis, and electron microscopy. It is well recognized that the skin of infants and children is more susceptible to blister formation than that of adults.

Hereditary blistering disorders

Epidermolysis Bullosa

The term *epidermolysis bullosa* (EB) refers to a group of inherited disorders characterized by bullous lesions that develop spontaneously or as a result of varying degrees of friction or trauma.[1–3] Approximately 20 phenotypes of inherited epidermolysis bullosa have now been delineated, as recently reclassified.[1] They may be divided into four major inherited forms, based on the presence or absence of scarring, the mode of inheritance, the level of skin cleavage, and the presence or absence of structural elements of skin (Fig. 13.1). The first three are the traditional EB subgroups: (1) *simplex*; (2) *junctional*; and (3) *dystrophic*. Plakophilin-1 deficiency is now considered a form of EB simplex and Kindler syndrome (discussed after therapy of EB), an autosomal recessive disorder, is the 4th subtype of EB.

In epidermolysis bullosa simplex (epidermolytic EB, EB simplex; EBS) the blister cleavage occurs within the epidermis and healing occurs without scarring. In junctional epidermolysis bullosa (JEB), the skin separates in the lamina lucida of the dermal-epidermal junction and blistering leads to atrophic scarring. In dystrophic (dermolytic) epidermolysis bullosa (DEB) the blister forms in the papillary dermis, below the basement membrane and patients form scars and milia. Bart syndrome (congenital localized absence of skin), although originally thought to be a distinct mechano-bullous syndrome,[4] is now known to be a phenotypic pattern that neonates with all major forms of epidermolysis bullosa may demonstrate at birth (Fig. 13.2),[5,6] although it most commonly is seen with dystrophic forms of EB. Neonates show congenital localized absence of skin, usually involving the lower extremities. Most affected babies also show blistering elsewhere of the skin and mucous membranes and congenital absence or dystrophy of the nails. EB acquisita is an acquired immune-mediated blistering disorder that can resemble DEB (see below).

Skin biopsy samples are required to confirm the diagnosis of EB and to determine the subtype. Biopsies are ideally performed at the edge of a lesion, freshly induced by rotating the skin with a moist Q-tip. Light microscopic evaluation of biopsy sections is not terribly useful, except for rare types (such as lethal acatholytic EB). Specimens are best placed in special transport medium and processed for immunofluorescence mapping studies. These studies allow determination of the level of cleavage based on the known localization of antigens with the skin, and the presence, attenuation, or absence of each structural protein for which the gene is mutated in EB. The underlying molecular basis for every major subtype of epidermolysis bullosa is now known, with mutations in 13 genes responsible for the clinical subtypes.[1]

The overall incidence of epidermolysis bullosa is 1 in every 50 000 births, although the simplex forms comprise the majority of cases. A national epidermolysis bullosa registry was established in the USA, which has generated data beneficial to many families who have children with epidermolysis bullosa. The Dystrophic Epidermolysis Bullosa Research Association (DEBRA), a national (www.debra.org) and international (www.debra-international.org) group, is dedicated to research and support for patients with all forms of epidermolysis bullosa and their families. DEBRA also has specific websites for several other countries.[1]

Epidermolysis Bullosa Simplex

EBS is characterized by blisters that develop in areas of trauma and most commonly results from defective keratin filaments.[7,8] Since the blister cleavage is intraepidermal, lesions tend to heal without scarring. The major clinical forms of epidermolysis bullosa simplex include localized EBS (formerly called Weber–Cockayne disease), generalized EBS (formerly called Koebner type), and EBS-Dowling–Meara (also called EBS herpetiformis); the common and unusual subtypes of EBS are listed in Table 13.1.[1] The vast majority of patients with EB simplex show autosomal dominant inheritance, although rare autosomal recessive forms of the Dowling–Meara and localized forms have been described.[9,10] The lethal acantholytic form, plakophilin deficiency, and bullous pemphigoid antigen 1 deficiency (the most recently recognized type) are autosomal recessive.

Epidermolysis bullosa simplex Dowling–Meara

Epidermolysis bullosa simplex Dowling–Meara (EBS herpetiformis) is the most severe form of EBS from keratin gene mutations (Table 13.2). During the newborn period, the generalized blisters tend to be large and may be difficult to distinguish from those of the severe dystrophic or junctional forms of EB, despite the relatively good overall prognosis of babies with the Dowling–Meara form (Fig. 13.3).[11] Many young infants also show a significant inflammatory reaction in association with blistering and the formation at sites of healed blisters of transient milia, a finding usually characteristic of the dystrophic forms. The characteristic small, clustered (herpetiform) blisters may be seen in neonates, especially on the proximal extremities or trunk, but are more commonly noted during infancy and later childhood (Fig. 13.4). Blistering tends to decrease during

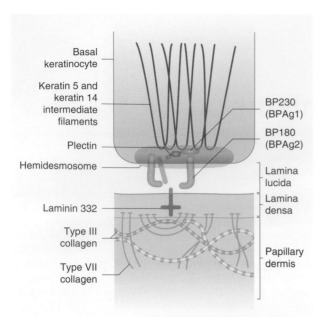

Figure 13.1 Schematic of the structural elements of the basal keratinocytes, basement membrane zone, and upper dermis.

Labels in figure:
- Basal keratinocyte
- Keratin 5 and keratin 14 intermediate filaments
- Plectin
- Hemidesmosome
- Laminin 332
- Type III collagen
- Type VII collagen
- BP230 (BPAg1)
- BP180 (BPAg2)
- Lamina lucida
- Lamina densa
- Papillary dermis

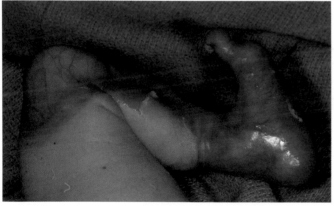

Figure 13.2 Epidermolysis bullosa. Congenital localized absence of skin, also known as Bart syndrome, is now known to be a pattern seen in any of the 3 major subsets of EB. This baby with 'Bart syndrome' has a form of junctional EB, but denudement at birth is most often seen in babies with dystrophic EB and, occasionally, EB simplex.

later childhood and adulthood, and hyperkeratosis of the palms and soles may develop by 6 or 7 years of age, especially in those younger children with significant palmoplantar blistering (Fig. 13.5). During the neonatal period and early infancy, the extensive blistering may prove life threatening. After this period, however, the blistering is rarely a threat to life. Nail involvement with sloughing is common in the Dowling–Meara form, but the nails regrow without dystrophy. Similarly, oral and esophageal mucosal blistering may occur, and cause problems with feeding and obtaining adequate nutrition, especially with the markedly increased caloric needs of more severely affected infants and younger children. Ocular mucosal blistering is less common. Natal teeth have been described in association with the Dowling–Meara form.

Other generalized epidermolysis bullosa simplex

The subtype that used to be called 'Koebner' EBS is now classified as *other generalized epidermolysis bullosa simplex* and is characterized

Table 13.1 Classification and causes of major forms of epidermolysis bullosa simplex (EBS)

Type	Inheritance	Gene defect
Suprabasal		
Lethal acantholytic EB	AR	Carboxy terminal of desmoplakin
Ectodermal dysplasia-skin fragility	AR	Plakophilin-1
EB superficialis	AD	?
Basal		
Localized (EBS-loc)	AD	KRT5, KRT14
Dowling–Meara (EBS–DM)	AD	KRT5, KRT14
Other, generalized	AD	KRT5
Mottled pigmentation	AD	KRT5, KRT14
Muscular dystrophy	AD	Plectin
Pyloric atresia	AR	Integrins α6 and β4, plectin
Autosomal recessive	AR	KRT5, KRT14
Bullous pemphigoid antigen	AR	Dystrophin
Ogna	AD	Plectin
Migratory circinate	AD	Tail of KRT5

Table 13.2 Characteristics of major forms of epidermolysis bullosa simplex (EBS)

Type	Clinical manifestations
EBS, localized	Easy blistering on palms and soles May be focal keratoderma of palms and soles in adults ~25% may show oral mucosal erosions Rarely show reticulated pigmentation, esp. on arms and trunk and punctate keratoderma (EBS with mottled pigmentation)
EBS, other generalized	Generalized blistering Variable mucosal involvement Focal keratoderma of palms and soles Nail involvement in 20% Improves with advancing age
EBS, Dowling–Meara	Most severe in neonate, infant; improves beyond childhood Large, generalized blisters; later, smaller (herpetiform) blisters Mucosal blistering, including esophageal Nails thickened, shed but regrow May have natal teeth
EBS with mottled pigmentation	Reticulated hyperpigmentation, especially on arms and trunk Punctate keratoses and keratoderma

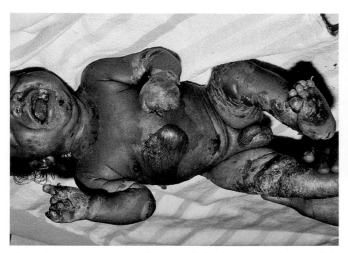

Figure 13.3 Dowling–Meara form of EB simplex. During the neonatal and early infantile periods the blistering is often severe and generalized, making distinction clinically from other forms of epidermolysis bullosa difficult. Note the thickening and sloughing of nails and the blistering of the oral mucosa.

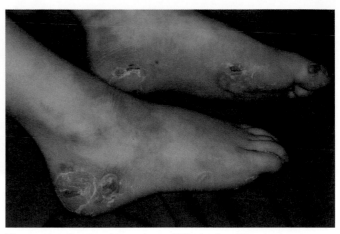

Figure 13.5 Dowling–Meara form of EB simplex. Blistering on the palms and soles may be severe, but palms and soles show thickening with advancing age that is likely protective.

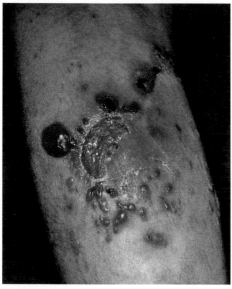

Figure 13.4 Dowling–Meara form of EB simplex. With advancing age, the blisters often become smaller and more clustered in this form of epidermolysis bullosa. Blisters may be hemorrhagic and quite inflamed.

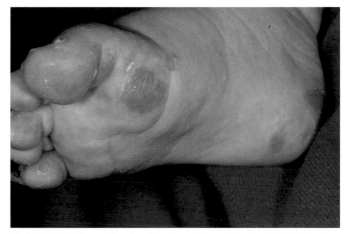

Figure 13.6 EB simplex, localized type. Note the superficial blistering with both intact bullae and denuded skin. This form tends to be limited to the palms and soles.

Localized epidermolysis bullosa simplex

Localized epidermolysis bullosa simplex (epidermolysis bullosa simplex of the hands and feet, the Weber–Cockayne variant) is the most common clinical variant (Table 13.2). A relatively high threshold of frictional trauma is required to induce blister formation. Bullae are usually confined to the hands and feet (primarily the palms and soles; Fig. 13.6); they are often first seen in infants, but may not appear until adolescence or early adulthood. The bullae are usually associated with trauma, occur more readily in hot weather with sweating of the feet, and do not tend to be seriously debilitating. Hyperhidrosis is common, and hyperkeratosis of the palms and soles, although often present, is usually mild. Lesions heal rapidly without scarring, nail involvement rarely occurs, and the mucous membranes do not tend to be involved. In young children, blisters may develop on the knees from the frictional trauma of crawling. In adolescents and young adults, blisters often occur on the feet after long hikes or dancing, or on the hands following a game of tennis or golf. *EBS with mottled pigmentation* is characterized by a mottled, reticulated pigmentation (Fig. 13.7), particularly of the trunk and neck, in association with mild acral blistering (Table 13.2). Patients often show verrucous papules of the hands and feet and palmoplantar keratoderma.[12]

by generalized blistering of skin, most notable at sites of friction (Table 13.2). Extensive blistering in the neonatal period and early infancy increases the risk of sepsis and may be life threatening. In general, the tendency toward blistering tends to improve with advancing age, particularly by teenage years. Hyperhidrosis is common, and mild to moderate hyperkeratosis of the soles is often present. Although erosions of the mucous membranes may be seen in the newborn as a result of vigorous sucking, mucosal involvement is generally mild and the nails are rarely affected. Involvement of the conjunctiva and cornea has rarely been described. The newly described *migratory circinate EBS* results from mutations in the tail domain of KRT 5, and is characterized by small blisters on the hands, feet and legs with migratory circinate erythema and post-inflammatory hyperpigmentation. There is no mucosal or nail involvement.

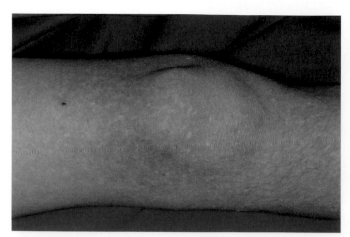

Figure 13.7 EB simplex with mottled pigmentation. The reticulated pigmentation may be bothersome to affected individuals, but the mild blistering, as seen proximal to the knee, is not.

Table 13.3 Classification and causes of major forms of junctional epidermolysis bullosa

Type	Inheritance	Gene defect
Herlitz	AR	Laminin 332
Other	AR	
Non-Herlitz, generalized	AR	Laminin 332
		Type XVII collagen
Non-Herlitz, localized	AR	Type XVII collagen
With pyloric atresia	AR	Integrin α6 β4
Inversa	AR	Laminin 332
Late onset	AR	?
LOC syndrome	AR	Laminin 332, α3 chain

LOC; laryngo-onycho-cutaneous syndrome

EBS of the Dowling–Meara, generalized, and localized forms results from mutations in the genes encoding keratin 5 and keratin 14 (the keratins expressed in basal cells). Keratins are the most abundant proteins of epidermal keratinocytes, and keratin pairs are critical for the filamentous network that provides integrity to epidermal cells. When a point mutation occurs in one of the keratin alleles, resulting in a change in one amino acid, the abnormal keratin protein is still able to form filaments, but these filaments are abnormal. The abnormal filaments do not provide adequate structural integrity to the cell and, as a result, the cell lyses. Cytolysis of epidermal basal cells is the essential histologic feature of all forms of EBS resulting from keratin gene mutations. Electron microscopic examination shows cleavage through the basal layer (above the periodic acid-Schiff-positive basement membrane of the epidermis). In the severe Dowling–Meara form, clumping of tonofilaments and displacement of nuclei are seen ultrastructurally. The risk of cell lysis and the trauma required to elicit the blistering depend on the site of the mutation and how critical that gene region is for resultant keratin function. The sites of mutations in the most severe Dowling–Meara form are most critical for keratin function (end terminal rod domains), whereas the sites mutated in the localized type are least critical. The mutations that lead to EBS with mottled pigmentation tend to be at the head region of *KRT 5* or *KRT14* (most often a mutation that changes the 25th amino acid of keratin 5)[13,14] suggesting that this site on the keratin protein is vital for the transfer of pigment from melanocytes to keratinocytes.

EBS superficialis is an erosive form with cleavage in the upper epidermis and stratum corneum in which patients heal with scarring and milia; although a type VII gene mutation has been shown, suggesting EBS superficialis to be a form of dominant dystrophic EB, the underlying genetic defect in the original cases remains unclear and it remains classified as EBS.[1,15] The *lethal acantholytic form of EB* (LAEB) presents at birth with generalized denudement and absence of hair and nails.[16,17] Frank blisters are not seen, but the skin peels in sheets. Mucosal sloughing is severe and affected neonates are born with teeth. All babies to date have died in the neonatal period. Cardiomegaly may be associated. Mutations have been described in the C-terminal domain of desmoplakin (*DSP*). *Plakophilin deficiency* (ectodermal dysplasia with skin fragility) results from mutations in the gene encoding plakophilin-1 (*PKP1*). Affected patients show generalized erythroderma at birth with blistering. The soles are often most disabling, with palmoplantar keratoderma and painful fissures. Superficial erosions and crusting are prominent in the perioral area, and tongue fissures have been described. The hair tends to be short and sparse, and the nails are thickened and dystrophic. Affected individuals show variable hypohidrosis, blepharitis, and growth retardation.[18] Plakophilin-1 is a structural component of the desmosomes that allows cell–cell adhesion; biopsies of affected skin show acanthosis, acantholysis, widening of the space between keratinocytes, and few, poorly-formed desmosomes.[19] The most recently described form of EBS is autosomal recessive and results from absence of two isoforms of the bullous pemphigoid antigen (BPAG1-e and -n).[20] The only affected individual to date experienced lifelong blistering and erosions, especially at the ankles and feet, in association with skin peeling, occasional hemorrhage, dyspigmentation and toenail dystrophy.

Three forms of EBS result from mutations in the gene-encoding plectin (*PLEC1*): EBS with muscular dystrophy, EBS-Ogna, and EBS with pyloric atresia.[21] *EBS with muscular dystrophy* presents in the neonatal or infantile period with generalized blisters, but the muscular dystrophy may not present until adulthood. Patients may show ptosis and granulation tissue with stenosis of the respiratory tract. *EBS-Ogna* mainly shows acral blistering, although more generalized blistering has been described; affected individuals characteristically bruise easily and may show onychogryphosis. *EBS with pyloric atresia* presents with the same generalized blistering and cutis aplasia and pyloric atresia as JEB with pyloric atresia. Malformed pinnae and nasal alae, joint contractures, and cryptorchidism are other shared features. Plectin interacts with α6β4 integin, providing a rationale for similar clinical manifestations. The mutations of EBS with muscular dystrophy cluster in exon 31, which is spliced out in one of the two isoforms of plectin, explaining the much milder phenotype of EBS with muscular dystrophy.[22]

Junctional Epidermolysis Bullosa

Junctional epidermolysis bullosa (JEB) is group of mechanobullous disorders in which the cleavage plane occurs in the lamina lucida at the junction of the epidermis and dermis (Table 13.3).[23,24] Encompassing a spectrum from severe life-threatening disease to relatively mild involvement, various subtypes of this disorder have been described, each transmitted in an autosomal recessive manner (Table 13.4). Recently, an autosomal dominant form of non-Herlitz JEB has been described.[25] In the most severe form, JEB-Herlitz (JEB-H), blistering begins at birth and death occurs in 40% by 1 year of age and 50% by 2 years of age.[26] Although early death is a risk during the first years of life in infants with the non-Herlitz types of

Table 13.4 Characteristics of major forms of junctional epidermolysis bullosa

Type	Clinical manifestations
Herlitz type	50% of patients die by 2 years old Blisters heal with atrophic scarring, but no milia Periungual and fingerpad blistering, erythema Blistering of oral and esophageal mucosae Laryngeal and airway involvement with early hoarseness Later, perioral granulation tissue with sparing of lips Anonychia Dental enamel hypoplasia, excessive caries Growth retardation Anemia
Non-Herlitz types, generalized	Less severe, but similar manifestations to Herlitz type, including dental, nail and laryngeal involvement Granulation tissue is rare Perinasal cicatricization Less mucosal involvement Alopecia Anemia, but not as severe as JEB–H
Non-Herlitz types, localized	Localized blisters without residual scarring or granulation tissue Minimal mucosal involvement Dental and nail abnormalities as in JEB–H
With pyloric atresia	Usually lethal in neonatal period Generalized blistering, leading to atrophic scarring May be born with large areas of cutis aplasia No granulation tissue Nail dystrophy or anonychia Pyloric atresia, GU malformations Rudimentary ears Dental enamel hypoplasia (survivors) Variable anemia, growth retardation, mucosal blistering

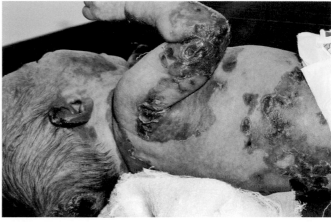

Figure 13.8 Junctional EB, Herlitz type. Generalized distribution of blisters and erosions at birth.

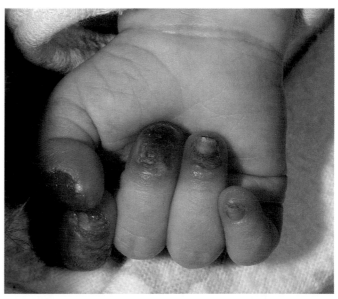

Figure 13.9 Junctional EB, Herlitz type. Blistering of the fingertips with periungual erythema and sloughing of the nails is characteristic of junctional EB.

JEB, the prognosis overall is better than that of JEB, Herlitz type (except with pyloric aresia). Survival into adulthood is common for the non-Herlitz types of JEB, but has been occasionally described for individuals with the Herlitz type of JEB.

JEB is characterized by the generalized distribution of blisters and large erosions (Fig. 13.8), mainly on the buttocks, perioral area, trunk, and scalp. Blistering is almost always present at birth (Fig. 13.2). Blistering of the fingertips with sloughing of the nails (Fig. 13.9) and perioral involvement (Fig. 13.10) with sparing of the lips are important, if not diagnostic, features of the junctional forms of EB. Granulation tissue, especially of the perioral region, is characteristic of JEB-H (and laryngo-onycho-cutaneous syndrome), and is usually present by a few years of age. Sites of healing tend to be atrophic, but without milia. The mucous membranes are affected, especially the oral mucosae (Fig. 13.11). The genitourinary and gastrointestinal tracts are less severely affected in the non-Herlitz types than in the Herlitz form. The teeth are dysplastic, and a cobblestone appearance to the dental enamel is characteristic, even in the mildest forms. Severe growth retardation and recalcitrant

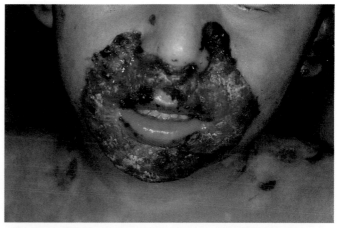

Figure 13.10 Junctional EB, Herlitz type. Perioral blistering with formation of granulation tissue is characteristic. Note that the lips are relatively spared, but the teeth show enamel dysplasia.

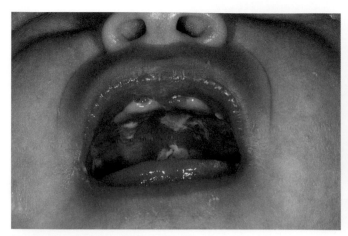

Figure 13.11 Junctional EB, non-Herlitz type. Oral mucosal sloughing during the neonatal period and infancy may make oral feeding difficult.

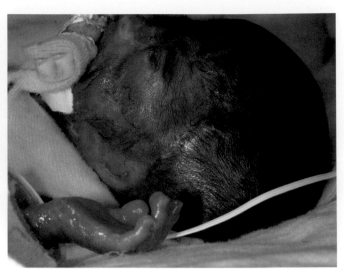

Figure 13.12 Junctional EB, pyloric atresia type. The rudimentary ears and extensive denudement of the extremities is typical of this type of EB. This baby had a mutation in the gene encoding integrin β4.

anemia are common with the Herlitz type, but are less of a problem with the non-Herlitz forms. Hoarseness and laryngeal involvement are common, and the involvement of the airway region may lead to death. Mutations in the Herlitz form always affect a gene encoding one of the three chains of laminin 332 (LAMA3, LAMB3, and LAMC2 encoding α3, β3, and γ2 chains, respectively).

Mutations in the α3 chain of laminin 332 also lead to *laryngo-onycho-cutaneous* (LOC; Shabbir's) syndrome.[27,28] LOC syndrome occurs most often in the Punjab region of India and Pakistan. It features excessive granulation tissue of the larynx (leading to hoarseness and potentially airway obstruction), conjunctival granulation tissue (leading to corneal scarring and potentially blindness), and erosive blisters most commonly on the face and neck. Death is common because of respiratory tract involvement. *JEB inversa* results from milder mutations a laminin 332 gene, and presents with blisters predominantly in intertriginous areas (axillary areas and groin). Mucosal blistering tends to be variable in extent, but less than in the generalized forms. The non-Herlitz forms most commonly affect the gene encoding BP180 (collagen XVII; *COL17A1*), but occasionally reflect at least one missense mutation in a gene encoding laminin 332.

JEB with pyloric atresia results from mutations in either α6 integrin (*ITGA6*) or its hemidesmosome partner, β4 integrin (*ITGB4*).[22] Blistering is generalized at birth, often with large areas of cutis aplasia. The presence of rudimentary and malformed ears is associated with pyloric atresia (Fig. 13.12) and usually genitourinary tract malformations, attesting to the important role of α6β4 integrin in the development of the ears, pylorus and genitourinary tract.[8] Less commonly, EB with pyloric atresia results from plectin abnormalities (see above). A *late onset form of JEB* has been described with onset in young adulthood or later; nails are dystrophic or absent and dental enamel is hypoplastic, but blistering is milder than in other junctional forms. Patients may have hyperhidrosis and absent dermatoglyphics.

Early diagnosis of the subtype of JEB is critical, and is based on immunomapping and detection of lamina lucida proteins by immunofluorescence staining. Immunomapping studies of sections from skin adjacent to a freshly induced blister show cleavage at the lamina lucida level. Electron microscopic evaluations reveal markedly reduced or absent hemidesmosomes, anchoring structures that span the lamina lucida of the basement membrane of skin and mucosae.

Table 13.5 Classification and causes of major forms of dystrophic epidermolysis bullosa

Type	Inheritance	Gene defect
Dominant		
Generalized	AD	Collagen VII
Acral	AD	Collagen VII
Pretibial	AD	Collagen VII
Pruriginosa	AD	Collagen VII
Nails only	AD	Collagen VII
Bullous dermolysis of the newborn	AD	Collagen VII
Recessive		
Severe generalized	AR	Collagen VII
Generalized other	AD	Collagen VII
Inversa	AR	Collagen VII
Pretibial	AR	Collagen VII
Pruriginosa	AR	Collagen VII
Centripetalis	AR	Collagen VII
Bullous dermolysis of the newborn	AR	Collagen VII

Dystrophic epidermolysis bullosa

The scarring (dystrophic) types of epidermolysis bullosa are predominantly divided into dominant and recessive forms (Tables 13.5, 13.6). The recessive forms have been further subdivided into the severe generalized and generalized other forms. The dominant disease is considerably less severe; affected individuals are generally healthy, are of normal stature, and show limited blistering of the skin. The severe generalized form of RDEB, conversely, is severe and incapacitating. Functional deformities of the hands and feet result from extensive scarring, growth and development are retarded, and profound anemia and hypoalbuminemia are standard. All forms of

Table 13.6 Characteristics of major forms of dystrophic epidermolysis bullosa

Type	Clinical manifestations
Dominant dystrophic	Onset at birth to early infancy
	Blistering predominates on dorsum of hands, elbows, knees, and lower legs
	Milia associated with scarring
	Some patients develop scar-like lesions, especially on the trunk
	80% have nail dystrophy
Recessive dystrophic, severe generalized	Present at birth
	Widespread blistering, scarring, milia
	Deformities: pseudosyndactyly, joint contractures
	Severe involvement of mucous membranes, nails; alopecia
	Growth retardation, poor nutrition
	Anemia
	Mottled, carious teeth
	Osteoporosis, delayed puberty, cardiomyopathy, glomerulonephritis, renal amyloidosis, IgA nephropathy
	Predisposition to squamous cell carcinoma in heavily scarred areas
Recessive dystrophic, generalized other	Generalized blisters from birth with milia, scarring
	Less anemia, growth retardation, mucosal but more esophageal issues with advancing age

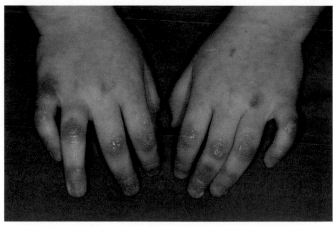

Figure 13.13 Dominant dystrophic EB. Note the blistering on the dorsum of the hand, predominantly over the knuckle areas with residual scarring and milia.

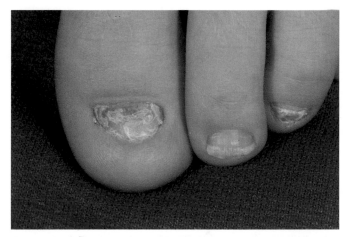

Figure 13.14 Dominant dystrophic EB. Nail dystrophy, especially of the toenails, is commonly seen in individuals with dominant dystrophic EB.

dystrophic EB affect anchoring fibrils, critical elements for epidermal-dermal cohesion, and result from mutations in type VII collagen.[29-31]

Dominant dystrophic epidermolysis bullosa

Dominant dystrophic epidermolysis bullosa (DDEB, generalized) generally presents at birth or shortly thereafter, although mild cases may not show blistering or nail changes until adulthood. The blisters and resultant scars and milia formation primarily involve the extensor areas of the extremities and the dorsum of the hands (Fig. 13.13). Nail thickening, dystrophy, or complete nail destruction are seen in 80% of cases (Fig. 13.14).[32] Although mucous membrane lesions appear in 20% of cases, they tend to be mild and not problematic. The teeth and hair are generally not affected, and physical development is normal. *DDEB, nails only* shows no blisters, but dystrophic or absent nails. An acral form (*DDEB acral*) shows blisters on the hands and feet only, whereas the pretibial form (*DDEB pretibial*) also shows lichen planus-like lesions of the pretibial area. *DEB pruriginosa* is characterized by typical DEB lesions (dominant or recessive) but an onset during childhood and severe associated pruritus.[33] *Bullous dermolysis of the newborn* (DEB-BDN, formerly called transient BDN) shows skin blistering, often extensive, at birth or in early infancy (Fig. 13.15). However, blistering dramatically improves during the first months to 2 years of life and, beyond mild residual atrophy, scarring and nail dystrophy and an increased risk of dental caries, ongoing blistering is not a problem. The disorder results from mild mutations in COL7A1, and can be inherited in a dominant or recessive manner.

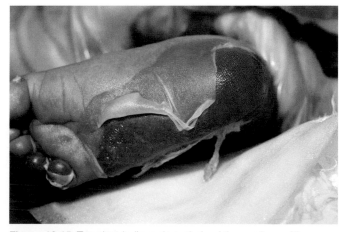

Figure 13.15 Transient bullous dermolysis of the newborn. After extensive blistering of the lower extremity at birth, no further blisters developed. Immunomapping showed the split to be in the upper dermis, and staining for type VII collagen was reduced.

Severe generalized recessive dystrophic epidermolysis bullosa

Children with severe generalized recessive dystrophic EB (RDEB) have a severe life-altering bullous disease characterized by widespread dystrophic scarring and deformity and by severe involvement of mucous membranes. RDEB may manifest as a less severe form ('generalized other RDEB') with less severe blistering of the skin and mucosae. Two other forms of RDEB have more localized cutaneous involvement. Blistering in *RDEB inversa* tends to involve the intertriginous axial, lumbosacral and acral sites in addition to extensive mucosal involvement, including esophageal strictures. *RDEB centripetalis* tends to show blistering, scarring and milia limited to the pretibial areas and nails (resembling DDEB), but patients also have mild to moderate mucosal blistering. Although any area of the skin may be involved in infants, the most commonly affected areas are the hands, feet, buttocks, scapulae, face, occiput, elbows, and knees. In older children the hands, feet, knees, elbows, and posterior neck/upper mid-back (Fig. 13.16) are most commonly involved. Bullae may be hemorrhagic, and large areas, especially on the lower extremities, may be completely devoid of skin. When a blister ruptures or its roof peels off, a raw painful surface is evident. The Nikolsky sign (production or enlargement of a blister by slight pressure or the production of a moist abrasion by slight pressure on the skin) is often positive. Fluid contained in bullae, although at first sterile, may become secondarily infected, which can lead to sepsis; *Staphylococcus aureus* and *Pseudomonas aeruginosa* are the most common organisms.

Bullae are often followed by atrophic scars and varying degrees of hyperpigmentation or hypopigmentation. Milia overlying the scars are characteristic. Occasionally, dark, irregular hyperpigmented patches develop that are worrisome dermoscopically,[34] but show benign nevi or increased basal pigment deposition histologically.[35,36] Pigmented lesions may clear spontaneously. The hands and lower aspects of the legs are particularly susceptible to severe blistering and scarring. The fingers and toes may become fused, with resultant pseudosyndactyly in which the digits become bound together by a glove-like epidermal sac, with resulting claw-like clubbing or mitten-like deformities (Fig. 13.17). The fingers and toes become immobile (usually during the first years of life), and the wrists, elbows, knees, and ankles may become fixed in a flexed position from contractures, leading to immobility and often confinement to a wheelchair.

Oral mucosal involvement occurs soon after birth, leading to dysphagia and limiting the ability to suck well. Erosions of the esophagus may at times result in segmental stenosis (most often in the upper third) with consequent difficulty in swallowing.[1] Gastroesophageal reflux disease frequently occurs, especially presenting as effortless vomiting. Constipation is common, and may be related to anal fissuring, inadequate dietary fiber, and administration of iron. Affected children are reluctant to eat and often fail to thrive, given their increased nutritional needs owing to loss of protein and other nutrients through wounds. As the child grows older there is a tendency for the disease to become less severe, but the affected individual soon learns to avoid hot drinks, rough foods, and large particles that might produce blistering of the mouth, pharynx, or esophagus. Typically, patients show microstomia, owing to intraoral scarring and a frenulum that is bound down. The eyes may develop blisters, with associated ocular inflammation and later corneal scarring, potentially leading to visual impairment.[37] Hoarseness, aphonia, and even laryngeal stenosis may result from laryngeal blistering and scarring. Bone mineralization is low in patients with EB, particularly in RDEB, probably owing to a combination of insufficient nutrition, reduced physical activity, and chronic inflammation.[2,38]

The teeth in RDEB are particularly susceptible to early and frequently severe caries. The progressive intraoral scarring leads to microstomia and decreased salivation.[2,39] Even routine dental care may cause the eruption of bullae and erosions on the lips, gingivae, and oral mucosa. The nails may show severe dystrophy or complete absence of nails. Scalp and body hair may be sparse, and there may be patches of cicatricial alopecia.[40]

In patients with the severe generalized form of RDEB, death may occur during infancy or childhood as a result of septicemia, pneumonia, or renal failure. Patients with RDEB (and rarely DDEB) have an increased risk of glomerulonephritis, renal amyloidosis, and IgA nephropathy.[2,41–43] The tremendous loss of fluid, blood, and protein through the skin coupled with malnutrition can lead to hypoalbuminemia and anemia. Dilated cardiomyopathy is an uncommon complication (4.5% by 20 years of age),[44] but may be fatal, especially in the presence of concurrent chronic renal failure. The cause of the cardiomyopathy may be multifactorial, including from transfusion-associated iron overload, viral myocarditis, and deficiency of selenium and carnitine. Other complications of RDEB include erosions and scarring of the anal area (often resulting in severe discomfort, chronic constipation, or soiling), urethral ste-

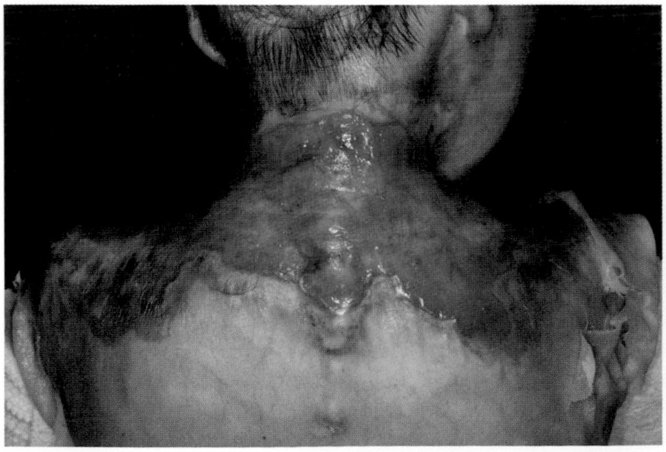

Figure 13.16 Recessive dystrophic EB. This young girl demonstrates the 'shawl sign' of RDEB. Despite haircuts, dressings, and vigorous protection, this area has continued to be blistering and open for the past 5 years.

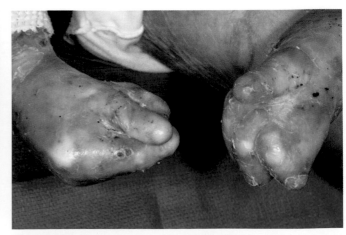

Figure 13.17 Recessive dystrophic EB. Pseudosyndactyly or mitten deformities of both hands in this 5-year-old girl with extensive atrophic scarring.

nosis, urinary retention, hypertrophy of the bladder, and occasionally hydronephrosis.[3,41]

Patients with RDEB (and to a lesser extent JEB, but not DDEB) show a progressively increasing risk of developing cutaneous squamous cell carcinomas (7.5%, 68%, 80%, and 90% by 20, 35, 45, and 55 years of age, respectively)[45] in heavily ulcerated and scarred areas of skin.[46] These lesions are predominantly over joints and on the distal extremities, and present as nodular lesions or non-healing ulcers.[47,48] Suspicious masses should be biopsied to distinguished SCCs from a benign lesion such as verruciform xanthoma.[49,50] Cutaneous carcinomas tend to be locally aggressive, often requiring amputation, and tend to metastasize, leading to death.

Death during childhood is most common with JEB (median age 4–6 months).[26] Sepsis, failure to thrive, and respiratory failure are the major causes of death during childhood. Children with RDEB generally survive the neonatal and infantile periods, but succumb to infect later during childhood or to aggressive cutaneous carcinomas during adulthood.

Treatment of epidermolysis bullosa

As in any inherited disorder, it is the responsibility of the physician to inform parents of the risks of transmitting genetic abnormalities.[53] When the condition is determined by a dominant gene (as in DDEB)[51,52] and a parent is affected, the risk of the disorder in siblings is 50%. In a family in which a child manifests abnormalities because of a recessive gene (as in RDEB), parents risk a 25% possibility with each pregnancy of the disorder occurring in future offspring. Appropriate genetic counseling, however, depends on accurate diagnosis. Since the clinical course of many forms of epidermolysis bullosa is variable, especially during the neonatal and infantile periods, it is recommended that patients be carefully evaluated as early as possible with immunofluorescent mapping, monoclonal antibody studies, and DNA analysis if appropriate in an effort to establish the correct diagnosis. Prenatal diagnosis of all forms of EB is now available using molecular techniques, but is easiest if the gene defect is known in that family.[54] Preimplantation diagnosis has been performed, and is an option that utilizes *in vitro* fertilization to ensure a normal fetus without the risk of abortion.[55,56]

The psychosocial effects of EB, especially the more severe forms, on the affected individual and family are among the most dramatic of any skin disease.[53] Affected children are concerned about having itchy skin; being in pain; having difficulty with participation; failing to understand others; and feeling different.[57] Parents of affected children worry about the child being different; the child suffering pain; feeling uncertain; restrictions on employment and leisure; problems with organizing care; being constantly on duty; family problems; the ignorance and lack of skills of alternative care providers; and resistance by the child to care.[58] These problems should be discussed and psychological support for patients and their families offered as part of optimal care.

The treatment of epidermolysis bullosa is palliative, with protection from friction or overheating, avoidance of abrasion and constriction, control of secondary infection, nutritional supplementation, and pain control. Since blisters result from mechanical injury, measures should be taken to relieve pressure and prevent unnecessary trauma. Clothing should be soft and worn inside-out. Labels that may rub the skin should be removed. Velcro closures are less traumatizing than other traditional closures. Mittens can be worn to minimize self-induced trauma. Shoes should be soft and fit well; leather shoes with leather linings, ideally with external seams (e.g., moccasins), are usually recommended.[53] During the summer, canvas shoes and jelly sandals are the best choices. Shoes should be large enough to accommodate dressings, and minimize friction. Insoles can be made from cooling gel, sheepskin, or protective dressings. Affected babies can be lifted and moved on a soft pad, and the bathtub can be lined with a thick towel. A cool environment and lubrication of the skin to decrease surface friction are helpful in the reduction of blister formation. When blisters occur, extension may be prevented by aseptic aspiration of blister fluid. The roofs of blisters should be left intact whenever possible to protect the underlying skin.

Keeping EBS palms and soles cool and dry helps to minimize blistering, especially during hot weather. Hyperhidrosis is often a concomitant feature, and measures to minimize the increased blistering associated with hyperhidrosis can be helpful. These include application of 20% aluminum chloride hexahydrate at night and gently dried with a cool hairdryer, wearing of socks that absorb moisture,[53] and sprinkling of affected areas with absorbent powder, such as Zeasorb. For extreme cases and in older patients with the localized form of EBS, injections of botulinum toxin A have been advocated.[59] Silver-impregnated socks can decrease infections and increase foot comfort.

A water mattress and a soft fleece covering will help to limit friction and trauma. Daily baths and topical application to eroded areas of protective petrolatum or, especially if slightly crusted, antibiotic ointments (usually bacitracin) are helpful. Protective dressings that do not adhere to wounds should be applied to eroded areas to promote healing but prevent further denudation when dressings are changed (e.g., petrolatum-impregnated gauze, Telfa, Mepilex, Mepilex Transfer, Mepitel, Restore).[60] In children with RDEB, dressings should be carefully placed between the digits to decrease the risk of pseudosyndactyly (Fig. 13.18). Sterile precautions must be taken when changing dressings to reduce the risk of bacterial infection. Tape and any significant pressure to skin must be avoided. Dressings can be held in place by rolled gauze (such as Kerlix) with tape only applied to the dressing itself or by stockinette

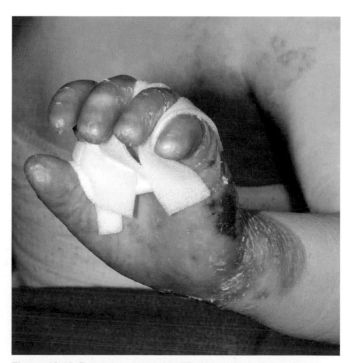

Figure 13.18 Recessive dystrophic EB. Non-adherent dressings should be placed between the fingers and toes of children with RDEB to reduce the risk of pseudosyndactyly. Note the scarred skin and anonychia.

(such as Surgifix or Spandage). Dressings with silver have helped patients with recurrent infections, but application of silver sulfadiazine has been associated with argyria.[61,62] Given the benefit of EB skin exposure to silver and the unknown significance of high blood levels of silver, many families consider the benefits in decreasing infection and promoting wound healing to outweigh the risk.[63] A variety of other topically applied preparations have been promoted or are in trials to encourage wound healing, such as thymosin beta 4[64] and medical grade honey.[65] Crusted or purulent areas should be cultured and treated based on the sensitivity of organisms. Topical application of mupirocin and/or gentamicin ointments may be useful for limited areas of crusting. More extensive involvement requires administration of systemic antibiotics. Excessive usage of systemic antibiotics, however, should be avoided because of the high risk of development of resistance. Gentamicin soaks (480 mg/L saline), acetic acid soaks (diluted white vinegar), and addition of small amounts of bleach to the bathwater (e.g., one-quarter to one-half of a cup per tub) have been used to decrease the overgrowth of pseudomonas and staphylococcal organisms. The risk of sepsis with cutaneous infection is high in neonates and infants, and patients should be monitored carefully. Topical and systemic steroids are generally not useful for patients with EB, and should be avoided in view of their promotion of infection and other side-effects. Limited application of potent topical steroid, however, or thalidomide has been helpful for the granulation tissue of laminin 332 defects.[66]

Pain control is an important component of EB care, especially in affected infants. The changing of dressings at blistered sites is excruciatingly painful for patients, yet must be performed from a few times weekly to up to twice daily, depending on the extent of drainage and the presence of infection. Methadone and liquid cough suppressants with dextromethorphan have been used to relieve discomfort in infants. For older children, acetaminophen with codeine, oral midazolam, or morphine has been used before dressing changes and baths to improve tolerance. Amitriptyline and cognitive behavioral techniques have also been suggested to relieve the chronic pain and discomfort.[67]

Nutritional supplementation is critical for patients with the more severe forms of EB to prevent failure to thrive, which has been linked to mortality in 20.5% of patients with JEB–H by 2 years of age. The loss of protein, iron, and blood through the open areas of skin leads to hypo-albuminemia and deficiency of iron and trace minerals. Furthermore, the chronic disruption of the epithelial lining of the small intestine leads to gross malabsorption of nutrients and the pain with ingestion of food decreases intake. Consultation with a nutritionist is important to maximize caloric and protein intake, and provide specific nutrients and vitamins, such as iron, zinc and vitamin D3. Oral iron may be poorly tolerated by the gastrointestinal tract and constipation is a potential issue; intravenous administration of iron or blood transfusions may be needed to maintain a Hgb of at least 8 g/dL in severely affected children. Soft nipples, such as the Haberman feeder, should be used, with the opening enlarged to minimize the need for sucking. The lips should be protected with petrolatum prior to initiating feeding. In general, nasogastric tube feeding should be avoided or, if necessary, a tube suitable for long-term feeding should be used. Placement of a button gastrostomy tube should be considered in infants who start to drop off of their growth curve, as a means of supplemental feeding to increase caloric intake and as an alternative route to oral feeding; early gastrostomy placement should be considered for JEB-H and RDEB. Regular dental intervention is essential to decrease caries; teeth can be cleaned with soft moist gauze and rinses of chlorhexidine.[68] Endosseous implants have been placed successfully in patients with EB.[69]

Dysphagia is the major symptom of esophageal involvement in RDEB.[70,71] It may result from a reversible inflammatory reaction or from a permanent stricture. Barium studies demonstrate esophageal lesions; endoscopy, however, is not recommended. Softening of the diet for several weeks may result in modest to marked improvement of symptoms. If conservative management fails to result in proper nourishment, esophageal dilatation, ideally through fluoroscopic guidance, should be performed, and may be repeated if stenosis recurs. Esophageal perforation is the most serious complication of dilatation. Surgery is an alternative, through colonic interposition and resection of localized strictures with end-to-end anastomosis, but the procedures carry a high risk. Gastroesophageal reflux may be exacerbated by esophageal dilatation, but responds to medical management with thickening of the milk, H_2-blockers, proton pump inhibitors or pro-motility agents. Constipation is usually managed by maintaining adequate fluid intake and dietary fiber, and administering laxatives such as polyethylene glycol 3350 (MiraLax). Restoration of function in severe fusion and flexion deformities of the hands and feet can often be helped by physiotherapy and appropriate plastic surgery. Healing in these 'degloving' procedures may be facilitated by application of 'biological dressings' with the tissue engineered skin substitutes and autologous epidermal grafts to the wounds (Fig. 13.19).[72–74] Anesthesia management for procedures is complicated, but may include mask anesthesia, endotracheal tube, intravenous sedation and local anesthetic blocks.[75,76]

With repeated blistering, ulceration, and scar formation, squamous cell carcinomas may sometimes develop on the involved skin or mucous membrane, particularly in RDEB and, to a lesser extent, JEB–H. Wounds that fail to heal or appear atypical, especially in affected adults, deserve biopsy to consider the possibility of squamous cell carcinoma. SCCs rarely appear on the tongue or esophagus. The accumulative risk in RDEB is 13% by 20 years of age, 57% by 35 years, and 87% by 45 years of age.[3] Melanoma may arise in children with RDEB, and the risk of developing basal cell carcinomas seems to be increased in adults with EBS–DM. Early intervention is key using full-thickness excision with wide margins.[77] Mohs surgery offers no long-term benefit in decreasing local recurrence, metastases or death. Amputation is required in 42% of patients with RDEB and SCC, with approximately equal outcomes on the hands and legs. Surgical debulking and radiation therapy are palliative to reduce pain or bleeding. Recently, cetuximab (EGFR antagonist) has controlled metastasized SCC in a patient.[78]

During the past few years, considerable research has shown the value of protein and gene replacement for the recessive forms of EB in animal models.[79] Transplantation of gene-corrected cultured epidermal stems cells from a patient with JEB-non-Herlitz led to

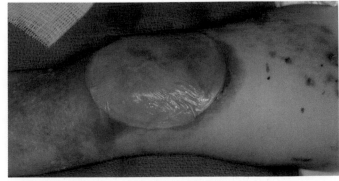

Figure 13.19 Biological dressings for EB. Biological dressings can be used selectively to promote healing of denuded areas.

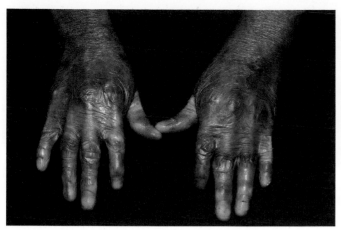

Figure 13.20 Kindler syndrome. This boy shows poikiloderma, cutaneous atrophy, webbing of the fingers, and nail dystrophy.

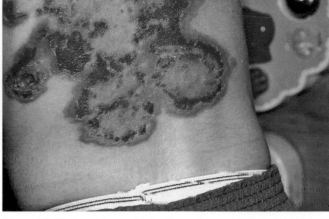

Figure 13.21 Pemphigus vulgaris. The cutaneous bullae and erosions are uncommon in children. The most common manifestation of pemphigus vulgaris is oral mucosal blistering. (Courtesy of Dr Moise Levy.)

normal-appearing skin for at least a year, but this approach used retroviral insertion.[80] Intradermal injection of allogeneic fibroblasts temporarily stimulated increased expression of type VII collagen from the patient (not donor) fibroblasts, especially in RDEB patients with less severe disease.[81] Most recently, several patients with RDEB have shown gradual improvement after stem cell transplantation;[82] further studies, including with reduced intensity conditioning regimens, are underway.

Kindler Syndrome

Kindler syndrome is characterized by generalized progressive poikiloderma, congenital acral skin blistering, diffuse cutaneous atrophy (Fig. 13.20), skin fragility, webbing of the fingers and toes, nail dystrophy, oral mucosal lesions, and photosensitivity, sometimes within minutes after exposure.[83,84] Other features are hyperkeratosis of the palms and soles; leukokeratosis; red friable hyperplastic gums; constipation and sometimes severe colitis; esophageal, laryngeal, anal, vaginal and urethral meatal stenosis; and phimosis.[85] Although the photosensitivity and the blister formation seem to decrease with age, the atrophic scarring and poikiloderma increase. The incidence of squamous cell carcinoma of the acral skin or mouth is increased. Treatment of this disorder requires the avoidance of trauma and the proper use of emollients, appropriate sun protection, and the judicious use of antibiotics to prevent secondary infection. Regular dental care and surveillance for early malignancies are important, as is iron replacement if anemic and management of the stenoses and colitis. The gene mutated in Kindler syndrome is *FERMT1* (formerly called *KIND-1*), which encodes fermitin family homolog 1 (FFH1) protein or Kindlin-1, a focal adhesion protein that links the actin cytoskeleton with the underlying extracellular matrix and controls lamellipodia formation in keratinocytes, thus regulating cell adhesion and motility.[86–88]

Immune-mediated blistering disorders

The chronic non-hereditary bullous diseases of childhood are a group of largely autoimmune disorders with autoantibodies directed against structural components of the skin. Diagnosis is based on clinical characteristics and histologic and immunofluorescent features of skin biopsy specimens. Treatment of autoimmune blistering disorders usually requires systemic immunosuppressive agents. In general, pemphigus, mucous membrane pemphigoid, and epidermolysis bullosa acquisita are more challenging to manage.

Pemphigus

Pemphigus is a term applied to a group of severe, chronic, sometimes fatal blistering disorders characterized by flaccid bullae that develop on normal-appearing skin and mucous membranes. Pemphigus can be classified into pemphigus vulgaris, pemphigus foliaceus, IgA pemphigus, drug-induced pemphigus, and paraneoplastic pemphigus. The blister formation in pemphigus results from acantholysis, which is loss of cohesion between epidermal cells owing to intercellular edema and the disappearance of intercellular bridges in the lower epidermis. The structural components against which autoantibodies are generated in pemphigus are all components of desmosomes.

Pemphigus vulgaris

Pemphigus vulgaris is a potentially life-threatening chronic vesiculobullous disease characterized by flaccid bullae and persistent erosions, with a predilection for middle-aged individuals. An extremely uncommon disorder of childhood, the prognosis is better in children than in adults.[89] The cutaneous lesions of pemphigus vulgaris favor the seborrheic areas (the face, scalp, neck, sternum, axillae, groin, and periumbilical regions) and pressure areas of the feet and back (Fig. 13.21). The oral mucosae are affected in 95% of patients and are the initial site in the majority of patients, often months before the appearance of skin lesions. Intact blisters are rarely seen on the oral mucosa, since they rupture soon after formation, leaving raw denuded painful erosions that heal slowly. Other mucosal surfaces, the anogenital areas, conjunctivae,[90] vermilion borders of the lips, pharynx, and the larynx, may be similarly involved. Pemphigus in children can involve the esophagus and ileum, leading to protein-losing enteropathy.[91] Since a majority of patients with proven pemphigus vulgaris present with painful oral erosions for weeks to months before they develop the characteristic bullous eruption (and the disease may be limited to mucosae), children with severe recurrent mucocutaneous lesions or chronic erosive mucous membrane disease should be examined carefully.[92] Mucosal biopsy should be performed if skin lesions are not present.

The primary cutaneous lesions of pemphigus vulgaris appear as vesicles or bullae that arise on erythematous plaques or normal-appearing skin. The initial lesions may remain localized to one area of the skin or mucous membrane for weeks or months before other areas of the skin are involved. With the onset of new lesions, the patient may experience some pruritus, burning, or local discomfort. Blisters generally measure 1 cm or less at onset but may increase by peripheral extension to several centimeters in diameter. Lateral pressure applied to the normal-appearing skin at the periphery of a lesion results in lesional extension and shearing of skin (the Nikolsky sign). This phenomenon, a manifestation of defective epidermal cohesion, is not pathognomonic of pemphigus, since the Nikolsky sign may also be seen in patients with epidermolysis bullosa, bullous pemphigoid, Stevens–Johnson syndrome, and toxic epidermal necrolysis. Vertical pressure may also produce peripheral extension of lesions. The blisters rupture easily, and the resultant erosions are painful, bleed easily, and heal slowly. Scaling and crusting are common, and patients frequently are misdiagnosed as having impetigo or infected seborrheic dermatitis.

A variant of pemphigus vulgaris, *pemphigus vegetans*, is differentiated by the hypertrophic granulomatous tissue (vegetations) after healing and the tendency for predilection for the face, flexural, and intertriginous areas. Patients frequently show small pustules at the periphery of ruptured bullae.[93]

Confirmation of the diagnosis of pemphigus vulgaris depends on histologic examination of new lesions, and immunofluorescent studies. The earliest histologic change is intercellular edema, with loss of cohesion between epidermal cells, resulting in the formation of clefts and bullae in a suprabasal location. The basal cells, although separated from one another, remain attached to the dermis, with a resultant 'row of tombstones' appearance. A rapid Tzanck smear will show acantholytic cells.[94] Direct immunofluorescent tests on biopsied samples show IgG and complement bound to intercellular areas of the epidermis. Indirect immunofluorescent studies of the serum of patients with pemphigus vulgaris show IgG antibodies binding to the intercellular spaces. Levels of circulating antibody correlate with disease activity; increases in titers may precede clinical flares and decreases in titer correlate with clinical responses. The targeted structural antigen in patients with only mucosal pemphigus is desmoglein 3, a desmosomal component expressed in the mucosa and lower region of the epidermis, and the presence of antibody can be tested by ELISA. Desmoglein 1 can compensate for desmoglein 3 in skin; antibodies against both desmogleins must be present for both mucosal and skin blistering to occur in pemphigus.

A transient form of pemphigus vulgaris, *neonatal pemphigus vulgaris*, may be seen in infants of pregnant women with circulating anti-desmoglein 3 antibodies, even without active mucocutaneous disease. Blistering subsides in affected neonates within a few weeks, concomitant with the catabolism of maternal antibodies.[95–97]

Pemphigus foliaceus

Pemphigus foliaceus (superficial pemphigus) is a more superficial form of pemphigus.[98] The disease most commonly affects middle-aged persons and, although rare in children, is more common than pemphigus vulgaris in prepubertal childhood. The disorder in children is more benign than that in adults, and the course is milder than that of pemphigus vulgaris.

Bullae, when seen, are usually small and flaccid. They rupture easily and, because of their superficial location, leave shallow erosions. Slowly spreading crusted plaques thought to be impetigo, but resistant to oral antibiotics, are the most common presenting manifestation (Fig. 13.22). Patients often show an arcuate configuration to lesions. Common areas of erosive involvement include the

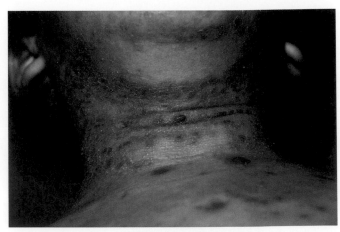

Figure 13.22 Pemphigus foliaceus. Children with pemphigus foliaceus are often thought to have impetigo and treated unsuccessfully with courses of antibiotics as a result; the target of this immunobullous disorder, desmoglein 1, is the same target as the exfoliatin produced by *Staphylococcus aureus* infection.

scalp,[99] face, upper chest, abdomen, and back. Bullae are more likely to be intact if located on the lower extremities. Patients generally are not severely ill but may rarely complain of pruritus, pain, and burning. At times, however, the clinical picture may progress to resemble that of a severe generalized exfoliative dermatitis. Oral lesions are rarely seen in pemphigus foliaceus and, when present, usually consist of small, superficial, often inconspicuous erosions.

Pemphigus erythematosus (Senear–Usher syndrome) is a variant of pemphigus foliaceus in which lesions often localize to the butterfly area of the face, the scalp, upper chest, and back. Patients may show detectable antinuclear antibodies.[100,101] *Fogo selvagem* (endemic pemphigus; Brazilian pemphigus) is a variant of pemphigus foliaceus found in tropical regions, but is clinically indistinguishable from sporadic pemphigus foliaceus.[102] Endemic in Brazil, and to a lesser extent in other South American countries, 15% of patients are children. The striking distribution of lesions on sun-exposed skin, its burned appearance, and the painful burning sensation in lesions (more so than in sporadic pemphigus foliaceus) are responsible for the name fogo selvagem (Portuguese, meaning 'wildfire'). In chronic cases hyperpigmentation, hyperkeratosis, and loss of hair over the scalp and body are prominent features of this disorder.

Histologic findings in pemphigus foliaceus are similar to those of pemphigus vulgaris and demonstrate epidermal bullae and intercellular acantholysis of the epidermis. The acantholysis seen in pemphigus foliaceus, however, is more superficial and occurs in the upper epidermis, usually in the granular layer or just beneath it, with resultant formation of clefts in a superficial, often subcorneal, location. Direct immunofluorescence shows an intracellular deposition of IgG and C[3] that is indistinguishable from that of pemphigus vulgaris. The targeted antigen is desmoglein 1, a desmosomal component localized to the suprabasal keratinocytes, which is also the target of bacterial exfoliative toxins in patients with bullous impetigo and staphylococcal scalded skin syndrome (Ch. 14).[103] IgG4 and IgM anti-desmoglein 1 antibodies have been described in association with fogo selvagem.[104,105] Although desmoglein 1 is also found in the mucosa, desmoglein 3 at this location provides stabilization and patients with pemphigus foliaceus, as a result, do not tend to have oral mucosal lesions.[106] Neonatal pemphigus has not been observed in infants born to mothers with active fogo selvagem, but has been described in babies of mothers with sporadic pemphigus foliaceus and high titers of anti-desmoglein 1 antibodies.[107,108]

Drug-induced pemphigus

Drug-induced pemphigus is particularly rare in children. The most commonly implicated agents are penicillamine and captopril (Table 13.7). Both of these medications have sulfhydryl groups that are thought to interact with the sulfhydryl groups in desmogleins 1 and 3, thus modifying the antigenicity of the desmoglein. In contrast to other types of drug reactions, drug-induced pemphigus often requires several months of exposure to the medication before onset. Initially, a nonspecific morbilliform, annular, or urticarial eruption may be seen, eventually evolving after a variable latency period into the blistering process. The disorder typically resembles pemphigus foliaceus more often than pemphigus vulgaris. Oral lesions are rare.

IgA pemphigus

IgA pemphigus, characterized by the intercellular deposition of IgA rather than IgG autoantibodies, has been divided into the subcorneal pustular dermatosis form and intraepidermal neutrophilic IgA dermatosis, based on the subcorneal or intraepidermal localization of the blister histologically. Both conditions clinically show vesicles, small bullae, and pustules overlying well-circumscribed erythema. IgA pemphigus resembling pemphigus vegetans has also been described.[109] The youngest reported patient was 1 month of age.[110] The autoantigen for the subcorneal pustular dermatosis form has been shown to be the desmosomal protein desmocollin 1.[111] Although circulating antibodies against either desmoglein 1 and desmoglein 3 have been identified in patients with intraepidermal neutrophilic IgA dermatosis, other patients have shown no identifiable autoantigen.[112–114]

The pustular form may be the same disorder as *subcorneal pustular dermatosis* (Sneddon–Wilkinson disease), a condition that rarely occurs in children, although it has been described in individuals as young as 7 weeks of age.[115] The disease generally begins with small pustules or vesicles on an erythematous base. Occasionally only vesicles may be present, but these soon change into sterile pustules. The pustules tend to appear in crops and spread to large parts of the body, forming large circinate or gyrate patterns that coalesce to form serpiginous patterns, especially on the abdomen, axillae, and groin. Individual lesions tend to last for periods of 5 days, with new lesions appearing as others disappear. As the pustules resolve they are replaced by a superficial leafy scale or crust. After the eruption resolves, a faint blotchy brown hyperpigmentation, without atrophy or scarring, remains. The condition is benign and is characterized by remissions and exacerbations that may last for 5–8 years. Histopathologic examination of an intact lesion of subcorneal pustular dermatosis reveals a subcorneal blister filled almost entirely with neutrophilic polymorphonuclear leukocytes, but immunofluorescence analysis shows no immunodeposits.

Paraneoplastic pemphigus

Paraneoplastic pemphigus, a rare autoimmune disorder associated with malignancy, has been described occasionally in children.[116] The majority of pediatric patients have underlying Castleman's disease, a lymphoproliferative disorder characterized by massive

Table 13.7 Causes of drug-induced pemphigus
Beta blockers
Captopril
Ceftazidime
Penicillamine
Penicillin
Progesterone
Rifampin

growth of lymphoid tissue, usually located in the retroperitoneum or mediastinum.[117] Sarcoma, T-cell lymphoblastic lymphoma, and myofibroblastic tumor may also underlie paraneoplastic pemphigus; occasionally, no underlying tumor is detected.

All patients tend to show intractable stomatitis, particularly involving the labial mucosa and resembling the labial manifestations of Stevens–Johnson syndrome. Two-thirds of patients show conjunctival involvement, sometimes leading to symblepharon and visual impairment. Skin changes can be bullous, and/or may resemble lichen planus or erythema multiforme. The trunk and extremities are most commonly involved. Palmoplantar involvement and paronychial inflammation, which may result in nail shedding, are frequently seen. Mucosae of the tracheobronchial system are also involved, and respiratory involvement with the development of bronchiolitis obliterans may be fatal.[118]

Biopsies show intraepithelial acantholysis, keratinocyte dyskeratosis, and basal cell vacuolar changes, combining the histologic features of pemphigus and Stevens–Johnson syndrome. Direct immunofluorescence is often negative, but immunoblots show several circulating autoantibodies directed against a variety of epidermal proteins, particularly of the plakin family (desmoglein 1 and 3, bullous pemphigoid antigen 1, desmoplakin, envoplakin and periplakin).

Paraneoplastic pemphigus must be distinguished from Stevens–Johnson syndrome, toxic epidermal necrolysis, pemphigus vulgaris, bullous and cicatricial forms of pemphigoid, lichen planus pemphigoides, and mucosal infections from herpes or candida. Once the diagnosis is suspected in a child or adolescent, evaluation for malignancy should be initiated. Complete physical examination, particularly of the liver, spleen, and lymph nodes, complete blood count, serum protein electrophoresis, and computerized tomographic scans of the chest, abdomen, and pelvis should be performed to seek evidence of malignancy.

Treatment of pemphigus

The treatment of choice for pemphigus vulgaris is systemic corticosteroid therapy, given either as high doses orally (1–2 mg/kg per day) or as intravenous pulses.[119] Dapsone[120] (see below) and, if not successful, mycophenolate mofetil (600–1200 mg/m^2 per day),[121] cyclosporine (5 mg/kg per day), azathioprine (2–4 mg/kg per day),[122] or high-dose intravenous immunoglobulin[123,124] are steroid-sparing agents that can be added to allow the corticosteroid to be tapered, although each of these agents has significant potential side-effects. The use of rituximab (monoclonal anti-CD20 antibody) should be reserved for treatment-resistant cases, given the high risk of side-effects.[125,126] Immunoadsorption is preferred to plasmapheresis because it clears the circulating antibodies without depleting other plasma proteins, such as clotting factors, hormones and albumin.[127]

Pemphigus foliaceus is a milder disorder. Suprapotent topical corticosteroids may be effective in some patients, but often treatment with dapsone, with or without systemic corticosteroids (initially 1 mg/kg per day), may be required for clearance. In all forms of pemphigus, therapy should be tapered gradually as tolerated when improvement is noted, which may require several months in severe cases. Although patients with Brazilian pemphigus (fogo selvagem) may respond to antimalarial therapy (quinine or quinacrine), systemic corticosteroids continue to be the treatment of choice. Once the disease has cleared, pemphigus foliaceus has a lesser tendency to recur than pemphigus vulgaris.

Drug-induced pemphigus usually clears with treatment of the pemphigus and withdrawal of the offending medication. IgA pemphigus in children usually responds to treatment with dapsone or sulfapyridine within 24–48 h, but tends to be more difficult to control with steroids and other systemic antiinflammatory agents.

Oral retinoids have been used in patients with IgA pemphigus who do not respond to systemic administration of corticosteroids and dapsone.[128]

Patients with paraneoplastic pemphigus often clear or improve significantly with surgical removal of the Castleman's disease, but not until 6–18 months after tumor removal. The prognosis is much worse with malignant neoplasms. The majority of patients succumb within months of the diagnosis, usually to respiratory failure or secondary infection. Aggressive treatment of the malignancy coupled with immunosuppressive therapy, e.g., the combination of systemic corticosteroids and cyclosporine, should be initiated, but may not affect the prognosis. A support group for patients with pemphigus can be accessed at: www.pemphigus.org.

Bullous Pemphigoid

Bullous pemphigoid (BP) is a blistering disorder characterized by large, tense, subepidermal bullae that appear on normal-appearing or erythematous skin. Although usually seen in elderly persons, BP may also occur occasionally in infants as young as 2 months of age[129] and in children,[130–132] the youngest reported being a 2-month-old infant.[132]

The disorder often starts as mild to moderate pruritus, with urticarial or erythematous plaques that evolve over weeks to months into large, tense, sometimes hemorrhagic bullae. Lesions may appear on normal skin or on an erythematous base. The blisters frequently occur at the periphery of annular or polycyclic erythematous plaques. Bullae typically measure 0.25–2.0 cm in diameter. The lower abdomen, anogenital region (including the vulva), and flexural areas of the arms and legs are most often involved, although bullae not uncommonly occur on the face in children. The Nikolsky sign is characteristically absent, and blisters do not extend or increase in size as they do in patients with pemphigus vulgaris. Blistering of the palms and soles is quite frequently seen in affected infants, whereas penile involvement is more common in older children.[129,132–134] The bullae tend to be more tense and inflamed than those of pemphigus vulgaris (Fig. 13.23), and the course of BP is more indolent than that of pemphigus vulgaris. Blisters resolve without scarring. Oral lesions are seen in approximately 25% of patients, especially in older children.

Variants include *cicatricial pemphigoid*, which affects mucosal surfaces, and a localized form (chronic pemphigoid of Brunsting–Perry), which is generally limited to the head and neck. The predominant localization of blisters in cicatricial pemphigoid is mucosal[135] (Fig. 13.24), with only 25% of patients showing skin involvement, particularly on the face, neck, and upper chest. Recurrent bullae are seen in the oral mucosa, conjunctivae, and other mucous membranes such as those of the nasopharynx, esophagus, larynx, genitalia,[136] and anus.[137] Oral involvement often takes the form of a desquamative gingivitis,[138] and ocular involvement may not occur until many years after the onset of the condition. Eye involvement often presents as dryness of the eyes with a feeling of chronic, intractable conjunctival irritation. Conjunctival involvement can lead to entropion, trichiasis (ingrowing eyelashes), symblepharon, dryness of the cornea, corneal ulceration, and, in 25% of patients, blindness. Esophageal lesions may result in stricture formation. Laryngeal lesions, when present, can be life threatening. Adhesions of the genitourinary region may lead to phimosis in boys and narrowing of the vaginal opening in affected girls. Lichen planus pemphigoides is an overlap disease in which the lichen planus develops first;[139] most cases respond to dapsone (see Ch. 4).

Biopsy specimens of cutaneous lesions show subepidermal blister formation, generally without papillary microabscesses (an important diagnostic feature of dermatitis herpetiformis). Eosinophils are often seen in sections, and peripheral eosinophilia is common. Direct immunofluorescence reveals deposition of C_3 and IgG at the lamina lucida of the basement membrane zone. Although indirect testing of serum for circulating IgG anti-basement membrane zone antibodies (IIF) is positive in 72% of children, antibody titers do not correlate with clinical disease activity. These circulating immune deposits bind to the roof of salt-split skin, in which the cleavage runs through the lamina lucida of basement membrane. Antibodies are most commonly directed against BP180 antigen, but may be directed against BP230.[133] ELISA assays have been shown to be more sensitive and just as specific as IIF.[140]

Potent topical corticosteroids may be effective for localized areas of involvement and in mildly affected patients.[141] In general, systemic corticosteroids are the mainstay of treatment (1–2 mg/kg per day). Sulfapyridine (2 mg/kg per day), dapsone (3–6 mg/kg per day), and azathioprine (4 mg/kg per day) have been used as steroid-sparing agents.[142] Erythromycin (50 mg/kg per day) with or without nicotinamide (40 mg/kg per day) has been beneficial in some children, presumably owing to its antiinflammatory effects. The disorder remits in most children within a year and has an excellent

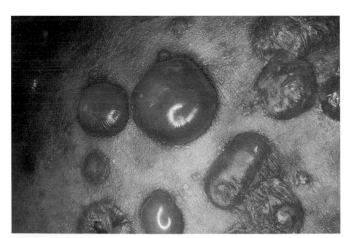

Figure 13.23 Bullous pemphigoid. Large tense bullae are seen on the lower region of the abdomen in this 13-year-old boy.

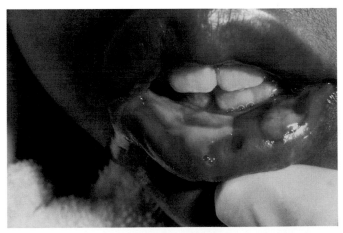

Figure 13.24 Cicatricial pemphigoid. This 3-year-old boy showed blistering of the oral and ocular mucosae. Early diagnosis is critical to prevent the scarring and permanent blindness. The minority of patients with this condition show cutaneous involvement.

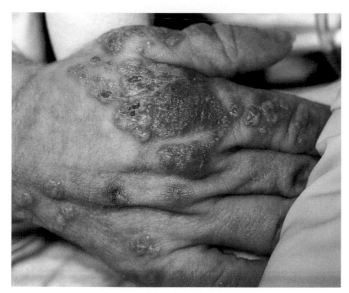

Figure 13.25 Pemphigus gestationis. Cutaneous involvement of the newborn has been noted in about 10% of infants born to mothers with this disorder. In the neonate the condition subsides within several weeks as maternal antibodies wane. (Courtesy of Moise Levy, MD.)

prognosis. Rarely, plasma exchange and extracorporeal photochemotherapy have been used for childhood bullous pemphigoid.[143]

Pemphigoid gestationis

Pemphigoid gestationis (formerly called herpes gestationis) usually presents during the second or 3rd trimester of pregnancy or in the immediate postpartum period. It occurs in 1 : 50 000 pregnancies. Skin lesions often start at the umbilical area and spread to the abdomen and thighs. Before the development of bullae, initial lesions may be pruritic, eczematous, or erythema multiforme-like erythematous papules and plaques. The disorder can start for the first time with any pregnancy, but then tends to recur in subsequent pregnancies. Although the eruption tends to clear in the majority of patients within a few days of delivery, it can persist for many months after delivery. Mild recurrences occasionally have been noted to appear at the time of menstruation, in women who take oral contraceptives, and in women with choriocarcinomas and hydatidiform moles. Cutaneous involvement of the newborn has been noted in about 10% of infants born to mothers with this disorder (Fig. 13.25); on the basis of immunofluorescent findings, a high percentage of newborns have been noted to have subclinical forms of pemphigoid gestationis as well.

The immunopathologic hallmark of pemphigoid gestationis is deposition of C_3, with or without IgG, distributed in a linear band along the basement membrane. The targeted antigens in skin are BP180 and, less commonly, BP230.[144]

The course of pemphigoid gestationis is characterized by alternating exacerbations and remissions. Systemic corticosteroids are the most reliable mode of therapy and, with certain precautions, are generally considered safe for both mother and fetus, especially after the first trimester of pregnancy. Alternate-day dosage, if possible, is preferable to daily treatment. To avoid fetal adrenal suppression, dosages should be reduced to a minimum during the final weeks of pregnancy. The cutaneous lesions in infants with this disorder generally remit within several weeks and do not require therapy. Although there may be an increased risk of prematurity or intrauterine growth restriction, pemphigoid gestationis does not result in an increased mortality risk for the mother or the fetus.

Dermatitis Herpetiformis

Dermatitis herpetiformis (Duhring's disease) is characterized by an intensely pruritic papulovesicular and, at times, bullous eruption that responds dramatically to orally administered doses of sulfones or sulfapyridine.[145] Although the disorder may affect infants and children, dermatitis herpetiformis generally occurs during the second to fifth decades of life. It is most common in individuals of Northern European descent, is rare in African-Americans, and, in contrast to many autoimmune disorders, affects males more frequently than females. Diagnosis of this disorder cannot be based solely on the morphologic aspects and distribution of lesions, but on the constellation of clinical appearance, histopathologic characteristics, immunofluorescent findings, serologic testing, and response to therapy.

Dermatitis herpetiformis tends to affect the extensor surfaces: the elbows, knees, sacrum, buttocks, and shoulders, and occasionally the face, eyelids, facial hairline, posterior nuchal area, and scalp. Lesions are usually grouped and symmetrical in distribution. In association with the onset of intense pruritus or burning, erythematous and, at times, urticarial lesions may develop. Characteristic of this disorder are minute, clear, relatively tense vesicles that measure from 0.3 to 4.0 mm in diameter. These vesicles rupture easily, either spontaneously or when scratched. Not uncommonly, the grouped ('herpetiform') vesicles and papules are seen amidst excoriated papules and postinflammatory hypo- and hyperpigmentation. The general course of this disorder is chronic (often lasting 5–10 years or more) with frequent exacerbations and remissions.

Dermatitis herpetiformis is generally manifested as a purely cutaneous disorder, and gastrointestinal complaints are rare. Studies have demonstrated, however, that 75–90% of patients with this disorder also have small bowel abnormalities, histologically indistinguishable from those seen in celiac-type gluten-sensitivity enteropathy.[146] Neurologic abnormalities are rarely described, but ataxia may be the presenting sign.[147] Some consider dermatitis herpetiformis to be a cutaneous manifestation of celiac disease. Both DH and celiac disease are strongly associated with HLA DR3 and DQw2.[148] As in patients with celiac disease, patients with DH may show circulating IgA autoantibodies to tissue transglutaminase (TG2) and to endomysium; however, autoantibodies against epidermal transglutaminase (TG3) have more recently been shown to be more sensitive and specific to DH and detection correlates with disease activity.[149–151]

Childhood DH can be confused with arthropod bites, dermatitis, urticaria, scabies, and pityriasis lichenoides et varioliformis acuta. Serum IgA anti-transglutaminase 3 levels have been proposed as a screening test for DH. Confirmation of the diagnosis requires lesional biopsy for routine histologic evaluation and, most importantly, perilesional biopsy for immunofluorescent analysis. Subepidermal microabscesses with accumulations of neutrophils and eosinophils are found at the tips of the dermal papillae by routine histology. IgA is seen at the tips of the dermal papillae in a granular pattern by immunofluorescent microscopy of perilesional skin.[152]

Sulfones (dapsone) and sulfapyridine are effective in relieving the symptoms and suppressing the eruption of dermatitis herpetiformis in children as well as adults. Dramatic relief from the use of these agents, frequently as early as 24–48 h after initiation, is often helpful in making the diagnosis. The recommended initial dosage for dapsone is 2 mg/kg per day. Once existing lesions have been suppressed, the dosage may be tapered to a minimal level (usually 12.5–50 mg/day). Baseline blood counts and glucose-6-phosphate dehydrogenase (G6PD) levels are important before initiating therapy. Blood counts should be repeated weekly for the first month, then monthly for the next 5 months. In addition to hemolytic anemia (especially seen in patients with G6PD deficiency, a contraindication to use), side-effects include methemoglobinemia (manifested by bluish discoloration of the face, mucous membranes, and nails), nausea, vomiting, headache, giddiness, tachycardia, psychoses, anemia, leukopenia, fever, exfoliative dermatitis, liver necrosis, lymphadenitis, and peripheral neuropathy. If at all possible, a gluten-free diet should be instituted. By gluten-free diet alone, children remit in approximately 11 months, emphasizing that dapsone is idea to control the inflammatory phase. It should be noted, however, that only highly motivated individuals will adhere to this diet. Support and information about dermatitis herpetiformis and gluten-free diets can be found online through the Gluten Intolerance Group (at: www.gluten.net) and the Dermatitis Herpetiformis Online Community (at: www.dermatitisherpetiformis.org.uk).

Linear IgA Bullous Dermatosis

Linear IgA bullous dermatosis of childhood (chronic bullous disease of childhood) is a subepidermal blistering disease that may be indistinguishable both clinically and histologically from bullous pemphigoid.[153,154] Its onset is usually in the first decade of life, particularly during preschool years. Spontaneous remission usually occurs after several months to 3 years, and almost always before the onset of puberty. IgA nephropathy is a rare complication.[155] Drugs, especially antibiotics such as vancomycin, amoxicillin-clavulanate, and trimethoprim-sulfamethoxazole, are occasional triggers.[156–158]

The eruption is characterized by large, tense, clear or hemorrhagic bullae measuring 1.0–2.0 cm in diameter on a normal or erythematous base. The eruption is widespread, and areas of predilection include the face, scalp, lower part of the trunk (including the genitalia and pubis), buttocks, inner thighs, legs, and dorsal aspect of the feet (Fig. 13.26). The bullae may form characteristic annular or rosette-like lesions composed of sausage-shaped blisters resembling a cluster of jewels surrounding a central crust, the 'string of pearls' sign (Fig. 13.27). Mucous membrane lesions occasionally occur. Pruritus is a variable feature and may be mild to moderate, intense and distressing, or completely absent.

Histologically, chronic bullous disease of childhood is characterized by subepidermal bullae with edema of adjacent dermal papillae and a dermal infiltrate of neutrophilic polymorphonuclear leukocytes, eosinophils, and mononuclear cells. The immunofluorescent findings of linear IgA deposits in the lamina lucida zone of the dermal-epidermal junction obtained from perilesional skin confirm the diagnosis; occasionally children show both IgA and IgG antibodies.[159,160] Circulating IgA basement membrane zone antibody is found in up to 80% of patients, and usually binds the epidermal side of salt-split skin. Antibodies are most commonly directed against a 97 kDa and/or 120 kDa fragment of BP180; the 120 kDa fragment is generated from BP180 by disintegrin-metalloproteinases (ADAMs), whereas the 97 kDa fragment is generated by plasmin from the 120 kDa fragment.[161] Some children with clinically typical chronic bullous disease of childhood show 'mixed immunobullous disease of childhood', in which both IgG and IgA autoantibodies are detected.

Response to therapy is generally favorable. Dapsone, as in dermatitis herpetiformis, is the drug of choice, although patients have responded to administration of erythromycin, dicloxacillin, or sulfonamides.[162–164] Responses to antibiotics, however, are often transient and their use has been advocated initially while awaiting results of diagnostic tests or in patients unable to take dapsone and sulfapyridine.[165] If response to dapsone or antibiotics is inadequate, sulfapyridine, systemic corticosteroids, and mycophenolate mofetil are alternative therapies.

Epidermolysis Bullosa Acquisita

Acquired epidermolysis bullosa (epidermolysis bullosa acquisita, EBA) is a subepidermal blistering disorder that usually takes on one of two forms: a generalized inflammatory eruption clinically indistinguishable from bullous pemphigoid and a non-inflammatory acral blistering disorder that results in scarring and milia formation (Fig. 13.28), reminiscent of dominant dystrophic EB. Approximately 40 cases in children have been described.[166] A neonate with EBA from transplacental transfer of antibody has recently been described (Fig. 13.29).[167] Blisters may be hemorrhagic or serous and tend to be localized to sites of trauma or pressure, especially on the extensor areas of the extremities. Oropharyngeal mucous membrane erosions are frequently seen; the conjunctival, esophageal, and anogenital mucous membranes are less commonly involved, although blindness may result. The nails may be dystrophic and scarring alopecia may be seen.

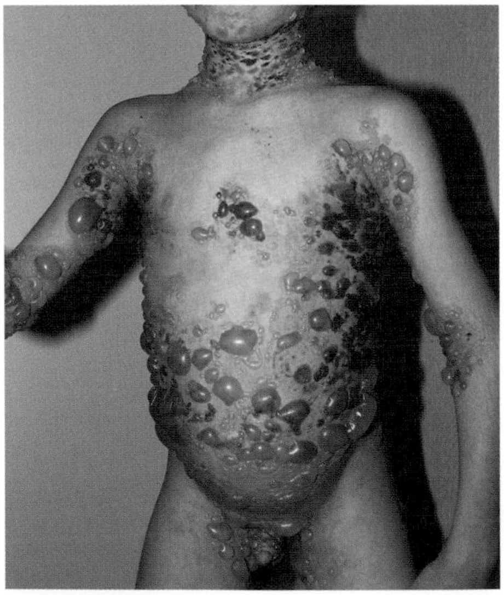

Figure 13.26 Chronic bullous disease of childhood. Large, tense, clear or hemorrhagic bullae are commonly found on the face, lower part of the trunk, and genitalia.

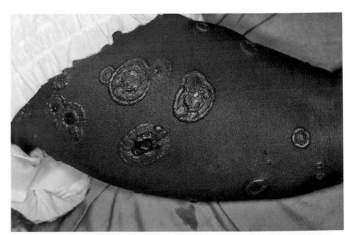

Figure 13.27 Chronic bullous disease of childhood. The bullae may form characteristic annular or rosette-like lesions resembling a cluster of jewels surrounding a central crust, the 'string of pearls' sign.

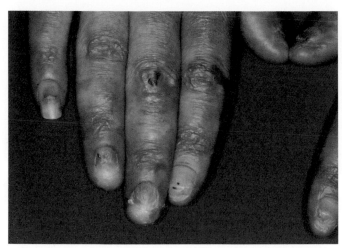

Figure 13.28 Epidermolysis bullosa acquisita. This disorder may be indistinguishable from bullous pemphigoid or may resemble dystrophic EB, as in this patient. Note the scarring, milia, and nail dystrophy. The immunodeposits in patients with EB acquisita are directed against collagen VII, the same protein missing or dysfunctional in patients with dystrophic EB.

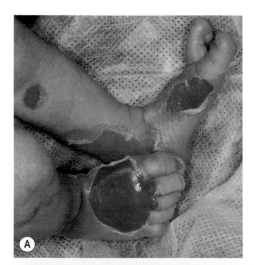

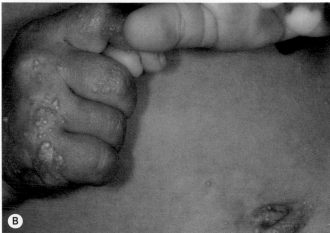

Figure 13.29 Epidermolysis bullosa acquisita. This baby developed EB acquisita by transplacental passage of maternal antibodies against type VII collagen. Tense blisters resulted in neonatal denudement (A) and subsequent milia formation (B), as in dystrophic EB.

The condition results from the deposition of IgG, and less commonly IgA,[168,169] autoantibodies directed against type VII collagen (Fig. 13.1). Type VII collagen is a structural component of anchoring fibrils that is missing or abnormal in children with recessive or dominant dystrophic epidermolysis bullosa, respectively. Immunofluorescence examination shows the linear deposition of IgG and sometimes C_3 at the lower lamina densa or sublamina densa zones of the basement membrane. Indirect immunofluorescence shows IgG binding to the dermal side of salt-split skin (e.g., beneath the lamina lucida). Immunoblotting analysis shows binding to a 290-kDa protein that corresponds to type VII collagen and recognition primarily of the NC1 non-collagenous domain of type VII collagen; however, children may show antibodies directed against additional domains, particularly children with EBA younger than 10 years of age with the inflammatory phenotype.[170]

EBA has a chronic course with flares, but seems to have a better prognosis in children than in adults. Dapsone and corticosteroids are first-line therapy and often lead to remission within about 2 years; mycophenolate mofetil may be steroid-sparing. Rituximab is now also used for treatment-resistant EBA.[171,172] Childhood IgA-mediated EBA has responded to mycophenolate mofetil.[169] Colchicine, infliximab, photophoresis and intravenous immunoglobulin have been helpful for some patients.[173] The recent demonstration that T cells are critical in initiation of EBA suggests that T cell-directed immunomodulatory strategies may be effective in the future.[174]

Bullous Systemic Lupus Erythematosus

Similar to patients with epidermolysis bullosa acquisita, patients with lupus erythematosus who manifest immune-mediated bullae show antibodies directed against type VII collagen.[175–177] However, the clinical manifestations more closely resemble those of bullous pemphigoid or dermatitis herpetiformis. African-American adolescents and young women are most frequently affected, with a mean age of onset of 22 years.[178] Occasionally, bullous SLE is the presenting sign of lupus,[179] but more typically it develops in a patient with known SLE (see Ch. 22). Typical lesions are pruritic vesicles and tense bullae with occasional erythematous macules and papules (Fig. 13.30). Lesions tend to leave post-inflammatory hypo- or hyperpigmentation. Sun-exposed areas are most commonly involved, but flexor and extensor skin surfaces, as well as oral

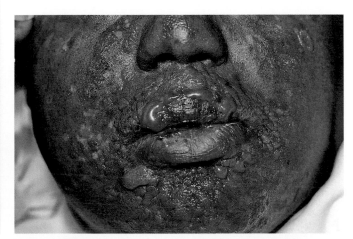

Figure 13.30 Bullous systemic lupus erythematosus. Pruritic vesicles and tense bullae develop, and may leave intense postinflammatory hypo- or hyperpigmentation. This adolescent responded to the combination of prednisone, azathioprine, and dapsone.

mucosae, may be affected. Bullous SLE in a linear pattern following Blaschko's lines has been described in a child.[180]

Immunofluorescence examination shows deposition of IgG, and sometimes IgM, IgA, or C_3, at the basement membrane and upper dermis. Granular, linear, and mixed patterns have all been described. Prognosis is usually favorable, and is largely determined by the course of the associated systemic lupus erythematosus. Most patients respond quickly to dapsone therapy (in contrast to EBA). Administration of systemic corticosteroids with or without additional immunosuppressive agents (e.g., methotrexate, mycophenolate mofetil, azathioprine, cyclophosphamide, or cyclosporine) has led to variable response.

Key References

Abrams ML, Smidt A, Benjamin L, et al. Congenital epidermolysis bullosa acquisita: vertical transfer of maternal autoantibody from mother to infant. *Arch Dermatol.* 2010 Nov 15. [Epub ahead of print].

Culton DA, Qian Y, Li N, et al. Advances in pemphigus and its endemic pemphigus foliaceus (Fogo Selvagem) phenotype: a paradigm of human autoimmunity. *J Autoimmun.* 2008;31:311–324.

Fassihi H, Eady RA, Mellerio JE, et al. Prenatal diagnosis for severe inherited skin disorders: 25 years' experience. *Br J Dermatol.* 2006; 154:106–113.

Fine JD, Eady RA, Bauer EA, et al. The classification of inherited epidermolysis bullosa (EB): Report of the Third International Consensus Meeting on Diagnosis and Classification of EB. *J Am Acad Dermatol.* 2008;58:931–950.

Fine JD, Johnson LB, Weiner M, et al. Cause-specific risks of childhood death in inherited epidermolysis bullosa. *J Pediatr.* 2008;152:276–280.

Fine JD, Johnson LB, Weiner M, et al. Epidermolysis bullosa and the risk of life-threatening cancers: the National EB Registry experience, 1986–2006. *J Am Acad Dermatol.* 2009;60:203–211.

Fine JD, Mellerio JE. Extracutaneous manifestations and complications of inherited epidermolysis bullosa: part I. Epithelial associated tissues. *J Am Acad Dermatol.* 2009;61:367–384; quiz 385–366.

Fine JD, Mellerio JE. Extracutaneous manifestations and complications of inherited epidermolysis bullosa: part II. Other organs. *J Am Acad Dermatol.* 2009;61:387–402; quiz 403–384.

Hull CM, Liddle M, Hansen N, et al. Elevation of IgA anti-epidermal transglutaminase antibodies in dermatitis herpetiformis. *Br J Dermatol.* 2008;159:120–124.

Kasperkiewicz M, Schmidt E. Current treatment of autoimmune blistering diseases. *Curr Drug Discov Technol.* 2009;6:270–280.

Ly L, Su JC. Dressings used in epidermolysis bullosa blister wounds: a review. *J Wound Care.* 2008;17:482, 484–486, 488 passim.

Bacterial, Mycobacterial, and Protozoal Infections of the Skin

14

The normal skin of healthy infants and children is resistant to invasion by most bacteria because the cutaneous surface provides a dry mechanical barrier from which contaminating organisms are constantly removed by desquamation. Under normal conditions the skin is sterile at delivery and for a short period thereafter. During the process of vaginal birth it acquires organisms from the birth canal, which gradually increase in number during the first 10 days of life. If the newborn is delivered by cesarean section, however, the cutaneous surface remains sterile until after delivery but soon becomes exposed to bacteria from human contactants and fomites.

Almost any organism may live on the cutaneous surface under appropriate conditions. A complete list of transient organisms accordingly would include virtually all microorganisms found in the human environment. The number of species composing the resident flora, however, is relatively small and consists predominantly of Gram-positive organisms and a few Gram-negative species, including *Propionibacterium acnes* (normally found in high concentrations about the pilosebaceous follicles of the face and less commonly the axillae and forearms), aerobic diphtheroids (*Corynebacterium minutissimum* and *Corynebacterium tenuis*), *Staphylococcus epidermidis* micrococci, and anaerobic Gram-positive cocci. Others include Gram-negative bacilli (*Escherichia coli*, *Proteus*, *Enterobacter*, and *Pseudomonas*, among others), found uncommonly on normal skin except in the moist intertriginous areas of the groin, axillae, and toe webs, and *Staphylococcus aureus*, a common pathogen that appears to usually be seeded from the carrier state in the anterior nares.

Since the cutaneous surface is continuously exposed to microorganisms, it is most helpful to distinguish among transient, resident, and pathogenic flora. The transient flora consists of multiple organisms that are deposited on the skin from the environment, presumably do not proliferate, and are removed easily by washing or scrubbing of the affected area. The resident flora consists of a smaller number of organisms that are found more or less regularly in appreciable numbers on the skin of normal individuals, multiply on the skin, form stable communities on the cutaneous surface, and are not easily dislodged. Pathogenic bacteria, not ordinarily a regular part of this flora, persist on the skin if there is continuous replacement from some internal or external source, or if the integrity of the skin is disrupted by injury or disease. It should be noted that the mere presence of potentially pathogenic bacteria in a cutaneous lesion does not necessarily prove the demonstrable organism to be a cause of bacterial infection.

Children have a more varied cutaneous flora than adults and often harbor soil bacteria on their skin. Prepubertal children lack sebum and accordingly have fewer diphtheroid organisms than adults. It is estimated that 10–30% of individuals are nasal carriers of *S. aureus*, and that 70–90% are transient carriers.[1,2] Such coagulase-positive staphylococci are not considered part of the normal cutaneous flora of glabrous skin in adults but are frequent transients acquired from carrier sites such as the anterior nares and perineum.

The introduction of a vast array of antibiotics and chemotherapeutic agents has affected striking changes in the management of bacterial infections. With increased use of these agents the focus of attention has shifted to identifying the specific bacterial cause and its antimicrobial sensitivity pattern, when feasible, permitting the appropriate choice of antibacterial agent(s). In purulent skin infections it is relatively easy to obtain adequate specimens for examination and culture. With dry or crusted lesions, the yield will be greatest if the crust is gently lifted off and cultures are obtained from the moist underlying surface. In nonpurulent infections like erysipelas or cellulitis, past recommendations were for aspiration of the most active zone (not the surrounding area of erythema) with a 25-gauge needle attached to a syringe containing sterile saline without added preservatives. This procedure, unfortunately, has a very high false negative rate and often the clinician in this setting is forced to rely on clinical features or other diagnostic findings.

Bacterial infections

Impetigo

Impetigo is a common, contagious superficial skin infection caused by streptococci, staphylococci, or both. Although seen in all age groups, the disease is most common in infants and children. Lesions may involve any body surface but occur most frequently on the exposed parts of the body, especially the face, hands, neck, and extremities.

There are two classic forms of impetigo, *bullous and non-bullous* (or crusted). Non-bullous impetigo accounts for >70% of cases.[3] It begins with a 1–2 mm erythematous papule or pustule that soon develops into thin-roofed vesicle or bulla surrounded by a narrow rim of erythema. The vesicle ruptures easily, with release of a thin cloudy yellow fluid that subsequently dries, forming a honey-colored crust, the hallmark of non-bullous impetigo (Fig. 14.1). The infection is easily spread by auto-inoculation (Fig. 14.2) through fingers, towels, or clothing, with resultant satellite lesions in either adjacent areas or other parts of the body. Individual lesions may extend peripherally with central clearing, resulting in annular or gyrate morphologies. Non-bullous impetigo historically was caused primarily by group A β-hemolytic streptococci (GABHS), but now appears to be most commonly caused by *S. aureus*.[3,4] Anaerobic organisms may also be recovered from lesions of non-bullous impetigo.[4]

Bullous impetigo, which is nearly always caused by *S. aureus*, presents as flaccid, thin-walled bullae or, more commonly, tender shallow erosions surrounded by a remnant of the blister roof (Fig. 14.3). Common locations include the diaper region (Fig. 14.4), face, and extremities. Lesions of bullous impetigo can be thought of as a localized form of staphylococcal scalded skin syndrome (see Staphylococcal Scalded Skin Syndrome, below), the characteristic lesions being the result of the same exfoliative toxin as implicated

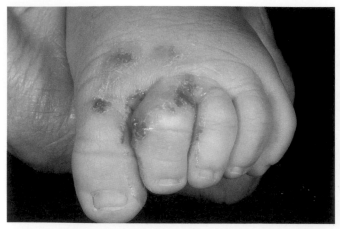

Figure 14.1 Non-bullous (crusted) impetigo. Erythematous papules with honey yellow-colored crusting.

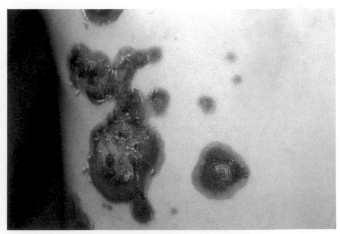

Figure 14.3 Bullous impetigo. Multiple tender, erythematous patches with a peripheral collarette, representing remnants of the blister roof.

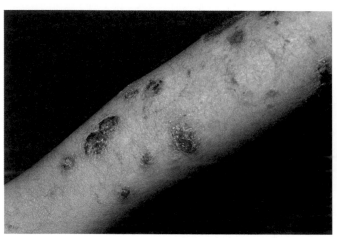

Figure 14.2 Non-bullous (crusted) impetigo. These multiple lesions have spread as a result of 'autoinoculation'.

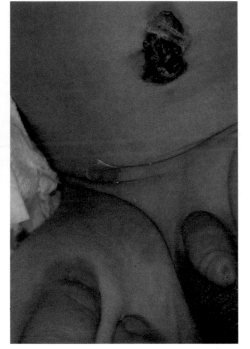

Figure 14.4 Bullous impetigo. Inguinal involvement in a newborn male. Lesions of bullous impetigo have a preference for this location in diapered infants.

in that condition. 'Neonatal pustulosis' (see Ch. 2), another condition favoring the diaper region and other fold areas in infants, is usually caused by *S. aureus* and presents with small pustules on an erythematous base which rupture easily upon swabbing.

Fever and regional lymphadenopathy may occur later in the course of impetigo, but appear to be more common with the non-bullous type caused by GABHS. Potential complications of both bullous and non-bullous impetigo include sepsis, osteomyelitis, septic arthritis, lymphadenitis, and pneumonia.[3] Cutaneous streptococcal disease may be associated with guttate psoriasis, scarlet fever, and poststreptococcal glomerulonephritis when a nephritogenic strain of GABHS is implicated.

An important reservoir for staphylococci is the upper respiratory tract of asymptomatic persons. Asymptomatic nasal carriage occurs in 20–40% of normal adults, and up to 80% of patients with atopic dermatitis. The perineum is another common site of carriage, albeit not as common as the nares. These carriers spread the agent to the skin of infants and young children, probably with their hands. The reservoir for streptococci involved in skin infections appears to be skin lesions of other individuals, not the respiratory tract of affected or asymptomatic persons. Factors such as trauma and insect bites probably contribute to the pathogenesis of this infection.

Treatment of impetigo depends on the clinical presentation. Untreated, the disorder may last for 2–3 weeks, with continuous spread and development of new lesions. In severe cases there may be large crusted vegetations with deep extension and ulceration. Gentle cleansing, removal of crusts, and drainage of blisters and pustules may help prevent local spread of disease. If crusts are firmly adherent, warm soaks or compresses are useful.

Topical antibiotics may be useful in the treatment of mild, localized disease due to *S. aureus*. With streptococcal or more severe staphylococcal infections, however, systemic antibiotics produce a swifter response and fewer failures. Bacitracin, polymyxin, gentamicin, and erythromycin are all effective topical agents and are relatively non-allergenic. Recent reports highlight bacitracin as a potential contact allergen, and this should be remembered in patients treated with this agent who develop worsening erythema and evidence of contact dermatitis.[5,6] Neomycin is another effective topical agent, although reports of contact allergy have traditionally appeared to be more common with this agent than with other topical antimicrobials (see Ch. 3). Mupirocin exerts a high level of bactericidal activity against a broad spectrum of Gram-positive organisms including *S. aureus* and GABHS, and has little or no potential for irritation, side-effects, resistance, or cross-reaction with other antibiotics. Some studies have demonstrated equal or greater effectiveness of mupirocin over oral erythromycin in the treatment of impetigo in children.[7,8] Nasal carriage of *S. aureus* may be reduced with the use of intranasal mupirocin, which should be considered in known carriers with recurrent impetigo or in the setting of epidemic outbreaks. Retapamulin, a newer pleuromutilin-class topical antibiotic for the treatment of skin and skin-structure infections, has been demonstrated effective against both *S. aureus* and GABHS and is another treatment option for localized impetigo.[9,10]

Oral therapy of impetigo should be with an agent that covers both *S. aureus* and GABHS, as distinguishing between these etiologies clinically is usually not possible. In areas with a low prevalence of erythromycin-resistant *S. aureus*, erythromycin ethylsuccinate or erythromycin estolate are reasonable options. If known, erythromycin resistance is present in the community, alternative oral agents with a good track record include a penicillinase-resistant penicillin (i.e., cloxacillin or dicloxacillin), amoxicillin plus clavulinic acid, a first- (i.e., cephalexin) or second- (i.e., cefprozil) generation cephalosporin, clindamycin, or in some cases, newer macrolide antibiotics (i.e., clarithromycin or azithromycin).

In severe or recalcitrant cases, skin swab for bacterial culture and sensitivity testing should be performed. The evolving epidemiology of community-associated methicillin-resistant *S. aureus* (CA-MRSA, see below) infection must be considered in this setting, as highlighted by several recent reports of the increasing prevalence of this pathogen. These patients frequently lack traditional risk factors for MRSA, and the isolates may be more susceptible to clindamycin and trimethoprim-sulfamethoxazole.[11,12]

Lesions of impetigo caused by GABHS are shallow and usually heal well, and rheumatic fever does not occur following streptococcal skin infection. In contrast, acute glomerulonephritis and scarlet fever can follow cutaneous streptococcal infection. As in the case of nephritis following streptococcal pharyngitis, only certain serologic types, different from those producing nephritis as a sequel of streptococcal pharyngitis, appear to result in this complication of cutaneous infection.[9] This complication is uncommon, except for certain epidemics due to nephritogenic strains of streptococci. Although systemic antibiotics help eliminate cutaneous streptococci, they do not appear to prevent glomerulonephritis due to streptococcal impetigo. In general, however, with the changing bacteriology and the fact that staphylococci are a more common cause of both types of impetigo, concerns about post-impetigo glomerulonephritis have been greatly reduced.

Methicillin-resistant *Staphylococcus Aureus* (MRSA) Infections

The epidemiology of *S. aureus* skin and soft tissue infections has changed over the last decade, with an increasing prevalence of community-associated methicillin-resistant *S. aureus* (CA-MRSA) infections observed in both the USA and elsewhere. Since the initial descriptions of children lacking predisposing risk factors with CA-MRSA infection in the late 1990s, marked increases in *S. aureus* isolates with this characteristic were observed, both in endemic and epidemic forms. By the mid-first decade of the twenty-first century, up to 50% of CA-*S. aureus* infections in many US centers were being identified as MRSA.[13]

MRSA originated after the introduction of a mobile genetic element, staphylococcal chromosomal cassette (SCC) carrying the *mecA* gene, into strains of methicillin-susceptible *S. aureus*. This gene encodes an altered penicillin binding protein.[14] In distinction to hospital-associated MRSA, CA-MRSA is generally classified as such when there is no history of prior MRSA infection or colonization, when the positive culture was obtained in the outpatient setting or isolated within 48 h of hospitalization, and when the patient lacks an exposure history (i.e., to a healthcare facility, chronic care facility, or indwelling catheter).[13,14] Molecular characteristics of the isolate are also useful in distinguishing the strains.

CA-MRSA infections seem to disproportionately affect children, young adults, and individuals from ethnic minority and low socioeconomic groups.[15] Spread is facilitated by crowding, skin-to-skin contact, skin compromise and shared personal hygiene items. Cutaneous CA-MRSA infections are common in athletes, most notably collegiate football players.[16,17] The potential clinical manifestations associated with CA-MRSA infection are listed in Table 14.1. Empiric outpatient therapy decisions for CA-MRSA infections should incorporate the type and site of infection, prevalence of the organism in the community, and local antibiotic susceptibility patterns.[15] Abscesses, which are collections of pus within the dermis and deeper skin layers, are a common manifestation of CA-MRSA infection. Incision and drainage of abscesses is often useful, and sometimes sufficient as monotherapy, for purulent uncomplicated infections. The most commonly utilized oral antibiotics in the USA are: trimethoprim-sulfamethoxazole, clindamycin, doxycycline, linezolid, rifampin, and the fluoroquinolones. Fusidic acid is also utilized in the UK, Australia and other countries.[18] Inducible clindamycin resistance has increased in recent years, and should be considered when testing reveals clindamycin susceptibility and

---

Table 14.1 Clinical associations with community-associated MRSA infection

Skin/soft tissue infections
  Folliculitis
  Furuncles
  Carbuncles
  Impetigo
  Pustulosis (neonates)
  Cellulitis
  Abscesses
  Paronychia
  Staphylococcal scalded skin syndrome
  Necrotizing fasciitis/myositis
Pneumonia/empyema
Lymphadenitis
Otitis media/externa
Osteomyelitis
Thrombophlebitis
Septic arthritis
Bacteremia
Pyelonephritis
Toxic shock syndrome
Endocarditis
Epidural abscess

Adapted from Miller and Kaplan (2009),[14] Paintsil (2007),[15] and Kirkland and Adams (2008).[17] MRSA, Methicillin-resistant *S. aureus*.

erythromycin resistance. In these instances, a 'D-test' should be performed and used to guide the choice of therapy. Management of colonization has been attempted with intranasal mupirocin and skin disinfection, with variable success.[19]

Ecthyma

Ecthyma is a deep or ulcerative type of pyoderma commonly seen on the lower extremities and buttocks of children, and caused most often by GABHS. It may occur as small punched-out ulcers or a deep spreading ulcerative process. The disorder begins in the same manner as impetigo, often following infected insect bites or minor trauma, but penetrates through the epidermis to produce a shallow ulcer. The initial lesion is a vesiculopustule with an erythematous base and firmly adherent crust. Removal of the crust reveals a lesion deeper than that seen in impetigo, with an underlying saucer-shaped ulcer and raised margin (Fig. 14.5). The lesions are painful and heal slowly over a few weeks, often with scar formation. When multiple, lesions of ecthyma may be confused with child abuse related to cigarette burns. *Staphylococcus aureus* (including MRSA) may occasionally be cultured from the lesions, and epidemic outbreaks have been reported, occasionally in association with post-streptococcal glomerulonephritis or other systemic sequelae.[20,21] Treatment consists of warm compresses and the appropriate systemic antibiotic.

Ecthyma gangrenosum is a cutaneous finding that may be seen in patients with *Pseudomonas aeruginosa* bacteremia. Most of the affected individuals have an underlying immunodeficiency (either congenital or acquired) or a history of cancer chemotherapy. There are reports of ecthyma gangrenosum in apparently healthy, immunocompetent children (often presenting with diaper-area involvement), but the diagnosis should prompt a thorough investigation for occult immunodeficiency.[22,23] Neutropenia may be a risk factor for ecthyma gangrenosum. The characteristic lesions are hemorrhagic papules with a pink or violaceous rim (Fig. 14.6) that progress to bullae, ulcers, and necrotic plaques. Eschar formation eventually occurs (Fig. 14.7), and old lesions heal with scarring. The diagnosis can be confirmed by Gram stain and bacterial culture of lesions or blood cultures, which are positive for *P. aeruginosa*. Treatment with appropriate antipseudomonal therapy (i.e., aminoglycoside and an antipseudomonal penicillin) should be instituted early.

Folliculitis

The term *folliculitis* refers to an infection of hair follicles. The clinical appearance varies according to the location and depth of follicular involvement. Deeper follicular infections (furuncles and carbuncles) are discussed later. Superficial folliculitis (Bockhart's impetigo), an infection of the follicular ostium, begins with superficial, small yellow-white pustules, often with a narrow red areola (Fig. 14.8) and a hair shaft protruding from the center of the lesion. It occurs most commonly in children and usually is seen on the buttocks (Fig. 14.9) and extremities, especially the thighs. Most lesions are painless, occur in crops, and heal over 7–10 days with postinflammatory hyperpigmentation. *Staphylococcus aureus* is by far the most common pathogen; other possible etiologies include streptococci, Gram negative organisms, and even dermatophytes. In immunocompromised children, commensal organisms may cause folliculitis, including *Pityrosporum* and *Demodex* (see Ch. 18). Superficial folliculitis is not always infectious in origin. 'Sterile folliculitis' may

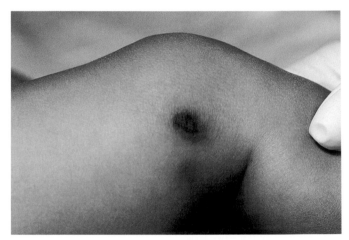

Figure 14.6 Ecthyma gangrenosum. These hemorrhagic, necrotic skin lesions were accompanied by Pseudomonas aeruginosa bacteremia in this immunosuppressed child being treated with chemotherapy.

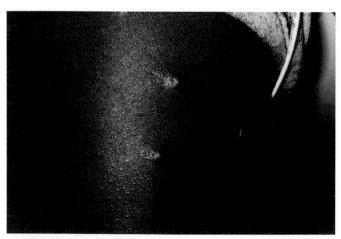

Figure 14.5 Ecthyma. Well-demarcated, punched-out ulcers on the thigh of this 10-year-old male.

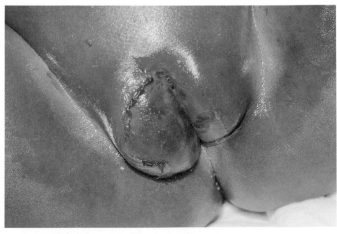

Figure 14.7 Ecthyma gangrenosum. This child with congenital immunodeficiency developed thick eschars, which required a diverting colostomy and eventual skin grafting.

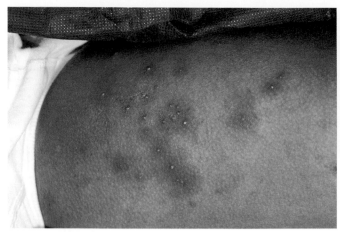

Figure 14.8 Bacterial folliculitis. Erythematous, follicular papulopustules.

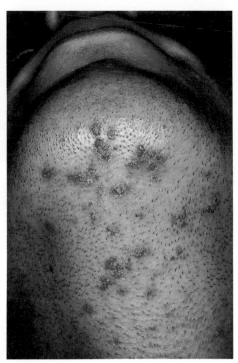

Figure 14.10 Folliculitis barbae. Follicular papules, pustules, and crusting with autoinoculation, and caused by shaving.

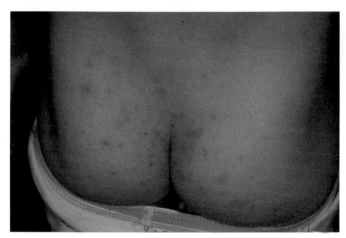

Figure 14.9 Bacterial folliculitis. Erythematous follicular papules and papulopustules on the buttocks of a young boy. This is the most common location for bacterial folliculitis in children.

be seen after skin contact with oil or other occlusive products, which result in follicular plugging and inflammation. A classic example of sterile folliculitis is the scalp pustulosis occasionally associated with application of hair oils.

Superficial folliculitis usually responds to gentle cleansing with antibacterial soaps and the application of topical antibiotics, such as clindamycin, erythromycin, or mupirocin. More extensive or resistant cases should be treated with a systemic antibiotic (a penicillinase-resistant penicillin or cephalosporin, depending on local resistance patterns). In such instances, bacterial culture should be obtained prior to the initiation of systemic therapy. Sodium hypochlorite (bleach) baths on a twice weekly basis may be useful for individuals or families with recurrent folliculitis or furunculosis (see below). The recommended concentration is ¼–½ cup of bleach dissolved in a full bathtub of water.

Folliculitis barbae

Folliculitis barbae (sycosis barbae) is a term used to describe a deep-seated folliculitis of the beard area involving the entire depth of the follicle and perifollicular region (Fig. 14.10). A pruritic papule is usually the initial lesion, with the process spreading from one follicle to another by trauma from scratching and/or shaving. The disorder is characterized by follicular papules and pustules and, with progression, erythema, crusting, and boggy infiltration of the skin. Although occasionally other bacteria may be isolated, the etiology is usually *S. aureus*. The use of an electric rather than traditional razor or complete avoidance of shaving can sometimes be helpful in prevention and treatment of this condition. Warm compresses and topical antibiotics are often sufficient to control minor forms of sycosis barbae. If the condition is severe or recurrent, several weeks of systemic antibiotics may be necessary.

Pseudofolliculitis barbae

Pseudofolliculitis barbae (PFB) (see Ch. 7) is a common non-infectious inflammatory disorder of the pilosebaceous follicles of the beard that may be confused with sycosis barbae. PFB (commonly referred to as 'razor bumps') is caused by shaved hairs that curve inward with resultant penetration of the skin, followed by an inflammatory foreign body reaction. This form of folliculitis is seen particularly in African-Americans and individuals with curly hair. Mild cases may be managed by careful shaving and occasionally by changing from a traditional to an electric razor. Close shaving, which promotes oblique penetration of hairs into the skin, should be avoided whenever possible. Other treatment options include chemical depilatory creams, topical retinoids or glycolic acid, or complete avoidance of shaving. Recently, epilation laser therapy (Ch. 7) has been demonstrated effective for the condition.[24,25]

Pseudomonal folliculitis (hot tub folliculitis)

Pseudomonal folliculitis is a form of folliculitis caused by *P. aeruginosa* that occurs following exposure to poorly chlorinated hot tubs, whirlpools, or swimming pools. It has also been reported in association with a contaminated water slide,[26] a contaminated loofah sponge,[27] and following shower/bath exposure.[28,29] It is characterized by erythematous, follicular pustules, and vesiculopustules, which occur most often on the trunk, buttocks, and legs (Fig. 14.11), especially in sites occluded by swimming garments. Lesions usually develop within 1–2 days after exposure. Mild constitutional symptoms may be present, including fever, malaise, headache, and arthralgias. More serious associations, including urinary tract infection and pneumonia, have also been reported.[30,31] Lesions of hot tub folliculitis generally subside spontaneously over 7–10 days. Anti-pseudomonal antibiotic therapy (i.e., with ciprofloxacin) may be necessary in severe cases. Preventive measures include maintenance of appropriate chlorination, frequent water changes, and thorough scrubbing of whirlpool baths and hot tubs with each water change.

Hot hand–foot syndrome (also known as *Pseudomonas hot foot syndrome*) presents with painful, erythematous palmoplantar nodules (Fig. 14.12) after exposure to water containing a high concentration of *P. aeruginosa*, and may be seen in conjunction with hot tub folliculitis.[32] When pustules are present, the organism can be easily cultured from skin swab material. An epidemic occurred in children exposed to the same community wading pool whose floor was coated with abrasive grit and which, along with the inlets and a drain, yielded *P. aeruginosa* on culture.[33] This disorder may be related to (or the same condition as) 'idiopathic palmoplantar hidradenitis of childhood' (see Ch. 20).

Eosinophilic pustular folliculitis

Eosinophilic pustular folliculitis (Ofuji's disease, EPF) is a dermatosis of unknown cause characterized by erythematous patches with follicular papules and pustules, often in an annular or serpiginous arrangement, with occasional peripheral eosinophilia and leukocytosis. It was classically reported in Japanese individuals, although it may be seen in people of diverse ethnic backgrounds, and men appear to be affected more than women.[34] Although this disorder is not bacterial in origin, it is included here, as it is in the differential diagnosis of folliculitis. EPF may involve any surface area, including the face, trunk, and extremities. A form of EPF is recognized as an extremely pruritic dermatosis in adult patients with human immunodeficiency virus (HIV) infection, usually presenting late in the course of infection.[35] A distinct form of EPF occurs in otherwise healthy infants and toddlers, presenting with recurrent crops of itchy follicular pustules of the scalp and extremities, with eventual spontaneous involution (see Ch. 2). Whereas adults tend to have annular, serpiginous, or polycyclic lesions, the prominent scalp involvement and failure to form annular rings appear to distinguish the infantile form. Occasionally, EPF may be a presenting feature of the hyperimmunoglobulin-E (hyper-IgE) syndrome (see Ch. 3).[36]

Treatment options for EPF include oral erythromycin, topical corticosteroids, dapsone, indomethacin, colchicine, topical tacrolimus, antihistamines and ultraviolet B phototherapy, which have each been used with variable success. The majority of patients respond to treatment with the former two agents. The other treatments have been demonstrated successful, but carry a greater risk of adverse effects.

Furuncles and Carbuncles

Furuncles (or 'boils') are painful, deep infections of the hair follicle in which purulent material extends into the dermis and subcutaneous tissues, forming perifollicular abscesses (see above). These lesions have a tendency toward central necrosis and suppuration. They are caused by *S. aureus*, and are seen most frequently in older children and adults. They usually develop from a preceding folliculitis, with deeper extension into the dermis and subcutaneous tissue. Chronic carriers of *S. aureus* are particularly predisposed.[37] Furuncles are most common in areas of skin that are hairy and subject to friction and maceration, particularly the back, axillae, thighs, buttocks, and perineum. They present as tender red nodules (Fig. 14.13), which gradually become fluctuant and, if untreated, may have a purulent blood-tinged discharge. There is a high rate of contagion in patients with furunculosis.

Carbuncles are larger, deep-seated staphylococcal abscesses composed of aggregates of interconnected furuncles that drain at multiple points on the cutaneous surface (Fig. 14.14). They are usually seen in males on the posterior neck, back, thighs, and buttocks, and extend into the deeper dermis and subcutaneous tissues, reaching a larger size than furuncles (up to 10 cm in diameter). They undergo necrosis and suppuration more slowly than furuncles, and may present with severe pain and constitutional symptoms. Several factors predispose to the development of furuncles and carbuncles (Table 14.2).

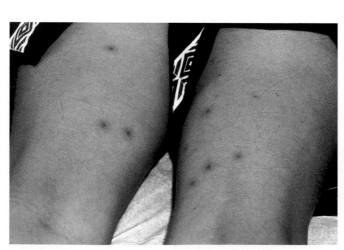

Figure 14.11 Pseudomonal (hot tub) folliculitis. Erythematous, follicular papules and papulopustules of the thighs, correlating with areas covered by the swim garment.

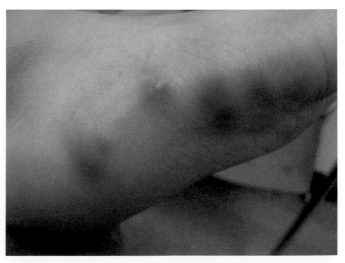

Figure 14.12 *Pseudomonas* hot foot syndrome. Tender papules and papulopustules on the plantar foot. Culture of a swab from one of the pustules grew out *Pseudomonas aeruginosa*. (Courtesy of John J. Van Aalst, MD.)

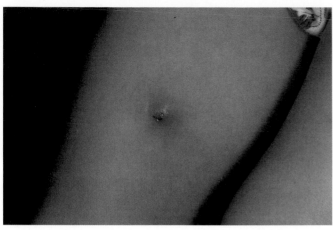

Figure 14.13 Furuncle. This tender, fluctuant papulonodule was located on the thigh, in the same patient with folliculitis shown in Figure 14.9.

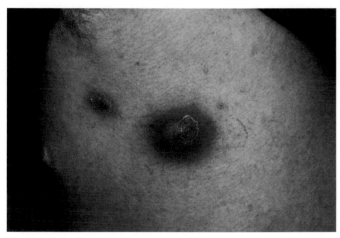

Figure 14.14 Carbuncle. Large, tender, erythematous nodule on the lateral trunk of this 14-year-old obese male. Note the adjacent, smaller furuncle.

Table 14.2 Predisposing factors for furuncles and carbuncles
Diabetes mellitus
Obesity
Scabies
Hematologic disorders
Immunodeficiencies, including hyper-IgE syndrome
Malnutrition
Chemotherapy
Corticosteroid therapy
Local skin trauma (abrasions, cuts, excoriations)
Debilitated state

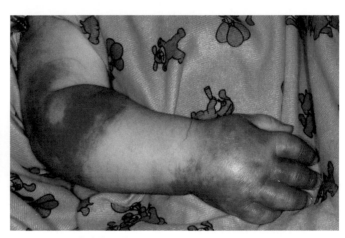

Figure 14.15 Cellulitis. Erythematous patches and plaques with edema, involving the arm of this 18-month-old male. Note the multifocal nature and partial clearing as a result of parenteral antibiotic therapy.

The treatment of furuncles and carbuncles depends on the extent and location of lesions. The mainstay of therapy is systemic antistaphylococcal antibiotics, with incision and drainage of fluctuant lesions. Cultures with sensitivity testing should be considered, especially in geographic areas with an increasing prevalence of staphylococcal resistance. Topical antibiotics (as discussed earlier for impetigo and folliculitis) are not sufficient for the treatment of furuncles and carbuncles given the depth of the process. Lastly, attention to predisposing factors with appropriate treatment or modification (as feasible) is indicated.

Cellulitis

Cellulitis is an acute infection of the skin, particularly the subcutaneous tissues, characterized by erythema, swelling, and tenderness. The borders of cellulitis are not elevated or sharply defined, which helps to contrast it from the more superficial form called erysipelas (see below).

Cellulitis usually occurs following some form of skin trauma, including puncture wounds, lacerations, dermatitis, burns, varicella, or dermatophyte infections. It presents with markedly red, tender, warm swelling of the skin with an infiltrated appearance (Fig. 14.15), and the most common location is the lower extremities. Constitutional symptoms including malaise and fever are often present. The most common causes of cellulitis are *S. aureus* and GABHS, although occasionally other bacterial agents may be implicated. In young children, particularly those under 2 years of age, *Haemophilus influenzae* type b (Hib) was traditionally implicated in a facial cellulitis termed *buccal cellulitis*, although this form is now less common since licensure of the conjugated Hib vaccine.[38] Buccal cellulitis characteristically reveals a dusky red to blue discoloration of the involved skin. Children with *H. influenzae* cellulitis may be quite toxic, with accompanying upper respiratory tract symptoms and bacteremia or septicemia. *Streptococcus pneumoniae* is another potential etiology of facial cellulitis in children, occurring especially in those under 36 months of age who are at risk for pneumococcal bacteremia. Since 96% of the serotypes (in one large series of *S. pneumoniae* facial cellulitis) are included in the heptavalent-conjugated pneumococcal vaccine now licensed in the USA, this cause of cellulitis will likely become significantly less relevant in years to come.[39] Lastly, in children younger than 3 months of age, cellulitis is most commonly caused by group B streptococci (GBS) and is more likely to be associated with invasive disease, including bacteremia and meningitis.[40] These children require blood, urine and cerebrospinal fluid sampling and cultures as part of their initial evaluation.

Periorbital cellulitis is a unique form of cellulitis that deserves special mention here, given the potential confusion with *orbital cellulitis* and the associated complications. Periorbital (preseptal) cellulitis is a form of the disease that presents with erythema and swelling of the periorbital tissues. It may follow skin trauma, in which case it is usually due to *S. aureus* or GABHS infection, or may result from cutaneous spread of pathogens from the paranasal sinuses or bloodstream, where it may result from Hib or *S. pneumoniae* infection. If the infection traverses the orbital septum (a continuation of the periosteum of the bony orbit to the margins of the upper and lower eyelids), it may result in orbital cellulitis, a more serious condition that may be complicated by abscess formation or cavernous sinus thrombosis.[41] Patients with orbital cellulitis may present with proptosis, ophthalmoplegia, and decreased visual acuity in addition to the cutaneous findings. CT and ophthalmologic examinations are indicated if orbital cellulitis is suspected. The microbiology of periorbital and orbital cellulitis have also changed with the advent of Hib immunization, and Hib is now a very uncommon cause of these disorders, being supplanted by streptococcal species (including *S. pneumoniae* and GABHS) and *S. aureus*.[42–44]

Treatment of cellulitis depends on the clinical presentation and knowledge (and identification, when possible) of the affecting organisms. The diagnosis of cellulitis is generally a clinical one, although fine needle aspiration with Gram stain and bacterial culture may be helpful when unusual organisms are suspected (i.e., the immunocompromised host).[37] Antibiotic therapy that covers for GABHS and *S. aureus* will be appropriate in most cases of routine, non-facial cellulitis. In geographic areas with high rates of CA-MRSA, antibiotic selection should include coverage against this organism. In children with facial or periorbital cellulitis, the possibility of *S. pneumoniae* and Hib infection should be considered in conjunction with the patient's age and immunization status, and antibiotics chosen accordingly. In infants younger than 3 months of age with cellulitis, GBS should be presumed as a potential etiologic agent and in these infants, as well as the patient with periorbital or orbital cellulitis who is young, toxic or presents with signs of meningeal irritation, laboratory evaluation for sepsis and meningitis should be performed. Hospitalization with parenteral antibiotic therapy (and ophthalmologic consultation in those with orbital cellulitis) is indicated in these latter settings.

Erysipelas

Erysipelas is a superficial cellulitis of the skin with marked lymphatic involvement, due in most cases to GABHS. The organism usually gains access by direct inoculation through a break in the skin, but occasionally hematogenous infection may occur. The initial lesion begins as a small area of erythema that gradually enlarges to reveal a characteristic warm, painful, shiny bright-red infiltrated plaque with a distinct and well-marginated border. The face, scalp, and hands are the most common sites of involvement, although erysipelas may involve any skin surface. Penicillin, or a macrolide antibiotic in patients with penicillin allergy, is the drug of choice for therapy. In occasional patients, *S. aureus* may be a copathogen, in which case antimicrobial therapy directed against this organism is necessary.

Perianal Streptococcal Dermatitis

Perianal streptococcal dermatitis (PSD, also known as perianal dermatitis, perianal cellulitis, perianal streptococcal cellulitis, and streptococcal perianal disease) is a well-defined entity that may be frequently overlooked. It presents as sharply circumscribed perianal erythema, with occasional fissures, purulent discharge, and/or functional disturbances.[45] GABHS is the etiology in most cases of PSD, although *S. aureus* and coliform bacteria have also been

recovered.[46,47] An epidemic outbreak in a day care center has been reported.[48]

The skin findings in PSD are variable, from a dry pink appearance to bright red erythema (Fig. 14.16), with a wet surface and occasionally the presence of a white pseudomembrane.[49] The surface is often tender to touch, and associated symptoms include rectal itching or discomfort, painful defecation, blood-streaked stools, and constipation. In males, balanoposthitis or, in females, vulvovaginitis may be present.[50] Fever is notoriously rare in patients with PSD. Streptococcal pharyngitis may concomitantly be present in patients with PSD, but the exact associations between pharyngitis, PSD, and streptococcal colonization is unclear.[49] There is some suggestion that specific GABHS isolates may have a tropism for perineal tissues, but the mechanism of infection is not yet clear.[50] Guttate psoriasis (see Ch. 4), which is classically associated with streptococcal pharyngitis,

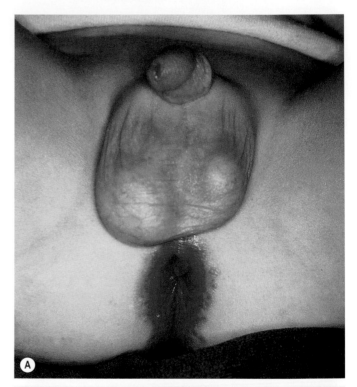

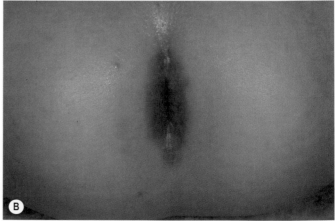

Figure 14.16 Perianal streptococcal dermatitis. Bright red erythema with a moist, tender surface (A) and pink maceration with mild exudate or pseudomembrane (B). Both patients were tender to palpation and had painful defecation.

may also be associated with PSD, and in any patient presenting with new onset guttate psoriasis, a thorough anogenital examination should be performed.

The differential diagnosis of PSD is broad and includes psoriasis, candidiasis, seborrheic dermatitis, cutaneous Crohn's disease, pinworm infestation, and sexual abuse. The diagnosis can be confirmed by bacterial culture of a perianal swab, but when performing cultures to confirm the diagnosis of PSD, it is important to notify the laboratory of the microbe (GABHS) in question, as several labs utilize media selective for enteric pathogens with rectal swabs. Treatment with oral penicillin V (or erythromycin for penicillin-allergic patients) is usually effective, with or without concomitant topical mupirocin. Oral cefuroxime was demonstrated more effective than penicillin in one study, and is another reasonable option.[51]

Blistering Dactylitis

Blistering dactylitis (also known as blistering distal dactylitis) is a unique bullous manifestation of GABHS infection or, only occasionally, other bacteria including *S. aureus* and group B streptococci.[52–54] In its classic form, blistering dactylitis presents as a painful, tense superficial blister on an erythematous base (Fig. 14.17), most often located over the volar fat pad of the distal phalanx of a finger or several fingers. It is most common in children between the ages of 2 and 16 years, although it is also reported in adults, most notably immunocompromised ones. The blisters may occasionally extend to involve the dorsal surfaces of the fingers. Systemic manifestations including fever are rare. The differential diagnosis of blistering dactylitis includes bullous impetigo, herpetic whitlow, traumatic blistering, burns, and epidermolysis bullosa. Coexistent whitlow and blistering dactylitis has been reported.[55] The diagnosis is confirmed by Gram stain and culture of blister fluid. If herpes infection is suspected, Tzanck smear, direct fluorescent antibody testing, or viral culture should be performed. Streptococcal blistering dactylitis is successfully treated with penicillin or erythromycin, but given reports of staphylococci as an etiology, antimicrobial therapy may need to be modified to cover for both organisms.

Necrotizing Fasciitis

Necrotizing fasciitis is a rapidly progressive, potentially fatal, necrotizing infection of the skin and subcutaneous tissues frequently associated with severe systemic toxicity. Over the years it has been known by several different names, including *hospital gangrene*, *acute infective gangrene*, *streptococcal gangrene*, *gangrenous erysipelas*, *synergistic necrotizing cellulitis* and *Meleney's ulcer*. A recently popular term is *flesh-eating bacteria disease*. Although usually due to GABHS, necrotizing fasciitis may be polymicrobial in nature, and has been reported in association with other streptococci, *P. aeruginosa*, *S. aureus*, *Klebsiella* spp., *Enterobacter cloacae*, *Serratia* spp., *Proteus* spp., enterococcus, a variety of anaerobic agents including *Clostridium* spp. and *Bacteroides* spp., and even *Vibrio* spp.[56–60] The disorder is most common in individuals with decreased local resistance (skin injury, surgery, varicella), malnutrition, or chronic disease. Necrotizing fasciitis is rare in children. In neonates, it has been observed in association with omphalitis, balanitis, mammitis, and fetal scalp monitoring.[61]

Necrotizing fasciitis usually presents on an extremity, and is characterized by pain, edema, and erythema with exquisite tenderness to palpation. These changes quickly progress through several sequential stages, including ecchymosis, bullae, necrosis (Fig. 14.18), gangrene, and with deep and extensive infection, overlying skin anesthesia.[57] The inflammation extends deeply along fascial planes, highlighting the importance of rapid diagnosis and surgical exploration. Laboratory findings include leukocytosis, elevated serum creatine kinase level, and bacteremia. The most serious complication of necrotizing fasciitis is streptococcal toxic shock syndrome (see below), which is characterized by hypotension, renal impairment, coagulopathy, liver abnormalities, respiratory distress, and a diffuse erythematous cutaneous eruption. Clinical clues that suggest necrotizing fasciitis over cellulitis include intense pain, rapid progression, bullae, necrosis, and lack of a rapid response to antibiotic therapy. Imaging studies may be useful in confirming the diagnosis, especially if soft tissue gas is present, although this is not a consistent finding. MR imaging may be useful in distinguishing necrotizing fasciitis from uncomplicated infective fasciitis.[62] Confirmation of infection can be accomplished with Gram stain and culture of blister fluid, lesion discharge or tissue, blood culture, and polymerase chain reaction (PCR) analysis for pyrogenic exotoxin B on tissue biopsy specimens.[58]

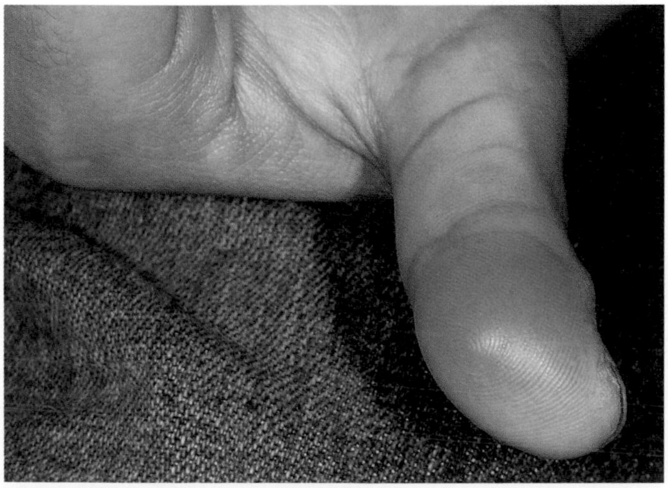

Figure 14.17 Blistering dactylitis. Edema and a tense bulla on the thumb of this 7-year-old girl. Culture of the blister fluid yielded *Staphylococcus aureus* rather than the more commonly seen group A β-hemolytic streptococcus (GABHS).

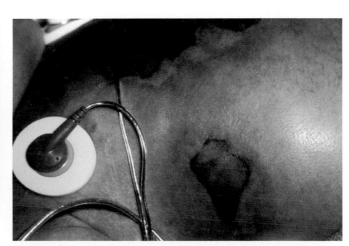

Figure 14.18 Necrotizing fasciitis. Erythema and necrosis of the abdominal wall are seen in this severely ill toddler.

Prompt, thorough surgical debridement of necrotic tissue is of prime importance in the management of patients with this disorder, as without exploration and debridement, the mortality rate approaches 100%.[63] Antimicrobial therapy should be initiated immediately, and the chosen agents should have activity against Gram-positive, Gram-negative, *Clostridium*, and anaerobic organisms.[57,60] Clindamycin, in particular, seems to be quite effective as part of the antimicrobial regimen, given its ability to suppress both toxin and M protein synthesis.[59] Antimicrobial therapy should be adjusted based on the results of Gram stain and bacterial cultures of the surgical specimen. In addition to these specific therapies, fluid resuscitation and blood pressure/blood product support are frequently indicated. The roles of hyperbaric oxygen therapy and intravenous immunoglobulin remain controversial, the latter being used primarily in the setting of GABHS infection with toxic shock syndrome.

Noma

Noma (cancrum oris, necrotizing ulcerative stomatitis) is a rare, progressive destructive infection usually involving the soft and hard tissues of the oral and para-oral structures. Most reported cases of noma are in severely malnourished or chronically debilitated children, and the disease tends to be most common in sub-Saharan Africa, South America, and Asia. The triad of malnutrition, poor oral hygiene, and periodontal disease contributes to the increased incidence in these locations.[64] It is usually caused by anaerobic organisms, including *Fusobacterium* spp., *Prevotella intermedia*, *Actinomyces* spp., *Peptostreptococcus micros*, and *Borrelia* spp., and is characterized by a gangrenous, ulcerative infection of the gingivae, buccal mucosa, and eventually the cheeks and jaw. The initial stage of noma is characterized by a painful, small purple-red lesion that becomes indurated and progresses to edema, necrosis, and ulceration. With expansion, underlying bone involvement occurs, with resultant loss of dentition. Bony sequestrations of the mandible or maxilla may occur. Patients may also have fever, tachycardia, tachypnea and anorexia, and their medical history may reveal recurrent fevers, diarrhea, and history or parasitic and/or viral infections.[65] Treatment of noma includes antibiotics, wound care, and debridement with eventual surgical reconstruction. Without treatment, the mortality rate is 70–90%, and survivors suffer the long-term sequelae of orofacial mutilation and functional impairment.[66] Rehydration, attention to electrolyte balance, and nutritional rehabilitation to correct protein and micronutrient deficiencies are other important aspects of therapy.[65]

Noma neonatorum is a gangrenous process of the nose, eyelids, oral cavity, and anogenital region in low-birthweight infants and usually caused by *P. aeruginosa*. Most patients also have *Pseudomonas* sepsis, and the mortality rate without antimicrobial therapy is extremely high. Noma neonatorum, which is also more common in developing countries, was so named because of the clinical and histologic similarity to noma. However, there is significant overlap with the clinical presentation of *ecthyma gangrenosum*. Although some of the reported infants had immunodeficiency, it was either absent or not tested for in the majority of published cases. Noma neonatorum may represent a neonatal form of ecthyma gangrenosum.[67]

Meningococcemia

Meningococcal infection, caused by the Gram-negative diplococcus *Neisseria meningitidis*, is a major world health problem in children under 5 years of age and is the leading cause of bacterial meningitis in children. Three serogroups of *N. meningitidis*, A, B and C, account for more than 90% of cases of meningococcal disease, and along with groups Y and W-135 are implicated most commonly worldwide as causes of invasive disease.[68,69] Person-to-person spread of *N. meningitidis* usually occurs through inhalation of droplets of infected nasopharyngeal secretions by direct or indirect oral contact.[70]

Acute meningococcemia may present in a variety of ways, from transient fever to fulminant disease. Following an upper respiratory prodrome, patients develop high fever and severe headache. If meningitis develops, stiff neck, nausea, vomiting, and coma may be present. Up to two-thirds of patients will develop a skin eruption, most classically a petechial rash of the skin and mucous membranes. Other cutaneous morphologies include macular, morbilliform, and urticarial eruptions, as well as a gray-colored acrocyanosis. The petechiae are usually small, stellate, and gray-purple with a raised border and slightly depressed, vesicular or pustular center.[71] The trunk and lower extremities (especially ankles and wrists) are common sites of predilection, whereas the palms, soles, and head tend to be spared. Mucosal surfaces including the palpebral and bulbar conjunctivae may be involved.[68] More extensive hemorrhagic lesions are seen in fulminant meningococcal infections, and a progressive increase on all areas of the body may be followed by coalescence of lesions to form large purpuric patches with sharply marginated borders (Fig. 14.19). These may progress to bullae, necrosis with sloughing, and eventual eschar formation. Autoamputation related to digital ischemic necrosis is a potential complication. Consumptive coagulopathy may be present, and when occurring in the setting of progressive cutaneous hemorrhage and necrosis, is termed purpura fulminans.[72] This finding is felt to portend a poor prognosis for the patient with meningococcemia.

Chronic meningococcemia is a rare form of meningococcal infection that is unusual in children. It is characterized by intermittent episodes of skin lesions in conjunction with fever, joint pain, myalgia, and episcleritis. The cutaneous lesions, seen in the majority of patients, appear in crops coincident with or after the fever. Individual lesions are usually macular, and occasionally purpuric or pustular. Because of potential confusion with other infectious or collagen vascular illnesses, a high index of suspicion is necessary.[73] Patients with complement deficiencies, especially the terminal complement system (C5–9), have an increased risk of both acute and chronic meningococcal infections.[74]

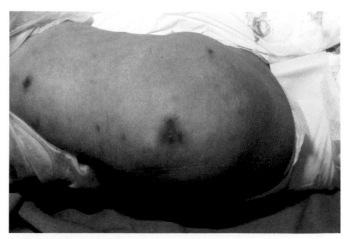

Figure 14.19 Meningococcemia. Erythematous macules and papules with petechiae, purpura, and early skin necrosis.

The differential diagnosis of meningococcemia includes gonococcemia, Henoch–Schönlein purpura, rickettsial diseases, enteroviral infections, erythema multiforme, atypical measles, hypersensitivity vasculitis, and other bacterial septicemias or meningitides. The diagnosis is confirmed by culture of the blood and cerebrospinal fluid. Isolation of meningococci from the nasopharynx is presumptive but not diagnostic, since asymptomatic carriage is not uncommon.[68] Petechial lesions can be smeared and examined for the presence of Gram-negative diplococci and may be cultured for organisms. Serologic assays that can detect *N. meningitidis* capsular polysaccharide antigen in CSF, urine, serum, and other bodily fluids are also available. A serogroup-specific polymerase chain reaction test to detect *N. meningitidis* is used routinely in the UK and may be useful in patients who receive antimicrobial therapy before cultures have been obtained.[69]

Meningococcal disease is treated with penicillin G, but at the time of presentation, the initial choice of antimicrobials should be based on the clinical differential diagnosis and local antibiotic susceptibility patterns. Antibiotics with more expanded coverage, such as cefotaxime or ceftriaxone, are often used initially in patients presenting with sepsis or meningitis until the diagnosis is confirmed.[68] In patients with a history of anaphylaxis to penicillin, chloramphenicol is recommended.[69] Supportive therapy with fluid, pressor, and blood product support, as indicated, is vital. Chemoprophylaxis of close contacts of patients with invasive meningococcal disease is recommended within 24 h of diagnosis of the index case. Selective immunization is recommended for children ≥2 years of age in high-risk groups (asplenia, terminal complement deficiencies, or travel to endemic or epidemic areas). Routine immunization with the licensed quadrivalent vaccine is recommended for adolescents at the 11–12-year visit and at high school entry or 15 years of age (whichever comes first), as well as entering college students who plan to live in dormitories and military recruits. However, routine childhood immunization is not recommended because of the low incidence of disease, the poor response in young children, the short-lived immunity and the potential impaired response to subsequent vaccine doses in some serogroups.[69,75]

Gonococcemia

Gonococcemia is associated with cutaneous lesions similar to those of meningococcemia and presents with fever, chills, arthralgia, and myalgia in patients with gonococcal septicemia. Symptoms of sexually transmitted gonococcal infection may or may not be present, including vaginitis, pelvic inflammatory disease, urethritis, proctitis, or pharyngitis. Hematogenous spread of *Neisseria gonorrhoeae* occurs in up to 3% of untreated persons with mucosal gonorrhea.[76] Skin lesions develop within 3–21 days of contact, are located primarily over joints of the distal extremities, and usually appear as petechiae, small erythematous or hemorrhagic papules, or vesiculopustules (Fig. 14.20). They usually heal spontaneously in 4–6 days.

The causative agent, *N. gonorrhoeae*, is a Gram-negative diplococcus and may be demonstrated by smear, culture, or immunofluorescence studies of skin lesions or by culture of the blood, anogenital tract, pharynx, or joint fluid on Thayer–Martin medium (chocolate agar with the addition of antibiotics to inhibit normal flora and non-pathogenic neisserial organisms). Nucleic acid amplification studies (i.e., PCR) are also available, and have a high sensitivity and specificity when performed on urethral or cervicovaginal swabs.[76]

The treatment of choice for gonococcemia is parenteral ceftriaxone or cefotaxime. Alternatives for individuals with β-lactam allergy include ciprofloxacin, ofloxacin, or spectinomycin. If concomitant infection with *Chlamydia trachomatis* is suspected, initial

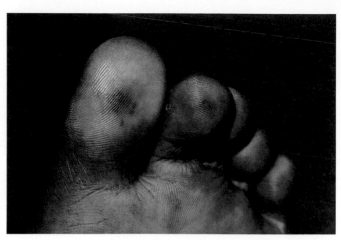

Figure 14.20 Gonococcemia. Hemorrhagic, erythematous papules and nodules involve the distal digits in this 17-year-old female with disseminated gonococcal infection and underlying systemic lupus erythematosus.

therapy should also include erythromycin, doxycycline, or azithromycin.

Staphylococcal Scalded Skin Syndrome

Staphylococcal scalded skin syndrome (SSSS) is a term used to describe a blistering skin disease caused by the epidermolytic toxin-producing *S. aureus*. It was previously known as Ritter's disease or pemphigus neonatorum, and tends to occur most often in neonates and young children. Its severity may range from mild, localized blistering to widespread exfoliation.

The pathogenesis of SSSS relates to the production of epidermolytic (or exfoliative) toxins (ET), of which there are two serotypes affecting humans, ETA and ETB. These toxins have high sequence homology and are both capable of cleaving the epidermis at the superficial level of the stratum granulosum. The pathogenic mechanisms of ETA and ETB have been clearly elucidated, and they have been shown to target desmoglein 1, a cell-cell adhesion molecule found in desmosomes of the superficial epidermis.[77–79] Desmoglein 1 is the same molecule targeted in the autoimmune blistering disease, pemphigus foliaceus.[77] There are two main theories for the observation that SSSS preferentially affects neonates and children – lack of protection from antitoxin antibodies, and decreased renal excretion of the toxin.[80] In adults, SSSS is quite rare and usually occurs in the setting of immunosuppression, malignancy, heart disease, or diabetes.[81]

Outbreaks of SSSS have been reported in neonatal intensive care units and well baby nurseries. In these settings, asymptomatic or clinically infected health care workers often act as carriers of the epidemic strain of *S. aureus*, and given the potential severity of infection in the premature infant, prompt recognition with institution of strict infection control strategies is vital to prevent further nosocomial spread.[82,83]

SSSS generally begins with localized infection of the conjunctivae, nares, perioral region, perineum, or umbilicus. Separation of perioral crusts often leaves behind radial fissures around the mouth, resulting in the characteristic facial appearance of SSSS (Figs 14.21, 14.22). Other infections that may serve as the initial nidus for SSSS include pneumonia, septic arthritis, endocarditis, or pyomyositis. Fever, malaise, lethargy, irritability, and poor feeding subsequently

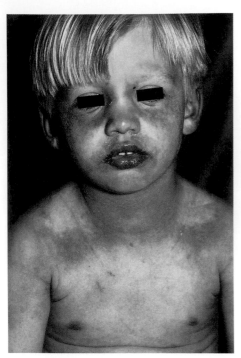

Figure 14.21 Staphylococcal scalded skin syndrome. Periorbital and perioral erythema, and erythema of the neck folds and upper trunk in this 4-year-old boy with early infection.

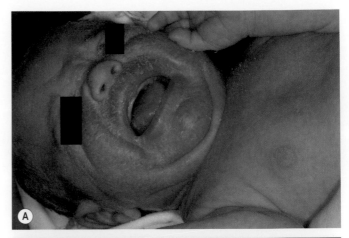

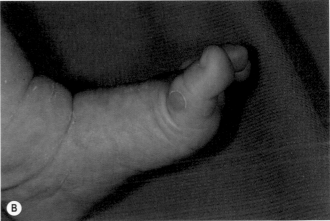

Figure 14.22 Staphylococcal scalded skin syndrome. Facial and neck fold erythema with desquamation, crusting and perioral radial fissures (A) and a distant ruptured bulla on the toe (B) of an infant girl with the disorder.

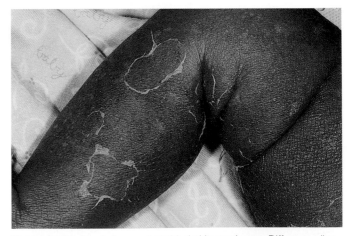

Figure 14.23 Staphylococcal scalded skin syndrome. Diffuse peeling and erythema in a 4-week-old African-American infant girl, who also had *S. aureus* isolated from her blood.

develop, and the generalized eruption begins. The rash is characterized by erythema that progresses to large, superficial fragile blisters that rupture easily, leaving behind denuded, desquamating, erythematous, and tender skin (Figs 14.22, 14.23). The eruption is most marked in flexural creases, but may involve the entire surface area of skin. The Nikolsky sign (progression of the blister cleavage plane induced by gentle pressure on the edge of the bulla) is positive. With extensive denudation of skin, patients may have decreased thermoregulatory ability, extensive fluid losses, and electrolyte imbalance, and are at serious risk for secondary infection and sepsis. With appropriate management, the skin heals without scarring given the superficial cleavage plane of the blisters.

SSSS is usually diagnosed based on the clinical presentation. The main differential diagnosis is toxic epidermal necrolysis (TEN), a severe exfoliative condition that is usually drug-induced and has a high mortality rate. The most helpful distinguishing feature of TEN is mucosal involvement, including of the mouth, conjunctivae, trachea, and genital mucosa, which is lacking in SSSS.[80] Other less common differential diagnoses include scalding burns, epidermolysis bullosa, graft-versus-host disease, nutritional deficiency dermatosis, and bullous ichthyosis (in the neonate). The diagnosis of SSSS is confirmed by isolation of *S. aureus*. It must be remembered that the majority of blisters in SSSS are sterile, as they are caused by the hematogenous dissemination of the bacterial toxin, not the bacteria itself. The organism is most easily recovered from pyogenic (not exfoliative) foci on the skin, conjunctivae, nares, or nasopharynx. When the diagnosis remains in question, differentiation from TEN can be made by microscopic examination of a skin snip of the blister roof or a skin biopsy. In SSSS, cleavage occurs in the superficial epidermis at the level of the granular layer; whereas in TEN the split occurs below the dermal-epidermal junction.

Treatment of SSSS is directed at the eradication of toxin-producing staphylococci, thus terminating toxin production. A penicillinase-resistant penicillin, first- or second-generation cephalosporin, or clindamycin are all appropriate initial choices, with modification based on sensitivity testing. In patients with MRSA infection, parenteral vancomycin or other agents (as dictated by local resistance patterns) would be indicated. As SSSS is usually a more mild disease in older children, ambulatory therapy may be an option in this population. In neonates, or in infants or children with severe infection, hospitalization is mandatory, with attention to fluid and electrolyte management, infection control measures, pain management, and meticulous wound care with contact isolation. In particularly severe disease, care in an intensive care or burn unit is required. Neutralizing antibodies that inhibit the binding of ETs to desmoglein 1 are under investigation, given concerns about the development of antibiotic-resistant, exfoliative-toxin-producing staphylococci.[84]

Toxic Shock Syndrome

Toxic shock syndrome (TSS) is an acute febrile illness characterized by fever, rash, hypotension, and multisystem organ involvement. Although classically described in menstruating women in relation to the use of superabsorbent tampons, TSS is now recognized in both menstrual and non-menstrual forms, the latter now being more common.[85] Non-menstrual TSS may occur in association with surgical procedures, nasal packing, the postpartum state, and a variety of *S. aureus* infections.

TSS is caused by toxin-producing strains of *S. aureus*. Manifestations of the disease are mediated primarily by the toxic shock syndrome toxin (TSST-1) and staphylococcal enterotoxins (SEA, SEB, SEC). These toxins are capable of widespread polyclonal activation of T cells, which results in massive cytokine release and in the clinical picture of TSS. Both TSST-1 and the staphylococcal enterotoxins are considered 'superantigens', given their ability to activate T cells without intracellular processing and via specific binding to MHC class II molecules.[86,87]

A prodrome of mild constitutional symptoms, including malaise, myalgias, and chills, often precedes the symptoms of TSS. Eventually fever develops, along with lethargy, diarrhea, chills, nausea, and altered mental status. Symptoms of hypovolemia, including hyperventilation, palpitations, and orthostatic dizziness, may be present.[88] Physical findings include high fever, hypotension, a diffuse rash, and pharyngitis with hyperemia of mucous membranes. The cutaneous eruption is a diffuse, macular erythroderma, occasionally reminiscent of the rash of scarlet fever. Accentuation of the eruption in skin folds is a common finding, and in rare cases, the inguinal or perineal regions may be the only skin surfaces involved.[89] Edema of the hands, feet, and face may be present, and desquamation of the affected skin surfaces (Fig. 14.24) eventually ensues. The nails may be shed, and telogen effluvium may occur up to several months later. Oral examination often reveals a strawberry tongue (Fig. 14.25), and palatal petechiae may be present. Diffuse myalgia is almost always present, and many patients complain of exquisite skin or muscle tenderness when they are touched or moved.

In addition to the fever, desquamating rash, and hypotension, evidence of multiorgan involvement is present. To meet the case definition of TSS, three or more of seven other organ systems must be involved (Table 14.3).[90] The diagnosis of TSS generally rests on clinical criteria, although isolation of *S. aureus* from a normally sterile site, especially if toxin production can be demonstrated, is supportive. Histopathologic findings on skin biopsy are not pathognomonic. The differential diagnosis of TSS includes streptococcal TSS (see below), Kawasaki disease, scarlet fever, drug reaction, atypical measles, Rocky Mountain spotted fever, and other exanthematous illnesses. The presence of shock and multiorgan involvement is unusual in the other entities, except for streptococcal TSS, which usually has some distinguishing features.

A neonatal TSS-like disease has been reported, and in some of these patients MRSA was recovered.[91] When studied, several of these

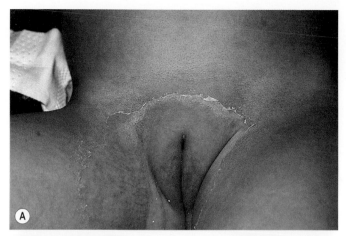
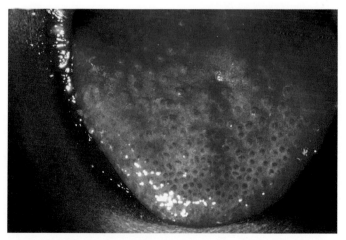

Figure 14.24 Desquamation in toxic shock syndrome. Mild perineal (A) and digital (B) desquamation in a 3-year-old female with toxic shock syndrome.

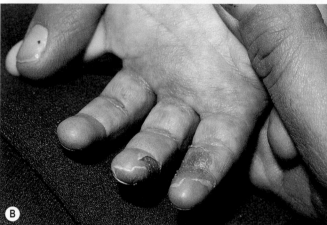

Figure 14.25 Strawberry tongue in toxic shock syndrome. Hyperemia with prominent lingual papillae.

MRSA isolates were positive for TSST-1 production. Most of the reported neonates had a mild course with a fairly rapid recovery.[91]

Since the late 1980s, a disease similar to TSS yet with some distinguishing features has been recognized. This disorder is associated with toxin-producing GABHS, and is now well recognized as *streptococcal toxic shock syndrome*. Although the pathogenic mechanisms

Table 14.3 Case definition of toxic shock syndrome

- Temperature >38.9°C (102.0°F)
- Diffuse macular erythroderma
- Desquamation, 1–2 weeks after onset, particularly of the palms and soles
- Hypotension
- Multisystem involvement (3 or more of the following):
  - Gastrointestinal (vomiting, diarrhea)
  - Muscular (severe myalgia, increased creatine phosphokinase level)
  - Mucous membrane (vaginal, oropharyngeal, or conjunctival hyperemia)
  - Renal (elevated serum urea nitrogen or serum creatinine level more than twice the upper limit of normal, or urinary sediment with >5 WBC per field in absence of UTI)
  - Hepatic (total bilirubin, AST or ALT greater than twice the upper limit of normal)
  - Hematologic (platelet count ≤100 000/mm^3)
  - Central nervous system (disorientation, altered consciousness without focal neurologic signs when fever and hypotension are absent)

Laboratory criteria: Negative results on the following tests (if obtained):
  - Blood, throat, or CSF cultures (except blood culture may be + for *S. aureus*)
  - Serologic tests for Rocky Mountain spotted fever, leptospirosis, or measles

'Probable' disease: meets laboratory criteria, and 4 of the 5 bulleted findings are present

'Confirmed' disease: meets laboratory criteria, and all 5 of the bulleted findings, including desquamation (unless patient expires before desquamation occurs)

Adapted from American Academy of Pediatrics. Toxic shock syndrome. In Pickering LK, Baker CJ, Long SS, McMillan JA, eds. Red Book: 2006 Report of the Committee on Infectious Diseases. 27th ed. Elk Grove Village, IL: American Academy of Pediatrics; 2006: pp. 660–665. © Copyright American Academy of Pediatrics. All rights reserved.[153] WBC, white blood cell; UTI, urinary tract infection; AST, aspartate aminotransferase; ALT, alanine aminotransferase; CSF, cerebrospinal fluid.

Table 14.4 Case definition of streptococcal toxic shock syndrome

Isolation of GABHS:
- from a normally sterile site (i.e., blood, CSF, peritoneal fluid, tissue biopsy)*

OR
- from a non-sterile site (i.e., throat, sputum, vagina)**

AND
- Hypotension or shock

AND
- At least 2 of the following:
  - renal impairment (creatinine >2 mg/dL or >twice the upper limit for age)
  - coagulopathy (DIC or thrombocytopenia)
  - hepatic involvement (AST, ALT or total bilirubin >twice the upper limit for age)
  - adult respiratory distress syndrome
  - generalized erythematous rash with or without desquamation
  - soft-tissue necrosis (i.e., necrotizing fasciitis or myositis or gangrene)

'Definite' case: * and both bulleted findings

'Probable' case: ** and both bulleted findings

Adapted from American Academy of Pediatrics CoID. Severe invasive group A streptococcal infections: A subject review. *Pediatrics* 1998;101(1):136–140; and Wolf JE, Rabinowitz LG. Streptococcal toxic shock-like syndrome. *Arch Dermatol* 1995;131(1):73–77. © 1995 American Medical Association. All rights reserved.[92,93] GABHS, group A beta-hemolytic streptococcus; CSF, cerebrospinal fluid; DIC, disseminated intravascular coagulopathy; AST, aspartate aminotransferase; ALT, alanine aminotransferase.

are not entirely clear, streptococcal pyrogenic exotoxins (SPEA, SPEB, SPEC), mitogenic factor, and streptococcal superantigen appear to be associated with the clinical findings.

Streptococcal TSS is similarly characterized by the acute onset of shock and multisystem organ failure, but unlike staphylococcal TSS, patients usually have a focal, invasive tissue or blood infection with GABHS (Table 14.4). Most patients with streptococcal TSS have pain localized to an extremity in association with necrotizing fasciitis or myonecrosis. This pain is usually out of proportion to the clinical findings on physical examination. Varicella is a particularly important risk factor for invasive GABHS infections in children, and in the child with varicella who becomes febrile after having been afebrile, or who has any fever beyond the fourth day of illness, GABHS infection should be considered.[92]

A prodromal illness with influenza-like symptoms is present in up to 20% of patients with streptococcal TSS. Subsequently, shock develops rapidly and often the patients develop renal impairment, disseminated intravascular coagulopathy, and an 'adult respiratory distress syndrome'-like illness. Physical examination reveals a diffuse macular erythroderma and mucous membrane findings, similar to those seen in staphylococcal TSS. Examination of the site of primary infection (usually an extremity) reveals localized swelling and erythema, with eventual development of vesicles and hemorrhagic bullae.[93] Laboratory aberrations include leukocytosis, anemia, thrombocytopenia, elevation of serum creatinine and creatine phosphokinase, hypocalcemia, abnormal liver function studies, and evidence of disseminated coagulopathy.

Management of TSS is similar for both staphylococcal and streptococcal disease. Supportive therapy, vasopressors, and antibiotics are the mainstays of therapy. Identification of sites of infection is vital, with appropriate drainage or, in the case of streptococcal TSS, aggressive and early surgical exploration and debridement as indicated. Many experts recommend combination antibiotic therapy including clindamycin, given its effects on protein (i.e., toxin) synthesis inhibition, although clindamycin should not be used alone.[92] Intravenous immunoglobulin (IVIG) may be beneficial when used in combination with antibiotics for TSS because IVIG blocks superantigen-induced T-cell activation. Use of IVIG should be considered in patients in whom there has been no clinical response within the first several hours of aggressive supportive therapy.[90,94]

Erythrasma

Erythrasma is a superficial bacterial infection of the skin caused by *Corynebacterium minutissimum*. It is characterized by asymptomatic, well-demarcated, reddish brown, slightly scaly patches in the groin, axillae, gluteal crease, or inframammary regions, and less often the interdigital spaces of the feet. Some 15% of cases occur in children between 5 and 14 years of age. Erythrasma is frequently confused with a dermatophyte infection (i.e., tinea corporis), with which it may occasionally co-exist. However, it can be differentiated from tinea infection by the characteristic coral red fluorescence seen when viewed under Wood's lamp illumination (due to the production of porphyrins by the corynebacteria). Erythrasma tends to be more common in overweight patients, the elderly and diabetics.[95] Culturing the organism is difficult and requires a special medium.

Erythrasma may be treated with topical antibiotics, including erythromycin or clindamycin. Antibacterial soaps may help prevent recurrence. Oral antibiotic therapy is very effective, including erythromycin, tetracycline, or newer macrolide agents.[96] *C. minutissimum* has rarely been associated with more severe disease, including cellulitis and bacteremia.[97]

Trichomycosis Axillaris

Trichomycosis axillaris (trichobacteriosis) is a superficial infection of the axillary and, less commonly, pubic hairs that results in adherent white or yellow concretions distributed irregularly along the hair shafts. *Corynebacterium tenuis* is the causative agent for this condition, and hence the traditional name trichomycosis axillaris, which implies a fungal infection, is a misnomer. The disorder usually occurs after puberty, owing to its association with axillary and pubic hair, but then occurs with equal frequency in all postpubertal age groups. The most frequent sign of trichomycosis axillaris is the presence of red-stained perspiration on the clothing, and individuals with hyperhidrosis frequently complain of a particularly offensive axillary odor. The nodules of trichomycosis axillaris consist of bacterial elements embedded in an amorphous matrix and Gram stain reveals threadlike Gram-positive bacteria. Affected areas only rarely fluoresce (as a pale yellow color) under Wood's light examination. Treatment consists of shaving the hairs of the affected areas, using antiperspirants (to help decrease hyperhidrosis and growth of Gram-positive flora), and the application of topical antibiotics such as clindamycin or erythromycin.

Pitted Keratolysis

Pitted keratolysis is another superficial corynebacterial infection, in this case involving the plantar feet, lateral aspects of the toes, and occasionally the palms. It is characterized by erythema with shallow round pits (Fig. 14.26), crateriform depressions, or shallow erosions, most commonly involving weight-bearing portions of the feet. Malodor is common, and although the condition is usually asymptomatic, painful, plaque-like lesions have been reported in children.[98] Pitted keratolysis is caused by *Corynebacterium* (*Kytococcus*) *sedentarius*, which produces extracellular enzymes capable of degrading human keratins.[99] The disorder has worldwide distribution and occurs most commonly in hot tropical climates and in populations (i.e., homeless individuals) who experience repeated skin exposure to moisture and environmental hazards.[100] The

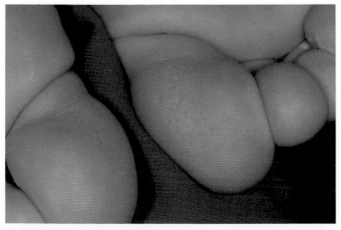

Figure 14.26 Pitted keratolysis. Shallow pits of the plantar great toes in this adolescent boy. Malodor was also present.

diagnosis is fairly straightforward and based on clinical findings, although Gram stain of stratum corneum shavings can be used if necessary. Culture is generally not helpful. Pitted keratolysis is treated with topical erythromycin, clindamycin, or mupirocin. Treatment of the hyperhidrosis component with prescription-strength aluminum chloride products or 40% formaldehyde in petrolatum ointment is also useful.

Erysipeloid

Erysipeloid is an infection of traumatized skin, particularly the fingers, hands, or arms of individuals who handle meat, raw saltwater fish, shellfish, or poultry. It is caused by *Erysipelothrix rhusiopathiae* (*insidiosa*), a Gram-positive bacillus that can survive for months in soil or decomposed organic material. Human infection with this organism can take one of three forms: the mild cutaneous infection erysipeloid, which may be confused clinically with erysipelas; a diffuse cutaneous form; and a serious systemic infection, usually septicemia or endocarditis.[101] Erysipeloid presents 1–7 days following inoculation as a painful, violaceous-red, sharply demarcated patch, usually on the hand. Burning, pain, or pruritus may be reported by the patient, and constitutional symptoms may occasionally be present. A diffuse, generalized eruption in regions remote from the site of infection, hemorrhagic vesicles, and regional lymphadenopathy may occasionally occur. Systemic complications are rare and include septicemia, endocarditis, septic arthritis, cerebral infarct, osseous necrosis, and pulmonary effusion. When endocarditis occurs, it tends to involve structurally damaged but native left-sided valves.[102]

The diagnosis of localized cutaneous erysipeloid can be difficult, as the organism does not grow well in culture and tissue biopsy findings are nonspecific. Blood culture may be useful when systemic infection is present. Although the vast majority of patients with untreated localized erysipeloid tend to recover spontaneously within 3 weeks, antibiotics such as penicillin, erythromycin, and doxycycline have been demonstrated to be effective.

Non-tuberculous ('atypical') mycobacterial infections

The non-tuberculous mycobacteria (NTM), which have traditionally been referred to as 'atypical mycobacteria', include those species different from *Mycobacterium tuberculosis*. These slender, non-motile, acid-fast organisms have a worldwide distribution and, usually, are non-pathogenic for humans. Infection tends to occur in immunocompromised individuals or, when in the immunocompetent host, following an episode of skin trauma.[103] Six major clinical syndromes have been identified, including lung infection, lymphadenitis, skin and soft tissue infection, disseminated infection, catheter-related infection, and chronic granulomatous infection of bones, joints and tendon sheaths.[104] Skin infection with NTM usually manifests as skin nodules, abscesses, papulopustules or ulcers.[105] Systemic spread most often occurs in immunocompromised hosts. The diagnosis of NTM infection is usually confirmed by histology and tissue culture.

The NTM include *Mycobacterium marinum*, *Mycobacterium ulcerans*, *Mycobacterium fortuitum*, *Mycobacterium chelonae*, *Mycobacterium abscessus*, *Mycobacterium kansasii*, *Mycobacterium avium-intracellulare* (*Mycobacterium avium complex*) and a variety of others that less commonly result in clinical infection. Those that will be discussed in this section are *M. marinum* (swimming pool granuloma), *M. ulcerans* (Buruli ulcer), and *M. fortuitum*/*M. chelonae*/*M. abscessus* (the 'rapid growers'). Cervical lymphadenitis due to NTM will also be briefly discussed.

Mycobacterium marinum may result in a skin infection termed 'swimming pool granuloma' or 'fish tank granuloma'. The organism resides in stagnant and seawater as well as in natural pools and some heated pools in temperate climates. Fish tank water exposure is a more recently described source for inoculation, and seems to be a fairly common mode of infection.[106,107] Abrasions from swimming pools or fish tanks, and at times cuts sustained from cleaning fish, may become infected with this NTM. Most lesions begin on an extremity, hand, or foot after an incubation period of 2–3 weeks. In some studies, the incubation period may be longer, up to 9 months after inoculation.[108] Infection begins with a nodule or pustule that eventually forms an ulcer or abscess. Multiple secondary lesions develop, often in a linear, lymphatic ('sporotrichoid') distribution (Fig. 14.27). Without therapy, the skin lesions resolve over 1–3 years with scarring. Potential associated complications include tenosynovitis, arthritis and osteomyelitis, and in immunocompromised individuals, severe disseminated infection may occur. The differential diagnosis includes cellulitis, sporotrichosis, syphilis, cutaneous leishmaniasis, tularemia, foreign body reaction, cat-scratch disease, neoplasia, and deep fungal infection. Skin biopsy reveals inflammation with tuberculoid granulomas, and culture of *M. marinum* from tissue confirms the diagnosis. Although PPD skin testing may be positive, it is not diagnostic of *M. marinum* infection.

When a patient presents with cutaneous lesions suggestive of *M. marinum* infection, a thorough exposure history should be pursued, and tissue biopsy performed. Although there is no completely satisfactory treatment for this infection, options that have been used with variable success include tetracycline, minocycline, doxycycline, clarithromycin, sulfamethoxazole-trimethoprim, and rifampin, alone or in combination with ethambutol.[103,106,109] Excision, curettage, and warm compresses are traditional treatment modalities that may be helpful for early or small lesions, but recurrences are common.

M. ulcerans may result in an ulcerating skin condition called Buruli ulcer, which is most common in Africa, Central and South America, and Asia. Buruli ulcer usually begins following a scrape by grass or a thorn, and presents initially as a painless nodule that progresses to abscess formation and, eventually, a shallow ulcer. The favored site of distribution is a lower extremity. The ulcer persists for months to years and eventually heals spontaneously with scarring and lymphedema.[103] Surgery, hyperthermic therapy, and systemic antimicrobials have all been used with variable success.

Mycobacterium fortuitum, *M. chelonae*, and *M. abscessus* are all referred to as 'rapid growers' given their distinctive ability to produce colonies in culture as soon as 5–7 days. They may result in clinical disease after trauma, the most notable association being abscess formation following surgery, especially within post-surgical scars.

Cervical lymphadenitis due to NTM should be mentioned, as it is the most common manifestation of infection with these agents in healthy, immunocompetent children. These patients usually present with unilateral cervical lymphadenopathy, although other sites may be involved, including the inguinal region, axilla, and lower limb.[110,111] There may or may not be a history of preceding local trauma, and the area may reveal overlying erythema (Fig. 14.28), violaceous discoloration, fluctuance or drainage. The most common of the NTM to cause cervical lymphadenitis is *M. avium-intracellulare*.[110,112] Treatment options include surgery, incision and drainage, and antimicrobial therapy including ethambutol, rifampicin and clarithromycin. Observation alone is another option, given the complete resolution seen in most patients within 9–12 months.[113]

Tuberculosis of the skin

The incidence of cutaneous tuberculosis, until recently, has been declining owing to the availability of effective antimycobacterial therapy, improvement in living standards, and vigorous preventative and therapeutic programs. However, it has re-emerged more recently in areas with a high incidence of HIV infection and multidrug-resistant pulmonary tuberculosis.[114] Cutaneous

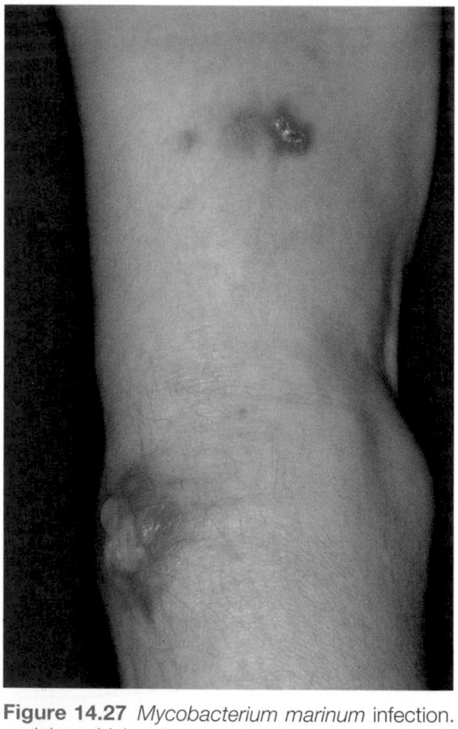

Figure 14.27 *Mycobacterium marinum* infection. This boy developed nodules which subsequently ulcerated, on the dorsal foot (superior lesion in photograph) and the medial ankle (inferior lesion in photograph). The family had a large fish tank which they routinely cleaned in the bathtub used by the patient.

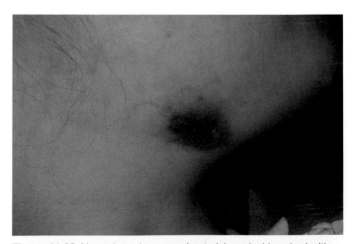

Figure 14.28 Non-tuberculous mycobacterial cervical lymphadenitis. This fluctuant, violaceous nodule developed in the inferior mandibular region of this otherwise-healthy 3-year-old girl. Occasional drainage had been noted by her parents, and the lesion improved gradually with clarithromycin therapy.

tuberculosis can be acquired either exogenously or via hematogenous spread of *M. tuberculosis* and may show a wide range of clinical presentations. The majority of cases of cutaneous tuberculosis are related to systemic involvement. In this section, several types of tuberculous skin lesions are reviewed. Of the lesions discussed, scrofuloderma and lupus vulgaris tend to be the most common types of cutaneous tuberculosis to occur in children.[115,116]

Primary tuberculous complex (*tuberculous chancre*) develops as a result of inoculation of *M. tuberculosis* into the skin (and occasionally the mucosa) of an individual who has not previously been infected or who has not acquired immunity to the organism. This disorder occurs on exposed surfaces at sites of trauma (i.e., abrasion, insect bite, puncture wound). The cutaneous lesion develops 2–4 weeks following inoculation, and the earliest lesion is a brown red papule that develops into an indurated plaque that may ulcerate. The edges of the ulcer are ragged and undermined, and thick adherent crusts may be present. When viewed through a glass slide producing pressure on the lesion (diascopy), these areas may have an 'apple jelly' yellow-brown color. Marked regional lymphadenopathy may be associated with the skin lesion,[117] and usually develops several weeks after the cutaneous lesion. Healing of the ulcer generally occurs over several weeks, but the regional lymphadenopathy may persist significantly longer, and after weeks to months, may soften and form sinuses that communicate with the skin surface (scrofuloderma).

Scrofuloderma refers to direct extension to the skin from underlying foci of tuberculous infection, and in addition to lymph nodes, may occur overlying infection of the bone or joint. It is manifested most commonly as painless swelling in the parotid, submandibular, supraclavicular, or lateral regions of the neck.[118] *Mycobacterium tuberculosis* can be easily identified by Gram stain and culture of the draining exudate. Untreated lesions of scrofuloderma may persist with little change for years, and eventually heal with cicatricial bands.

Tuberculosis verrucosa cutis (warty tuberculosis) is an externally acquired, relatively uncommon inoculation type of tuberculosis in individuals who have had previous contact with *M. tuberculosis* and thus have some degree of immunity. The inoculation usually occurs at sites of minor wounds or abrasions, and it occurs most often in adults with occupations that require the handling of tuberculous patients or tissues, including pathologists ('prosector's wart') and butchers ('butcher's wart'). Lesions usually occur on the dorsal hands, fingers, or lower extremities. They begin as small violaceous papules that become hyperkeratotic and warty. Multiple lesions may occur, but the majority of lesions of tuberculosis verrucosa cutis are solitary.

Lupus vulgaris is the most common form of cutaneous tuberculosis. It is a chronic, smoldering form of the infection, and usually occurs in individuals with a high degree of sensitivity. Although lupus vulgaris can arise at the site of a primary inoculation, in the scar of scrofuloderma, or at the site of a bacillus Calmette–Guérin (BCG) vaccination, it generally appears in previously normal areas of skin. The most common location of involvement is the face, and regional lymphadenopathy may be present in over half of the patients.[116] Lupus vulgaris presents as small, soft brown-red papules that enlarge and coalesce to form larger patches with elevation and intensification of their brownish color (Fig. 14.29). As in tuberculous chancre, the lesion shows a characteristic apple-jelly color on diascopy. The natural history of lupus vulgaris is marked by slow and limited growth over years or, occasionally, decades. Ulceration and atrophy may occur.[115,118] When ulceration occurs, it may be complicated by scarring and disfigurement, especially with nose and nasal cartilage involvement. The differential diagnosis of lupus

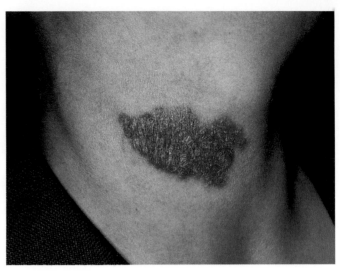

Figure 14.29 Lupus vulgaris. Elevated, brown-red plaque composed of coalescing papules. (Courtesy of Department of Dermatology, Yale University School of Medicine.)

vulgaris includes sarcoidosis, cutaneous lymphoid hyperplasia, lupus erythematosus, halogenoderma, leishmaniasis, leprosy, deep fungal infections, and cutaneous malignancy.

Orificial tuberculosis is a rare manifestation of cutaneous tuberculosis occurring usually in debilitated or immunocompromised individuals. It affects the mucocutaneous junctions of the orifices (nose, mouth, anus, urinary meatus, and genital) and is caused by autoinoculation of tubercle bacilli from secretions. Lesions present as shallow, painful ulcers with a granulating base and undermined edges, with swelling, edema, and inflammation of the surrounding mucosa. Painful ulcers of the mouth or other mucosal membranes in patients with visceral tuberculosis should arouse suspicion of this disorder.

Miliary tuberculosis of the skin (tuberculosis cutis miliaris disseminata) is an extremely rare manifestation of fulminating pulmonary or meningeal tuberculosis. It is quite uncommon in children, and in recent times is seen most often in the setting of adult HIV infection.[119,120] When present, the eruption is due to hematogenous dissemination of *M. tuberculosis* to the skin in addition to multiple internal organs. Cutaneous lesions present as minute, symmetrically distributed, erythematous, red-brown macules, papules, or vesiculopustules. Purpuric lesions may occasionally be present. The course of miliary tuberculosis is usually fulminating, and the mortality rate high.

Diagnostic options for cutaneous tuberculosis include smears, stains, and cultures of skin swabs, aspirates, and biopsy tissue. The Mantoux intradermal tuberculin test is frequently positive, but the reactivity does not correlate with disease activity.[116] PCR amplification of *M. tuberculosis* DNA is a rapid, sensitive, and accurate technique for diagnosis and may be applied to paraffin-embedded skin biopsy tissue.[121,122]

The treatment of all forms of cutaneous tuberculosis is similar to that used for active pulmonary tuberculosis. Current recommendations of the American Academy of Pediatrics include a 6-month regimen consisting of isoniazid, rifampin, and pyrazinamide for 2 months followed by 4 months of isoniazid and rifampin (with ethambutol or streptomycin added if drug resistance is a concern), or a 6-month regimen (for hilar adenopathy only) of isoniazid and rifampin.[123] Tuberculous meningitis is treated with a four-drug regimen for 2 months followed by isoniazid and rifampin for 7–10 more months.[123]

The tuberculid disorders

The tuberculids are hypersensitivity reactions to *M. tuberculosis*, and classically include erythema induratum, papulonecrotic tuberculid, and lichen scrofulosorum. Originally felt to be related to toxins or an allergic response to tubercle bacilli, they are currently believed to be the result of hematogenous dissemination of organisms from an internal focus to the skin, where they incite a cutaneous inflammatory response. *Lupus miliaris disseminatus faciei* (formally described as a tuberculid) is probably more aptly described as a granulomatous disorder of the pilosebaceous units (see Ch. 8). A deep nodular form presenting on the lower extremities has been termed *nodular tuberculid*, and seems to represent a hybrid between papulonecrotic tuberculid and erythema induratum.[124]

Erythema induratum of Bazin is a chronic, recurring panniculitis (inflammation of the fat) that typically occurs on the calves of girls and young women. Although the association with tuberculosis has historically been controversial, the clinical and histopathologic features, ability to identify *M. tuberculosis* on PCR studies, and response to antituberculosis therapy seem to support a tuberculous etiology.[125–129] Lesions present as symmetrical, tender deep-seated nodules that develop into red-purple masses that tend to ulcerate. The ulcers are irregular and shallow and heal with an atrophic scar. Erythema induratum tends to be chronic and recurrent; many patients have a personal or family history of tuberculosis. The tuberculin skin test is positive, but mycobacteria are seldom recovered from lesions by standard culture techniques. Recently, PCR analysis of skin biopsy specimens has been found to be rapid and sensitive in the diagnosis of this disorder.[127–129] Treatment of erythema induratum with combination antituberculous therapy is usually successful, although in untreated patients the lesions usually involute spontaneously over a period of years.

Papulonecrotic tuberculid is the most common tuberculid seen in children, although it is rarely seen in the USA. It is characterized by symmetric crops of dusky red, small papules and nodules with central necrosis or ulceration, which heal with superficial scarring. Sites of predilection for papulonecrotic tuberculid include the extensor extremities (particularly the knees and elbows), the buttocks, and the lower trunk. Ear involvement may also be common, and pulmonary tuberculosis is usually present.[130] The lesions may clinically resemble those of varicella. As with erythema induratum, recovery of the organism from standard tissue culture is of low yield. Patients usually have a positive intradermal tuberculin skin test reaction, and gene-amplification PCR performed on skin biopsy tissue is useful in confirming the diagnosis.[131] Papulonecrotic tuberculid usually responds promptly to antituberculous therapy.

Lichen scrofulosorum is characterized by clusters of lichenoid papules on the trunk of children or young adults, usually in association with tuberculosis of lymph nodes and/or other organs. Lesions are firm, 1–5 mm, flesh-colored to reddish brown flat-topped papules. They tend to be asymptomatic and slowly undergo spontaneous involution.

Leprosy

Leprosy (Hansen's disease) is a chronic infectious disorder of worldwide distribution in which the acid-fast bacillus *Mycobacterium leprae* has a special predilection for the skin and nervous system. Although the worldwide incidence of leprosy has decreased significantly, likely in response to multidrug therapy (MDT), widespread BCG vaccination, and public health initiatives, it is still somewhat prevalent in certain areas, including India, China, and South-east Asia. Leprosy is rare in the USA, with around 85% of diagnosed cases occurring in immigrants, and the disease may mimic many common dermatological and neurological disorders.[132]

Although there is no universal agreement on the classification of leprosy, the disorder is usually divided into several clinical subtypes, depending on the patient's degree of immunity to *M. leprae* (Table 14.5). At one end of the spectrum is the lepromatous (LL) form of the disorder, the disfiguring disease most familiar to the public. In this variant patients are anergic to *M. leprae* and develop widespread disease involving the skin (Fig. 14.30), upper respiratory tract, sensory and motor nerves, eyes (superficial keratitis), testes, lymph nodes, and bone. Many bacilli are present in the tissues. Nodules or diffuse infiltrates, especially on the face and earlobes, produce the characteristic 'leonine facies'. Loss of eyebrows and eyelashes may also occur. At the opposite pole is tuberculoid leprosy (TT), a form that occurs in patients with a very high degree of immunity against *M. leprae*. In this variant, patients have only a single or occasionally a few large well-defined macules or infiltrative plaques that show hypopigmentation and loss of sensation. The peripheral nerves, most commonly the ulnar, external popliteal, and great auricular, are thickened and palpable, and patients may develop trophic disturbances and paralyses. Between these ends of the

Table 14.5 Classification of leprosy (in order of decreasing host resistance)

Group	Clinical features
Tuberculoid (TT) (mildest; high resistance)	A single or few localized anesthetic macules or plaques; hair loss within lesions; few if any organisms; peripheral nerve involvement common
Borderline tuberculoid (BT)	Lesions similar to TT but more numerous; satellite papules around larger lesions (at times); hair and sensation diminished (but not absent) within lesions; peripheral nerve involvement common
Borderline borderline (BB)	Features of both TT and LL; more lesions than BT; borders more vague; nerve involvement and satellite lesions common; many bacilli usually present
Borderline lepromatous (BL)	Multiple non-anesthetic asymmetrically distributed annular plaques; may be surrounding papules; late neural lesions; leonine facies
Lepromatous (LL) (most severe; low or no resistance)	Generalized involvement (skin, mucous membranes, upper respiratory tract, reticuloendothelial system, adrenal glands, and testes); no neural lesions until late; no sensory or hair growth impairment; many bacilli in tissue
Indeterminate	Small number of hypopigmented macules; no thickened nerves or sensory impairment

Note: The three intermediate forms (BT, BB, and BL) are clinically unstable and may pass from milder to more severe states and vice versa.

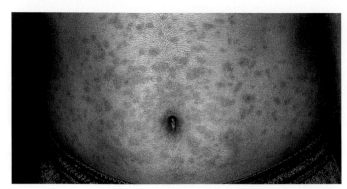

Figure 14.30 Lepromatous leprosy. Erythematous, infiltrative patches and plaques that revealed many acid-fast bacilli in the skin biopsy specimen.

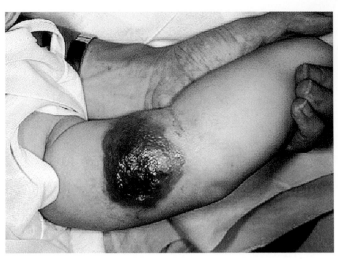

Figure 14.31 Cutaneous anthrax in a child. Erythematous plaque with necrosis and eschar formation in a 7-month-old male. Anthrax bacilli were detected in biopsy tissue. (Reprinted with permission from Roche KJ, Chang MW, Lazarus H. Images in clinical medicine. Cutaneous anthrax infection. N Engl J Med 2001; 345(22):1611. © 2001, Massachusetts Medical Society. All rights reserved.)

spectrum, borderline forms of the disorder are seen. Patients with borderline lepromatous leprosy tend to have the most extensive involvement of nerves. Owing to the decreased sensation in affected areas, these patients are at risk for secondary infections and digital ulceration. Blindness occurs in around 5% of patients with leprosy.[133]

The incubation period of leprosy is typically very long and ranges from 3 months to 40 years (average, 2–4 years).[132] Early childhood disease often presents with solitary lesions, which may occur on any exposed area of the skin, and childhood disease is most commonly indeterminate or at the tuberculoid end of the spectrum. The mode of transmission of leprosy remains unclear, although an upper respiratory route is suggested.

Leprosy should be suspected in any patient from a leprosy-endemic area (or immigrants from such regions) presenting with chronic hypopigmented or infiltrative skin lesions, skin anesthesia, thickened nerves, or eye complaints. The diagnosis is confirmed by the identification of acid-fast bacilli in skin smears or biopsy material, and the histologic picture reveals a granulomatous infiltrate containing large foamy histiocytes (lepra cells) in the epidermis. Treatment should be directed by a clinician experienced in the care of the leprosy patient, and preferably in a Hansen's disease center, where feasible. Although therapeutic recommendations of the past called for monotherapy with dapsone, given increasing resistance to this approach MDT is now recommended and includes other agents such as rifampin and clofazimine. In treated patients, 95% of all nerve function impairment develops within 2 years, supporting a decreased frequency for neurologic follow-up in patients without neurologic findings by that time.[134]

Leprosy reactions are fairly commonplace during treatment for the disease, and are related to immune-mediated inflammation. These reactional states, which include reversal reactions and erythema nodosum leprosum (ENL), may result in worsening of neural and skin lesions and significant tissue damage. These reactions are often treated with systemic corticosteroids and, in the case of ENL, thalidomide is a very effective agent.[135] Although at this point there is no effective vaccination for leprosy, BCG vaccination has been demonstrated to be effective at protecting some populations from infection.[132,136]

Anthrax

Anthrax, an infection caused by the Gram-positive *Bacillus anthracis*, is occasionally transmitted to humans through contact with infected animals or animal products, such as hides or wool. Whereas this mode of infection usually results in cutaneous anthrax, inhalation disease ('woolsorters' disease') has occurred in settings such as factories where processing of these products takes place.[137] Anthrax has long been considered a potential agent of biologic warfare, the significance of which was magnified by the events of September 11, 2001, and the following apparent bioterrorism involving the spread of B. anthracis via bioengineered spore-containing letters within the US postal system. These events highlight the importance of adequate education in, and recognition of, this infection and other potential biologic weapons of mass destruction.

Clinical infection with *B. anthracis* usually takes one of three forms: *inhalational*, *cutaneous*, or *gastrointestinal*. The cutaneous form ('malignant pustule') is responsible for 95% of the cases in the USA, and is usually an occupational disease of farmers, butchers, veterinarians, and individuals who process animal products.[138] The spore is introduced via an abrasion or cut in the skin, and develops into the primary lesion, which is a painless, pruritic papule. This papule progresses to develop small surrounding vesicles surrounded by a brawny, non-pitting edema. The vesicles rupture with the development of necrosis, and eventually a black eschar forms (Fig. 14.31) and overlies an ulcer. Low-grade fever, malaise, and headache are often present, and regional lymphadenopathy early in the course is common. Without therapy, this form is fatal in 20% of cases.[139] Cutaneous anthrax is rare in children, and may be accompanied by anthrax meningitis or systemic spread of disease. Microangiopathic hemolytic anemia, hyponatremia, and coagulopathy were reported in a 7-month-old infant with cutaneous infection.[140]

Gastrointestinal anthrax forms following ingestion of undercooked meat from infected animals. In this case, the characteristic eschar forms in the gastrointestinal tract, usually the terminal ileum or cecum, and patients present with fever, nausea, vomiting, and anorexia. Severe abdominal pain (presenting as an acute abdomen), bloody diarrhea, sepsis, and death may ensue, with a >50% mortality.

Inhalational anthrax is the most severe form of infection, and is traditionally associated with a very high (>95%) mortality rate. Patients present with flu-like symptoms, and progress to dyspnea, stridor, fever, and cyanosis. Meningitis, coma, and death may ensue.

The diagnosis of anthrax can be confirmed by Gram stain and culture of a skin lesion, cerebrospinal fluid, or blood. Confirmatory studies are usually performed in a reference laboratory. Nasal swabs are used epidemiologically but are not a reliable method of diagnosis.[137,139] Serologic testing is useful only from a retrospective standpoint, and requires acute and convalescent samples. Histopathologic examination of a skin biopsy specimen may also be useful, especially with the concomitant use of a tissue Gram stain.

Penicillin has been the drug of choice for anthrax for many decades, with penicillin resistance found only rarely in naturally occurring strains. Other antimicrobials with good activity against *B. anthracis* include ciprofloxacin, tetracyclines, macrolides, clindamycin, and cephalosporins. Some of these other agents may be more concentrated in the phagocyte and therefore may be more desirable.[141] Postexposure prophylaxis is recommended in situations where there is a credible threat of exposure to spores, and ciprofloxacin (alternative doxycycline) is recommended for a full 60 days in this setting.

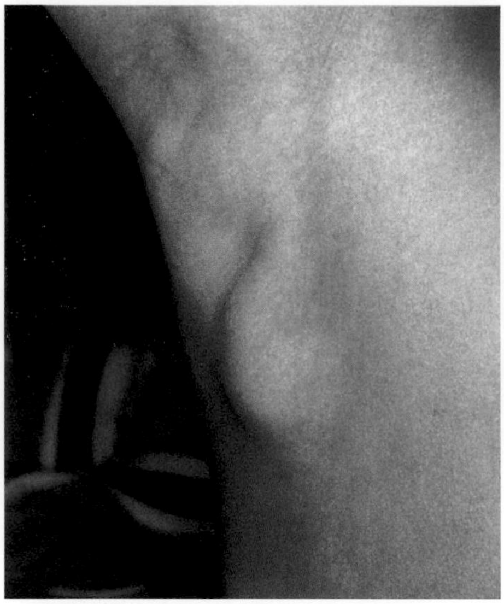

Figure 14.32 Cat-scratch disease. Axillary lymphadenopathy in a 2-year-old boy with a crusted red papule at the primary inoculation site on the chest.

Cat-scratch disease

Cat-scratch disease (CSD) is an acute, self-limited infection of children and young adults caused by the pleomorphic Gram-negative bacillus *Bartonella henselae*. *Bartonella* species, which are Gram-negative bacilli, result in a variety of diseases in humans, including Carrion disease, prolonged fever of unknown origin, encephalopathy, ocular disease, trench fever and endocarditis. CSD is a benign cause of lymphadenitis in children, and is usually transmitted from infected kittens to humans by means of a scratch or bite that is often recalled only in retrospect.[142] The domesticated house cat is the most important natural reservoir for *B. henselae*, and stray cats and kittens are more likely to be infected than are pet or adult cats.[143] It is estimated that up to half of domestic cats have antibodies to *B. henselae*, testing seropositive for the bacteria.[144] This organism has also been linked to bacillary angiomatosis (see Ch. 12), a vascular proliferative disease seen most commonly in HIV-infected individuals. CSD is most common in areas with warm climates, and occurs most often in the fall and winter.[145]

The most common clinical presentation of CSD is lymphadenopathy. However, the infection usually begins with a small papule or nodule within the original cat-scratch line 3–10 days following the trauma. Over the following 1–2 weeks, the regional lymph nodes draining the region begin to enlarge (Fig. 14.32), reaching the point of maximal enlargement around 1 month after the initial injury.[146] Often, the initial wound at the site of contact with the animal has resolved by the time the patient pursues medical care. The enlarged lymph nodes gradually decrease in size over a period of a few months, in the absence of therapy. In up to 10% of patients, lymph nodes will become erythematous and fluctuant, occasionally requiring needle aspiration.[145] In 85% of patients, there is only a single lymph node involved.[144] Common locations for the lymphadenopathy of CSD include the neck, axillary, and inguinal regions.[147] In one large series, the most common sites of lymphadenopathy (in order of decreasing frequency) were the axilla, epitrochlear region, cervical region, submandibular region, and groin.[148] Biopsy of lymph nodes, when performed, reveals granulomas with multiple microabscesses.

Other features that may be present in patients with CSD include fever, headache, and malaise. *Parinaud oculoglandular syndrome* consists of unilateral granulomatous conjunctivitis at the site of inocu-

lation, with concomitant ipsilateral preauricular lymphadenopathy, and represents the most common form of atypical CSD. This presentation appears to occur as a result of indirect inoculation of the organism into the eye, rather than by direct contact through a cat scratch, as is typical of CSD. Other less common associations include neuroretinitis (presenting as acute onset unilateral vision loss), encephalopathy, endocarditis, seizures, generalized lymphadenopathy, or prolonged fever. Immunocompromised individuals with *B. henselae* infection may develop a disseminated, invasive form of infection that involves multiple organs. *Bacillary peliosis* is the term used to describe reticuloendothelial organ involvement, including the liver (peliosis hepatis), spleen, abdominal lymph nodes, and bone marrow.[145]

Cat-scratch disease is usually diagnosed based on the characteristic clinical presentation in combination with a history of recent contact with a cat. Diagnostic confirmation is provided by positive serologic studies for antibodies to *B. henselae* (either >1:64 antibody titer or a four-fold titer elevation between acute and convalescent sera). Serology remains the most practical diagnostic tool for the laboratory detection of *B. henselae* infection.[144] Blood and tissue can be cultured, but the organism is slow growing and may be difficult to isolate. Identification of the organism in tissue samples stained with the Warthin-Starry silver stain lends further support to the diagnosis and may be useful in some settings. The most sensitive test available is *B. henselae* DNA sequence detection via PCR, but this modality is not readily available.[146]

Treatment of CSD in the immunocompetent host with uncomplicated disease is not always necessary, as it is a self-limited disease and studies demonstrating a significant advantage of therapy are lacking. However, treatment may shorten the period of symptomatic illness, and may promote more rapid resolution of the clinical abnormalities.[146] *Bartonella henselae* has been demonstrated to be susceptible to a variety of antimicrobial agents, including azithromycin (the recommendation of many clinician-researchers), clarithromycin, rifampin, doxycycline, ciprofloxacin, gentamicin, and trimethoprim-sulfamethoxazole. Disease in immunocompromised patients may be more serious, and thus therapy is usually recommended with a macrolide, rifampin, or doxycycline for at least 6 weeks.[142] Surgical removal of lymph nodes is generally not indicated, except in rare patients in whom the diagnosis is in doubt, in whom repeated aspirations fail to relieve pain, or in whom the inflammatory process persists without involution.

Disorders due to fungus-like bacteria

Actinomycosis and nocardiosis are disorders caused by actinomycetes, which are Gram-positive organisms that may resemble fungi both microscopically and macroscopically. Although these infections can occur at any age, they most often occur in adults. Although primary skin infection is rare, involvement of the cutaneous and subcutaneous tissues may result from contiguous spread from other sites or secondary infection of traumatized or injured skin, particularly in debilitated or immunodeficient individuals.

Actinomycosis

Actinomycosis is a chronic suppurative infection caused by *Actinomyces israelii*, an anaerobic Gram-positive saprophyte of the tonsillar crypts, carious teeth, and female genital tract, and rarely by other *Actinomyces* spp. Infection is often associated with dental procedures, trauma, or surgery.[149] This disorder is clinically characterized by the production of 'sulfur granules' from multiple draining sinuses. It tends to occur in one of three areas: the cervicofacial region (most common), lungs, or intestinal tract. Cervicofacial actinomycosis, seen most often in individuals with poor oral hygiene and carious teeth, begins when the infecting organism invades a traumatized oral mucous membrane. This form presents as soft tissue swelling, usually over the mandibular region. It increases to form a brawny, erythematous nodule that discharges serosanguineous or purulent material through multiple sinus tracts, from which the characteristic sulfur-yellow granules consisting of masses of organisms can be demonstrated. Destruction of bone with periostitis and osteomyelitis may occur, and absence of regional lymph node involvement is characteristic.

Aspiration of the organism causes pulmonary infection, which progresses through the pleura, causing draining sinus tracts of the chest wall. It may occur following esophageal disruption during surgery or non-penetrating trauma, or may occur as a manifestation of extension of cervicofacial infection.[150] The abdominal form develops from the ileum, cecum, or appendix (in association with appendicitis) and is seen as draining sinuses, tracts, or subcutaneous abscesses, extending to either the abdominal wall or the perineum. Primary infection of other body sites may affect the urinary tract, central nervous system, bones, and joints. A localized form, known as mycetoma, occurs most frequently on the feet or ankles of individuals who walk around barefoot (see Ch. 17).

Actinomycosis is diagnosed by isolation and identification of the causative organism in anaerobic culture. It may also be confirmed by observation of the highly characteristic 'sulfur' granules (groups of delicate filaments, frequently with club-shaped ends) in purulent or biopsied materials. The course of actinomycosis is prolonged and characterized by closure of one sinus tract and the opening of another. Treatment is with intravenous penicillin G for 4–6 weeks, followed by oral penicillin in high doses for 6–12 months.[150] Surgical incision and drainage of abscesses and excision of fibrotic, avascular tissue are occasionally necessary. Alternative antibiotics for penicillin-allergic patients include tetracyclines, erythromycin, or clindamycin.

Nocardiosis

Nocardiosis is a severe, primarily pulmonary infection caused by an aerobic Gram-positive, partially acid-fast fungus-like organism, *Nocardia asteroides*. It is less often caused by *Nocardia braziliensis* or other species. Nocardiosis primarily affects men in the 30- to 50-year age group, although it has been increasingly recognized in infants and children. Disseminated disease has a significant morbidity and mortality, and is more likely in immunosuppressed hosts.

Nocardiosis may occur with several different presentations, including pulmonary, systemic, CNS, and cutaneous/subcutaneous forms. It generally occurs through inhalation of contaminated dust, and the clinical picture is usually that of a primary pulmonary disease that resembles tuberculosis in its clinical and radiographic findings. These primary pulmonary infections may result in blood vessel erosion with subsequent hematogenous dissemination to other organs, including the skin. In those instances in which the skin is involved (<15% of cases), the most common lesions are abscesses of the chest wall with granulomatous lesions surrounding draining sinuses.[151] Primary cutaneous or subcutaneous nocardiosis is usually the result of traumatic implantation of foreign objects into the skin.[149] Once inoculated into the skin, it may present in a lymphocutaneous syndrome mimicking sporotrichosis, as a cellulites-like picture, or as a mycetoma (large, draining mass).[152] Disorders which may predispose to invasive disease include chronic granulomatous disease, organ transplantation, human immunodeficiency virus infection, or diseases requiring long-term systemic steroid therapy.[153]

Nocardiosis should be considered in obscure pulmonary and meningeal syndromes and chronic suppurative disorders of the bones or skin. The diagnosis is established by the presence of organisms in smears or cultures of sputum, aspirated material collected from lesions, or biopsy material. Unfortunately, the diagnosis is seldom established until the disease is far advanced. The cornerstone of therapy for nocardiosis is sulfonamides and trimethoprim-sulfamethoxazole. Imipenem, third-generation cephalosporins, amoxicillin-clavulanate, amikacin, minocycline, and fluoroquinolones may be other options.[152]

Treponemal infections

Syphilis

Syphilis is an infectious disease caused by the spirochetal organism *Treponema pallidum*. It is transmitted primarily by sexual contact, with the next most common mode being vertical transmission across the placenta, which may result in congenital syphilis (see Ch. 2). After a steady decline in the number of cases of syphilis in the early 1970s, the incidence of syphilis has fluctuated with peaks and troughs occurring in approximately 10-year cycles, with the overall trend being toward increasing rates.[154] Syphilis continues to be an important health problem throughout the world, and left untreated may result in long-term neurologic, cardiovascular, and other systemic sequelae, as well as congenital syphilis in offspring of infected mothers. Some 15–40% of untreated patients will develop recognizable late complications.[154] Currently, more than 60% of new cases of syphilis occur in men who have sex with men, and the HIV co-infection rate is high (up to 60% in some geographic locations) among patients with syphilis in the USA.[155,156]

Untreated acquired syphilis is characterized by a series of clinical stages, which are summarized in Table 14.6. There may be considerable overlap of symptoms in the various stages, and the early stages may pass by undiagnosed. The incubation period for syphilis ranges

Table 14.6 Clinical stages of syphilis

Stage	Clinical manifestations
Primary	Painless papule or ulcer at site of inoculation
	Regional lymphadenopathy
Secondary	Generalized macular/papular rash, involves palms/soles
	Condyloma lata in intertriginous areas
	Mucous patches
	Constitutional symptoms
	Occasional aseptic meningitis
Latent	No symptoms, but specific antibody tests positive
Tertiary	
Cardiovascular	Aortic aneurysm
Neurosyphilis	CVA, paresis, psychiatric symptoms, ataxia, autonomic dysfunction, cranial nerve palsies, optic neuritis
Gumma	Inflammatory infiltrates in multiple organs

CVA, cerebrovascular accident.

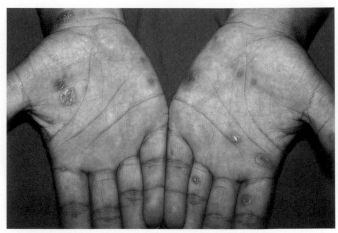

Figure 14.34 Secondary syphilis. Crusted, hyperkeratotic, erythematous papules and plaques of the palms.

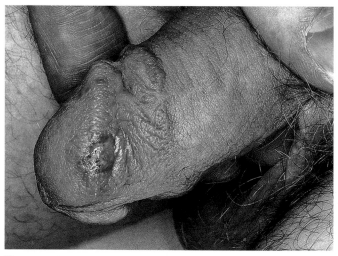

Figure 14.33 Primary syphilis. Eroded chancre of the glans penis in a male with primary infection.

from 5 to 90 days. Patients with early syphilis (primary, secondary, and the first year of latent syphilis) are considered infectious. The late latent (after the first year) and late stages, conversely, are considered non-infectious, rarely relapse, and tend to be destructive and scarring.

Primary syphilis usually manifests as a single, painless genital papule or more commonly ulcer, occurring on the labia or vaginal wall in females and the glans penis (Fig. 14.33) in males. In homosexual men, anorectal ulcers are most common. Painless regional lymphadenopathy is often present, although there may occasionally be tenderness to palpation. The differential diagnosis of the primary syphilitic chancre includes other sexually transmitted diseases, including herpes simplex virus infection and chancroid (caused by *Hemophilus ducreyi*), which both tend to be differentiated by painful ulcers. Extragenital ulcers occur infrequently in primary syphilis, and when present occur most commonly on the fingers, tongue

borders, or anus. If left untreated, the ulcer of primary syphilis heals spontaneously over 4–6 weeks.

Secondary syphilis develops 2–8 weeks after exposure in untreated individuals, and is more common in females given the increased number of asymptomatic or undiagnosed primary lesions compared to men.[157] The primary chancre may still be present at the time of diagnosis of secondary syphilis. The classic cutaneous findings of this stage are characterized by a widespread macular and papular skin eruption, which may occasionally be follicular or pustular. Examination reveals pink to erythematous, slightly scaly macules and papules that often involve the palms and soles, as well as flanks and arms. In dark-skinned individuals the lesions tend to be hyperpigmented. The palm and sole lesions may appear as macular or hyperkeratotic red-brown papules or plaques (Fig. 14.34), and are often helpful in the differentiation between secondary syphilis and the primary differential diagnosis, pityriasis rosea. Other entities in the differential diagnosis include drug eruption, lichen planus, acute exanthems, tinea versicolor, sarcoidosis, Mucha–Habermann disease (pityriasis lichenoides), nummular eczema, and psoriasis.

Other mucocutaneous lesions seen in secondary syphilis include alopecia, mucous patches, and condyloma lata. Patchy alopecia may be present in up to 7% of patients, and classically has a 'moth-eaten' appearance. Mucous patches occur on the tongue, buccal mucosa, and lips and present as erythematous patches, often with associated erosion and a silvery-gray membrane. Condyloma lata are smooth, gray plaques found in warm and moist intertriginous zones in up to 20% of patients. These lesions are highly infectious and must be differentiated from genital warts (condylomata acuminata).

Systemic symptoms may also be present, and include fever, headache, malaise, pharyngitis, and arthralgias. Ocular inflammatory conditions (including episcleritis, keratitis, and uveitis) may occur, as may aseptic meningitis, painless lymphadenopathy (especially epitrochlear), and hepatitis. A particularly aggressive form, termed lues-maligna, has been observed most frequently in the HIV-infected population.[158]

Cutaneous lesions of secondary syphilis usually heal without scarring, even in the absence of therapy, within 2–10 weeks. Residual hyper- or hypopigmentation may be present. Residual hypopigmentation on the skin of the neck has been termed the *necklace of Venus* (leukoderma colli).

Latent syphilis is a stage of the disease during which there are no clinical signs or symptoms or during which there are mild but generally unrecognized nonspecific symptoms such as malaise, anorexia, headache, sore throat, arthralgia, and low-grade fever. A diagnosis of latent syphilis is usually established on the basis of a positive serologic test after other stages of syphilis have been ruled out by physical and cerebrospinal fluid examination. This stage is arbitrarily divided into early latent syphilis (occurring within 1 year of infection) and late latent syphilis (occurring after 1 year). Patients with early latent syphilis are considered to be infectious.

Tertiary syphilis is divided into late benign syphilis (gumma), neurosyphilis, and cardiovascular syphilis (Table 14.5). It appears in around 10–40% of untreated patients, and after a latent period of 3–30 years or longer. Tertiary syphilis is extremely rare in children.

The hallmark lesions of late benign syphilis are the 'gummas,' and the skin is one of the most common organs of involvement, other common sites being the bone and liver. The cutaneous lesions present as superficial nodules or noduloulcerative plaques that may result in punched out ulcers. Common sites of involvement include the extremities, face, scalp, sternum, and the sternoclavicular joints. Upon healing, hyperpigmentation and atrophic scarring may persist. When the palate or nasal mucosa is affected, destruction is often pronounced and may lead to perforation of the affected areas. Large gummas may have several perforations, and as the intervening bridges of skin break down and necrose, lesions tend to produce arched or scalloped margins with arciform and geographic patterns. Bone lesions occurring in this stage are marked by periostitis involving the cranial bones, tibia, and clavicle, and present with nocturnal pain and local swelling.[154]

The diagnosis of syphilis depends on the combined findings from history, clinical examination, tissue examination, and serologic studies. *T. pallidum* cannot be cultured. Dark-field microscopy is the gold standard diagnostic method for primary syphilis, although it is not always readily available. Direct fluorescent antibody testing for *T. pallidum* has also been described for the diagnosis of primary syphilis. Both of these approaches, however, have been supplanted by serologic diagnostic methods, which are also the mainstay of laboratory diagnosis for secondary, latent, and tertiary syphilis.

Serologic tests, which provide only indirect evidence of infection, are divided into non-treponemal and treponemal categories. The non-treponemal tests detect an antibody against cardiolipin that is present in the sera of many patients with syphilis. These examinations include the Venereal Disease Reference Laboratory (VDRL) slide test and the Rapid Plasma Reagin (RPR) card test. These examinations are inexpensive, rapid, and convenient, but may result in false positive reactions (i.e., with advanced age, malignancies, Lyme disease, chronic liver disease, pregnancy, systemic lupus erythematosus, and some viral or bacterial infections) and are limited in their sensitivity. The treponemal tests include the fluorescent treponemal antibody absorption (FTA-ABS) test, the microhemagglutination test for *T. pallidum* (MHA-TP), and the *T. pallidum* immobilization (TPI) test. Although the TPI test has been the standard against which all subsequent tests have been compared, it is rarely used today since it is difficult, expensive, and only available in a few laboratories. Treponemal tests measure specific antibodies formed by the host in response to infection with *T. pallidum*. They have a higher sensitivity and specificity than non-treponemal tests and are used as confirmation of diagnosis. Treponemal tests establish the high likelihood of a treponemal infection either at the present time or at sometime in the past.[159] Newer treponemal tests are under evaluation, including the latex agglutination test for *T. pallidum* (TPLA) and enzyme immunoassays.[160]

Parenteral penicillin G is the mainstay of treatment for all forms of syphilis, with dosing regimens and duration of therapy varying based on stage of disease and the clinical manifestations that are present.[161] In patients with penicillin allergy, doxycycline is the preferred alternative, and others include tetracycline, erythromycin, or ceftriaxone. Azithromycin has been investigated for its utility in treating patients with early disease.[162] The treatment of choice for congenital syphilis or neurosyphilis is aqueous crystalline penicillin G.[161] Patients under therapy for syphilis are generally assessed for response to therapy by serial quantitative non-treponemal tests. Patients with early syphilis and congenital syphilis should have repeat quantitative, non-treponemal testing at 1, 3, 6, 12, and 24 months after treatment, and patients with late disease should be evaluated at 12 and 24 months. Patients with neurosyphilis require close follow-up clinical and CSF examinations done at 6-month intervals for at least the first 2 years after diagnosis.

Pinta

Pinta, a non-venereal treponemal infection caused by *Treponema pallidum* subsp. *carateum*, occurs almost exclusively among the dark-skinned population of Central and South America and Cuba. It is transmitted by direct contact and is frequently seen in children of affected parents. Although transmission by insects is possible, this mode of exposure is considered to be exceedingly rare. Pinta is the only spirochetal disease that results only in cutaneous manifestations.

There are three basic forms of pinta, termed *primary*, *secondary*, and *late*. The primary stage, seen on uncovered areas such as the face, arms, and legs, begins 1–8 weeks after inoculation as red papules, which enlarge into oval or round erythematous scaly plaques measuring up to 10 cm in diameter. Small papules frequently become surrounded by satellite macules or papules that coalesce to form configurative patterns. Regional lymphadenopathy is common. After several months to years, secondary lesions (referred to as 'pintids') appear as small, scaly papules that coalesce into large scaly plaques. Their color is initially red to violaceous, with progression to slate-blue, brown, gray, or black hue.[163] In this stage, widespread involvement is present, with coalescence of lesions. The differential diagnosis may include psoriasis, eczema, tinea corporis, syphilis, or leprosy. Lesions of primary and secondary pinta are highly infectious.

The late phase develops in 3–10 years and is characterized by irregular pigmentation with a range of different shades (correlating with the site of deposition of melanin in the dermis), resulting in a spotted and highly characteristic appearance. These lesions have an insidious onset, usually during adolescence or young adulthood, and are eventually replaced by depigmented patches closely resembling vitiligo. The most common sites of involvement are the bony prominences, including wrists, elbows, and ankles. Periarticular skin atrophy and extensor surface hyperkeratosis is also common during this phase.[164]

The diagnosis of pinta is made by identification of *T. carateum* on dark-field examination or, more commonly, serologic testing. The serologic studies utilized for the diagnosis of pinta are the same as those utilized for venereal syphilis, and these diseases are immunologically and serologically indistinguishable.[165] Penicillin is the treatment of choice, with options similar to those of syphilis for penicillin-allergic patients.

Yaws

Yaws, which is caused by *Treponema pallidum* subsp. *pertenue*, is a non-venereal treponemal disease endemic in many tropical regions that typically begins in childhood (usually before puberty). It is also transmitted by direct skin contact, and has been divided into *primary*, *secondary*, and *tertiary* stages. The primary stage is characterized by an erythematous papule that occurs, within 2–4 weeks, at the site of inoculation (the 'mother yaw'), usually the legs, feet, or buttocks. It enlarges and becomes confluent with surrounding satellite nodules, with eventual ulceration. This stage is occasionally accompanied by constitutional symptoms, arthralgias, and lymphadenopathy. Spontaneous healing of the skin lesion eventually occurs with scarring, although it may take up to 6 months.[166]

Weeks to months following the primary lesion, secondary yaws occurs, presenting as smaller, widespread cutaneous papules (daughter yaws or 'framboesias'), which tend to occur adjacent to body orifices. These lesions ulcerate and secrete infectious treponemes. This stage is characterized also by palmoplantar lesions, bone involvement, lymphadenopathy, and occasional neurologic and ophthalmologic abnormalities. Hyperkeratotic involvement of the palms and soles with painful fissuring is common. The latter may cause patients to walk on the sides of their feet, producing a characteristic gait known as 'crab yaws.'

Although the disorder generally terminates with the secondary stage, 10% of patients develop a late tertiary stage in which gummatous lesions occur. These lesions, which present 5–10 years after inoculation, may be locally destructive and lead to skin ulceration as well as deforming bone and joint sequelae. Late neurologic or ophthalmologic manifestations may occasionally present during the tertiary stage, but are not typical.

Yaws is usually diagnosed based on the characteristic clinical findings in an endemic region, combined with dark-field microscopy or serologic studies. Again, the same serologic examinations used to diagnose venereal syphilis and pinta are utilized. Treatment is the same as that for pinta.

Lyme Disease

Lyme disease is the most common vector-borne disease in the USA. It was first recognized in south-eastern Connecticut in 1975 and is an immune-mediated multisystem disorder caused by the spirochete *Borrelia burgdorferi*. Lyme disease is transmitted by *Ixodes* species ticks, primarily *Ixodes scapularis* (the deer tick) in the USA. It occurs most commonly in areas where deer ticks are abundant and *B. burgdorferi* carriage common, especially the coastal north-eastern, mid-Atlantic, and northern central regions of the USA, as well as much of Europe and Northern Asia.[167] Lyme disease is rare in the Pacific states because of the low infection rate of *Ixodes pacificus* (the Western black-legged tick) with *B. burgdorferi*.[168] When cases occur in the western states, they are most common in northern California and Oregon. In Europe, the vector is most often *Ixodes ricinus*, and the pathogenic *Borrelia* species are *Borrelia afzelii* and *Borrelia garinii*.[169] There is a bimodal age distribution of Lyme disease, with the initial peak occurring in children between the ages of 5 and 14 years.[170]

There are several factors associated with the risk of transmission of *B. burgdorferi* from ticks to humans. Because organisms often remain dormant in the tick until multiplication and migration occur during feeding, the risk of transmission is low if the tick is removed within 24 h of attachment. In addition, the proportion of infected ticks varies according to geographic location, and hence the risk of disease is low outside of endemic regions.

The clinical findings of Lyme disease were originally described as occurring in three stages, although now they are generally divided into two stages: early (divided into early localized or early disseminated) and late (Table 14.7). The onset of clinical manifestations usually occurs from 3 days to 4 weeks following the tick bite. However, because of the small pencil-point size of the *Ixodes* tick, only about 30% of patients recall having had a tick bite.

Table 14.7 Clinical manifestations of Lyme disease

Stage of disease	Clinical findings
Early localized	Erythema migrans (single)
	Constitutional symptoms (headache, myalgias, arthralgias, fatigue, fever)
	Lymphadenopathy
Early disseminated	Erythema migrans (multiple)
	Lymphadenopathy
	Constitutional symptoms (headache, myalgias, arthralgias, fatigue, fever)

	Neurologic
	  Facial palsy
	  Meningitis
	  Other neuropathies

	Cardiac
	  AV conduction defects
	  Congestive heart failure
	  Myocarditis

	Rheumatologic Arthritis

Late	Neurologic
	  Encephalopathy
	  Encephalomyelitis
	  Peripheral neuropathy

	Rheumatologic Arthritis

	Cutaneous
	  Lymphocytoma cutis
	  Acrodermatitis chronica atrophicans

AV, atrioventricular.

Early localized Lyme disease

The earliest manifestation of Lyme disease is usually a single skin lesion termed *erythema migrans* (*EM*). It is felt that at this stage the spirochetal infection is restricted to the skin in most patients. EM begins with a red papule at the site of the bite and progresses to become a flat, erythematous patch. With peripheral expansion, there may be central clearing (although not always), resulting in an annular patch (Fig. 14.35). This lesion usually is non-palpable, and it is most commonly asymptomatic. Occasional variations include vesicular, urticarial, scaly, and purpuric presentations.[171] Systemic symptoms may be present, and include fatigue, fever, chills, headache, myalgias, and arthralgias. Lymphadenopathy may also occur. Although EM may occur anywhere on the cutaneous surface, the thighs, groin, and axillae are particularly common sites of involvement. The lesions can be differentiated from those of tinea corporis and nummular eczema by rapid peripheral expansion, lack of scaling, and lack of pruritus. The eruption of EM resolves spontaneously over several weeks even without therapy. Multiple EM lesions may be seen, and usually correlate with spirochetemia and disseminated disease (see below).

Early disseminated Lyme disease

As the organism disseminates, patients may show additional signs or symptoms, including multiple lesions of EM (Fig. 14.36). The individual lesions are similar to the original EM lesion, although they tend to be less inflamed and do not extend as aggressively.[172] Multiple EM lesions occur in around 25% of infected children in the USA.[168] Constitutional symptoms are common during this stage usually mono- or oligoarticular, and tends to involve the knees most commonly, although migratory and small joint involvement may be seen. The presentation may simulate that of juvenile rheumatoid arthritis or an acute septic arthritis, and confusion with the latter may be compounded by the finding of markedly elevated joint fluid leukocyte counts.[173] The most common neurologic sequelae of late disease are encephalopathy, encephalomyelitis, and sensorineural peripheral neuropathy, although late neurologic disease tends to be rare in children.

Other cutaneous manifestations that have been potentially linked to *B. burgdorferi* infection include linear morphea, lichen sclerosis et atrophicus, and lymphocytoma cutis (cutaneous lymphoid hyperplasia). In Europe, *B. burgdorferi* infection has also been associated with Bannworth's syndrome (localized radicular pains accompanied by motor or sensory changes and occasionally lymphocytic meningitis), atrophoderma of Pasini and Pierini, eosinophilic fasciitis, and progressive facial hemiatrophy. Acrodermatitis chronica atrophicans (ACA) is reported primarily in Europe as a late manifestation of disease. It is characterized early by violaceous plaques followed by induration, hyperpigmentation, and atrophy of the skin on the distal extensor extremities, and may be associated with concurrent arthritis and neuropathy.[172]

Chronic Lyme disease (also known as post-treatment chronic Lyme disease) is a challenging and controversial entity from both a diagnostic and therapeutic standpoint. Two syndromes to occur in this context have been reported. The first consists of patients who continue to have symptoms similar to the pre-treatment period despite appropriate therapy, especially joint complaints. The second syndrome to occur in this setting is similar to chronic fatigue syndrome or fibromyalgia, and patients present with complaints of extreme fatigue, myalgias, headache, polyarthralgias, and mood disturbances. Some patients are more symptomatic than others, possibly reflecting some sort of genetic influence, and although the disease does not tend to be destructive or progressive, its effects can be quite debilitating.[174]

The diagnosis of Lyme disease relies upon clinical findings suggestive of the disease in combination with confirmatory laboratory testing. Antibody determinations are the most commonly utilized diagnostic examinations, and include indirect immunofluorescence assays and ELISA assays. Both can assess for IgM and IgG antibodies to *B. burgdorferi*. It must be remembered that patients with early localized Lyme disease are frequently seronegative for antibodies, and hence the diagnosis in that setting requires astute clinical judgment. Serologic studies may also be limited by cross-reactivities with other organisms and high rates of seropositivity among asymptomatic persons in endemic areas.[175] Immunoblotting or Western blotting allows for more specific detection of antibodies and maybe used in conjunction with the above-mentioned assays. Culture of *B. burgdorferi* is possible from tissue or fluid, but it is slow and difficult and requires special media that are not readily available. PCR studies for Lyme disease have been applied to a variety of tissues and fluids, but in general, are neither approved nor widely available for this purpose and may result in false positive results. Lyme urinary antigen capture tests are unreliable and should not be used.

The treatment of Lyme disease depends on the type of presentation and the age of the patient. In patients in whom the diagnosis of early Lyme disease is strongly suspected, treatment is initiated based on clinical findings, given the potential delays in laboratory confirmation. Doxycycline for 14–21 days is the treatment of choice for early localized disease in children >8 years of age. For those <8 years, amoxicillin or cefuroxime for the same time period is indicated.[176] Alternatives include erythromycin or clarithromycin.[171] Early disseminated and late disease is treated with the same oral regimen, but for 21 days. Persistent or recurrent arthritis, carditis,

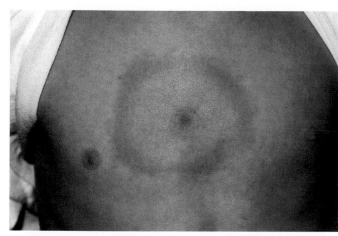

Figure 14.35 Erythema migrans of Lyme disease. Expanding, erythematous, annular patch of early localized Lyme disease. A small red papule is seen centrally at the site of the tick bite.

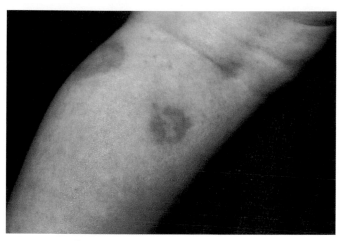

Figure 14.36 Erythema migrans, multiple lesions. Multiple erythematous macules and patches were present in this child with early disseminated Lyme disease.

of infection. Neurologic manifestations of early disseminated Lyme disease include peripheral neuropathy (especially cranial nerve VII palsy) and lymphocytic meningitis. Facial palsy is the most characteristic neuropathy, and is reported in 40–50% of patients with neurologic involvement. Bilateral facial palsy, a quite rare presentation, should be highly suspicious for Lyme disease, especially when occurring in an endemic area. The facial palsy of Lyme disease usually resolves in 2–8 weeks with or without treatment. Other cranial and peripheral mononeuropathies are possible, albeit more common in adults than children,[171] and a Guillain–Barré-like syndrome has been reported. Migratory arthralgia or frank arthritis may also occur, as may cardiac involvement. The latter is marked by first-, second-, or third-degree atrioventricular conduction defects or bundle branch blocks, and less commonly carditis or congestive heart failure.[171]

Late Lyme disease

The primary features of late Lyme disease, which occurs in 60% of untreated cases, are arthritis and neurologic disease. Fortunately, with better and earlier recognition of this disorder, manifestations of late disease have become much less common.[167] Cutaneous manifestations during late disease include lymphocytoma cutis and acrodermatitis chronica atrophicans (see below). The arthritis is meningitis, or encephalitis are treated with parenteral ceftriaxone or penicillin for 14–28 days.[176] Occasional patients may develop intensification of symptoms during the first 24 h of antibiotic therapy (a Jarisch–Herxheimer-like reaction), presumably caused by the host immune response to dying organisms. This reaction usually disappears in 1–2 days and is not an indication for discontinuation of therapy.

The hallmark of prevention for Lyme disease is tick avoidance. Simple measures to this end include avoidance of tick-infested areas, tucking pant legs into socks, and inspection for ticks after high-risk activities or exposures in endemic areas. The judicious use of chemical repellents such as N,N-diethyl-3-methylbenzamide (DEET) or permethrin (see Ch. 18) on skin or clothing is also helpful. Since the *Ixodes* tick must be attached to the skin for at least 24 h before infection is transmitted, daily inspection should be performed on individuals following exposure to potentially infested areas, and prompt tick removal by grasping the tick with a forceps, tweezers, or gloved fingers will help prevent transmission of the disease.[177] Removal should be performed without crushing the tick and an effort made to leave no body parts behind.

Most experts recommend against serologic testing or prophylactic antibiotic therapy after a tick bite, especially for patients who have had ticks attached for <24 h.[167] Most deer ticks, even in highly endemic areas for Lyme disease, are not infected with *B. burgdorferi*, and the overall risk of infection after a recognized deer tick bite in such an area is only around 1.4%.[178] A vaccine for Lyme disease was available and approved by the US Food and Drug Administration for individuals between 15 and 70 years of age, but was subsequently withdrawn in 2002 and is no longer available.

Protozoal disorders

Leishmaniasis

The term *leishmaniasis* refers to three different diseases caused by the protozoan parasite of the genus *Leishmania*: cutaneous leishmaniasis (oriental sore, Delhi boil, Balkh sore), mucocutaneous leishmaniasis, and visceral leishmaniasis (kala-azar). These infections are characterized by diversity and complexity, and the majority of cases occur in Afghanistan, Algeria, Iran, Iraq, Saudi Arabia, and Syria (in the 'Old World') and Brazil and Peru (in the 'New World').[179] Leishmania is present in most tropical and subtropical countries, owing to characteristics of the sandfly vector (see below). Travelers can become infected even after short stays in leishmania-endemic areas,[180] and the increase in travel to endemic regions of South and Central America has led to an increase in the number of cases diagnosed in the USA.[181] Although there may be overlap in clinical presentations caused by specific species, in general Old World cutaneous leishmaniasis is caused by *Leishmania tropica* or *Leishmania major*, New World cutaneous disease by *Leishmania braziliensis* or *Leishmania mexicana*, mucocutaneous disease by *L. braziliensis*, and visceral disease by *Leishmania donovani*. There are, however, multiple other less common species of *Leishmania* as well.

Leishmaniasis is transmitted by the sandfly (*Phlebotomus* or *Lutzomyia* sp.), which lives in dark and damp places. Sandflies fly silently and are most active in the evening and at night. The infection is transmitted to humans (an accidental host) by the bite of the sandfly, which itself becomes infected after a blood meal from infected mammals (primarily rodents and dogs).[179,182] An important epidemiologic observation of recent note is the increasing incidence of visceral leishmaniasis among AIDS patients in southern Europe and a few other endemic areas.[182,183] *Leishmania* spp. are obligate intracellular parasites of macrophages, by which they are phagocytosed following inoculation into the skin. They subsequently

replicate within macrophages and spread throughout the reticuloendothelial system of the host.

Cutaneous leishmaniasis has a variety of clinical presentations, although the most common is an indolent skin ulcer. There are an estimated 1.5 million new cases of cutaneous disease each year, and the incidence may be increasing.[184] The incubation period following the bite of the sandfly is usually 1–12 weeks, and occasionally the infection may remain subclinical. The initial lesion is a papule, which enlarges to form a painless ulcer with a raised margin and necrotic base (Figs 14.37, 14.38). Most often there are one to two lesions, although multiple lesions have been observed and some patients may show a lymphangitic distribution similar to that of sporotrichosis.[180] Regional lymphadenopathy and secondary

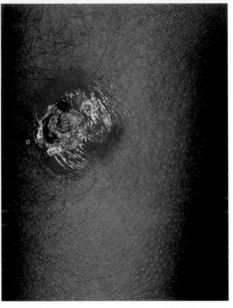

Figure 14.37 Cutaneous leishmaniasis. An erythematous crusted plaque in a 4-year-old child. (Courtesy of William Burrows, MD.)

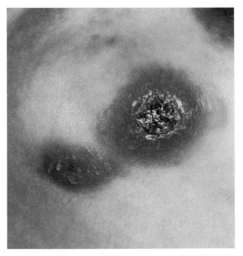

Figure 14.38 Cutaneous leishmaniasis. Multiple erythematous papules and plaques with necrosis and crusting were present in this 2-year-old female. *Leishmania tropica* was confirmed by PCR analysis. (Courtesy of Ayelet Shani-Adir, MD.)

bacterial infection may occur, the latter of which is often associated with pain.[179] Most lesions of cutaneous leishmaniasis heal over months to years, leaving an atrophic scar.

Other presentations of cutaneous leishmaniasis include a dry ulcerative form that appears as a brown nodule that ulcerates more slowly and reveals an adherent crust; *leishmaniasis recidivans*, which is manifested by red to yellow-brown papules that appear in or close to a scar of an old lesion of cutaneous leishmaniasis; and a non-ulcerating generalized form that may resemble lepromatous leprosy. Patients with this form of leishmaniasis present a public health hazard, since the skin is heavily infested and may act as a reservoir for transmission by the *Phlebotomus* fly.

The differential diagnosis of cutaneous leishmaniasis includes foreign-body reactions, tropical or traumatic ulcers, superinfected insect bites, myiasis, impetigo, fungal and mycobacterial infections, sarcoidosis, and neoplasms.[179,180] The diagnosis of leishmaniasis is usually made on the basis of the typical lesion(s) combined with a history of exposure or travel to an endemic region. Confirming the diagnosis can be challenging. Tissue biopsy for culture, smear, and histologic evaluation is useful. An impression smear is made by gently pressing the fresh biopsy tissue against a glass microscope slide, staining with Giemsa or hematoxylin and eosin (H&E) stain, and examining for amastigotes (intracellular organisms). Tissue specimens for culture must be plated on special culture, and the organisms can be typed by isoenzyme analysis in a reference laboratory, although the procedure is quite time-consuming.[184] Alternative methods for diagnosis include needle aspirates, slit-skin smears, monoclonal antibody tissue stains, and molecular techniques based on kinetoplast (a small portion of extranuclear material) DNA analysis. Serologic studies, which may be helpful in visceral or disseminated cutaneous disease, are usually of no value for localized cutaneous leishmaniasis. PCR-based diagnosis is also possible, and is particularly useful in cases with a low parasite load (i.e., mucosal leishmaniasis).

Mucocutaneous leishmaniasis results from hematogenous or lymphatic dissemination of organisms from skin to the nasopharyngeal mucosa. It often manifests years following resolution of cutaneous lesions of leishmaniasis.[180] Mucocutaneous leishmaniasis presents with chronic nasal symptoms and is followed by progressive nasopharyngeal destruction. Secondary bacterial infections with regional adenitis and lymphangitis are common, and occasionally the mucocutaneous lesions may be nodular and vegetative. Destruction of the nasal septum and nasopharynx may result in soft tissue and cartilage erosion, with resultant deformities of the nose, lips, cheeks, pharynx, larynx and palate that are often cosmetically debilitating.[185]

Visceral leishmaniasis may present with varied clinical findings and severity of illness. It infects an estimated 500 000 new individuals in less-developed countries each year, and may occur in large-scale epidemics, especially in east Africa and India.[186,187] The classic kala-azar syndrome, caused by *L. donovani*, results in fever, cachexia, hepatosplenomegaly, pancytopenia, and progressive deterioration. If left untreated, visceral leishmaniasis is often fatal. A common complication following therapy for kala-azar is 'post-kala-azar dermal leishmaniasis'. This disorder is characterized by macular,

papular, and nodular skin lesions that usually begin around the mouth and subsequently generalize.[188]

Treatment of leishmaniasis depends upon the clinical presentation, and in fact there is no single optimal therapy for all forms. When considering treatment for cutaneous disease, it is important to remember that this form of leishmaniasis tends to heal spontaneously, but that *L. braziliensis* has the potential to progress to mucocutaneous disease.[184] Therefore, any patient with *L. braziliensis* confirmed as the etiologic agent, or with a history of contracting the infection in an area endemic for this organism, should receive adequate systemic therapy. The goals of therapy are to reduce scarring and prevent parasite dissemination.

Pentavalent antimonial drugs, i.e., sodium stibogluconate (Pentostam) and meglumine antimonate (Glucantime) remain the mainstay of systemic therapy. These agents are generally administered in the hospital, although controlled outpatient management is an acceptable alternative in some situations. Pentostam is available in the USA from the Drug Service of the Centers for Disease Control. Potential toxicities related to the antimonial agents include electrocardiographic abnormalities, hepatic toxicity, pancreatitis, and pneumonitis. Amphotericin B and its lipid formulations have shown efficacy in the treatment of leishmaniasis, especially in India where antimonial resistance has been an increasing concern.[182,186] Other treatments utilized with varying degrees of success have included cryosurgery, surgical excision, topical paromomycin ointment, intralesional sodium stibogluconate, and pentamidine. More recently, other potentially promising treatments for visceral leishmaniasis have been studied, including the anticancer alkylphosphocholines miltefosine, edelfosine, and ilmofosine.[189,190]

Key References

 The complete list of 190 references for this chapter is available online at **www.expertconsult.com**. See inside cover for registration details.

Amagai M, Yamaguchi T, Hanakawa Y, et al. Staphylococcal exfoliative toxin B specifically cleaves desmoglein 1. *J Invest Dermatol*. 2002;118:845–850.

Bratton RL, Whiteside JW, Hovan MJ, et al. Diagnosis and treatment of Lyme disease. *Mayo Clin Proc*. 2008;83(5):566–571.

Cainzos M, Gonzalez-Rodriguez FJ. Necrotizing soft tissue infections. *Curr Opin Crit Care*. 2007;13:433–439.

Dodiuk-Gad R, Dyachenko P, Ziv M, et al. Nontuberculous mycobacterial infections of the skin: A retrospective study of 25 cases. *J Am Acad Dermatol*. 2007;57:413–420.

Florin TA, Zaoutis TE, Zaoutis LB. Beyond cat scratch disease: Widening spectrum of Bartonella henselae infection. *Pediatrics*. 2008;121(5):e1413–e1425.

Gorwitz RJ. Community-associated methicillin-resistant Staphylococcus aureus. Epidemiology and update. *Pediatr Infect Dis J*. 2008;27(10):925–926.

Lappin E, Ferguson AJ. Gram-positive toxic shock syndromes. *Lancet*. 2009;9:281–290.

Miller LG, Kaplan SL. Staphylococcus aureus: A community pathogen. *Infect Dis Clin N Am*. 2009;23:35–52.

15

Viral Diseases of the Skin

Viruses are ultramicroscopic organisms that grow only within living cells. The antigenic material responsible for viral immunologic reactions is present in the outer protein membrane (capsid) of the virus. The nucleoprotein core is composed of either deoxyribonucleic acid (DNA) or ribonucleic acid (RNA). Lacking ribosomes, viruses depend on the use of the host cells' enzyme systems, blending with metabolic material of the host cell and frequently remaining undetected until some stimulus incites the production of new viral particles.

Viral infections of the skin may present with varied morphologies, including papules, vesiculobullous lesions, ulcers, and tumors. This chapter will include a discussion of herpes simplex virus (HSV) infections, herpes zoster, viral-like disorders of the oral mucosa, and warts. Some poxvirus infections will be discussed, including molluscum contagiosum, cowpox, pseudocowpox (milker's nodules), orf, and smallpox. Although human immunodeficiency virus (HIV) infection does not result in primary skin disease, a brief discussion of acquired immunodeficiency syndrome (AIDS) in children and its skin disease associations is included. Neonatal herpes infection is discussed in Chapter 2.

Herpes simplex virus infection

The herpesvirus family includes the herpes simplex virus (HSV), Epstein–Barr virus, cytomegalovirus, varicella-zoster virus, and human herpesviruses 6–8. Aside from HSV, the other herpesviruses are implicated primarily in exanthematous illnesses. HSV infections are quite prevalent in both children and adults. HSV-1 and HSV-2 are double-stranded DNA viruses that primarily infect the epidermis or mucosal surfaces. After acute infection, the virus rapidly replicates and establishes latent infection in regional nerve ganglia, from which it occasionally reactivates.[1,2]

HSV-1 is primarily associated with oral and labial lesions, and HSV-2 with genital lesions, although the predilection of a specific viral serotype to a particular anatomic site appears to be changing.[3] Primary HSV-1 infection is largely a childhood disease that affects the oral mucosa, pharynx, lips, and occasionally the eyes.[2] HSV-2 is primarily implicated in genital tract disease, with spread occurring via sexual contact, or in neonates, most commonly by passage through an infected birth canal (Ch. 2). Although the mucocutaneous lesions caused by HSV-1 and HSV-2 are clinically indistinguishable, differentiation between the two serotypes can be made by viral culture, Western blot serologic testing, HSV antigen detection with monoclonal anti-HSV antibodies, or polymerase chain reaction (PCR) studies.

Infection with HSV is classified as primary or recurrent. Primary infections occur in individuals without circulating antibodies, and result from direct contact with infected secretions or actual mucocutaneous lesions. Following an incubation of days to weeks, they may present as sub-clinical infection characterized only by the development of antibodies, as a localized or generalized cutaneous eruption, or as a serious systemic infection with central nervous system or disseminated involvement. Most primary HSV infections are asymptomatic. Recurrent HSV infection occurs in individuals who were previously infected, either clinically or subclinically. It is characterized by repeated episodes of mucocutaneous lesions at the same site or sites.

Topical and systemic antiviral agents commonly used to treat HSV infections are summarized in Table 15.1.

Herpetic Gingivostomatitis

Herpetic gingivostomatitis most commonly occurs in children between the ages of 10 months and 5 years, although it may occur at any age. It presents with small vesicles on an erythematous base, which evolve into painful, shallow gray erosions and ulcerations (Fig. 15.1). The lesions most often involve the palate, tongue, and gingivae. Gingival swelling and easy bleeding may occur. Perioral lesions involving the lips, cheeks, and chin (Fig. 15.2) occur in up to three-quarters of patients.[4] Other common features include fever, drooling, eating and drinking difficulties, foul breath odor, and irritability. Cervical and submandibular lymphadenopathy is also quite common. Secondary bacteremia with group A β-hemolytic streptococci, *Staphylococcus aureus* or other organisms may occasionally be a complication.[5]

The differential diagnosis of herpetic gingivostomatitis in a child includes herpangina, hand-foot-and-mouth disease, aphthous stomatitis, and Stevens–Johnson syndrome. The diagnosis can be confirmed by viral culture or direct fluorescent antibody studies, when necessary. Although gingivostomatitis is usually caused by HSV-1, HSV-2 may cause a similar syndrome, usually in adolescents and young adults who engage in oral–genital contact.[1] Such primary HSV-2 infection results in similar symptoms of gingivostomatitis and pharyngitis, which in some patients may be difficult to differentiate from bacterial pharyngitis. Adolescents and young adults may also present with primary HSV-1 gingivostomatitis.[6,7]

Although herpetic gingivostomatitis tends to be self-limited over 10 days to 2 weeks, dehydration may result from poor oral intake and excessive fluid losses, especially in younger children. In some patients, hospitalization may be required for intravenous hydration and pain control. Ambulatory treatment measures include supportive therapy with fluids and use of topical analgesics, anesthetics or coating agents, including lidocaine, diphenhydramine, Milk of Magnesia, Maalox or Kaopectate.[8] Specific antiviral therapy with acyclovir is advocated by some, seems most effective when started within 3 days of disease onset, and may prevent the development of new lesions and diminish difficulties with eating and rates of hospitalization in young children.[9–11]

Ocular Herpes Infection

Primary HSV infection of the eye can result in a severe purulent conjunctivitis with edema, erythema, and vesiculation, with

Table 15.1 Topical and oral antiviral medications used for HSV infections[a]

Drug	Supplied	Regimen	Indication/Comment
Topical			
Acyclovir	5% cream (2 g, 5 g)	Apply 5 times/day	Recurrent HL; A: ≥12 years; Rx
	5% ointment (3 g, 15 g)	Apply 6 times/day	Initial GH, localized HSV; A: adults; Rx
Penciclovir	1% cream (1.5 g)	Apply q. 2 h (awake)	Recurrent HL; A: ≥12 years; Rx
Docosanol	10% cream (2 g)	Apply 5 times/day	HL; A: ≥12 years; OTC
Oral (all Rx)			
Acyclovir	200 mg capsule		A: ≥2 years
	400 mg, 800 mg tablet		
	200 mg/5 mL susp		
		200 mg 5 times/day	Initial GH; 10 days
		200 mg 5 times/day	Recurrent GH; 5 days
		400 mg 2 times/day	Suppression, recurrent GH; up to 12 months, then re-evaluate
Famciclovir	125, 250, 500 mg tablet		A: ≥18 years
		1500 mg single dose	Recurrent HL
		1000 mg twice daily	Recurrent GH; 1 day
		250 mg 2 times/day	Suppression, recurrent GH; up to 12 months
Valacyclovir	500 mg, 1 g caplet		A: adults
		1 g 2 times/day	Initial GH; 10 days
		500 mg 2 times/day	Recurrent GH; 3 days
		500 mg–1 g once daily	Suppressive GH
		2 g 2 times/day	HL; 1 day

[a]Approved indications and regimens listed; often used off-label. HSV, herpes simplex virus; HL, herpes labialis; A, approved; Rx: by prescription; GH, genital herpes; OTC, over-the-counter.

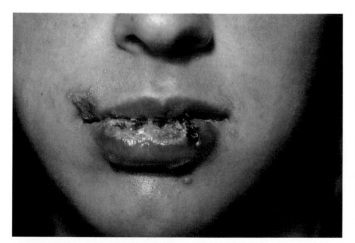

Figure 15.1 Herpetic gingivostomatitis. Multiple erosions with crusting. Note the associated lesions involving the chin.

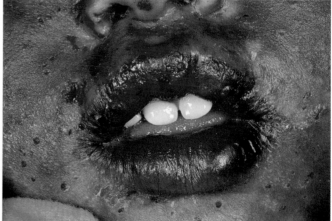

Figure 15.2 Herpetic gingivostomatitis. Lip erosions with multiple perioral herpetic lesions.

superficial erosion or ulceration of the cornea (epithelial keratitis). Ocular HSV infection is a leading cause of recurrent keratoconjunctivitis with associated corneal opacification, and one of the chief causes of corneal blindness in the USA.[1,8] This infection results from recurrent viral shedding from the trigeminal nerve reactivation, and is more often due to HSV-1. Patients with keratoconjunctivitis present with pain, photophobia, lacrimation, and eye discharge. There may also be involvement of the eyelid (blepharitis). Deeper involvement of the cornea (stromal keratitis) or anterior uvea (iritis) may occur, and both are more serious and associated with a greater risk of visual loss. Ocular HSV infections may be unilateral or bilateral; patients with bilateral involvement tend to have a more protracted clinical course and recurrences are more common.[12] Bacterial superinfection of herpetic keratoconjunctivitis is common.

The diagnosis of herpetic keratoconjunctivitis can be confirmed with viral culture. Nested PCR studies, where available, seem to be superior to culture and can be performed on tear film or corneal scrapings.[13] Ophthalmology referral is indicated, and treatment includes topical antiviral ophthalmic ointments or solutions and oral antiviral agents. Topical antiviral agents include trifluridine, vidarabine, and idoxuridine. Most cases of primary superficial herpetic keratoconjunctivitis heal over 2 weeks, without permanent corneal damage.

Herpes Labialis

Herpes labialis refers to herpetic infections occurring on the lips, most often the vermilion border. This is the most common type of recurrent herpes infection, and represents the classic 'cold sore'. As with other types of recurrent infection, it occurs following reactivation of latent HSV in the cells of the trigeminal ganglia. Herpes labialis often presents initially with prodromal symptoms such as tingling, burning, or itching. At 1–2 days later, the cutaneous eruption appears as a localized cluster of small vesicles or erosions on an erythematous base (Fig. 15.3). Occasionally, other areas of the face may be involved, and in immunocompromised individuals, oral mucosal and/or severe involvement (Fig. 15.4) may be noted (see below). Topical and oral antiviral agents are useful in treating herpes labialis, especially when initiated within 1–2 days of the disease onset. Prophylaxis with oral agents is advocated by many for patients with a history of multiple recurrences of herpes labialis.

Genital Herpes

Genital herpes (herpetic vulvovaginitis, herpes progenitalis) is one of the most widespread sexually transmitted diseases (STDs) in the developed world, with an increasing incidence.[14,15] HSV-2

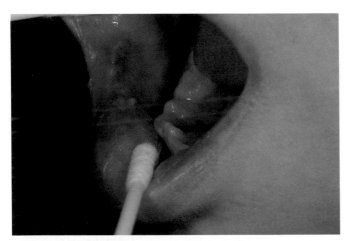

Figure 15.3 Herpes labialis. Erythematous erosions clustered on the right lower lip in a patient with labial herpes. This young girl also had herpes-associated erythema multiforme (see Ch. 20).

is primarily responsible for genital tract herpetic infections, and seroprevalence studies reveal rates as high as 60–90% in developing countries, and 20–22% of the general population in developed countries.[2,16] The proportion of HSV-1 isolates in genital herpes is also increasing, especially in young adults and college students.[17] Risk factors that directly correlate with HSV-2 infection include race (higher risk in African-Americans and Hispanics), age, years of sexual experience, lower family income, lower education level, number of sexual partners, and other STDs.[2] The diagnosis of genital HSV in a child should raise the suspicion of sexual abuse.[18] Maternal–fetal transmission of HSV may result in neonatal herpes, which is discussed in Chapter 2.

The majority of HSV-2 infections are subclinical and go unrecognized by the host.[8] Symptomatic primary genital herpes presents with lesions 2–8 days following contact with an infected individual. In distinction, first episode, non-primary genital herpes (i.e., the initial episode of genital herpes in a host with a past history of nongenital herpes) may not present with signs or symptoms for several months.[15] The lesions of primary genital HSV are painful vesicles clustered on an erythematous base (Fig. 15.5), and distributed on the vulva, labia, vagina, perineum, penile shaft, glans penis, urethra, and less often the scrotum. In females, cervical involvement, intense soft tissue swelling, and severe pain may be present. The vesicles rupture rapidly, leaving behind painful erosions or ulcers that may be associated with pruritus, dysuria, vaginal and urethral discharge, and tender inguinal lymphadenopathy. Pustules may occasionally be present. Systemic signs and symptoms may include fever, malaise, headache, and myalgias. Herpetic sacral radiculomyelitis, with urinary or fecal retention and neuralgias, may occur, as may aseptic meningitis.[1,8] Less common features of HSV infection include endometritis and salpingitis in women and prostatitis in men. The symptoms of genital HSV usually improve over 5–7 days, and the cutaneous lesions heal over 2–4 weeks without therapy.

Genital herpes may show a heterogeneous clinical spectrum. Extragenital involvement may be seen, with lesions most commonly involving the buttocks, anal region, thighs, mouth, and fingers (see below).[2,14] Atypical morphologies may also be present, including deep and tender ulcers, single erosions, erosive urethritis, vulvar fissure, and penile edema.[14] A high index of suspicion must be maintained, especially in the immunocompromised host or in patients with features of other STDs.

Recurrent genital HSV infection is characterized by less severe cutaneous lesions, which are usually preceded by a prodrome of pain, tenderness, itching, tingling, or paresthesia. The vesicles are

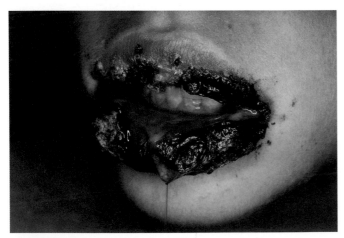

Figure 15.4 Herpes labialis. Severe crusting and lip edema in a patient receiving cancer chemotherapy.

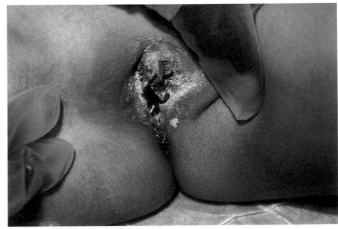

Figure 15.5 Genital herpes. Vesicles on an erythematous base involving the right labia minora in a childhood victim of sexual abuse.

fewer in number, and recurrent disease may be less common with HSV-1 versus HSV-2 disease. Triggering factors for recurrent disease may include physical or emotional stress, febrile illness, and menstruation. Recurrence rates tend to be highest for the first years following the initial infection.[19] Asymptomatic ('subclinical') HSV shedding is another feature of genital herpes, and among women with genital HSV-2 infection, occurs on an average of 2% of days.[20] The risk of subclinical shedding increases with the frequency of symptomatic recurrences.

The diagnosis of genital herpes can be confirmed by viral culture, Tzanck preparation (cannot distinguish between HSV-1 and HSV-2), direct fluorescent antibody testing, Western blot serologic testing, or PCR. Treatments for genital herpes include supportive care and antiviral therapy (Table 15.1). Supportive measures include warm sitz baths, topical anesthetics, topical antibacterial ointments to prevent secondary infection, and oral analgesics. Education regarding the nature and risks of HSV infection and safe sex practices should be offered, and evaluation for other STDs considered when appropriate. An effective vaccine against HSV is highly desirable, and research toward this end is ongoing. A glycoprotein-D-subunit vaccine has shown benefit in females who are seronegative for both HSV-1 and HSV-2.[21]

The choice of antiviral therapy depends on the host immune status and the nature of the infection (primary or recurrent). Oral acyclovir, famciclovir, and valacyclovir may all help to speed healing, decrease symptoms, and decrease viral shedding. Long-term suppressive therapy in patients with frequent recurrences is useful in reducing both the frequency and duration of flares. Although topical acyclovir ointment may offer some benefit for initial genital herpes infections, it offers little in recurrent infections.

Cutaneous Herpes and Eczema Herpeticum

Cutaneous HSV infection can occur on any body surface area. Involvement of the finger (herpetic whitlow) is discussed in the next section. Non-orolabial, non-genital involvement presents in a similar fashion, with clustered vesicles or erosions on an erythematous base (Figs 15.6, 15.7). The lesions maybe misdiagnosed as impetigo or herpes zoster. Occasionally, recurrent cutaneous HSV may present only with prodromal symptoms followed by skin erythema and edema, but without the characteristic vesiculation. In some instances, patients with recurrent cutaneous HSV may develop associated secondary bacterial infection or lymphangitis.

Eczema herpeticum (EH, Kaposi's varicelliform eruption, see also Ch. 3) is a severe, disseminated HSV infection that occurs in individuals with atopic dermatitis or other chronic skin disease, including pemphigus, Darier disease, burns, and others.[22] Although the etiology of EH has not been clearly established, the impaired skin barrier associated with these diseases is believed to create a more permissive environment for viral invasion and binding to cellular receptors.[22] Patients present usually with the abrupt onset of fever, malaise, and a widespread eruption of monomorphous vesicles and erosions (Figs 15.8, 15.9 and see Ch. 3, Figs 3.24, 3.25). The lesions are most prominent in areas of active dermatitis, but especially tend to involve the head, neck, and trunk.

Complications of EH include keratoconjunctivitis, secondary bacterial superinfection, fluid loss, and viremia. The mainstay of treatment for EH is systemic antiviral therapy, which for the majority of patients is most appropriately administered via intravenous

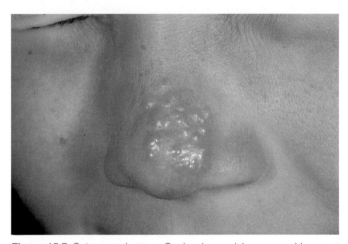

Figure 15.7 Cutaneous herpes. Coalescing vesicles on a red base over the distal nose.

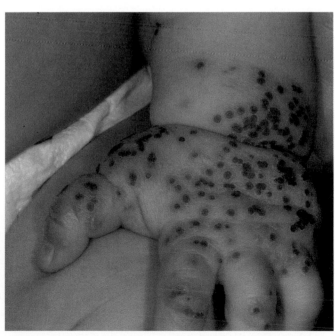

Figure 15.8 Eczema herpeticum. This toddler with chronic atopic dermatitis had an explosive onset of fever and widespread vesicles with crusting in eczematous areas. Note the monomorphous nature and clustering of these crusted papules on the dorsal hand, with a few intact small vesicles.

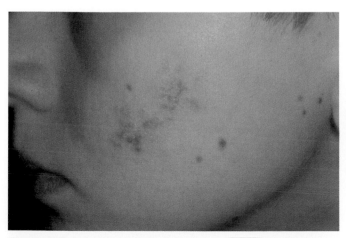

Figure 15.6 Cutaneous herpes. Resolving vesicles and crusted papules overlying an erythematous base, on the left cheek.

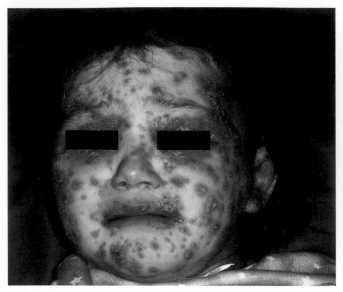

Figure 15.9 Eczema herpeticum. These coalescing vesicles progressed rapidly in this young girl with atopic dermatitis.

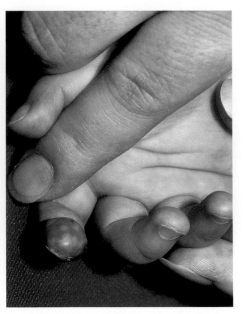

Figure 15.10 Herpetic whitlow. Clustered, tender, deep-seated vesicles of the distal phalanx.

delivery in the hospital. Other treatment considerations include hydration with attention to electrolyte balance, antibiotic therapy for secondary bacterial infection, and pain control. Meticulous skin care should be performed, with bland emollients applied during the early phase of barrier recovery, and the later addition of anti-inflammatory agents for the dermatitis once healing is well under way. In addition, ophthalmologic evaluation is indicated when facial involvement is present.

Erythema multiforme (see Ch. 20), an acute, self-limited reactive skin disease, has been associated with HSV infection in both children and adults. In prepubertal children with erythema multiforme, especially the recurrent type, HSV DNA was detected by PCR studies on skin biopsy specimens taken from the target lesions.[23,24] This finding was noted both in patients with a known history of HSV and in those without any such history. Prophylactic acyclovir may thus be useful in abrogating recurrences of erythema multiforme in children.

Herpetic Whitlow

Herpetic whitlow is a unique form of HSV infection involving the pulp of the distal phalanx (or multiple phalanges). It is seen most often in physicians, dentists, dental hygienists, and nurses who have contact with the mouth or genital regions of patients with herpetic lesions. It may also occur as a result of autoinoculation in patients with herpes labialis, herpes stomatitis, or genital herpes.[25] The virus is inoculated onto the skin of one or more fingers, resulting in a deep-seated, painful vesicular or bullous eruption with erythema (Fig. 15.10). Spontaneous resolution usually occurs over 3 weeks if the condition is left untreated. The differential diagnosis of herpetic whitlow may include blistering dactylitis, burns, and impetigo. The diagnosis is confirmed by viral culture or direct fluorescent antibody testing, and treatment with oral acyclovir or other antiviral agents may result in alleviation of pain and more rapid healing.

Herpes Gladiatorum

Herpes gladiatorum is a term used to describe a widespread primary inoculation HSV infection occurring in contact sports enthusiasts, such as wrestlers or rugby players. It may occur at some time in up to one-third of wrestlers, and is characterized by grouped vesicles on an erythematous base. The most common locations for herpes gladiatorum are the head, neck, and upper extremities.[26,27] In addition to widespread cutaneous lesions, affected individuals may have fever, malaise, sore throat, anorexia, headache, weight loss, and regional lymphadenopathy. The cutaneous lesions of herpes gladiatorum may occasionally lack classic vesicles, in which case the differential diagnosis may include tinea corporis gladiatorum, impetigo, and atopic dermatitis.[27]

Herpes gladiatorum can be effectively treated with oral acyclovir, famciclovir, or valacyclovir. The duration of therapy necessary before allowing the athlete to return to competition is controversial, and evidence-based recommendations do not exist. Sharing of equipment and towels should be discouraged, and appropriate cleaning of wrestling mats encouraged. Seasonal antiviral prophylaxis has been advocated by some in an effort to suppress recurrent outbreaks and reduce the risk of spread to susceptible teammates or opponents.[28,29]

Herpes in the Immunocompromised Host

Severe, chronic, and recalcitrant HSV infections may be seen in the setting of immunodeficiency. These settings include individuals with hematologic malignancy, those with a history of bone marrow or solid organ transplantation, and those with HIV infection. Although these patients may develop common forms of HSV infection, their lesions may be more widespread and extensive. Persistent or recurrent ulcers are a common manifestation of HSV infection in patients with AIDS.[1] Large, persistent ulcers in HIV-infected patients should arouse suspicion for HSV although the differential diagnosis may include syphilis and chancroid. Less common locations are also more likely to be involved in these patients, such as the buttocks and back.[14] HSV lesions in immunocompromised hosts may also be verrucous, pustular, markedly crusted (Fig. 15.11), necrotic (Fig. 15.12), or exophytic.

In addition to cutaneous lesions, disseminated HSV may be noted in this patient population. Oropharyngeal involvement, esophagitis, tracheobronchitis, pneumonitis, hepatitis, pancreatitis, adrenal necrosis, and gastrointestinal tract and bone marrow

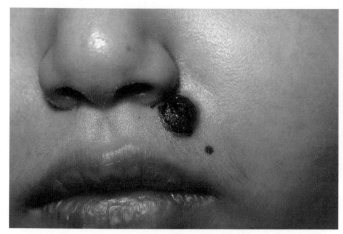

Figure 15.11 Herpes in the immunocompromised host. This large, crusted plaque was culture-positive for *H. simplex* in this 6-year-old female receiving chemotherapy for leukemia.

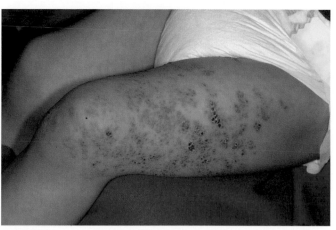

Figure 15.13 Herpes zoster. Confluent vesicles and crusted vesicles with erythema in a dermatomal distribution on the left thigh. This boy was otherwise healthy with no identifiable underlying predisposition.

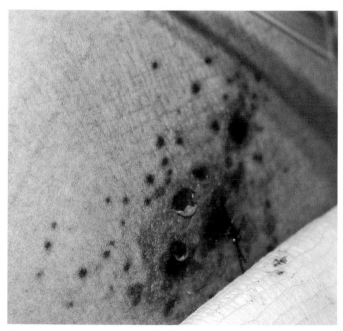

Figure 15.12 Herpes in the immunocompromised host. Vesicles rapidly progressed to necrotic plaques in this young girl status post-bone marrow transplantation.

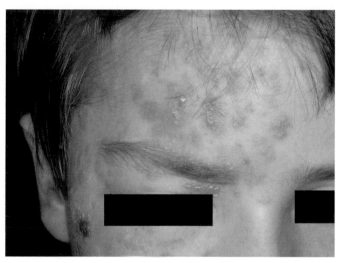

Figure 15.14 Herpes zoster. Edema with erythema and vesiculation, distributed in a V1 and partial V2 distribution. Corneal involvement may occur with this presentation.

involvement may occur.[1] These severe and/or disseminated infections may be caused by either HSV-1 or HSV-2.

Herpes zoster

Herpes zoster (HZ, 'zoster', shingles) is an acute vesicular eruption caused by reactivation of a latent infection with varicella-zoster virus (VZV) in the sensory ganglia. Although it is most often seen in elderly or immunosuppressed individuals, it may also occur in children. Although pediatric zoster is most common in immunocompromised children or those who had a primary intrauterine infection or acute varicella within the first year of life,[30] it may occasionally occur in children without any of these risk factors. Neonatal herpes zoster has rarely been reported, presumably in association with exposure to varicella zoster *in utero*. Since licensure

of the live attenuated Oka strain varicella vaccine, it has become clear that HZ may be caused by reactivation of latent vaccine virus, even in children.[31,32] Studies of HZ incidence since implementation of the vaccination program in 1995 have yielded conflicting results, showing both increased incidence and no increase, and suggesting that there may be other unidentified risk factors for HZ that are changing over time.[33]

Herpes zoster is characterized by vesicles and erythema clustered in a dermatomal distribution of one or more sensory nerves (Fig. 15.13). The most frequently affected dermatomes are the second cervical to lumbar nerves (C2 to L2) and the fifth (Fig. 15.14) and seventh cranial nerves. Patients often complain of hyperesthesia, pain, and tenderness to light touch in the affected area(s), usually before any cutaneous findings are present. Although the eruption is usually unilateral with a sharp demarcation at the midline, occasional contralateral involvement is seen. It is not unusual to see a few randomly scattered vesicular lesions beyond the primary dermatomal involvement, and such scattered lesions do not necessarily constitute disseminated zoster.

Successive crops of new lesions with extension of the process may occur for up to 1 week, followed by crusting of the vesicles and healing over 1–2 weeks. In children, the disorder tends to be more mild, and healing often occurs rapidly, within a few days to 1 week.[34] In addition, in otherwise healthy children, post-herpetic neuralgia (PHN, a delayed phenomenon of chronic pain and paresthesias in an area previously affected by HZ) is rare. PHN is more common in elderly patients, and in those with a history of ophthalmic HZ (see below).[35]

Immunocompromised children with HZ may have more extensive involvement with a higher risk of viremia and visceral dissemination.[34] This may include pneumonia, encephalitis, hepatitis, and disseminated intravascular coagulopathy.[34,36] These patients may also have disseminated cutaneous involvement, presenting in a fashion more typical of acute varicella and with no obvious dermatomal component.[36] 'Abdominal zoster' refers to the presentation of HZ as severe abdominal pain that precedes the development of cutaneous lesions. These patients are often explored surgically, and the condition is associated with a high incidence of abdominal visceral involvement. Children infected with HIV may have chronic or relapsing HZ, or HZ with unusual cutaneous lesions (i.e., hyperkeratotic papules, ulcers, or necrotic plaques).

Infection associated with the ophthalmic branch of the fifth (trigeminal) nerve may involve the cornea with keratitis and uveitis and may lead to permanent damage. This presentation (termed *herpes zoster ophthalmicus*) occurs when the nasociliary branch is involved and, accordingly, presents with cutaneous involvement of the nasal tip (Hutchinson's sign).[37] This important sign should not be overlooked, and should prompt rapid diagnosis, referral, and institution of therapy.

HZ of the maxillary division of the trigeminal nerve produces vesiculation of the palate, uvula, and tonsillar area. Involvement of the mandibular division produces vesicular involvement of the anterior aspects of the tongue, floor of the mouth, lips, and buccal mucous membranes. Involvement of the geniculate ganglion produces lesions on the tongue, ear, and skin of the auditory canal. When accompanied by Bell's palsy and disturbances of hearing and equilibrium, it is part of the *Ramsay Hunt syndrome*.

The diagnosis of HZ is often a clinical one, and in typical cases further evaluations are generally unnecessary. In patients in whom diagnostic confirmation is indicated, direct detection with fluorescent antibody stains of vesicle base scrapings is useful. Viral culture can be used, but VZV may take up to 1 week to induce cytopathic changes. PCR studies are not available on a widespread basis for clinical use, and serologic studies are generally not useful in this setting.

Treatment for HZ consists of symptomatic measures and specific antiviral therapy (Table 15.2). Symptomatic care includes wet compresses, drying lotions (i.e., calamine), antihistamines, and analgesics. High-dose acyclovir decreases vesicle formation, time to crusting, and days of pain when instituted within 72 h of onset of the exanthem. Acyclovir should be administered via the intravenous route in immunocompromised patients, given their greater severity of disease, or in any patient with disseminated or severe infection. Other antiviral options in immunocompetent patients or those with uncomplicated HZ include valacyclovir and famciclovir. A herpes zoster vaccine is approved for adults 60 years of age and older, with widespread vaccination desirable to help in the prevention of HZ and PHN in this population, and in reducing the health and financial costs of HZ.[38,39]

Viral-like disorders of the oral mucosa

Aphthous Stomatitis

Recurrent aphthous stomatitis (RAS, aphthous ulcers, canker sores) is one of the most common painful diseases affecting the oral mucosa of children. It has been reported in 5–25% of the general population.[40] The etiology is not well understood, and treatment has traditionally been symptomatic. Aphthous stomatitis presents with single or multiple shallow erosions or ulcerations (Fig. 15.15) on the labial and buccal mucosa, gingivae, tongue, floor of the mouth, palate, or pharynx. Prior to the onset of the lesions,

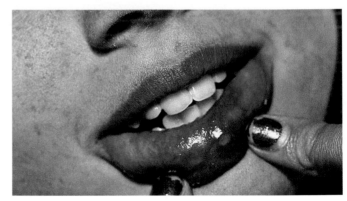

Figure 15.15 Aphthous stomatitis. Multiple shallow erosions of the labial mucosa.

Table 15.2 Systemic antiviral medications used for herpes zoster[a]

Drug	Supplied	Regimen	Indication/comment
Acyclovir	200 mg capsule		A: ≥2 years
	400 mg, 800 mg tablet		
	200 mg/5 mL susp	800 mg 5 times/day	Adult dose; 7–10 days
			Pediatric HZ dosing: NE
	500 mg/10 mL IV	60 mg/kg per day	IC <12 years; divide every 8 h; 7–10 days
		30 mg/kg per day	IC ≥12 years; divide every 8 h; 7 days
Famciclovir	125, 250, 500 mg tablet	500 mg 3 times/day	A: ≥18 years; 7 days
Valacyclovir	500 mg, 1 g caplet	1 g 3 times/day	A: adults; 7 days

[a]Approved indications and regimens listed; often used off-label. A, approved; HZ, herpes zoster; NE, not established; IV, intravenous preparation; IC, immunocompromised.

a tingling sensation may be present. At 24–48 h later, a focal erythema develops, followed soon thereafter by tiny, superficial gray-white erosions. Usually there are 1–3 lesions (*minor RAS*; 80–85% of cases), and the area of erosion increases and evolves into one or more sharply defined shallow ulcers covered by gray membranes and surrounded by sharp borders and slightly elevated, bright red areolae. Lesions usually measure 3–6 mm in diameter and, if left untreated, persist for 8–12 days (sometimes longer) and heal without scarring. Occasional patients develop larger ulcerations, up to several centimeters in size, with prolonged pain, fever, and healing with scarring. This variant has been termed *major RAS* (10% of cases; formally known as Sutton disease), and may be associated with dysphagia, malaise, and HIV infection.[41] Another form of aphthae, *herpetiform RAS*, occurs in 5–10% of aphthae patients and presents as clusters of pinpoint ulcers that simulate, but are not due to, infection with HSV.[42]

Aphthous stomatitis is believed to be multifactorial in origin, and may occur in response to a variety of triggering factors, including stress, trauma, hormonal changes, and infection. Cytokines are felt to play an important role, and polymorphisms in the genes for interleukins (IL)-lb and -6 may increase a patient's individual risk of RAS.[43] HLA-B52 and -B44 antigens were found to be strongly associated with RAS in Israeli Arab youths.[44] Drug-induced RAS has also been suggested, especially in association with nonsteroidal anti-inflammatory drugs and beta blockers.[45] Both Epstein–Barr virus and cytomegalovirus have been hypothesized as potential infectious causes of RAS.[46,47] In the vast majority of cases, the etiology remains unknown.

The differential diagnosis (and/or potential associations) of RAS includes Behçet syndrome (Ch. 25), inflammatory bowel disease (Ch. 25), cyclic neutropenia, gluten-sensitive enteropathy, herpes simplex infection, candidiasis, vitamin/nutritional deficiencies, and the syndrome of periodic fever, aphthous stomatitis, pharyngitis, and cervical adenitis (PFAPA, Marshall's syndrome; Ch. 25). PFAPA is characterized by periodic high fevers (up to 41°C), aphthous ulcers, pharyngitis (which is usually culture-negative), and cervical adenitis. Associated symptoms include headache, nausea, vomiting, and abdominal pain.[42,48] The syndrome usually occurs in patients <5 years of age, and flares recur at 21–42-day intervals. The fevers resolve over 24–48 h spontaneously, and often drop dramatically after even a single dose of oral corticosteroids. Other reportedly effective therapies have included cimetidine and tonsillectomy.[48] Overall, patients with PFAPA do well with spontaneous resolution of the episodes within 3–5 years and without any long-term sequelae.

Treatments for RAS include primarily topical corticosteroids and topical and/or oral analgesics. Topical clobetasol propionate, a potent corticosteroid, in a denture paste or oral analgesic base and applied two to three times daily often results in remission and symptomatic relief.[49] Mixtures of diphenhydramine elixir and Kaopectate or Maalox have been used successfully, as have a variety of medical mouthwashes (i.e., chlorhexidine, or Peridex, antibacterial oral rinse). Patients with severe manifestations of RAS may respond to oral colchicine, thalidomide, or dapsone.

Acute Necrotizing Gingivitis

Acute necrotizing gingivitis (trench mouth, Vincent's stomatitis, Vincent's angina) is a painful ulcerative disorder that chiefly affects adolescents and young adults. Although formerly common in schools and military establishments, it is quite rare in the USA and Western Hemisphere, perhaps owing to improved oral and dental care. The cause of acute necrotizing gingivitis is often a mix of bacterial pathogens, including *Fusobacterium*, *Prevotella*, and spirochetes.

The condition occurs most frequently in patients with predisposing conditions such as malnutrition, poor oral hygiene, or immunosuppression.

Clinical findings consist of painful gingivae that bleed easily and an inflamed, eroded, hemorrhagic oropharynx. Ulcerations are most common at the gingival margins and interdental papillae. The ulcers are covered by a grayish white slough or pseudomembrane that can be removed, leaving behind a raw bleeding surface. Single or multiple papillae may be involved, and the ulceration can be very extensive. Associated features include lymphadenopathy pain, bleeding of the gums, fever, and a foul breath odor. Treatment of acute necrotizing gingivitis consists of debridement by a dentist or periodontist and broad-spectrum antibiotic therapy. Chlorhexidine or saltwater oral rinses may help to alleviate discomfort. Attention to good oral hygiene and nutritional rehabilitation (where indicated) are important steps in prevention.

Warts

Warts (verrucae) are a common viral infection of the skin and mucosae caused by the human papillomavirus (HPV). These benign intraepidermal tumors most commonly occur in children and young adults, and their incidence has been estimated at 10%.[50,51] Although harmless and frequently self-involuting over years, warts are occasionally painful and may carry a negative social stigma. In addition, HPV may be associated with cutaneous and genital oncogenesis, particularly in immunosuppressed individuals.

There are four basic types of warts: verruca vulgaris, verruca plana, verruca plantaris, and condyloma acuminatum. Each of these will be discussed individually in the following sections. Most warts occur on the hands, fingers, elbows, and plantar surfaces of the feet. Patients with warts frequently autoinoculate themselves inadvertently, with the subsequent appearance of multiple secondary lesions. A classic feature of cutaneous warts is that of *koebnerization*, whereby a linear constellation of lesions develops along the path of excoriation (Fig. 15.16).

HPV is transmitted via skin-to-skin contact or from fomites, where recently shed viruses may survive if the environment is warm and moist (i.e., locker room floors, pool decking, showers, etc.). The entry site is often an area of recent trauma or a skin region with subclinical abrasion or fissuring. The incubation period from inoculation to development of the wart may range from 1 to 6 months

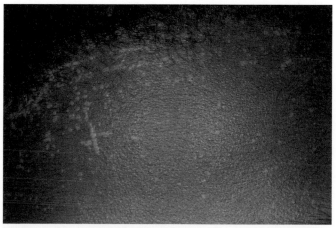

Figure 15.16 Warts with koebnerization. Multiple small, verrucous papules with a linear clustering (Koebner phenomenon) were present on this child's forehead.

or more. Although the duration of warts is variable, one study documented that two-thirds of lesions resolve spontaneously within 2 years.[52] The most important mechanism in wart regression appears to be cell-mediated immunity, with cytokines released by keratinocytes or immune system cells and inducing an immune response against HPV.[53]

Over 130 HPV types comprise this family of small double-stranded DNA viruses, and the various HPV types have been divided into two groups: cutaneous and mucosal.[54,55] Mucosal types are recovered mainly in the genital tract, although other mucosae may be infected, including the respiratory tract, nose, conjunctiva, and mouth. Although the same HPV virus can cause various types of warts, there is often a correlation between the virus type and the clinical/morphologic characteristics of the lesions it causes. For instance, HPV types 1, 2, 4, and 7 are often associated with common warts (verrucae vulgaris); type 1 with deep palmar and plantar warts; types 3, 10, 28, and 41 with flat warts; types 5, 8, 17, and 20 (among others) with the autosomal recessive disorder epidermodysplasia verruciformis (see later); and types 6 and 11 with respiratory, conjunctival, and genital infection.[54] In addition, high-risk cervical cancer-associated HPV types include 16, 18, 31, 33, 35, 39, and 45, among others. HPV types 16 and 18 are the most frequent 'high-risk' types found in the female anogenital system and are seen in up to 70% of women with cervical cancer. Laboratory diagnosis of HPV skin infection is usually unnecessary, and the diagnosis usually straightforward. In instances where identification of the HPV type is necessary, options include nuclear acid hybridization assays via Southern blotting, dot blots, RNA and DNA probes, and PCR studies.

Verrucae Vulgaris

Verrucae vulgaris (common warts) occur predominantly on the dorsal surface of the hands or periungual regions, but may be seen anywhere on the cutaneous surface. Occasionally they may also occur on the oral mucosa. Common warts may occur as single or multiple lesions. They clinically present as flesh-colored, verrucous (rough surfaced) papules that may be dome-shaped (Fig. 15.17), exophytic (Fig. 15.18), or filiform (i.e., having a stalk, Fig. 15.19). Individual lesions may coalesce into larger plaques (Fig. 15.20). 'Ring warts' may occur following overly-aggressive therapies, and are another example of koebnerization (Fig. 15.21). Oral lesions present as small, pink-white, soft papules and plaques of the labial, lingual (Fig. 15.22), buccal, or gingival mucosa. In *Heck's disease*,

multiple verrucous papules occur in a similar mucosal distribution (Fig. 15.23).

Periungual and subungual verrucae (Figs 15.24, 15.25) occur around and beneath nail beds, particularly on the fingers of cuticle-pickers and nail biters. These lesions, because of their location and

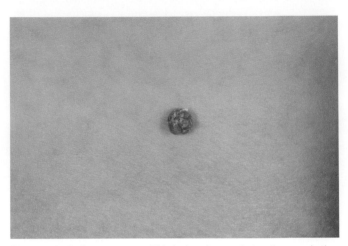

Figure 15.18 Common wart. This lesion demonstrates the exophytic type of verruca vulgaris.

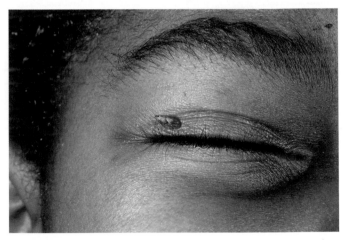

Figure 15.19 Common wart. This lesion has a stalk, and is termed a filiform wart.

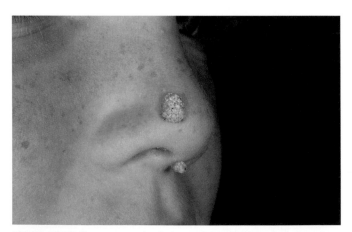

Figure 15.17 Common warts. A dome-shaped lesion of the lateral nose and a filiform lesion of the columella.

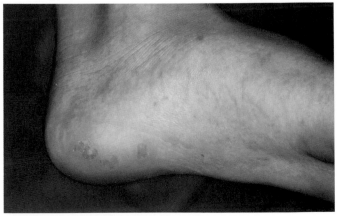

Figure 15.20 Common warts. Multiple lesions coalesce into a mosaic plaque on the plantar surface.

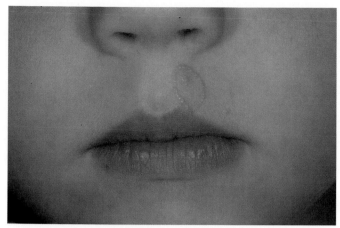

Figure 15.21 Ring warts. This annular plaque composed of small verrucous papules developed following a marked blister response to therapy of a single wart above the upper lip.

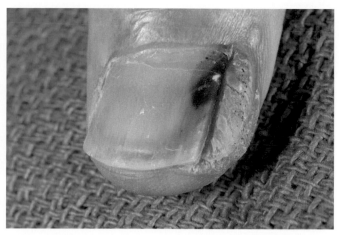

Figure 15.24 Periungual warts. Verrucous papules of the lateral nail fold. Note adjacent subungual hemorrhage.

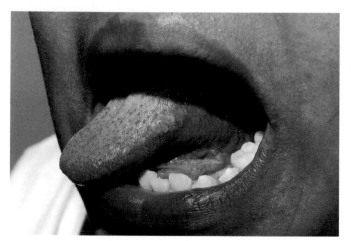

Figure 15.22 Common warts affecting mucosa. This tongue lesion presented as a soft, verrucous papule.

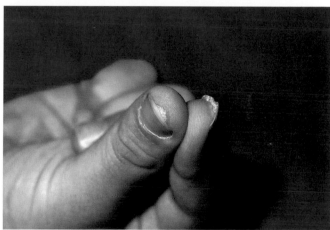

Figure 15.25 Subungual warts. Verrucous papules of the distal thumb and index finger, with extension under the nail plate.

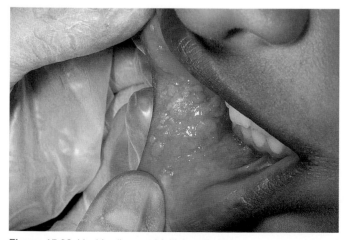

Figure 15.23 Heck's disease. Multiple soft, pink verrucous papules of the inner lip mucosa.

susceptibility to trauma, frequently become irritated, infected, or tender and are often more resistant to therapy. Satellite lesions may appear, particularly near warts that have been irritated, manipulated, or incompletely treated. When the diagnosis of verruca is in doubt, gentle paring with a No.15 scalpel blade will reveal characteristic punctate black dots that represent thrombosed capillaries (Fig. 15.26).

Verrucae Plana

Verrucae plana (flat warts) occur primarily on the face, neck, arms, and legs. They are usually seen as smooth, flesh-colored to slightly pink or brown, flat-topped papules measuring 2–5 mm in diameter (Figs 15.16, 15.27, 15.28). They vary from a few lesions to several hundred in any given individual. In the bearded areas of men, and on the legs of women, irritation from shaving tends to cause their spread. Contiguous warts may coalesce to form larger, plaque-like lesions. Again, linear arrangements of the papules in areas of scratching (koebnerization) are characteristic (Figs 15.16, 15.29).

Verrucae Plantaris

Verrucae plantaris (plantar warts) occur on the plantar surfaces of the feet and tend to be the most symptomatic type of warts, as well as a therapeutic challenge. They usually occur on the weight-bearing areas of the heels, toes, and mid-metatarsal areas (Fig. 15.30). Because of the pressure of walking, the lesions often develop an 'endophytic' component and are very painful and tender.

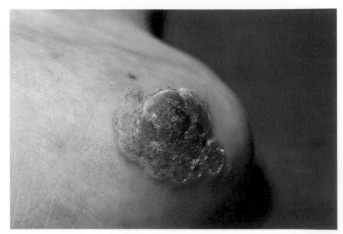

Figure 15.26 Wart with thrombosed capillaries. Note the multiple 'black dots' within this large mosaic plantar wart.

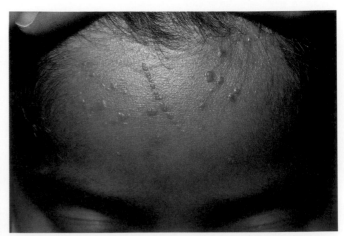

Figure 15.29 Flat warts with koebnerization. Flat papules on the forehead, with a linear configuration (Koebner phenomenon) at sites of autoinoculation.

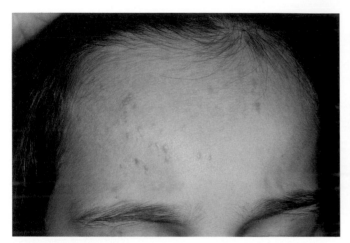

Figure 15.27 Flat warts. Flat, verrucous papules.

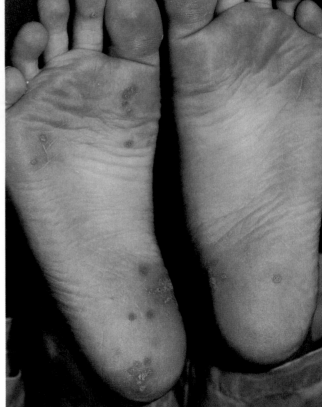

Figure 15.30 Plantar warts. Verrucous papules on the plantar surfaces.

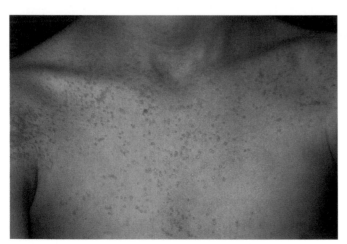

Figure 15.28 Flat warts. Multiple disseminated flat papules in a patient infected with human immunodeficiency virus.

Coalescence of multiple lesions may result in *mosaic warts* (Fig. 15.31). It may occasionally be difficult to differentiate plantar warts from corns or calluses. *Corns* are localized hyperkeratoses that form over interphalangeal joints as the result of intermittent pressure and friction. Penetrating corns often appear at the base of the second or third metatarsal-phalangeal joint. They can be distinguished from plantar warts by the lack of thrombosed capillaries after paring and by their characteristic hard core. *Soft corns* are macerated hyperkeratotic lesions that persist at points of friction and pressure in intertriginous areas. They are usually seen on the lateral aspect of the toes, or in the web spaces between the fourth and fifth toes.

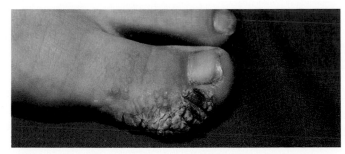

Figure 15.31 Plantar warts, mosaic. Multiple verrucous papules coalesced into this giant, painful verrucous plaque.

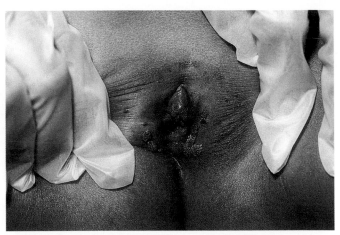

Figure 15.33 Condylomata acuminata. Verrucous papules of the labial surfaces, with a large, vegetative lesion protruding from the vagina. This toddler had been sexually abused.

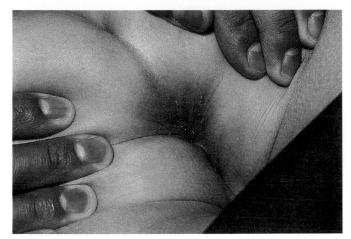

Figure 15.32 Condylomata acuminata. Verrucous, brown papules in a perianal distribution.

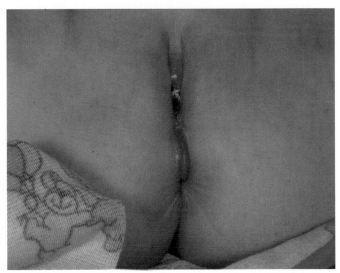

Figure 15.34 Infantile perianal pyramidal protrusion. Pyramidal-shaped, fleshy papule of the midline raphe.

Black heel (talon noir, calcaneal petechiae) is a common condition frequently confused with plantar warts. In this disorder, superficial dermal capillaries are ruptured by the shearing action associated with sudden stops in athletic individuals, usually tennis, racquetball, or basketball players. Clinically, it is characterized by clusters of brown or blue-black, pinpoint petechial macules in the horny layer along the backs or sides of the heels or lateral edges of the feet. Gentle paring of the surface with a No.15 scalpel blade can help differentiate this condition from malignant melanoma, calluses, corns, and plantar warts.

Condylomata Acuminata

Condylomata acuminata (anogenital warts) are HPV-induced lesions of the anogenital tract, and one of the most common sexually transmitted diseases. The diagnosis of condylomata acuminata in a child is fraught with anxiety for parents and practitioners alike, and the implications regarding sexual abuse versus benign transmission are controversial and often unclear. Although condylomata often occur after sexual contact, other modes of acquiring the infection include vertical (perinatal) transmission, benign (non-sexual) heteroinoculation, and autoinoculation. In addition, fomite spread is another potential mode of transmission.[56]

Condylomata acuminata present most commonly in the perianal area as flesh-colored, soft, verrucous papules (Fig. 15.32) measuring 1–5 mm in diameter. The lesions are usually multiple, and 'mirror image' lesions may be noted on each side of the anus. Other areas of involvement include the glans penis, penile shaft, scrotum, and vulva. Vaginal and cervical involvement are appreciable only with internal examination. Occasionally, lesions may enlarge rapidly and present as large, exophytic, cauliflower-like masses (Fig. 15.33). Childhood condylomata lesions are usually incidentally noted during diaper changes, toileting, bathing, or physical examinations.[57] The lesions are usually asymptomatic, but irritation, bleeding, and pain may occur. The differential diagnosis of condylomata acuminata includes molluscum contagiosum, epidermal nevus, skin tag, and pseudoverrucous papules and nodules. *Infantile perianal pyramidal protrusion* is a pyramidal-shaped, flesh-colored to pink soft tissue swelling (Fig. 15.34) that appears in the medial raphe of girls, and may represent a peculiar form of lichen sclerosus et atrophicus.[58,59] The distribution, appearance, and solitary nature of this lesion should distinguish it from condylomata.

The diagnosis of condylomata acuminata in a child should prompt consideration for the possibility of sexual abuse. However, it should be remembered that anogenital warts occur in large numbers of children as a result of innocent (non-sexual) or vertical transmission or from autoinoculation. Although HPV DNA typing is occasionally considered, it does not help in the differentiation between the various modes of transmission.[56,57] Although innocent autoinoculation or heteroinoculation from hand warts is common, and the finding of such hand lesions in an adult contact or caretaker might be reassuring, fondling is a form of sexual abuse commonly seen in younger children and thus the possibility of sexual abuse must still be considered.[60]

When a child is diagnosed with anogenital condylomata, a directed history should include the age of onset, history of maternal infection (genital warts or abnormal Pap smear), and personal or family history of warts, as well as inquiries about the child's social environment and all caregivers.[60] Physical examination should be focused on findings suggestive of sexual abuse, and laboratory evaluation for other sexually transmitted diseases performed if non-innocent HPV transmission is suggested. A behavioral and social assessment by a skilled professional should be considered. The literature contains significant disagreement with regard to the prevalence of sexual abuse in children with condylomata, with estimates ranging variably from 4% to 91%.[57] Although sexual transmission of HPV may occur at any age, the risk seems greater in children over 3–4 years of age.[61,62] The Committee on Child Abuse and Neglect of the American Academy of Pediatrics considers the presence of anogenital warts in children 'suspicious' and recommends reporting to a child protective agency.[18]

The authors' personal approach is to consider non-sexual transmission of HPV if the child is under 3 years of age; if lesions developed within the 1st year of life; if the patient has other non-genital warts; if warts are present in close contacts, especially genital warts (or history of abnormal Pap smear) in the mother; and when there are no findings to suggest sexual abuse. If there is any suspicion of sexual abuse, referral to child protective services is initiated. In patients in whom there is uncertainty or where the situation is ambiguous, a social worker from the protective services team should be enlisted early on in the evaluation. Although the diagnosis of sexual abuse must never be missed, 'reflexive reporting' to child welfare authorities should be avoided given the emotional devastation and destruction that may result. If the practitioner evaluating the patient is uncomfortable in the evaluation, referral should be made to a clinician with expertise for further evaluation.[57]

Treatment of condylomata acuminata in children (see below) is challenging for many reasons. In an interesting study of the natural history of these lesions in children, spontaneous resolution occurred in 54% of patients within 5 years of the diagnosis, suggesting that nonintervention is a reasonable initial approach to managing this condition.[63]

Treatment of common warts and condylomata acuminata

No specific antiviral therapy exists for HPV infections, and most wart treatments rely on destruction of the affected area of epidermal proliferation. Some newer methods of therapy are immunomodulatory in nature. As spontaneous involution of warts may occur, watchful waiting is an appropriate consideration, especially in younger patients in whom destructive therapies are traumatic and poorly tolerated. When considering therapy for warts, every effort should be made to avoid overly aggressive or scarring therapies. Table 15.3 lists some of the treatment options for common, plantar, and planar warts and for condylomata acuminata. Several are discussed here in more detail.

Patients and parents must be reminded that even with apparent 'cures' of warts or condylomata, latent HPV infection in grossly normal appearing squamous epithelium beyond the areas of treatment may persist and results in a fairly high risk of recurrence. Whether warts should be treated depends on the patient's and parents' desires, and the nature of the lesions. Those patients with warts that are painful, extensive, enlarging, subject to trauma, or cosmetically objectionable are most likely to be interested in therapy. If treatment is to be given, it should be harmless to the child, and if a painful therapy is being utilized, the child should be old enough

Table 15.3 Treatments for warts and condylomata acuminata in children

Treatment	Comment
Warts	
Watchful waiting	Especially appropriate in young children
Topical salicylic acid	Available OTC; may be more effective when combined with duct tape occlusion
Cryotherapy	Both in-office and OTC available
Manual paring or filing	May minimize pain from plantar warts
Immunotherapy:	
Oral	Cimetidine; OL use (see text)
Topical	Imiquimod (home use; OL); squaric acid dibutylester
Laser therapy	Pulsed dye laser potentially useful; CO2 laser useful but scarring may result
Injection therapy	i.e., *Candida* antigens, bleomycin, interferon; rarely utilized in children
Curettage, electrocautery	Rarely utilized in children
Topical retinoids	May be useful for flat warts; OL
Topical chemotherapy:	
5% 5-fluorouracil	OL use; may be useful for facial flat warts
2% 5-fluorouracil + 17% salicylic acid	Available OTC from compounding pharmacy; useful for plantar warts; applied nightly with tape occlusion
Condylomata	
Watchful waiting	Especially appropriate in young children
Chemovesicants	Podophyllin, TCA, podofilox
Immunotherapy:	
Oral	Cimetidine; OL use (see text)
Topical	Imiquimod; OL if <12 years
Cryotherapy	
Laser therapy	Rarely used for this indication in children
Surgery	Rarely used for this indication in children

OTC, over-the-counter; OL, off-label; CO2, carbon dioxide; TCA, trichloroacetic acid.

to consent to the therapy. Parents occasionally request painful therapies (i.e., cryotherapy) for young children; this decision should be made only after a thorough discussion of the therapy, the pain involved, and its risk-to-benefit ratio. It should be emphasized that some modalities used for the treatment of warts in adults are neither feasible nor desirable for the treatment of warts in children. The choice of therapy will depend on the age and personality of the patient, and the number, size, and location of the lesions.

Salicylic acid is available commercially under a variety of brand names, including Duofilm, Occlusal, Wart-Off, Clear Away, and Mediplast. It comes as liquids, gels, plasters, and pads. Salicylic acid preparations are applied directly to the wart surface, and may be left on continuously or overnight. An effective form of combination therapy is to apply a salicylic acid liquid to the wart(s), and after drying occurs (5 min) to occlude the surface with duct tape. This treatment is placed on at bedtime, and the duct tape is removed the following morning. With removal of the tape, gradual debridement of the wart is performed, and the application is repeated nightly until the warts have resolved. Salicylic acid therapy may take from 2 to 12 weeks for complete wart resolution. A potential side-effect of this therapy is maceration and irritation of the skin surrounding the wart. If this occurs, therapy should be held for 2–3 days to allow for resolution, and then it is resumed. A compounded product of 17% salicylic acid and 2% 5-fluorouracil (WartPEEL, NuCara Pharmacy, Coralville, IA) is available and quite effective when applied to plantar warts nightly under tape occlusion.

Cryotherapy is a highly effective therapy for warts, albeit one that is painful and that may be unacceptably traumatic for younger patients. The most effective cryogen appears to be liquid nitrogen, which has a vaporization temperature of −196°C.[60] Other agents, such as dimethyl ether and propane (Histofreezer) and chlorodifluoromethane (Verruca-Freeze) achieve temperatures in the range −40 to −80°C, and appear to be less effective.[64] Liquid nitrogen is applied to the wart, with a cotton-tipped applicator or via a spray gun, for 10–20 s. The number of applications per treatment session depends on multiple factors, including the size of the wart, its location, past responses, and style of the physician. The goal is to induce blister formation above the dermal-epidermal junction, without causing a deep ulcer or significant necrosis to surrounding tissue. Therapy is often repeated at 3–4-week intervals, and may be more effective when preceded by gentle debridement of warty tissue with a No.15 scalpel blade. Cryotherapy may be extremely uncomfortable, and some children will not accept this mode of therapy. Although the child can be held down for the procedure, this is an undesirable approach in most instances, and alternative treatments should be considered. Several over-the-counter cryotherapy wart removal products (i.e., Wartner, Compound W Freeze Off, Dr Scholl's Freeze Away) are available, and use the combination of dimethyl ether and propane to freeze to −57°C. The cryogen is delivered by a foam pad attached to an applicator, and held on the wart for 10–20 s.

Immunologic forms of wart therapy rely on the host immune system to mount a response against the HPV-induced lesions. Although these forms of therapy are not uniformly efficacious, they offer another option in the treatment of patients with warts. The most common form of oral immunotherapy is treatment with cimetidine, which is believed to possess immunomodulatory activity including the ability to inhibit suppressor T-cell function, activate Th1 cells, and stimulate production of IL-2 and interferon-γ.[65,66] In one study, 32 children with warts were treated with cimetidine, 25–40 mg/kg per day divided into three or four doses, with an 81% clearance rate after 2 months of treatment.[65] Other studies of cimetidine and warts have shown conflicting results.[67–70] When utilized, most experts recommend 30–40 mg/kg per day divided into twice daily doses.

However, the treatment is usually well tolerated with few if any side-effects, and when effective, recurrences are rare.

Imiquimod is a topical immune response modifier, approved for the treatment of genital and perianal warts in patients 12 years of age or older. It is marketed in a 5% cream (Aldara), and is applied to those lesions thrice weekly on nonconsecutive days. Imiquimod has its therapeutic effect via induction of interferon-α and other cytokines in the skin.[71,72] Studies have suggested that the off-label use of this agent, with more frequent application schedules (once daily for 5 weeks to twice daily applications), may be useful in the treatment of common warts.[73,74]

Topical immunotherapy with squaric acid dibutylester (SADBE) is another option in the treatment of recalcitrant warts. Topical immunotherapy was initially described with dinitrochlorobenzene (DNCB), and subsequently with diphenylcyclopropenone (DCP). These agents are less desirable because of mutagenicity associated with the former and local side-effects associated with the latter.[75] With SADBE immunotherapy, sensitization of (unaffected) skin is followed by the application of the solution to non-facial warts. The therapy is painless and often effective, with complete clearance rates ranging from 58% to 84% in open label studies.[75–77]

Side-effects of this treatment include allergic contact dermatitis (at either sensitization or treatment sites) and rarely urticaria. The hypothesized mechanism of action of this form of immunotherapy is generation of a delayed-type hypersensitivity reaction at the site of the wart, and possibly a systemic antiviral effect since even untreated lesions at distal sites may occasionally resolve.[75]

Pulsed-dye laser therapy is another option for the treatment of recalcitrant warts. This laser, which is most often utilized in the treatment of vascular birthmarks, works by selectively destroying the blood vessels found within warts.[78] This therapy has a large advantage over carbon dioxide laser therapy in that it is non-scarring and the period of postoperative recovery is significantly shorter. Pulsed-dye laser therapy has been demonstrated to be quite effective in the treatment of warts, including common, plantar, and periungual types.[50,78,79] Its use, however, is best limited to lesions that are recalcitrant and have failed other therapeutic modalities.

Flat warts may be treated with a variety of modalities, although their small size, frequent location on the face, and occurrence in groups make aggressive therapies impractical. Treatment options for these lesions include light cryotherapy, imiquimod, topical retinoids (i.e., tretinoin or adapalene cream), oral cimetidine, topical chemotherapy (i.e., 5-fluorouracil cream) or topical immunotherapy.

Therapies for condylomata acuminata have been poorly studied in children. As mentioned, a significant portion of anogenital warts in the pediatric population may spontaneously involute over several years, and thus watchful waiting is an appropriate consideration. When therapy is desired, a commonly used regimen is that of either podophyllin or trichloroacetic acid (or the two in combination), which are applied in the office. These agents cause cytotoxic effects with resultant necrosis of the affected cells, and their use may be limited by local irritation. Podofilox solution or gel (Condylox) is a closely related compound marketed for application in the home setting. Podofilox, which is approved for use in adult patients, is applied twice daily for three consecutive days, although more limited regimens (i.e., once daily) are often recommended for children to try and avoid local irritation. Self-treatment with podofilox has shown greater efficacy and cost-effectiveness than office therapy with podophyllin.[80] Imiquimod, applied three times weekly on non-consecutive days, is another option that has been demonstrated effective in the treatment of external genital and perianal warts.[81] This treatment is also occasionally limited by local irritation. Other treatments utilized occasionally for condylomata acuminata include cryotherapy, laser therapy,[82,83] oral cimetidine, topical immunotherapy,[84] 5-fluorouracil cream, and surgical ablation.

Epidermodysplasia Verruciformis

Epidermodysplasia verruciformis (EV) is a rare autosomal recessive disorder characterized by a genetically determined susceptibility to widespread and persistent infection of the skin with specific HPV types.[85] Infections begin in early childhood and malignant transformation (non-melanoma skin cancer) occurs in approximately half of patients during adulthood. The predisposition to HPV infection is believed to be the result of an immunogenetic defect associated with generation of cytokines, which down regulate cell-mediated immunity, and possibly with low levels of IL-10.[86] The role of environmental factors (most notably UV irradiation) also appears to be important in the pathogenesis of the HPV-associated malignancies.[87] Recently, EV was found to be caused by inactivating mutations in two adjacent, related genes, EVER1/TMC6 and EVER2/TMC8. These genes encode transmembrane proteins located in the endoplasmic reticulum.[88,89] EV may represent a primary deficiency of intrinsic immunity to the EV-specific HPVs (betapapillomaviruses) or in innate immunity, or both.[89]

Patients with EV present during childhood with widespread tinea versicolor-like, hypopigmented macules and/or flat 'verruca plana'-like papules. These papules are red to red-brown, and may coalesce into larger plaques. The most common locations for the warty lesions are the hands, extremities, and the face, whereas the tinea versicolor-like lesions occur predominantly on the trunk.[87] When skin malignancy (usually squamous cell carcinoma) develops during adulthood, it is most often at sun-exposed sites, and these tumors are most often associated with HPV types 5 and 8. There is no specific therapy for EV. Protection from UV radiation with protective clothing and sunscreens and sun avoidance are vital. Close clinical surveillance for squamous cell carcinoma is recommended, with early surgical excision as needed. Experimental therapies have included interferon, imiquimod, cimetidine, photodynamic therapy and systemic retinoids.[87,90]

Recurrent Respiratory Papillomatosis

Recurrent respiratory papillomatosis (RRP, laryngeal papillomatosis) is a disorder of HPV-associated benign tumors of the larynx, and at times other portions of the aerodigestive tract. RRP is the most common benign neoplasm of the larynx in children, and is usually caused by HPV types 6 and 11, which are both common genital tract HPV types.[91] Although the exact method of HPV acquisition in patients with RRP is not well established, it is most likely caused by maternal–fetal transmission (ascending *in utero* infection or direct contact in the birth canal), and less likely via postnatal acquisition.[92,93] However, even given the potential links among cervical HPV, vaginal delivery, and RRP, the utility of elective cesarean sections in mothers with genital tract HPV infection as a preventive measure remains controversial.[93–95]

In fact, very few children who are exposed to genital HPV at birth develop symptoms of RRP.

Although the tumors of RRP are benign, significant morbidity may result from obstruction of the airway and potential malignant degeneration. RRP is usually diagnosed before the age of 5 years, and the clinical presentation often includes the triad of stridor, progressive hoarseness, and respiratory distress.[91] Patients may be initially diagnosed with asthma, croup, or bronchitis. In some, the condition may go undiagnosed until frank respiratory distress develops, with the resultant need for emergent tracheotomy. The condition is diagnosed with direct airway endoscopy, and the mainstay of therapy for RRP is surgery or laser therapy. Adjuvant treatments include interferon, photodynamic therapy, and antiviral therapy. Intralesional cidofovir in combination with surgery has been advocated as an effective therapeutic combination.[96,97] It also appears that aggressive control of gastroesophageal reflux disease, when present, is vital since it may contribute to the severity of RRP.[91,98]

Molluscum contagiosum

Molluscum contagiosum (MC) is a common cutaneous viral infection in children caused by a member of the poxvirus family (molluscum contagiosum virus, or MCV). Although MC is frequently a sexually transmitted infection or associated with immunodeficiency (especially HIV infection) in adults, childhood disease tends to lack these associations. There has been a dramatic increase in MC over recent decades in the USA, with an 11-fold increase in patient visits for the disorder reported for one 18-year period.[99] In children, the infection is also becoming more prevalent, as the spread of virus through skin-to-skin contact and fomites is rapid and easy. MC occurs most often in school-age children, and especially those under 8 years of age. Although controversy still exists, epidemiologic data suggest that MC may be transmitted via swimming pools, as well as via fomites such as sponges and towels and in beauty parlors.[100–103]

Autoinoculation of the virus is a common mode of spread in affected patients. MC lesions tend to spread more rapidly in children with atopic dermatitis, possibly related to suppressed helper T-cell responses. Congenital MC have been reported, and likely represent vertical transmission of MCV.[104]

MC presents as pearly, flesh-colored to pink papules that often appear translucent (Figs 15.35–15.37). The range in size is from 2

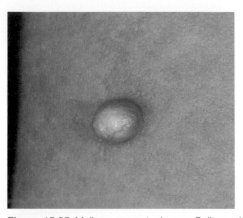

Figure 15.35 Molluscum contagiosum. Solitary, dome-shaped pearly papule. Note the capped white plug.

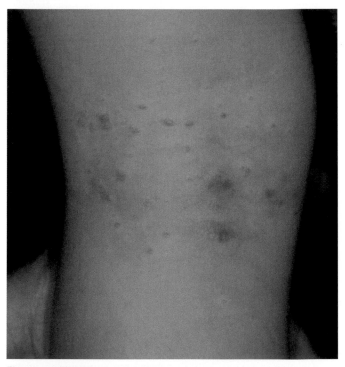

Figure 15.36 Molluscum contagiosum. Multiple pearly translucent papules in the popliteal fossa. Note erythema and flattening of some lesions, representing the host immune response and early involution.

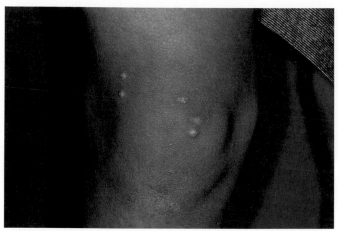

Figure 15.37 Molluscum contagiosum. Pearly, umbilicated papules around the knee.

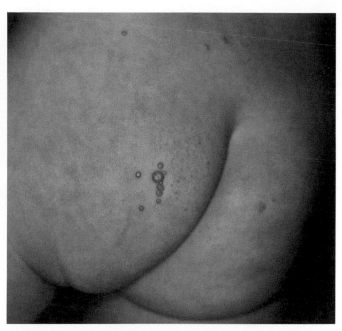

Figure 15.39 Molluscum contagiosum with koebnerization. Linear configuration of lesions along a line of autoinoculation.

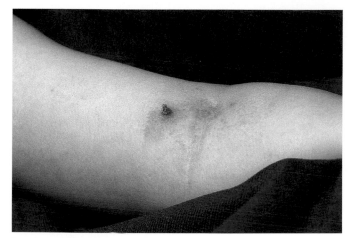

Figure 15.38 Molluscum contagiosum. This solitary lesion, with surrounding dermatitis, demonstrates the central excrescence that may be present in some mollusca.

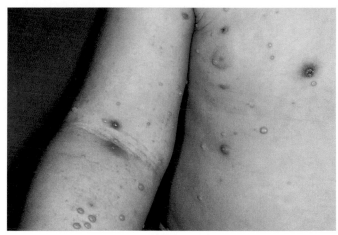

Figure 15.40 Molluscum contagiosum with host immune response. The bright red appearance of several of the lesions is typical once an immune response is being mounted by the host. The inflamed lesions usually resolve over 2–3 weeks.

to 8 mm. A small central dell or depression may or may not be evident, and occasionally excrescences protrude from this central region (Fig. 15.38). Although single lesions may occur, MC most often presents with numerous clustered papules, and linear configurations (from koebnerization) may be present (Fig. 15.39). Although MC may occur on any area of the skin surface, they are most common in areas of skin rubbing or moist regions, including the axillae, popliteal fossae, and groin. Genital and perianal lesions are also common, even in children, in whom the disorder is nearly always transmitted in a benign (non-sexual) fashion. Lesions may develop significant erythema (Fig. 15.40), which usually represents a host immune response against MCV, and often heralds spontaneous involution. Occasionally, childhood MC may be marked by very high numbers of lesions (Fig. 15.41) or a giant size (Fig. 15.42). The latter may occasionally be confused with other causes of 'cutaneous pseudolymphoma' (see Ch. 10). Surrounding dermatitis around MC lesions ('molluscum dermatitis') is common (Fig. 15.43), and may propagate the cycle of infection when the patient scratches and subsequently autoinoculates the virus to other regions. Complications of MC are rare, but include secondary bacterial infection (Fig. 15.44), which is often secondary to scratching-induced impetiginization. In some patients with eyelid lesions, chronic conjunctivitis or superficial punctate keratitis may develop.

Spontaneous clearing of MC often occurs over years, but parents and patients may request therapy for several reasons. These include the cosmetic significance of the lesions, pruritus, and epidemiologic concerns of other parents, teachers, or school nurses. In addition, in patients with an underlying atopic diathesis, the lesions may be more extensive and autoinoculation more significant given the extensive pruritus. Traditional therapies (and those utilized in adults), such as curettage or cryotherapy, rely on destructive measures and may be traumatic for pediatric patients. Although curettage is not a preferred method of the authors, the pain of the procedure may be reduced by pretreatment of the lesional areas with topical anesthetic (lidocaine or lidocaine/prilocaine) cream. Care must be exercised, however, given reports of the latter (lidocaine/prilocaine, eutectic mixture of local anesthetics, EMLA) cream in association with adverse events including methemoglobinemia, hypoxemia, and seizures.[105,106] In these reports, however, the topical anesthetic

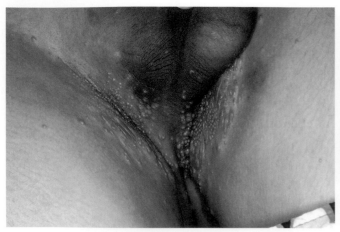

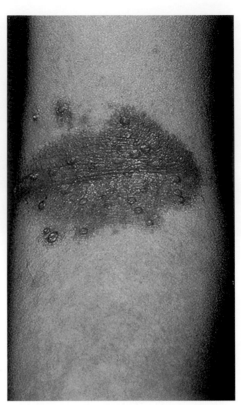

Figure 15.41 Molluscum contagiosum in an immunocompromised host. This young boy receiving cancer chemotherapy had disseminated mollusca contagiosa, including multiple recalcitrant lesions in the groin.

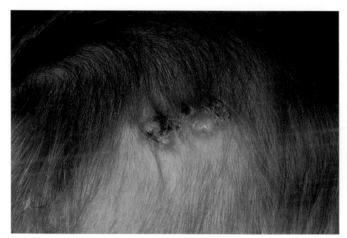

Figure 15.43 Molluscum contagiosum with molluscum dermatitis. Note the intensely erythematous, scaly plaque surrounding multiple mollusca in the antecubital fossa.

Figure 15.42 Giant molluscum contagiosum. These two nodular plaques of the scalp turned out to be giant molluscum lesions. This pattern of presentation may be confused with other causes of cutaneous pseudolymphoma (see Ch. 10).

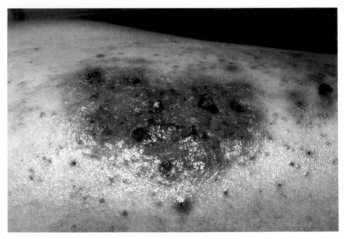

Figure 15.44 Molluscum contagiosum with secondary bacterial infection. This patient with mollusca developed an associated dermatitis and eventual secondary infection with *S. aureus*.

had been applied in excess of the recommended use. The maximum dose and application area recommendations suggested by the manufacturer of EMLA cream are listed in Table 15.4.

A highly effective and well-tolerated therapy for MC is the in-office application of cantharidin. Cantharidin is an extract from the blister beetle, *Cantharis vesicatoria*, and is known to induce vesiculation of the epidermis upon application to human skin.[107] Although concerns regarding the safety of cantharidin therapy have tempered its use for some, with appropriate application and patient education it is usually very well tolerated and effective.[107–109]

A concentration of 0.7% or 0.9% cantharidin is usually used, and guidelines for the safe and effective use of this agent for treatment of MC are listed in Table 15.5. Treatment results in blister formation within 24–48 h, with healing over several days to 1 week. The extent of blistering is minimized by having the patient (or parent) rinse treated areas after a specified time following application, usually 2–6 h.[109] Treatment of perioral or periocular facial lesions, mucosal sites or occluded areas (i.e., diaper region) with this agent is not generally recommended. Cantharidin should be applied in the office only, by a physician or other qualified and well-trained health

professional. If molluscum dermatitis is present, it should be cleared by use of a topical corticosteroid ointment prior to commencing with cantharidin therapy. At the time of this writing, the US Food and Drug Administration is critically re-evaluating the utilization of cantharidin, which currently requires compounding by a pharmacy. Although considered a first-line treatment for molluscum contagiosum by many practitioners, access to cantharidin in the USA may become very limited or completely unavailable.

Other methods of therapy that have been reported for MC include imiquimod cream, topical tretinoin cream, salicylic acid, α-hydroxy

Table 15.4 Maximum recommended EMLA dose and application areas

Age and body weight[a]	Maximum total dose of EMLA (g)	Maximum appl. area (cm^2)	Maximum appl. time (h)
0–3 months or <5 kg	1	10	1
3–12 months and >5 kg	2	20	4
1–6 years and >10 kg	10	100	4
7–12 years and >20 kg	20	200	4

[a]If patient is older than 3 months of age and does not meet minimum weight requirement, the maximum total dose of EMLA should be based on the patient's *weight*.

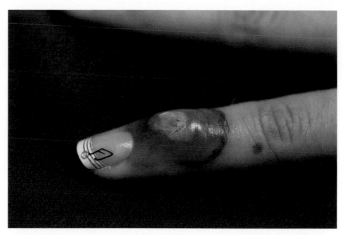

Figure 15.45 Orf. An inflammatory nodule with superficial vesiculation and oozing on the distal index finger of a 16-year-old female. She had been bitten by a goat 3 weeks prior while visiting a petting zoo.

Table 15.5 Guidelines for treatment of molluscum contagiosum with cantharidin

Patient and parent education (handouts useful)
Avoid treating lesions in the following sites:
   Facial
   Mucosal
   Occluded
Treat 20–30 lesions maximum per treatment session
Application of cantharidin (0.7% or 0.9%):
   Use applicator stick or blunt (wooden) end of cotton-tipped
      applicator
   Apply single droplet to each lesion
   Avoid 'painting'
   Let area dry for at least 2 min before patient gets dressed
   Do not occlude treated sites
Have patient bathe/rinse off all treated sites in 2–6 h (may vary
   based on past response; 4 h good starting point with first
   treatment; may rinse sooner if significant discomfort or if
   vesiculation is noted)
Acetaminophen administered by parent if needed for pain
Bacitracin ointment applied to blisters twice daily until areas heal
Therapy repeated at 3–4-week intervals as needed

acids, tape stripping, pulsed-dye laser therapy, 5% potassium hydroxide, topical cidofovir, oral cimetidine, and silver nitrate paste.[73,100,107,110–119]

Imiquimod cream has been used with different treatment regimens, from three times weekly to application on a daily basis, with variable results. Topical tretinoin cream is a commonly used method for treating facial molluscum contagiosum, although its use may be limited by its irritation potential.

Cowpox and pseudocowpox

Cowpox is a rare zoonotic infection caused by a DNA orthopoxvirus that is similar to the vaccinia and smallpox viruses. It is transmitted by contact with infected animals, which may include cattle (from whom it may be transmitted as an occupational infection) and wild rodents, which serve as its natural reservoir.[120] Following an incubation period of 1–3 weeks, a localized crusted nodule with ulceration or vesiculation forms, and evolves through several stages to ultimately heal with a scar over several weeks. Flu-like symptoms may

occasionally be present, and lymphadenopathy is common. Immunocompromised hosts may develop severe generalized infection. Although there is no accepted standard for therapy, cidofovir and some novel antiviral agents have been studies for patients with severe involvement, and measures to prevent secondary bacterial infection (i.e., wound care, topical and oral antibiotics) are recommended.[120]

Pseudocowpox (milker's nodule, paravaccinia) is a parapox virus infection seen worldwide and usually occurring in dairy farmers and new milkers. The infection is acquired from contact with the infected teats of cattle infected with the virus, and children may occasionally acquire it. Clinically, pseudocowpox is characterized by a single or several papules on the hands or fingers, which progress through several stages: a macular or papular lesion becomes a vesicular lesion, then subsequently progresses to a nodular stage with weeping, then to a papillomatous or verrucous (warty) stage, and finally a dry crust develops and healing occurs over 4–8 weeks. Typically, no scarring results. Secondary bacterial infection may occur in some patients. Occasionally, an erythema multiforme-like secondary eruption may occur.[121] Treatment is similar to that discussed above for cowpox.

The diagnosis of cowpox or pseudocowpox is usually made by the combination of the history of exposure and clinical examination. The differential diagnosis may include herpetic whitlow or other poxvirus infections (i.e., orf). If confirmation of the diagnosis is necessary, virus isolation and serologic studies may be useful. In addition, light or electron microscopic examination of skin biopsy tissue is useful, the latter showing characteristic brick-shaped viral particles.[120,122]

Orf

Orf (ecthyma contagiosum) is another parapox virus infection that normally infects sheep and goats (scabby mouth, sore mouth, contagious pustular dermatosis) and, occasionally, humans. Transmission is via contact with infected lesions in animals or fomites, including barn doors, fences, troughs, and shears.[122] Clinically, orf usually presents with a solitary lesion (Fig. 15.45), although several lesions may be present. The clinical stages of the skin lesions are identical to those described previously for cowpox and pseudocowpox. Associations include secondary bacterial infection, lymphadenopathy, lymphangitis, erythema multiforme-like eruptions, and recurrences in immunocompromised hosts.[123,124] Giant lesions of orf are occasionally reported.[125] Diagnostic modalities are the same as those for discussed above, and in addition, a PCR method for diagnosis has been described.[126] Treatment is supportive, and the lesions involute spontaneously over 4–8 weeks, without scarring. Antibiotics should be given if secondary bacterial infection is present.

Smallpox

Smallpox (variola major) is an exanthematous disease, but is included here with other poxvirus infections. The last case of endemic smallpox occurred in Somalia in 1977, and the disease was declared eradicated in 1980.[127] Variola virus, the etiologic agent of smallpox, has been maintained since that time in two high-security laboratories, the Centers for Disease Control and Prevention (CDC) in Atlanta and the Vektor Institute in Novosibirsk, Russia. However, concerns that some virus may exist outside of these laboratories and that it could potentially be used for a widespread bioterrorism attack remain. Routine vaccination for smallpox ended after the eradication declaration in 1980 and, as such, a large population of susceptible persons now exists. The remaining protection of individuals who had received past vaccination is unclear.

Smallpox begins with entry of the virus from respiratory droplets via the respiratory tract. It then travels to regional lymph nodes, where replication occurs. Viremia develops, and after an incubation period of 7–17 days, symptoms develop. These include high fever, malaise, severe headache, and backache. The temperature may be as high as 40°C. An enanthem precedes the exanthem, and presents as erythematous macules on the oral mucosae, including the palate, tongue, and pharynx. The characteristic exanthem begins 1–2 days later with erythematous macules that progress to papules, then vesicles and eventually pustules (Fig. 15.46) over 4–7 days. All lesions tend to be in the same stage of development, which is a useful feature in distinguishing smallpox from varicella (Ch. 16) (Table 15.6). Skin lesions begin on the face and extremities, with subsequent spread to the rest of the body and eventual widespread involvement. Crusting then begins around day 8 or 9, followed by healing with scarring. Complications of smallpox include secondary bacterial infection (usually associated with a second fever spike during the exanthem phase), pneumonia, arthritis, encephalitis, and death. Mortality in the past was as high as 30%, although it

would probably be lower in developed countries with the availability of modern-day medical intervention. In survivors, blindness may occur because of viral keratitis or bacterial eye infection.

Variants of smallpox include hemorrhagic and malignant forms. In the hemorrhagic form, which is uniformly fatal, patients have high fever, abdominal pain, and then petechiae and hemorrhage of skin and mucous membranes.[128] The malignant form is similar, but without progression of the rash from vesicles to pustules. *Variola minor* (*alastrim*) is a less severe variant of smallpox, with fewer lesions and a milder course occurring in individuals with partial immunity.[128] These patients have a longer incubation period, milder prodrome, and lower mortality rate.[129]

Rapid diagnosis of smallpox is vital, as a single confirmed case could result in an international epidemic. State health officials should be contacted, and the tissue submitted to a Biological Safety Level 4 laboratory for processing.[127] The CDC should also be notified. Airborne and contact precautions should be strictly followed. Vesicular or pustular fluid, crusts (scabs), blood samples, and throat swabs should be collected as directed by regional or national health authorities. Methods for confirming the diagnosis of smallpox include cell culture, PCR, electron microscopy, serologies, and immunohistochemical stains. Collection of epidemiologic data is vital, and contacts must be identified so that vaccination can be administered. The administration of vaccine within 4 days of exposure may diminish the severity of the illness.

Therapy for smallpox consists first and foremost of isolation of the patient, who will remain infectious until approximately 10 days

Table 15.6 Distinguishing features of smallpox and varicella		
	Smallpox	**Varicella**
Prodrome	High fever, headache, backache, malaise	Mild fever, constitutional symptoms
Skin examination	Centrifugal distribution; pustules all in same stage of development; deep involvement	Central distribution; vesicles and crusted papules in different stages at one time; superficial
Scarring	Common; often severe	Occasional; usually mild (unless secondary bacterial infection)
Complications	Bacterial infection, pneumonia, arthritis, encephalitis, blindness, death	Bacterial infection; rarely pneumonia, encephalitis, arthritis

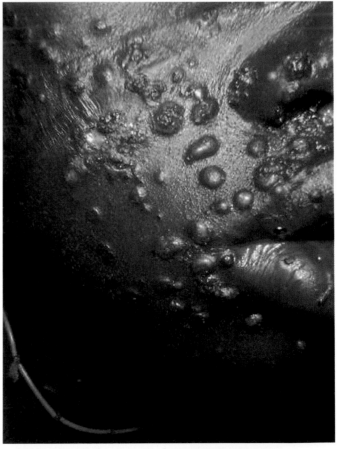

Figure 15.46 Smallpox. Multiple, tense pustules of the face in a patient from Ghana with smallpox. (Courtesy of the CDC, Dr J Noble Jr.).

from the onset of the rash. Vaccination should be given, and meticulous skin and eye care, as well as hydration and nutrition support, is vital. No specific antiviral therapy exists for smallpox, although cidofovir has shown some benefit in the postexposure prevention of other poxvirus infections.[130,131]

The issue of smallpox vaccination has received much attention with the resurgence of interest in this disease. Dryvax (Wyeth Laboratories) is a purified product made from the skin of calves infected with the vaccinia virus, another orthopoxvirus. Although production was discontinued in 1983, some vaccine has remained in storage at the CDC, and vaccination has been recommended only for laboratory workers with a high probability of exposure to orthopoxviruses.[132] In light of world events in the twenty-first century, several groups of individuals have received smallpox vaccination, including physicians from the CDC and eligible first responders and healthcare workers. New production of smallpox vaccine has again been initiated, this time in tissue cell culture. The current recommended vaccination strategy is known as 'ring vaccination,' and also referred to as surveillance and containment. In this strategy, if a single case of smallpox occurs, infected patients would be immediately isolated, and contacts would be identified and immunized by specially trained (and vaccinated) healthcare teams.

Complications of smallpox vaccination include local vaccination site reactions and more widespread reactions, such as fever, generalized vaccinia, urticaria, erythema multiforme, encephalitis and rarely death. Local reactions are common and include pustules at the vaccination site, bacterial superinfection, and lymphadenitis. In addition, pustular reactions at sites distant from the vaccination site occasionally occur from autoinoculation. *Eczema vaccinatum* is a serious, potentially life-threatening side-effect of smallpox vaccination, occurring in individuals with atopic dermatitis or less commonly other skin disorders. It is due to widespread dissemination of vaccinia, and can occur in patients with either active or quiescent dermatitis.[133] The barrier disruption in these patients permits viral implantation, with subsequent spreading from cell to cell and, occasionally, a viremic phase.[134] The lesions are similar in appearance to those associated with primary vaccination, but with extensive involvement they may become confluent (Fig. 15.47). Bacterial superinfection, shock, and death may occur, especially without the prompt administration of vaccinia immunoglobulin (VIG). Scarring is common. Because of the risks of eczema vaccinatum, individuals

with this disease should not receive elective vaccination if there is no risk of exposure to smallpox, and individuals who have regular contact with persons with atopic dermatitis should not receive vaccination unless they can avoid person-to-person contact until the scab separates from the vaccination site.[134] In addition to administration of VIG, patients with eczema vaccinatum may require treatment with cidofovir, ST-246 or other potent antivirals. Importantly, patients with eczema vaccinatum may shed large amounts of virus, and viable vaccinia virus may be present on inanimate objects in their environment, potentially causing inadvertent infection in other susceptible individuals exposed to those items.[135]

Childhood smallpox vaccination is a topic that has received considerable attention as part of the 'pre-event' vaccination program. Of concern is the fact that children under the age of 5 years have historically had the highest rates of complications, especially for the most severe reactions.[127] In response to this and other data, the Advisory Committee on Immunization Practices does not recommend routine smallpox vaccination for children and adolescents <18 years of age, and the Committee on Infectious Diseases of the American Academy of Pediatrics has strongly endorsed further vaccine development and testing in children as well as adults.[129,136]

Acquired immunodeficiency syndrome in children

Infection with human immunodeficiency virus (HIV) type 1 occurs worldwide in adults and children, with the majority of new pediatric cases occurring in children living in sub-Saharan Africa (up to 2000 new cases per day). The number of children with acquired immunodeficiency syndrome (AIDS) is decreasing in the USA owing to better prevention of perinatal transmission and the availability of effective therapies.[137] HIV-1 is an RNA retrovirus that infects CD4+ T lymphocytes, as well as other cells of the immune system. With the subsequent depletion of CD4+ T cells, progressive immunocompromise occurs, leaving the patient at risk for a wide variety of infections, inflammatory conditions, and malignancies. AIDS is diagnosed when an infected patient has an opportunistic or other unusual or persistent infection as well as a CD4+ T cell count <200 cells/μL.

More than 90% of infant and childhood HIV-1 infections in the USA are due to perinatal (mother-to-child) transmission. The remaining children acquire the infection from blood product exposure, sexual abuse, or unknown sources. It is estimated that, in the absence of antiretroviral therapy, approximately 30% of HIV-1 infected women transmit the virus to their infants.[138] This can occur *in utero*, during delivery, or via breast-feeding after delivery. Maternal plasma viral load is one of the strongest predictors of perinatal transmission.[139] Infection with herpes simplex virus type 2 or other sexually transmitted diseases resulting in cervical or vaginal ulcers also increase the risk of transmission.[140] When infants acquire the infection via breast-feeding, it tends to occur within the first several months of life.[141] Formula feeding, therefore, is a desirable choice in this setting. The availability of treatments and the global commitment to prevent mother-to-child transmission have positively impacted the epidemiology of childhood HIV infection. In the USA, the number of infected infants per year has decreased from approximately 1800 to fewer than 100.[142]

Adolescents, on the other hand, are a population with a markedly increasing rate of HIV-1 infection. Some of these patients acquired the infection perinatally and because of improved medical care, are living longer than in the past. Vertically infected adolescents will increase dramatically in numbers over the years to come.[143] In others, high-risk behaviors such as intravenous drug abuse and

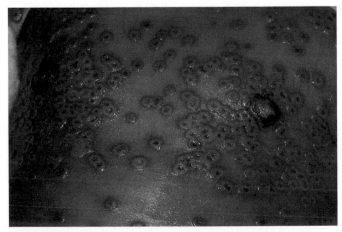

Figure 15.47 Eczema vaccinatum. Extensive umbilicated papulopustules involving the chest and nipples of a 2-year-old hospitalized male. He had a history of atopic dermatitis and was exposed to vaccinia virus via household contact with a relative who had recently received smallpox vaccination. (Courtesy of Sarah Stein, MD.)

unprotected sexual intercourse place them at increased risk. Those at highest risk are homeless youth and those living in poverty. Sexual abuse victims are another population of adolescent youth at high risk for HIV-1 infection. A high index of suspicion of HIV-1 infection should be maintained when an at-risk adolescent presents with a mononucleosis-like illness or persistent adenopathy.[137]

HIV-1 infection may present differently depending upon the child's age. Although a detailed discussion of the clinical features is beyond the scope of this section, a brief review is included. Importantly, cutaneous and/or mucosal findings are often significant in the patient with HIV-1 infection or AIDS. These are listed in Table 15.7.

Acute HIV-1 infection may present with several non-specific features, known as *acute HIV infection syndrome*. Symptoms may include fever, myalgias, fatigue, pharyngitis, weight loss, and headache, and because of the nonspecific nature of many of these, the infection often goes unrecognized.[144] Dermatologic features that may be seen during acute HIV infection syndrome include a mononucleosis-like, erythematous eruption, desquamation of palms and soles, urticaria, and alopecia. In addition, gastrointestinal symptoms are common during this acute illness, and include abdominal pain, vomiting, and diarrhea.

In infants with HIV-1 infection, the most common features include *Pneumocystis carinii* pneumonia (PCP), lymphoid interstitial pneumonitis (LIP), failure to thrive, recurrent infections (especially bacterial and candidal), and encephalopathy.[137] LIP occurs in the setting of Epstein–Barr virus (EBV) infection, with chronic lymphoid pulmonary infiltrates and a 'honeycomb' pattern on chest

Table 15.7 Mucocutaneous manifestations of HIV-1/AIDS

Class	Type	Comment
Infections	Bacterial	Syphilis
		Staphylococcus aureus: impetigo, folliculitis, ecthyma, abscess
		Pseudomonas aeruginosa: folliculitis, ecthyma gangrenosum, abscess
		Bartonella: bacillary angiomatosis
	Mycobacterial	MAC: nodules, ulcers, pustules, folliculitis
		TB: scrofuloderma, papules, vesicles, ulcers, nodules, pustules, abscess
		Atypical mycobacteria: various skin findings
	Viral	HSV: typical or atypical (deep ulcers, thick crusts)
		VZV: primary varicella, herpes zoster
		CMV: perianal ulceration, vesicles, purpura, nodules
		EBV: oral hairy leukoplakia
		HPV: common warts, condylomata acuminata
		Molluscum contagiosum: often genitals/face or widespread; recalcitrant
	Fungal	*Candida albicans*: cutaneous, oral, esophageal, vulvovaginal
		Pityrosporum ovale: tinea versicolor
		Dermatophytes: tinea infections, onychomycosis
		Deep fungal infections: histoplasmosis, cryptococcosis, coccidioidomycosis, *Penicillium mameffei*: various skin findings
	Protozoal	*Pneumocystis carinii*: occasional skin lesions
Infestations	Scabies	Classic findings or severe, crusted (Norwegian) form
	Amoeba	*Acanthamoeba, Naegleria* spp.: papules, nodules, ulcers
	Demodicidosis	*Demodex folliculorum*: folliculitis (often facial)
Inflammatory	Psoriasis	May be severe, widespread
	Reactive arthritis	NG urethritis, arthritis and skin changes: keratoderma blennorrhagicum, balanitis, oral ulceration
	Seborrheic dermatitis	More severe, more widespread
	Eosinophilic folliculitis	Sterile, pruritic follicular papules and pustules
	Drug eruption	May be severe; most often secondary to trimethoprim/sulfamethoxazole, penicillins, antituberculous medications; morbilliform eruption
Idiopathic	Pruritus	Absence of primary cutaneous findings; may be severe
	Papular eruption	Pruritic, nonfollicular papules
	Ichthyosis	An acquired form of the disorder
	Xerosis	Severe skin dryness
Malignant	Kaposi sarcoma	Skin and mucosal nodules, plaques; may metastasize; mainly homosexual/bisexual men; association with HHV-8
	Cutaneous lymphoma	Usually T-cell, less commonly B-cell non-Hodgkin lymphoma
	Other skin cancers	Basal cell, squamous cell carcinoma; malignant melanoma

Adapted from Moylett and Shearer (2002);[144] Brodie et al. (1999);[145] McClain (2001);[146] Majaliwa et al. (2009);[147] Shingadia and Novelli (2003);[148] Forsyth (2003);[149] Oleske (2003);[150] Van der Linden et al. (2009);[151] Safrit (2003);[152] Leonard and McComsey (2003),[153] and Rico et al. (1997).[154] HIV-1, human immunodeficiency virus type 1; AIDS, acquired immunodeficiency syndrome; MAC, *Mycobacterium avium* complex; TB, *Mycobacterium tuberculosis*; HSV, herpes simplex virus; VZV, varicella zoster virus; CMV, cytomegalovirus; EBV, Epstein–Barr virus; HPV, human papillomavirus; NG, non-gonococcal; HHV, human herpesvirus.

radiography. It may represent a unique immune response to coinfection with EBV and HIV,[145,146] and it usually responds to therapy with oxygen and steroids. Patients with LIP have a better prognosis than those with PCP, the latter of which is the most common AIDS-defining illness in children. The acute HIV infection syndrome may be absent in infants with HIV-1 infection.[143] Infants infected with HIV-1 are prone to gastrointestinal infections, enteropathy, and malabsorption. They may also have hepatosplenomegaly and lymphadenopathy. Primary infection with cytomegalovirus (CMV) may result in hepatitis, bone marrow failure, pneumonitis, or encephalitis. Perinatal HIV infection may also result in endocrine dysfunction with growth failure and pubertal delay.[147]

In children (i.e., those between 2 and 6 years of age), the most common features of HIV-1 infection are recurrent episodes of otitis media and sinusitis, recurrent bacterial infections, LIP, and encephalopathy. Other serious infections, including meningitis and osteomyelitis, may occur. Invasive disease caused by *Streptococcus pneumoniae* may occur, although this may become less common with the advent of routine pneumococcal immunization. Again, hepatomegaly and lymphadenopathy are common, and problems with weight gain and linear growth may be seen.

In older children and adolescents with HIV-1 infection, the most common signs and symptoms include *Candida* infections (i.e., oral thrush, vulvovaginitis, esophagitis), herpes zoster, recurrent herpes simplex infection, parotitis, cryptosporidiosis, and infections with cytomegalovirus and atypical mycobacteria. Nonspecific signs following acute HIV infection are common, and may simulate those of EBV infection. Poor growth, pubertal delay, and HIV-associated wasting may all occur.

There are multiple other associations with HIV-1 infection. Metabolic disturbances may result in hyperlipidemia, body fat redistribution (with resultant lipodystrophy or lipoatrophy), insulin resistance, and hyperglycemia. Lipodystrophy appears to be propagated by the use of combination antiretroviral therapy (cART, see below), which contributes to altered lipid metabolism.[144] Ocular manifestations include retinopathy, keratoconjunctivitis, keratitis, iridocyclitis, and retinal microvasculopathy Infectious retinitis may be caused by CMV, VZV, *Toxoplasma*, or other agents. Cardiac manifestations of HIV-1 infection include effusion, myocarditis, endocarditis, dilated cardiomyopathy, and pulmonary hypertension. In addition to HIV-associated encephalitis, or AIDS encephalopathy, other neurologic complications include aseptic meningitis, peripheral neuropathy, Guillain–Barré-like syndrome, and myelopathy. Patients may also have genitourinary, rheumatologic, gastrointestinal, and hematologic manifestations, and have an increased risk of malignancy, especially non-Hodgkin lymphoma. Tuberculosis occurs with increased frequency in patients infected with HIV-1, and has important epidemiologic significance both within the community and for the world at large. In fact, the incidence of tuberculosis worldwide has been increasing, owing primarily to the incidence of HIV infection.[148] Psychological effects of HIV infection can be profound, and may relate to the degree of illness, the threat of death, the association with substance abuse, and the social stigma associated with the disease.[149]

The diagnosis of HIV infection is based on clinical, immunologic, and serologic findings and the exclusion of other causes of immunodeficiency. Antibody-based tests include enzyme-linked immunosorbent assays (ELISAs), second-generation ELISAs, and confirmatory Western blotting. Direct detection assays include p24 antigen capture ELISA and DNA/RNA assays via PCR, *in situ* hybridization, or other hybridization assays. In infants under 18 months of age, anti-HIV antibody may be transplacental and therefore is not diagnostic of HIV infection (although a negative result suggests that the infant is uninfected). The diagnostic method of choice in infants, therefore, is HIV DNA PCR on peripheral blood lymphocytes.[143] Other laboratory tests that may be useful in the evaluation for HIV infection include complete blood cell counts with platelets, CD4+ lymphocyte counts, serum chemistries, and urinalysis. Plasma HIV RNA (viral load) studies are useful in monitoring response to therapy, and are the best indicator of risk for disease progression in children.[150]

The mainstays of therapy for patients with HIV infection are a combination of medications encompassing one to three main categories. These categories include nucleoside and nucleotide analogue reverse transcriptase inhibitors (NRTIs or NtRTIs, including AZT, didanosine or ddI, stavudine or d4T, lamivudine or 3TC, zalcitabine or ddC, abacavir or ABV, emtricitabine, zidovudine, and tenofovir), non-nucleoside analogue reverse transcriptase inhibitors (NNRTIs, including nevirapine, efavirenz, and etravirine), and HIV protease inhibitors (PIs, including atazanavir, darunavir, fosamprenavir, nelfinavir, ritonavir, indinavir, saquinavir, tipranavir, lopinavir/ritonavir, and lopinavir).[137,151] Fusion inhibitors (enfuvirtide, maraviroc) interfere with the penetration of HIV into the target cells, and integrase inhibitors (raltegravir) block the viral integrase and insertion of the DNA copy of the viral genome into the host cell chromosome.[151] In addition, HIV vaccines intended to boost immunity toward the virus have been studied,[152] and adjunctive therapies such as intravenous immune globulin and cytokine therapy are occasionally utilized.

Special considerations in treating young children infected with HIV include differences in body size, composition, and drug metabolism, distribution and elimination. (Updated treatment guidelines for pediatric HIV infection can be found at: www.aidsinfo.nih.gov/guidelines.) In infants, the best outcome is seen when antiretroviral therapy is immediately initiated after diagnosis. In older children or adolescents, the decision to start therapy is based on the viral load, CD4+ lymphocyte count, and clinical status. Survival in HIV-infected children has improved notably with the introduction of cART, with a decrease in disease progression and mortality.[153] However, children seem to be more likely than adults to develop metabolic side-effects of therapy, including lipodystrophy, dyslipidemia, insulin resistance, mitochondrial toxicity with lactic acidemia, and decreased bone mineral density. Interestingly, HIV-associated growth retardation, manifested by muscle wasting and decreased linear growth, appears to be minimized with the use of cART in children, although the long-term significance of these findings is unclear.[154]

Key References

Fatahzadeh M, Schwartz RA. Human herpes simplex virus infections: epidemiology, pathogenesis, symptomatology, diagnosis and management. *J Am Acad Dermatol.* 2007;57:737–763.

Mammas IN, Sourvinos G, Spandidos DA. Human papilloma virus (HPV) infection in children and adolescents. *Eur J Pediatr.* 2009;168:267–273.

Nasser M, Fedorowicz Z, Khoshnevisan MH, Shahiri Tabarestani M. Acyclovir for treating primary herpetic gingivostomatitis. *Cochrane Database Syst Rev.* 2008 Oct 8;4:CD006700.

Paintsil E, Andiman WA. Update on successes and challenges regarding mother-to-child transmission of HIV. *Curr Opin Pediatr.* 2009;21(1):94–101.

Reynolds MA, Chaves SS, Harpaz R, et al. The impact of the varicella vaccination program on herpes zoster epidemiology in the United States: a review. *J Infect Dis.* 2008;197(Suppl 2):S224–S227.

16 Exanthematous Diseases of Childhood

Several viral and bacterial illnesses may be accompanied by localized or generalized skin eruptions called *exanthems*. These eruptions may be the first manifestation of a disorder, and frequently are the reason for parents and patients to pursue medical evaluation. Prompt recognition and diagnosis of exanthems is desirable and may dictate that other examinations be performed to assess for systemic associations. Although identification of the exact infectious agent is not always practical or possible, knowledge of the most common causes of the various exanthems is important from an epidemiologic perspective. For instance, when diagnosing a child with a parvovirus B19-related exanthematous disease, consideration of at-risk contacts (i.e., gravid females, individuals with hemolysis or conditions resulting in decreased red blood cell production) is vital.

The majority of childhood exanthems are caused by viruses, and less often by bacterial or rickettsial agents. Most childhood exanthems are diagnosed and managed by primary care providers, and thus a thorough familiarity with both classic and atypical exanthems is desirable for the pediatric primary care practitioner. When evaluating the patient with an exanthem, several features should be considered, including the morphology of individual lesions, the distribution pattern, prodromal and concurrent symptoms, known exposures, associated enanthem (eruption of the mucous membranes), local epidemiology, and the findings of a thorough review of systems and physical examination. Whereas some exanthematous processes present with a characteristic patterning of lesion morphology and distribution, others may reveal no pathognomonic features, and the cutaneous findings must be taken into consideration along with the overall presentation of the patient. Exanthems may be divided into erythematous, vesicular, and papular forms, and have also been invariably described as morbilliform ('measles-like'), rubelliform ('rubella-like'), scarlatiniform ('scarlet fever-like'), or urticarial.[1] Pustular and petechial changes may occasionally be noted.

The classic childhood exanthems are listed in Table 16.1. These disorders were originally classified with a numerical designation in the early 1900s. Since then, much has been learned about the etiologic agents of the classic exanthems, and several newer exanthematous disorders have been described. This chapter includes a discussion of the classic exanthems, varicella, infectious mononucleosis, and exanthems due to enteroviruses, *Mycoplasma*, and rickettsial agents. In addition, nonspecific viral exanthems will be discussed, as will some 'atypical' exanthems, including papular acrodermatitis of childhood, unilateral laterothoracic exanthem, and papular-purpuric gloves and socks syndrome. Kawasaki disease, which may have clinical overlap with multiple exanthematous disorders, is discussed in Chapter 21. Acute generalized exanthematous pustulosis (AGEP), another exanthematous disorder, is discussed in Chapter 20.

Varicella (chickenpox)

Varicella-zoster virus (VZV) is a member of the herpesvirus family, and the causative agent of both varicella (chicken pox) and herpes zoster (shingles, Ch. 15). Varicella results from primary infection with VZV, and is a highly communicable human disease. Once acquired, VZV becomes permanently established in the sensory ganglia in a latent form, with intermittent reactivation in a dermatomal distribution, resulting in herpes zoster.[2] Although acute varicella is usually a self-limited infection, prior to extensive use of the varicella vaccine most children had upward of 250–500 skin lesions, approximately 9000–11 000 children were hospitalized annually, and up to 100 individuals per year died of the disease or its complications.[3,4]

VZV is found worldwide, and annual epidemics occur most often during late winter and spring.[5] Varicella is highly contagious, and is usually spread in the period between the prodrome and the first 3 days of the skin eruption.[6] VZV is transmitted via respiratory droplets, then enters regional lymph nodes and, eventually, a viremia ensues with more widespread dissemination. Primary infection elicits a humoral immune response, with production of IgA, IgM, and IgG anti-VZV antibodies, the latter of which help to protect against reinfection.[5] Patients are considered contagious until at least 5 days after onset of the rash, or until all existing lesions are dry and crusted.

A live attenuated varicella vaccine (Oka strain) was introduced in 1995, and in 1996 the Advisory Committee on Immunization Practices (ACIP) recommended universal 1-dose vaccination of all children at age 12–18 months, with catchup vaccination of all susceptible children before age 13 years.[4] The ACIP and the American Academy of Pediatrics (AAP) have expanded their recommendations to include use of the vaccine for postexposure prophylaxis and for some immunocompromised children.[3] The vaccine is also indicated in adults who are susceptible to varicella. Overall, the vaccine has been quite effective in decreasing the overall incidence of varicella, and in vaccinees who develop breakthrough disease, the disease tends to be milder with fewer lesions that may remain papular rather than becoming vesicular.[3] In a 6-year case–control study of the effectiveness of the varicella vaccine over time, the effectiveness in the year after vaccination (97%) was greater than in years 2–8 after vaccination (84%), although most cases of breakthrough disease in vaccinees were mild.[7] Another study of the effectiveness of a one- versus two-vaccination regimen revealed high

Numerical designation	Name(s)	Agent(s)	Comment
1	Measles, rubeola	Measles virus (paramyxovirus)	Declining incidence with vaccination; occasional epidemics of imported cases in USA
2	Scarlet fever, scarlatina	GABHS	Toxin-mediated
3	German measles, rubella	Rubella virus (togavirus)	Rare with vaccination
4	Filatow–Dukes disease	?SA	No longer considered a distinct entity
5	Erythema infectiosum, fifth disease, slapped cheek disease	Parvovirus B19	Patients not contagious once rash is present
6	Exanthem subitum, roseola infantum, sixth disease	HHV-6 and HHV-7	Diffuse rash appears after abrupt defervescence

Table 16.1 The 'classic' childhood exanthems

GABHS, Group A β-hemolytic streptococcus; SA, *Staphylococcus aureus*; HHV, human herpesvirus.

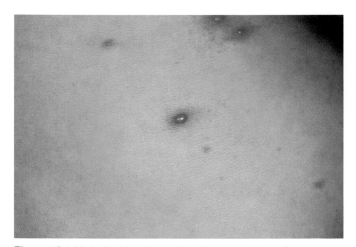

Figure 16.1 Varicella. Note the early lesions, consisting of erythematous macules and papules, and the well-developed vesicular lesion.

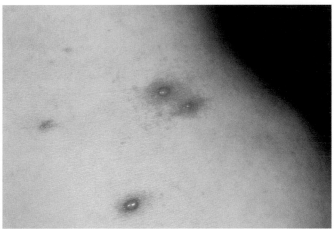

Figure 16.2 Varicella. These well-developed lesions demonstrate why they have been likened to 'dewdrops on a rose petal'.

vaccine efficacy over 10 years for both groups (94.4% and 98.3%, respectively), and again, breakthrough disease was mild.[8] A decline in varicella-related hospitalizations for invasive group A β-hemolytic streptococcal (GABHS) infections has been documented between the period of the pre-vaccine era and that of widespread vaccine use.[9] Although some studies have demonstrated lower effectiveness of the varicella vaccine than expected, overall, the data appear to support its universal use. In 2006, because of insufficient population immunity to prevent community transmission, the ACIP and AAP changed the varicella vaccine policy, recommending a universal 2-dose vaccination program.[10]

Primary varicella begins with a prodrome of fever, chills, malaise, headache, arthralgia, and myalgia. At 24–48 h later, the earliest skin lesions become evident, initially as a red macule or papule (Fig. 16.1) that progresses rapidly to a vesicular phase. The fully developed lesion has been likened to a 'dewdrop on a rose petal' (Fig. 16.2). Varicella lesions present initially on the scalp, face, or trunk and then spread to the extremities. Older lesions crust over and new lesions continue to develop, resulting in the pathognomonic finding of lesions in various stages being present at the same time (Fig. 16.3). New lesions continue to develop for 3–4 days, and by day 6, most lesions have crusted over. Patients with sunburn or dermatitis may develop a more severe exanthem. An associated enanthem may be present, consisting of painful erosions in the oropharynx, conjunctivae, or vaginal mucosae. The lesions of

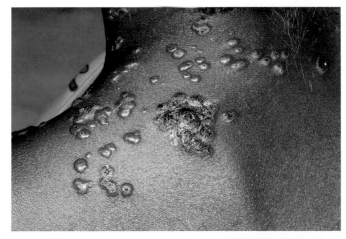

Figure 16.3 Varicella. Various stages are present in this HIV-infected patient with varicella, including vesicles and crusted papules.

varicella heal with hypopigmentation (Fig. 16.4) and scarring (Fig. 16.5), especially at sites of the initial lesions.

Varicella tends to be a mild, self-limited disease in most immunocompetent hosts. Complications, however, may occur. The most common complication is secondary bacterial superinfection,

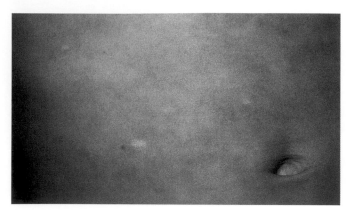

Figure 16.4 Varicella scarring. Hypopigmented macules and scars are present in this patient with a history of varicella.

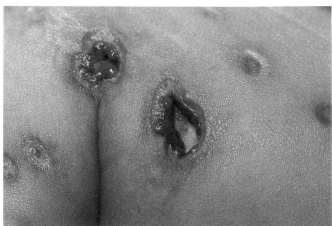

Figure 16.6 Varicella, complicated. Deep, ulcerative lesions occurred in this young girl with underlying immunodeficiency and secondary infection of the skin with *Streptococcus pyogenes*.

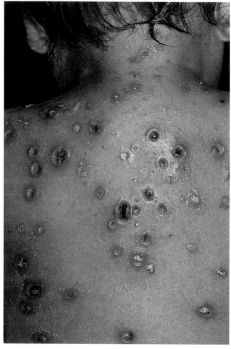

Figure 16.5 Varicella scarring. Large, deep scars are present in this patient who had secondary bacterial infection of her primary varicella lesions.

usually due to *Staphylococcus aureus* or GABHS.[11] Invasive GABHS infections, including streptococcal toxic shock syndrome and necrotizing fasciitis, may rarely occur. Secondary bacterial infection usually presents as isolated secondary fever or localized symptoms, such as bulla (large blister) formation or cellulitis. *Varicella gangrenosa* is diagnosed when an area reveals rapidly progressing erythema, induration, and pain.[5] Peripheral gangrene may occur in the distal extremities.[12] Other skin-related complications include deep ulcerative lesions (Fig. 16.6), subcutaneous abscesses, and regional lymphadenitis. Patients under the age of 5 years who live in a household with older children, seem to be at greatest risk for bacterial complications.[11] In patients who develop secondary bacterial infection, bacteremia may occur, as may pneumonia, arthritis, or osteomyelitis.

Second to bacterial superinfection, the most frequent complication in patients with primary varicella is neurologic involvement. This may present as encephalitis, meningoencephalitis, cerebellar ataxia, transverse myelitis, or Guillain–Barré syndrome. Reye syndrome was a fairly common complication of varicella in the past, before the association with salicylates was identified. Reye syndrome (acute encephalopathy and fatty degeneration of the viscera) presents with decreased level of consciousness, vomiting, and abnormalities in liver function. The incidence of this complication has fallen dramatically over recent years. Varicella pneumonia is the most common serious complication in adults, but is rare in healthy children.[2,5] When it occurs during the course of childhood varicella, it is usually bacterial in origin. Thrombocytopenia, arthritis, uveitis, nephritis, myocarditis, pancreatitis, and hepatitis may also occasionally occur. Purpura fulminans is a rare and life-threatening complication of varicella, and disseminated intravascular coagulopathy may occasionally occur.

Immunocompromised hosts with varicella, including those with leukemia, lymphoma, or HIV infection, those receiving corticosteroids, and those with a history of organ or bone marrow transplantation, may have more serious disease and a higher incidence of complications. These individuals have an increased risk of disseminated varicella, lung disease, thrombocytopenia, and other organ involvement. Bacterial superinfection may also occur with increased frequency, and hemorrhagic complications of the disease are more common. Varicella during pregnancy poses an increased risk of serious disease to both the mother and the fetus (see Ch. 2). Pregnant females have a higher incidence of varicella pneumonia, and mortality from the disease is increased.

The diagnosis of primary varicella is usually based on the history and clinical findings. Laboratory confirmation, when desired, can be performed by either virologic or serologic methods. Virologic methods include direct and indirect immunofluorescence studies, which are performed on tissue (i.e., cells scraped from the base of a fresh vesicle, or organ biopsy tissue in patients with disseminated disease). These studies have the advantages of being both rapid and sensitive.[13,14] Tzanck smears on skin scrapings identify multinucleated giant cells and confirm the diagnosis of herpesvirus infection, but are not specific for VZV. Cell culture is unequivocally confirmatory, but not ideal for VZV given the prolonged time necessary for cytopathic effects to appear. Other virologic methods include hybridization and PCR assays. Serologic studies for diagnosing VZV infection include acute and convalescent IgM and IgG antibody titers.

The treatment of varicella in otherwise-healthy children is usually symptomatic, with the goals being control of pain and pruritus, and prevention of secondary superinfection. Supportive therapies include oral antihistamines for pruritus, acetaminophen for fever or pain, and topical care. Useful topical regimens may include cool compresses, oatmeal baths, and application of topical products such as bacitracin ointment, calamine lotion, pramoxine-containing preparations, or menthol-camphor (Sarna) lotion. Antibiotics should be given if secondary bacterial infection is present.

The decision regarding the use of antiviral therapy for primary varicella depends on several factors, including host immune status, the extent of the infection, and timing of the diagnosis. Acyclovir, famciclovir, and valacyclovir are antiviral agents licensed for treatment of VZV infections, although the latter two are not approved for primary varicella. Oral acyclovir has been suggested in some studies to decrease the severity of primary VZV infection, including a decrease in the days of fever, number of days of new lesion formation, total number of lesions, and pruritus. In immunocompetent hosts, however, antiviral therapy for primary varicella is generally not recommended for routine use. In a review of published studies on acyclovir treatment of varicella in otherwise healthy children and adolescents, a reduction in the number of days with fever was noted, but the results were inconsistent with respect to the number of days to no new lesions, maximum number of lesions, and number of days to relief of itching.[14] In addition, no differences in the incidence of varicella complications between acyclovir and placebo groups were consistently noted.[15] Oral acyclovir should be considered, however, for healthy individuals who are at risk for moderate or severe disease, such as those over 12 years of age, those with chronic skin or lung disorders, and those receiving chronic therapy with salicylates or corticosteroids.[16] When used in the treatment of varicella in otherwise healthy patients, acyclovir should be started within 24 h of the appearance of the rash. The use of oral acyclovir for pregnant females with uncomplicated varicella remains controversial, although some experts recommend its use for those who develop it during the 2nd or 3rd trimesters.

In immunocompromised children, intravenous antiviral therapy with acyclovir should be administered, and is most effective when initiated early in the course of the disease (within 24–72 h of the onset of the rash). Some experts endorse high-dose oral acyclovir in selected immunocompromised individuals who are perceived to be at a lower risk for severe disseminated varicella.[16] In susceptible individuals with a known exposure to VZV, options include administration of varicella-zoster immune globulin (VariZIG) or varicella vaccine. VariZIG is a high-titer preparation of VZV immunoglobulin (IgG), and which is given via the intramuscular route. It is recommended for susceptible high-risk individuals and pregnant females who have been exposed to VZV (Table 16.2). VariZIG is best given within 48 h of the exposure, but can be given up to 96 h later.[5,16]

Rubeola (measles)

In the pre-vaccine era, more than 500 000 cases of measles, or rubeola, were reported annually in the USA. After introduction of a live-virus vaccine in 1963, a significant reduction in the incidence of infection was noted. However, a dramatic resurgence occurred from the period of 1989–1990, and during this period, the highest mortality since 1977 was noted.[17,18] Those affected most during the measles resurgence were preschool-age children from the inner-city areas, especially unvaccinated, low-income patients. A majority of the deaths occurring from measles infection during this period

Table 16.2 Indications for varicella-zoster immune globulin (VariZIG)

Types of exposure to VZV:
 Residing in same household as infected patient
 Playmate: face-to-face indoor play
 Hospital: varicella in roommate, face-to-face contact with infected staff member or patient, visit by a person deemed contagious with varicella; intimate contact with person deemed contagious with zoster
 Newborn: onset of varicella (not herpes zoster) in mother from 5 days or less before delivery or within 48 hours after delivery

Candidates for VariZIG:
 Immunocompromised child without history of varicella or varicella immunization
 Susceptible pregnant female
 Newborn infant whose mother develops varicella (see above)
 Hospitalized premature infant:
  ≥28 weeks' gestation, if mother lacks reliable history of varicella or serologic evidence of antibodies
  <28 weeks' gestation or birthweight 1000 g or less, regardless of maternal history of varicella or serologic status

Adapted from American Academy of Pediatrics (2009).[16] VZV, varicella-zoster virus.

occurred in children aged 5 years or younger.[18] Other target populations during the measles resurgence included vaccinated school-age children and college students, probably owing to the insufficiency of a single vaccine dose and waning immunity.

In response to the measles resurgence of the 1980s, the Committee on Infectious Diseases of the American Academy of Pediatrics (AAP) and the Advisory Committee on Immunization Practices (ACIP) recommended an amendment to the prior vaccination schedule, and suggested two doses of measles vaccination rather than one.[18,19] The current recommendation for measles vaccination calls for a two-dose schedule, with the first given at 12–15 months and the second at 4–6 years of age, and re-vaccination of children 11–12 years of age or older who received only one previous dose of measles vaccine.[20] Changes in the measles vaccination strategy resulted in a markedly diminished incidence of the disease in the USA, with 100 cases reported in 1999.[21] Although the incidence in the USA declined to extremely low levels compared with the pre-vaccine era, measles continues to be a major health problem worldwide, with the World Health Organization estimating around 700 000 deaths per year from the disease.[22] Of the 100 cases reported in the USA in 1999, 33% were imported from other countries.[21] In developing countries, infants under 9 months of age, who are too young to have received vaccination, have a high incidence of measles with more multisystem involvement and a greater risk of death.[22] Importantly, sporadic epidemics of primarily importation-associated measles in the USA continue to occur. During January–July 2008, 131 measles cases were reported to the Centers for Disease Control, and these occurred primarily in unvaccinated school-aged children.[23] The majority of these children were eligible for vaccination, but had parents who chose not to have them vaccinated.

Measles is caused by a single-stranded RNA virus in the family Paramyxoviridae. Infection begins in the nasopharyngeal epithelium, and less commonly through the conjunctivae. From the initial site of infection, the virus enters the lymph nodes and lymphatics and multiplies within the reticuloendothelial system, with a subsequent viremia.[22] The virus is then disseminated to multiple lymphoid tissues and other organs, including the skin, liver, and gastrointestinal tract.[24] Measles immunity includes cell-mediated, humoral and mucosal responses. Measles antibodies are responsible for protection from future infection or reinfection.[22]

Measles classically presents with fever and the three Cs: cough, coryza, and conjunctivitis. The pathognomonic enanthem, Koplik spots, usually occurs during this prodromal period and presents with punctuate, gray-white to erythematous papules distributed on the buccal mucosa (Fig. 16.7). The skin eruption of measles usually begins 2–4 days following the prodrome. It begins on the face (Fig. 16.8), especially the forehead, hairline, and behind the ears, and spreads downward onto the trunk (Fig. 16.9) and extremities. The lesions are erythematous to purple-red macules and papules, which may become confluent and which fade in the same order as their appearance, leaving behind coppery macules and desquamation.

Complications of measles include pneumonia, bronchitis, otitis, gastroenteritis, myocarditis, and encephalitis.

Modified measles is measles occurring in a previously vaccinated individual. In this situation, the prodrome is milder and of shorter duration, the exanthem is less prominent, and Koplik spots may be absent.[25] This presentation of measles may pose a diagnostic challenge given the non-pathognomonic presentation. *Atypical measles* occurs rarely in contemporary times, and is seen in individuals exposed to natural measles following vaccination with the killed measles vaccines. These vaccines were utilized for a short period in the 1960s in the USA, and for more variable periods of time in other countries, including Canada and Sweden.[25] It has occasionally been reported in children who received the live attenuated vaccine.[26] Atypical measles presents with high fever, headaches, and myalgias, and eventually the measles rash and often pneumonia. Hemorrhagic features may be present and the exanthem may be confused with Rocky Mountain spotted fever. Subacute sclerosing panencephalitis is a delayed neurodegenerative disease characterized by seizures, personality changes, coma, and occasionally death. It occurs many years later in 1 in 100 000 patients with measles.[27]

The diagnosis of measles is traditionally made based upon clinical presentation, with laboratory confirmation if necessary. Acute and convalescent serologic studies documenting a fourfold increase in titer confirm the diagnosis of measles.[28] Polymerase chain reaction (PCR) and semi-quantitative real-time PCR assays have been developed, the latter being quite sensitive and specific and potentially useful in situations where early and rapid diagnosis is vital.[29] The treatment of uncomplicated measles is largely supportive, as specific antiviral therapies do not exist. Ribavirin, a synthetic nucleoside analogue useful in the treatment of other paramyxovirus (i.e., respiratory syncytial virus) infections, has been utilized in severely ill or immunocompromised patients.[27,30] Antibiotics are useful only

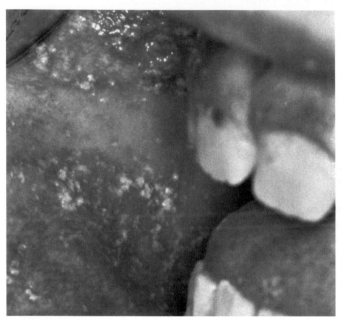

Figure 16.7 Koplik spots. Gray-white papules of the buccal mucosa in a patient with measles.

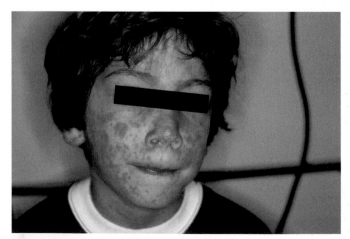

Figure 16.8 Rubeola (measles). Erythematous macules and patches of the face early in the course of the disease.

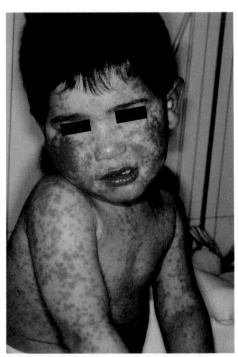

Figure 16.9 Rubeola (measles). Intensely erythematous patches of the face with cephalocaudad spread onto the trunk and extremities.

in patients with secondary bacterial infections, such as otitis media or bacterial pneumonia. Vitamin A supplementation has been recommended by the World Health Organization and the United Nations International Children's Emergency Fund for children with measles who reside in areas where vitamin A deficiency is a recognized problem, or where the measles case fatality rate is 1% or greater.[31] In these instances, vitamin A appears to reduce mortality and ameliorate the severity of diarrhea, possibly through a protective action on the epithelial lining of the gastrointestinal tract, increased mucus secretion, and enhanced local barriers to infection.[32] Hospitalized patients with measles should be kept in respiratory isolation for 4 days from the onset of the rash. Most patients will recover completely without sequelae, and have lifelong immune protection against reinfection.

Scarlet fever

Scarlet fever (scarlatina) is a bacterial exanthem that may, at times, be confused with a variety of viral exanthematous diseases. It is caused by GABHS, and is primarily a disease of children between the ages of 1 and 10 years. It is very rarely diagnosed in infants. Transmission of GABHS is usually via respiratory secretions. Epidemiologic changes over time in the types of streptococcal pyrogenic exotoxin (SPE) produced by the organism have been associated with changes in the severity of this disease. The shift from SPE-A- to SPE-B- and SPE-C-producing strains, which was seen early in the twentieth century, has paralleled the decrease in morbidity and mortality from scarlet fever, as well as the decline in incidence and severity of rheumatic fever in the USA.[33] However, a more recent resurgence in acute rheumatic fever has been observed in the USA, with several epidemics of disease occurring among focal segments of the population, and isolates in these outbreaks revealed more virulent organisms rich in mucin and M protein expression.[34]

Scarlet fever presents with fever, throat pain, headache, and chills, along with cutaneous findings. It is less commonly associated with streptococcal skin infection rather than pharyngitis. The primary distinction between streptococcal pharyngitis and scarlet fever is the accompanying exanthem present in the latter. Oropharyngeal inspection reveals tonsillopharyngeal erythema, exudates, and petechial macules of the palate. During the first few days of illness, the tongue may reveal a white coating with red and edematous papillae projecting through (white strawberry tongue). By the 4th or 5th day, the coating peels off, leaving behind a red, glistening tongue studded with prominent papillae (red strawberry tongue).

The differential diagnosis of streptococcal pharyngitis includes infection with viral agents (especially mononucleosis), *Mycoplasma*, *Chlamydia*, and *Arcanobacterium haemolyticum*. In adolescents, the differential diagnosis should include groups C and G *Streptococcus* sp. and *Neisseria gonorrhoeae*,[35] and in developing countries *Corynebacterium diphtheriae* may be implicated. *Arcanobacterium haemolyticum*, formerly known as *Corynebacterium haemolyticum*, is a Gram-positive bacillus that most often infects adolescents and young adults, and may result in a syndrome of pharyngitis and a scarlatiniform exanthem.[36] The pharyngitis in these patients is usually severe (occasionally mistaken for diphtheria), and the exanthem may also occasionally mimic toxic shock syndrome, measles, urticaria, or erythema multiforme.[37,38]

Tender anterior cervical adenopathy is frequently present in patients with scarlet fever, and rhinorrhea and cough are usually absent. Some experts argue that presence of the latter two findings is a negative factor for the diagnosis of GABHS infection.[35] The exanthem of scarlet fever presents as a fine, erythematous, macular and papular eruption (Fig. 16.10) that has been described as

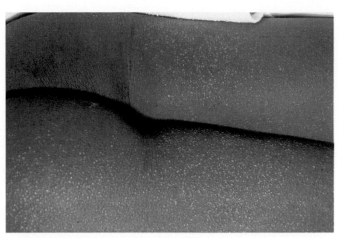

Figure 16.10 Scarlet fever. Diffuse erythema with small, punctuate papules. This eruption has a sandpapery texture to palpation.

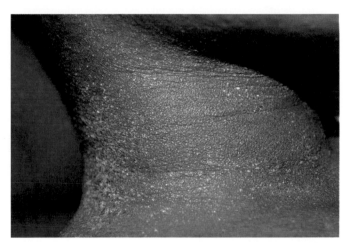

Figure 16.11 Scarlet fever in dark-skinned patient. The rash in this patient resembles 'gooseflesh'. Note the early desquamation at some sites.

'sandpapery'. It involves the trunk and extremities, and may be accentuated in flexural areas with a petechial component ('Pastia's lines'). In darker-skinned individuals, the exanthem of scarlet fever may be more difficult to recognize, and may consist only of punctate papules resembling cutis anserina (goose flesh) (Fig. 16.11). Circumoral pallor may be a useful clinical sign, and is visualized as a rim of pallor encircling the perioral area. The exanthem generally resolves over 4–5 days, and may heal with thick sheets of desquamation, especially over the hands, feet, toes, and fingers (Fig. 16.12). An interesting observation is that the SPEs produced by GABHS contribute to the exanthem by their ability to stimulate a delayed-type hypersensitivity response, which requires prior exposure of the host to the organism.[39]

Scarlet fever is diagnosed based on the clinical presentation in conjunction with results of laboratory testing. The gold standard laboratory examination is throat culture with growth of GABHS. Rapid antigen detection ('rapid strep' testing), when properly performed, has a high sensitivity and specificity.[35] In addition, antistreptococcal serologies may occasionally be useful. Complications of scarlet fever include pneumonia, pericarditis, meningitis,

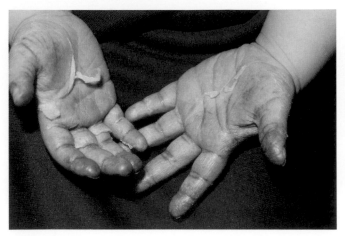

Figure 16.12 Post-scarlet fever desquamation. Extensive peeling of the hands and digits occurred in this patient following treatment for scarlet fever.

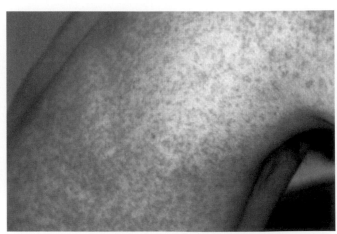

Figure 16.13 Rubella. Nonspecific, 'rose-pink' macules and papules on the trunk of an adolescent male with German measles.

hepatitis, glomerulonephritis, and rheumatic fever. Although the symptoms of streptococcal pharyngitis and scarlet fever will often improve spontaneously, treatment more rapidly alleviates symptoms and, more importantly, is the primary mode of prevention for the subsequent occurrence of acute rheumatic fever (ARF). The prevailing theory regarding ARF prevention is that antimicrobial therapy should be started within 9 days from the onset of symptoms of GABHS pharyngitis.[35,40]

The drug of choice for treatment of scarlet fever is penicillin V. Although amoxicillin or ampicillin is frequently used, they have no microbiologic advantage over penicillin.[40] In penicillin-allergic patients, erythromycin or another macrolide (i.e., clarithromycin or azithromycin) is indicated. Other options include a first-generation cephalosporin (although the possibility of cross-reaction in penicillin-allergic patients must be considered) or intramuscular penicillin G, which has the advantage of not being compliance-dependent, but the disadvantage of being painful during administration.[40]

Rubella (German measles)

Rubella, or German measles, is a viral exanthematous disease with a worldwide distribution. The incidence of rubella has greatly decreased since widespread rubella vaccination began in the USA in 1969. Before that time, epidemics occurred every 6–9 years, and major epidemics or pandemics occurred every 10–20 years.[41] The primary goal of the rubella vaccination program was to prevent fetal infection, which may have various effects including miscarriage, stillbirth, and congenital rubella syndrome (see Ch. 2). Although reported rubella cases in the USA are now quite low, outbreaks still occur, primarily among Hispanic adults, most of whom were born outside of the country and are unvaccinated.[42] In 2005, the USA was the first country in the Americas to declare elimination of endemic rubella virus transmission, and the Pan American Health Organization continues to pursue its goal of rubella elimination in all of the Americas and the Caribbean.[43]

Rubella is caused by an RNA virus in the Togaviridae family. Humans are the only source of infection, and postnatal disease is spread through direct or droplet contact from nasopharyngeal secretions. Up to 50% of cases of rubella are asymptomatic, and mild, self-limited disease is common. The incubation period ranges from 14 to 23 days.

Prodromal symptoms may occur, especially in adolescents and adults, and include low-grade fever, headache, malaise, eye pain, myalgias, sore throat, rhinorrhea, and cough. The prodrome usually presents 2–5 days before the exanthem appears. The skin eruption consists of erythematous to 'rose-pink' macules and papules (Fig. 16.13), which tend to become confluent and which most commonly involve the face and trunk. The eruption spreads in a cephalocaudad manner, and begins to involute after 1–3 days, fading in the same order in which it appeared. After severe rubella eruptions, a fine flaky desquamation may be observed in areas of maximum involvement.

Generalized lymphadenopathy often occurs, especially in the suboccipital, postauricular, and cervical regions. Although this pattern of lymph node enlargement is highly characteristic of rubella, it is not pathognomonic, and may occur in other disorders including measles, varicella, adenovirus infection, and mononucleosis. Arthralgias and arthritis are common, especially in females in whom they occur up to 52% of the time.[44] The most common joints affected are those of the fingers, wrists, and knees. Complete resolution of the joint symptoms may take up to several weeks, and chronic arthritis occasionally develops. A characteristic enanthem, Forschheimer spots, may be present in patients with rubella and presents with erythematous and petechial macules on the soft palate.[45] Other complications of rubella include encephalitis (which occurs in 1 in 6000 patients), myocarditis, pericarditis, and hepatitis.[28] Anemia, neutropenia, and thrombocytopenia may also occur, as may hemolytic-uremic syndrome.

A clinical diagnosis of rubella is difficult to make, given the potential overlap with multiple other exanthematous diseases. Serologic tests are most useful in confirming the diagnosis of rubella. The presence of rubella-specific IgM antibody indicates recent infection, as does a fourfold or greater increase in titer between acute and convalescent serum taken 1–2 weeks apart.[28,46] The virus can be isolated from nasal specimens plated onto appropriate cell culture media. The treatment of postnatal rubella is generally supportive. Hospitalized patients require contact isolation (and non-hospitalized children should be excused from school or day care) for 7 days following onset of the rash.

The ongoing efforts of global rubella eradication campaigns will hopefully result in eventual worldwide elimination of the disease. Continued efforts to ensure the immunity of women of childbearing age will help to decrease the incidence of vertical transmission and congenital rubella syndrome.

Dukes' disease

In 1900, Dukes described what was believed to be a unique exanthem and contrasted it from rubella and scarlet fever.[47] This disorder was termed 'fourth disease,' and subsequently became known as Filatow–Dukes' disease given a similar description by Filatow 15 years prior. The exanthem was described as bright red papules with a diffuse distribution, skin tenderness, and fever, and there was significant overlap with other exanthematous diseases, including staphylococcal scalded skin syndrome, scarlet fever, and rubella. Significant controversy followed the initial descriptions of fourth disease, and some authors propose that a distinct disorder never existed.[48] The possibility that epidermolytic toxin-producing staphylococci were the etiologic agent for the disorder described in the original reports has been suggested.[49] In general, researchers and practitioners alike have abandoned the idea of Filatow–Dukes' disease representing a distinct entity.

Erythema infectiosum

Erythema infectiosum (EI, fifth disease) is a common childhood exanthematous illness caused by parvovirus B19 (B19). Although parvoviruses are ubiquitous in nature and may cause significant disease in a wide range of animals, B19 is the only one resulting in human disease.[50] Several disorders have been linked to B19 infection in humans (Table 16.3), including EI, arthritis, aplastic crises, and fetal hydrops. B19 infection is common in most countries, and in the USA, 60% of adults are seropositive for the virus.[51] Infection is most common in school-age children.

In patients with classic EI, B19 infection is transmitted via the respiratory tract, and is followed by a viremia that ends after 5–7 days with the production of IgM anti-B19 antibody. Prodromal symptoms such as headaches, fever, and chills are common during the viremic phase.[52] Respiratory symptoms may also be present. IgG antibody appears during the third week of illness and coincides with the appearance of the rash and arthralgias, and hence patients with the cutaneous findings of EI are not considered infectious. Outbreaks of EI occur primarily during the winter and spring.

EI is the most recognizable B19-associated manifestation. It is also known as 'slapped cheek' disease given the characteristic fiery-red facial erythema (Fig. 16.14) that occurs 2–3 days following the prodromal symptoms. The cheeks are most prominently affected, with the nasal bridge and perioral areas usually being spared. This phase of the illness has been termed the first stage, and is subsequently followed by stages two and three. The differential diagnosis of the initial eruption of EI includes phototoxic reaction and systemic lupus erythematosus.

During stage two, the patient develops a lacy, reticulated eruption on the extremities and trunk 1–4 days following the facial rash. This eruption may be pruritic, and is often evanescent. It often begins with a confluent pattern, followed by central clearing, which results in the lacy and reticulated appearance (Figs 16.15, 16.16). The palms and soles are usually spared. The rash of the second stage of EI tends to fade over 2–3 weeks, but may intermittently recur in response to environmental stimuli, including sunlight, warm temperatures (i.e., a hot bath), or physical activity. This intermittent waxing and waning represents the third stage of EI, and the duration is variable, usually 1–3 weeks.

Joint symptoms occur in 8–10% of children with EI, but in up to 60% of adults with primary B19 infection, especially females.[50,53,54] The most commonly involved joints include the metacarpophalangeal joints, proximal interphalangeal joints, knees, wrists, and ankles. For most patients, the joint symptoms are transient and self-limited. Occasionally, affected children develop a chronic arthritis.[55] Some experts have suggested a potential association between B19 infection and rheumatic arthritis or other connective tissue diseases, although the strength of this association remains unclear.

B19 has a remarkable affinity for erythroid precursors, binding to a receptor known as P antigen (globoside).[56] Direct infection of the red blood cell precursors results in a transient arrest in red blood cell production and resultant transient anemia. Transient aplastic crises may occur in patients suffering from disorders of decreased red blood cell production or increased red blood cell destruction or loss. Predisposing disorders include iron deficiency anemia, spherocytosis, sickle cell disease, thalassemia, glucose-6-phosphate dehydrogenase deficiency, and pyruvate kinase deficiency. Although these episodes may be asymptomatic, with spontaneous recovery, severe involvement may result in chills, pallor, weakness, fatigue, vasoocclusive crises, or congestive heart failure. Treatment with red blood cell transfusions may be indicated and, for some patients, is life-saving.

Table 16.3 Clinical associations with parvovirus B19 infection
Asymptomatic infection
Exanthematous disorders
Erythema infectiosum (fifth disease)
Papular-purpuric gloves and socks syndrome
Asymmetric periflexural exanthem
'Bathing trunk' exanthem
Petechial exanthems
Other disorders
Arthritis
Transient aplastic crises
Chronic anemia
Refractory anemia following solid organ or stem cell transplantation
Fetal hydrops
Vasculitis
Neurologic disease
Rheumatologic disease

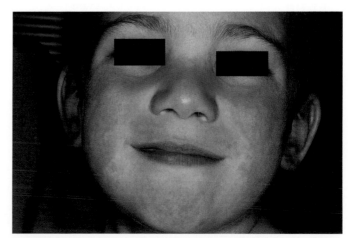

Figure 16.14 Erythema infectiosum. Erythema of the bilateral cheeks, which has been likened to a 'slapped cheeks' appearance.

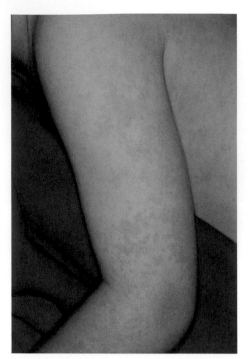

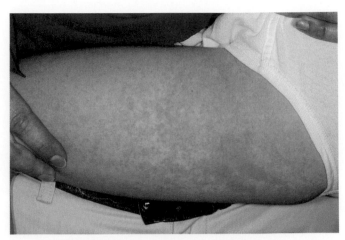

Figure 16.16 Erythema infectiosum. Patchy erythema with reticulate changes of the inner thigh in a patient with erythema infectiosum.

Figure 16.15 Erythema infectiosum. Reticulate erythema on the upper arm of a patient with erythema infectiosum.

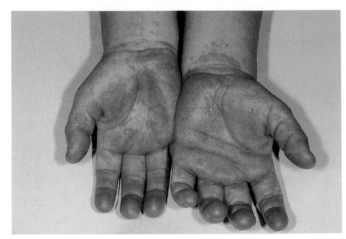

Figure 16.17 Papular-purpuric gloves and socks syndrome. Petechial purpura of the palms in a patient with parvovirus B19 infection.

Because B19 can cross the placenta, fetal infection is possible in nonimmune females with acute infection. With time it has become clear that B19 may result in a variety of fetal effects, occasionally even death. This epidemiologic consideration is important in caring for pediatric patients with B19-associated disorders. Fetal effects of B19 infection may include anemia (ranging from mild and self-limited to severe), high-output congestive heart failure, hydrops fetalis (generalized edema with ascites, pleural effusions, and poly-hydramnios), and intrauterine fetal demise. The majority of preg-nant women with B19 infection are asymptomatic, which makes the true incidence of fetal involvement difficult to determine.[52,57] It is estimated that 30–66% of adult females are immune to B19 infection,[57–60] and therefore their fetuses are not at risk. In the majority of fetuses who acquire acute infection *in utero*, the infec-tion is self-limited and they are delivered asymptomatic and at term.[61] The greatest risk appears to be when infection is acquired before 20 weeks' gestation, and most fetal losses occur between 9 and 28 weeks' gestation.[57,62] The overall risk of B19-related fetal loss in pregnancies complicated by B19 infection is estimated around 1–9%.[57,60,63] Surviving infants tend to be healthy, with normal devel-opment and neurologic outcome.[63,64] B19-related teratogenicity has only rarely been reported.[64,65] The diagnosis of B19 infection during pregnancy can be confirmed by maternal B19 IgM and IgG antibod-ies or PCR assay (see also below). These studies are usually corrobo-rated with findings on prenatal ultrasonography, most often evidence of fetal anemia and hydrops.[66] Management of severely afflicted fetuses with B19 infection includes fetal digitalization and *in utero* blood transfusions.

Papular-Purpuric Gloves and Socks Syndrome

Papular-purpuric gloves and socks syndrome (PPGSS) is another viral exanthematous illness, which in many (but not all) cases has

been documented to be caused by B19. This rare disorder presents most often in young adults, less often in children, and is usually diagnosed during the spring and summer months.[67,68] Patients with PPGSS present with the acute onset of rapidly progressive, sym-metric swelling and erythema of the hands and feet, often with a petechial or purpuric component (Figs 16.17, 16.18). The eruption has a sharp demarcation at the wrists and ankles, and is usually quite pruritic. A more diffuse, papular exanthem may occur else-where on the body. An associated enanthem consisting of hypere-mia, petechiae, and erosions is often present, and affects the soft and hard palate, pharynx, tongue, and inner lips.[67,69]

Associated symptoms include fever, arthralgias, malaise, and res-piratory or gastrointestinal complaints. Hematologic complica-tions, including leukopenia and thrombocytopenia, are rarely observed.[67,69–71] Mononeuritis multiplex has been described, in association with perineuritis noted on skin biopsy.[72] PPGSS resolves spontaneously over 1–2 weeks, and recurrences are rare. Impor-tantly, the antibody response to B19 seen in PPGSS may differ from that observed in patients with EI, such that patients with the exan-them of PPGSS may still be viremic, and therefore, infectious.[67,69]

The diagnosis of B19 infections is often made clinically in patients presenting with classic EI. In immunocompetent children who are

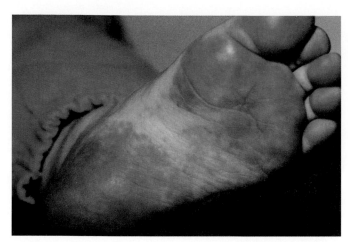

Figure 16.18 Papular-purpuric gloves and socks syndrome. Erythema and petechiae of the plantar feet were accompanied by pruritus and sore throat in this young girl with parvovirus B19 infection.

Table 16.4 Some clinical associations with HHV-6 and HHV-7 infection

Condition	HHV-6, -7, or both	Comment
Roseola infantum	Both	HHV-6 more common
Fever	Both	Infants mainly
Febrile seizures	Both	In young infants
Otitis media	6	
Meningitis	6	
Encephalitis	Both	
Hepatitis	Both	
Lymphadenopathy	Both	
Lymphoproliferative disease	6	Proposed but unproven
Infections in transplant pts	6	Viral reactivation
Hemophagocytic syndrome	6	Transplant patients
Drug hypersensitivity syndrome	Both, but mainly 6	Proposed as complex interplay between drug reaction and HHV infection
HIV-1 cofactor	Both	Proposed but unproven
Pityriasis rosea	7	Controversial
Mononucleosis	Both	In adults
Multiple sclerosis	6	In adults; controversial

Adapted from Leach (2000);[76] Kimberlin (1998);[78] Braun et al. (1997);[80] Levy (1997);[81] Tohyama et al. (2007);[82] Dharancy et al. (2008),[83] and Mitani et al. (2005).[84] HHV, human herpesvirus; HIV-1, human immunodeficiency virus.

otherwise well, laboratory confirmation of B19 infection is usually unnecessary. Instances in which such confirmation may be indicated, however, include atypical presentations, immunocompromised hosts, individuals with hematologic diseases, and those who have been exposed to gravid females. Serologic studies including enzyme immunoassays and radioimmunoassay are useful in detecting anti-B19 IgM and IgG antibodies, and other useful tests include direct hybridization with DNA probes, *in situ* hybridization, and PCR studies.[50,56,73] In a pregnant female who has been exposed to B19, serologic testing for IgM and IgG antibodies should be performed, and if acute infection is documented, serial fetal ultrasonography is usually indicated. Maternal and fetal serum PCR techniques may be useful, especially when serologic study results are unclear.[74] B19 antigen detection in amniotic fluid samples has also been described.[75]

Roseola infantum

Roseola infantum (exanthem subitum, sixth disease) is a common childhood disease caused by human herpesvirus (HHV) type 6 or 7. HHV-6 and -7 are ubiquitous members of the Herpesviridae family. These DNA viruses preferentially infect activated T cells, resulting in enhancement of natural killer cell activity and induction of numerous cytokines.[76] As with other herpesviruses, they become latent following primary infection, and may reactivate during times of altered immunity.[77] Serologic studies have demonstrated that most children have been infected with HHV-6 before 3 years of age, and with HHV-7 by 6–10 years of age.[76–78]

Transmission of HHV-6 and -7 is believed to be primarily via saliva, and horizontal transmission between mother and child is well documented.[77] Persistent or intermittent excretion of HHV-6 in saliva and stool has been documented in parents of children who had documented primary infection.[79] Although most newborns have transplacentally acquired antibodies, by 6 months nearly all have become seronegative and are therefore susceptible to infection.[76] HHV-6 has been divided into two variants, HHV-6A and -6B. Most childhood infections are ascribed to the HHV-6B variant, and HHV-6A may be more frequently implicated in immunocompromised hosts.[80]

A broad range of conditions has been potentially linked to infection with HHV-6 and -7 (Table 16.4). By far, however, the best-recognized association for both agents is that of roseola infantum. Roseola is a mild exanthematous illness that most often occurs in children under 3 years of age. The classic presentation is that of high fever (101–106°F), which lasts for 3–5 days, in an otherwise well infant. With normalization of the temperature, the classic exanthem appears, initially on the trunk and eventually spreading to involve the extremities, neck, and face. The skin eruption is composed of fairly nondescript, erythematous, blanchable macules and papules (Fig. 16.19) that occasionally display a peripheral halo of vasoconstriction. The exanthem usually resolves over 1–3 days.

Associated signs and symptoms may include irritability, diarrhea, bulging fontanelle, cough, cervical lymphadenopathy, and edematous eyelids.[85] Periorbital edema is quite common and, when present in a febrile but otherwise well-appearing child, may be a useful clue to the diagnosis during the pre-exanthematous stage. Nagayama spots are erythematous papules involving the mucosa of the soft palate and uvula, and represent the enanthem that occurs in up to two-thirds of patients.[80,85] The differential diagnosis of the skin eruption in roseola infantum may include measles and rubella, although the temporal characteristics (rash following abrupt defervescence) are usually suggestive of roseola.

Primary HHV-6 infection may also be asymptomatic, or may present in a manner distinct from classic roseola infantum. Nonspecific fever in infants with or without otitis media may frequently

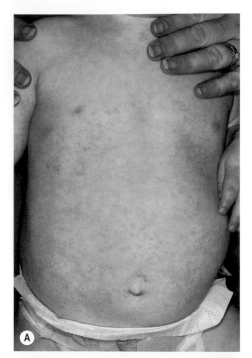

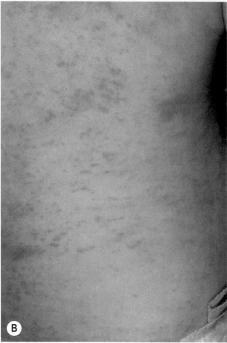

Figure 16.19 Roseola infantum. Erythematous, blanchable macules and papules (A) in an infant who had a high fever for 3 days preceding the skin eruption. On closer inspection (B), some lesions reveal a subtle peripheral halo of vasoconstriction.

be due to HHV-6 infection.[86,87] First febrile seizures in young children may also frequently be associated with primary HHV-6 infection.[86,88] Other potential central nervous system complications include encephalopathy and encephalitis, which tend to occur during the pre-exanthematous stage and which may be associated with long-term neurologic morbidity.[89] HHV-6-associated encephalitis has occurred in both immunocompetent and immunocompromised patients. Solid organ and bone marrow transplant recipients

are at increased risk of reactivation disease, which may be asymptomatic or present with rash, fever, encephalitis, pneumonitis, hepatitis, or bone marrow suppression.[90,91] In some patients, the clinical presentation of HHV-6 reactivation may mimic that of acute graft-versus-host disease.

Treatment for roseola infantum is unnecessary, and the illness usually spontaneously resolves without long-term sequelae. Although *in vitro* studies or clinical observations have suggested anti-HHV activity of ganciclovir, foscarnet and cidofovir, these agents are rarely used clinically for patients with HHV-6 or -7 infection. However, further research to identify effective treatment options is desirable given the wide array of complications that may be associated with severe infection or infection in the immunocompromised host.

Other viral exanthems

Nonspecific Viral Exanthems

Although several exanthematous eruptions may present with characteristic features, such as lesion morphology or distribution, the majority are somewhat nonspecific and may be difficult to distinctly categorize. These eruptions may be hard to distinguish from drug reactions or, in some younger patients, miliaria rubra (prickly heat). Unique defining characteristics, such as an associated enanthem or symptom complex, may be absent. Most nonspecific exanthems fall into the erythematous and/or papular categories, presenting with blanchable red macules and papules with a diffuse distribution (Fig. 16.20). Associated symptoms, which are generally nonspecific as well, may include fever, headache, myalgias, fatigue, and respiratory or gastrointestinal complaints.[92] Most nonspecific exanthems resolve without treatment over 1 week without long-term sequelae.

Common causes of nonspecific exanthems include non-polio enteroviruses (see below) and respiratory viruses (i.e., adenovirus, rhinovirus, parainfluenza virus, respiratory syncytial virus, influenza virus). Other potential agents include Epstein–Barr virus (EBV), HHV-6 and -7, and parvovirus B19, although these agents more often result in distinct exanthematous illnesses as discussed elsewhere in this chapter. In general, the majority of nonspecific exanthems occurring in the winter months are caused by the respiratory viruses, and those occurring during the summer months are most often caused by the enteroviruses.

Papular Acrodermatitis of Childhood

Papular acrodermatitis of childhood (PAC, Gianotti–Crosti syndrome) was initially described in 1955 by Gianotti as an erythematous papular eruption symmetrically distributed on the face, buttocks, and extremities of children. A subsequent description by Crosti and Gianotti was made in 1956, and since then the disorder has been commonly known as Gianotti–Crosti syndrome. A viral etiology was suspected early on following the description of the disorder, and subsequently the notion of hepatitis B virus as a cause was hypothesized. It is currently well accepted that PAC is a distinct viral exanthem that may occur following infection with any of several viral agents, with hepatitis B being one possible (but uncommon) cause in certain parts of the world, especially Italy and Japan.[93]

PAC occurs predominantly in children between the ages of 1 and 6 years. Prior to the appearance of the exanthem, upper respiratory symptoms, fever, and lymphadenopathy may be present. The eruption is characterized by edematous, erythematous, monomorphous papules and occasionally papulovesicles, distributed symmetrically

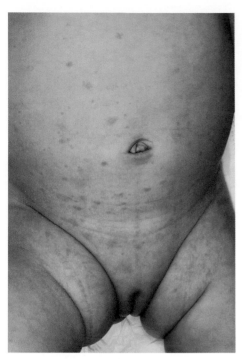

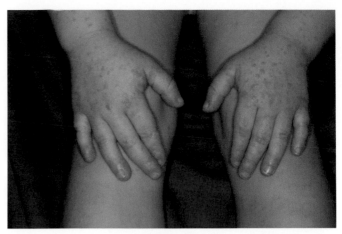

Figure 16.22 Papular acrodermatitis of childhood. Monomorphous, erythematous papules of the dorsal hands in a young girl who had similar lesions on the face and the extensor surfaces of her arms and legs.

Figure 16.20 Nonspecific viral exanthem. Nondescript erythematous macules and papules in an infant with a nonspecific symptom complex.

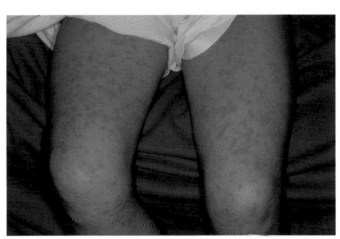

Figure 16.23 Papular acrodermatitis of childhood. Erythematous, edematous papules of the thighs and knees in a patient with Gianotti–Crosti syndrome.

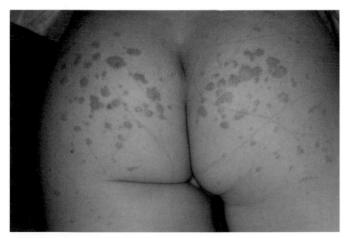

Figure 16.21 Papular acrodermatitis of childhood. Erythematous, edematous papules symmetrically distributed on the bilateral buttocks.

over the face, buttocks (Fig. 16.21) and extensor surfaces of the upper (Fig. 16.22) and lower (Fig. 16.23) extremities. Occasionally, the papules coalesce into larger, erythematous plaques (Fig. 16.24). Hemorrhagic changes or localized purpura (Fig. 16.25) may occasionally be present. The trunk is usually (but not always) spared in patients with PAC.[94] In most patients, the skin eruption is asymptomatic, although mild pruritus may be present.

A viral etiology has long been suspected as the cause of PAC. In 1970, two independent groups confirmed the association with hepatitis B infection.[95,96] In these patients, the exanthem was accompanied by acute anicteric hepatitis. In patients with hepatitis-associated PAC, hepatitis B surface antigen subtype *ayw* has been most classically implicated. Another term, *papulovesicular acrolocated syndrome* (PVAS), was traditionally used to describe a similar presentation with a more vesicular component. It was once believed that this presentation was distinct based on the presence of pruritus and the lack of both hepatitis and a hepatitis B association. In a review of 308 cases of Gianotti–Crosti syndrome in Italy, however, distinction between PAC and PVAS was not clinically possible, nor was there a significant difference in the presentation or course as related to the etiologic agent (i.e., hepatitis B versus other viruses).[97]

Subsequently, multiple viral agents have been implicated in causing PAC. These include EBV which is believed to be the most common etiology in the USA, as well as cytomegalovirus, Coxsackie viruses, respiratory viruses (adenovirus, respiratory syncytial virus, parainfluenza virus), parvovirus B19, rotavirus, and HHV-6.[93,97–104] A possible association with immunizations has also been suggested.

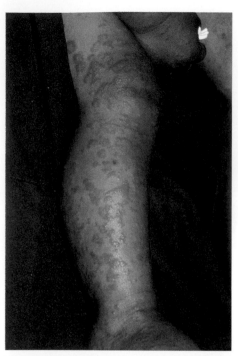

Figure 16.24 Papular acrodermatitis of childhood. Erythematous papules coalesced into larger, edematous plaques in this patient.

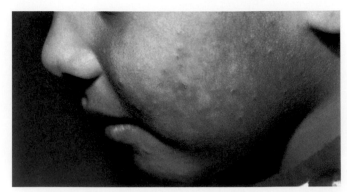

Figure 16.26 Papular acrodermatitis of childhood. Post-inflammatory hypopigmentation. These post-inflammatory changes are most common in patients with darker native complexions.

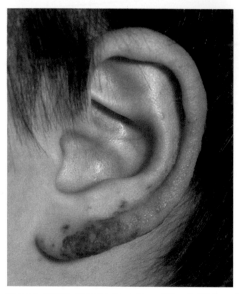

Figure 16.25 Papular acrodermatitis of childhood. Localized purpura of the ear lobe occurred in this patient with the disorder.

Vaccination reports have included measles-mumps-rubella, *Haemophilus*, oral polio, diphtheria-pertussis-tetanus, Japanese B encephalitis, and hepatitis B vaccines.[105–110] PAC seems to be a distinct exanthem occurring in response to a variety of viral agents and possibly vaccinations, with hepatitis B being an extremely rare cause in the USA.

Treatment for PAC is supportive. Although the eruption is self-limited, it may take 8–12 weeks to resolve completely. Post-inflammatory hypopigmentation (Fig. 16.26) may occasionally persist for several months following resolution of the exanthem. Routine laboratory studies for hepatitis are generally not warranted. However, a thorough history (including potential risk factors for

hepatitis) and physical examination (with attention to the presence or absence of hepatosplenomegaly and lymphadenopathy) should be performed. Hepatitis serologies and liver function studies should be performed only in patients in whom there is a clinical suspicion.

Unilateral Laterothoracic Exanthem

Unilateral laterothoracic exanthem (ULE, asymmetric periflexural exanthem of childhood) was initially described by Bodemer and de Prost in 1992 as a distinct exanthem presenting initially in a unilateral, localized fashion.[111] It was probably described years earlier when Brunner et al. described a 'new papular exanthem of childhood' in 1962,[112] and in 1986 when Taieb et al. reported five children with a 'localized erythema' similar to that described in ULE.[113]

ULE is most common in patients between 1 and 5 years of age. It usually occurs during the winter or spring, although it has been described year round.[112,114,115] In most patients, onset of the skin eruption is unilateral and on the trunk (Fig. 16.27), often with extension toward the axilla (Fig. 16.28), and less often around the inguinal region or on an extremity (Fig. 16.29). The lesions spread in a centrifugal fashion, and often become bilateral, although they maintain a predominance on the initial side of involvement. The skin lesions in ULE may show various morphologies, including macules, papules, eczematous changes, and morbilliform, scarlatiniform, annular, or reticulate patterns. Some have described early lesions as consisting of a red papule surrounded by a pale halo.[114] Pruritus occurs in around 50% of patients. Vesicles and purpuric changes are rare. Desquamation is common during the healing stage, and postinflammatory pigment changes may also be present. Although skin biopsy is usually unnecessary, when performed it has revealed a lymphocytic infiltrate with notable clustering around the dermal eccrine ducts.[114,116] The most common initial misdiagnosis is that of contact dermatitis. The clinical differential diagnosis of ULE may also include nonspecific exanthem, pityriasis rosea, scarlet fever, miliaria, erythema infectiosum, tinea, and papular acrodermatitis of childhood.

Associated features may include a prodrome consisting of low-grade fevers and respiratory or gastrointestinal symptoms. Fatigue and conjunctivitis may also be present. Enlarged axillary and/or inguinal lymph nodes are occasionally noted, and hepatosplenomegaly is generally absent. An associated enanthem has not been described with ULE.

The etiology of ULE remains unclear, although most favor a viral etiology. Early reports suggested *Spiroplasma* infection,[113] although this has not been confirmed in subsequent studies. In a prospective,

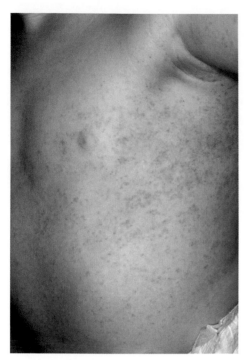

Figure 16.27 Unilateral laterothoracic exanthem. Erythematous macules and papules of the lateral trunk. The eruption eventually generalized.

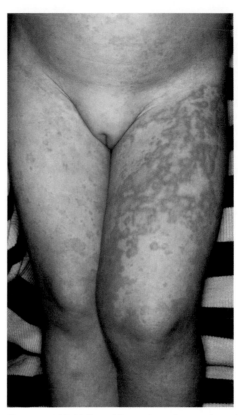

Figure 16.29 Unilateral laterothoracic exanthem. The thigh was the initial site of involvement in this patient, whose lesions demonstrate an erythema infectiosum-like morphology. (Courtesy of Dr Sarah Chamlin.)

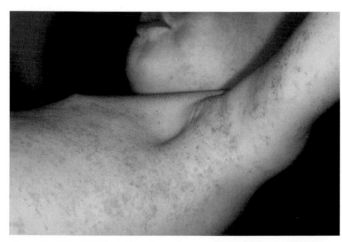

Figure 16.28 Unilateral laterothoracic exanthem. Early involvement shows localization to the lateral trunk, axilla, and proximal inner arm in this patient.

case-controlled study using throat, stool, blood, and skin samples, several microbiologic investigations were performed for viral and bacterial infection. No differences between cases and controls were noted, and no consistent etiologic agent was identified.[117] Although parainfluenza virus and adenovirus infection were diagnosed in six patients in one series, confirmation of a causal role is lacking.[115] ULE appears to be a distinct presentation pattern in response to a variety of potential infectious agents.

The lesions of ULE resolve spontaneously, but similar to those of papular acrodermatitis of childhood, may be delayed. Most often, ULE resolves over 3–4 weeks, although in some patients it may take up to 8 weeks. Treatment is supportive.

Enteroviral Exanthems

Enteroviruses, a subgroup of the picornaviruses, may cause a variety of clinical syndromes with associated exanthems. Human enteroviruses are small, single-stranded RNA viruses that include echovirus (31 serotypes), coxsackievirus A (23 types), coxsackievirus B (6 types), enterovirus 68–71 (4 types), and polioviruses (3 types).[118] The majority of enterovirus infections seen in practice are benign and manifested by fever alone or distinct syndromes, including hand-foot-and-mouth disease, herpangina, hemorrhagic conjunctivitis, and pleurodynia.[119] However, severe or life-threatening infections may also result from enteroviral infection, including meningitis, encephalitis, myocarditis, neonatal sepsis, and polio. Infections in neonates are often disseminated, and may be difficult to differentiate from bacterial processes.[120] Non-polio enteroviruses are the leading cause of viral meningitis.[119,121] Spread of enteroviruses occurs person-to-person via the fecal–oral route and occasionally common source exposure (i.e., swimming pool water).[122] Enteroviral infections tend to predominate during the summer and fall, although sporadic cases may be seen throughout the year.

Nonspecific exanthems due to non-polio enteroviruses are common, and may present as macular and papular, non-pruritic eruptions with or without petechiae. When a petechial component is present, the clinical presentation may be confused with that of more serious infections such as meningococcemia. This diagnostic confusion may be exacerbated by the concomitant presence of aseptic meningitis, which may accompany enterovirus, coxsackievirus, or echovirus infections.[25] Other exanthem patterns may include urticarial, scarlatiniform, zosteriform, and vesicular forms.[118]

Table 16.5 lists some exanthem/enanthem associations with the nonpolio enteroviruses. Several are discussed in the following in more detail.

Hand-foot-and-mouth disease (HFMD) is the best-recognized enteroviral exanthem. It is a disorder of young children, most commonly affecting those between 1 and 4 years of age. HFMD has been linked to several non-polio enteroviruses, including coxsackieviruses A5, A7, A9, A10, A16 (most common), B1, B2, B3, and B5, echovirus 4,[134] and enterovirus 71.[92] Patients present with fever, malaise, and the characteristic exanthem, which consists of gray-white, vesicular lesions on the palms (Fig. 16.30) and soles (Fig. 16.31), and less often involving the dorsal or lateral surfaces of the hands and feet. A less specific macular and papular erythematous eruption may be present on the buttocks, thighs, and external genitalia. Occasionally, a more diffuse vesicular eruption, with lesions in areas other than the palms and soles, may be present (Fig. 16.32). The enanthem of HFMD consists of vesicles and erosions of the buccal surfaces, palate, tongue (Fig. 16.33), uvula, gingivae, and anterior tonsillar pillars. These lesions are painful and lead to anorexia and, occasionally, dehydration. Cervical and submandibular lymphadenopathy may occasionally be present in patients with HFMD.

Although the course of HFMD is most often benign and treatment is supportive, epidemics of enterovirus 71 infection in Taiwan highlight the potential seriousness of the infection. In these epidemics, severe disease was seen most often in children under 5 years of age, with the majority of deaths occurring secondary to pulmonary edema or pulmonary hemorrhage.[135] Other complications included encephalitis, aseptic meningitis, acute flaccid paralysis, and myocarditis.[135,136]

Herpangina is a characteristic enanthem that may be caused by a variety of non-polio enteroviruses, especially coxsackieviruses A and B. It presents with fever, sore throat, and malaise, usually in children between 3 and 10 years of age. Inspection of the oral mucosa reveals gray-white vesicles and erythematous erosions involving the palate, uvula, and tonsillar pillars. Although it may occasionally be confused with acute herpetic gingivostomatitis, labial and skin involvement is much more common with herpes simplex virus infection. Treatment for HFMD or herpangina consists of pain control and ensurance of adequate fluid intake in order to prevent dehydration. The lesions spontaneously resolve over 1 week.

Echovirus exanthems have been variably described with a number of presentations and morphologies. Some of these include macular, vesicular, urticarial, and petechial eruptions, erythema multiforme, HFMD, and roseola-like exanthems.[25] Echovirus 6 has been associated with a dermatomal, vesicular eruption mimicking herpes zoster.[123] Echovirus type 9 infection may result in an illness with aseptic meningitis and a petechial eruption that may mimic meningococcemia.[137] Echovirus 16 was classically associated with a roseola-like exanthem referred to as 'Boston exanthem,' which was one of the initial exanthems to be described and virologically confirmed. Approximately one-third of individuals with echovirus infection may develop a rubelliform eruption consisting of discrete pink-red macules that spread from the face and neck to the upper trunk and extremities. Some patients also have yellow or gray-white lesions on the oral mucous membranes that may resemble Koplik

Table 16.5 Some reported exanthem/enanthem associations with enteroviruses	
Exanthem	**Comment**
Hand-foot-and-mouth disease	Most common; coxsackievirus A or B, enterovirus 71
Herpangina	Oral lesions and fever; coxsackievirus A or B
Hemorrhagic conjunctivitis	Eyelid edema, lacrimation, pain; coxsackievirus A24 and enterovirus 70
Nonspecific exanthem	Any enterovirus
Gianotti–Crosti syndrome	Coxsackievirus A or B
Henoch-Schonlein purpura	Coxsackievirus B1
Still's-like disease	Coxsackievirus B4
Zoster-like eruption	Echovirus 6
EI-like eruption	Echovirus 12
Congenital skin lesions	Coxsackievirus B3
Eruptive pseudoangiomatosis	Echovirus
AGEP	Coxsackievirus B4
Nail matrix arrest (Fig. 16.34)	Patients with preceding hand-foot-and-mouth disease

Adapted from Meade and Chang (1979);[123] Cherry et al. (1969);[124] Prose et al. (1993);[125] Mancini and Bodemer (2003);[126] Costa et al. (1995);[127] Sauerbrei et al. (2000);[128] Roberts-Thomson et al. (1986);[129] Feio et al. (1997);[130] Clementz and Mancini (2000);[131] Bernier et al. (2001),[132] and Balfour et al. (1972).[133] EI, erythema infectiosum; AGEPD, acute generalized exanthematous pustulosis.

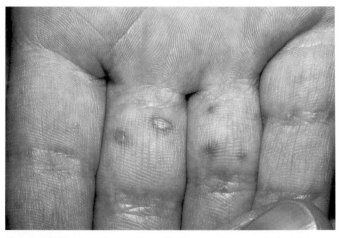

Figure 16.30 Hand-foot-and-mouth disease. Deep-seated vesicles with erythema involving the palmar surface of the fingers.

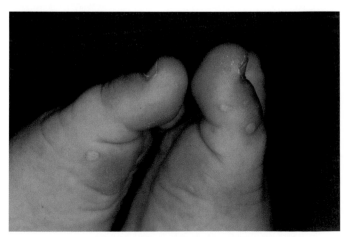

Figure 16.31 Hand-foot-and-mouth disease. Erythematous deep-seated and superficial vesicles involved the plantar surface in this infant with erosions of the palate and uvula.

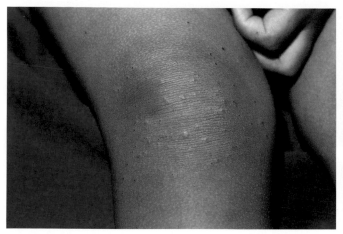

Figure 16.32 Hand-foot-and-mouth disease. Red to purple vesicles involved the knees and elbows in this patient with classic lesions involving the mouth, palms, and soles.

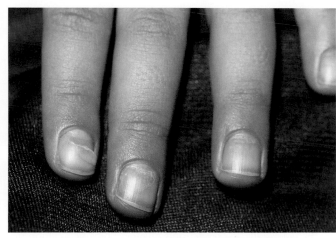

Figure 16.34 Nail matrix arrest following hand-foot-and-mouth disease. Transverse ridging and eventual nail shedding occurred in this 5-year-old male 2 months after having the enteroviral infection. The nails spontaneously grew back normally within several months.

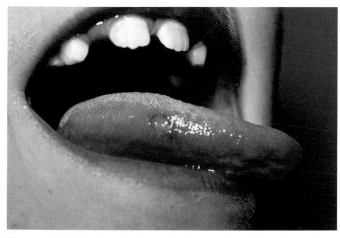

Figure 16.33 Hand-foot-and-mouth disease. A painful erosion of the lateral aspect of the tongue.

Table 16.6 Some disease associations with Epstein–Barr virus (EBV)
Asymptomatic infection
Infectious mononucleosis
Lymphoproliferative disorders
X-linked lymphoproliferative syndrome
EBV-associated hemophagocytic syndrome
Lymphoproliferative disorders in immunocompromised patients
Gianotti–Crosti syndrome
Chronic EBV infection
Oral hairy leukoplakia
Neoplastic disorders
Burkitt lymphoma
Nasopharyngeal carcinoma
B- or T-cell lymphoma (including AIDS-associated B cell lymphomas)
Extranodal NK/T cell lymphoma, nasal type
Hodgkin disease
Hepatocellular carcinoma

spots. Other symptoms that may be associated with echovirus infection include fever, gastrointestinal complaints, upper respiratory symptoms, and conjunctivitis.

Eruptive pseudoangiomatosis is an exanthem consisting of the acute onset of hemangioma-like lesions, and possibly related to echovirus infection.[138] Cherry et al., in 1969, originally described four children with acute echovirus infection (two with echovirus 25 and two with echovirus 32) who developed such lesions, with resolution occurring over 2–6 days.[124] Other affected children were subsequently described, all of whom presented with the acute onset and spontaneous resolution of angioma-like papules during the course of a viral illness.[125,139] The disorder has also been observed in adults.[140,141] The angiomatous papules in eruptive pseudoangiomatosis are often surrounded by a rim of blanching, and histopathologic evaluation, when performed, has revealed dilated dermal blood vessels and plump endothelial cells, without any increase in the number of blood vessels.[125,142] Associated symptoms have included fever, malaise, headache, diarrhea, and respiratory complaints. Although echoviruses have not been confirmed as the etiology by other investigators, a viral cause continues to seem most likely.

Infectious Mononucleosis

Infectious mononucleosis (IM) is a common infection occurring during adolescence, and usually associated with EBV infection. Although most cases of IM are related to EBV infection, not all primary EBV infections manifest as IM.[143] The spectrum of disorders linked to EBV infection is shown in Table 16.6. Other etiologic agents of IM-like illness include cytomegalovirus (CMV), hepatitis A, adenovirus, group A β-hemolytic streptococcus, HHV-6, rubella virus, HIV, and *Toxoplasma gondii*.[144,145] Malignancy and drug reactions may also result in IM-like illnesses.[143]

Confirmation of EBV as the major cause of IM occurred in the late 1960s.[143,145] EBV is a member of the Herpesviridae family, and as such is a large, DNA-containing virus with the ability to become latent following primary infection, and with the potential for subsequent reactivation. The virus has tropism for both lymphocytes (especially B cells) and epithelial cells, with infection beginning in the oropharyngeal epithelial cells, which may shed the virus for up to 18 months following primary acquisition.[145,146] The primary transmission route is via saliva.

Primary EBV infection in infancy is mostly asymptomatic, or presents with very mild, nonspecific symptoms such as upper respiratory tract symptoms, pharyngitis, lymphadenopathy, and fever. Epidemiologic studies suggest that most children have acquired EBV by 5 years of age in underdeveloped countries or lower socioeconomic classes, while primary infection occurs later in life (i.e., between 10 and 30 years) in developed countries and higher socioeconomic classes.[143,147] Older children and adolescents are more likely to develop clinical symptoms of IM, following an incubation period of 2–7 weeks.

IM is generally a benign, self-limited illness characterized by fever, exudative tonsillopharyngitis, and lymphadenopathy. Malaise, fatigue, and headache are also common. The temperature may reach 40°C and is often prolonged, lasting for 1–2 weeks. Physical examination may reveal splenomegaly, hepatomegaly, eyelid edema, palatal petechiae, jaundice, and a skin eruption. The lymphadenopathy is typically nontender and involves both the anterior and posterior cervical chains. Diffuse adenopathy is occasionally present. Historically, IM was divided into three syndromes: *anginose*, characterized by the classic triad of fever, pharyngitis, and lymphadenopathy; *typhoidal*, characterized by prolonged high fever; and *glandular*, characterized by mild pharyngitis, low-grade fever, and marked lymphadenopathy.

The skin eruption of IM is nonspecific, occurs in around 5% of patients, and may present as a macular, petechial, scarlatiniform, urticarial, or erythema multiforme-like rash.[145,147] Following the administration of ampicillin or amoxicillin, however, 90–95% of patients develop an erythematous macular and papular eruption (Fig. 16.35), which may be related to ampicillin-antibody immune complexes resulting from B cell activation.[148] This reaction occurs about 5–9 days after starting the antibiotic, and does not appear to represent a true drug allergy.

Useful laboratory evaluations in patients with IM include hematologic and hepatic panels and serologic analysis. Complete blood cell counts often reveal an absolute lymphocytosis, often with >10% atypical lymphocytes (representing activated T cells). Other aberrations may include thrombocytopenia and neutropenia, the latter developing 1–2 weeks into the illness. Autoimmune hemolytic anemia is uncommon, occurring in around 3% of cases.[148] Mild hepatitis may be manifested by elevations in the hepatic transaminases, alkaline phosphatase, and LDH. Coagulopathy is usually absent. The most useful confirmatory examination is the serologic assay for heterophil antibodies. These IgM antibodies can be readily measured with a variety of rapid test kits, and have high specificity. Although up to 15% of patients with IM may initially be negative for heterophile antibodies, many become positive on repeat testing performed during the 2nd or 3rd week of the illness.

Virus-specific serologies should be used to diagnose IM in children under 4 years of age (who are often heterophile antibody negative), patients with atypical presentations, or those with severe or prolonged illness.[145] EBV serology interpretations are shown in Table 16.7. Detection methods for EBV-related proteins or DNA are also available.

Complications of IM include splenic rupture, upper airway obstruction, chronic fatigue, and neurologic findings. Subcapsular splenic hemorrhage with rupture is fortunately quite rare (<0.5% of cases in adults). It presents as an abrupt onset of left upper quadrant abdominal pain, and may be treated by splenectomy or non-operative management. Upper airway obstruction may result from tonsillar hypertrophy and is treated as an inpatient with close observation, maintenance of the airway, hydration, and occasionally systemic corticosteroids.[148] Neurologic complications include cranial nerve palsies, meningoencephalitis, and seizures. Other less common complications include pneumonia (which is often related to coinfection with a bacterial or another viral agent), electrocardiographic abnormalities, rhabdomyolysis, and chronic liver disease.[145,148]

The management of IM is primarily supportive. Bed rest, fluids, and analgesics are commonly recommended. Patients with splenomegaly are counseled to avoid strenuous exercise and contact sports to prevent the complication of splenic rupture. These activities should be avoided for the duration of splenomegaly, usually 1 month following onset of symptoms.[143] Amoxicillin and ampicillin should be avoided in patients with suspected IM. Corticosteroids are generally recommended only for patients with complications such as marked tonsillar hypertrophy with the potential for airway obstruction, massive splenomegaly, myocarditis, hemolytic anemia, or hemophagocytic syndrome.[149] Acyclovir, which may show *in vitro* activity against EBV, is of no proven value in the treatment of EBV associated IM or lymphoproliferative syndromes.[143,149]

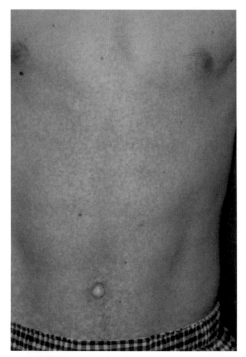

Figure 16.35 Infectious mononucleosis. A diffuse, erythematous macular and papular eruption occurred in this adolescent male after receiving amoxicillin therapy.

Table 16.7 Epstein–Barr virus-specific serology interpretation				
	Viral capsid antigen (VCA)			
Status	IgG	IgM	EA	EBNA
No past infection	−	−	−	−
Acute IM	+	+	±	−
Convalescent IM	+	±	±	±
Past infection	+	−	Low + or −	+
Reactivated/chronic	++	±	++	±

Kawa (2000).[146] EA, early antigen; EBNA, Epstein–Barr virus nuclear antigen; IM, infectious mononucleosis.

Exanthems associated with *Mycoplasma pneumoniae* infection

Mycoplasmas are a distinct class of bacteria that lack rigid cell walls and are thus insensitive to antibiotics that inhibit cell wall synthesis, such as penicillins. The best-recognized agent in this class is *Mycoplasma pneumoniae*, a prominent etiology of atypical pneumonia in school-age children, adolescents, and adults. This infection generally presents with the insidious onset of fever, malaise, headache and cough, and may be associated with skin findings in up to one-third of patients.[150] A variety of cutaneous eruptions have been linked to *M. pneumoniae* infection. These include nonspecific erythematous macular and papular eruptions,[151–153] erythema nodosum,[150] urticaria,[150] erythema multiforme minor,[154] Stevens–Johnson syndrome,[155,156] and subcorneal pustular dermatosis.[157,158] Stevens–Johnson syndrome is the most significant cutaneous association with *M. pneumoniae* infection, and is discussed in detail in Chapter 20.

Rickettsial diseases

Although the use of molecular technology has resulted in some reclassifications of agents included in the order Rickettsiales, these organisms are all included in this section. These genus groups include *Bartonella*, *Coxiella*, *Ehrlichia* and *Rickettsia*. Table 16.8 is a summary of several rickettsial organisms and their disease associations. Bacillary angiomatosis, caused by *Bartonella henselae* and *Bartonella quintana*, is discussed in Chapter 12. Cat-scratch disease, caused by *B. henselae*, is discussed in Chapter 14. Some other rickettsial disorders are discussed here.

Rickettsial infections are arthropod-borne diseases caused by microorganisms that occupy an intermediate position between bacteria and viruses. Spread by blood-sucking insects such as the body louse, fleas, and ticks, the various rickettsial diseases that occur in the USA include endemic or murine typhus, rickettsialpox, Rocky Mountain spotted fever, and Q fever. Human granulocytic ehrlichiosis and human monocytic ehrlichiosis cases have also been reported with an expanding geographic distribution.

Endemic Typhus

Endemic (murine) typhus is caused by *Rickettsia typhi* and is transmitted by the rat flea, *Xenopsylla cheopis*. It occurs worldwide, especially in warm climates with heavy populations of rats or opossums.[159] Although endemic typhus occurs most often in developing nations, it continues to occur in the USA, especially in Gulf Coastal areas and Texas.[160] Adults are most often affected, but children have constituted up to 75% of infections in some outbreaks.[159] Clinical manifestations most commonly include fever and headache, with rash occurring in around two-thirds of patients. The eruption is variably characterized as macular, papular, and occasionally petechial. Other features may include nausea, vomiting, malaise, myalgias, diarrhea, arthralgia, lymphadenopathy, conjunctivitis, and pneumonitis. Effective treatments include tetracycline and chloramphenicol.

Rickettsialpox

Rickettsialpox, caused by *Rickettsia akari*, is transmitted to humans by the house mouse mite *Liponyssoides sanguineus*. Although rickettsialpox is infrequently reported or diagnosed, it remains endemic in certain regions of the USA, particularly New York City.[161] The disorder begins with the bite of an infected mite, which results in a black eschar and, subsequently, other symptoms. The classic triad of rickettsialpox consists of fever, eschar, and rash. The skin eruption presents as numerous, monomorphous red papules with a small, central vesicular component. Although it may occasionally be confused with varicella, the rash of rickettsialpox is characterized by fewer lesions, less pruritus, monomorphous nature, and lack of an eschar.[161] Other features include myalgias, gastrointestinal symptoms, arthralgias, and lymphadenopathy. Although rickettsialpox is self-limited over 7–10 days, treatments of choice include doxycycline or chloramphenicol.

Rocky Mountain Spotted Fever

Rocky Mountain spotted fever (RMSF) is caused by *Rickettsia rickettsii*, and is the most common rickettsial illness in the USA. In one

Table 16.8 Some rickettsial organisms and their disease associations

Organism	Disease association(s)	Vector
Bartonella		
Bartonella henselae	Bacillary angiomatosis, CSD, endocarditis, bacillary peliosis	?Cat flea
Bartonella quintana	Trench fever, bacillary angiomatosis, endocarditis, bacillary peliosis	Human body louse
Coxiella		
Coxiella burnetii	Q fever, endocarditis	Ticks
Ehrlichia		
Ehrlichia chaffeensis	Human monocytic ehrlichiosis	Lone star tick
Anaplasma phagocytophilum	Human granulocytic ehrlichiosis	Deer tick, dog tick
Rickettsia		
Rickettsia akari	Rickettsialpox	House mouse mite
Rickettsia conorii	Mediterranean spotted fever	Dog ticks
Rickettsia prowazekii	Epidemic typhus	Human body louse
Rickettsia rickettsii	Rocky Mountain spotted fever	Wood tick, dog tick
Rickettsia typhi	Endemic typhus	Rat flea

CSD, cat-scratch disease.

4-year period during the mid-1990s, the average annual RMSF incidence was 2.2 cases per million persons, with the highest incidence confirmed among children 5–9 years of age (3.7 per million).[162] Of 4800 cases reported to the CDC between 1990 and 1998, 20% of cases and 15% of reported deaths were in children under 10 years of age.[163] Among children living in the southeastern and south central USA, 12% had positive *R. rickettsii* antibody titers in one serologic survey, and hence exposure to the agent may be more common than indicated by reports of disease.[164] Because of the rapid progression of disease and the high mortality rate that may be seen without appropriate therapy, prompt diagnosis and initiation of specific treatment is vital in children with RMSF. Despite the name of this disease, it has been reported throughout the continental USA, except for in Maine and Vermont.[163,165] The highest incidence is in Oklahoma, Tennessee, Arkansas and the South Atlantic region; the most important factor in transmission of the disease is the prevalence of infected ticks.[166,167]

RMSF is transmitted by the bite of the wood tick (*Dermacentor andersoni*) in the Western USA and Canada, and the dog tick (*D. variabilis*) in the Eastern USA. Most cases occur during the spring and summer months. Even in areas considered to be highly endemic for the disease (i.e., Virginia, North Carolina, Oklahoma), only a small fraction of ticks are infected with *R. ricketsii*.[168] Up to 40% of individuals diagnosed with RMSF do not recall a history of tick bite.[168] Importantly, ticks may attach to any body site (some of which are difficult to observe), often have a painless bite, and commonly go unnoticed.[166]

Patients with RMSF usually report symptoms within 14 days of the tick bite. The initial prodromal symptoms include headache, gastrointestinal symptoms, malaise, and myalgias. These are followed by fever and rash. The classic triad of RMSF consists of fever, headache, and rash, but many patients with the disease do not present in this classic fashion. Headache is a very prominent feature, may be severe, and is usually accompanied by severe myalgias. Patients with GI complaints may have nausea, vomiting, and generalized or focal abdominal pain, occasionally mimicking an acute abdomen.[168] Neurologic findings may include meningismus, seizures, and psychiatric complaints. Photophobia may also be present.

An exanthem occurs in up to 90% of patients with RMSF, and usually appears around day 3–5 of the illness. It begins as discrete erythematous, blanching macules and papules, which begin in a peripheral fashion and spread centrally (centripetally). Common locations for early lesions include the ankles, wrists, palms, and soles. With time, the skin lesions evolve into petechial macules and papules (Fig. 16.36). Occasionally, they become hemorrhagic and focal areas of necrosis may occur. Larger areas of purpura may be present, and in some patients, the skin eruption mimics that of meningococcemia. Skin necrosis and gangrene may occasionally

result. Some patients have a delayed appearance of the rash, and in up to 10%, the rash is completely absent ('spotless' RMSF).[168] These patients seem to have the same course as patients with a rash, and the index of suspicion must be higher in them, incorporating clinical and epidemiologic clues, when present. Other mucocutaneous features may include hyperpigmentation, jaundice and mucosal erosions.

Laboratory findings in RMSF may include a left shift with a normal to low white blood cell count, thrombocytopenia, liver function abnormalities, and decreased serum sodium. A lymphocytic cerebrospinal fluid pleocytosis is often noted. The differential diagnosis of RMSF includes other rickettsial diseases, meningococcal disease, measles, and other viral exanthems. The diagnosis is usually made on a clinical basis, and if the disease is even remotely suspected, prompt institution of a tetracycline-class antibiotic should occur. Biopsy of skin lesions reveals endothelial cell damage with a perivascular and interstitial mononuclear cell infiltrate and small vessel vasculitis, as well as extravasation of red blood cells and fibrin thrombi within vessels.[169,170] The indirect fluorescent antibody (IFA) test is the most widely used diagnostic examination, and detects anti-*R. rickettsii* IgM and IgG antibodies, which are usually present 10–14 days following acute infection. ELISA testing has also been utilized.[171]

The treatment of choice for RMSF is doxycycline, which is preferable to other tetracycline agents because of its reliable absorption, twice-daily dosing schedule, and broader spectrum of coverage for other tick-borne diseases.[166,168] If RMSF is strongly suspected, treatment should be promptly initiated and not delayed while waiting for laboratory confirmation. Chloramphenicol is also effective, but is generally used only for patients in whom a contraindication to doxycycline is present (i.e., pregnancy). In an analysis of risk factors for fatal RMSF, evidence for the superiority of tetracyclines was demonstrated, even when compared with chloramphenicol therapy.[172] It should be noted that the risk of dental staining, which may be associated with doxycycline therapy in children under 8 years of age, is generally far outweighed by the risk of RMSF going untreated. Doxycycline therapy is recommended by the American Academy of Pediatrics and by the Centers for Disease Control and Prevention as the treatment of choice in both RMSF and ehrlichiosis (see below).[173] Dental staining appears to be dose- and duration-related, and is unlikely to occur in children treated with short courses of tetracyclines.[167,174] Therapy should be continued until the patient demonstrates clinical improvement and is afebrile for at least 3 days. Most patients are treated for 7–10 days.

Useful measures in preventing RMSF include wearing long clothing when outdoors (especially when in high-risk areas for tick bites), use of insect repellents effective against ticks (see Ch. 18), and frequent inspection for ticks with tweezer removal when necessary. It seems that transmission of the organism probably cannot occur until after 24 h of tick attachment.[175]

Q Fever

Q fever, caused by the rickettsia *Coxiella burnetii*, is a worldwide zoonosis affecting domestic animals, birds, and arthropods.[176] It is transmitted to humans through contact with infected domestic animals, including cattle, sheep, and goats, or the products of these animals.[169] The primary route of human infection appears to be via inhalation of contaminated aerosols, and since the organism has a low respiratory infective dose, there is concern over its potential use as an agent of biologic warfare.[176] Tick bites are an unusual source of transmission of *C. burnetii* to humans.

The presentation of Q fever in humans is variable. It may present as a nonspecific flu-like illness, atypical pneumonia, or hepatitis.

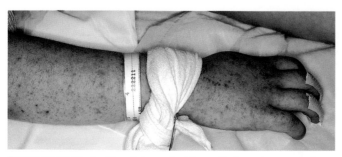

Figure 16.36 Rocky Mountain spotted fever. Erythematous macules and petechiae involving the hand and forearm.

Other clinical manifestations may include fever, myocarditis, pericarditis, osteomyelitis, and central nervous system infection.[177] Malaise is common, and may persist for months after the acute symptoms have disappeared. Rash is reported in up to 20% of patients, and does not appear to have distinguishing features. Erythematous macules, petechiae, purpura, urticaria, vesicles, livedo reticularis, and erythema nodosum have been reported.[169] The diagnosis of Q fever is confirmed by serologic studies or PCR, and treatment with doxycycline, fluoroquinolones, or co-trimoxazole is effective. In several patients, Q fever is a self-limited disease that is diagnosed retrospectively.[176] A history of recent contact with farm animals and pets, in the presence of consistent clinical findings, should prompt investigation for *C. burnetii*.[177]

Ehrlichiosis

Ehrlichia are obligate intracellular bacteria that belong to the family Rickettsiae. The two forms of disease of most concern in the USA are human monocytic ehrlichiosis and human granulocytic ehrlichiosis, both of which are transmitted by tick bites and have similar clinical manifestations.

Human monocytic ehrlichiosis (HME) is caused by *Ehrlichia chaffeensis*, and occurs primarily in the south-eastern and south-central USA. The most common vector is the Lone Star tick (*Amblyomma americanum*), and the distribution of disease closely parallels the endemic regions for this arthropod.[178] Most cases of HME occur during late spring and summer.

Human granulocytic ehrlichiosis (HGE) is caused by *Anaplasma phagocytophilum*, which was previously known as 'the agent of human granulocytic ehrlichiosis'.[179] This infection is caused by bites from infected deer ticks or dog ticks, and is seen with a broader geographic distribution in the USA. Most cases of HGE occur between the months of April and September.

There may be considerable overlap of the clinical manifestations in patients with HME and HGE. Nonspecific symptoms of both disorders include fever, fatigue, headache, malaise, chills, myalgia, nausea, and rash. Hematologic aberrations may include progressive leukopenia, thrombocytopenia, and anemia. Some patients have elevation of liver transaminases, alkaline phosphatase, and lactate dehydrogenase, and hyponatremia may also be present. Hepatosplenomegaly and systolic murmur are common examination findings in patients with HME.[178] Shock necessitating pressor support and mechanical ventilation has been reported in patients with HME.[180]

The incidence of rash in patients with HME or HGE is not well established, but seems to occur less often than that seen in patients with RMSF. It has been described as macular, papular, or petechial. Other less commonly reported patterns include vesicular, nodular, purpuric, vasculitic, and ulcerated types.[169] The distribution is variable, and the onset of the cutaneous eruption is most often within the first 3–10 days of the illness. The skin lesions seen in patients with HGE may predominate in the vicinity of the tick bite. The differential diagnosis of ehrlichiosis is broad, including septic shock, meningococcemia, thrombotic thrombocytopenic purpura, toxic shock syndrome, Rocky Mountain spotted fever, Lyme disease, murine typhus, tularemia, babesiosis, and other tick-borne fevers.

Diagnostic options for ehrlichiosis include examination of peripheral blood smears, immunohistology, PCR assay, isolation of the organism, and serologic studies.[181] The most clinically relevant laboratory study is that of paired serologies (often via indirect immunofluorescence assay), which often need to be performed by a reference laboratory. Western blotting has also been utilized.[182] The treatment of choice for ehrlichiosis is doxycycline, and chloramphenicol is also a useful agent.[169,178,183] Rifampin has been successfully used in children with HGE and may be another option for patients with non-life-threatening disease.[81] Efforts to reduce contact with ticks are also useful in lowering the risk of ehrlichiosis.

Key References

The complete list of 183 references for this chapter is available online at **www.expertconsult.com.**
See inside cover for registration details.

Marin M, Meissner HC, Seward JF. Varicella prevention in the USA: A review of successes and challenges. *Pediatrics*. 2008;122:e744–e751.

Morbidity and Mortality Weekly Report. Update: Measles – USA, January–July 2008. *MMWR Weekly*. 2008;57(33):893–896.

Morbidity and Mortality Weekly Report. Progress toward elimination of rubella and congenital rubella syndrome – the Americas, 2003–2008. *MMWR Weekly*. 2008;57(43):1176–1179.

Pasquinelli L. Enterovirus infections. *Pediatr Rev*. 2006;27(2):e14–e15.

Schalock PC, Dinulos JGH. Mycoplasma pneumoniae-induced cutaneous disease. *Int J Dermatol*. 2009; 48:673–681.

17

Skin Disorders due to Fungi

Fungi are a group of simple plants that lack flowers, leaves, and chlorophyll, and get their nourishment from dead or living organic matter, thus depending on plants, animals, and humans for their existence. Fungal infections that affect humans may be superficial, deep, or systemic, and can occasionally be fatal. Although they do not rank as pathogens with the bacteria or viruses, a number of species once thought to be ubiquitous and harmless have been implicated in various diseases, and with the increasing use of broad-spectrum antibiotics, corticosteroids, and potent cytotoxic agents and the increasing incidence of acquired immunodeficiency, deep mycoses have become increasingly significant.

The pathogenic fungal diseases are divided into superficial and deep infections. The superficial infections are those limited to the epidermis, hair, nails, and mucous membranes. Deep fungal infections are those in which the organisms affect other organs of the body or invade the skin through direct extension or hematogenous spread.

Superficial fungal infections

There are three common types of superficial fungal infection: dermatophytosis, tinea versicolor, and candidiasis (moniliasis). Those caused by dermatophytes are termed *tinea*, *dermatophytosis*, or, because of the annular appearance of the lesions, *ringworm*. In addition, tinea nigra, a superficial infection of the stratum corneum caused by a yeast-like fungus and frequently misdiagnosed as a melanocytic lesion, and piedra, an asymptomatic infection of the hair shaft, may be noted in both children and adults.

The dermatophytes are a group of related fungi that live in soil, on animals, or on humans. They digest keratin and invade the skin, hair, and nails, producing a diverse array of clinical lesions. Depending on the involved site, the infection may be termed *tinea capitis*, *tinea faciei*, *tinea barbae*, *tinea corporis*, *tinea manuum*, *tinea pedis*, *tinea cruris*, or *tinea unguium* (*onychomycosis*, tinea of the nails). The diagnosis and management of fungal diseases of childhood have become easier in the past decade owing to the development of more effective diagnostic techniques and therapeutic agents.

Diagnosis of Fungal Infections

Tests for fungal infection are rewarding procedures readily available to all physicians, not merely those trained in dermatology. Diagnosis of ringworm of the scalp may be aided by the presence of fluorescence under a Wood's light examination, although the changing epidemiology of this infection in the USA has made this exam clinically irrelevant in most cases. Other diagnostic studies that may be useful include direct microscopic examination of skin scrapings or infected hairs and fungal culture. These tests can be performed simply, inexpensively, and rapidly, in the office. Laboratory confirmation of fungal infection is useful in confirming the diagnosis, in detecting the asymptomatic carrier state, and, in the case of tinea

capitis, in demonstrating a mycologic cure when clinical symptoms have resolved. Dermatophyte identification may also provide useful epidemiologic information (i.e., human-to-human versus animal-to-human transmission) and may help guide the clinician's choice of antifungal therapy.

Wood's light examination

The discovery in 1925 that hair infected by certain dermatophytes would fluoresce when exposed to ultraviolet light filtered by a Wood's filter led to a helpful but occasionally improperly used diagnostic tool. When Wood's light examination is performed, it must be remembered that infected hairs, not the skin, fluoresce when exposed to light rays emitted by this lamp. Although the nature and the source of the fluorescent substance in infected hairs are not fully understood, this phenomenon is believed to be the result of a substance, perhaps pteridine, emitted when the fungus invades the hair.

Optimally, a powerful Wood's lamp should be used in a completely darkened room. The usefulness of Wood's lamp examination depends on the pattern of arthroconidial formation and hair invasion. Organisms that result in ectothrix infection (i.e., *Microsporum audouinii* and *Microsporum canis*) result in brilliant green fluorescence with this exam. However, those organisms associated with endothrix infection (i.e., *Trichophyton tonsurans* and *Trichophyton violaceum*), where organisms are present within the hair shaft, show no fluorescence. *Trichophyton schoenleinii*, the cause of favus (see below), produces a pale green fluorescence on Wood's lamp examination. Sources of error in Wood's light examinations include an insufficiently darkened room; the blue or purple fluorescence produced by lint, scales, serum exudates, or ointments containing petrolatum; and failure to remember that it is the infected hair and not the skin that fluoresces.

Potassium Hydroxide Wet-mount Preparations

Microscopic examination of skin scrapings is an important but frequently overlooked aid in the diagnosis of suspected fungal infection of the skin or hair. This examination will yield rapid results but requires considerable experience, as false positive interpretations are common. Material for mycologic study should be taken by gently scraping outward from the active border of a suspected lesion with a No.15 scalpel blade or the edge of a glass slide. Moistening the skin with alcohol before performing the scraping may be useful in adhering the skin debris to the blade before it is smeared on a slide. Cut hairs, nail scrapings, subungual debris, and material from the edge of an affected nail may also be used for wet-mount examination. The material is placed on a glass microscope slide with care and spread out flat and evenly in a single layer. A coverslip is applied, and a few drops of 10–20% potassium hydroxide (KOH) are added at the side of the coverslip until the entire space between coverslip and slide is filled. Gentle heating of the preparation (with care to prevent boiling of the KOH, as this will cause crystallization) should be performed until the horny cells and debris are rendered translucent. If the potassium hydroxide solution contains dimethylsulfoxide (DMSO), the slide should not be heated since heating a DMSO-KOH preparation will dissolve fungi as well as epidermal cells.[1]

After collection and preparation of the specimen, gentle pressure is applied to the coverslip. This will improve the preparation by forcing out trapped air and thinning the specimen, thus allowing better visualization of fungi. The light of the microscope condenser should be dimmed, to enhance contrast between branched hyphae and epidermal elements, and the specimen viewed under low power. A positive KOH examination reveals branching fungal hyphae with septations (Fig. 17.1).

Fungal culture

Although direct microscopic examination of skin scrapings will often confirm the suspicion of tinea, definitive identification rests on isolation of the fungus by the gold standard, fungal culture. There are several types of fungal culture media, but the most popular are Sabouraud's dextrose agar or Mycosel (Mycobiotic) agar containing cycloheximide and chloramphenicol, which suppresses growth of common saprophytic and bacterial contaminants, respectively.[2] Dermatophyte Test Medium (DTM) agar is another commonly used media, which also contains antibiotics (cycloheximide, gentamicin, and chlortetracycline), which inhibit saprophytic fungi and bacteria. DTM also contains a color indicator that changes from yellow to orange to red in the presence of dermatophytes. This medium is particularly useful for physicians who lack detailed knowledge of fungus colony morphology and simply require confirmation of dermatophyte infection. However, one disadvantage of DTM is that the addition of the color indicator precludes laboratory identification of the exact dermatophyte because it may obscure some colonial features used to distinguish these organisms.

Specimens for fungal culture may be obtained via a variety of collection procedures. Traditional methods include plucking broken hairs or scraping scale, but these procedures may be frightening or painful for younger children. Other modalities include use of a sterile toothbrush, wet gauze, cytobrushes, and adhesive tape. Use of a cytobrush has demonstrated very high sensitivity when compared with the traditional method of scraping the scalp.[3] Recently,

the simplicity and reliability of a cotton swab technique has been confirmed.[4] In this method, a sterile cotton tip applicator moistened with tap water (or culturette swab in transport medium) is rubbed vigorously and rotated over the affected area of the scalp, then inoculated onto the appropriate fungal medium. This technique is atraumatic, readily available, and both sensitive and specific, even with delays between collection and plating of the sample.[4]

The Dermatophytoses

Tinea capitis

Tinea capitis, the most common dermatophytosis of childhood, is a fungal infection of the skin and hair of the scalp characterized by scaling and patchy alopecia. It is generally a disease of prepubertal children, especially those between the ages of 3 and 7 years, although infants and adults are occasionally affected. A variety of dermatophytes may cause tinea capitis, especially *T. tonsurans* (the most common etiology in the USA, where it causes >90% of infections), *T. violaceum*, *M. canis*, and *M. audouinii*. These organisms may be anthropophilic (spread from humans, i.e., *T. tonsurans* and *T. violaceum*); zoophilic (spread from animals, i.e., *M. canis* and *M. audouinii*); or geophilic (spread from soil). Dermatophytes have a short incubation period (generally 1–3 weeks) and infect boys more commonly than girls. Predisposing factors for tinea capitis include large family size, crowded living conditions, and low socioeconomic class.[2] In addition to transmission from other humans or animals, dermatophyte spread via fomites (hairbrushes, combs, hats, and contaminated grooming instruments) is well documented. The reason for increased resistance to tinea capitis infection after puberty is unknown, but may be related to a higher content of fungistatic fatty acids in the sebum of postpubertal individuals. Hair care practices (styling, frequency of washing, use of oils or grease, etc.), traditionally believed to play a significant role in the acquisition of tinea capitis, appear to not play a major role.[5]

Asymptomatic scalp carriage of dermatophytes varies and tends to correlate with the amount of tinea capitis in a community.[6] Such carriers constitute a major reservoir for transmission of the organisms causing the disease. Asymptomatic carriage is most common with the anthropophilic organisms *T. tonsurans* and *T. violaceum*, and most carriers are African-American, Afro-Caribbean, or black children in Africa.[2] Household contacts may be a significant source of asymptomatic carriers, and co-sleeping and comb sharing seem to be important factors in the spread of disease in this setting.[7] Varied treatment options have been suggested for the carrier state, although there is a paucity of well-designed clinical studies.

The clinical manifestations of tinea capitis are varied, and are summarized in Table 17.1. It may present in a 'seborrheic dermatitis' pattern, with diffuse scaling and minimal inflammation (Fig. 17.2). One or multiple patches of alopecia may be present (Fig. 17.3), and at times tinea capitis may present in a fashion similar to alopecia areata. 'Black dot' tinea presents with alopecic areas with small black dots within them, representing the ends of broken off hair shafts (Fig. 17.4). This form is most commonly seen with endothrix infections, such as *T. tonsurans*. It should be noted that the black dot sign is probably overemphasized and, although present, may frequently be relatively inconspicuous.

Scalp pustules may be present, and need to be distinguished from bacterial or sterile folliculitis. 'Kerion' (Fig. 17.5) is a markedly inflammatory presentation of tinea capitis, and reveals a boggy plaque with alopecia, pustules, and often purulent drainage from the surface. These lesions represent a vigorous host immune response to the dermatophyte, and are caused most often by *M.*

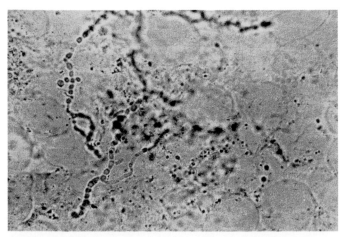

Figure 17.1 Potassium hydroxide examination in tinea. Note the septated fungal elements (hyphae). (Courtesy of Alfred W. Kopf, MD.)

Table 17.1 Clinical manifestations of tinea capitis in children

Clinical feature	Comment
Scalp	
Alopecia	One or multiple patches; may simulate alopecia areata
Scaling	May be minimally inflammatory; may mimic seborrheic dermatitis
Erythema	Localized or widespread
Pustules	Differential diagnosis includes sterile folliculitis or bacterial folliculitis
'Black dots'	Alopecia with hair shafts broken off at surface of skin
Kerion	Boggy, tender plaque with pustules and purulent discharge; represents a vigorous host immune response
Scarring	Rarely seen when untreated; usually follows kerion
Favus	Yellow, cup-shaped crusts around the hair
Other	
Lymphadenopathy	Common; cervical or occipital
'Id' reaction	Widespread, papular or papulovesicular eruption; extremity-predominant; usually seen after initiation of therapy; must be recognized as distinct from true drug reaction

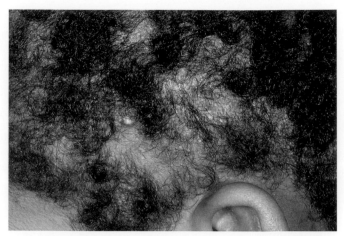

Figure 17.3 Tinea capitis. Multiple patches of alopecia with erythema and scaling. Note the presence of pustules.

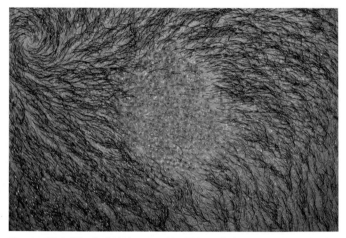

Figure 17.4 'Black dot' tinea capitis. This well-demarcated patch of alopecia is composed of numerous broken-off hair shafts ('black dots').

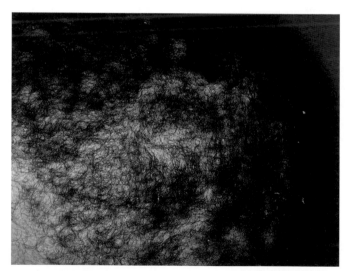

Figure 17.2 Tinea capitis. Diffuse scaling with minimal erythema and patchy alopecia.

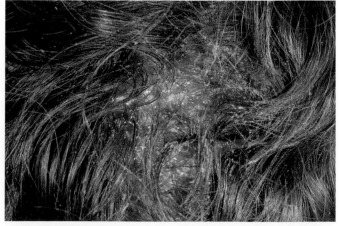

Figure 17.5 Kerion. This fluctuant, erythematous, boggy, and crusted plaque was exquisitely tender to palpation. *T. tonsurans* was isolated in fungal culture.

canis and *T. tonsurans* (and in rural areas by *Trichophyton verrucosum*). Although kerions may heal spontaneously, aggressive therapy is desirable as the severe inflammatory response may result in permanent scarring alopecia (Fig. 17.6).

Lymphadenopathy, especially cervical or suboccipital, is very common in symptomatic patients with tinea capitis. In one study, presence of lymphadenopathy was highly suggestive of a positive fungal culture in children who were suspected of having tinea capitis, especially those with the concomitant presence of alopecia or scaling.[8]

Favus, a severe chronic form of tinea capitis rarely seen in the USA, is caused by the fungus *T. schoenleinii*. This disorder is

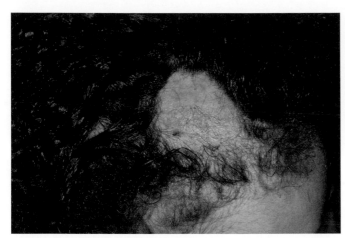

Figure 17.6 Scarring alopecia following kerion. This patch of alopecia persisted following therapy for a severe kerion.

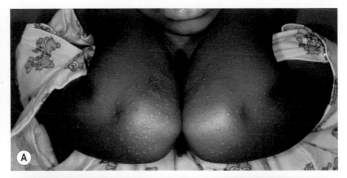

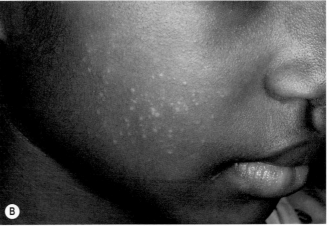

Figure 17.8 Dermatophytid ('id') reaction. These flesh-colored, pruritic papules developed on the extensor extremities (A) and face (B) after initiating oral therapy for tinea capitis.

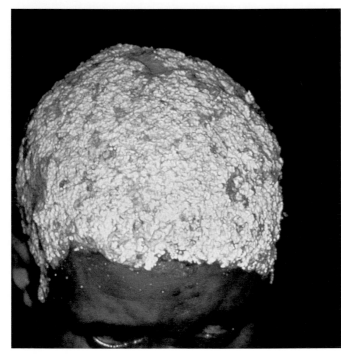

Figure 17.7 Favus. This severe form of tinea capitis is caused most often by *T. schoenleinii*. (Courtesy of Israel Dvoretzky, MD and Benjamin K. Fisher, MD.)

characterized by scaly erythematous patches with yellow crusts or 'scutula,' representing hairs matted together with hyphae and keratin debris (Fig. 17.7). Such infections frequently result in scarring and permanent alopecia.[9]

A widespread papular hypersensitivity or dermatophytid ('id') reaction may occur in patients with tinea capitis. This usually presents as tiny lichenoid papules on the scalp, trunk, and extremities (Fig. 17.8), which may be pruritic. This reaction is commonly seen after initiation of antifungal therapy, and needs to be differentiated from a drug reaction so as to avoid the unnecessary discontinuation of therapy for the tinea. Although this distinction may not always be straightforward, drug reactions tend to be morbilliform, more widespread, and more erythematous. Id reactions represent an immune response to the dermatophyte, and are best

treated symptomatically with topical corticosteroid preparations and oral antihistamines as needed.

The differential diagnosis of tinea capitis includes seborrheic dermatitis, psoriasis, alopecia areata, trichotillomania, folliculitis, impetigo, lupus erythematosus, and a variety of less common scalp dermatoses. Confirmation of the diagnosis is desirable, and the gold standard is fungal culture, as discussed earlier. Wood's light examination may be useful if the infection cause is an 'ectothrix' organism, but this is less common in the USA. Demonstration of the fungus by potassium hydroxide wet-mount preparations of broken hairs or black dots, collected with a forceps, or of skin scrapings from scaly areas may be useful. Microscopic examination of an infected hair (Fig. 17.9) will reveal tiny arthrospores surrounding the hair shaft in *Microsporum* infection (ectothrix infection) and chains of arthrospores within the hair shaft (endothrix infection) in *T. tonsurans* and *T. violaceum* infections.

The color change in a DTM-plated fungal culture may begin within 24–48 h for fast-growing dermatophytes and appears as a pinkish or red zone around the developing colony. The color will intensify as growth proceeds, with full color development for most cultures in 3–7 days (Fig. 17.10). When DTM medium is used, however, the culture should not be evaluated for color after 10 days, since contaminant fungal growth may cause color change by that time, thus leading to false-positive results. It must be remembered that fungi grow best at room temperature and require oxygen. Accordingly, the culture media should be left at room temperature, and the tops of the culture tubes or bottles should be left slightly unscrewed (or the tubes maybe covered only with a cotton plug) to allow aeration of the preparation.

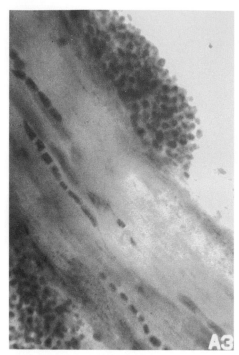

Figure 17.9 Potassium hydroxide examination of hair. Note multiple spores surrounding the hair shaft ('ectothrix') in this patient with *Microsporum* infection. (Courtesy of Alfred W. Kopf, MD.)

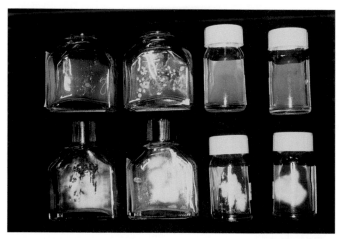

Figure 17.10 Fungal cultures. Cultures plated on Sabouraud's agar (upper panel, two on left) and dermatophyte test medium (DTM, upper panel, two on right) reveal fungal growth and color change (yellow to red on DTM, lower panel), confirming the presence of a dermatophyte.

Tinea capitis requires systemic therapy since the drug needs to penetrate the hair follicle. For decades, the treatment of choice for tinea capitis has been griseofulvin, and this drug remained the only agent approved by the US Food and Drug Administration (FDA) for the treatment of this disorder in children until recently. Terbinafine oral granules are now approved by the FDA for treatment of tinea capitis in children ≥4 years of age. Several other agents, including the azole antifungals (fluconazole, itraconazole, and ketoconazole) have been increasingly evaluated as alternative approaches to therapy. Hence, although griseofulvin remains the 'gold standard',

newer treatment options continue to be explored and may, in the near future, lead to a modification of the traditional approach to therapy. In some instances, these newer agents may be preferable given similar efficacy to griseofulvin and shorter treatment durations.[10]

Griseofulvin is a well-tolerated and safe drug that has been extensively used worldwide for this indication. Although in the past doses of 10 mg/kg per day were utilized, most experts currently recommend 20–25 mg/kg per day of microsize griseofulvin for 6–8 weeks (10–15 mg/kg per day if the ultramicrosize form is used). Absorption of griseofulvin is enhanced by a fatty meal, which should be recommended to the patient and parents. Treatment failures are reported, and may represent increasing resistance of dermatophytes, although non-compliance with therapy or repeat exposure to infected contacts are probably more common reasons for treatment failure.

Side-effects of griseofulvin are rare, and include headache, gastrointestinal disturbance, photosensitivity and rare morbilliform drug reactions. Hematologic and hepatic toxicity is very uncommon, and routine laboratory monitoring is generally not recommended. Although potential cross allergy with penicillins or cephalosporins is frequently mentioned, in reality this risk is quite low. Concomitant therapy with an antifungal shampoo, such as ketoconazole or selenium sulfide, twice to thrice weekly is desirable, as these agents may aid in removing scales and eradicating viable spores, which may help decrease the potential spread of infection.[11,12] This recommendation should be made regardless of the choice of the systemic agent.

Contraindications to griseofulvin therapy include pregnancy, hepatic failure, and porphyria (especially acute intermittent, variegate, and porphyria cutanea tarda). The drug has rarely been implicated in causing exacerbations of lupus erythematosus or lupus-like syndromes.[13] Drug interactions include warfarin-type anticoagulants, barbiturates, and oral contraceptives, and in addition, a disulfiram-like reaction may occur with alcohol ingestion.

Terbinafine is a newer allylamine antifungal agent that seems to hold significant promise as a standard therapy for tinea capitis. It is currently approved for onychomycosis and, as noted above, was more recently approved for treatment of tinea capitis in children 4 years of age and older (in the 'oral granules' formulation). Comparative studies between terbinafine and griseofulvin have demonstrated that treatment with the former for 4 weeks is at least as effective as griseofulvin for 8 weeks.[14,15] In a comparison of terbinafine oral granules to griseofulvin oral suspension, the former resulted in greater rates of clinical cure and mycologic cure for patients infected with *Trichophyton tonsurans* (but not *Microsporum canis*).[16] Studies have evaluated a variety of treatment regimens and durations, including continuous therapy for 1–10 weeks (current package recommendation for terbinafine granules: 6 weeks) and pulsed dosing, somewhat similar to that described for itraconazole (see below). Suggested dosing regimens for terbinafine include 3–6 mg/kg per day or a schedule based on patient weight. According to this schedule, the granules (which come in packets of either 125 mg or 187.5 mg) are dosed as follows: <25 kg: 125 mg/day; 25–35 kg: 187.5 mg/day; >35 kg: 250 mg/day.[17] Some authors have suggested that the 'weight-scheduled' dosing may underdose individuals at the high-end of the weight range. In a duration-finding study of terbinafine in the treatment of tinea capitis, a 2- or 4-week regimen was found to be clinically superior to a 1-week regimen.[18] Higher doses of terbinafine or a longer course of therapy may be necessary for *M. canis* infections.[19,20]

Side-effects related to terbinafine therapy are rare, and include gastrointestinal symptoms, dizziness, headache, and, uncommonly, drug reactions (see Chs 20 and 22). Elevated hepatic transaminases are occasionally seen, and some drugs, including cimetidine, terfenadine, and cyclosporine, may interact.

Ketoconazole, a broad-spectrum azole antifungal compound, has good activity against dermatophytes, especially *Trichophyton* species. However, given the potential risk of hepatotoxicity and the lack of a liquid formulation, this drug is not a favorable alternative to griseofulvin. Other azole antifungal agents, such as fluconazole and itraconazole, seem to offer more promise as alternative agents in the treatment of tinea capitis.

Fluconazole, which is currently approved for systemic mycoses, has been demonstrated effective in tinea capitis, and as with the other newer agents, may require a shorter treatment duration. It has an excellent safety profile, is usually well tolerated, and is available in a liquid suspension for children (10 and 40 mg/cc). Fluconazole has shown efficacy against both *Microsporum* and *Trichophyton* species. Most studies have evaluated dosing of 3–6 mg/kg per day for 2–4 weeks.[21-23] Once weekly, pulse dosing for 8–12 weeks has also been demonstrated effective.[24] Potential adverse effects of fluconazole include gastrointestinal symptoms, headache, or drug reaction. Hematologic and hepatic toxicity may occasionally occur.

Itraconazole is another azole antifungal agent that has been studied for use in tinea capitis, where it has been demonstrated effective in most (but not all) studies. It is currently approved for onychomycosis and some systemic mycoses, and in studies has shown efficacy against both *Microsporum* and *Trichophyton* species. Itraconazole is effective in a 100 mg capsule and a 10 mg/cc oral solution. The dosing recommended for this agent is 3–5 mg/kg per day, with the lower end of the dosing schedule utilized when the oral solution is used. There are numerous studies evaluating itraconazole as a therapy of tinea capitis, and it has been demonstrated effective both in continuous dosing for 2–12 weeks and in a variety of 'pulsed' dosing regimens. One such pulsed regimen consists of a daily dose for 1 week, followed by repeat pulsing for 1 week given 2 weeks later, and a third pulse given 3 weeks after the second pulse.[25] In this regimen, the decision to administer the second or third pulse was determined by the response of the patient at that point in the therapy. Side-effects of itraconazole therapy include headache, gastrointestinal complaints, and occasional hepatic dysfunction. The oral solution seems to be associated with an increased incidence of gastrointestinal side-effects. Multiple drug interactions are possible, and hence all concomitantly ingested medications should be carefully referenced before considering itraconazole therapy. Concurrent administration of non-sedating antihistamines such as astemizole and terfenadine is contraindicated because of the risk of cardiac toxicity.

An important consideration in the child with tinea capitis is school attendance and the issue of contagiousness. It is not practical to keep children with tinea capitis out of the classroom, since spore shedding may continue for months, even after adequate therapy.[26] Appropriate therapy should be instituted, and children receiving treatment should be allowed to attend school.[27] Measures should be taken, where feasible, to avoid transmission between susceptible hosts, including no sharing of combs, brushes, hats, or hooded jackets. In patients in whom appropriate therapy has not led to improvement in symptoms, siblings and close contacts should be examined and fungal cultures performed.

The treatment of kerion deserves special mention. These markedly inflammatory reactions not uncommonly result in permanent scarring alopecia, and therefore rapid institution of aggressive therapy is indicated. In addition to antifungal therapy, systemic antibiotics should be considered, especially in the presence of significant crusting. Skin swab for bacterial culture and sensitivity may be useful in this setting to guide the choice of antimicrobial. Oral corticosteroids are recommended by many in the treatment of kerions, in a dose of 0.5–1 mg/kg per day for 2–4 weeks, although good controlled studies are lacking. Anecdotally, this approach is associated with more rapid resolution of the inflammation and reduction of pain.

Tinea faciei

Dermatophyte infection of the face is referred to as tinea faciei. Although it often presents in a similar fashion to tinea corporis (see below) with annular, scaly plaques (Fig. 17.11), tinea faciei may sometimes be quite subtle clinically, especially if topical corticosteroids have been used. In these instances, it is referred to as 'tinea incognito' (Fig. 17.12), which may also occur in non-facial areas (Fig. 17.13). Although localized mild involvement may respond to topical antifungal therapy, systemic treatment (as described for tinea capitis) is often required to completely clear these lesions.

Tinea barbae

Tinea barbae is an uncommon fungal infection of the bearded area and surrounding skin of adolescent and adult males. Since the most common etiologic agents are zoophilic species of *Trichophyton mentagrophytes* and *T. verrucosum* (occasionally *T. violaceum* and *Trichophyton rubrum*), it occurs primarily among individuals from rural areas in close contact with cattle or other domestic animals.

The infection is usually confined to one side of the face and may consist of a solitary lesion or multiple areas of involvement. The majority of infections are characterized by highly inflammatory purulent papules, pustules, exudate, crusting, and boggy nodules. The hairs within the infected areas are loose or absent, and pus may be expressed through the follicular openings. Spontaneous resolution may occur, or the lesions may persist for months with resultant alopecia and scar formation. Occasionally, a less inflammatory

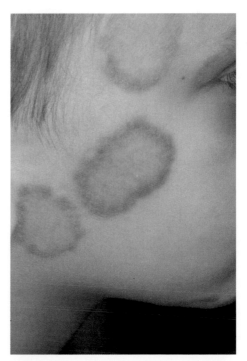

Figure 17.11 Tinea faciei. Annular, erythematous scaly plaques of the face.

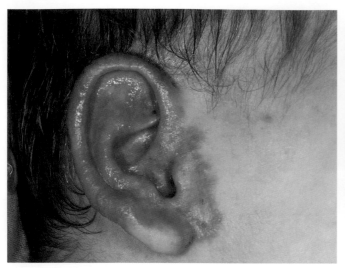

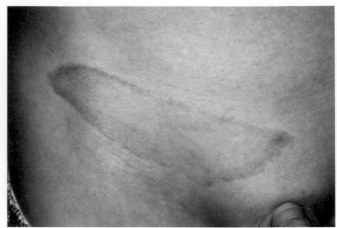

Figure 17.14 Tinea corporis. An expanding, erythematous, annular plaque.

Figure 17.12 Tinea 'incognito'. This markedly inflamed ear had been treated with a variety of topical preparations (including topical corticosteroids, following which the annular border developed) prior to the diagnosis of tinea.

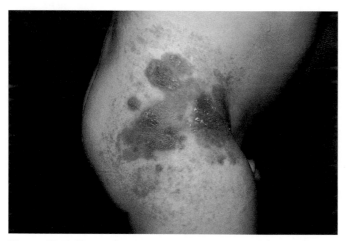

Figure 17.13 Tinea incognito. This impressive dermatitis involving the diaper region ultimately cleared following systemic antifungal therapy. Fungal culture revealed *T. mentagrophytes*.

superficial variety may occur, characterized by mild pustular folliculitis, erythematous patches with broken-off hairs, and a vesiculopustular border with central clearing similar to that seen in tinea corporis.

Tinea barbae must be differentiated from bacterial folliculitis of the bearded area (sycosis barbae), contact dermatitis, herpes zoster, or severe herpes simplex. Sycosis barbae is distinguished by the presence of papular and pustular lesions pierced in the center by a hair that is loose and easily extracted. Herpes simplex or herpes zoster usually presents with clusters of vesicles or erosions on an erythematous base, and the diagnosis is confirmed by Tzanck preparation, direct fluorescent antibody examination, or viral culture. Tinea barbae can be confirmed by microscopic examination of a potassium hydroxide wet-mount of skin scrapings for fungal elements, and/or fungal culture.

Treatment of tinea barbae consists of warm compresses (which help to remove crusts), and topical or oral antibiotics for the frequent secondary bacterial infection. The mainstay of therapy is an oral antifungal agent. With appropriate therapy, resolution occurs over 4–6 weeks.

Tinea corporis

Superficial tinea infections of the skin are termed *tinea corporis*. Sites of predilection include the non-hairy areas of the face (particularly in children; see Tinea faciei, above), the trunk, and extremities, with exclusion of ringworm of the scalp (tinea capitis), bearded areas (tinea barbae), groin (tinea cruris), hands (tinea manuum), feet (tinea pedis), and nails (onychomycosis). Contact with other individuals, such as is seen in high school and college wrestlers ('tinea corporis gladiatorum'), and domestic animals, particularly young kittens and puppies, is a common cause of the affliction in children. The causative organism in young children is frequently *M. canis*, and occasionally *M. audouinii* or *T. mentagrophytes*. In older children and adults, *T. rubrum*, *T. verrucosum*, *T. mentagrophytes*, or *T. tonsurans* are more likely to be responsible. In children with infection caused by *T. rubrum* or *Epidermophyton floccosum*, parents with tinea infection (especially tinea pedis or onychomycosis) are commonly the source of infection.

Tinea corporis tends to be asymmetrically distributed and is characterized by one or more annular, sharply circumscribed scaly plaques with a clear center and a scaly, vesicular, papular, or pustular border (hence the term, *ringworm*) (Figs 17.14, 17.15). When multiple lesions are present, they may become coalescent, resulting in bizarre polycyclic configurations (Fig. 17.16). Although tinea corporis may occur in people of all ages, it is most commonly seen in children, in individuals in warm humid climates, and in patients with systemic diseases such as diabetes mellitus, leukemia, or immunodeficiency.

Tinea corporis is frequently manifested as classic ringworm with annular, oval, or circinate lesions. The pattern may, however, be variable, and it may mimic a variety of other dermatoses, including the herald patch of pityriasis rosea, nummular eczema, psoriasis, contact dermatitis, seborrheic dermatitis, tinea versicolor, vitiligo, erythema migrans (Lyme disease), granuloma annulare, fixed drug eruption, and lupus erythematosus. The use of topical corticosteroids may mask the diagnosis by altering the presenting features while the infection persists. Presentations that may occur in this setting include tinea incognito (as described above) and Majocchi's granuloma. This perifollicular granulomatous disorder, which also occurs on the legs of women with tinea who shave,

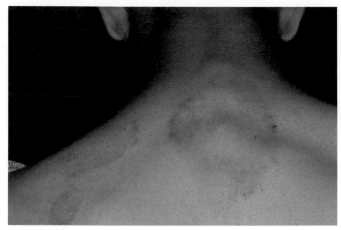

Figure 17.15 Tinea corporis. Multiple annular, erythematous, scaly plaques, with hyperpigmentation of the upper back and shoulders of a teenaged boy.

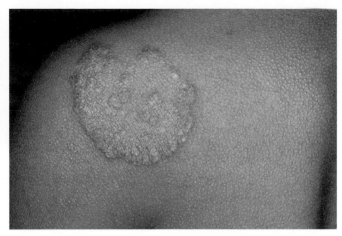

Figure 17.17 Majocchi's granuloma. This annular plaque developed follicular papules following treatment with topical corticosteroids.

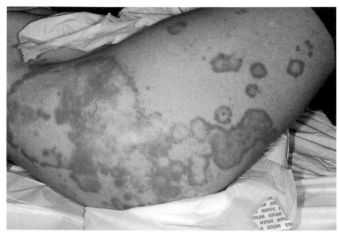

Figure 17.16 Tinea corporis. Multiple annular erythematous plaques with confluence and a polycyclic configuration occurred in this immunocompromised patient.

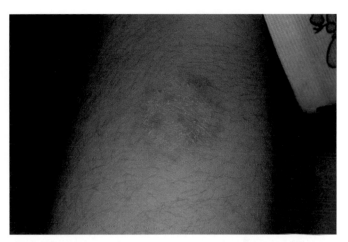

Figure 17.18 Majocchi's granuloma. An annular plaque studded with multiple small pustules. This lesion developed after treatment with topical corticosteroids.

is a distinctive variant of ringworm and essentially represents a granulomatous folliculitis and perifolliculitis caused by *T. rubrum* or *T. mentagrophytes*. It presents with erythematous plaques or patches that reveal scattered papules, papulonodules or pustules studding the surface (Figs 17.17, 17.18). If observed early in the course of the process, a hair may be noted in the center of the papular or pustular lesions.

Tinea corporis can frequently be diagnosed based upon the clinical presentation. Diagnostic examinations include potassium hydroxide wet-mount examination of skin scrapings and fungal culture, as described earlier for tinea capitis. Wood's lamp examination is usually not useful for diagnosing tinea corporis.

Confusion often exists among non-dermatologists regarding the classification and management of 'cutaneous fungal infections'. By definition, this term incorporates disorders due to either dermatophyte or *Candida* infection. It must be recognized, however, that dermatophytes and *Candida* are not synonymous, and that although nystatin is an effective agent against candidal infection, it is inappropriate and ineffective in the treatment of tinea (dermatophyte) infections. Conversely, some antifungal preparations that are active

against dermatophytes, such as tolnaftate and terbinafine, seem to be minimally effective agents for treating candidal infections.

Topical antifungal therapy is generally effective for superficial or localized tinea corporis. These agents are usually applied twice daily, are well tolerated, and have very few side-effects aside from occasional instances of irritant or allergic contact dermatitis. Table 17.2 lists some commonly used topical antifungal agents for dermatophyte infections. Although clinical improvement and relief of pruritus may be seen within the first week of therapy, treatment should be continued for 2–3 weeks to ensure complete resolution.

If a patient shows no clinical improvement after several weeks of therapy, the diagnosis should be reconsidered or, if confirmed and the patient has recalcitrant disease, a course of systemic therapy may be required. In certain situations, systemic antifungal therapy (similar to that described for tinea capitis) may be necessary from the start. These may include disseminated or severe disease, infection in an immunocompromised host, and Majocchi's granuloma, in which case the depth of infection within the hair follicle requires the degree of penetration permitted only by a systemic agent.

Table 17.2 Some commonly used topical antifungal agents for tinea

Generic name	Trade name (select)	Type	OTC/Rx
Butenafine	Mentax	C	Rx
Ciclopirox	Loprox, Penlac	C, I, G, NL	Rx
Clotrimazole	Lotrimin, Mycelex, Desenex	C, L, S, P	Both
Econazole	Spectazole, Ecostatin	C	Rx
Ketoconazole	Nizoral, Nizoral AD	C, Sh	Both
Miconazole	Monistat, Zeasorb AF, Micatin	C, L, R S	OTC
Naftifine	Naftin	C, G	Rx
Oxiconazole	Oxistat	C, L	Rx
Sulconazole	Exelderm	C, S	Rx
Terbinafine	Lamisil	C, S	Both
Tolnaftate	Tinactin, Zeasorb AF, Fungicure	C, G, R S	OTC

Adapted from Lesher and Woody (2003).[28]
OTC, over-the-counter; Rx, by prescription; C, cream; L, lotion; G, gel; NL, nail lacquer; S, solution; P, powder; Sh, Shampoo.

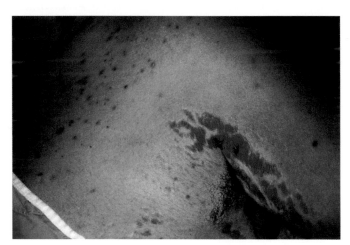

Figure 17.19 Steroid-induced striae. These lesions developed in the axilla of this patient following long-term therapy with betamethasone dipropionate in combination with clotrimazole. (Courtesy of Leonard Milstone, MD.)

Combination antifungal/corticosteroid preparations (i.e., 1% clotrimazole/0.05% betamethasone dipropionate) are widely used by non-dermatologists in the treatment of superficial fungal infections, but care should be exercised with these products as their use may result in persistent or worsening infection.[29,30] In addition, some of these products contain a fairly potent corticosteroid, and hence their indiscriminate use can result in topical corticosteroid toxicities, including skin atrophy, telangiectasia, striae (Fig. 17.19), or systemic absorption. In some instances, such as severe tinea manuum or tinea pedis, however, such a combination product may be useful, but should be applied for no longer than 2–4 weeks. This combination product should never be used in the diaper area, on the face, in fold areas, or under occlusion, and it is not recommended for children younger than 12 years of age.

Tinea corporis gladiatorum, which can impact an individual wrestler's ability to compete as well as have an effect on entire wrestling squads, may require systemic therapy, especially when extensive. Many have advocated different approaches for prevention, although well-designed clinical trials have been minimal. In one study, 100 mg of oral fluconazole given once weekly resulted in a significantly decreased incidence of infection when compared with placebo.[31]

Tinea imbricata

Tinea imbricata, which is caused by *Trichophyton concentricum*, is a superficial dermatophyte infection seen primarily in tropical regions of the Far East, South Pacific, South and Central America, and parts of Africa. It is characterized by concentric rings of scaling that form extensive patches with polycyclic borders. With time, the lesions spread peripherally and form large plaques, which may cover almost the entire skin surface, although the scalp, axillae, palms, and soles are usually spared. When fully developed, the concentric rings are seen as parallel lines of scales overlapping each other, resembling tiles or shingles (*imbrex* means 'shingle') on a roof. Diagnosis is based on the characteristic clinical presentation, microscopic demonstration of interlacing septate hyphae, and identification of the organism by fungal culture. Although treatment with a systemic antifungal agent will usually clear the eruption within 2–4 weeks, there is a tendency for recurrence when treatment is discontinued.

Tinea cruris

Tinea cruris ('jock itch') is an extremely common superficial fungal infection of the groin and upper thighs. It is seen primarily in male adolescents and adults, and occurs less commonly in females. Tinea cruris is most symptomatic in hot, humid weather and is most frequently noted in obese individuals or those subject to vigorous physical activity and chafing. Tight-fitting clothing such as athletic supporters, jockey shorts, wet bathing suits, and panty hose may contribute to this condition as well. The three most common dermatophytes to result in tinea cruris are *E. floccosum*, *T. rubrum*, and *T. mentagrophytes*. Tinea pedis is a common co-existing condition, possibly related to autoinoculation of the dermatophyte with clothing that comes into contact with the feet.

Tinea cruris presents as sharply marginated, erythematous plaques with an elevated border of scaling, pustules, or vesicles. It is usually but not always bilaterally symmetric, and involves the intertriginous folds near the scrotum, the upper inner thighs (Fig. 17.20), and occasionally the perianal regions, buttocks and abdomen. The scrotum and labia majora are usually spared, and if they are involved or satellite papulopustules are present, the diagnosis of candidiasis (Fig. 17.21) should be considered. The lesions of tinea cruris may vary in color from red to brown, and central clearing may be present. In chronic infection the redness and scaling may be slight, the active margin may be subtle or ill defined, and lichenification may be present.

Tinea cruris must be differentiated from intertrigo, seborrheic dermatitis, psoriasis, irritant contact dermatitis, allergic contact dermatitis (generally due to therapy), or erythrasma (a superficial dermatosis caused by the diphtheroid *Corynebacterium minutissimum*). A characteristic coral-red fluorescence under Wood's light examination is helpful in distinguishing erythrasma (see Ch. 14). The diagnosis of tinea cruris can be confirmed by a potassium hydroxide wet-mount microscopic examination of cutaneous scrapings or by fungal culture.

Topical therapy (as discussed for tinea corporis) usually suffices for tinea cruris, and is applied for 3–4 weeks. Other useful measures include reducing excessive chafing and irritation by the use of loose-fitting cotton underclothing, drying thoroughly following bathing

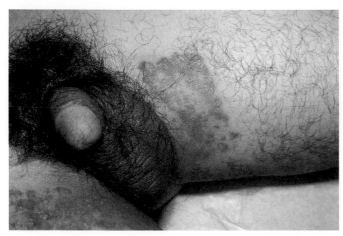

Figure 17.20 Tinea cruris. Scaly, erythematous plaques involving the bilateral medial thighs.

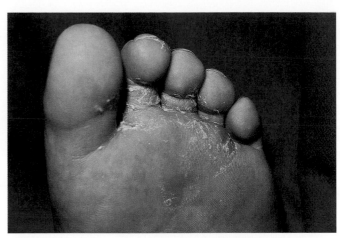

Figure 17.22 Intertriginous tinea pedis. Scaling, erythema, and maceration of the plantar foot and toe web spaces.

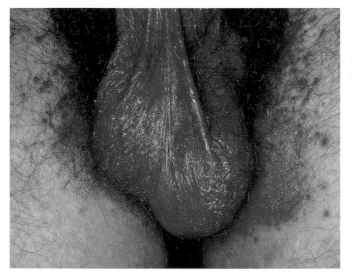

Figure 17.21 Genital candidiasis. Erythema and scaling of the scrotum, with involvement of the adjacent thigh regions. Note the associated satellite papules.

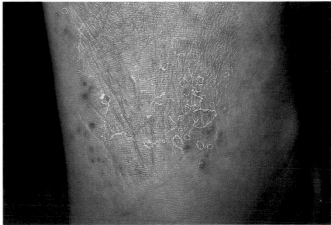

Figure 17.23 Vesicular tinea pedis. Erythema and scaling are accompanied by intensely pruritic, deep-seated vesicles on the plantar surface.

or perspiration, and weight loss. The use of an absorbent antifungal powder (i.e., Micatin, Tinactin, or ZeaSorb-AF) is sometimes helpful, and oral antifungal therapy is occasionally indicated for severe or recalcitrant disease. Tinea pedis, if present, should also be adequately treated as a preventative measure.

Tinea pedis

Tinea pedis, or 'athlete's foot', is relatively uncommon in young children but quite common in adolescents and adults, in whom it represents the most prevalent type of ringworm infection. Although children are not completely immune, most instances of athlete's foot in prepubertal individuals actually represent misdiagnosed cases of foot dermatitis, dyshidrotic eczema, contact dermatitis, or other dermatoses.[32,33] The differential diagnosis of tinea pedis also includes psoriasis, juvenile plantar dermatosis, erythrasma, and secondary syphilis. Associated conditions or complications include onychomycosis (see Tinea unguium (onychomycosis), below), secondary bacterial superinfection, id reaction, and cellulitis.

The etiologic agents most often responsible for tinea pedis are *T. rubrum* and *T. mentagrophytes*, and less often *E. floccosum*

or (especially in children) *T. tonsurans*. The disorder may present clinically in a variety of different ways. The *intertriginous* type, which is the most common presentation, reveals inflammation, scaling, and maceration in the toe web spaces (Fig. 17.22), especially the lateral ones. The inflammatory or *vesicular* type shows inflammation with vesicles (Fig. 17.23) or larger bullae, and usually results from *T. mentagrophytes* infection. This type occurs most often in summer, and an immune response to fungal elements may be reflected by a vesicular id eruption on the hands, extremities, and trunk. *Moccasin-type* tinea pedis presents with erythema, scaling, fissuring, and hyperkeratosis on the plantar surfaces (Fig. 17.24), often extending to the lateral foot margins. Contrary to the eruption seen in foot eczema, the dorsal aspects of the toes and feet are usually spared, although they may occasionally be involved (Fig. 17.25). This form may be resistant to topical therapy, thus requiring an oral antifungal medication.

The diagnosis of tinea pedis is based upon the clinical picture, with confirmation by potassium hydroxide examination and fungal culture. Treatment may be challenging, and efforts to protect the feet from commonplace sites of exposure to the organisms (i.e., public showers, gyms, locker rooms, pool decking, etc.) and to keep the feet dry are both important. Such efforts might include

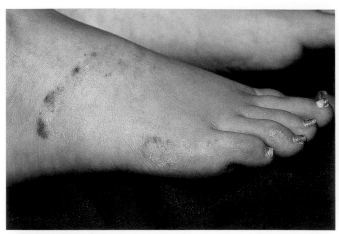

Figure 17.24 Moccasin-type tinea pedis. Erythema and scaling with involvement of the lateral foot borders. Note the associated onychomycosis.

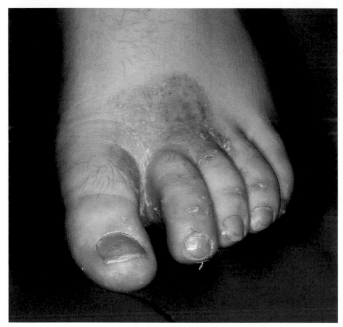

Figure 17.25 Tinea pedis. Involvement of the dorsal surface of the foot is occasionally noted. Note the toe web involvement.

thorough drying of the feet after bathing, avoidance of occlusive footwear or non-breathable socks, and the use of sandals or other footwear in high-risk areas. Absorbent antifungal powders or sprays may be used once or twice daily in individuals prone to these infections, especially following physical exertion and bathing. Those prone to hyperhidrosis can use 6.25–20% aluminum chloride (i.e., Certain Dri, Drysol, or Xerac AC) in an effort to decrease recurrent infection.

The usual treatment of choice for tinea pedis is a topical antifungal preparation applied twice daily. Acute vesicular lesions are best treated with wet compresses applied for 10–15 min two to four times daily, in addition to the antifungal therapy. In patients with severely inflammatory disease, or those with underlying chronic medical conditions such as diabetes or immunosuppression, oral antifungal therapy should be considered. The choices for oral

therapy are similar to those discussed for tinea capitis, and a review of the literature reveals that terbinafine may be one of the more effective agents for this indication.[34]

In instances in which the diagnosis is indeterminate, a topical antifungal agent and a corticosteroid formulation may both be used for a short period (2–4 weeks), at which time a fungal culture performed at the initiation of therapy can generally confirm or refute the diagnosis of tinea. If the diagnosis of tinea pedis is confirmed, the topical corticosteroid can be discontinued. Moccasin-type tinea pedia may require the addition of a keratolytic agent (i.e., lactic acid or urea) in addition to the antifungal, in order to treat the hyperkeratosis and accentuate penetration of the antimicrobial. Id reactions, when present, are best treated with topical corticosteroids and oral antihistamines (if needed), and generally improve with eradication of the primary infection.

Tinea manuum

Ringworm infection of the palmar hand (tinea manuum) is uncommon in childhood and, when present, is generally seen in postpubertal individuals. When ringworm occurs on the dorsum of the hand, it is referred to as tinea corporis rather than manuum. Tinea manuum is usually unilateral and is caused by the same fungi responsible for tinea pedis: *T. rubrum*, *T. mentagrophytes*, and *E. floccosum*. It may be seen in association with tinea pedis, and when occurring on only one hand, presents in a fashion that has been termed 'two-foot, one-hand syndrome'.

Clinical manifestations include a diffuse hyperkeratosis of the fingers and palm and a less common patchy inflammatory or vesicular reaction. Involvement of the fingernails (onychomycosis, see below) frequently occurs, and may be a clue to the diagnosis. When onychomycosis is present, it usually involves some but not all of the nails on the affected hand. Total nail involvement, if present, should suggest the possible diagnoses of psoriasis or lichen planus. The differential diagnosis of tinea manuum includes psoriasis, allergic or irritant contact dermatitis, dyshidrosis, and an id reaction. Unilateral involvement may be another clue to the diagnosis, which can be confirmed by potassium hydroxide microscopic examination or fungal culture.

The management of tinea manuum is essentially the same as that recommended for tinea pedis, and when the latter infection is simultaneously present, it should be appropriately treated as well.

Tinea unguium (onychomycosis)

Onychomycosis is a general term that refers to a fungal infection of the fingernails or toenails. 'Tinea unguium' is a term that specifically implies dermatophyte infection of the nails. However, the two terminologies are often used interchangeably in clinical practice, and for the purposes of the discussion, 'onychomycosis' will refer to dermatophyte nail infections caused usually by *T. rubrum*, *T. mentagrophytes*, and *E. floccosum*. Periungual infection due to *Candida albicans* is discussed below in the section on candidiasis. Onychomycosis is more common in adults, although it does occur in children, often in association with tinea pedis or tinea manuum but also as a primary infection. The overall prevalence of onychomycosis in children has been estimated to be between 0 and 2.6%.[35,36] The lower incidence in children has been attributed to faster nail growth, smaller surface area for invasion, less nail trauma, lower incidence of tinea pedis, and less time spent in environments prone to infected fomites, such as locker rooms.[37] The majority of prepubertal children with onychomycosis have a 1st-degree relative with onychomycosis and/or tinea pedis.

Onychomycosis is classified into several different patterns, including distal subungual, proximal subungual, and white superficial. The *distal subungual* type is the most common, and is characterized by invasion of the underlying nail bed and inferior portion of the nail plate, which leads to onycholysis (detachment of the nail plate from the nail bed) and thickening of the subungual region, which takes on a discolored yellow-brown appearance[38] (Fig. 17.26). Toenails are affected more frequently than fingernails. *Proximal subungual* onychomycosis is relatively uncommon, and occurs when the invasion of the nail unit starts at the proximal nail fold (the area near the cuticle). Clinically, destruction of the proximal nail plate is seen along with similar changes to the distal subungual type (Fig. 17.27). This form of onychomycosis is most common in HIV-infected individuals, and it is considered by some an early marker for this infection. *White superficial* onychomycosis occurs with superficial infection of the nail plate, and presents as well-delineated white plaques on the dorsal nail plate.

The diagnosis of onychomycosis is confirmed by direct microscopy of potassium hydroxide wet-mount preparations and fungal culture. Material for examination should be taken from the subungual debris, underside of the nail plate, nail clippings, or nail bed,

when necessary. Confirmation of the diagnosis is important, since many cases of nail dystrophy are not fungal in origin and are instead the result of another diagnosis, such as psoriasis, post-dermatitis onychodystrophy, chronic paronychia, trauma, drug-induced onycholysis, pachyonychia congenita, lichen planus, or a variety of other conditions (see Ch. 7). It must be remembered that onychomycosis is seldom symmetrical and that it is common to find involvement of only one, two, or three nails of only one hand or foot. In patients who have involvement of all nails, an alternative diagnosis should be highly suspected.

In general, topical agents tend to be relatively ineffective for the treatment of onychomycosis, in large part because of poor penetration through the nail plate. Topical antifungal therapy, however, is an important consideration as adjunctive therapy when tinea pedis is concomitantly present, in which case it may lower the relapse rate for onychomycosis. In addition, a newer agent, ciclopirox 8% nail lacquer solution, has shown promise as an effective topical agent for onychomycosis, occasionally as monotherapy or, more commonly, as an adjunctive treatment.[39,40] Definitive therapy for onychomycosis in most patients, however, is achieved only with the use of oral antifungal agents. When considering therapy for this condition in children, many factors need to be incorporated into the equation, including the results of diagnostic studies, severity of the infection, age of the patient, and risk-to-benefit ratio of the treatments being considered. Parents of younger children should be given the appropriate information regarding therapy and be allowed to make an informed decision. In many instances, a trial of topical therapy with further consideration of systemic therapy if needed down the road may be a desirable option for parents.

Griseofulvin has traditionally been the treatment of choice for systemic therapy of onychomycosis. However, this agent requires long-term administration and is associated with low cure rates and high relapse rates. Newer antifungal agents, including fluconazole, itraconazole, and terbinafine, appear promising as therapies for this condition, and the latter two medications are FDA-approved for this indication in adults. All of these agents have high affinity for keratin, another advantage over griseofulvin, and all remain concentrated in the nails for months after discontinuation of therapy.[38] In addition, they seem to result in much lower relapse rates.

The newer antifungal agents have been dosed in a variety of fashions in studies of onychomycosis. Fluconazole has usually been given as a weekly dose, but may require 12–26 weeks of treatment.[41] Itraconazole and terbinafine appear to be effective with a more convenient dosing regimen. Itraconazole 'pulse therapy' (given daily for 1 week/month for 3–4 months) is a preferred strategy in adults with onychomycosis. This approach has been studied in pediatric patients and appears to be effective and relatively safe,[37,42] although adequately randomized trials are lacking. Terbinafine has demonstrated significant effectiveness in the treatment of onychomycosis. This agent is usually given as a daily dose for 3–4 months, and several studies have suggested superior efficacy and cost-effectiveness over the other antifungal drugs.[43–45]

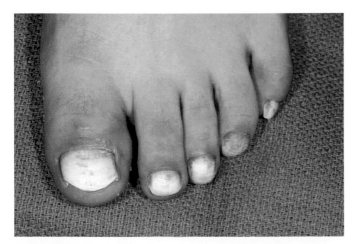

Figure 17.26 Onychomycosis, distal subungual type. Yellow-white discoloration and thickening, with the distal nail surfaces most involved.

Tinea Versicolor

Tinea versicolor (pityriasis versicolor) is an extremely common superficial fungal disorder of the skin characterized by multiple scaling, oval macules, patches, and thin plaques distributed over the upper portions of the trunk, proximal arms, and occasionally the neck or face. It is caused by the yeast forms of the dimorphic fungus *Malassezia furfur*, which are referred to as *Pityrosporum orbiculare* and *Pityrosporum ovale*. This organism is part of the normal cutaneous flora. The disorder occurs worldwide, and the majority of cases present in adolescents, possibly in relation to the lipophilic nature

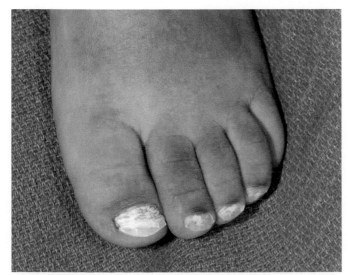

Figure 17.27 Onychomycosis, proximal subungual type. White discoloration of the nail plate, with the process originating at the proximal nail fold regions.

of the organism and the sebum-rich environment of the affected regions. Tinea versicolor only occasionally occurs in prepubertal children. Although *Malassezia* is part of the normal flora, in immunocompromised hosts this yeast may be associated with opportunistic infections, including catheter-related fungemia, peritonitis, septic arthritis, pulmonary infection and sinusitis.[46]

The diagnosis is usually made clinically based on the characteristic presentation. Lesions may be most appreciated during summer months, when sun exposure leads to increasing discrepancies in skin pigmentation between affected and unaffected areas. Examination reveals thin, scaly papules and plaques distributed on the chest, back (Fig. 17.28), and less commonly on the face and neck (Fig. 17.29). They may be hypopigmented or hyperpigmented, depending on the patient's complexion and history of sun exposure, and sometimes mild erythema is present. Scalloping of the borders is common, and lesions may be so numerous that they coalesce into larger patches. Lower extremities and genitals are rare sites of involvement. Interestingly, azelaic acid is a dicarboxylic acid produced by *M. furfur* that inhibits the dopa–tyrosinase reaction, which may result in the hypopigmentation seen in this disorder. This acid is marketed as an acne therapy product for acne-induced hyperpigmentation (see Ch. 8).

The differential diagnosis of tinea versicolor includes vitiligo, pityriasis alba, postinflammatory hypo- or hyperpigmentation, pityriasis rosea, tinea, psoriasis, and confluent and reticulate papillomatosis of Gougerot and Carteaud (see Ch. 23). Distinguishing clinical features are usually sufficient to differentiate these various conditions. Vitiligo presents with *depigmentation* rather than *hypopigmentation*, with well-demarcated patches most often localized around orifices and bony prominences. Pityriasis alba presents with hypopigmented patches, but these lesions are usually limited to the face, occur in atopic individuals, and are only rarely as extensive as one would expect for tinea versicolor. The diagnosis can be confirmed by a potassium hydroxide wet-mount of cutaneous scrapings, which reveals the highly characteristic short fungal hyphae and spores in grape-like clusters (the 'spaghetti-and-meatballs' pattern) (Fig. 17.30) on microscopic examination. Fungal culture is generally not useful, as the organism is difficult to grow on culture media and *M. furfur* is part of the normal skin flora.

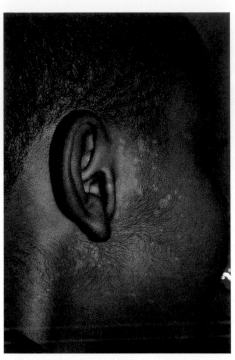

Figure 17.29 Tinea versicolor. Occasional involvement of the face and/or neck is noted, especially in darkly pigmented individuals.

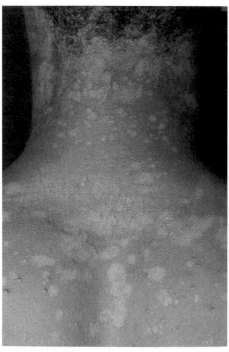

Figure 17.28 Tinea versicolor. Hypopigmented, minimally scaly macules and patches of seborrheic areas of the trunk.

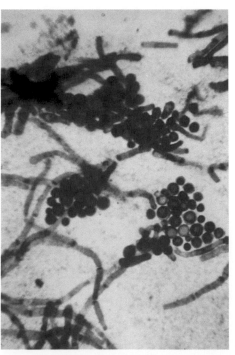

Figure 17.30 Potassium hydroxide preparation of tinea versicolor. Short, blunt-ended hyphae and clusters of spores are present in the classic 'spaghetti-and-meatballs' pattern in scrapings from a patient with tinea versicolor.

Tinea versicolor may respond to a variety of topical preparations. However, because the course of the disorder is usually chronic, recurrences are common, and the pigmentary changes may take months to years to revert, adequate patient education and setting appropriate expectations are vital. Selenium sulfide 2.5% shampoo is a convenient, inexpensive, safe, and relatively effective mode of therapy, especially for younger patients. It is applied in a thin layer for 10 min prior to rinsing for 1–2 weeks. Less frequent intermittent applications (i.e., every other week or monthly) are then useful for maintenance. Ketoconazole 2% shampoo has also been recommended, and was shown effective when applied as a single application or daily for 3 days.[47] More recently, terbinafine 1% spray has become available, and is applied once to twice daily for 1–2 weeks. Topical antifungal creams are also effective, but their use is often impractical given the wide surface area of skin usually involved.

Oral therapy is desirable in patients with severe disease or recurrent disease or in those in whom topical therapies have failed. A variety of oral antifungal agents, including ketoconazole, fluconazole, itraconazole, and terbinafine, have been proposed for this condition. Multiple dosing regimens have been advocated, including continuous, intermittent, and single-dose approaches. A favorite systemic regimen for tinea versicolor is single-dose (400 mg) ketoconazole, followed by physical activity to promote secretion of the drug onto the skin via sweating. The patient then delays showering or rinsing for 10–12 h, and repeats the therapy in 1 week. Itraconazole single-dose therapy (400 mg) was compared to a 7-day continuous therapy (200 mg daily dose), and both regimens were found to be equally effective.[48] In another randomized prospective study, single- and multiple-dose regimens of ketoconazole and fluconazole were compared, and single-dose 400 mg oral fluconazole provided the best clinical and mycological cure rates with no relapse during 12 months of follow-up.[49] In a study of extensive tinea versicolor, single dose ketoconazole (400 mg) was compared with two doses of fluconazole (300 mg) with a 2-week interval between doses. Similar clinical response was noted in both groups (81.5% improvement for fluconazole, 87.9% for ketoconazole), with no significant adverse events in either group.[50] There is no current consensus or 'gold standard' of care for systemic therapy of tinea versicolor, although the authors favor the single dose ketoconazole regimen. This treatment has been clinically demonstrated to be safe, without the concerns (i.e., hepatotoxicity) typically considered when treating with ketoconazole daily and for prolonged periods.

Tinea Nigra

Tinea nigra is a superficial fungal infection of the stratum corneum caused by the black yeast-like mold *Phaeoannellomyces* or *Hortaea werneckii* (formerly called *Cladosporium* or *Exophiala werneckii*). Since it is not caused by a dermatophyte fungus, 'tinea' (as with tinea versicolor) is a misnomer. This infection occurs most often in warm humid areas of Central or South America, Africa, Asia, and occasionally the coastal southern USA. It presents as an asymptomatic, light to dark brown or black, sharply marginated macule or patch, usually involving the palm and less likely the dorsal surface of the hand or plantar foot. Visible scaling is rare. The most important aspect of tinea nigra is the potential misdiagnosis as malignant melanoma. Other misdiagnoses may include post-inflammatory hyperpigmentation, fixed drug eruption or chemical stain.[51] Direct microscopic examination of a potassium hydroxide wet-mount preparation of skin scrapings reveals gray-brown to green hyphae and budding yeast cells, and fungal culture is confirmatory. Tinea nigra is treated with a topical antifungal preparation, such as miconazole, clotrimazole, or terbinafine cream. The application of

keratolytic agents such as salicylic acid or Whitfield's ointment (6% benzoic acid and 3% salicylic acid) or 10% thiabendazole solution is another therapeutic option.

Piedra

Piedra is an asymptomatic fungal infection of the hair shaft caused by *Piedraia hortae* (black piedra) or *Trichosporon cutaneum* (formerly known as *Trichosporon beigelii*; white piedra). Black piedra is seen most commonly in tropical areas of South America, the Far East, and the Pacific Islands. It is characterized by small, hard, and adherent brown-black nodules on the hair shafts of the scalp, which, on hair microscopy, are composed of honeycomb-like masses of fungal asci and ascospores. These nodules contain phosphorus, sulfur, and calcium, which are all part of the extracellular material involved in the organization of the fungus.[52] Fungal culture usually confirms the diagnosis. Traditional therapy consists of hair removal by clipping or shaving, and oral terbinafine may be useful.[53]

White piedra, caused by *T. cutaneum* but also a variety of other *Trichosporon* species, is seen in temperate climates of South America, Europe, Asia, Australia, and the southern USA. It may affect the scalp as well as eyelash, eyebrow, beard, axillary, or pubic hair. White piedra may be underreported in the USA, with recent reports in children from the northeastern states, several of whom were immigrants. This observation suggests that cases in the USA may be primarily imported and, hence, influenced by immigration trends.[54] It is characterized by asymptomatic, soft, white-tan elongated nodules on the hair shaft that may be mistaken for the nits of head louse infestation or hair casts. Microscopic examination of a hair mount reveals yeast-like cells completely encircling the hair shaft and occasional hyphae perpendicular to the hair shaft. The organism can be recovered from a fungal culture. Again, clipping or shaving the hair is usually curative. Oral itraconazole and fluconazole have been demonstrated effective in open-label studies, but recurrence may be noted.[54,55] Concomitant use of an azole (i.e., ketoconazole) shampoo has been advocated as adjunctive therapy.

Although the etiologic agent of white piedra usually results in this benign hair condition, disseminated infection may occur in immunocompromised hosts, especially those with neutropenia and HIV-infected individuals.[56,57] Low birthweight neonates are another population at risk for fungal septicemia with this organism.[58] Cutaneous lesions may occur with disseminated disease, and consist of purpuric papules, nodules, and necrosis. Therapy of *Trichosporon* sepsis/multiorgan dissemination is difficult, as many isolates are resistant to amphotericin B, and the mortality rate is high.

Candidiasis

Candidiasis (moniliasis) is an acute or chronic infection of the skin, mucous membranes, and occasionally internal organs caused by yeast-like fungi of the *Candida* genus. Although several candidal species may be associated with human infection, *C. albicans* is by far the most frequent cause. *Candida albicans* is not a normal cutaneous saprophyte, but usually exists in the microflora of the oral cavity, gastrointestinal tract, and vagina. It becomes a cutaneous pathogen when there is an alteration in host defenses, either localized or generalized, which allows the organism to become invasive.

Factors that predispose to candidiasis include endocrinologic disorders (i.e., diabetes mellitus, hypoparathyroidism, and Addison's disease), genetic disorders (i.e., Down syndrome, acrodermatitis enteropathica, and chronic mucocutaneous candidiasis), malignancy (especially leukemia or lymphoma), and certain systemic medications (i.e., antibiotics, corticosteroids, and immunosuppressive agents).

Newborns and infants are physiologically susceptible to candidal infection, which may be commonly manifested as oral candidiasis (thrush), diaper candidiasis, or intertrigo. Other presentations of candidal infection in childhood include vulvovaginitis, angular cheilitis (perlèche), and nail involvement (paronychia). Neonatal, congenital, systemic, and chronic mucocutaneous candidiases are additional patterns of infection with *Candida*. Candidiasis in the infant is frequently traceable to an infected mother who may be a vaginal or intestinal carrier of the organism. These infants may harbor *C. albicans* in the mouth or intestinal canal, and the infected saliva or stools constitute a focus for cutaneous infection. The presence of *Candida* spp. in the mouths of children has been proposed as a possible factor contributing to dental caries.[59] There follows a review of several types of mucocutaneous candidiasis in children, including a discussion of congenital and neonatal candidiasis and risk factors for severe disease. (Diaper candidiasis is discussed in detail in Ch. 2.)

Oral Candidiasis (Thrush)

Oral candidiasis (thrush) is a painless or painful *Candida* infection of the tongue, soft and hard palates, and buccal and gingival mucosae. It is characterized by white to gray, friable, pseudomembranous patches or plaques overlying a reddened mucosa (see Ch. 2, Fig. 2.22). Thrush may be acquired at the time of delivery during passage through an infected birth canal, during nursing from the skin of the mother's breast or hands, or from imperfect sterilization of feeding bottles.[60] Diagnosis is often clinical, and it can be confirmed by gentle attempts to remove the curd-like plaques that, in distinction to milk or formula residue, adhere to the underlying oral mucosa. Removal is accomplished by gently rubbing the area with a cotton applicator or tongue blade, which results in an underlying inflammatory mucosal erosion. The organism may be identified by microscopic evaluation of a potassium hydroxide wet-mount preparation of these materials or by fungal culture. Although most infants with oral thrush do not experience impairment of appetite or feeding, severe disease may be associated with such complications as well as significant pain. Immunocompromised infants often have a severe expression of oral candidiasis.

The usual approach to therapy, and one that is usually effective, is the administration of nystatin oral suspension, one dropperful in each cheek given four times daily. Massage of the suspension on the mucosa by the parent is useful following administration, and the medication is used for 7–14 days. Nystatin is unabsorbed from the gastrointestinal tract, as are some other topical therapies that have been used, including gentian violet, amphotericin B, miconazole, and clotrimazole. Options for older children include nystatin and clotrimazole tablets or troches. Although it has been suggested that clotrimazole or nystatin troches or suppositories may be inserted into the tip of a slit pacifier or nipple for the treatment of infants with oral candidiasis, these approaches have not been evaluated in controlled studies and the possibility of aspiration must be considered.[60,61] When treating infants with persistent or recurrent oral candidiasis, asymptomatic maternal vaginal candidiasis and candidal contamination of nipples or pacifiers should be considered as possible reservoirs for reinfection.[62] Oral antifungal agents, most notably fluconazole, have been demonstrated quite effective in the treatment of oral candidiasis in immunocompromised children.[63,64] In general, absorbable antifungal therapy should be used primarily if there is risk of dissemination or widespread disease is present.[65]

Intertrigo

The moist warm conditions found in intertriginous areas favor the development of candidal infection. Intertrigo (see also Ch. 3) refers to a condition marked by intense erythema in skin folds, including the axillary regions, anterior neck fold (Fig. 17.31), posterior auricular regions, and inguinal creases. Although it does not always represent a fungal process, *C. albicans* infection is common, and secondary bacterial (i.e., *Staphylococcus aureus*) infection may occasionally be present. *Streptococcal intertrigo* refers to intertrigo in association with group A β-hemolytic streptococcal (GABHS) infection.[66] It presents with intertriginous inflammation that is well demarcated, weeping and superficially eroded (Fig. 17.32). It is often associated with a foul odor, and lacks the satellite papules and papulopustules that are characteristic of candidal intertrigo.

Treatment of intertrigo with a topical antifungal agent (i.e., clotrimazole, econazole, or ketoconazole cream) applied two to three times daily is usually sufficient. More severe cases may require the addition of a low-strength topical corticosteroid or, when bacterial

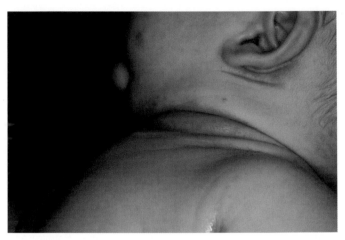

Figure 17.31 Intertrigo. Erythema and maceration of the anterior neck fold. Note the peripheral satellite papules and involvement of the auricular crease. Skin swab from this patient was positive for *C. albicans*.

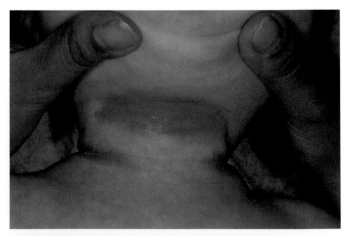

Figure 17.32 Streptococcal intertrigo. This infant presented with well-demarcated erythema with erosive changes, weeping and a foul odor. *S. pyogenes* was isolated on bacterial culture. Note the absence of satellite papules or pustules which are characteristic of candidal intertrigo.

infection is suspected, an appropriate oral antibiotic with activity against both *S. aureus* and GABHS.

Candidal Vulvovaginitis

Candida albicans is a common inhabitant of the vaginal tract, and its incidence increases in diabetes and pregnancy and in females taking antibiotics or oral anovulatory preparations. When vulvovaginitis occurs, the labia become edematous and red, white patches appear on an erythematous mucosal surface, and leukorrhea develops. The resultant symptoms include painful itching, burning, and dysuria. The infection may spread to the perineum, perianal region, gluteal folds, and upper inner aspects of the thighs as well. Although vulvovaginitis is more common in adults, it occurs in premenarchal as well as adolescent females. It accounted for nearly 62% of all gynecological problems seen during childhood and adolescence in one large study.[67] The differential considerations of candidal vulvovaginitis include bacterial infection, foreign body, poor hygiene, and sexual abuse.[68] The most common bacterial causes appear to be groups A and B β-hemolytic streptococci and enterococci.[67,69,70]

The diagnosis of candidal vulvovaginitis is established by the clinical signs and symptoms and by demonstration of the fungus by potassium hydroxide wet-mount examination and/or fungal culture. Treatment options include antifungal vaginal tablets, cream, or suppositories (i.e., clotrimazole, miconazole, nystatin, terconazole) used daily for 3–7 days (up to 14 days for nystatin). A single-dose regimen using a 500 mg vaginal tablet of clotrimazole was also found to be clinically efficacious.[71] A single-dose regimen of fluconazole 150 mg is quite effective in adolescents and adults.

Perlèche

Perlèche (angular cheilitis) is a common disorder characterized by fissuring and inflammation of the corners of the mouth (Fig. 17.33), with associated maceration and exudate. This condition appears to be related to moisture collecting at the mouth angles, and does not usually have any association with nutritional or vitamin deficiency. Whereas in adults it is often related to ill-fitting dentures, perlèche in children may be seen in conjunction with dental malocclusion, the presence of orthodontic appliances, and lip licking. Therapy is best accomplished by correction of the underlying predisposing factor; e.g., the condition often improves following the completion of orthodontia or following modification of lip-licking behavior.

Treatment consists of the application of a low-strength (i.e., class 6 or 7) topical corticosteroid ointment 2–3 times daily. A topical antifungal preparation (i.e., econazole or clotrimazole) should be added for more severe presentations, as *C. albicans* is often present, and if secondary bacterial infection is present, topical or oral antibiotic therapy is indicated.

Chronic Paronychia

Chronic paronychia (see also Ch. 7) is usually associated with *C. albicans* infection, and presents with transverse ridging of the nail plate, loss of the cuticle, and mild proximal/lateral periungual erythema (Fig. 17.34). It is distinguished from acute paronychia not only by the natural history (acute paronychia is more sudden in onset), but by lack of the marked edema, pain, and pustule formation, which are classically seen in the acute (bacterial) type. Chronic paronychia in children may be related to repeated finger or thumb sucking. Therapy with a topical antifungal cream applied twice daily is usually effective, although the nail plate may take several months to grow out normally. Oral fluconazole may also be effective for severe or resistant involvement. Attempts to decrease moisture of the affected digits will accentuate the response to therapy and help to minimize recurrences.

Erosio Interdigitalis Blastomycetica

Erosio interdigitalis blastomycetica (derived from Latin meaning 'an erosion between digits caused by a budding fungus') is a red, itchy, and occasionally slightly painful eruption of the web spaces between the fingers or toes. It is most common in individuals whose hands or feet are exposed to moisture frequently, and most commonly involves the lateral two web spaces (i.e., between the third and fourth and between the fourth and fifth digits). Erosio interdigitalis blastomycetica presents with erythema, maceration, and peeling of the affected region (Fig. 17.35), with a scaly and occasionally vesicular border. It seems to be due to infection with *C albicans* and, occasionally, there may be an associated Gram-negative infection (see Ch. 14). Treatment of erosio interdigitalis blastomycetica consists of keeping the hands and feet as dry as possible, and the use of a topical antifungal and (when needed) antibacterial preparation.

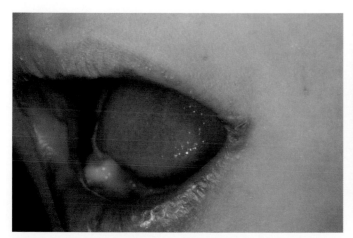

Figure 17.33 Perlèche (angular cheilitis). Erythema, fissuring, and exudate of the mouth angle.

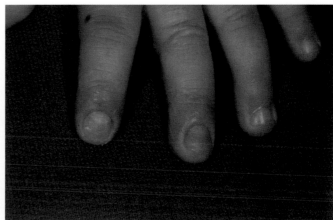

Figure 17.34 Chronic paronychia. Nail plate ridging, mild periungual erythema, and cuticle loss are seen involving the 1st and 2nd fingers in this patient with chronic Candida infection. Note the normal appearance of the 3rd and 4th fingers.

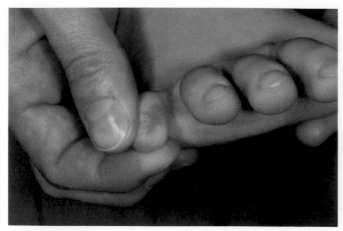

Figure 17.35 Erosio interdigitalis blastomycetica. Erythema, maceration and peeling of the fourth toe web space. This eruption cleared rapidly with topical azole antifungal therapy.

Black Hairy Tongue

Black hairy tongue is a term used to describe a disorder primary affecting adults and occasionally adolescents, and characterized by hypertrophic, elongated filiform papillae, which form a dense black to blue-black surface on the midportion of the dorsal tongue. It occurs less often in young children, but has been observed in an infant as young as 2 months of age.[72] The etiology is unknown, but it is frequently attributed to *C. albicans* or bacterial infection and is often associated with the prolonged use of antibiotics. Treatment consists primarily of improved oral hygiene, and gentle brushing of the dorsal tongue with a soft toothbrush and a small amount of toothpaste two to three times daily is usually effective.

Neonatal and Systemic Candidiasis

Two types of candidiasis in the newborn period have been reported: a *congenital* form in which the skin lesions are present at birth or within the first 6 days of life, and a *neonatal* form commonly seen after the 1st week of life. Neonatal candidiasis develops as a result of infection acquired by passage through an infected maternal birth canal. This perinatal or postnatal acquisition of *Candida* encompasses several clinical presentations, including localized disease (i.e., oral thrush and diaper dermatitis), systemic infection related to invasive procedures and infected indwelling devices, and 'invasive fungal dermatitis' seen in extremely low birthweight neonates. Although *C. albicans* is the primary pathogen, *Candida parapsilosis* is becoming a more significant pathogen in the neonatal setting, and *Candida glabrata* has been reported following *in vitro* fertilization and embryo transfer.[73–77]

Congenital candidiasis is acquired *in utero* and may be associated with premature labor, especially in instances where a foreign body (i.e., IUD or cervical sutures) is present. A history of maternal candidal vulvovaginitis is common in infants with congenital candidiasis, although the former is present in a high percentage (up to 25%) of pregnant women and in most instances is not associated with this neonatal infection.[78] Congenital candidiasis tends to run a more benign course in full-term infants without risk factors, but may result in serious systemic infection in premature neonates, especially those of extremely low birthweight. Other risk factors for invasive candidal infection include extensive instrumentation in the delivery room and invasive procedures utilized during the neonatal period.

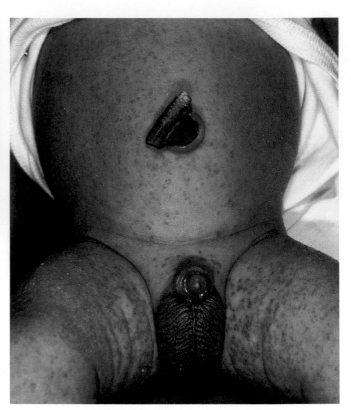

Figure 17.36 Congenital cutaneous candidiasis. Widespread erythematous papules and pustules in a 10-day-old male. This otherwise-healthy child had involvement limited to the skin and no risk factors for dissemination. His mother reported a history of vulvovaginal candidiasis during the last trimester of pregnancy.

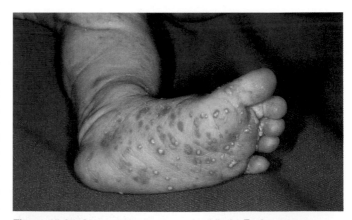

Figure 17.37 Congenital cutaneous candidiasis. Erythematous papules, papulovesicles, and pustules were present at birth in this full-term infant male. No extracutaneous involvement was noted.

Congenital cutaneous candidiasis (CCC) presents with multiple, widespread erythematous macules, papules, and pustules (Fig. 17.36), and occasionally bullae. In full-term infants, this form of candidiasis is often limited to the skin and resolves over 1–2 weeks.[74] The most common locations of involvement are the back, extensor surfaces of the extremities, and skin folds, with relative sparing of the diaper area.[79] Pustules on the palms and soles (Fig. 17.37) are a common and useful diagnostic finding. Oral thrush is uncommon in this setting, but nail changes (yellow discoloration, thickening, paronychia) (Fig. 17.38) are occasionally present. Such

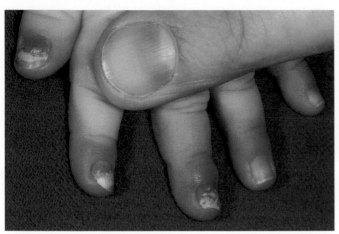

Figure 17.38 Congenital candidiasis. Yellow discoloration with ridging and nail plate separation in a newborn male with no other manifestations of *Candida* infection.

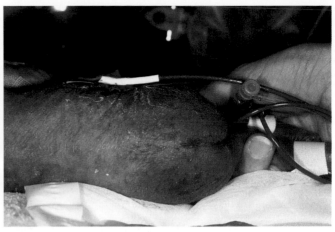

Figure 17.40 Invasive fungal dermatitis. Erythema with maceration, crusting, and peeling in an extremely low birthweight newborn with candidiasis. (Courtesy of Moise Levy, MD.)

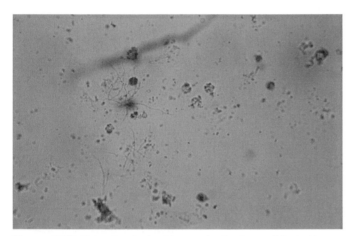

Figure 17.39 Potassium hydroxide examination in candidiasis. Spores and pseudohyphae as noted on microscopic examination of skin scrapings from a patient with candidiasis.

nail changes may be the sole manifestation of congenital candidiasis. The clinical findings in CCC may resemble erythema toxicum neonatorum, bacterial folliculitis, bullous impetigo, and congenital herpes, varicella, or syphilis. The definitive diagnosis of CCC is made by the microscopic finding of spores and pseudohyphae on skin scrapings (Fig. 17.39), or culture of the organism. Another useful diagnostic modality is examination of the placenta, which may reveal typical changes of candidiasis (including funisitis, abscesses, or chorioamnionitis).[79,80] In patients with CCC limited to the skin and without risk factors for disseminated disease, topical antifungal therapy often suffices.

Systemic candidiasis occurs primarily in very low birthweight infants and is typically seen between the 2nd and 6th weeks of life. The immature immune defenses of this population contribute to this propensity toward systemic disease.[79] Common features include apnea, hyperglycemia, temperature instability, lethargy, hypotension, and increasing respiratory requirements.[77] The skin surface may or may not be involved. These patients may have candidal septicemia, meningitis, urinary tract infection, or disseminated disease. Since the kidneys act as a filter for *Candida*, spores may be present on microscopic examination of urine samples.[80] Renal pelvis fungus balls may be seen in up to 42% of these infants, and

endocarditis, septic arthritis, endophthalmitis, and osteomyelitis may also occur. The diagnosis is confirmed by isolation of *Candida* from blood, urine, cerebrospinal fluid, or other normally sterile sites. Systemic candidiasis requires parenteral antifungal therapy, is associated with a high mortality rate, and may result in permanent neurodevelopmental deficits in long-term survivors.

'Invasive fungal dermatitis' refers to a clinical entity seen in extremely low birthweight infants, consisting of a distinct cutaneous presentation of *Candida* infection in combination with a high risk for internal dissemination.[78] The affected infants develop lesions after several days of life. Skin involvement is characterized by erosive and ulcerative lesions (Fig. 17.40) with extensive crusting. Vesicles, bullae, and 'burn-like' erythema may also be present, and desquamation and widespread denudation are common. A high index of suspicion should be maintained in extremely low birthweight infants with any of these findings, as disseminated infection is common, including fungemia, meningitis, urinary tract infection, and other organ involvement. Potential risk factors for this form of candidiasis include vaginal birth, postnatal steroids, and prolonged hyperglycemia.[78] The immature skin barrier function seen in extremely premature infants is believed to be pathogenic, with skin serving as the portal of entry for this infection.[78,81]

Chronic Mucocutaneous Candidiasis

Chronic mucocutaneous candidiasis (CMC) is characterized by recurrent infections of the skin, nails, and mucosae with *Candida* species, usually *C. albicans*. This disorder appears to be a common phenotype for a variety of defects in the immune response, most notably in the cellular branch of the immune system, and mainly the specific responses to antigens of *Candida* species.[82] CMC is often sporadic, although it may be familial, and has been reported in both autosomal dominant and recessive forms. It frequently presents during childhood. Associated conditions include hypothyroidism, polyendocrinopathy (autoimmune polyendocrinopathy–candidiasis–ectodermal dystrophy or APECED syndrome (see Ch. 23), hyper–IgE syndrome, thymoma, and chronic keratitis.[83] It has also been reported in association with elevated gliadin antibodies and a celiac disease-like presentation, with weaning of the antibodies during anti-candidal therapy.[84]

The clinical features of CMC are marked by the mucocutaneous findings. Oral candidiasis (thrush), candidal diaper dermatitis, candidal intertrigo, and paronychia that are persistent and recalcitrant to therapy are all common. Angular cheilitis (perlèche) is also seen. Generalized, scaly, erythematous, and crusted papules and plaques may be present, especially on the scalp, where they may lead to scarring alopecia. Nail involvement is notable for nail plate thickening and discoloration, and chronic paronychia may be present. Systemic candidiasis does not usually occur in patients with CMC. Dental enamel dysplasia occurs in some patients with APECED syndrome (see below), and at times may be so severe that it leads to early loss of dentition. Other infections may occur with increased frequency in these patients as well, most commonly tinea, pyogenic skin infection, sinusitis, pneumonitis, and urinary tract infection.

The most common endocrinopathies noted in association with CMC are hypoparathyroidism, hypoadrenalism (Addison disease), and gonadal failure. These endocrine abnormalities commonly do not appear until adolescence or adulthood, and therefore serial evaluations for endocrine function are indicated in patients with CMC, especially those with one endocrinopathy or with family members affected with APECED.[85] APECED, which is also known as *autoimmune polyendocrinopathy syndrome type I* (*APS1*), is an autosomal recessive disorder caused by mutations in the autoimmune regulator (AIRE) gene.[86,87] Besides the candidal infections and endocrine abnormalities, patients have ectodermal dystrophy manifested most commonly as alopecia areata, as well as nail dystrophy and dental enamel defects. Other observed defects may include vitiligo, chronic active hepatitis, growth hormone deficiency, thyroid disease, diabetes mellitus, pernicious anemia, keratopathy, celiac disease and iridocyclitis.[86,88] The autoimmune diathesis also is responsible for the candidal infections. Patients have been shown to have neutralizing autoantibodies directed against IL-17 and IL-22, cytokines that are important in immune responses to the candidal organism.[89,90]

The immune defects associated with CMC are quite variable and include severe combined immunodeficiency, decreased cytokine production, selective antibody deficiencies (i.e., IgG2, IgG4, IgA) and depressed natural killer cell activity.[82,84–92]

Treatment of CMC includes addressing the immunodeficiency status (and augmenting or correcting it, when feasible) and administration of topical and/or oral antifungal medications. Topical antifungal creams are useful for treatment of localized cutaneous lesions. Oral or vaginal candidiasis may benefit from oral troches or suspensions and vaginal creams or suppositories, respectively. The mainstays of therapy for CMC, however, are the oral antifungal agents, including ketoconazole, fluconazole, and itraconazole. When these agents are used as ongoing therapy for this indication, the possible side-effects, potential for drug interactions, and risk-to-benefit ratio must all be taken into consideration.

Deep fungal disorders

In contrast to the superficial dermatophytes, which are confined to dead keratinous tissue, certain mycotic infections have the capacity for deep invasion of the skin or subcutaneous tissues as well as the potential for systemic infection, especially of the lungs and reticuloendothelial system. There follows a review of several deep fungal infections, which have been divided into the subcutaneous, systemic, and opportunistic mycoses.

Subcutaneous Mycoses

The subcutaneous mycoses are a group of disorders caused mainly by fungi that exist as soil saprophytes and are normally of low virulence, but may result in infection involving the skin and subcutaneous tissues. Although these infections are found most often in adults with occupational exposure to soil and plants, all age groups are potentially susceptible. Rhinosporidiosis, which has been classified variably as a fungus or a protozoan parasite, has been included in this category and usually affects the nasal, nasopharyngeal, and ocular mucosae.

Sporotrichosis

Sporotrichosis is a granulomatous fungal infection of the skin and subcutaneous tissues caused by *Sporothrix schenckii*, a dimorphic fungus of worldwide distribution commonly isolated from soil and plants. It occurs in patients of all ages but is observed most commonly in adult males who, because of their occupation or leisure-time activities, are likely to be exposed to contaminated soil or vegetation (farmers, florists, gardeners, forestry workers, miners, and individuals who work with contaminated packing material). Childhood infection, although significantly less common, does occur and may go undiagnosed without a high index of suspicion.[93] Although human transmission can occur after close contact with suppurative wounds of sporotrichosis, the majority of clustered cases are most likely related to simultaneous inoculation from the same source.[94,95] Although disease is usually limited to the skin and subcutaneous tissues, disseminated sporotrichosis with fungemia may occur, especially in the setting of HIV infection.[96]

The clinical presentation of sporotrichosis is variable. The *lymphocutaneous* form is most common in adults, and presents with a painless, erythematous papule or nodule that begins on exposed areas of skin, most commonly the upper extremity. The initial lesion often follows a penetrating injury, such as that inflicted by a splinter, thorn, grain, rock, piece of glass, or cat scratch (cats are perhaps the only animals capable of transmitting this disorder[97]) contaminated with the organism. The lesions are often solitary, and enlarge over several weeks. Secondary discrete lesions may develop, and often progress toward more proximal sites, a pattern that has been referred to as 'sporotrichoid'[98] (Fig. 17.41). Regional lymphadenopathy and lymphadenitis are common. The skin lesions may ulcerate centrally and heal with scarring, although spontaneous clearing is unusual. In a series of 25 children with sporotrichosis, 60% had lesions on an extremity (followed by the face as the next most common site), and the majority had the lymphocutaneous form of the infection.[99] Epidemic sporotrichosis related to transmission from infected cats was reported in 1998–2004 in Brazil, and affected humans, cats and dogs.[100]

The *fixed cutaneous* form of sporotrichosis is characterized by localized skin lesions without lymphatic involvement. The skin

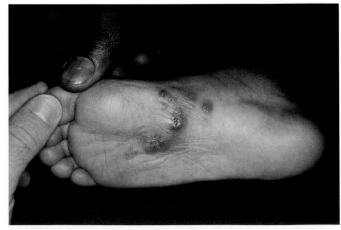

Figure 17.41 Sporotrichosis. Erythematous papules and nodules on the plantar surface, with early lymphangitic ('sporotrichoid') spread.

findings range from scaly papules to verrucous, ulcerated plaques or nodules, with or without satellite lesions. This form seems more common in children, and there may be a delay in diagnosis given the lack of a typical sporotrichoid distribution pattern.[93] It has been hypothesized that children manifesting fixed cutaneous forms may possess host factors that limit the infection to the inoculation site, even if the strain is capable of producing the more classic lymphocutaneous form commonly seen in adults.[101] This form of sporotrichosis was reported in a 3-week-old neonate, in whom the source of infection was unknown.[102]

Disseminated sporotrichosis is rare and usually occurs in individuals with immunologic defects or chronic disease. In these patients the cutaneous lesions may be widespread and develop after hematogenous spread of the infection from a primary focus in the skin or an occult pulmonary focus. Multiple additional organs may be involved, including the bones, joints, and central nervous system. This form of sporotrichosis may mimic tuberculosis (especially with upper lung radiographic lesions), and is associated with significant morbidity and mortality. *Multifocal cutaneous ulcers* have also been reported in sporotrichosis, in association with misuse of topical corticosteroids and self-inoculation.[103]

The differential diagnosis of cutaneous sporotrichosis includes atypical mycobacterial infection, bacterial abscess or ecthyma, *Nocardia*, foreign body granuloma, chromoblastomycosis, cutaneous manifestations of systemic mycoses, leishmaniasis, anthrax, and tularemia. The 'Gold Standard' for diagnosis is fungal culture of a skin biopsy specimen. Direct examination of smears or biopsy material is usually nonspecific.

The traditional treatment of choice for cutaneous sporotrichosis in adults has been orally administered saturated solution of potassium iodide (SSKI), 5 drops three times daily, increased to a maximum of 30–35 drops TID. Infants and young children are treated with 1–2 drops per year of age TID. SSKI therapy may be associated with increased lacrimation or salivation, metallic taste, gastrointestinal discomfort, diarrhea, and headache. Treatment is continued until 4–6 weeks after clinical resolution of lesions.

Newer data suggest that the treatment of choice for sporotrichosis is itraconazole for 3–6 months, with a reported success rate of 90–100% for cutaneous or lymphocutaneous disease.[104] In children, the recommended dose is 5 mg/kg daily. Fluconazole is another option, although it may be less effective. Terbinafine and local hyperthermia are other potential therapies for nondisseminated disease, and amphotericin B is indicated for patients with life-threatening, disseminated, or extensive infection.

Chromoblastomycosis

Chromoblastomycosis (chromomycosis) is an uncommon chronic fungal infection of the skin and subcutaneous tissue caused by a variety of dematiaceous fungi (filamentous fungi with melanin-type pigment in the fungal wall). At least five organisms are implicated in the disease, including species of *Phialophora*, *Fonsecaea*, or *Cladosporium*, all of which are common inhabitants of decaying wood and soil. Several cases have been reported following penetrating wounds of the skin, especially from splinters and thorns.[105] The disease is rare during childhood, and is seen most commonly in tropical and subtropical climates.[106]

Chromoblastomycosis is characterized initially by the formation of small scaly papules that may expand into nodules. The lesions, which are most often confined to the lower leg or foot, coalesce into larger nodules and plaques, and characteristically develop a very verrucous (warty) surface. There may be purulent drainage, and the lesions may be painless or tender. The surface may be studded with multiple 'black dots'. Longstanding lesions may result in edema of the extremity and scarring.

The differential diagnosis of chromoblastomycosis includes other deep fungal, mycobacterial, and bacterial infections, as well as cutaneous tuberculosis, leishmaniasis, leprosy, and tertiary syphilis. The diagnosis is confirmed by microscopic recognition of the organism in potassium hydroxide wet-mount preparations or tissue biopsy specimens, and by fungal culture. When the disease is localized, the treatment of choice is surgical excision of the affected tissue. Several destructive modalities, including cryotherapy, heat therapy, and radiation therapy, have been used. In more advanced cases, surgical or destructive approaches are not feasible and medical therapy is necessary. Systemic agents utilized for chromoblastomycosis include itraconazole (which appears to be the most effective[107]), terbinafine, thiabendazole, ketoconazole and 5-flucytosine.[106] Amphotericin B tends to be less effective.

Mycetoma

Mycetoma, also called *Madura foot*, is a chronic granulomatous infection of the subcutaneous tissues along with invasion of the fascia, muscles and bone and, when an extremity is involved, enlargement of the affected area. Although the majority of lesions are seen on the lower extremity, they may also occur on the hand, shoulder, buttocks, knees, or other regions of the body. The organisms that cause mycetoma are usually introduced by skin trauma. Mycetoma is endemic in Latin America, the Indian subcontinent, Africa, and between the latitudes of 15°S and 30°N around the Tropic of Cancer (the so-called 'mycetoma belt').[108]

Mycetoma may be caused by various species of true fungi ('eumycotic mycetoma'), including *Pseudoallescheria boydii*, *Madurella mycetomatis*, *M. grisea*, and *Phialophora verrucosa*. It may also be caused by anaerobic fungus-like bacteria, the actinomycetes ('actinomycotic mycetoma'), usually by species of *Nocardia*, *Actinomadura*, or *Streptomyces*. These organisms exist as saprophytes in soil or on vegetable matter. The most common agent worldwide is *Nocardia brasiliensis*. Mycetoma is uncommon in childhood and relatively rare in the USA, occurring most commonly in young adults and workers in rural tropical and subtropical areas who walk barefoot and are thus more readily exposed to the organisms.

The infection begins as one or more small, firm papules that gradually evolve into subcutaneous nodules with sinus tracts, draining abscesses, edema, and enlargement of the affected extremity. Purulent drainage is common and 'grains' of various colors may be visible in the exudate, the color depending on the infecting organism. Eventually, crusting and granulation tissue may develop, and the infection may extend to the deeper tissue levels and bone. A preliminary diagnosis can be made by microscopic examination of the granules to identify their actinomycete or fungal nature, but tissue culture is generally necessary for confirmation. Treatment of mycetoma depends on the causative agent. Therapeutic options for actinomycotic mycetoma include sulfonamides, streptomycin, tetracyclines, rifampicin, ciprofloxacin, amikacin, penicillin, imipenem and dapsone. Treatment of eumycotic mycetoma is more difficult and usually a combined approach of medical and surgical therapy. Small lesions may be best treated with complete excision. Medical therapies include the azole antifungals (especially ketoconazole and itraconazole) and amphotericin B.[109] Unfortunately, there is no single drug that gives consistently good results, and longstanding cases with extensive tissue destruction and fibrosis are frequently resistant to all forms of therapy.

Rhinosporidiosis

Rhinosporidiosis is a rare disorder caused by the organism *Rhinosporidium seeberi*. It occurs throughout the world, but is most common in the tropics, especially in India and Sri Lanka. It has been occasionally reported in the USA, especially the southern portion. Although rare in children, a cluster of pediatric cases was reported in rural north-east Georgia between 1981 and 1994.[110] Studies have suggested a possible link to swimming or bathing in freshwater ponds, lakes, or rivers.[111] Although *R. seeberi* was originally thought to be a protozoan parasite, it has most consistently been classified as a fungus, given its microscopic appearance and identification with fungal stains. Recent information supports its classification as a novel group of aquatic protistan parasites.[111]

Rhinosporidiosis is characterized by papules, nodules, and pedunculated vascular polypoid growths on the mucous membranes of the nose, nasopharynx, soft palate, and conjunctivae. Other potential sites of involvement include the upper respiratory passages, lacrimal sacs, skin, larynx, genitalia, or rectum. The surface often has a raspberry-like appearance and is studded with tiny white or yellow nodules. The lesions may become hyperplastic and may reach enormous size, and symptoms are often associated with physical obstruction. Diagnosis is confirmed by microscopic examination, and the organism is notoriously difficult to isolate in culture. Fine needle aspiration cytology may reveal the sporangia and spores of *R. seeberi*.[112] Treatment generally consists of electrosurgical destruction or surgical removal of lesions, when feasible. Antimicrobial agents, most notably dapsone, have been reportedly effective in some patients.

Systemic Mycoses

The systemic mycoses comprise a group of fungal disorders that arise from internal foci, usually the lungs or upper respiratory tract. When the skin lesions result from dissemination of the infection, the prognosis is generally poor. Primary inoculation disease of the skin occasionally occurs with these infections. Disorders in this group include blastomycosis, coccidioidomycosis, paracoccidioidomycosis, and histoplasmosis. Actinomycosis and nocardiosis, although frequently included under the group of disorders because of true fungi, are actually caused by fungus-like Gram-positive bacteria, and are discussed in the section on bacterial infections (see Ch. 14).

Blastomycosis

Blastomycosis (North American blastomycosis, Gilchrist's disease, Chicago disease) is a systemic granulomatous infection caused by the dimorphic fungus, *Blastomyces dermatitidis*. It occurs most often in the southeastern and south central states that border the Mississippi and Ohio Rivers, and the Great Lakes states. Blastomycosis occurs in three forms: pulmonary, disseminated (systemic), and primary cutaneous inoculation, which is quite rare. It has been cultured from soil, which is believed to be the reservoir for infection in humans.[113] Blastomycosis is rare in children, especially those under 1 year of age.[114] South American blastomycosis is a chronic granulomatous disease caused by *Paracoccidioides brasiliensis*, and is also known as paracoccidioidomycosis. It is discussed briefly later in this chapter.

Primary infection usually involves the lungs, and patients may present with nonspecific flu-like symptoms, cough, low-grade fever, night sweats, hemoptysis, or minimal symptomatology. Chest radiography is often nonspecific during acute infection. Many patients with acute pulmonary blastomycosis may go undiagnosed and thus untreated. The disorder may heal spontaneously, progress to chronic pulmonary disease with or without cavitation, or disseminate, primarily to skin, subcutaneous tissues, bones, and joints. Acute respiratory distress syndrome (ARDS) may occasionally occur.[115] Other potential sites of dissemination are the gastrointestinal tract, liver, spleen, genitourinary tract, and central nervous system.

Skin involvement in North American blastomycosis is most frequently associated with disseminated disease, and only occasionally because of primary inoculation. Primary cutaneous blastomycosis

is extremely rare in children, and often presents with a localized chancroid-like ulcer.[116] The primary types of skin changes noted in all forms of cutaneous blastomycosis are verrucous (warty) lesions and cutaneous ulcers.[117] Verrucous lesions present with heaped-up hyperkeratosis with a surrounding erythematous or violaceous color (Fig. 17.42). They may be confused with multiple other cutaneous infections or squamous cell carcinoma. The ulcerative lesions begin as papules or pustules and progress to superficial ulcers with granulation tissue (Fig. 17.43). Cutaneous lesions disseminated from a primary pulmonary focus are usually symmetrical and generally appear on the exposed areas of the body (the face, wrists, hands, and feet). In patients with primary cutaneous inoculation blastomycosis, the skin lesions occur with focal lymphadenopathy or

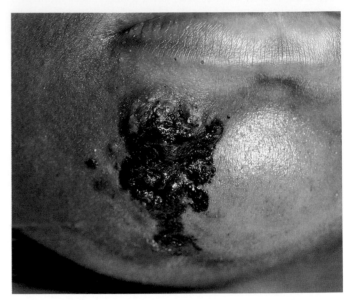

Figure 17.42 Cutaneous blastomycosis. Verrucous, crusted, erythematous plaque on the chin in a 15-year-old male with respiratory symptoms and bone pain. (Reprinted with permission from Cummins RE, Romero RC, Mancini AJ. Disseminated North American blastomycosis in an adolescent male; A delay in diagnosis. *Pediatrics* 1998;102(4):977–979. © Copyright American Academy of Pediatrics. All rights reserved.[118])

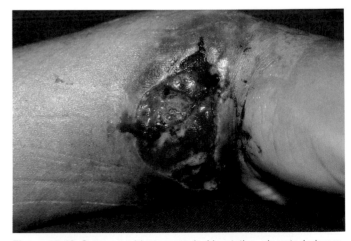

Figure 17.43 Cutaneous blastomycosis. Vegetative, ulcerated plaque of the volar wrist in the same patient shown in Figure 17.42. (Reprinted with permission from Cummins RE, Romero RC, Mancini AJ. Disseminated North American blastomycosis in an adolescent male; A delay in diagnosis. *Pediatrics* 1998;102(4):977–979. © Copyright American Academy of Pediatrics. All rights reserved.[118])

lymphangitis, but without evidence for systemic involvement.[119] Sources for primary inoculation disease include clinical exposures (i.e., laboratory or morgue, primarily in adults), animal bite or scratch, and other forms of skin trauma. The skin lesions of blastomycosis heal eventually (even without therapy), often resulting in permanent scarring.

North American blastomycosis is diagnosed by identification of the thick-walled, broad-based budding yeast cells in tissue samples or growth in fungal culture. Serologic studies are not useful, and enzyme immunoassays are sensitive but not available on a widespread basis. Cytologic examination of specimens (i.e., sputum) may be useful.[120] Urine antigen detection may be useful in children for both diagnosis and for following response to therapy.[121] A high index of suspicion must be maintained in the patient presenting with cutaneous ulcers or verrucous skin lesions, especially if other symptoms of systemic disease are present, most notably those referable to the lungs or bones, and if the patient resides in (or has traveled to) an endemic area. A delay in diagnosis is common, especially in children.[118]

Treatment depends upon the extent of disease and immune status of the patient. Whereas observation alone may be an option for mild pulmonary or primary inoculation skin disease, most patients require therapy, especially those with severe disease or immunocompromised or disseminated involvement. Local excision has been utilized for small lesions limited to skin. Systemic therapeutic options for blastomycosis include itraconazole, ketoconazole, fluconazole, and amphotericin B. Azole antifungal therapy should be continued for at least 6 months, and for at least 1 year in patients with blastomycotic osteomyelitis.[122,123] Life-threatening, CNS, or disseminated disease, as well as infection in the immunocompromised host, should be treated initially with amphotericin B, and therapy can be switched over to itraconazole after clinical stabilization.[122,123]

Coccidioidomycosis

Coccidioidomycosis is a deep fungal infection caused by *Coccidioides immitis*, a soil saprophyte endemic in the hot, arid desert areas of the south-western USA (especially the San Joaquin Valley in California), Mexico, and parts of South America. Inhalation of airborne arthroconidia results in infection, which in many cases is asymptomatic. Rare fomite transmission has been reported.[124] Periodic epidemics of coccidioidomycosis have been seen, often following severe dust storms and even, in 1994, following a California earthquake.[125]

Coccidioides immitis infection is often asymptomatic, or may present with influenza-like symptoms of fever, cough, chest pain, headache, sore throat, and fatigue.[126] Erythema nodosum or erythema multiforme may develop. Generalized arthralgias may accompany these acute symptoms, and this syndrome is referred to as 'desert rheumatism' or 'Valley fever'. Acute pulmonary infection, which accounts for 98% of cases, usually resolves without therapy over several weeks.[127] Around 5% of patients will have asymptomatic residual lesions in the lungs, usually nodules or thin-walled cavities.[127]

Extrapulmonary disease occurs in a minority of patients, and in this case, the organism disseminates hematogenously to any of several organs, including the meninges, bones, joints, skin, and soft tissues. Disseminated disease is most common in African-Americans, Filipinos, and Native Americans, as well as in patients with immunosuppression.[126] More recently, *Coccidioides* species have become significant opportunistic pathogens in patients infected with HIV and in organ transplant recipients.[128]

Skin involvement in coccidioidomycosis may be seen in the setting of acute disease or disseminated disease and, rarely, as a primary inoculation infection. During the acute phase of infection, a generalized erythematous macular exanthem may appear within the first 1–2 days of illness. As mentioned earlier, erythema multiforme or erythema nodosum lesions may also present during this phase of the illness, as may Sweet's syndrome (see Ch. 20) or an entity referred to as 'interstitial granulomatous dermatitis'. The latter refers to a granulomatous dermatitis that may occur in the setting of a variety of infectious, inflammatory or autoimmune disorders.[128] In addition to these 'parainfectious' cutaneous stigmata, infectious skin lesions may present (primarily with disseminated disease) as single or multiple verrucous, granulomatous papules and plaques (Fig. 17.44), subcutaneous abscess, acneiform papules and pustules. Cutaneous findings in coccidioidomycosis are not specific, and as with many deep fungal disorders, may suggest a variety of potential diagnoses in the differential. Primary cutaneous inoculation is relatively rare and occurs through injury by contaminated splinters or thorns or by accidental inoculation in laboratory or autopsy rooms. This form of coccidioidomycosis is usually characterized by a painless ulcerated plaque with lymphangitis and lymphadenopathy (similar to that seen in sporotrichosis or blastomycosis). Although healing usually takes place within a few months, there are rare reports of patients with primary cutaneous inoculation developing systemic dissemination.[129]

The diagnosis of coccidioidomycosis can be confirmed by demonstration of the characteristic large, thick-walled mature spherules with endospores in tissue biopsy specimens. Fungal culture of materials such as pus, sputum, or aspirates will often grow *C. immitis*, but since the organism is highly infectious, special precautions are necessary to prevent laboratory accidents due to air-borne spread of arthrospores. Serologic and skin testing are also useful in making the diagnosis of coccidioidomycosis. The coccidioidin skin test usually becomes positive soon after the development of symptoms in patients with primary infection, although anergy may be present in progressive disease.[127] IgM and IgG (complement fixation) antibodies may be present, the latter appearing between 4 and 12 weeks after infection and disappearing several months later if disease resolution occurs. Changes in the antibody titer may be useful for following disease activity and response to therapy. A high titer of complement fixation antibody denotes severe extensive disease and a poorer prognosis; complement fixation antibodies in cerebrospinal fluid indicate the presence of central nervous system infection. *In situ* hybridization and PCR techniques may also be useful in confirming the diagnosis.[128]

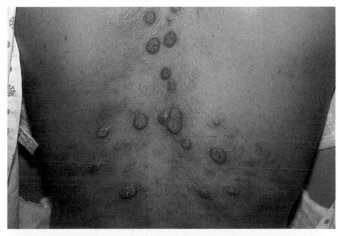

Figure 17.44 Cutaneous coccidioidomycosis. Multiple verrucous papules and plaques in a patient with cutaneous coccidioidomycosis, disseminated from a primary pulmonary infection.

The majority of infections with coccidioidomycosis are self-limiting, go undetected, and do not require specific therapy. Disseminated disease, however, may follow a fulminant course or persist for several years. The choice of the therapeutic agent and decisions regarding length of therapy depend on the immune status of the host, the seriousness of the infection, and the organs involved. Therapeutic options include amphotericin B, ketoconazole, itraconazole, and fluconazole. Amphotericin B is the recommended initial therapy for severe or progressive infection, and fluconazole is recommended for CNS infections.[130] Patients with CNS infection with *C. immitis* may require amphotericin B infusions into the cerebrospinal fluid. Pulmonary resection has a role in managing severe hemoptysis, sequestrations, or lung cavitations.

Paracoccidioidomycosis

South American blastomycosis (paracoccidioidomycosis) occurs almost exclusively in South and Central America, and is caused by infection with the dimorphic fungus, *P. brasiliensis*. The disorder is endemic in Brazil (where the majority of cases occur), Venezuela, Colombia, Ecuador, Argentina, and Peru. It may occur many years after relocation out of an endemic region.[131] More recently, paracoccidioidomycosis has become an opportunistic infection in HIV-infected individuals. It is most common in adults, and uncommon in childhood, when it is referred to as the 'acute juvenile form'. It is thought that the organism lives as a saprophyte on vegetation or in soil, and that the infection is acquired by direct implantation into the skin or mucous membranes, possibly through the practice of cleaning the teeth with small pieces of infected vegetation or, in pulmonary lesions, by direct inhalation of the organism.

Paracoccidioidomycosis may present with a wide spectrum of involvement, ranging from asymptomatic pulmonary infection to symptomatic infection involving one or several organs, which may progress in a fulminant fashion. The most common organs of involvement are the lungs, skin, mucosae, lymph nodes, and bone. Mucocutaneous involvement presents with infiltrative, ulcerative lesions on the lips and in the mouth, pharynx, or nasal cavity. The ulcerative and verrucous plaques may extend and ultimately progress to destroy the nose, lips, and facies. Pain and dental loss may occur. Hematogenous or lymphatic spread results in subcutaneous abscesses, and the lymph nodes draining the affected areas are palpable, painful, and adherent to the overlying skin, occasionally progressing to form chronic sinuses and suppurative plaques. Primary cutaneous infection is rarely reported.[132] The juvenile form tends to be more aggressive and involve primarily the reticuloendothelial system.[131]

Paracoccidioidomycosis is diagnosed by recognition of the typical yeast forms in tissue specimens, fungal culture, serologic studies (mainly in immunocompetent hosts) or newer molecular methodologies such as PCR, which may be useful in following response to therapy.[131] Treatment usually consists of azole antifungals or amphotericin B.

Histoplasmosis

Histoplasmosis is another deep fungal infection caused by a dimorphic fungus, in this case, *Histoplasma capsulatum*. This organism is endemic in the Americas, especially in Ohio and the Mississippi river valley, and is more concentrated in places where the soil is enriched by bird excreta or bat guano.[133] Infection is usually acquired by inhalation of fungal microconidia, and may result in various manifestations, from asymptomatic infection to disseminated, progressive disease. Transmission from fomites, direct inoculation, organ transplantation and sexual contact have also been reported.[134] Histoplasmosis affects infants and children as well as adults.

The manifestations of histoplasmosis are quite varied. Primary infection is asymptomatic or produces very mild symptoms in up to 95% of patients. Many patients manifest pulmonary symptoms, including cough and chest pain, along with fever and malaise. A chronic pulmonary form may resemble tuberculosis both clinically and radiographically. Involvement of the reticuloendothelial system may occur, and accounts for most of the signs of progressive disseminated histoplasmosis (PDH). PDH tends to occur in patients with compromised cell mediated immunity. Bone marrow involvement with pancytopenia is common, as are hepatosplenomegaly and lymphadenopathy.[135] Gastrointestinal bleeding, meningitis, adrenal gland involvement, and endocarditis may also occur with disseminated histoplasmosis. Disseminated disease occurs in <1% of those infected. Cardiac tamponade may develop in up to 25% of pulmonary histoplasmosis patients.[134]

Skin involvement is uncommon in histoplasmosis, but may be seen in the disseminated form, and rarely in a primary inoculation form. The morphologic characteristics include papules, pustules, purpura, abscesses, severe dermatitis, and verrucous lesions. Erythema multiforme and erythema nodosum may both occur, usually in the setting of acute pulmonary infection. The characteristic ulcerative, mucocutaneous lesions of the nose, mouth, pharynx, larynx, genitals, and perianal region are seen in chronic disseminated disease and in patients with immunodeficiency. Lesions in these regions may present as superficial or deep ulcerations with heaped up borders, nodular masses or verrucous plaques.[136]

Children with histoplasmosis tend to have more disseminated disease. In fact, 20% of apparently immunocompetent patients with disseminated infection are children.[133] A disseminated form of histoplasmosis in infants may be associated with transient hyperglobulinemia and T-cell deficiency and, when occurring after exposure to a large inoculum of the pathogen, has a high mortality rate.[137] In children with histoplasmosis, the frequency of extensive ulcers along the gastrointestinal mucosa that give rise to diarrhea and other gastrointestinal disturbances suggests that organisms may be ingested rather than inhaled in these individuals.

The 'gold standards' for diagnosing histoplasmosis are identification of the small intracellular yeast-like organisms in tissue specimens, sputum, or peripheral blood, and fungal culture. The usefulness of the histoplasmin skin test is quite low, given its non-specificity especially in endemic areas.[135] *Histoplasma* serologies (including complement fixation and immunodiffusion precipitin bands) are available but hampered by high rates of false-positives and false-negatives. Detection of *Histoplasma* antigen in urine may be useful, but also has the disadvantage of many potential causes for false-positive results, especially other endemic mycoses.[136] An enzyme-linked immunosorbent assay (ELISA) against *H. capsulation* circulating antigens has good sensitivity and excellent specificity,[138] although it may not be readily available. PCR assays are also being developed, although none is currently commercially available.

In mild cases of histoplasmosis, treatment may not be necessary, and the disorder runs a benign, self-limited course. For severe or widespread disease, systemic antifungal therapy with amphotericin B is usually indicated. For more localized or less severe disease (i.e., chronic pulmonary histoplasmosis), oral azole antifungal therapy is an option. Various regimens have been reported in pediatric patients. Disseminated childhood histoplasmosis has been treated successfully with itraconazole for 3–12 months, as well as with parenteral amphotericin B followed by oral ketoconazole for 3 months.[133,137] In patients with AIDS and severe histoplasmosis, amphotericin B is indicated, whereas itraconazole may be appropriate therapy for mild disseminated disease.[139] Fluconazole is less effective than the other azole antifungal agents, and clinical data on the newer azoles, voriconazole and posaconazole, are limited.[136]

Opportunistic Mycoses

With the spread of AIDS and advancements in cancer chemotherapy, bone marrow and solid organ transplantation, and both routine and intensive medical care, certain patient populations who are vulnerable to potentially fatal deep fungal infections have emerged. These organisms are generally non-pathogenic, but in certain at-risk individuals who have an alteration or breakdown of host defenses, may result in severe disseminated infection. The 'opportunistic mycoses' to be discussed here include aspergillosis, cryptococcosis, fusarium, and mucormycosis.

Aspergillosis

Aspergillosis is an uncommon opportunistic fungal disease of the respiratory tract and other sites caused by a variety of *Aspergillus* species. Although *Aspergillus fumigatus* is the most commonly identified pathogen, *Aspergillus niger*, *Aspergillus flavus* and an increasing number of other species have been reported in recent years. Invasive aspergillosis is most often seen in patients with prolonged neutropenia and in transplant recipients.[140]

Aspergillus species are ubiquitous and are normally nonpathogenic. When pathogenic, they primarily cause infection in the lung, although the skin, eyes, CNS, bones, gastrointestinal tract, liver, spleen, lymph nodes, nasopharynx, and genitourinary tract may also be affected. In children, the highest risk groups are those with AIDS, leukemia, corticosteroid or immunosuppressive therapy, chronic granulomatous disease, and severe combined immunodeficiency.[141] Neonates appear to be another population at risk for invasive aspergillosis. Neonatal aspergillosis risk factors include corticosteroid use, prematurity, prolonged hospitalization, and skin trauma from tape adhesive in relation to prolonged use of arm boards.[142] Despite aggressive therapy, invasive aspergillosis in children is associated with a mortality rate as high as 85%.[143]

One of the most common characteristic manifestations of aspergillosis is the pulmonary intracavitary fungus ball. This is composed of colonies of *Aspergillus*, inflammatory exudate, cells, and fibrin in the form of a sphere, which may measure from 1 to 5 cm in diameter. Although it occasionally causes hemoptysis, most patients with fungus balls are asymptomatic. Another form of pulmonary disease is invasive pulmonary aspergillosis, which may be necrotizing and is often associated with multiorgan dissemination.

Cutaneous aspergillosis may occur in two forms, primary or secondary. Primary cutaneous aspergillosis usually occurs at sites of skin injury, such as intravenous catheter insertion sites, burns, surgical wounds, or sites covered by various products including occlusive dressings and tape. Secondary cutaneous aspergillosis occurs with direct extension to the skin from underlying soft tissue infection or hematogenous dissemination.[144] Less commonly, an opportunistic infection of the paranasal sinuses may result in mucopurulent or blood-tinged nasal discharge, headache, periorbital neuralgia, and rhinitis. With extension of this process, the face may become erythematous, swollen, warm, and tender, suggesting a diagnosis of cellulitis or erysipelas.

Cutaneous aspergillosis may initially present as nondescript erythematous macules, papules, or plaques. Common secondary findings include hemorrhagic bullae and necrosis (Fig. 17.45), which may extend rapidly. Eschar formation is often seen. In patients with hematogenous dissemination, embolic lesions present as widespread erythematous to purpuric macules and papules, with ulceration and necrosis, and may simulate the lesions of ecthyma gangrenosum (caused by *Pseudomonas aeruginosa*). Pustules overlying an erythematous patch are a common finding in the early cutaneous lesions of neonates, often progressing to ulceration, necrosis, and eschar formation.[145]

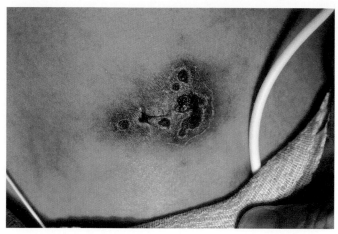

Figure 17.45 Cutaneous aspergillosis. Erythematous plaque with necrosis and eschar formation in a young immunosuppressed female with disseminated *Aspergillus fumigatus* infection.

The diagnosis of cutaneous aspergillus can be confirmed by tissue biopsy for histopathology and fungal culture. A deep skin biopsy is desirable in order to visualize the dermal and subcutaneous blood vessels, given the angiotropic nature of *Aspergillus* spp. Fungal stains applied to the biopsy material will reveal large fungal hyphae with 'acute angle' branching, and this method will enable a more rapid diagnosis than awaiting results of the fungal culture. Blood cultures are rarely positive. ELISA and polymerase chain reaction (PCR) testing are available in some centers and may offer a more rapid and reliable means of diagnosing disseminated aspergillosis, especially in immunocompromised children.[141] Diagnosis via newer antigen tests, such as the galactomannan assay, has not yet been clearly validated for pediatric patients.[142]

The treatment of aspergillosis depends on the underlying immune status of the patient and risk factors for disseminated infection. In most cases, systemic therapy is indicated. Occasionally, surgical approaches may suffice (i.e., primary cutaneous aspergillosis in a burn patient without underlying risk factors for disseminated disease). Although amphotericin B has been the mainstay of systemic therapy for years, in some patients this agent is associated with untoward side-effects and in others it may result in a suboptimal response.[140] Azole antifungal agents such as itraconazole have also been used with mixed results. The newer broad-spectrum triazole, voriconazole, has been evaluated and demonstrated effective in adults and children with invasive aspergillosis, although the numerous drug interactions may limit its usefulness in some patients.[140,146,147] Caspofungin therapy has also been studied in salvage therapy for invasive aspergillosis, and a body-surface area dosing calculation is preferred over a weight-based regimen for treating children with this agent.[148]

Cryptococcosis

Cryptococcus neoformans is a ubiquitous encapsulated fungus capable of causing severe disease in immunocompromised individuals, especially those with AIDS. Disseminated disease has been rarely observed in immunocompetent children.[149] Whereas it is well established as the most common cause of life-threatening fungal infection in HIV-infected adults, infection in HIV-infected children may occur in up to 1% of those with AIDS.[150] The organism has been found in various fruits, soil, pigeon excreta, and cow's milk. It is believed to be acquired via inhalation of aerosolized particles from the environment, and recent data suggest that *C. neoformans* may infect many immunocompetent children early in life, resulting in either asymptomatic infection or nonspecific 'viral' symptoms.[151] The incidence of cryptococcosis has declined in the past decade, largely because of the improvements in HIV care and the use of highly active antiretroviral therapy (HAART).[152]

Cryptococcal infection most commonly presents as meningitis, meningoencephalitis, or sepsis. Infection may be localized to the lungs, producing focal pneumonia, patchy infiltrates, solitary nodules, abscesses, or pleural effusion. Pulmonary symptoms, however, may be absent or minimal and, although pulmonary involvement may be progressive, in most instances CNS manifestations predominate and infection is detected only after dissemination, which may include the skin. Cutaneous lesions may present months prior to other signs of systemic infection.[153] They may occasionally occur following trauma or extension from bony involvement, but are usually the result of hematogenous spread from a pulmonary focus.

Skin lesions, which occur in 6–15% of patients with systemic infection, present most commonly on the head and neck, where they may often mimic the lesions of molluscum contagiosum. They begin as painless, firm, pink to red papules, pustules, or acneiform lesions. The molluscum-like lesions may be umbilicated or contain a tiny central hemorrhagic crust, and may be multiple.[153] Surrounding inflammation is usually absent. As the lesions enlarge they may form infiltrated plaques, nodules, abscesses, or ulcers, often with raised papillomatous borders.

The diagnosis of cryptococcosis is confirmed by demonstration of the characteristic organism (surrounded by a polysaccharide capsule and with characteristic budding seen in India ink preparations) in cerebrospinal fluid, skin lesions, sputum, or tissue sections. Definitive diagnosis relies on isolation of the organism from biopsy tissue or bodily fluids.[154] Serologic studies, immunoblotting, and ELISA or latex agglutination assays for the cryptococcal polysaccharide are other diagnostic modalities. The recommended therapy for cryptococcosis is amphotericin B with 5-flucytosine or fluconazole, as combination therapy appears to be superior to amphotericin monotherapy.[155] Fluconazole suppression is recommended after completion of the primary therapy.[154]

Fusarium infection

Fusarium species are molds that are normally found in soil and the air, and which may result in localized infections in the nail (fusarium onychomycosis or paronychia) or in burn sites or surgical wounds. However, invasive fusarium infection (or 'fusariosis') is an increasingly prevalent, serious opportunistic fungal infection that occurs especially in patients with hematologic malignancy undergoing cytotoxic chemotherapy or bone marrow transplantation. Prolonged neutropenia seems to be the main risk factor for this infection. Skin lesions are common in patients with disseminated *Fusarium* infection, and may serve as the portal of entry for more widespread involvement. Cutaneous involvement may be mistaken for aspergillosis, given the potential clinical overlap in presentation.

Immunocompromised patients with *Fusarium* infection may present with refractory fever, skin lesions, sinusitis, myalgias, or pneumonia. Endophthalmitis may occur from hematogenous seeding, as opposed to the fusarial endophthalmitis that occurs in immunocompetent hosts as a complication of advanced keratitis or following ophthalmologic surgery.[156] Fungemia with multi-organ involvement is possible, and the organism is more often cultured from the blood than is *Aspergillus*. Disseminated infection is often notable for skin lesions, which occur in up to 80% of these patients.[157] Skin lesions of fusariosis may include paronychia, tinea pedis, onychomycosis, digital ulcers, or widespread lesions most

often involving the extremities. The disseminated lesions present most often as painful, red to gray macules or papules, with purpura, necrosis, and eschar formation.[158] They may mimic the lesions of ecthyma gangrenosum.[159,160] Pustules, cellulitis, abscesses, bullae, and subcutaneous nodules may also occur, and 'target lesions' have been described.[160,161]

Fusariosis is usually diagnosed via microscopic examination of skin biopsy specimens, with confirmation by fungal culture of tissues and/or blood. Treatment is difficult, and includes regular or lipid formulations of amphotericin B, itraconazole, and correction of the neutropenia with G-CSF or GM-CSF-stimulated granulocyte transfusions.[160] Newer antifungal agents such as voriconazole or posaconazole may also have a role in the treatment of this serious infection.[161,162]

Mucormycosis

Mucormycosis (also known as zygomycosis or phycomycosis) is an opportunistic fungal infection caused by a group of organisms in the class Mucorales (previously referred to as Zygomycetes). Infection of the immunocompetent host is extremely rare, despite continual exposure to these organisms. Mucormycosis occurs mainly in immunocompromised individuals and in patients with debilitating diseases (i.e., diabetes mellitus, anemia, heart or liver disease, burns, leukemia, or lymphoma), and is among the most acute, fulminant, and fatal of all fungal infections.[163] It may involve any organ of the body but most commonly affects the skin, lungs, meninges, gastrointestinal tract, and structures of the head and neck. Up to 10% of cases of mucormycosis may occur in immunocompetent individuals without identifiable predisposing factors.[164]

The causative fungi of mucormycosis include species of *Mucor*, *Rhizopus*, *Absidia*, and *Rhizomucor*. These organisms are saprophytic and grow on decaying organic materials such as vegetation, fruit, and bread.[165] The portal of entry for these infections varies with the site of the disease. Rhinocerebral mucormycosis is the most common form, and affects primarily diabetics as well as patients with immunocompromise.

Cutaneous or subcutaneous infections are rare and occur most frequently in diabetics with recurrent acidosis or in patients with a history of skin trauma or severe burns. This form of infection is characterized by hemorrhagic or necrotic papules and plaques, chronic indolent ulcers, and slowly enlarging dusky nodules. The initial lesion is often a small area of macular discoloration or dusky erythema, which gradually enlarges and ulcerates. Necrosis may be marked, and there may be a foul-smelling purulent exudate. A gangrenous form results in rapid ulceration and necrotizing fasciitis-like tissue destruction. The skin lesions of cutaneous mucormycosis are not pathognomonic, and may be confused with lesion of ecthyma gangrenosum, aspergillosis, deep fungal infections, other soft tissue infections, pyoderma gangrenosum, or vasculitis.[163,166] The skin lesions may be primary or secondary, in which case they are related to hematogenous dissemination of the organism from a primary infection in another organ.

The rhinocerebral form is usually characterized by a suppurative necrotizing infection of the paranasal sinuses with periorbital pain, swelling, edema, proptosis, extraocular muscle paresis, and decreased visual acuity. This form is uniformly fatal within weeks when there is extensive involvement, and combined treatment with surgical debridement/resection and systemic antifungals is warranted.[167] An angioinvasive form of mucormycosis has been described in neonates, usually those with the risk factors of prematurity, low birthweight, broad-spectrum antibiotic or corticosteroid therapy, and history of local skin trauma.[168]

The diagnosis of mucormycosis relies on tissue biopsy and histologic examination. Broad, non-septated, thick-walled hyphae are seen, and may be noted to be invading cutaneous blood vessels. Fungal culture is confirmatory. Therapy is difficult and often requires a combination of surgical debridement, treatment of the underlying disease process, and intravenous amphotericin B. Lipid formulations of amphotericin B appear to be more efficacious in treating central nervous system mycormycosis.[169] Posaconazole may be a reasonable option for those who are resistant to, or intolerant of, amphotericin.[169]

Key References

 The complete list of 169 references for this chapter is available online at **www.expertconsult.com.**
See inside cover for registration details.

DiCaudo DJ. Coccidioidomycosis: A review and update. *J Am Acad Dermatol.* 2006;55:929–942.

Ginter-Hanselmayer G, Weger W, Smolle J. Onychomycosis: a new emerging infectious disease in childhood population and adolescents. Report on treatment experience with terbinafine and itraconazole in 36 patients. *J Eur Acad Dermatol Venereol.* 2008;22:470–475.

Honig PJ, Frieden IJ, Kim HJ, Yan AC. Streptococcal intertrigo: An underrecognized condition in children. *Pediatrics.* 2003;112:1427–1429.

Sethi A, Antaya R. Systemic antifungal therapy for cutaneous infections in children. *Pediatr Infect Dis J.* 2006;25(7):643–644.

18

Infestations, Bites, and Stings

Parasites are a fascinating and important cause of skin disease in children. They produce their effects in various ways: mechanical trauma from bites or stings, injection of pharmacologically active substances that induce local or systemic effects, allergic reactions in a previously sensitized host, persistent granulomatous reactions to retained mouth parts, direct invasion of the epidermis, or transmission of infectious disease by blood-sucking insects.

Arthropods

Arthropods are elongated invertebrate animals with segmented bodies, true appendages, and a chitinous exoskeleton. Those of dermatologic significance are the eight-legged arachnids (mites, ticks, spiders, and scorpions) and the six-legged insects (lice, flies, mosquitoes, fleas, bugs, bees, wasps, ants, caterpillars/moths, and beetles).

Arachnids

The term *mite* refers to a large number of tiny arachnids, many of which live at least part of their lives as parasites upon animals or plants or in prepared foods. Of greatest clinical significance are itch mites (*Sarcoptes scabiei*), grain mites, and harvest mites (chiggers). Avian mite dermatitis has also been recognized with increased frequency in recent years. Mites attack humans by burrowing under or attaching themselves to the skin, where they inflict trivial bites and cause associated dermatitides.

Scabies

Scabies is a common skin infestation caused by the mite, *S. scabiei*. This mite is an obligate human parasite, residing in burrowed tunnels within the human epidermis. Mites of all developmental stages may burrow into skin, depositing feces in their tracks. The female mite also lays eggs in these burrows, which serves to further propagate the infestation. The adult female mite has a lifespan of around 15–30 days, measures around 400 μm, and lays 1–4 eggs/day, which hatch in 3–4 days.[1,2] After hatching, the larvae mature into adult mites in 10–14 days, and the duration of the whole life cycle is 30–60 days.

Scabies is transmitted most often by direct contact with an infested individual, although acquisition from fomites such as bedding and clothing is also possible. The survival time for a mite separated from the human host is estimated at several days. Scabies disproportionately affects women and children, as well as individuals with certain predisposing conditions, including immunocompromise, severe mental or physical handicap, and HIV infection. Scabies is seen worldwide in infants and children, and in the USA, there seems to be a fairly high incidence in foreign-born adoptees, especially those from Asia or Latin America.[3,4] This latter observation is likely related to the high frequency of infestation seen in orphanages.

The incubation of classic scabies is around 3 weeks, with reinfestation resulting in more immediate symptoms.[5] The initial symptom of scabies is usually pruritus, which is often evident well before the clinical signs become apparent. Patients with scabies usually complain of worsening pruritus during night-time hours. Infants and young children may also experience irritability and poor feeding. The skin findings include papules, nodules, burrows, and vesiculopustules (Figs 18.1–18.5). The most common locations for scabies lesions are the interdigital spaces, wrists, ankles, axillae, waist, groin, palms, and soles. Burrows on the palms may reveal a pattern of scale reminiscent of the wake left on a water surface by a moving boat, and has been termed the 'wake sign'.[6] In infants, lesions may also be seen on the head (Fig. 18.6), which is rarely involved in older patients. Infants commonly have involvement of the palms, soles, and axillae. In older children and adolescents, the most common sites of involvement are the wrists, interdigital spaces, and waist. Although bullous lesions are uncommon in scabies, vesicles are often found in infants and young children, owing to the predisposition for blister formation seen in this age group. Occasionally, the Darier sign may be positive and hence the diagnosis of urticaria pigmentosa may be considered.[7] Genital involvement, presenting as papules, crusted papules or nodules (Figs 18.7, 18.8), and areolar lesions are other classic presentation patterns. Excoriations are commonly noted.

Scabies nodules are red-brown nodules (Figs 18.9, 18.10), which represent a vigorous hypersensitivity response of the host. They occur most commonly on the trunk, axillary regions, and genitalia, and are seen primarily in infants. Although they eventually resolve, scabies nodules may be present for several months. They are occasionally misdiagnosed (both clinically and histologically) as signs of a neoplastic disorder (i.e., leukemia or lymphoma cutis).

Crusted or Norwegian scabies is a form of the disorder that presents as scaly, dermatitic papules or plaques. Crusted scabies may be localized or generalized, and occurs primarily in immunocompromised patients (especially those with HIV infection) and in those who are mentally retarded or physically incapacitated.[5] The lesions of this disorder may mimic eczema (Fig. 18.11), psoriasis, warts or a drug reaction, and nail dystrophy may be present. Crusted scabies is frequently misdiagnosed and mismanaged.[8] The lesions may become heavily crusted and hyperkeratotic, and often are minimally pruritic. Crusted scabies is extremely contagious, given the large numbers of mites (thousands) that may be present. In classic scabies, only around 12 mites on average are present. Patients with crusted scabies are often the source for large epidemics within hospitals, given the lack of recognition and subsequent delay in diagnosis.

Complications of scabies are generally mild. They include secondary bacterial infection, impaired skin integrity, pain, and, rarely, debilitation related to limitations in movement secondary to pain. Secondary infection is most commonly due to *Staphylococcus aureus* or group A β-hemolytic streptococci, and presents as crusting, oozing, pustules or vesiculopustules. Bullous lesions have been

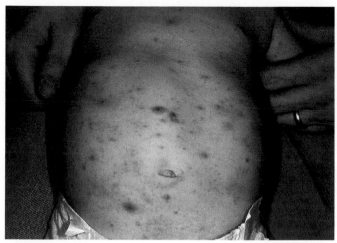

Figure 18.1 Scabies. Erythematous papules with crusting in an infested male infant.

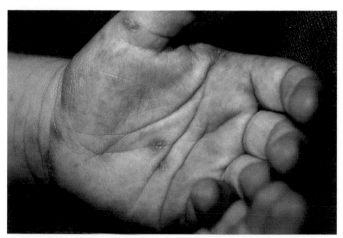

Figure 18.2 Scabies. Erythematous papules and burrows involving the palm and wrist. Scrapings of lesions from the palmar creases have a high yield on microscopic examination.

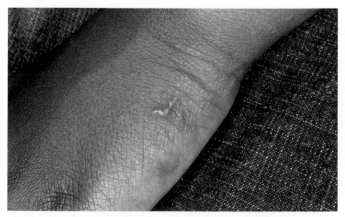

Figure 18.3 Scabies. Curvilinear burrow of the lateral hand.

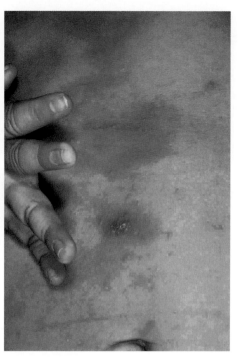

Figure 18.4 Scabies. Crusted papule of the abdomen in an infant with scabies.

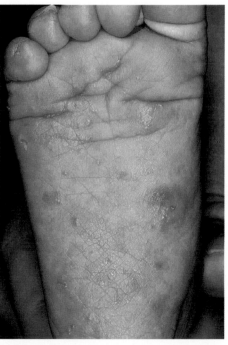

Figure 18.5 Scabies. Erythematous papules and linear burrows of the plantar surface of the foot.

described, primarily in older adults, which on occasion may simulate (or possibly evolve into) the autoimmune blistering disorder, bullous pemphigoid.[9,10] Necrotizing vasculitis in the presence of lupus anticoagulant has also been reported.[11]

Animal-transmitted scabies, which is *Sarcoptes* infestation transmitted from domestic animals, usually results in a short-lived infestation with spontaneous resolution in the human host. The close relationship of humans with dogs makes the canine form of animal scabies (*S. scabiei var. canis*) the most common type transmitted to humans.[12,13] Canine scabies, or sarcoptic mange, causes patchy loss of hair with scaling in the dog. It is seen most commonly in undernourished, heavily parasitized puppies, and a presumptive diagnosis can be made on the basis of exposure to a pet with a pruritic eruption, alopecia, and the characteristic mouse-like odor of animals with extensive sarcoptic infestation. In children with

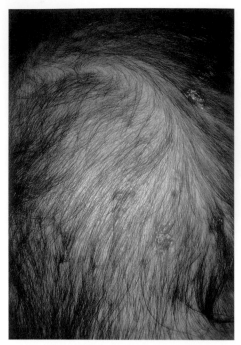

Figure 18.6 Scabies. Erythematous papules and crusted papules of the scalp in an infant.

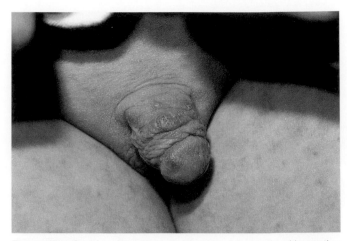

Figure 18.7 Scabies. Erythematous papules of the penis with crusting of the glans penis. These findings are highly suggestive of scabies infestation.

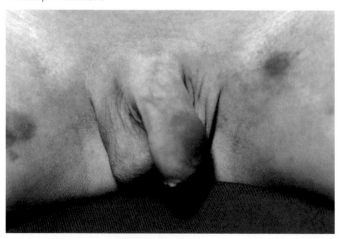

Figure 18.8 Scabies. Nodules of the penis and inguinal regions in a young male recently treated for scabies.

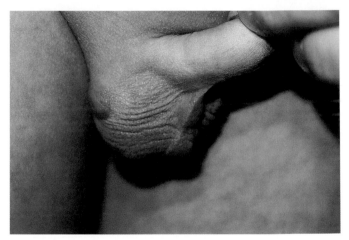

Figure 18.9 Scabies nodules. These infiltrative nodules persisted for 6 months after effective treatment for scabies.

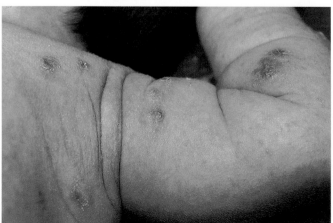

Figure 18.10 Scabies nodules. Early scabies nodules developing at sites of crusting; these lesions persisted long after adequate therapy for the infestation.

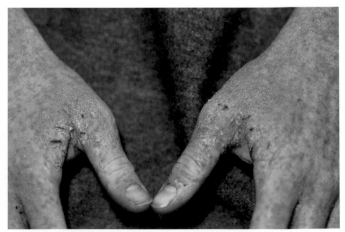

Figure 18.11 Crusted scabies. This heart transplant recipient had eczematous, crusted plaques in a widespread distribution, which was resistant to topical corticosteroid therapy. Mineral oil preparation revealed many live scabies mites.

canine scabies the papular eruption most commonly involves the forearms, lower region of the chest, abdomen, and thighs. The distribution differs from that of human scabies in that it tends to spare the interdigital webs and the genitalia, and burrows are absent. The mite of canine scabies does not reproduce on human skin, and therefore the infestation is usually self-limited, clearing spontaneously over several weeks.

The diagnosis of scabies is suggested in the child with pruritus, a papular or papulovesicular eruption with burrows, and the characteristic distribution pattern. However, the differential diagnosis may be broad, and includes atopic dermatitis, contact dermatitis, seborrheic dermatitis, Langerhans cell histiocytosis, impetigo, pyoderma, viral exanthem, papular urticaria, arthropod bites, and acropustulosis of infancy. The latter, which may represent a post-scabietic hypersensitivity response, is discussed in detail in Chapter 2. A definitive diagnosis of scabies is made via mineral oil examination (Table 18.1), with the microscopic identification of mites (Fig. 18.12) or their eggs or feces (scybala) (Fig. 18.13). Ideal skin lesions for sampling include burrows and fresh papules. In young patients in whom skin scrapings might be difficult, obtaining samples from adult contacts (i.e., parents) with lesions is a consideration. Skin biopsy is rarely necessary. High-magnification videodermatoscopy is a non-invasive technique for diagnosing scabies.[14]

Therapeutic options for scabies are listed in Table 18.2, and a few are discussed here in more detail. The treatment of choice for scabies is 5% permethrin cream, which is applied from the neck down and left on for 8–14 h, followed by thorough rinsing. Permethrin, a synthetic pyrethroid, is a neurotoxin and an excellent scabicide with low potential for toxicity. There appears to be little, if any, resistance of scabies to permethrin, and overall the response rate to treatment is excellent. A second treatment with permethrin, 1 week following the first, is often recommended, although studies suggest a relatively high cure rate after a single application.[1,15] Treatment of all close contacts is also recommended, in an effort to minimize ongoing propagation of the infestation. In a systematic review and meta-analysis of scabies therapies, permethrin was demonstrated to be the most effective treatment.[16]

Permethrin should be applied in a thin, even coat and rubbed in well to all skin surfaces. In infants, application should include the scalp and face, with care to avoid the regions around the eyes and mouth. Special attention should be paid to applying the medication to web spaces, the umbilicus, the genitals, and the gluteal cleft. Fingernails and toenails should be trimmed short and the medication applied as well as possible to the region under the nail edge. Permethrin is not recommended for infants <2 months of age or for pregnant (pregnancy Class B) or nursing women. It is vital for

patients and parents to understand that, following appropriate therapy, signs and symptoms of scabies may not clear for 2–6 weeks following successful treatment, since the hypersensitivity state does not cease immediately after eradication of the infection.[17] The family should have this information before starting therapy, and it may be useful to provide a topical corticosteroid and oral antihistamine for symptomatic relief during this period.

Lindane 1% lotion was, for years, the primary therapy for scabies prior to the development of permethrin and escalating reports of lindane-related toxicities. Lindane is applied to the skin for 8–12 h, with reapplication in 1 week. Although the majority of untoward effects attributed to the use of lindane have been associated with inappropriate, prolonged, or repetitive use, true toxicity potential does exist, and becomes more relevant in infants and small children owing to a relatively greater skin surface and possibly higher blood level accumulations in this age group. When *in vitro* percutaneous absorption of 5% permethrin was compared to 1% lindane, it was shown that human skin was 20-fold more permeable to lindane. In addition, *in vivo* guinea pig blood and brain levels of lindane were four-fold greater than permethrin levels following a single

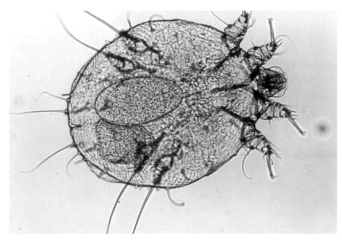

Figure 18.12 Scabies mite. Note the eggs within the body of the mite. (Live scabies mite ×40 magnification.)

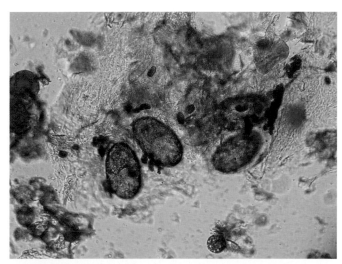

Figure 18.13 Scabies preparation. This mineral oil preparation (performed on scrapings from the patient in Fig. 18.5) reveals multiple eggs (larger, oval bodies) and smaller fecal pellets ('scybala,' the dark brown circular concretions).

Table 18.1 Performing a mineral oil examination for scabies
1. Apply a drop of mineral oil to the lesion(s) to be scraped
2. Scrape through the lesion with a No.15 scalpel blade (a small amount of bleeding is expected with appropriately deep scrapings)
3. Smear contents of scraping on a clean glass slide
4. Add a few more drops of mineral oil
5. Place cover slip over oil and examine under microscope at low power

Criteria for a positive mineral oil examination:
Scabies mite
  or
Ova (eggs)
  or
Scybala (feces)

Table 18.2 Treatment options for scabies

Name	Instructions for use	Comment
Permethrin 5% cream (Elimite, Acticin)	Apply from neck down; rinse in 8–14 h	Not for use under 2 months of age; may repeat in 1 week if necessary; treat scalp in infants
Lindane 1% lotion	Apply from neck down; rinse in 8–12 h	Not recommended for infants; not first-line therapy; potential CNS toxicity
Sulfur 6% ointment	Apply from neck down for 3 consecutive nights; rinse 24 h after last application	Older therapy; malodorous; compounded in petrolatum; safe in infants, pregnant females
Crotamiton cream (Eurax)	Apply from neck down for 2 consecutive nights; rinse 48 h after last application	High failure rate; may require up to 5 daily applications
Benzyl benzoate	Apply nightly or every other night for 3 applications	Not available in the USA
Ivermectin (Stromectol)	200 μg/kg per dose given orally for 2 doses, 2 weeks apart	Off-label use; consider for severe infestations, crusted scabies, IC patients, scabies epidemics; should not be used under 5 years of age

CNS, central nervous system; IC, immunocompromised.

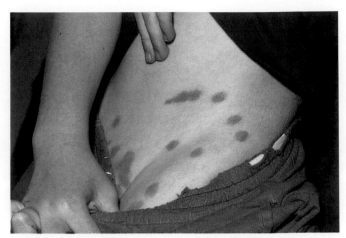

Figure 18.14 Chigger bites. Multiple itchy, edematous, urticarial papules. Some revealed a small hemorrhagic punctum.

Regardless of the treatment used for scabies, environmental decontamination is important given the possibility of spread of scabies from fomites. Clothing, bed linens, and towels should be machine washed in hot water and dried using a high-heat setting. Clothing or other items (i.e., stuffed animals) that cannot be washed may be dry cleaned or stored in bags for 3 days to 1 week, as the mite will die when separated from the human host. In addition, systemic antibiotic therapy should be given if secondary bacterial superinfection is present. Scabies nodules can be treated symptomatically with topical or intralesional corticosteroids.

Other mites

Mites are small arachnids with mouthparts capable of puncturing and feeding on host tissue fluids. A variety of food and animal mites may result in pruritic dermatoses in exposed humans, and may also be vectors of infectious diseases. Mite bites should be considered in the patient with an unexplained, itchy papular skin eruption.

Harvest mites (chiggers, jiggers, 'red bugs') are a member of the American harvest mite family and are commonly found in the southern USA. Also known as *Trombicula alfreddugesi*, the chigger is distinct from other mites in that only the larva is parasitic to humans and animals. The eight-legged adult and nymphal stages are spent in a non-parasitic existence. Chiggers live in grain stems, in grasses, or in areas overgrown with briars or blackberry bushes, where they exist and feed on vegetable matter, minute arthropods, and insect eggs. The six-legged larva clings to vegetation, awaiting the passage of an unsuspecting host and then attaches to the skin when the host brushes against the foliage.[31] The mite then injects an irritating secretion that causes itching, and then drops to the ground to molt (or is scratched off) within a few days. The lesions of chigger bites present as urticarial, erythematous papules (Fig. 18.14). They occasionally reveal a hemorrhagic punctum, and in some patients, there may be more diffuse erythema, vesicles or bullae. Pruritus tends to be intense. The 'summer penile syndrome' refers to a seasonal acute hypersensitivity reaction to chigger bites, and presents with penile swelling, pruritus, and occasional dysuria.[32] Most patients have a history of recent exposure to woods, parks, or lawns.

Treatment of chigger bites consists of antihistamines, cool baths or compresses, and topical corticosteroids. Secondary infection should be treated with systemic antibiotics. Household vinegar (5% acetic acid) has been suggested as a useful measure for postexposure prophylaxis and treatment of pruritus.[31] Chiggers may be disease

application.[18] Reactions attributed to the use of lindane have included eczema, urticaria, aplastic anemia, alopecia, muscular spasms, and central nervous system toxicity, manifested by irritability, nausea, vomiting, amblyopia, headache, dizziness, and convulsions.[19–26] Lindane-resistant scabies has also been an increasing problem in the USA and Central America. This agent, which is recommended as a second-line therapy, is banned in California.

Ivermectin has been reported with increasing frequency as a treatment option for scabies. This agent has been used extensively in veterinary medicine since 1981, for a wide variety of parasitic infestations in farm and domestic animals.[27] Oral ivermectin (Stromectol) is approved for the treatment of strongyloides and onchocerciasis in adult humans. It is also effective for the treatment of loiasis and bancroftian filariasis.[28] Ivermectin acts by blocking chemical transmission across invertebrate nerve synapses that utilize glutamate or γ-aminobutyric acid (GABA), resulting in paralysis and death. It has selective activity against human parasites because of its high affinity for the channels found in the peripheral nervous system of invertebrates.[29] Several studies have evaluated the role of ivermectin (as an off-label agent) in the treatment of scabies, and found it very effective in either a single- or two-dose regimen of 200 μg/kg per dose. Ivermectin is especially useful in immunocompromised patients with scabies and patients with crusted scabies, where it may be used alone or in combination with topical scabicides or keratolytic agents. Topical 1% ivermectin, which is not readily available, has reportedly been effective as well.[30]

vectors for scrub typhus, hemorrhagic fever with renal syndrome, hantavirus pulmonary syndrome, and ehrlichiosis.[33]

Grain mites (*straw itch mite*, *Pyemotes ventricosus*) feed on the larvae of insects, seeds, grains, and plant stems. Persons coming into contact with infested straw and grain are particularly susceptible to this form of dermatitis.[34] This seasonal eruption presents as severely pruritic, pale pink to bright red macules, papulovesicles, or pustules followed by urticarial wheals. Occasionally, a purpuric eruption develops. In severe cases, constitutional symptoms and fever may be present, and the presentation may be mistaken for acute varicella. The eruption is self-limited and treatment, as with chigger bite reactions, is supportive.

Avian mites (*fowl mites*, *bird mites*) are divided into two genera, *Dermanyssus* and *Ornithonyssus*. They are known to infest humans accidentally, resulting in a pruritic, widespread papular dermatitis. 'Gamasoidosis' is the term used to describe the human skin disorder resulting from non-burrowing, blood sucking mites from birds and other animals.[35] The diagnosis of avian mite dermatitis is often overlooked, due to lack of awareness and the small size of the mites.[36] Common causes include *Dermanyssus gallinae* (chicken mite), *Dermanyssus americanus* (American bird mite), *Ornithonyssus sylviarum* (northern fowl mite), and *Ornithonyssus bursa* (tropical fowl mite). *Dermanyssus gallinae*, the most common cause, infects various birds including chickens, parakeets, pigeons, canaries, and starlings. Although the mite remains on the bird at night, during the day it may migrate to the nest and can survive without feeding for several months. When birds leave their nest, such as in the spring or early summer, the mites search for other hosts and human infestation may be the result. Clinical examination reveals papules (Fig. 18.15), vesicles, and urticarial lesions without burrows, as the mite does not burrow into the skin. The diagnosis of avian mite dermatitis is confirmed by identification of the mites found in pillows, bed sheets, clothing, nests, birds, and, only rarely, humans. Special attention should be given to potential sites for nesting, such as porches, attics, eaves, air conditioning systems, and ventilation ducts. Pet gerbils were the source for *O. sylviarum* and *D. gallinae* in one report.[37] Treatment for avian mite dermatitis, as with other mite bites, is symptomatic.

Other mites may result in similar, nonspecific, pruritic papular eruptions in the human host. The rat mite, *Ornithonyssus bacoti*, is found in rats and extermination is often necessary for eradication.[38] It has also been reported in pet hamsters.[39] *Cheyletiella* mites are

large, animal-specific non-burrowing mites that include *Cheyletiella blakei* (found on cats), *Cheyletiella yasguri* (found on dogs), and *Cheyletiella parasitivorax* (found on rabbits). When these mites are in close proximity to a human host, they bite quickly and run, returning to their animal host.[40] They are very difficult to visualize with the human eye. Skin lesions include grouped pruritic papules, urticarial wheals and bullous lesions. In pets infested with *Cheyletiella*, the pet exhibits patches of fine, powdery scale ('walking dandruff'). Other mites of potential human concern include house-dust mites (*Dermatophagoides* species), the snake mite (*Ophionyssus natricis*), and the house-mouse mite (*Liponyssoides sanguineus*).

Demodex mites are present normally in adult human hair follicles and sebaceous glands of the face, where they are considered to be 'commensal ectoparasites'.[41] They are less commonly present in childhood skin. The two species are *Demodex folliculorum* and *Demodex brevis*. 'Demodex folliculitis' presents as a very itchy papular and pustular eruption on the face, usually in children with leukemia or HIV infection.[41,42] There may be an accentuation in the perioral regions. Reported topical therapies have included 5% permethrin cream, metronidazole, sulfur and sodium sulfacetamide.

Ticks

Ticks are large, globular arachnids with short legs, hard leathery skin, and mouthparts adaptable for sucking blood from mammals, birds, and reptiles. They are important vectors of diseases such as relapsing fever, rickettsial infections (Rocky Mountain spotted fever, Mediterranean spotted fever, Q fever, and ehrlichiosis; see Ch. 16), Lyme disease (see Ch. 14), babesiosis, Colorado tick fever, and tularemia. Although tick bites may be painful, the majority are painless and may go unnoticed.

Ticks are classified into three family groups: hard ticks (Ixodidae), soft ticks (Argasidae), and Nuttalliellidae.[43] They are found in grass, shrubs, vines, and bushes, from which they attach themselves to dogs, cattle, deer, and humans. Ticks penetrate human epidermis with distal mouthparts called chelicerae (Fig. 18.16), and then insert another part called the hypostome through which they feed on blood and deposit a variety of agents, including anticoagulant and antiinflammatory agents. Both acute and chronic dermatoses may result from tick bites. Acute changes include erythema, papules, nodules, bullae, ulceration, and necrosis. Multiple pruritic papules caused by infestation with tick larvae have also been reported.[44] Chronic changes include granulomas, alopecia, and secondary bacterial infection. Localized foreign body-type reactions may result from retained mouthparts or improper tick removal, and occasionally persist for months to years. T- or B-cell cutaneous lymphoid hyperplasia may also be noted, often with copious numbers of eosinophils when tissue biopsies are analyzed histologically. The B-cell type may be difficult to distinguish from true B-cell lymphoma.[45]

Non-dermatological findings that may result from tick bites include anaphylaxis, fever, headache, flu-like symptoms, abdominal pain, and vomiting. Tick paralysis is a reversible disorder characterized by ascending motor weakness and flaccid paralysis. It is believed to be due to a neurotoxin injected into the victim while the tick is engorging, and it appears that the tick must feed for several days before paralysis occurs. Bulbar paralysis, dysarthria, dysphagia, and death from respiratory failure may occur. Most cases of tick paralysis occur in children, and removing the tick results in rapid resolution of the signs and symptoms.[46]

Various methods of prevention for tick-borne diseases have been advocated. Avoidance of tick habitats may reduce risks, but this is not always feasible. Recommendations for clothing include wearing light-colored, long-sleeved clothes and footwear, tucking pants into socks and taping exposed edges.[43] Insect repellents containing

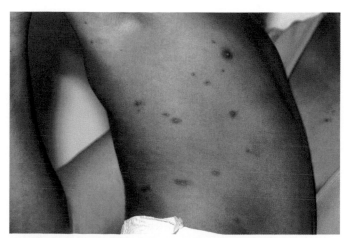

Figure 18.15 Avian mite dermatitis. Multiple papules and papulovesicles, which were very pruritic. Upon investigation, a bird's nest was noted near the window in this patient's bedroom, and was believed to be the source of the infestation.

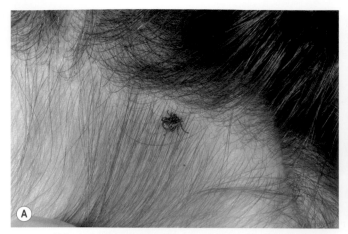

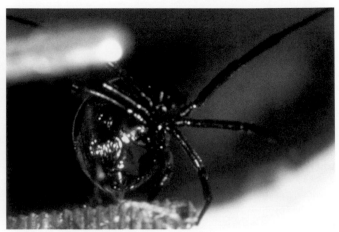

Figure 18.17 Black widow spider. Note classic red hourglass marking on the underside of the abdomen. (Courtesy of Dirk M Elston, MD.)

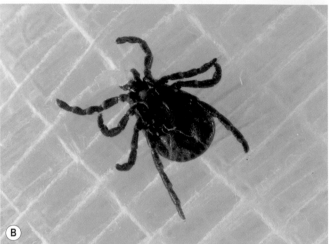

Figure 18.16 Tick bite. (A) This tick was found on clinical examination of the scalp of this 9-year-old male, who came to the office for an unrelated matter. He had been playing in a forested area in Michigan 3 days previously. (B) The tick, following gentle manual removal.

N,N-diethyl-3-methylbenzamide (DEET) or picaridin applied to exposed areas of skin, and permethrin applied to clothing, are both effective parts of prevention (see below). Frequent examination of skin for ticks is also important in high-risk areas and during high-risk seasons.

Prompt tick removal is also important in reducing the transmission of disease. The entire tick must be removed completely, including the mouthpart and the cement the tick secretes to secure attachment.[47] A variety of commercial tick-removal devices are available, and are quite successful. Manual extraction of a tick is performed with blunt, medium-tipped forceps. The tick is grasped as close to the skin as possible, and perpendicular traction is used to gradually extract the entire tick, taking care not to twist the forceps.[47] Should a portion of the tick be retained, a cutaneous punch biopsy will effectively remove it.

Spiders

Spiders, because of their menacing appearance, are frequently blamed for more damage than they actually create. Virtually all of the serious spider bites on the North American continent are caused by the black widow spider and the brown recluse spider. Bites of the former tend to have milder outcomes, whereas bites of the latter often result in more severe sequelae.[48] Children are more vulnerable to the effects of spider bites. Patients reporting spider bites are often

diagnosed in emergency departments as having skin or soft-tissue infection.[49] The gold standard for diagnosing spider bites is collection and proper identification of the biting spider, although this rarely occurs.

The black widow spider, or *Latrodectus mactans*, is a potentially dangerous spider found mainly in southern Canada, the USA, Cuba, and Mexico. It is recognized by its coal-black color and globular body (1 cm in diameter) with a red or orange hourglass marking on the underside of its abdomen (Fig. 18.17). A webspinner (in contrast to burrowing spiders), it lives in cool dark places in buildings and little-used structures and often spins its web across outdoor furniture. Consequently, a significant number of bites in the southern USA occur around the genitalia and buttocks.

The black widow spider bites humans only in self-defense. The female spider is more dangerous than the male as a result of her larger size and more potent neurotoxin.[50] α-Latrotoxin, the potent black widow neurotoxin, triggers synaptic vesicle release from presynaptic nerve terminals, and results in its effects via exocytosis of neurotransmitters.[51] Two red, punctate marks and local swelling are often seen, and burning or stinging develops at the site of the envenomation. This is followed, usually within 10 min to an hour, by severe cramping abdominal pain and spasmodic muscular contractions, which peak in around 3 h. Irritability, sweating, and agitation are common in children. Hypertension within the initial hours following the bite occurs in 20–30% of patients,[50] and, although it may be severe, it is often asymptomatic in children.[52] Although the bite may be fatal, most children recover spontaneously in 2–3 days.

Treatment options for black widow spider bites include benzodiazepines, calcium gluconate, and specific antivenin. Diazepam is the most commonly utilized benzodiazepine. Intravenous opioids are also utilized, and seem very effective in providing symptomatic relief.[53] Antivenin therapy has been demonstrated useful, even when given as late as 90 h after the bite.[54] Although specific antivenin may not be available in some parts of the world, redback spider (*Latrodectus hasseltii*) antivenin has also been shown to be effective in neutralizing *L. mactans* venom in mouse models.[55,56]

Spiders of the *Loxosceles* family cause cutaneous and subcutaneous injury primarily via the enzyme sphingomyelinase D (see below). There are roughly 100 species of *Loxosceles* spiders, with 80% of them being found in the Western hemisphere.[57] The brown recluse spider, or *Loxosceles reclusa*, is the one of the most dangerous spiders in the USA. This spider is indigenous to the area spanning eastward from southeastern Nebraska and the eastern half of Texas to the western part of Georgia.[58] The northern boundary includes southern Missouri, Illinois, Indiana, and Ohio, and the southern boundary is the Gulf of Mexico. In non-endemic areas, such as the western USA, physician overdiagnosis of brown recluse bites (also known as loxoscelism) is common.[59]

The brown recluse spider has an oval, tan to dark brown body, about 1 cm in length and 4–6 mm in width. A dark-brown violin-shaped marking extends dorsally from the eyes back to the distal cephalothorax (Fig. 18.18), and there are three pairs of eyes, rather than the four seen in other spiders. The brown recluse spider thrives in human-altered environments, such as attics, basements, and boxes.[58] When in the house, the spider is often found in storage closets (among clothing); when outdoors, it generally resides in grasses, rocky bluffs, and barns. Because of its normal shyness and predilection for dark recesses, it bites only in self-defense when approached.

The venom of *L. reclusa* contains numerous enzymes, most notably sphingomyelinase D2 (SMD), as well as alkaline phosphatase, esterase, ATPase and hyaluronidase. SMD may result in many effects, including lysis of red blood cells, complement activation, platelet activation, and thrombosis.[60] Activation of neutrophils results in the classic cutaneous necrosis seen, as a result of neutrophil secretion with subsequent endothelial damage, thrombosis, and ischemia. The local effect on tissues seems to be directly related to the amount of venom injected. Systemic findings may also occur and are more common in children.

The clinical presentation of loxoscelism begins within 6 h of the bite, usually with pruritus, pain, and/or erythema at the site. Within 24 h, a red ring develops, followed by blue-purple discoloration (Fig. 18.19) with an increase in pain. Ultimately, gangrenous ulceration with necrosis and eschar formation occurs (Fig. 18.20),

occasionally with bulla formation. Anesthesia is often present in the center of the affected area. A generalized petechial or morbilliform eruption may also be present.[57] Systemic findings may include chills, fever, nausea, and joint pain. Rare findings include severe hemolysis, renal failure, and pulmonary edema. Necrotizing fasciitis has also been reported.[61] Lymphangitis is not uncommon when the bite occurs on an extremity. In mild cases, *L. reclusa* bites may result only in a mild urticarial reaction.

Brown recluse spider bites heal very slowly, and scarring frequently results. Progression to pyoderma gangrenosum-like ulcers has been reported, but is rare. For the majority of small, uncomplicated bite reactions, spontaneous healing is the rule. Conservative treatment measures for these patients include rest, ice compression, and elevation (RICE) of the affected area. Antibiotics should be considered if secondary bacterial infection is suspected. Aspirin, antihistamines (most notably cyproheptadine), and tetanus vaccination may be considered, and dapsone therapy has been utilized but must be closely monitored given the toxicity profile.[58] Dapsone is felt, by some, to be effective when administered early in the course of the bite reaction, and may have its therapeutic effects via suppression of neutrophil chemotaxis. However, side-effects including dose-related hemolysis, agranulocytosis, cholestasis, and methemoglobinemia limit its widespread use. When systemic signs and

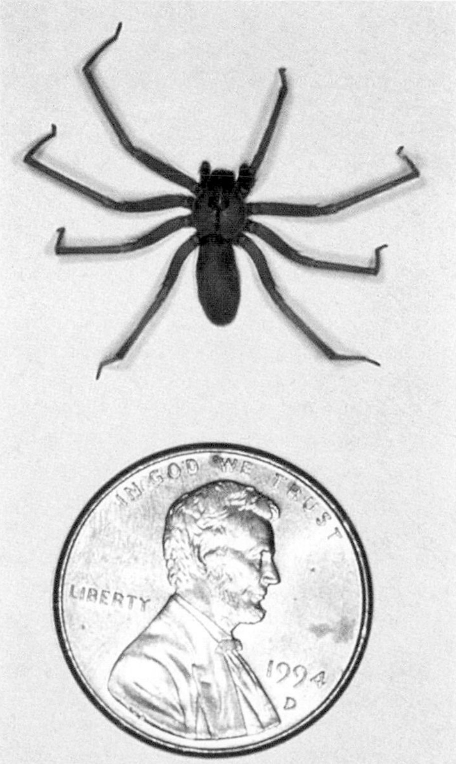

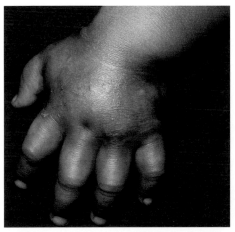

Figure 18.19 Brown recluse spider bite reaction. Swelling and mild erythema are noted early in the course following a brown recluse spider bite.

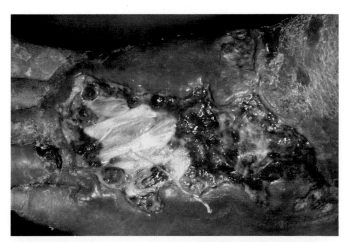

Figure 18.20 Brown recluse spider bite reaction. Massive deep ulceration with eschar formation. (Courtesy of Brooke Army Medical Center teaching file.)

Figure 18.18 Brown recluse spider. Note the brown, violin-shaped marking on the dorsal surface. The adjacent penny gives a size reference. (Courtesy of Dirk M Elson, MD.)

symptoms are present, fluid support should be given and systemic corticosteroids may be considered. Other reported therapies have included hyperbaric oxygen, vasodilators, heparin, nitroglycerin, electric shock, curettage and surgical excision.[57]

Scorpions

Scorpions are tropical photophobic arachnids that hide by day and hunt by night. They differ from other arachnids in that they have an elongated abdomen ending in a stinger (Fig. 18.21A). Scorpions are found worldwide, particularly in the tropics, and in North America they are generally seen in the southern USA and Mexico. The Buthidae family are the most toxic of scorpions, and are found mainly in India, Spain, the Middle East, and northern Africa.[50] The major scorpion offender in the USA is *Centroides exilicauda*.

Although the majority of scorpion stings in the USA are not severe and do not warrant significant medical therapy, children seem to be at greater risk of developing severe scorpion envenomation. Hence, stings in children should be watched carefully, particularly during the first 4 h, to assess for a more serious reaction. The venom apparatus of the scorpion is carried in its curved stinger at the tip of the tail, which is swung over the scorpion's head to penetrate the victim's skin. During the day scorpions hide in shoes, closets, clothing, and crevices. Some species of ground scorpions, however, may burrow and hide in gravel or children's sandboxes. They rarely attack humans but will do so when accidentally

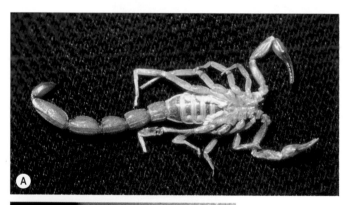

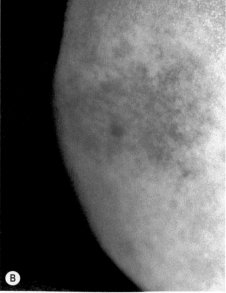

Figure 18.21 Scorpion (A) and scorpion sting, early reaction (B). Painful burning and erythema was present shortly following the sting.

disturbed, brushed against, or stepped upon. The effect of the sting depends upon the amount of envenomation and the age and size of the individual. The majority of published reports of severe or fatal envenomation have been in children less than 10 years of age.[62,63]

During a sting, the scorpion releases two noxious agents: a localized hemolytic toxin and a dangerous neurotoxic venom. The hemolytic toxin may cause a painful burning sensation, with pronounced redness (Fig. 18.21B), swelling, discoloration, severe necrosis, lymphangitis, and, in some patients, disseminated intravascular coagulation or renal failure. The neurotoxic venom, which reaches the systemic circulation primarily via the lymphatics, may produce local numbness and a severe generalized reaction consisting of sweating, salivation, tightness in the throat, abdominal cramps, cyanosis, convulsions, and, particularly in small children, respiratory paralysis and death. Tachycardia and hypertension are common, and may persist for several hours. Pulmonary edema, with or without hemoptysis, and shock may develop. Local cutaneous reactions may vary, and include erythema, petechiae, purpura, bullae, edema, induration, necrosis, and ulceration.[64]

Treatment for scorpion envenomation is difficult, without consensus on one gold standard of care. Immediate measures include application of a tourniquet above the area of the sting and the application of ice or cold water. Serotherapy, which refers to administration of scorpion antivenom, has been advocated by some but has been found ineffective by some investigators, and does not prevent the development of cardiac problems.[50,65–67] Fluid resuscitation, sedation, and treatment of hypertension may be indicated. Prazosin therapy has been shown to decrease the development of acute pulmonary edema.[68] A large series of severe scorpion envenomation in children suggested that the beneficial effects of antivenom and/or prazosin is questionable when hospital admission is delayed.[63] Continuous intravenous midazolam infusion has also been utilized to control agitation and involuntary motor activity.[69] Although intravenous high-dose corticosteroid therapy was once recommended, it appears to offer no significant benefit in terms or mortality, duration of hospital stay, or cost.[70] Intravenous administration of scorpion-specific F(ab')(2) antivenom was found to reverse the neurologic effects of scorpion envenomation in critically ill children within 4 h, with reduced need for midazolam sedation.[71]

Insects

Insects are the class of arthropods characterized by division into three parts (a head, thorax, and abdomen). Noxious insects are ubiquitous, affecting all humans in some manner at one time or another. The insects of medical significance include lice, mosquitoes, flies, fleas, bed bugs, bees, wasps, ants, caterpillars/moths, and beetles.

Lice (pediculosis)

Lice have plagued humans since ancient times. Infection is most common during times of stress, such as war, or in crowded environments such as schools, camps, or institutions. Following widespread use of DDT after the end of the Second World War, there were relatively few reports of pediculosis in the USA. Subsequent restrictions on the use of DDT in the USA since 1973, however, resulted in an increase in the number of cases, particularly pediculosis capitis and pediculosis pubis. Lice occur wherever there are humans. They spend their entire life as ectoparasites, depending on human blood for sustenance. Their existence independent of humans is generally not possible. All lice feed by pressing their mouth against the host's skin, piercing the surface, and injecting an anticoagulant to facilitate the blood flow during feeding.

Lice are small, six-legged, wingless insects with translucent, gray-white bodies that become red when engorged with blood. They measure 1–4 mm in size, and are visible to the naked eye on close inspection. Three species of lice infest humans:

1. *Pediculus humanus corporis* (the body louse)
2. *Pediculus humanus capitis* (the head louse)
3. *Phthirus pubis* (the pubic, or 'crab' louse).

Body lice and head lice (Fig. 18.22) are very similar in appearance, with elongated bodies and three pairs of claw-like legs. Pubic lice, on the other hand, have short bodies and resemble crabs in appearance. The body louse is the only louse that can carry human disease, including louse-borne relapsing fever, trench fever, and epidemic typhus. Body and head lice are transmitted by close contact or via fomites, including clothing (body louse) and combs, brushes, and hats or other headgear (head louse). Pubic lice are transmitted by intimate physical contact, and are considered in most cases to be a sexually transmitted disease. Non-sexual transmission of pubic lice may occur, though, and probably accounts for most cases of infestation involving the eyebrows and/or eyelashes in children, although the possibility of sexual abuse should always be considered in this setting.

Lice egg cases are called nits, and are firmly attached to the hair shaft with a cement that makes them difficult to remove. They are gray to yellow-white in color, and are seen as tiny pinhead specks measuring 0.3–0.8 mm (Fig. 18.23). The nits of head lice are attached to the hair shaft at a more acute angle than those of pubic lice.[72] Head lice nits are usually laid within 1–2 mm of the scalp, and in general, attached nits further from the scalp are more likely to be non-viable. Nits are usually easily distinguished from hair casts or dandruff by the inability to remove them from the hair shaft and, if necessary, microscopic evaluation. The differential diagnosis of nits is shown in Table 18.3. Nits incubate for about 1 week, and then young lice hatch, passing through several nymph stages and growing into adult lice over 1–2 weeks. *Pediculosis corporis* (body lice) most commonly occurs in homeless individuals, refugees, victims of wars and natural disasters, and those living in crowded conditions.[73] The nits of the body louse attach firmly to clothing fibers, where they may remain viable for weeks. The louse itself is rarely observed on the skin. It obtains its nourishment by clinging to the patient's clothing and intermittently piercing the skin. The primary lesion is a small, red macule, papule, or urticarial wheal with a hemorrhagic central punctum. Primary lesions may be difficult to visualize due to excoriations related to scratching, and secondary impetiginization may be present. The diagnosis of body lice is confirmed by finding lice or nits in clothing, often in seams. Treatment consists primarily of thorough deinfestation of all clothing and bedding. Treatment of the patient with 5% permethrin cream or lindane 1% lotion may also be useful, as an occasional louse may remain and return to feed.

Pediculosis pubis (pubic lice, crab lice) involves primarily the pubic area, but may also involve the scalp, eyebrows and eyelashes, beard, and other hairy areas. Live lice and nits are usually seen. Itching may be the initial symptom, but in persistent cases eczematization or secondary infection may occur. A characteristic skin finding is maculae ceruleae, which are gray-blue macules on the abdomen and thighs. They are felt to represent hemosiderin deposition in the deep dermis as a result of the bites. Treatment of pubic lice is generally similar to that used for head lice (see below), as well as laundering of all clothing and bed linens. Eyelash involvement is usually treated with an occlusive agent, such as petroleum jelly.

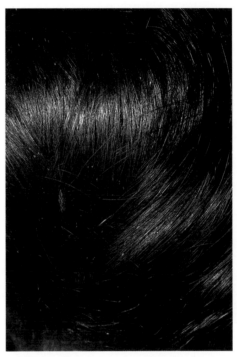

Figure 18.23 Nits. These eggs are seen as tiny, gray-white specks attached firmly to hair shafts.

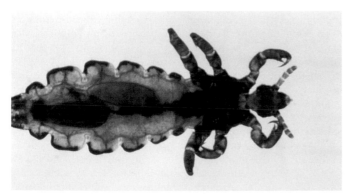

Figure 18.22 Head louse. Note the elongated body, three pairs of legs, and nits (eggs) within the body of the louse.

Table 18.3 Differential diagnosis of nits	
Diagnosis	**Comment**
Nits	Firmly adherent to hair shaft; not easily removed with fingers
Seborrheic dermatitis (dandruff)	Diffuse scalp scaling; scales occasionally adhere to hair, but easy to remove; scalp erythema may be present
Hair casts	Keratin protein which encircles hair shaft; easily removed
Piedra	Fungal infection of hair; firm nodules attached to hair shafts, white or black in color
Psoriasis	Thick silvery scales, often present overlying red plaques on the scalp
Hair products	i.e., hairspray, mousse, gel

Pediculosis capitis (head lice) is by far the most common form of lice to affect children, and usually affects those between 3 and 12 years of age. As mentioned, it is spread through head-to-head contact and fomites, including headgear, combs, brushes, towels, and upholstery. The transmission from fomites contributes to the increasingly challenging cycle of head lice infestation. All socioeconomic groups are affected, although African-Americans are less often infested with head lice, possibly related to the diameter, shape or twisted nature of their hair shafts (which makes grasping of the shaft more difficult for the louse).[72,74–76] The clinical findings consist primarily of pruritus, with secondary excoriation and occasional secondary bacterial infection. Cervical and suboccipital lymphadenopathy may be present. Head lice do not transmit other infectious disease agents. The diagnosis is confirmed by finding live lice (Fig. 18.24) or viable nits on the scalp. In patients in whom the diagnosis is based only on nits, their viability can be confirmed by mounting them on a glass slide and performing microscopic evaluation at low power. Viable nits have an intact operculum (cap) on the non-attached end and a developing louse within the egg (Fig. 18.25).

Although the clinical syndrome of head lice infestation is not serious, it is a cause of significant psychosocial distress, embarrassment, and lost school and work days. Since non-viable nits may persist on hair shafts for several months, the potential exists for

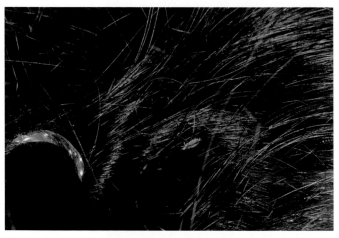

Figure 18.24 Pediculosis capitis. Note the live head louse, easily seen with the naked eye.

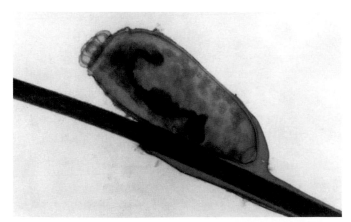

Figure 18.25 Nit. This ×40 magnification light microscopy image shows a nit firmly attached to the hair shaft by a cement-like substance. Note the intact cap (operculum) and the developing louse within the egg.

misdiagnosing active infestation when in fact there is none. It has been tradition in some communities for 'no nit' policies to be enforced, in which children with nits are excluded from school until they are adequately treated and all visible nits have been removed. Such policies may lead to unnecessary exposure to pediculicidal agents, missed school, and loss of parental work time.[77] The American Academy of Pediatrics recommends against no-nit policies, since they have not been effective in controlling head lice transmission.[78] Misidentification of non-lice non-nit debris (such as dandruff, fibers, dirt, scabs, hair casts) may also result in the over-diagnosis and consequent mismanagement of head lice.[79] Pediculicidal agents should be used only when viable nits or live lice are observed. In general, nits located close to the scalp are viable and unhatched, although in warmer climates, viable ones may be found several inches away from the scalp.

Treatment options for head lice are summarized in Table 18.4. Head lice therapy is recommended for individuals diagnosed with an active infestation, and prophylactic therapy is recommended for bedmates and immediate members of the household of the infested index patient. The standard of care is application of 1% permethrin cream rinse to mildly damp hair, followed by rinsing 10 min later. Although permethrin is both pediculicidal and ovicidal, many physicians recommend a second treatment 7–10 days following the initial therapy. This agent is FDA approved for children as young as 2 months of age, and is recommended as first-line therapy by the American Academy of Pediatrics.[78] Increasing resistance concerns have been reported with permethrin (see below).

Lindane (or gamma benzene hexachloride) is a slow-acting pesticide that has been used frequently in the past. This agent is stored in fat and nerve tissues, and concerns regarding absorption and neurotoxicity have resulted in many recommending against its use, although most reported toxicities occurred with incorrect usage. Lindane use has been banned in the state of California since 2002.[80] The synergized pyrethrins (i.e., pyrethrin + piperonyl butoxide) include extracts from the *Chrysanthemum* family. These agents are pediculicidal only, and treatment failures are more common.

Malathion is a weak organophosphate cholinesterase inhibitor that had been unavailable in the USA for several years. This agent has more recently been reintroduced and approved for use in children 6 years of age and older. It is not considered a first-line therapy. Malathion is both pediculicidal and ovicidal, and resistance is quite rare. The isopropanol-containing vehicle contributes to its effectiveness, but also its flammability.[72] Malathion 0.5% lotion is applied to dry hair and rinsed after 8–12 h.

Benzyl alcohol 5% lotion is a newer addition to the prescription lice therapy market in the USA. It is FDA-approved in children 6 months of age and older. This agent is a non-neurotoxic product that kills lice via blockage of their respiratory mechanism. Although head lice have evolved the ability to temporarily close their breathing 'spiracles' (holes), benzyl alcohol 5% lotion stuns the spiracles open, while the mineral oil vehicle obstructs them, killing the lice via asphyxiation.[81] This product provides an alternative for parents who are concerned about the use of neurotoxic pediculicidal agents. Repeat therapy is necessary, and benzyl alcohol 5% lotion is not ovicidal.

Other, less conventional therapies have been used with variable success. These include 5% permethrin, oral trimethoprim-sulfamethoxazole, oral ivermectin, greasy preparations (i.e., olive oil, mayonnaise and petroleum jelly, which are believed to work via occlusion of the respiratory spiracles of the adult louse), and styling gels.[72,76,82] None of these agents have been studied scientifically and their true effectiveness remains unclear. Trimethoprim-sulfamethoxazole is believed to kill symbiotic bacteria present in the louse gut, and was shown in one study to work synergistically

Table 18.4 Treatments for pediculosis capitis (head lice)

Name	Instructions for use	Comment
Permethrin 1% cream rinse (Nix)	Apply to damp hair after shampooing; leave on for 10 min, then rinse	Pediculicidal and ovicidal; repeat treatment in 7–10 days; OTC
Pyrethrin + piperonyl butoxide (RID, Pronto, A-200)	Apply to dry hair; leave on for 10 min, then rinse	Pediculicidal only; repeat treatment in 7–10; derived from chrysanthemum; OTC
Lindane 1% shampoo, lotion (Kwell)	Apply to dry hair; leave on for 4 min (shampoo) or overnight (lotion), then rinse	Stored in nerve/fat tissue; possible CNS toxicity (although usually observed with incorrect usage) and resistance concerns; low ovicidal activity; should not be first choice therapy; Rx
Benzyl alcohol 5% lotion (Ulesfia)	Apply to dry hair, leave on for 10 min, rinse; repeat in 7 days	Kills lice by asphyxiation; contains no neurotoxic pesticide; Rx
Malathion 0.5% lotion (Ovide)	Apply to dry hair, rinse after 8–12 h; repeat in 7–10 days	Approved for children 6 years and older; ovicidal and pediculicidal; not first-line therapy; flammable; Rx
Trimethoprim-sulfamethoxazole (Bactrim)	8–10 mg/kg per day divided BID for 10 days	Occasionally used off-label (not FDA-approved for lice); purportedly kills symbiotic bacteria in louse gut; risk of severe allergic reactions; Rx
Ivermectin, oral (Stromectol, 3 or 6 mg tablets)	200 µg/kg single dose, repeat in 1–2 weeks	Occasionally used off-label for resistant cases or crusted scabies; FDA-approved for strongyloidiasis, onchocerciasis; side-effects include headache, dizziness, nausea, vomiting; Rx
Manual nit removal	Comb with fine-toothed nit removal comb	Difficult, tedious (see text)
Permethrin 0.5% spray (RID)	Spray on inanimate objects	For furniture and bedding; not for use on skin; OTC
Occlusive agents (petrolatum, olive oil, mayonnaise, others)	Applied and typically left on overnight, then rinsed out	Therapeutic goal is suffocation of lice; potentially limited by ability of lice to temporarily close breathing spiracles; no evidence-based data to support efficacy

OTC, over-the-counter; CNS, central nervous system; Rx, by prescription; BID, twice daily.

with 1% permethrin cream rinse when the two were used in combination.[83] The potential for severe allergic reaction to this agent makes it less desirable as a lice therapy. Ivermectin has been used as an off-label oral therapy in the same dose (200 µg/kg) as that discussed for scabies infestation. Thirty-minute applications of hot air have been studied as a potential therapy for head lice.[84] Spinosad, a non-synthetic fermentation product of the soil bacterium *Saccharopolyspora spinosa*, has been found useful as a creme rinse, with better efficacy than permethrin in one report.[85]

Manual lice and especially nit removal is a tedious task, which is unlikely to prevent spread of the infestation unless performed by professional nit-removing salons. Nits, given their firm adherence to the hair shaft, remain in place long after the viable louse has left the casing. It should be recalled that viable nits are deposited on hair close to the scalp (usually within 1–2 mm), and most nits that are further out than 5–7 mm are no longer viable. However, in some instances, nit removal is desirable, such as for aesthetic purposes or in response to societal pressures. This is accomplished with manual removal and with fine-toothed 'nit combs', which are widely available and occasionally packaged with pediculicidal agents. 'Wet combing' refers to use of the nit comb on damp hair, which is believed to slow down live lice and facilitate removal of nits. A variety of agents have been used in an effort to loosen the 'cement' that attaches the nit to the hair shaft. These include vinegar, 8% formic acid (Step 2), and a variety of vinegar-based products.

The issue of drug resistance has emerged over the years, and clearly appears to be a significant consideration in certain communities. Before assuming true drug resistance, however, other reasons for therapeutic failure should be considered. These include incorrect diagnosis, repeat infestation, and non-compliance with therapy. True resistance has been documented to permethrin, lindane,

synergized natural pyrethrins, and malathion.[86–90] Malathion appears to be the agent with the least documented resistance, especially in the USA.[86,87] Lack of susceptibility to pyrethroid insecticides (permethrin, pyrethrins) is usually attributed to an amino acid substitution in a protein that confers 'knockdown resistance', which subsequently desensitizes cholinergic nerves to the activity of these toxins.[91,92]

Regardless of the method of therapy, other family members and close contacts should be examined and those with evidence of infestation should also be treated. Play areas and furniture can be vacuumed, and bedding, clothing, and headgear should be machine washed in hot water and dried on a high-heat setting. Items that cannot be washed may be dry-cleaned or placed in sealed plastic bags for 2 weeks. Hats, combs, brushes, grooming aids, towels, school lockers and hooks, and other items that come into contact with the head or head coverings should not be shared. Combs and brushes may be coated with the pediculicide for 15 min or soaked in rubbing alcohol for 1 h, followed by washing in hot soapy water. Alternatively, these items can be discarded and replaced with new ones.

Information for patients regarding management and control of head lice is available from the National Pediculosis Association at: www.headlice.org.

Mosquitoes and flies

Flies and mosquitoes belong to the order Diptera. One of the largest orders of insects, it includes the two-winged biting flies, gnats, and mosquitoes. Of these, mosquitoes are the most important from the standpoint of human health. They are seen worldwide and may be vectors of many important diseases, such as encephalitis (including West Nile encephalitis), malaria, yellow fever, and filariasis. In the

USA, the most common insect bites of infants and children are those of mosquitoes.

Mosquitoes are attracted to bright clothing, heat, humidity, and human odors, particularly those of young children. Carbon dioxide, released mainly in the breath but also from the skin, is a long-range attractant for mosquitos and can be detected from up to 36 m away.[93] In unsensitized individuals, the ordinary mosquito bite produces only mild, local irritation. This manifests as a slight stinging sensation and a small, pruritic erythematous papule. In sensitized individuals, however, mosquito bites produce itching; urticarial wheals, which may last for several hours to several days; or firm papules or nodules (Fig. 18.26), which may persist for longer periods of time. Occasionally, and particularly in the young, mosquito bites may produce blisters or hemorrhagic lesions. Excoriation of these lesions may result in secondary eczematization and impetiginization. Systemic Arthus-type reactions and anaphylaxis are rare, but do occur. Hypersensitivity to mosquito bites has also been associated with Epstein–Barr virus-associated lymphoproliferative disorders.[94,95]

Although the diagnosis of insect bites is often obvious, differentiation from other papular, vesicular, and pruritic eruptions may also be suggested by the characteristic grouping of lesions, a central punctum when present, the acute nature of most reactions, and their seasonal incidence. Treatment of mosquito bites includes oral antihistamines, cool compresses, and topical antipruritic agents such as calamine lotion and topical corticosteroids. When topical corticosteroids are used, stronger preparations (i.e., class II–V) are most effective, with caution exercised not to apply these agents to the face, groin, or fold areas. Topical diphenhydramine should be avoided given risks of allergic contact sensitization. Cetirizine or loratadine, taken prophylactically have both been shown to decrease immediate whealing and pruritus as well as delayed pruritus.[96,97]

Prevention is most effectively accomplished by the use of insect repellents (see below). Another important measure, especially during high-risk activities or exposure times, is the use of protective clothing (hats, socks and shoes, and long-sleeved shirts tucked into pants). Scented hairsprays, pomades, soaps, lotions, powders, colognes, and perfumes may attract all forms of stinging insects, and should be avoided unless necessary. Although some have suggested that thiamine hydrochloride taken orally may help to repel insects, this measure remains unproven. Efforts at reducing mosquito populations include ultrasonic electronic devices, for use by the consumer, and insecticide spraying programs, which have been adopted by several communities.

Various species of biting flies (sandflies, gnats, black flies, deerflies, horseflies) are known to attack the exposed areas of the face, neck, arms, and legs, with the production of painful or pruritic papules or nodules, often with vesiculation. Although lesions often disappear in a few hours, they may persist for several days and can be quite annoying, particularly in small children. Treatment consists of the prophylactic use of insect repellents and treatment of symptoms with acetaminophen, antihistamines, calamine lotion, or topical corticosteroids.

Non-biting flies, including common houseflies, tend to feed at open wounds, exudates, and cutaneous ulcers and may produce *myiasis*, a far less common but significant skin disorder. Myiasis is usually a travel-associated dermatosis, and is caused most often by infestation with *Dermatobia hominis* (human botfly). It is most common following travel to Central and South America.[98] In this disorder, the adult female lays eggs on other arthropods (flies, mosquitoes, ticks, etc.) and this vector then transmits the larvae to the skin of the human host. The larvae penetrate skin, mature in the dermis and subcutaneous tissues, and eventually reach such a size (Fig. 18.27) that they are unable to spontaneously emerge. Clinically, patients present with furuncular nodules (Fig. 18.28), which

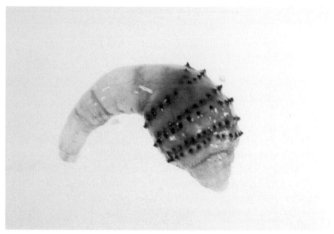

Figure 18.27 Botfly larva. Note the posterior spines and odd shape of the second stage larva, which makes it difficult to dislodge through the overlying tiny skin orifice.

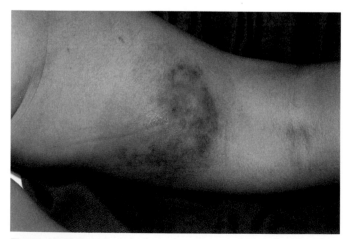

Figure 18.26 Severe mosquito bite reaction. An indurated, firm, edematous plaque with secondary petechiae from rubbing.

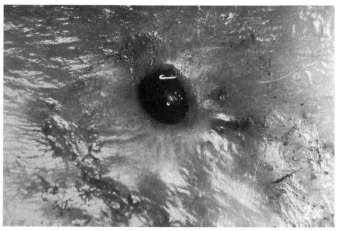

Figure 18.28 Myiasis. A furuncular nodule with a small, central opening. Note the visible tip of the larva within the opening.

may drain and often have a central opening (sinus tract), which serves as a site for respiration and excretion. The patient may report a sensation of 'crawling in the skin.' Treatments include extraction of the larvae through suffocation (petroleum jelly, butter, paraffin, oil) or surgical removal.[98,99]

Fleas

Fleas (Siphonaptera) exist universally among animals and humans. Those that most commonly attack humans in the USA are the human flea (*Pulex irritans*), the cat flea (*Ctenocephalides felis*), and the dog flea (*Ctenocephalides canis*). The eruption produced by a flea bite in a sensitized individual is an urticarial wheal or papule (Fig. 18.29), often with a centrally located hemorrhagic punctum. In highly susceptible individuals, particularly young children, wheals may progress and develop into tense bullae (Figs 18.30, 18.31). Flea bites are often multiple and grouped together in linear or irregular clusters on the arms, forearms, or legs or on areas where clothing fits snugly (thighs, buttocks, waist, and lower abdomen). Bites in a linear configuration (the 'breakfast, lunch, and dinner' sign, Fig. 18.32) are common, and relate to their tendency to jump and crawl but not fly. Treatment is similar to that described for mosquito bites.

Elimination of fleas by treatment of suspected animal carriers and cleaning/spraying of carpets, floors, crevices, and other potentially infested areas should be considered. It should be noted that for every flea seen on the pet there are many more in the environment, that flea collars are not completely effective, and that animal flea sprays and powders, if used, must be repeated every 2 weeks during the summer months to be effective.[100]

Tungiasis is a skin infestation caused by the gravid sand flea, *Tunga penetrans* (chigoe flea, jigger flea). It is endemic in South and Central America, parts of Africa, India and Pakistan. Tungiasis is rare in the USA, and usually seen in those who have traveled to an endemic region.[101] In tungiasis, the female flea attaches herself to the warm-blooded host, burrows through the epidermis into the dermis, and gradually enlarges. Clinical lesions are red nodules with a central

punctum or ulceration, occasionally resembling an abscess. Treatment consists of flea removal, wound care, tetanus prophylaxis and, when necessary, treatment of secondary bacterial infection.[101]

Bed bugs

Bed bugs are a member of the order Hemiptera, which also includes reduviid bugs. The most common species to parasitize humans is *Cimex lectularius*. Bed bugs are red-brown, blood-sucking, nocturnal insects that are 3–5 mm in size. They are wingless, with flattened oval bodies and three pairs of legs (Fig. 18.33). The female bug deposits eggs on rough surfaces, cracks, and crevices. They avoid light, hiding out during the day in cracks in walls and floors and in furniture, and responding to warmth and carbon dioxide (which are both present in sleeping humans) at night. Bites present as erythematous papules, and the breakfast, lunch, and dinner sign may again be present. Bullous lesions may also occur.[102] Bed bug bites most commonly occur on exposed areas of the face, neck, arms, or hands.

Systemic reactions which may possibly be attributable to bed bug bites include urticaria, angioedema, asthma, and anaphylaxis. The bed bug is capable of traveling long distances in search of food, often from one house to another, and has been known to survive without food for up to 6 months to a year. It has been suggested

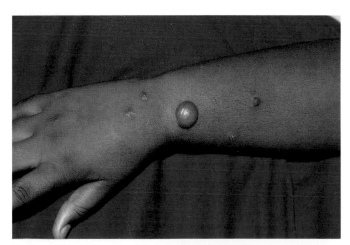

Figure 18.30 Bullous flea bite reaction. Tense bulla and surrounding crusted papules in a patient with a hypersensitivity to flea bites.

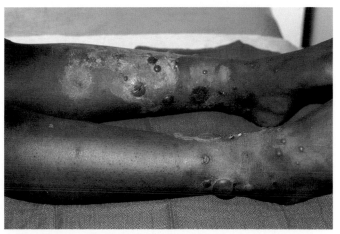

Figure 18.31 Bullous flea bite reaction. Multiple tense bullae and secondary bacterial impetiginization in a patient with flea bite hypersensitivity.

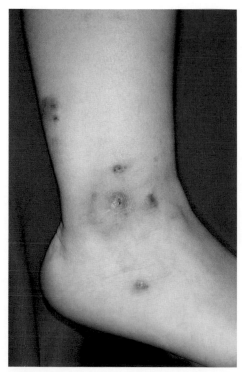

Figure 18.29 Flea bites. Multiple excoriated, clustered red papules.

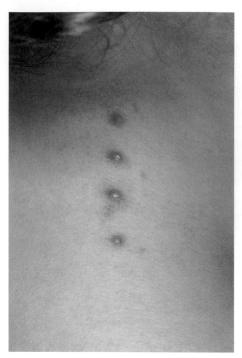

Figure 18.32 Flea bites. The classic linear configuration of flea bites (the 'breakfast, lunch, and dinner' sign), caused by the tendency of fleas to jump and crawl rather than fly.

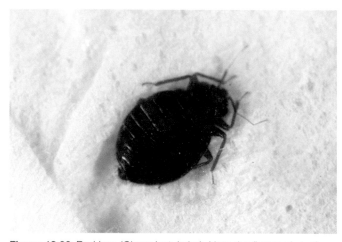

Figure 18.33 Bed bug (*Cimex lectularius*). Note the flattened, oval body and three pairs of legs. The family that brought it in had been complaining of itchy, red bite reactions for several months.

that bed bugs may be vectors for hepatitis B, human immunodeficiency virus, plague, yellow fever, tuberculosis, relapsing fever, leprosy, leishmania, filariasis or trypanosomiasis, although there is currently little evidence to support that they are vectors for any communicable diseases.[103-105] Since 1980, bed bug infestations have been observed increasingly in homes, apartments, hotel rooms, dormitories and hospitals in the USA.[105]

Treatment is directed at elimination of the bug from the environment with insecticides, and eliminating potential hiding sites. Although individual lesions require no direct therapy, oral antihistamines, topical corticosteroids, or calamine lotion may be used for symptomatic relief. Systemic corticosteroids have occasionally been utilized. Preventive measures that have been advocated for bed bug bites includes wearing pajamas that cover the majority of skin,

covering bedposts with petrolatum, and manual inspection of hotel headboards and mattresses.[106] Once infestation has occurred, useful measures for eradication may include vacuuming of exposed hiding locations, washing all linens in hot water and drying on low heat, steam cleaning, use of mattress and box spring encasements, discarding of furniture, placement of insect growth regulators, and pesticide spraying.[105,106]

Bees, wasps, and ants

Bees, wasps, and ants belong to the order Hymenoptera, a large order of insects that contains about 100 000 species. Like most other insects, they have three pairs of legs and four wings and are recognized by the narrow isthmus separating the abdomen from the thorax. Hymenoptera venom allergy can result in life-threatening allergic reactions, and is responsible for at least 40 deaths per year in the USA.[107,108] The three families of stinging insects in the order Hymenoptera include Vespidae (yellow jackets, wasps and hornets), Apidae (honeybees and bumblebees), and Formicidae (stinging ants).

Bees, the only insects that produce food eaten by humans, live in almost every part of the world except the North and South Poles. Honeybees live and work together in large groups and do not sting unless frightened or injured. Africanized ('killer') honeybees are hybrid honeybees (from interbreeding of African and domestic honeybees in South America) that tend to attack in swarms, and which have gradually been migrating into the USA. Wasps, among the most interesting and intelligent of insects, may live together in cooperative fashion, as seen with the so-called social wasps (hornets and yellow jackets), or may live as solitary insects. Most wasps are beneficial to humans, since they destroy large numbers of flies, caterpillars, and other insects that may be harmful. As with bees, wasps ordinarily do not sting humans unless they are bothered or frightened. However, yellow jackets and hornets tend to be quite aggressive, especially when near their nest or if disturbed.[108]

Symptoms of bee or wasp stings vary from mild local pruritus, pain, and edema to general anaphylactic reactions with associated difficulty in breathing and swallowing, hoarseness, slurred speech, gastrointestinal disturbances, abdominal pain, dizziness, weakness, confusion, generalized edema, cardiovascular collapse, and, occasionally, sudden death.

Ants, like bees and wasps, have large glands at the tip of the abdomen from which they introduce venom into wounds produced by their bites. The fire ant (*Solenopsis richteri and invicta*) is originally from South America and has spread rapidly in the southern USA, where it has become an agricultural pest and a health hazard.[109] It produces a venom more potent than that of other members of the order Hymenoptera. The fire ant was named for the extreme burning pain inflicted by its sting, and tends to attack without warning.[110] During one bite cycle, the fire ant may inflict seven to eight stings in a circular pattern. The immediate reaction is characterized by a painful wheal and flare response, with vesicles developing over several hours. Pustular changes eventually occur, and some patients develop large, local erythematous reactions. Anaphylaxis is a common cause of significant morbidity, and may be fatal.

The treatment of ordinary bee, wasp, or ant stings consists of local application of antipruritic shake lotions (i.e., calamine lotion), cool compresses or cool baths, and oral antihistamines. A papain solution made of one part meat tenderizer to four parts water may help to relieve local symptoms of pain or discomfort. Severe allergic reactions are treated with epinephrine, antihistamines, oxygen, and systemic corticosteroids. Patients known to be at risk for severe systemic reactions to bee, wasp, hornet, yellow jacket, or fire ant stings should be given an epinephrine pen kit and be educated in its proper use in an emergency. Preventative techniques include education on practical avoidance measures and referral to an allergist for consideration of allergen testing and immunotherapy.

Allergen immunotherapy is an effective form of prevention for certain individuals at risk for severe insect sting reactions. Commercial venoms for both skin testing and immunotherapy are available for yellow jackets, white faced hornet, yellow hornet, wasp, and honeybee, and the cDNA of most major allergens of bee and vespid venoms has been cloned and is available in a recombinant form.[107,108] Sequential bee-sting challenge tests can be used as a diagnostic tool to assess the need for venom immunotherapy in bee-venom allergic children.[111] For fire ant immunotherapy, imported fire ant whole-body extract is the main reagent used.[110] The therapeutic goals of immunotherapy are to prevent life-threatening reactions, reduce morbidity from such stings, and decrease insect sting anxiety.

Blister beetles

Blister beetles (*Cantharis vesicatoria*, order Coleoptera) contain cantharidin, a vesicant most concentrated in the beetles' genitalia, and the active principle of the purported aphrodisiac Spanish fly.[112] The lesions produced accidentally by crushing blister beetles, by discharge of their body fluid on the skin, or by external therapeutic use of cantharidin (as in the treatment of molluscum contagiosum) consist of slowly forming blisters that involve the outer layers of the skin. Treatment depends on the extent and location of lesions. Simple aseptic drainage of large bullae and cool compresses generally give adequate relief of symptoms. If vesicles are not traumatized, they usually resolve in 3–4 days, with subsequent desquamation and healing. Blister beetle ingestion, when reported, may result in oral mucosal blistering, abdominal pain, vomiting, hematuria, oliguria, and renal failure.[113]

Papular urticaria

Papular urticaria is a common condition of childhood characterized by a chronic or recurrent, papular eruption caused by hypersensitivity to a variety of bites, including those of mosquitoes, fleas, bed bugs, and mites. It is often pruritic and uncomfortable, and the resultant scratching may result in open erosions and secondary bacterial superinfection. One of the most challenging aspects of papular urticaria is convincing parents that the lesions are related to a bite reaction, and identifying and eradicating the source of the offending insect.[114]

Papular urticaria presents with multiple urticarial, 3–10 mm papules (Fig. 18.34). Lesions are frequently grouped or clustered, in a fashion similar to acute bite reactions. They may be excoriated or crusted (Fig. 18.35), and a central punctum may be visible overlying each papule. Papular urticaria is most common in the summer and late spring, and flea bites are the most common cause. Individual lesions tend to resolve over 1–2 weeks, and may heal with post-inflammatory erythema or hyperpigmentation. Recurrent episodes are common, especially if there is ongoing exposure to the offending insects.

The differential diagnosis of papular urticaria includes ordinary urticaria, pityriasis lichenoides et varioliformis acuta (PLEVA), papular acrodermatitis of childhood (Gianotti Crosti syndrome), and lymphomatoid papulosis. Histopathologic examination of skin biopsy specimens reveals spongiosis (epidermal edema), subepidermal edema, and a mixed inflammatory infiltrate that often includes eosinophils.[115] Skin biopsy is useful both in confirming the diagnosis and in persuading the parents regarding the nature of the condition. Symptomatic treatment includes oral antihistamines and topical corticosteroids, as well as topical antipruritic preparations containing menthol, camphor, or pramoxine. Environmental control measures are also desirable, when feasible.

Insect repellents

Protection from insect bites includes several measures, such as avoiding infested areas, wearing protective clothing, and controlling insect populations, when possible. However, the most effective avoidance measure in most situations is the application of insect repellent to the skin. Several types of repellents are commercially available, and include both synthetic chemicals and plant-derived essential oils.

DEET (N,N-diethyl-3-methylbenzamide, formerly N,N-diethyl-m-toluamide) has traditionally been the most effective and most widely used repellent.[116] DEET is a broad-spectrum insect repellent that is effective against mosquitoes, biting flies, chiggers, fleas, and ticks.[117] Higher concentrations of DEET result in longer-lasting protection, although these effects seem to plateau at concentrations >50%. In the USA, DEET is available in variable concentrations in multiple vehicles, including solutions, lotions, creams, gels, pump sprays, sticks, roll-ons, wristbands, and impregnated towelettes.[93,116] The mechanism of action of DEET is to provide a vapor barrier which deters the biting insect from coming into contact with human skin.[118] Firm guidelines or recommendations for choosing an appropriate DEET concentration are not available. However, it is generally accepted that products with 10–35% DEET will provide adequate

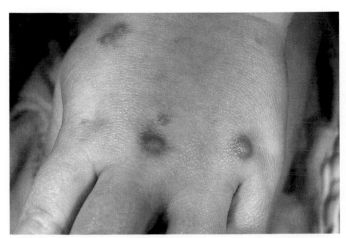

Figure 18.34 Papular urticaria. These edematous, red papules would intermittently swell and become itchier.

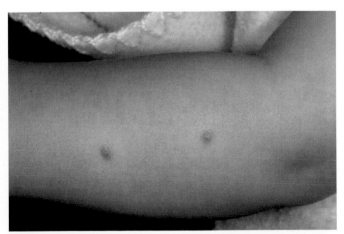

Figure 18.35 Papular urticaria. These edematous, pruritic red papules continued to intermittently enlarge for many months.

protection in most circumstances.[93] Some general recommendations for the use of DEET-containing products are listed in Table 18.5.

The use of DEET in young children has been a source of some concern, given rare reports of potential neurologic toxicity. Small amounts of DEET may be absorbed through the skin, yet seems to be completely eliminated (along with its metabolites) within 4 h of application in adults.[119] Although the pharmacokinetics are not as well understood in children, reports of neurologic toxicity are rare and, in fact, in one study of data collected by the American Association of Poison Control Centers, infants and children had lower rates of severe adverse events than did adults.[120] Many of the reports of DEET-related toxicity involved long-term, heavy, frequent, or whole-body application of DEET, and in some, the product was orally ingested.[117,121] The Environmental Protection Agency, in 1998, completed a re-registration eligibility decision for DEET, and in this process included a review of acute, subacute, and chronic toxicity data. The agency concluded that normal use of insect repellents containing DEET poses no significant risks to children or adults, that product labeling would be modified to include recommendations for safe use, and that child safety claims on labels were prohibited, given the lack of appropriate scientific data to support such claims.[117,121,122] Human health risk assessments were conducted for DEET and picaradin (see below), and found no significant toxicological risks from typical use of these repellents.[123] The American Academy of Pediatrics, in the Red Book discussion of mosquito bite prevention, recommends repellents with DEET concentrations not exceeding 30%, and following such practical application guidelines as those outlined in Table 18.5.[124]

DEET-containing insect repellents should be carefully applied as they may damage plastics, rayon, leather, spandex, and other synthetic fabrics. They are not damaging, however, to cotton or wool. In addition, it should be remembered that DEET-containing products are flammable. Combination products containing DEET and sunscreen are not recommended, given the potentially decreased effectiveness of the sunscreen, and the different recommended application frequencies of these two products. Questions about the safety of DEET can be addressed by the EPA-sponsored National Pesticide Telecommunications Network at: www.ace.orst.edu/info/nptn.

Picaridin is a newer insect repellent that is effective against mosquitoes, biting flies and ticks. It is usually used in a concentration of up to 20%. Picaridin is reportedly of similar efficacy to DEET, is odorless, and will not damage plastics or fabrics.[118] Prior to its launch in the USA, picaridin was used fairly extensively in Europe and Australia. No serious adverse events have been reported to date. Another synthetic insect repellent available in the USA and Europe is IR3535, which fared poorly in an 'arm-in-cage' study when compared to DEET.[117]

Plant-derived repellents may have repellent activity, but none compare to the effectiveness and duration of action of DEET.[93] These products usually contain essential oils from any of several plants, including citronella, cedar, eucalyptus, lemongrass, and soybean. Citronella is the active ingredient in most 'natural' repellents marketed in the USA. It has a lemony scent, and is available in an oil and in candles. However, in areas with epidemics of mosquito-borne diseases (such as West Nile virus) or in high-risk settings, these products should not be relied upon as the sole protection from bites. When compared to DEET, a blend of the top three performing essential oils was found to offer some protection against various species of mosquitoes, but significantly less so than the chemical repellent.[125]

Other approaches to mosquito repellency include ingested garlic or vitamin B_1 and treated wristbands, each of which has less consistently demonstrated effectiveness. Permethrin, marketed in a 0.5% concentration (Permanone, Duranon, Cutter Outdoorsmen Gear Guard, Sawyer Clothing Tick Repellent, 3M Clothing and Gear) as a tick repellent, is also available and is sprayed on tents, clothing, and sleeping bags. This product is also effective against mosquitoes, flies, and chiggers, and works as a contact insecticide, resulting in central nervous system toxicity to the insect.

Caterpillars and moths

Caterpillars represent the larval stage of butterflies and moths of the order Lepidoptera. The hairs of certain moths and caterpillars are known to produce dermatitis, which can be severe and incapacitating to both children and adults. In the USA, the most frequently seen and most irritating of these are those due to the hairs of the brown-tail moth (usually seen in the north-eastern part of this country) and the puss caterpillar (the larva of the 'flannel' moth, *Megalopyge opercularis*), seen from Virginia southward to the states bordering the Gulf of Mexico.[126–128] Contact with the oak processionary caterpillar (*Thaumetopoea processionea*), found especially in oak forests in European countries, may result in multiple symptoms, including pruritus, dermatitis, conjunctivitis, pharyngitis, and respiratory distress.[129]

Reactions produced by contact with the hairs and spines of these moths and caterpillars appear to be associated with the release of histamine and other vasoactive substances and mechanical irritation by caterpillar hairs that become imbedded in the pores of affected individuals. They may be focal or more widespread. Examination typically reveals erythematous macules and papules, vesicles, urticaria, or even necrosis. Other reactions may include severe local pain, nausea, fever, swelling, numbness, muscle cramps, headache, seizures, and shock. The diagnosis of moth or caterpillar dermatitis can be confirmed by microscopic examination of tape strippings or scrapings of involved areas with demonstration of offending hairs. Although the disorder is self-limiting, relief can be obtained with the use of oral antihistamines, topical corticosteroids, ice packs, and topical antipruritic agents. In patients with severe reactions, fluid support, narcotics, and systemic corticosteroids may be necessary.

Table 18.5 Guidelines for the safe use of insect repellents in children
Do not apply to infants under 2 months of age.
Read and follow all package directions and precautions.
Use just enough repellent to lightly cover the skin; do not saturate the skin.
Apply only to exposed skin; do not use on clothing or apply under clothing.
Apply sparingly to the face, and avoid contact with the eyes and mouth.
Do not apply to the hands of small children.
Do not allow young children to apply products themselves.
Do not use sprays in enclosed areas or near food.
If self-applied, rinse palms to avoid inadvertent contact with eyes and mouth.
Do not use on open skin, cuts, wounds, or inflamed areas.
Once inside, wash all treated areas with soap and water.
Keep repellents out of the reach of children.
Use a separate sunscreen; avoid using combined insect repellent-sunscreen products as clinical data are limited.

Other cutaneous parasites

Cutaneous Larva Migrans (Creeping Eruption)

Cutaneous larva migrans (CLM, creeping eruption) is a self-limited skin eruption due to the larval stages of the dog and cat hookworms, *Ancylostoma caninum* and *Ancylostoma braziliensis*, respectively. *Uncinaria stenocephala* has also been implicated. CLM is one of the most frequent skin diseases among travelers returning from tropical countries.[130] In the USA, most cases of CLM are contracted in the southeastern states, most notably Florida and Georgia.[131] Worldwide, the disorder is most common in Mexico, Central and South America, Africa, South-east Asia, and the Caribbean.[131,132] The adult hookworms release eggs while in the intestines of their definitive hosts (dogs or cats), and these eggs are passed along with stool onto sandy, warm soil. Humans become incidental hosts when larvae burrow through intact skin that comes into contact with the infested soil. The disorder is quite common in children because of high-risk behaviors (i.e., playing in the sand) seen in this age group. It occurs sporadically or in small epidemics in high-income countries and in tourists who have visited the tropics.[133] The most commonly involved areas are the extremities (especially feet), buttocks, and genitalia. The incubation period for CLM may be prolonged for weeks to months.[134]

In the human host, the hookworm larvae are unable to complete their natural life cycle, and remain confined to the upper levels of skin, wandering aimlessly and producing the characteristic cutaneous findings. Initially, skin findings may be limited to one or a few erythematous papules. Ultimately, serpiginous, raised, sharply demarcated plaques develop (Figs 18.36, 18.37), and may advance up to 1–2 mm/day. Follicular involvement with folliculitis may also occur.[130,135] Vesicular or bullous lesions are rare. Without treatment, the larva eventually die, but this may take several months. The lesions of CLM are extremely pruritic, and may be complicated by pain and secondary bacterial infection. Although systemic dissemination of the parasite does not generally occur, eosinophilia is common and pneumonitis (Löffler syndrome) may occasionally be present.

The differential diagnosis of CLM may include other larval infestations, such as *Strongyloides stercoralis* and *Gnathostoma spinigerum*. Scabies, jellyfish stings, and phytophotodermatitis may also mimic CLM.[132] Treatment options for creeping eruption include liquid nitrogen cryotherapy (which was a traditional mainstay of treatment) and oral antihelminthic agents. Cryotherapy is rarely effective and is traumatic for most young children; hence it should be avoided for this indication. Oral agents demonstrated to be effective include thiabendazole, albendazole, and ivermectin. Thiabendazole is given at a dose of 25 mg/kg per day, divided into two doses, for 2–5 days. Potential side-effects include headache, dizziness, and gastrointestinal upset. Alternatively, topical thiabendazole (500 mg/5 mL) can be applied four times daily, and is often effective. Oral albendazole seems to be one of the most effective and well-tolerated therapies. It is given at a dose of 200–400 mg twice daily for 5–7 days.[136–138] Side-effects are rare with this agent, which has been used in nematode and cestode infestations. Use of these agents in young children has not been well studied. Ivermectin, an agent used primarily for onchocerciasis and other nematodes, has also been anecdotally reported as effective in open-label studies.[130] It is given as a single dose (200 µg/kg), and repeated in 1–2 weeks if necessary.

Cercarial Dermatitis (Swimmer's Itch)

Cercarial dermatitis (swimmer's itch) is an itchy, inflammatory dermatosis that results from penetration of human skin by non-human schistosome parasites. It occurs after swimming or wading in freshwater lakes, especially in the mid-western USA, and has more recently been demonstrated in the south-western USA.[139] The most clinically relevant organisms are the *Trichobilharzia* spp. The adult schistosomes reside in the mesenteric blood vessels of birds and mammals, and following passage from the blood to the intestine, eggs are deposited in water along with the host feces. Subsequently, miracidiae hatch and penetrate the intermediate host, usually snails.[140] Within the snail, they develop into cercariae, which leave the snails and reside in the upper levels of lakes until they can again infest the definitive host. However, they may also infest accidental hosts such as humans.

Swimmer's itch occurs on exposed areas of skin, which are the sites most readily available to the cercariae. Since humans are not

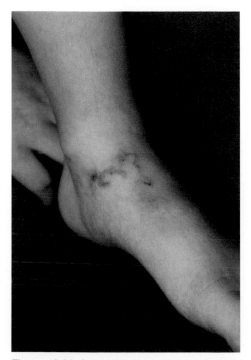

Figure 18.36 Cutaneous larva migrans. A serpiginous, migratory plaque on the dorsal foot.

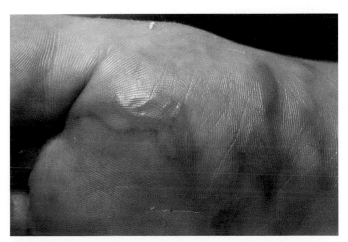

Figure 18.37 Cutaneous larva migrans. The plantar surface of this young boy revealed a very itchy, linear plaque that was noted to continuously extend over the several days prior to diagnosis.

the definitive host, the cercariae die within hours following skin penetration, and the host immune response results in the clinical eruption.[141] Often, the initial infestation does not result in a reaction but causes sensitization, which results in the clinical eruption following subsequent exposures.[140] Examination of the skin usually reveals nonspecific, erythematous papules and papulovesicles (Figs 18.38, 18.39). Excoriation may be present, and secondary bacterial superinfection is an occasional complication. Post-inflammatory hyperpigmentation is common.

The distribution of the lesions, combined with the history of exposure to a freshwater lake, will combine to suggest the diagnosis of swimmer's itch. Activities that involve more extensive contact with lake water (i.e., wading, working on the dock, and swimming)

are more likely to be associated with the disorder than other activities like boating, skiing, and tubing.[141] Aquariums containing snails may also be a source of swimmer's itch.[140,142] Water analysis via filtration and PCR detection may be useful if confirmation is required, and snails cannot be found.[143] Treatment is supportive, and consists of topical corticosteroids, topical antipruritic agents, oral antihistamines, and, rarely, systemic corticosteroids for severe cases.

Seabather's eruption

Seabather's eruption, also known as 'sea lice', is not a true parasitic infestation but is commonly confused with cercarial dermatitis, and is therefore included in this section. It results from a hypersensitivity reaction to the stinging nematocyst of a cnidarian larva, which includes jellyfish, Portuguese man-of-war, sea anemone, or fire coral (see below).[144] Most often, it has been associated with exposure to the larval form of the thimble-sized jellyfish, *Linuche unguiculata*.[144,145] Seabather's eruption occurs most commonly in marine saltwaters off of Florida, in the Gulf of Mexico, and in the Caribbean. (A discussion of traditional jellyfish stings can be found in the following section.)

The skin lesions of seabather's eruption, which tend to be limited to areas covered by the swimming garment, include erythematous papules, pustules, and papulovesicles (Figs 18.40, 18.41). Urticarial plaques may also be present, and pruritus is usually severe. Other symptoms may include fatigue, fever, chills, headache, and nausea. Many patients recall having seen 'thimble sized' jellyfish in the waters, or tiny 'black dots' along the water surface.[144] Symptoms may begin while in the water or when exiting, although in the majority of patients they begin several hours later. Longer swim times appear to increase the risk of seabather's eruption; in one report of 38 patients, the median duration of water exposure was 2.5 h (range 1–8 h).[146] Since freshwater is known to stimulate nematocyst discharge of toxins, removal of the bathing garment is recommended before rinsing, especially in areas where seabather's eruption warnings are posted.

The diagnosis of seabather's eruption is primarily a clinical one. It should be suspected in the patient presenting with an itchy, papulovesicular eruption limited to covered areas of skin, and occurring after exposure to saltwater. Skin biopsy[144] and serologic assays[144,147] have been used, but are generally unnecessary. Treatment is symptomatic, as discussed earlier for swimmer's itch.

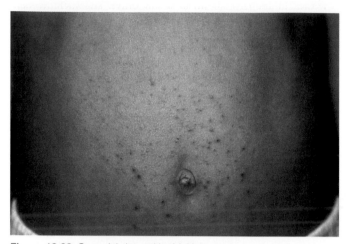

Figure 18.38 Cercarial dermatitis. Multiple pruritic, excoriated papules and papulovesicles on exposed surfaces of the skin. The patient had been swimming in a freshwater lake along with family members, several of whom developed similar lesions.

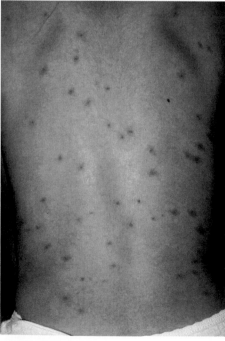

Figure 18.39 Cercarial dermatitis. Itchy, excoriated papules and papulovesicles, occurring on exposed areas of skin.

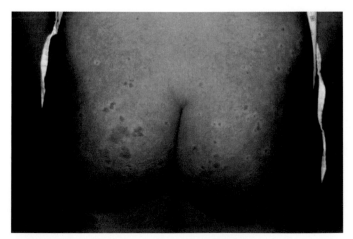

Figure 18.40 Seabather's eruption. These edematous, erythematous papules were limited to sites covered by the swimming garment.

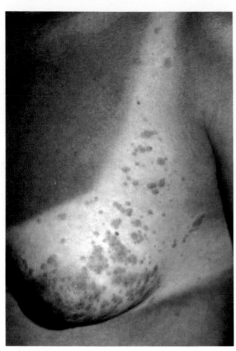

Figure 18.41 Seabather's eruption. Erythematous papules and papulovesicles limited to sites covered by the swimming garment, following a vacation in the Caribbean.

Jellyfish stings

Cnidarians (Phylum Cnidaria) are a group of aquatic animals which includes jellyfish, corals, sea anemones, and hydras. The cnidarian body consists of a gastrovascular cavity with a single opening, through which food is ingested and waste is released. Cnidarians have tentacles encircling their mouth, and bodies that are radially symmetrical. The Phylum Cnidaria consists of four classes: Hydrozoa (Portuguese man-of-war), Scyphozoa (true jellyfish), Cubozoa (box jellyfish or sea wasps), and Anthozoa (sea anemones and corals).

Jellyfish are marine invertebrates which are found both in the ocean and in fresh water. They are responsible for the most common ocean-related envenomations acquired by humans, and which may result in three types of responses, including immediate allergic, immediate toxic, and delayed allergic reactions.[148] The surface of jellyfish bodies and tentacles is covered in specialized cells called cnidoblasts, which contain in their cytoplasm a nematocyst, which is a capsule filled with a toxic fluid that is injected into human skin at the time of contact.[149] Cutaneous reactions to jellyfish stings may include urticarial wheals, burning, pruritus and tenderness. Papules and papulovesicles often occur, in linear and wispy patterns, and more chronic post-inflammatory pigmentary changes, scarring (including keloids) and lichenification may occur. Occasionally observed findings include thrombophlebitis, tender regional lymphadenopathy, angioedema, papular urticaria and distant hypersensitivity-type skin reactions (i.e., an id reaction). Fatal anaphylactic reactions are rare, but when they occur, are more common in children.[150] A persistent lichen planus-like eruption has been reported following jellyfish sting.[148] *Seabather's eruption* refers to a papulovesicular eruption occurring in covered areas of skin, in response to contact with nematocysts from thimble-sized jellyfish larvae (see above).

Treatment for jellyfish stings is supportive, and includes pain control, compression, application of vinegar (thought to help in deactivation of the nematocysts), avoidance of fresh water exposure (which may trigger firing of nematocysts), oral antihistamines, and manual removal of tentacles, when visible. Medical attention should be sought. Cardiopulmonary resuscitation and use of an epinephrine pen (when available) may be necessary if anaphylaxis occurs. Useful preventive measures include wearing protective swim- or diving-wear, and avoidance of areas known to be infested with jellyfish.

Key References

The complete list of 150 references for this chapter is available online at: **www.expertconsult.com.**
See inside cover for registration details.

Diamantis SA, Morrell DS, Burkhart CN. Treatment of head lice. *Dermatol Ther.* 2009;22(4):273–278.

Goddard J, deShazo R. Bed bugs (Cimex lectularius) and clinical consequences of their bites. *J Am Med Assoc.* 2009;301(13):1358–1366.

Hicks MI, Elston DM. Scabies. *Dermatol Ther.* 2009;22:279–292.

Katz TM, Miller JH, Hebert AA. Insect repellents: Historical perspectives and new developments. *J Am Acad Dermatol.* 2008;58:865–871.

McClain D, Dana AN, Goldenberg G. Mite infestations. *Dermatol Ther.* 2009;22:327–346.

Suchard JR. 'Spider bite' lesions are usually diagnosed as skin and soft-tissue infections. *J Emerg Med.* 2009; Nov 23 (Epub ahead of print).

Swanson DL, Vetter RS. Loxoscelism. *Clin Dermatol.* 2006;24:213–221.

Photosensitivity and Photoreactions

Reactions to the sun's rays have become increasingly common in recent years, owing not only to the ever-expanding number of photosensitizers in the environment, but also to much of the public's obsession with sunbathing. Sunlight emits a wide spectrum of radiation energy, extending from radiowaves through infrared, visible, and ultraviolet (UV) light, to X-rays. The wavelength range of visible light is 400–800 nm and is relatively harmless, except for individuals with photosensitivity disorders, such as porphyria, solar urticaria and polymorphous light eruption. The infrared range is 800–1800 nm. It is the UVA and UVB wavelengths (290–400 nm) that cause most cutaneous reactions. Wavelengths <220 nm are absorbed by atmospheric gases, including oxygen and nitrogen, and those <290 nm are absorbed by the atmospheric ozone layer. The remaining middle-wavelength (UVB, 290–320 nm) and long-wavelength (UVA1, 340–400 nm; UVA2, 320–340 nm) UV radiation can reach Earth and be absorbed by biological molecules, thereby damaging them. The skin is quite effective at protection from UV penetration, but the depth of penetration depends upon the wavelength. UVA easily reaches the deeper dermis, whereas UVB is absorbed in the epidermis and little reaches the upper dermis.

UV light also reaches the skin through reflection from snow (80–85%); sand (17–25%); water (5%, but up to 100% when the sun is directly overhead); sidewalks, and turf. UV exposure also increases by 4% for every 1000 foot elevation above sea level. It must be remembered that on a bright, cloudy day with thin cloud cover, it is possible to receive 60–85% of the amount of UV radiation present on a bright clear day. Hats and parasols provide only a moderate degree of protection, and surfaces with reflectivity greatly increase sunlight exposure.

Tanning and sunburn reactions

The visible short-term effects of UV exposure are sunburn (Figs. 19.1, 26.14) and tanning. The ability to cause sunburn markedly declines with increasing wavelength. UVA light at 360 nm is 1000-fold less effective in causing skin erythema (sunburn) than UVA light at 300 nm. Thus, UVB light is largely responsible for sunburn, with peak induction 6–24 h after exposure. Sunburns gradually fade during the next 3–5 days, as the skin starts to desquamate. Reactivity to UVB light may range in severity from a mild asymptomatic erythema to a more intense reaction, with redness accompanied by tenderness, pain, edema, and, at times, vesiculation and bulla formation, particularly the day after the sunburn first appears. If the sunburned area is extensive, constitutional symptoms may include nausea, malaise, headache, fever, chills, and even delirium. Sunburn during childhood correlates with a higher risk of developing melanocytic nevi,[1] as well as UV-induced skin cancers.

Tanning is also wavelength-dependent and is biphasic. Immediate pigment darkening results primarily from exposure to UVA light, is caused by alteration and redistribution of melanin, and fades in 6–8 h. Delayed tanning usually results from exposure to UVB and

peaks at about 3 days after exposure. Fair skin (type II, Table 19.1) is only able to tan with UVB dosages about the erythema threshold (i.e., a sunburn is required), whereas darker skin types (i.e., type III and higher) can tan significantly without burning (at suberythemogenic doses). Sunburn causes apoptosis (cell death) of keratinocytes ('sunburn cells') or, if the dosage is high enough, induces cell cycle arrest, allowing the cell to undergo repair of their DNA template before proliferating. Sunburn also depletes the protective Langerhans cells, causes epidermal thickening (which reduces exposure of the basal keratinocytes to UV radiation) as a protective mechanism, stimulates release of inflammatory cytokines, and induces the formation of antioxidative enzymes (which reduce oxidative DNA damage). The tan induced by UVB involves increased melanin synthesis, increased numbers of melanocytes, and increased transfer of melanosomes to keratinocytes.

The long-term effects of chronic sun exposure include photoaging, photocarcinogenesis, and immunosuppression. Given its potential to penetrate more deeply into the dermis, UVA light is thought to play a particularly important role in photoaging. UVA, but not UVB, is able to penetrate through window glass. Thus, individuals who sit in offices exposed to UVA through windows or drive cars extensively, can show significant asymmetry in UVA damage on the face. UVA light is also the light used in indoor tanning, a practice prevalent particularly among older female adolescents.[2–4] This practice promotes skin damage, leading to an increased risk of skin cancer and photodamage, but no increased protection against sun exposure.[5] The danger of using tanning facilities has led to legislation to control use by minors and limitations of exposure in several states. In addition, many facilities now offer 'safe' tanning, in which an artificial tan is produced by dihydroxyacetone (DHA). DHA is a sugar that interacts with the stratum corneum proteins to produce a brown pigment called melanoidins.[6] The brown color resists washing, but provides minimal and transient sun protection.

Prevention of sunburn depends primarily on the utilization of measures that reduce exposure to strong sunlight. This is especially important for fair-skinned individuals, particularly blue-eyed persons, redheads, blonds, and those with freckles who withstand actinic exposure poorly, burn easily, and, over the years, tend to suffer chronic effects of light exposure. Prophylactic measures to reduce the impact of harmful UV rays include timing of outdoor activities to avoid peak UV light exposure between 10 a.m. and 3 p.m. in the warmer seasons of the year; wearing broad-rimmed hats, sun protective clothing, and sunglasses; and staying in the shade. Light-textured materials such as T-shirts (especially when wet) give only partial protection. Clothes with a tighter weave are commercially available (e.g., www.sunprecautions.com; www.collibar.com; www.solumbra.com), or clothes can be laundered with a chemical that provides sun protection (SunGuard).

Sunscreens occupy an important position in the management of UV light exposure.[7–10] The lifetime use of sunscreen and sun-avoidance has been calculated to reduce the lifetime risk of

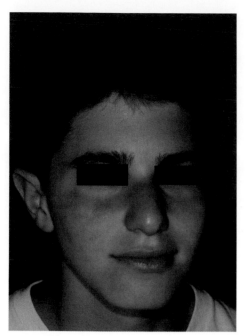

Figure 19.1 Sunburn. This adolescent became more sensitive to ultraviolet light exposure while taking isotretinoin.

Table 19.2 Common sunscreen filters and UV protection

Sunscreen filter	Wavelength protection
Organic sunscreens	
PABA group	UVB
Padimate O	
Salicylate	UVB
Octisalate	
Homosalate	
Cinnamate	UVB
Octinoxate	
Benzophenone	UVB, some UVA
Oxybenzophenone	
Avobenzone (Parsol 1789)	UVA
Bis-ethylhexyloxyphenol methoxyphenol triazine	UVA and UVB
Drometrizole trisiloxane	UVA and UVB
Methylene-bis-benzotriazolyl tetramethylbutylphenol	UVA and UVB
Terephthalylidene dicamphor sulfonic acid	UVA and UVB
Inorganic sunscreens	
Titanium dioxide	UVA and UVB
Zinc oxide	UVA and UVB

Table 19.1 Skin types and photosensitivity

Skin type	Reactivity to sun	Examples
I	Very sensitive: always burn easily and severely, tan little or not at all	Individuals with fair skin; blond or red hair, blue or brown eyes, and freckles
II	Very sensitive: usually burn easily, tan minimally or lightly	Individuals with fair skin; red, blond, or brown hair; and blue, hazel, or brown eyes
III	Moderately sensitive: burn moderately, tan gradually and uniformly	Average white individuals
IV	Moderately sensitive: burn minimally, tan easily	Individuals with dark brown hair, dark eyes, and white or light brown skin
V	Minimally sensitive: rarely burn, tan well and easily	Brown-skinned (Middle Eastern and Hispanic) individuals
VI	Deeply pigmented: almost never burn, tan profusely	Blacks and others with heavy pigmentation

developing UV-induced skin cancer by 78%.[11] The most common misconception (particularly among teenagers) is the belief that certain sunscreens can induce or promote a suntan. Sunscreens are topical preparations designed to protect the skin from the effects of UV light. The most common sunscreen components and their absorbance capacity are listed in Table 19.2. These inorganic sunscreens (titanium dioxide and zinc oxide) protect skin by reflecting and scattering UV and visible light (290–700 nm). These so-called 'inorganic' sunscreens frequently contain one or both of these agents. Organic sunscreens absorb light at particular wavelengths into specific chemical UV filters, and re-emit the energy as insignificant quantities of heat. Newer organic sunscreen components now absorb in both the UVA and UVB spectrum, thus providing protection against the damaging effects of the broad spectrum of UV light. These newer sunscreens are photostable (in contrast to avobenzone), and include bis-ethylhexyloxyphenol methoxyphenol triazine (anisotriazine, Tinosorb S), drometrizole trisiloxane (sila-triazole or Mexoryl XL), methylene-bis-benzotriazolyl tetramethyl-butylphenol (Tinosorb M), and terephthalylidene dicamphor sulfonic acid (Mexoryl SX). Ideally, organic sunscreens should be applied 20–30 min before the onset of sun exposure, so that there is adequate time to bind to the stratum corneum and show effectiveness; the inorganic sunscreens can be applied immediately before sun exposure. Sunscreens should be reapplied after swimming, periods of excessive perspiration, frequent washing, or showering. Oral sunscreens containing antioxidants (e.g., lycopene, vitamins C and E) and botanicals (e.g., polyphenols, such as green tea and flavonoids, such as genistein) are now commercially available. They provide some protection against acute sun damage, but they are not as effective as topical sunscreens in preventing sunburns,[8] their long-term protective effects are not clear, and they should not replace other forms of photoprotection for children.

Traditionally, protection against UVB light has been rated based on the sun protective factor (SPF). The SPF rating can be determined by dividing the least amount of time it takes to produce erythema on sunscreen-protected skin by the time it takes to produce the same erythema without sunscreen protection. Thus, individuals using a sunscreen with an SPF of 15 who normally burn following unprotected sun exposure, can theoretically stay out 15 times longer before getting the same degree of erythema. It should be recognized, however, that this SPF rating is only a reflection of protection against sunburn from UVB light and does not measure protection from the non-erythema effects, especially from UVA light, including immune suppression, photoaging, and skin cancer.

Thus, sunscreens that protect against exposure to UVA light should be chosen in addition to the SPF rating of the sunscreen. A new 4-star grading system has been proposed by the FDA to rate UVA-based on *in vitro* and *in vivo* testing.

In order to be effective, adequate amounts of sunscreen must be applied to all UV-exposed areas and the sunscreen must be reapplied every few hours. It is critical that individuals continue sensible sun protection by means other than sunscreens and not increase their exposure because of sunscreen availability.

The degree to which a person sunburns or tans depends on genetic factors and the natural protection of the skin. Skin types, accordingly, are ranked from skin type I, the most sensitive, to skin type VI, the least sensitive to sun damage (Table 19.1). Since sun damage begins in children and is cumulative, it is strongly recommended that everyone adopt a program of sun protection and daily sunscreen use, preferably with an SPF of 15 or greater, from infancy on. Individuals with extreme photosensitivity should use sunscreens with levels of SPF 30 or higher. For black-skinned individuals, who already have protective melanin levels, sunscreens with an SPF of 6 or 8 may be adequate, but black skin can burn as well, and the increased melanin is not totally protective.

Considerable media attention has focused on the need for UV-induced vitamin D synthesis in the skin as a rationale for sun exposure. In fact, UV exposure that stimulates vitamin D_3 production in the skin is inseparable from UV exposure that is carcinogenic. Although sunscreens do markedly reduce the capacity of skin to produce vitamin D (and greater vitamin D deficiency has been linked to darker skin color), sunscreen use has not been linked with deficiency, and oral administration of vitamin D likely suffices. The American Academy of Pediatrics has recently recommended increasing the minimum daily intake of vitamin D for infants, children and adolescents to 400 IU/day, beginning shortly after birth.[12] Patients who require strict photoprotection as treatment should be monitored for possible vitamin D deficiency and provided dietary supplementation.[13]

Treatment of sunburn consists of cool compresses or cool tub baths in colloidal oatmeal (such as Aveeno), baking soda, or cornstarch; topical formulations with pramoxine or menthol; mild topical corticosteroid formulations; an emollient cream; and systemic preparations with analgesic and antiinflammatory properties, such as NSAIDs. When symptoms are severe, a short course of systemic corticosteroids (oral prednisone, or its equivalent, in dosages of 1 mg/kg per day, with tapering after a period of 4–8 days) will abort severe reactions and afford added relief.

Certain disorders predispose individuals to the adverse effects of ultraviolet light. For example, children with alopecia totalis (see Ch. 7), just as adults with androgenetic alopecia and balding at the vertex, have a higher risk of developing skin cancer at the exposed site if not protected. Patients with diminished or absent melanin, as in oculocutaneous albinism (see Ch. 11), or with defective DNA repair mechanisms, as in xeroderma pigmentosum (see below) have an increased tendency to develop UV-induced DNA damage and cutaneous malignancy. Individuals with nevoid basal cell carcinoma syndrome (see Ch. 9), which predisposes to the early onset of numerous basal cell carcinomas, have mutations in the *PTCH* gene, a gene that can also be mutated by UV light exposure in sporadic basal cell carcinomas. Sunlight can also exacerbate or trigger certain dermatoses, among them acne, herpes simplex infection, lupus, dermatomyositis, Darier disease, pemphigus, and bullous pemphigoid.

Photodermatoses

Photosensitivity is a broad term used to describe abnormal or adverse reactions to sunlight energy in the skin.[14-18] Photodermatoses must be distinguished from reactions to sunlight from exaggerated exposure, which is a normal response. Photosensitivity in a child should be suspected if the child develops a sunburn reaction, swelling, or intense pruritus after limited exposure to sunlight or shows a rash or scarring predominantly in sun-exposed areas (face, V of the neck, and dorsal surface of the arms and hands). The history in a patient with a photosensitivity disorder is of great importance in determining the cause (Table 19.3). Examination should focus on the distribution of lesions, including the areas of sparing. In a photosensitivity disorder, the upper eyelids, postauricular and submental areas, area under the chin, nasolabial and neck folds, volar aspect of the wrist, and the antecubital fossae generally tend to be spared. The morphology of the lesions may be helpful as well (urticarial versus papular versus vesicular, and the presence of lichenification, which suggests chronicity).

Phototesting can be helpful in determining the cause of an acquired photodermatosis. Exposure to UV light of different wavelengths may replicate the lesion, offer the opportunity to see morphology if not present at the time of the examination, confirm the suspicion of photosensitivity, and determine the UV range that triggers the disorder.[19] Further laboratory investigations, such as antibody testing for suspected collagen vascular disease (such as ANA, anti-ds DNA, anti-Ro, and anti-La antibodies), blood and 24-h urine porphyrin levels, and photopatch testing in patients with suspected photoallergy, may be necessary. Performing a biopsy is rarely useful, except for suspected lupus erythematosus.

Idiopathic Photodermatoses

Solar urticaria

Solar urticaria is a relatively uncommon type I IgE-mediated type of sensitivity characterized by a sensation of pruritus or burning and erythema.[20,21] Typically affected areas are the arms, legs, and upper chest; areas with regular sun exposure, such as the hands and face, are less commonly involved. It appears either during or within 30 min of sunlight exposure and is followed almost immediately by a localized urticarial reaction confined to the exposed areas and

Table 19.3 Evaluation for potential photosensitivity disorders	
History	Age of onset; exposure to potential photosensitizers; season of the eruption; time of onset after exposure to the sun; duration of eruption; effect of window glass and exposure to other light sources, including tanning booths; history of atopy and other medical problems; response to medications and use of sunscreens; family history
Examination	Distribution and morphology
Phototesting	Action spectrum, time to onset, minimal urticarial dose, inhibition and augmentation spectra
Photopatch testing	If photoallergy is suspected
Laboratory	Complete blood count, metabolic panel, erythrocyte sedimentation rate, autoantibodies, esp. antinuclear antibody, porphyrins
Biopsy	Useful for lupus and possibly porphyrias, but not for other photodermatoses. Fibroblast cultures for XP testing

XP, xeroderma pigmentosum.

an irregular flare reaction that extends onto unexposed skin. After several hours, the involved skin returns to its normal appearance and new lesions will not develop for 12–24 h, even if subsequent exposure to sunlight occurs. *Fixed solar urticaria*, characterized by recurrent eruptions on the same body parts, is rare and less severe than typical solar urticaria.[22] Delayed fixed solar urticaria, occurring 6 h after exposure, has been described.[23] Although the reaction is generally transient, scratching and rubbing may lead to secondary eczematization with persistent cutaneous changes. The disorder usually does not manifest until the 3rd or 4th decade of life, and females are affected three times more often than males. It has been reported, however, as early as 1 week of age.[24] The condition persists for more than a decade in the majority of affected individuals and often for a lifetime. Systemic signs have occasionally been reported in association, including headache, nausea, wheezing, dizziness, syncope and rarely shock.

The cause of solar urticaria is unclear. Often phototesting can confirm the diagnosis and determine the wavelength range that causes the photosensitivity. If positive, whealing generally occurs within minutes. In some patients, the sensitivity involves the UVB range through the visible light range; the majority of patients react within the range of 290–480 nm. A negative phototest occurs in many patients, and does not exclude the diagnosis. In patients with mild forms of solar urticaria (those in whom the threshold is high), the disorder may be controlled simply by appropriate sunscreens and avoidance of prolonged unprotected sun exposure. Those individuals highly sensitive to sunlight, however, must completely avoid daytime exposure. Non-sedating antihistamines,[25] antimalarials, corticosteroids, intravenous immunoglobulin[26] and plasmapheresis have been beneficial. In some individuals, sun tolerance may be established by carefully metered exposures to natural or artificial light or the oral administration of a psoralen followed by UVA (PUVA).

Polymorphous light eruption

Polymorphous light eruption (PMLE) is the most common of the idiopathic disorders associated with photosensitivity.[27–29] It is predominantly a disorder of females in the second and third decades of life, and is estimated to occur in 10–15% of the US population. It occurs more often in individuals with lighter skin types. Although its etiology remains unknown, PMLE has been hypothesized to involve a failure of normal UV-induced immunosuppression.[30] An autosomal dominantly inherited form of polymorphic light eruption has been described in Native Americans of both North and South America.[31] Onset of this hereditary form is in childhood, and female patients outnumber male patients 2:1.

Often referred to as 'sun allergy' or 'sun poisoning', the clinical eruption consists of a group of pleomorphic or polymorphic lesions that usually occur 1–2 days after intense sunlight exposure, often while on vacation. In some individuals, the eruption is first seen in the spring and persists with continued sun exposure, but may improve later in the summer as the skin 'hardens' from UV light exposure. The lesions may range from small papular (Fig. 19.2), urticarial (Fig. 19.3), vesicular, or eczematous reactions to large papules, plaques, or patterns resembling erythema multiforme. A 'pinpoint' variant that resembles lichen nitidus clinically and histologically occurs more often in individuals with darker skin colors.[32,33] The areas of the body most commonly involved include the face, the sides of the neck, and sun-exposed areas of the arms and hands. In children, it most commonly begins on the face as an acute, erythematous, eczematous eruption with small papules. Pruritus may be severe. Lesions usually involute spontaneously in 1–2 weeks, provided no additional exposure to sunlight occurs.

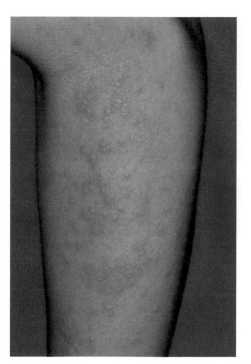

Figure 19.2 Polymorphous light eruption. Papular lesions occurred 2 days after intense sun exposure.

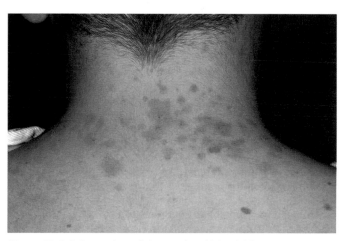

Figure 19.3 Polymorphous light eruption. Urticarial form.

Juvenile spring eruption is considered a subset of PMLE, and is characterized by photo-induced dull-red edematous papules that are largely confined to the helix of the ears (Fig. 19.4). Lesions may become vesicular and crusted, and occasionally appear on the dorsal aspects of the hands and on the trunk. Juvenile spring eruption occurs more commonly in boys than in girls, and particularly between the ages of 5 and 12 years. Protuberant ears and lack of hair cover have been strongly associated,[34] but skin color and use of sunscreen have not. Lesions heal within a week, without scarring, unless secondary infection develops. Lesions are more difficult than PMLE to reproduce by exposure to ultraviolet light.[35]

The diagnosis of polymorphous light eruption is suggested by the character of the lesions, their distribution, and their relationship to sun exposure. The diagnosis can be confirmed by phototesting, which leads to a reaction that, in contrast to that of solar urticaria, occurs within hours rather than minutes, lasts for days rather than hours, and is not urticarial. Some patients with SLE

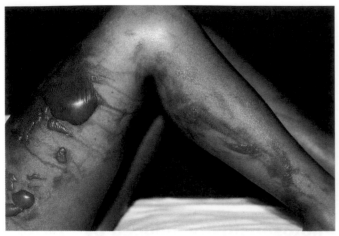

Figure 19.8 Phytophotodermatitis. Severe blistering associated with linear patterns of erythema and hyperpigmentation in a girl who had rinsed her hair with lime juice, then had intense sun exposure.

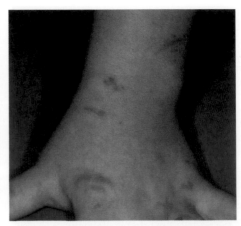

Figure 19.10 Phytophotodermatitis. This child had been playing outside and was exposed to photosensitizing plants.

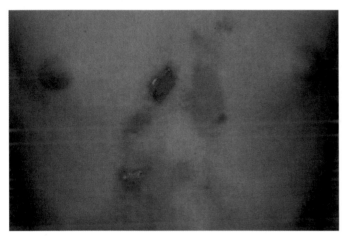

Figure 19.9 Phytophotodermatitis. Linear streaks of erythema and erosions on the trunk.

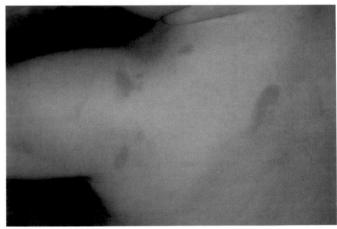

Figure 19.11 Phytophotodermatitis. Intense hyperpigmentation in geometric patterns on the back of young girl whose mother had been squeezing citrus fruit before picking her up on a vacation to the Caribbean.

At times, only the hyperpigmented streak appears without prior erythema (Fig. 19.11). The purple coloration of skin and bizarre patterning can be mistaken for child abuse and the blistering for herpes simplex infection.[69–71] Streaks on the trunk have been noted after dripping of lime juice (sometimes used as a hair rinse or in drinks) and thumbprint-shaped macules on the lateral aspects of the trunk may be described after a parent with furocoumarins on the fingers picks up a child. No treatment is necessary, once the diagnosis is made. The often-intense hyperpigmentation fades spontaneously during a period of weeks to months.

Systemic photosensitizers that may cause phototoxicity include systemic antibacterial agents (predominantly doxycycline; Fig. 19.12) and rarely other tetracyclines, sulfonamides, nalidixic acid, and fluoroquinolones;[72] antifungal preparations (griseofulvin and voriconazole);[73] phenothiazine derivatives, particularly chlorpromazine; sulfonylurea hypoglycemic agents; anovulatory drugs; lamotrigine; antihistamines (particularly the phenothiazine congeners); furosemide; non-steroidal anti-inflammatory preparations (see Pseudoporphyria, below); the antiarrhythmic drug amiodarone; quinine; isoniazid; thiazide diuretics; and certain dyes (acridine, methylviolet, and eosin).[74,75] Photo-onycholysis most

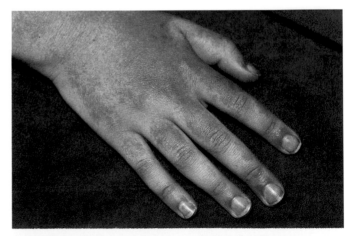

Figure 19.12 Photosensitivity from medication. Severe sunburn reaction despite sunscreen application in a teenager taking doxycycline for acne.

commonly occurs after administration of doxycycline[76] (see Ch. 8, Fig. 8.16). The phototoxicity from voriconazole, used to prevent fungal infections in transplant patients, can be confused with graft-versus-host disease.[73]

Photoallergy

Photoallergy is relatively uncommon and presumably is a form of cell-mediated delayed hypersensitivity.[77,78] The individual must first be sensitized to the allergen, which can require 7–10 days. When exposed to UV light, the light is absorbed by the photoantigen, which is thought to cause a change in the molecule. Instead of sunburn-type reactions, photoallergic responses are generally characterized by immediate urticarial or delayed papular or eczematoid lesions that are not followed by hyperpigmentation. After the first sensitization, subsequent photoallergic reactions generally appear within 24 h, even after very brief periods of exposure. Sunscreens with chemical components (especially benzophenones) are the leading cause because of their extensive use, although the risk of reaction with sunscreens containing these agents is <1% of allergic contact dermatitis.[79,80] In the past, children showed photoallergic reactions to salicylanilides (antimicrobial agents formerly in soaps but now only in industrial cleaners) and fragrances (musk ambrette, oil of Bergamot). These chemicals are no longer used in personal products. However, children or adolescents have been known to find a cologne with oil of Bergamot, apply it to the skin, and develop *Berloque* (*berlock*) *dermatitis* after UV exposure.[81] The reaction manifests as hyperpigmentation that might resemble a drop or a pendant, hence the name *berloque* (misspelled from the French word *breloque*) or *Berlock* (German), meaning trinket or pendant. This dermatitis is seen most frequently on the sides of the neck and in the retroauricular areas, shoulders, upper trunk, hands, or face. Promethazine hydrochloride cream and topical non-steroidal anti-inflammatory agents have caused photoreactions.

Suspected photoallergic contact dermatitis may be confirmed by photopatch testing. Photopatch testing is similar to traditional testing for contact dermatitis (see Ch. 3), except that two sets of patch tests are placed on the back. Twenty-four hours later, one set is uncovered and irradiated with UVA light. The following day a comparison is made of the covered and irradiated sites. A positive test reproduces the clinical eczematous lesion at the phototest site.

Therapy is treatment with topical antiinflammatory agents and avoidance of exposure to the offending antigen.

Genetic disorders associated with photosensitivity

Photosensitivity is a prominent feature of several genetic disorders. Some of these are described elsewhere in this text, such as Kindler syndrome (Ch. 13), trichothiodystrophy (Ch. 7), and ataxia-telangiectasia (Ch. 12).

Xeroderma Pigmentosum

Xeroderma pigmentosum (XP) is a rare autosomal recessive disease characterized by cutaneous photosensitivity, a decreased ability to repair DNA damaged by UV radiation, and the early development of cutaneous and ocular malignancies.[82,83] The disorder is estimated to occur in a frequency of one in a million individuals in the USA and Europe, and with a frequency in Japan as high as one in 40 000 persons. The risk of developing cutaneous malignancy does not diminish in patients with darker skin types.[84] Seven complementation groups (XP-A–XP-G) have been described based on *in vitro* cell fusion studies (Table 19.4).[85,86]

The basic abnormality is an absence of a component of the nucleotide excision repair complex. Complementation groups XP-C and XP-E recognize, and bind to, damaged DNA.[87–89] XP-A may help to assemble the DNA machinery around the damaged DNA site. This binding signals the XP-B and XP-D proteins to unwind the DNA in the damaged region and to allow DNA transcription. The XP-F and XP-G nucleases cut the DNA and allow excision of the UV-induced pyrimidine dimers. DNA repair rates may range from 0 to 50% of normal levels. A variant form has been described (XP-V). In the variant group, post-replication repair is defective, but excision repair is normal.

The cardinal features of this disorder include sensitivity to light, primarily at wavelengths 290–340 nm, premature aging of the skin accompanied by dystrophy, pigmentary changes, and the development of epithelial neoplasms; severe eye involvement; progressive neurologic degeneration in some patients; and malignancy.[90] In 75% of cases the first symptoms appear between 6 months and 3

Table 19.4 Subtypes of xeroderma pigmentosum (XP)

Group	Enzyme	Frequency	Skin disease	Neoplasia	Neurologic change	Comments
XP-A	DDB1	Esp. in Japan	+++	+++	+ to +++	Lowest repair activity
XP-B	ERCC3	Very rare	++ to +++	+++	+++	CS (two kindreds)
						One case of TTD
XP-C	Endonuclease	Most common	++ to +++	++; melanoma	Rare	
XP-D	ERCC2	20% of cases	++	+	Late onset or none	Tremendous variability in phenotype; TTD; XP-CS
XP-E	DDB2	Rare	+	Rare	None or mild	Mild phenotype
XP-F	ERCC4	Fairly rare	++	Few to none	Usually none	
XP-G	Endonuclease	Very rare	+++	Few or none	Cockayne type	CS has been associated
XP-variant	Polymerase eta	30% of cases	++ to +++	Later onset	++ in a few	

CS, Cockayne syndrome; DDB, DNA damage-binding protein; ERCC, excision repair cross-complementing genes; TTD, trichothiodystrophy; XP-CS, xeroderma pigmentosum-Cockayne complex; +, mild; ++, moderate; +++, severe.

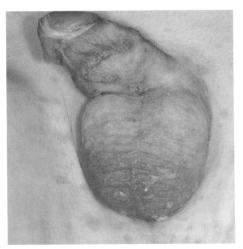

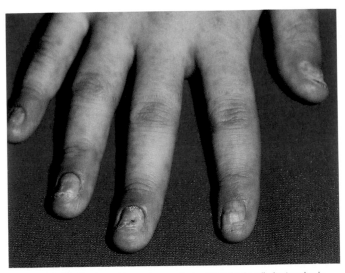

Figure 20.24 Toxic epidermal necrolysis. Note the discrete bullae on the scrotum sloughing of mucosae at the glans. The sloughed skin resembles wrinkled, wet tissue paper.

Figure 20.26 Toxic epidermal necrolysis. Residual nail dystrophy in an adolescent girl who also had widespread postinflammatory hyperpigmentation.

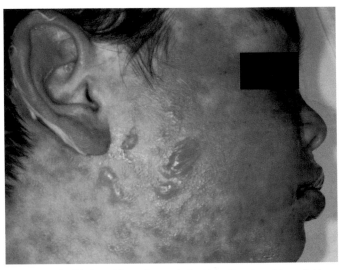

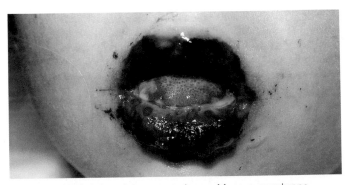

Figure 20.27 Stevens–Johnson syndrome. Mucous membrane involvement with severe swelling and hemorrhagic crusting of the lips.

Figure 20.25 Toxic epidermal necrolysis. Note the sloughing of skin on the ear, which is exacerbated by gentle stroking of the area (positive Nikolsky sign). The mucosal involvement in this boy originally was typical of SJS, but he progressed to the extensive denudement of TEN.

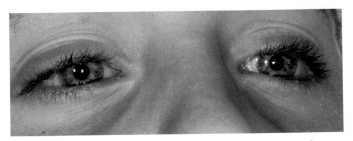

Figure 20.28 Stevens–Johnson syndrome. This boy shows early ophthalmic involvement with conjunctival injection, eyelid edema, erythema and exudative crusting.

typical of TEN). The early macular erythema of TEN may be localized, but more often is an extensive, painful erythroderma. After exerting light mechanical pressure with a finger to an area of erythema, the epidermis in patients with either SJS or TEN becomes wrinkled and peels off like wet tissue paper (Fig. 20.25), the characteristic *Nikolsky sign*. The Nikolsky sign may be seen in patients without clinical evidence of epidermal detachment, and can be a useful diagnostic tool. In addition to SJS and TEN, however, the Nikolsky sign may be seen in a variety of other bullous disorders (especially pemphigus, epidermolysis bullosa (see Ch. 13) and the staphylococcal scalded skin syndrome (SSSS; see Ch. 14)). Histopathologic examination of affected skin demonstrates necrosis of the lower epidermal cells with a sparse mononuclear cell infiltrate and, in the case of TEN, extensive necrosis with a subepidermal split. The epidermal necrosis correlates with the dusky blue coloration of lesions.

Cutaneous dyschromia is the most common sequela and may persist for years. Persistent nail dystrophy or anonychia is also frequently reported (Fig. 20.26), but cutaneous scarring is rare unless the patient develops secondary infection.[113]

The mucosal manifestations of SJS tend to occur 1–2 days before cutaneous manifestations. In SJS (and less prominently in TEN) the mucous membranes of the lips, tongue, buccal mucosae, eyes, nose, genitalia, and rectum may show extensive bullae with grayish white membranes, characteristic hemorrhagic crusts, and painful superficial erosions and ulcerations (Figs 20.27, 20.28). Uncommonly, the esophageal and respiratory epithelial mucosae are affected. By definition, two or more mucosal surfaces are involved. The oral mucosa is always affected, resulting in inability to drink or eat and leading to a risk of dehydration. Genital area lesions lead to painful micturition and defecation. Although lesions of the oral mucosae tend to heal without scarring, strictures or stenosis of esophageal, vaginal, urethral, and anal mucosae have been described as sequelae.

Severe purulent conjunctivitis with photophobia is the typical ocular manifestation (Fig. 20.28). Corneal ulcerations, keratitis, uveitis, and panophthalmitis may also occur. Sequelae occur in 40% of patients[114] and may be grave, with a possibility of keratoconjunctivitis sicca, corneal ulceration or neovascularization, trichiasis, symblepharon, and partial or even complete blindness.[113] The severity of the acute ophthalmologic manifestations does not correlate with long-term complications. Pulmonary involvement may occur as an extension from the oropharynx and tracheobronchial tree or may be due to pneumonitis associated with an initiating viral infection or secondary infection. In extreme cases, renal involvement with hematuria, nephritis, and, in some cases, progressive renal failure may result. Esophageal or tracheal ulceration, pyoderma, lymphadenopathy, hepatosplenomegaly with elevated transaminase levels, myocarditis, arthritis and arthralgias, and/or septicemia may also complicate the disorder (Table 20.5).

SJS is most often confused with Kawasaki disease. However, the conjunctivitis of Kawasaki disease lacks exudation, and the mucosal erythema and dryness is not associated with hemorrhagic crust and mucosal denudation[115] (see Ch. 21). The targetoid cutaneous lesions of SJS may resemble the target lesions of erythema multiforme (see Erythema multiforme, below), a disorder usually attributed to herpes simplex infection in children; erythema multiforme may also show blistering of the lip and oral mucosae that resembles SJS, although the blisters of erythema multiforme are usually fewer and less symptomatic.[116,117] The cutaneous lesions of erythema multiforme are more often found on the extremities and/or face, whereas the atypical target or purpuric lesions of SJS are more commonly located on the trunk.[117] Children with the rare immunobullous disorder, paraneoplastic pemphigus, may exhibit the mucocutaneous manifestations of SJS/TEN; the presence of epidermal acantholysis in biopsy specimens and the demonstration of antibody deposition in indirect immunofluorescence testing or immunoblot evaluation of serum allows paraneoplastic pemphigus to be distinguished (see Ch. 13). Other immunobullous disorders may also be confused with TEN (see Ch. 13). TEN and SSSS are usually easily distinguished; the blisters of TEN lead to denudement, whereas the desquamation of SSSS is superficial and associated with periorificial rather than true mucosal crusting. TEN can be distinguished from severe acute graft-versus-host disease by the history, other clinical findings, and the histologic findings.

Although mild cases of SJS may show significant improvement within 5–15 days, the course of SJS or TEN is often protracted, and may last more than a month. Epidermal detachment may be extensive, leading to massive fluid loss, similar to that of a patient with burns. Bacterial superinfection with sepsis, impairment of temperature regulation, severe dehydration, electrolyte imbalance, excessive energy expenditure, and alteration in immunologic function are the usual complications. End-organ failure can be severe, despite adequate supportive therapy. In adults, the mortality rate of SJS is 5%, transitional SJS-TEN 10–15%, and TEN 30–35%. Rates in children have been lower. A composite score (SCORTEN) has been used in adults to predict mortality,[118] but has not been evaluated in pediatric patients.

Drugs are the most frequent cause of TEN in children (Table 20.6), although Stevens–Johnson syndrome is much less frequently caused by a medication in a pediatric patient than in an adult.[1,119] Mycoplasma infection is the most likely infectious trigger of SJS in pediatric patients,[120] and may be associated with less severe disease than drug-induced SJS.[121] Other infections,[122,123] neoplasia, autoimmune disorders, and vaccination[124] have also been implicated, particularly H. simplex virus, which is more typically linked to erythema multiforme. The occurrence of these drug reactions is almost always within the first 8 weeks of drug use, but rarely within the first few days of drug administration. Most patients show evidence of SJS or TEN 7–21 days after the first drug exposure. Children with an earlier onset (mean 2–3 days) have been previously exposed to the drug or a cross-reacting analogue. Although >200 medications have been implicated as potential triggers of SJS-TEN, sulfonamides, penicillins, phenobarbital, carbamazepine, and lamotrigine have been most strongly associated with SJS-TEN.[125] Aromatic anticonvulsants (phenobarbital, phenytoin, and carbamazepine) tend to cross-react and cannot substitute for each other. Drugs with longer half-lives are associated with a higher incidence than those related but with shorter half-lives. NSAIDs, including ibuprofen,[126] and acetaminophen[127,125] have more recently been implicated as triggers and possibly exacerbants with other drugs, and are best avoided during hospitalization for SJS-TEN. Lymphocyte transformation tests have helped to identify the causative agents in some affected children but, in contrast to those for children with DRESS syndrome, need to be performed during the first week of the disorder.[107] The risk of developing SJS and TEN is significantly increased in patients with

---

Table 20.5 Features of Stevens–Johnson syndrome and toxic epidermal necrolysis

Constitutional
  Fever
  Dehydration

Mucocutaneous
  Stomatitis with hemorrhagic crusts
  Oral and genital erosions
  Dysphagia
  Purulent conjunctivitis with photophobia
  Occasionally esophageal and pulmonary mucosal sloughing
  Dusky erythematous macules, targetoid lesions, bullae, and skin
    sloughing

Visceral
  Lymphadenopathy
  Hepatosplenomegaly with hepatitis
  Uncommonly, pneumonitis, arthritis, myocarditis, and nephritis

Laboratory abnormalities
  Increased erythrocyte sedimentation rate (100%)
  Leukocytosis (60%)
  Eosinophilia (20%)
  Anemia (15%)
  Elevated hepatic transaminase levels (15%)
  Leukopenia (10%)
  Proteinuria, microscopic hematuria (5%)

Table 20.6 Most common pharmacologic triggers of SJS and TEN

Allopurinol
Barbiturates
Carbamazepine
Lamotrigine
NSAIDs
Penicillins
Phenytoin
Sulfonamides

HIV infection and who have a decreased capacity to detoxify reactive intermediate drug metabolites (e.g., slow acetylators or individuals with defects in epoxide hydrolase-mediated detoxification).

SJS and TEN are life-threatening disorders, and patients should be hospitalized. If possible, all drugs administered within 2 months before onset of the eruption should be discontinued,[128] and infectious causes should be sought and treated. Severe oropharyngeal involvement often necessitates frequent mouthwashes and local application of a topical anesthetic. When ocular involvement is present, ophthalmologic consultation should be obtained. Most recently short-term use of potent topical corticosteroids and application of amniotic membrane to the entire ocular surface has been advocated to preserve visual acuity and an intact ocular surface.[129-131] Patients should receive intravenous fluids and either a liquid diet if tolerated or parenteral nutrition; the measured resting energy requirement in pediatric SJS/TEN is increased by 30%.[132] A mouthwash containing Maalox, elixir of diphenhydramine, and viscous lidocaine (mixed 1:1:1) can be soothing and decrease pain. Oral histamines such as hydroxyzine or diphenhydramine can be beneficial, and more vigorous pain control is often necessary. Of note, TEN has also been associated rarely with acetaminophen ingestion in children.[133]

If damage to the epidermis is extensive, patients should be admitted to an intensive care unit or burn unit to allow special attention to fluid requirements, electrolyte balance, intravenous caloric replacement, and avoidance of secondary infection. Manipulation should be avoided but, if necessary, should be performed in a sterile fashion. Intact areas of skin should be kept dry. Open wounds should be cleansed daily. Detached areas should be covered with non-adherent, moist dressings (such as petrolatum-impregnated gauze) until re-epithelialization occurs. Periorificial areas can be treated with antibiotic ointment (such as bacitracin or mupirocin). Biologic dressings or skin equivalents may be considered for patients with extensive denudation.[134]

The response to supportive care alone has been excellent in the majority of children.[135] The administration of systemic medications as treatment is controversial, and there is little evidence-based data to support its use, especially in pediatric patients. Short-term administration of intravenous systemic corticosteroids (4 mg/kg per day) or pulsed intravenous steroids is sometimes advocated if started within the first 2–3 days of a drug-induced reaction.[136,137] However, several anecdotal reports and open-label, non-comparative trials have not demonstrated efficacy.[138] Continuing use of systemic steroids may increase morbidity and mortality from secondary infection, prolonging wound healing, masking early signs of sepsis, and triggering gastrointestinal bleeding. Intravenous immunoglobulin (IVIG) has been promoted as treatment of SJS and particularly TEN, based on the demonstrated role of Fas-mediated apoptosis in SJS-TEN and the demonstration that IVIG blocks Fas-mediated keratinocyte cell death *in vitro*.[139] Peak concentrations of serum soluble Fas ligand are noted at the onset of disease with a rapid diminution within 5 days of onset.[140] In addition, *FasL* gene polymorphisms have been shown to be associated with the risk of SJS-TEN.[141] In early studies, some children with SJS or TEN demonstrated shorter duration of fever and decreased development of new blisters if intravenous immunoglobulin was administered within 24–48 h[142-144] and 2.5–3.0 mg/kg per day for 3 days, has more recently been recommended. More recent studies have shown no benefit to the use of IVIG,[145] including for pediatric disease.[146,147] Double-blind, randomized, controlled trials have not been performed. Cyclosporine, cyclophosphamide, and plasmapheresis[148] have also been used anecdotally with good results. Thalidomide administration has been linked to increased mortality in a randomized placebo-controlled trial.[149]

Sun exposure should be avoided and sunscreens used liberally for at least a few months because of the potential for ultraviolet light-induced worsening of the residual dyspigmentation. Artificial tears and lubricants may be required for several years after diagnosis, if not lifelong, since ocular disease tends to progress after hospital discharge. Late ocular complications include dry eye syndrome (59%), subjunctival fibrous scarring (33%), corneal erosions (29%) and, in fewer than 25% trichiasis, symblepharon and visual loss.[150]

Fixed drug eruption

Fixed drug eruption is a term used to describe a sharply localized, circumscribed round or oval dermatitis that characteristically recurs in the same site or sites each time the offending drug is administered.[151] The persistent residual hyperpigmentation leads to the name of the eruption. In one series, fixed drug eruption was second in frequency to exanthematous reactions to drugs, and occurred in 22% of children with cutaneous reactions to drug ingestion.[152] Lesions first occur 1–2 weeks after initial ingestion of the drug, but within 30 min to 8 h after repeat ingestion subsequently. Fixed drug eruptions are type IV immune reactions, and have recently been shown to result from CD8+ memory T cells that persist intraepidermally at site of involvement and, upon stimulation by drug, release IFN-γ, leading to inflammation. Fas-Fas ligand interactions lead to the demonstrated basal keratinocyte apoptosis.

Lesions are solitary at first, but with repeated attacks new lesions usually appear and existing lesions may tend to increase in size to more than 10 cm in diameter. Not uncommonly, lesions recur at the same site(s). The lesions tend to be erythematous, edematous, and dusky at their onset with well-defined borders. At times they may become bullous (Fig. 20.29), with subsequent desquamation or crusting and a residual hyperpigmentation that may persist for months (Fig. 20.30). Lesions can occur anywhere on the body, but have a predilection for the perioral area, lips, hands, trunk, and genital region.[153,154] In a series of affected boys with genital involvement, the clinical presentation usually consisted of swelling and erythema of the penis and/or scrotum associated with pruritus or burning, restlessness, urinary retention, and painful micturition.[154]

By far the most common trigger of fixed drug eruptions in children is cotrimoxazole and other sulfa drugs. Acetaminophen, ibuprofen,[155] and, less commonly, loratadine[156] and pseudoephedrine have also been causative, and a careful history of administration of

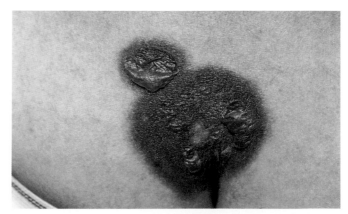

Figure 20.29 Fixed drug eruption. Well-defined, dusky erythematous plaques that may be bullous.

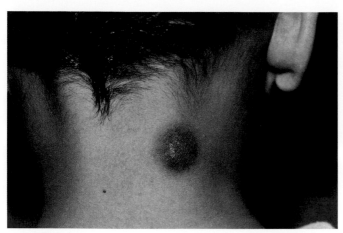

Figure 20.30 Fixed drug eruption. The residual hyperpigmentation at the site of a fixed drug eruption may persist for months.

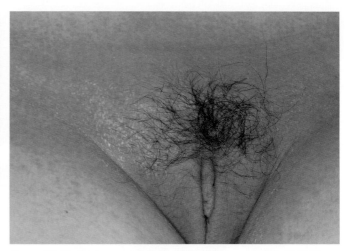

Figure 20.31 Acute generalized exanthematous pustulosis (AGEP). Affected individuals show large areas with erythroderma topped with small non-follicular tiny sterile pustules, usually in association with fever. Although often triggered by a virus or vaccination in children, this adolescent was taking an anticonvulsant medication.

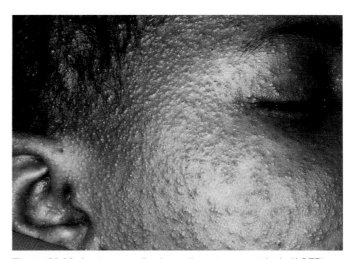

Figure 20.32 Acute generalized exanthematous pustulosis (AGEP). Pinpoint sterile papulopustules overlying erythroderma. No medication was associated, and the condition was attributed to a virus.

over-the-counter products is of key importance. Although phenolphthalein was a common cause in the past, its elimination from over-the-counter laxatives has markedly diminished its culpability. Other causative preparations include phenytoin, ciprofloxacin, metronidazole, penicillin, tetracycline, erythromycin, teichoplanin,[157] quinine and its derivatives, salicylates, potassium iodide, and metronidazole. Fixed food eruptions have been described after ingestion of various food substitutes and flavorings (especially tartrazine, as in artificially colored cheese crisps),[158] as well as licorice, cashews, lentils, and asparagus.

The diagnosis of fixed drug eruption is often missed, leading to repeated ingestion of the medication and recurrence. Lesions may be mistaken commonly for insect bites, urticaria, and, if more extensive, erythema multiforme or in their stage of hyperpigmentation for erythema dyschromicum perstans. Biopsy can aid in the diagnosis of fixed drug eruption, especially in the early stage in which a lichenoid infiltrate with necrotic keratinocytes may be seen. Avoidance of the offending agent is key, but the associated pruritus can be controlled by application of medium-strength to potent topical corticosteroids. If necessary, challenge with the drug usually confirms the causative agent within 30 min to 8 h, but theoretically can trigger a more severe reaction. Patch testing at the site of a previous lesion can lead to a positive result in up to 30% of patients.[159]

Acute generalized exanthematous pustulosis

Acute generalized exanthematous pustulosis (AGEP) is characterized by the acute onset of a generalized erythroderma topped with small nonfollicular sterile pustules, usually in association with fever (Figs 20.31, 20.32). The condition usually resolves spontaneously after 4–10 days with a characteristic pattern of desquamation. AGEP has been described in several children,[160,161] although it is much more common in adults. Medication has been the usual trigger in adults and can cause AGEP in children,[162,163] but the majority of children are administered no medication, suggesting that the condition is often triggered in response to viral infection or possibly vaccine administration.[161]

Erythema multiforme

Erythema multiforme (EM) is a specific self-limited hypersensitivity syndrome with a distinctive clinical pattern, the hallmark of which is the erythematous ring (the so-called iris or target lesion). The condition can occur at any age, but is most frequently seen in young adults; 20% of cases occur in children. The majority of cases of EM in children are precipitated by herpes simplex virus (HSV) type 1 infection,[164] although HSV type 2 infection has been described in affected adolescents.[165,166] Approximately 50% of cases follow herpes labialis infection, usually by 3–14 days, although concurrent infection and EM have been noted. HSV DNA has been detected in the early erythematous papules or the peripheral area of target lesions in 80% of patients with EM,[165] despite the low recovery of herpes simplex in cultures of lesions.[167] When associated with HSV, the disorder has been termed 'herpes-associated EM', or HAEM. Other viral disorders, including varicella,[168] orf and Epstein–Barr virus infection, have been implicated, and histoplasmosis has been associated in endemic areas. Erythema multiforme in association with high fever can be a sign of Kawasaki disease, especially in infants[169] (see Ch. 21; Fig. 21.30).

The diagnosis of erythema multiforme can generally be made by the clinical features and distribution of lesions (Table 20.7). The

Table 20.7 Clinical features of erythema multiforme
Acute, self-limited, recurrent course
Duration of 1–4 weeks
Symmetrically distributed, fixed lesions
Concentric color changes in at least some lesions (iris or target lesions)
If present, mucosal involvement limited to the mouth
In children, most likely cause for recurrent disease is herpes simplex virus

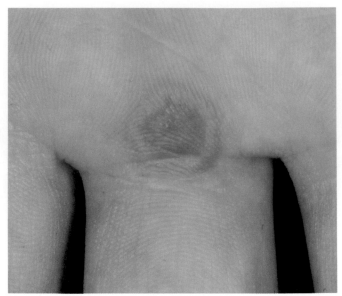

Figure 20.34 Erythema multiforme. Classic target lesion in this girl with recurrent herpetic lesions.

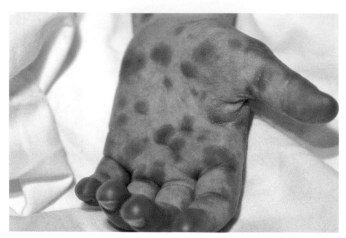

Figure 20.33 Erythema multiforme. Round erythematous swollen plaques and target lesions on the palms.

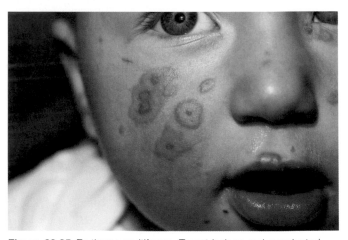

Figure 20.35 Erythema multiforme. Target lesions and marginated wheals with central vesicles are characteristic.

eruption is symmetric and may be noted on any part of the body, with a predilection for the palms and soles (Figs 20.33, 20.34), backs of the hands and feet, and extensor surfaces of the arms and legs. Lesions may be grouped, especially at the elbows and knees. As the disorder progresses during 72 h (and occasionally as long as a week), lesions may extend to the trunk, face, and neck. Once present, lesions are fixed for at least 7 days.

The primary lesion of erythema multiforme develops abruptly without a prodromal period. It is a dull red to dusky flat macule, or a sharply marginated wheal, in the center of which a papule or vesicle develops, thus creating the multiformity of lesions. The central area then flattens and develops dusky clearing, the result of epidermal cell necrosis. As a result it is not unusual to see iris or target lesions consisting of concentric circles whose bright red rings alternate with cyanotic or violaceous ones (Figs 20.35, 20.36). Lesions may also become bullous (*bullous EM*) (Fig. 20.37). Careful inspection of the eruption in erythema multiforme may disclose fine petechiae. Most lesions are asymptomatic, but itching or burning has been described. The isomorphic response (koebnerization) appears to participate in the development of lesions, with trauma and ultraviolet light injury as triggers.

Oral lesions are seen in 25–50% of children, usually in conjunction with cutaneous lesions. They initially appear as bullae that break soon after formation, accompanied by swelling and crusting of the lips and erosions of the buccal mucosa and tongue. Gingival involvement is rare, which helps to distinguish EM from primary herpes simplex infection of the mouth (Fig. 20.38). Most children with mucosal involvement have a few lesions and are mildly symptomatic; however, patients with extensively crusted lips and large bullous target lesions that may mimic Stevens–Johnson syndrome have been described.[116,117] Systemic manifestations, when present,

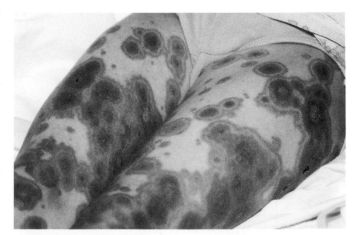

Figure 20.36 Erythema multiforme. Extensive target lesions on the thighs of a 12-year-old girl. The recurrent reaction was suppressed by administration of oral acyclovir.

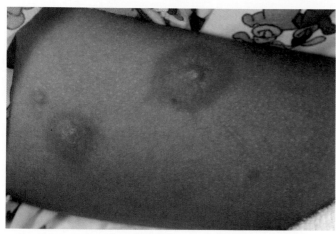

Figure 20.37 Erythema multiforme, bullous. If central epidermal necrosis is extensive, the center of the lesion may become bullous.

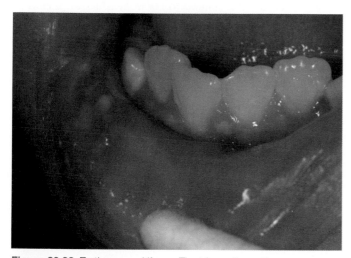

Figure 20.38 Erythema multiforme The trigger for erythema multiforme in children is frequently *H. simplex* inspection, which often precedes but may be detectable at the time when the erythema multiforme is present.

are mild and consist of low-grade fever, malaise, and, in rare cases, myalgia or arthralgia.

Biopsy of skin lesions is usually not needed to make a diagnosis of erythema multiforme. It should be performed only to consider other conditions, such as lupus erythematosus or vasculitis.[170] Focal liquefaction degeneration of epidermal keratinocytes and exocytosis of mononuclear cells in the epidermis are seen.

Most episodes of EM heal within 2–3 weeks without sequelae. Recurrences a few times yearly, however, are common. Symptomatic treatment with oral antihistamines usually suffices. Given the association with herpes simplex virus, however, prophylactic therapy with oral acyclovir (20 mg/kg per day) for 6–12 months should be considered for patients with recurrent disease.[165] Episodic therapy with acyclovir is not useful. Administration of immunosuppressive agents, such as oral corticosteroids, leads to longer and more frequent episodes.

Annular erythemas

The annular erythemas (erythema marginatum, erythema annulare centrifugum, erythema migrans, and annular erythema of infancy)

represent a group of reactive vascular dermatoses that are distinguished primarily by their oval, annular, arcuate, circinate, polycyclic, reticular, or serpiginous configurations with individual characteristics that allow differentiation into distinctive clinical categories.[171] They must be distinguished from other annular lesions seen in children, especially tinea, erythema multiforme and serum sickness-like reaction, annular pityriasis rosea, neonatal and subacute lupus erythematosus, granuloma annulare, and the annular lesions of erythrokeratodermia variabilis (see Ch. 5).

Erythema Marginatum and Rheumatic Fever

Erythema marginatum is a distinctive form of annular erythema that occurs on the trunk (especially on the abdomen) and the proximal extremities of patients with active rheumatic fever.[172,173] It is seen more frequently in children than in adults with rheumatic fever, but still only occurs in 6% of affected children.[174] The occurrence of erythema marginatum frequently follows the onset of migratory arthritis by a few days, but at times may also occur many months after the carditis.

Often easily overlooked, lesions are evanescent pink macules or papules that fade centrally in a few hours to several days, leaving a pale or sometimes pigmented center. They spread rapidly to form nonpruritic rings or segments of rings with elevated reticular, polycyclic, or serpiginous borders and may recur in crops in different areas. Lesions are frequently seen more easily in the afternoon, and coalescence of polycyclic lesions often results in a characteristic chicken-wire-like appearance. Gentle warming of the skin tends to enhance visualization of pale or barely perceptible lesions. Although the eruption seldom lasts more than several weeks, occasionally it may recur at sporadic intervals for several months to years.

Erythema marginatum presents a clinical picture that characteristically resembles a variety of dermatoses, including urticaria, erythema multiforme, and other transient figurate erythemas.[175] Unlike the characteristic rash of juvenile idiopathic arthritis (see Ch. 22), lesions of erythema marginatum are larger, spread centrifugally with central clearing, and are limited to the trunk and sometimes the proximal limbs. Histologic features of a neutrophilic perivascular infiltrate in the papillary dermis aid in diagnosis.

The most common associated features are carditis (76–93% of patients), fever (62%), congestive heart failure (44%), and arthritis (39–53% of patients). Sydenham's chorea is rarely seen. Approximately 2% of patients show urticarial lesions without annular rings[176] and up to 2% have subcutaneous nodules, usually a late manifestation. The nodules of rheumatic fever are smaller than those seen in juvenile idiopathic arthritis and usually clear within a month. They tend to occur in crops, are symmetrically distributed, are nontender, and are more readily felt than seen, requiring a careful search. Differentiation of subcutaneous nodules of rheumatic fever from rheumatoid nodules and granuloma annulare is not possible on clinical or histologic grounds alone, and requires the presence of other features.

Currently accepted criteria for the diagnosis of rheumatic fever include two major or one minor manifestation and evidence of recent group A streptococcal disease. The major manifestations include erythema marginatum, carditis, polyarthritis, chorea, and subcutaneous nodules. The minor manifestations include fever, arthralgias, previous rheumatic fever or rheumatic heart disease, leukocytosis, elevated erythrocyte sedimentation rate or positive C-reactive protein, and prolonged PR interval. Typical erythema marginatum has also been described in a patient with psittacosis.[177]

Erythema Annulare Centrifugum

Erythema annulare centrifugum (EAC) is an eruption characterized by persistent erythematous annular lesions, each with a clear center and a raised, thin, wall-like border that slowly enlarges centrifugally. Synonyms for erythema annulare centrifugum include *gyrate erythema* and *erythema perstans*.

Primary lesions of EAC tend to be single or multiple erythematous, edematous papules with a predilection for the trunk, buttocks, thighs, and legs (Figs 20.39, 20.40). They are asymptomatic except for occasional mild pruritus. The rings extend peripherally, usually slowly, 1–3 mm/day, sometimes up to 4 cm in a week. New lesions may form within the original circle. The resulting overall shape may be irregular, oval, circinate, semiannular, target-like, or polycyclic. The borders may eventually reach a size of 10 cm or more in diameter. The duration of the disease is extremely variable and may go on for weeks or months and, with new lesions appearing in successive crops, frequently for years.

At times the palpable border of the expanding ring may be topped by microvesicles or may show a fine collarette of scale on its trailing edge, suggesting a diagnosis of tinea corporis. Fungal infections can be distinguished by their more pronounced epidermal changes, with vesiculation or scaling or both at the edge of the lesions, by microscopic examination of skin scrapings, and by fungal culture. When the diagnosis is uncertain, histopathologic examination of cutaneous lesions showing focal infiltration of lymphocytes around the blood vessels and dermal appendages in a 'coat sleeve' arrangement may help to establish the diagnosis.

The etiology of EAC is unknown. Although it often occurs without apparent cause, most cases appear to be related to hypersensitivity to drugs, fungi, molluscum poxvirus,[178,179] certain foods, blood dyscrasia, autoimmune endocrinopathies or hepatitis,[180] or neoplastic disease (lymphomas).

Since EAC represents a hypersensitivity reaction, treatment depends on the determination and removal of the underlying cause. Antihistamines produce variable and usually incomplete relief; topical corticosteroids tend to be ineffective. Although systemic corticosteroids may aid the temporary resolution of lesions, unless the underlying cause is removed, the disorder frequently recurs as soon as medication is discontinued. Cases with onset during the neonatal period or early infancy and persistence into adulthood have been described (Fig. 20.41).[181,182] The eruption in these cases clears with febrile episodes or subcutaneous administration of interferon-α.

Annular erythema of infancy

Annular erythema of infancy may be a subset of erythema annulare centrifugum or a distinct entity in which infants have cyclic eruptions of urticarial annular erythema without a demonstrable underlying cause.[183] Lesions of classic annular erythema of infancy last for only a few days, in contrast to the more persistent lesions of erythema annulare centrifugum. This benign disorder is asymptomatic. It may resolve spontaneously after 3–11 months.[183] Neonatal

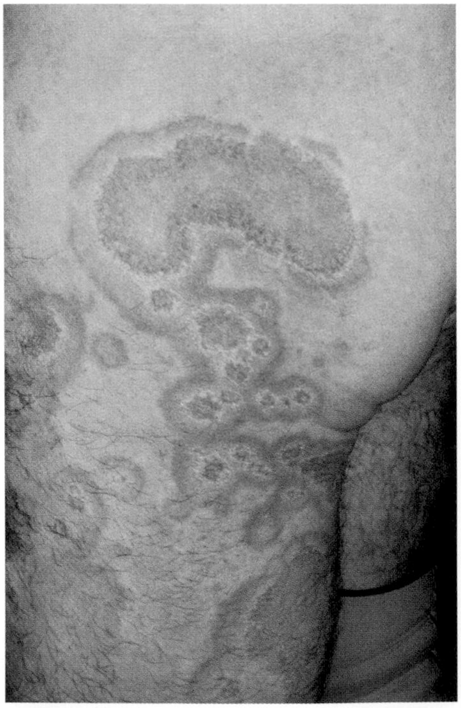

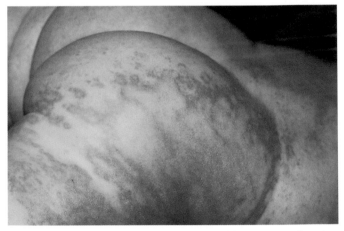

Figure 20.40 Erythema annulare centrifugum. No cause was found for the recurrent annular lesions in this infant.

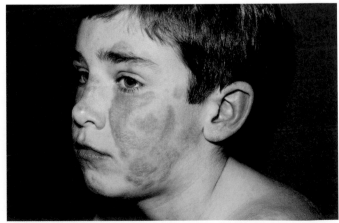

Figure 20.41 Erythema annulare centrifugum. This 10-year-old boy has had chronic, transitory annular plaques on the face, trunk, and extremities since the first weeks of life. They only clear transiently with febrile episodes.

Figure 20.39 Erythema annulare centrifugum (EAC). Slowly expanding annular lesions have dusky centers and palpable scaly erythematous borders. Although the annular rings showed no evidence of fungus, the EAC was thought to result from the patient's underlying tinea pedis.

lupus (see Ch. 22) must be considered. *Neutrophilic figurate erythema of infancy* is considered a neutrophilic variant of annular erythema of infancy, although the recurrences of the annular erythema may continue beyond infancy.[184]

Erythema Migrans

Erythema migrans (erythema chronicum migrans), the earliest sign of Lyme disease, is a cutaneous eruption that follows a tick bite and is characterized by single or multiple erythematous expanding lesions with advancing indurated borders and central clearing (see Ch. 14). Erythema migrans is caused by the tick-borne spirochete *Borrelia burgdorferi* (see Figs 14.35, 14.36).

Panniculitis

Panniculitis is a term to describe a group of disorders in which the major focus of inflammation is in the subcutaneous fat (Table 20.8).[185,186] The pathomechanism of most of these disorders is poorly understood. The most common subgroup is erythema nodosum (see below), which is frequently associated with streptococcal infection in children, but is considered a hypersensitivity disorder seen with several systemic disorders. Other forms of panniculitis are also commonly linked to systemic disorders, particularly collagen vascular disorders (see Ch. 22), Behçet syndrome (Ch. 25), lymphomas (see Ch. 10), diabetes (see Ch. 23), thyroid disease, α1-antitrypsin or pancreatic enzyme deficiency, and in association with generalized lipodystrophy. Disorders of the dermis, such as

leukocytoclastic vasculitis and granuloma annulare, may show subcutaneous involvement, but would not be considered primarily panniculitides. Infection may also lead to panniculitis, e.g., especially with tuberculosis and erythema induratum of Bazin and less commonly with atypical mycobacterial infection[187–189] (see Ch. 14). Particularly in immunocompromised children, lobular panniculitis can be a feature of deep fungal infection (candidiasis, fusariosis,[190] aspergillosis, cryptococcosis, histoplasmosis, sporotrichosis, and chromomycosis) or bacterial infection (e.g., *N. meningitidis*, *S. pyogenes*, *S. aureus*, *Klebsiella*, and *Pseudomonas* and *Nocardia* spp.).[191] (Subcutaneous fat necrosis of the newborn and sclerema neonatorum are discussed in Ch. 2.)

Classification of the panniculitides may be difficult, and several previous subtypes, such as Weber–Christian disease and Rothman–Makai syndrome, are no longer considered to be separate entities. Histopathologic evaluation of a biopsy large enough to include subcutaneous fat is often required to confirm the diagnosis of a specific form of panniculitis. Sections may show primarily septal involvement, as in erythema nodosum, or lobular, as in the panniculitis associated with α1-antitrypsin disease. A largely lobular form with needle-shaped clefts within lipocytes are characteristic of subcutaneous fat necrosis of the newborn, sclerema neonatorum, and poststeroid panniculitis,[192] whereas necrosis is an early finding of the panniculitis induced by pancreatic enzymes.[193,194]

Cold panniculitis, which is most common in infants and children, is characterized by painful poorly defined erythematous plaques or subcutaneous nodules that develop in areas exposed to cold (Fig. 20.42). Lesions appear several hours to 3 days after exposure and subside spontaneously, generally after a few weeks to a few months, leaving temporary residual pigmentation. The development of cold panniculitis in children appears to be related to the fact that subcutaneous fat solidifies more readily at lower temperatures in infants and young children than it does in adults. Cold panniculitis is often seen on the cheeks of toddlers and young children who suck popsicles (*popsicle panniculitis*),[195] at sites of contact with ice bags, cooling blankets before cardiac surgery or in treatment of arrhythmias,[196] and on the thighs and buttocks of young equestrians (*equestrian panniculitis*). Affected children are otherwise usually healthy and no intervention is necessary.

Table 20.8 Classification of the subtypes of panniculitis
Erythema nodosum

Infection
  Bacterial
  Mycobacterial (erythema induratum of Bazin)
  Fungal

Enzymatic disorders
  α1-Antitrypsin disease
  Pancreatic disease

Poststeroid

Malignant panniculitis
  Cytophagic histiocytic panniculitis
  Subcutaneous panniculitis-like T-cell lymphoma
  Edematous, scarring vasculitic panniculitis (hydroa-like
    lymphoma)

Lipoatrophic panniculitis
  Associated with autoimmune disorders: systemic lupus
    erythematosus, deep morphea, juvenile dermatomyositis
    (usually subclinical), polyarteritis nodosa
  Lipophagic panniculitis of childhood
  Atrophic connective tissue panniculitis of the ankles
  Recurrent lobular panniculitis

Physical agents
  Cold panniculitis (popsicle, equestrian)
  Injections, including factitial
  Blunt trauma

Subcutaneous fat necrosis of the newborn
Sclerema neonatorum

Selected syndromes
  H syndrome
  CANDLE syndrome

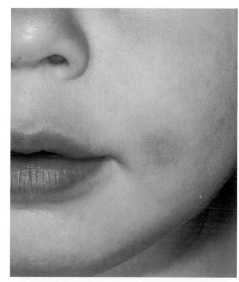

Figure 20.42 Popsicle panniculitis. This subtle erythematous macule resulted from cold panniculitis of the cheek after sucking on a popsicle. At times, the erythema is much more intense.

The red or purple-red nodules of *factitial panniculitis* result from the injection of foreign substances into the subcutaneous tissue. Diagnosis requires a high index of suspicion, but can be confirmed if foreign material is found in biopsy sections. For example, polarized light microscopic examination may show birefringent particles or, as in the case of injected silicone, oily substances with a characteristic Swiss cheese-like picture of oil cysts surrounded by fibrosis and inflammation. Milk, feces, mineral oil, and paraffin are among other substances that may be injected, leading to factitial panniculitis. In young children, these factitial lesions raise the possibility of Munchausen syndrome by proxy (see Ch. 26).

Poststeroid panniculitis, a rare entity of childhood, is characterized by small, sometimes pruritic or painful subcutaneous nodules on the cheeks, arms, trunk, and buttocks of young children. These generally develop within 2–4 weeks after the sudden discontinuation of systemic corticosteroid therapy.[197] Lesions tend to regress spontaneously without scarring.

Panniculitis can be a feature of malignancy, particularly lymphoma. *Subcutaneous panniculitis-like T-cell lymphoma* has occasionally been described in pediatric patients, especially adolescents (see Ch. 10).[198–201] Patients develop skin-colored to erythematous, often painful subcutaneous nodules or hemorrhagic plaques. Fever, mucosal ulcerations, hepatosplenomegaly with hepatic failure, pancytopenia, and intravascular coagulopathy are associated features. Biopsy sections show often atypical lymphocytes and, in about 50% of cases in children, evidence of hemophagocytosis, which portends a poor prognosis. In children, in contrast with adults, the face is frequently affected and systemic involvement is more common. Molecular genetic analysis and immunophenotyping should be performed. Suggested treatment includes initial administration of cyclosporine and prednisone for the inflammatory component,[111] followed by combination chemotherapy for the lymphoma. *Cytophagic histiocytic panniculitis* is characterized by chronic panniculitis in association with fever, hepatosplenomegaly, and pancytopenia because of bone marrow hemo cytophagocytosis. Histologically, the finding of cytophagic histiocytic panniculitis represents a reaction pattern that may be benign (in association with infection, especially EBV) or may prove to be associated with subcutaneous T cell lymphoma (see above). Panniculitis in association with vasculitis is a feature of hydroa-like lymphoma associated with EBV infection (see Ch. 19).

Alpha1-antitrypsin is a protease inhibitor made by the liver. Most normal individuals carry the MM genotype (i.e., both alleles are M), and have normal levels of α1-antitrypsin. Heterozygotes with one S or Z allele have a moderate deficiency of the inhibitor; individuals who are homozygous for the Z allele have a severe α1-antitrypsin deficiency. The clinical manifestations of *α1-antitrypsin deficiency* in children or adults may be cirrhosis, emphysema, pulmonary effusions, pulmonary embolism, membranous proliferative glomerulonephritis, pancreatitis, arthritis, vasculitis, angioedema, and panniculitis.[202] The panniculitis is usually seen in homozygotes, but has been described in heterozygotic pediatric patients, including the MS phenotype.[203] It is characterized by erythematous to purple tender nodules or plaques most commonly seen on the lower trunk, buttocks, and proximal, extremities after trauma. Deep necrotic ulcerations may develop and discharge an oily material. Lesions are often persistent and resistant to therapy, but eventually heal with scarring and atrophy. Replacement of α1-antitrypsin by intravenous infusion is the most effective therapy and can lead to rapid clearance of the panniculitis.

Patients with *cutaneous polyarteritis nodosa* (PAN), a form of deep dermal and subcutaneous vasculitis, have painful or tender subcutaneous nodules with overlying erythema or purple discoloration (see Ch. 21, Figs 21.16 and 21.17).[204–206] A streptococcal pharyngitis may precede the eruption.[207] Although the cutaneous features may manifest as an isolated benign form, the multisystemic form of polyarteritis nodosa should be considered, and may show weight loss, fever, abdominal pain, musculoskeletal signs, renal disease, and peripheral neuropathy. Typical lesions of cutaneous PAN show oval or linear nodules surrounded by livedo reticularis and often stellate necrosis.

Other forms of panniculitis include pancreatic panniculitis, a disorder that probably results from breakdown of subcutaneous fat caused by enzymes released into the circulation from a nodular or neoplastic pancreatic disease; erythema induratum, a deep-seated subcutaneous infiltration of the lower legs, especially the posterior calves, that often ulcerates before healing and results in atrophic scars (see Ch. 14); and traumatic panniculitis, a disorder consisting of hard, indurated, inflamed nodules following injury (Fig. 20.43). Lobular panniculitis may also lead to lipoatrophy.[208–210] Most often seen with systemic lupus erythematosus,[211] deep morphea and juvenile dermatomyositis[212] may also manifest with panniculitis that resolves with lipoatrophy (see Ch. 22). Residual lipoatrophy at the ankles in association lobular panniculitis and lipophages has been described with and without autoimmune disorders of other types, particularly thyroiditis and diabetes mellitus.[213,214] Panniculitis and lipoatrophy (particularly of the buttocks) are also features of *H syndrome*, an autosomal recessive disorder with panniculitis resulting from mutations in *SLC29A3*, a nucleoside transporter.[215–218] H syndrome is characterized by *h*yperpigmentation (often with induration) and *h*ypertrichosis of the inner thigh and usually spreads to involve the middle and lower parts of the body with conspicuous sparing of the knees and buttocks. Patients also show *h*epatosplenomegaly, *h*eart anomalies, and *h*ypogonadism. Panniculitis with vasculitis and atypical cells is also a feature of CANDLE (*c*hronic *a*typical *n*eutrophilic *d*ermatosis with *l*ipodystrophy and *e*levated temperature) syndrome.[219]

Erythema nodosum

Erythema nodosum is a hypersensitivity reaction characterized by red, tender, nodular lesions.[220] Occurrence peaks during adolescence and is rare under 2 years of age. During childhood girls are affected slightly more than boys, in contrast to adults, in which women are affected three to four times more often than men. The disease has its greatest incidence in the spring and fall and is less common in summer.

Lesions are most often is seen on the pretibial surfaces (Fig. 20.44), but occur more frequently in affected children on the thighs, arms, trunk and face than in adults.[221] They are most often 1–5 cm

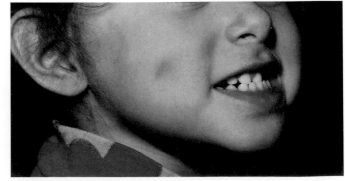

Figure 20.43 Traumatic fat necrosis. The panniculitis occurred after blunt trauma to the cheek and led to lipoatrophy.

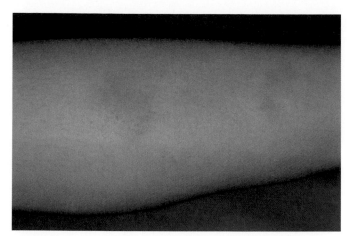

Figure 20.44 Erythema nodosum. Tender red oval nodules on the extensor aspect of the legs. Note that several have darkened and resemble bruises.

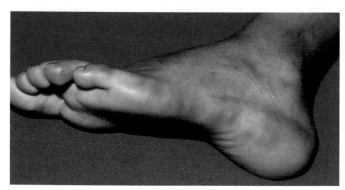

Figure 20.45 Erythema nodosum. These inflamed nodules proved to be a hypersensitivity reaction to Group A β-hemolytic streptococcal infection.

Table 20.9 Underlying causes of erythema nodosum
Idiopathic (~50%)
β-Hemolytic streptococcal infection, especially pharyngitis (most common detectable cause)

Other Infections
    Common: Mycoplasma, upper respiratory viruses (Epstein–Barr virus), mycobacteria (tuberculosis and atypical), coccidiomycosis in endemic areas
    Uncommon: *T. mentagrophytes, Yersinia, Shigella*, hepatitis B, brucellosis, meningococcosis, Neisserial infection, cat-scratch disease, HIV infection, chlamydia, blastomycosis, histoplasmosis, sporotrichosis, syphilis, pertussis, *Escherichia coli*, leprosy

Inflammatory
    Sarcoidosis
    Inflammatory bowel disease
    Behçet disease

Malignancy (especially leukemia)
Drugs   Oral contraceptives, sulfonamides, penicillins
Pregnancy

in diameter and are symmetrically distributed. Lesions are occasionally located on the knees, ankles, thighs, extensor aspects of the arms, the face, and neck. They are rarely found on the palms or soles (Fig. 20.45). Initially they appear as bright to deep red, warm and tender, oval, slightly elevated nodules. After a few days they develop a brownish red or purplish bruise-like appearance that is characteristic. Lesions do not ulcerate or leave scars.

Despite investigation, no underlying cause is found in most pediatric patients. Although possible etiologic causes are numerous (Table 20.9), the most common in the pediatric patient is β-hemolytic streptococcal infection. The list of other associated disorders is long, especially other infectious diseases (including tuberculosis, *Yersinia* infection, *T. mentagrophytes*[222,223] and infectious mononucleosis,[224–229] administration of oral contraceptives, inflammatory bowel disease, and sarcoidosis. In patients with coccidiomycosis, the presence of erythema nodosum suggests a positive prognostic sign and decreased risk of dissemination. Erythema nodosum leprosum shows panniculitis with leukocytoclastic vasculitis in biopsy sections.[230]

The eruption usually lasts 3–6 weeks but may recede earlier. Recrudescences may occur over a period of weeks to months, but attacks are seldom recurrent. Arthralgias may precede, coincide with, or follow the eruption in as many as 90% of cases. In the 10% of patients in whom the condition may present as a recurring disorder, recurrences are frequently associated with repeated streptococcal infection.

Erythema nodosum has a characteristic clinical picture, and diagnosis generally can be made on the basis of physical examination alone. Although diagnosis is usually not difficult, common bruises, cellulitis or erysipelas, deep fungal infections (such as Majocchi's granuloma or sporotrichosis), insect bites, deep thrombophlebitis, angiitis, erythema induratum, and fat-destructive panniculitides can be confused with this disorder. Eccrine hidradenitis can resemble erythema nodosum on the palms or soles.[231] When the diagnosis is in doubt, bacterial and fungal cultures and histologic examination of skin biopsy specimens generally will help clarify the diagnosis.

The management of erythema nodosum is directed at identification and treatment of the underlying cause. Minimal evaluation usually involves obtaining a CBC, throat culture, an ASO/ DNase B titer, chest radiograph, and tuberculin testing. Bed rest, with elevation of the patient's legs, helps reduce pain and edema. When pain, inflammation, or arthralgia is prominent, NSAIDs can be prescribed. Salicylates, colchicine, potassium iodide and, if severe, a short course of systemic corticosteroids are the most commonly used alternative therapies. In chronic or recurrent cases, detailed investigations must be performed to uncover the underlying cause. Intralesional corticosteroids frequently cause rapid involution of individual lesions, and in persistent or recurrent eruptions oral corticosteroids may be beneficial.

Cutaneous reactions to cold

A variety of conditions can occur when one is exposed to cold. Frostbite is caused by exposure to extreme cold. Trench foot and immersion foot are caused by a combination of cold and wetness. Perniosis (chilblains) represents an exaggerated response to cold and dampness in a predisposed individual. Individuals may also develop cutaneous changes after exposure to cold with dysproteinemia, such as with cryofibrinogenemia or cryoglobulinemia.

Frostbite

Frostbite is a disorder caused by the actual freezing of tissue at temperatures of extreme cold (−2°C to −10°C).[232] The duration of exposure, wind velocity, dependency of an extremity, application of emollients, and factors such as fatigue, injury, immobility, and general health potentiate the effects of the cold.[233] Frostbite is caused by direct cold injury to the cell, vascular insufficiency (constriction and vasoocclusion), and damage from inflammatory mediators. The vasoconstriction that occurs is an effort to conserve core body temperature at the expense of the distal extremities. Frostbite generally affects exposed areas, such as the toes, feet, fingers, nose, cheeks, and ears. Rarely, frostbite has resulted elsewhere from application of an ice pack[234] or from improper use of commercially available cryotherapy devices for wart removal.[235]

Four degrees of severity have been described. Frostnip, or first-degree frostbite, shows redness, edema, and transient discomfort. In mild cases, the affected area returns to normal within a period of a few hours with at most mild desquamation. Second-degree frostbite presents with marked erythema and swelling; the numbness is replaced by burning pain and, in a period of 24–48 h, vesicles and bullae appear. Although healing occurs, patients may show continuing sensory neuropathy and cold sensitivity. In third-degree frostbite hemorrhagic bullae or waxy, mummified skin is seen, consistent with extensive tissue loss. Full-thickness involvement of the skin, muscle, tendon, and bone occurs in fourth-degree frostbite; although recovery is possible, amputation (either surgical or autoamputation) results in most patients.[236]

The current goal of treatment is rapid rewarming to prevent further cold exposure and restore circulation.[237] The water bath temperature should be at least 40°C (104°F). Slow rewarming, use of dry heat, and rubbing with ice are all contraindicated. Pain during the thawing and immediately after thawing should be treated with potent analgesics and sedatives. Core warming and fluid resuscitation are also important in hypothermic patients. Other measures include wound care, administration of tetanus toxoid, avoidance of pressure and even light contact with the affected area, and vigorous treatment of infection when present. Thrombolytic therapy with intra-arterial infusion of tissue plasminogen activator can improve perfusion.[237] If surgical measures are required, they should be delayed as long as possible. Since the prediction of tissue loss is difficult, amputation of necrotic tissue is best deferred for a period of at least 60–90 days to allow time for contracture, shrinkage, and the formation of a definitive line of demarcation between necrotic and viable tissue.

Trench Foot (Immersion Foot)

Trench foot is a cold-induced non-freezing injury of the extremities that occurs in individuals constantly exposed to a wet and cold environment. The disorder resembles a mild to moderate frostbite, has predominantly been noted in the homeless,[238] and is uncommon in children.

During exposure there is usually an initial uncomfortable feeling of coldness followed by virtually no discomfort and, at times, a feeling of warmth as the nerves become sensitive. The limb becomes cold, numb, blue, swollen, and pulseless. The pain is aggravated by heat and relieved by cold. The ischemic tissue is prone to infection. In severe cases there is muscle weakness, joint stiffness, and gangrene that usually heals without tissue loss. A form of immersion foot has also been described in patients exposed to warm water for long periods of time. This disorder, characterized by a wrinkling, blanching, and maceration of the skin on the plantar and lateral aspects of the feet, has largely been reported in military personnel in tropical areas and in individuals who wear insulated boots for long periods of time. This form is generally reversible, leaving no residual disability.

Prevention is the best treatment. The skin should be rapidly dried should the condition occur. In the warm water form of immersion foot, the application of a silicone grease prior to water immersion may be helpful.

Perniosis

Perniosis (chilblains) is an exaggerated response to cold in predisposed individuals.[239] In pediatric patients, it largely is seen in teenagers, but has been described in younger children.[240] It has been noted in several adolescents with anorexia nervosa,[241] and may relate to impaired thermoregulation. Wet linings in shoe boots have also been blamed. Characterized by the occurrence of localized cyanosis, erythematous nodules, or ulcerations on exposed extremities in cold and damp weather, the disorder is most common in Northern Europe and the northern USA. Perniotic lesions may also be seen in patients with lupus erythematosus (see Ch. 22), hemolytic anemia, and chronic myelomonocytic leukemia.[242] Chilblain-like lesions on the fingers and toes are seen in 40% of children with Aicardi–Goutieres syndrome, a genetic disorder that is almost always associated with microcephaly and severe neurologic disease with developmental delay. Affected infants usually show the chilblain-like lesions in the first year and may develop digital ischemia. Biopsies may resemble lupus erythematosus[243] and autoimmune antibodies may be present. This autosomal recessive disorder results from mutations in genes encoding the DNA exonuclease TREX1 (AGS1) or components of the RNASEH2 endonuclease complex (AGS2, AGS3, AGS4).[244] Familial chilblain lupus has also been linked to heterozygous mutations in TREX1.

Mild cases of perniosis are manifested by an initial blanching, and then by ill-defined erythematous macules that become infiltrated and vary from a dark pink to a violaceous hue. In most cases the disorder is characterized by edematous patches of erythema or cyanosis that appear 12–24 h after exposure to cold. Initially patients are usually unaware of the disorder. With time the areas become edematous and bluish red, and eventually develop numbness, tingling, pruritus, burning, or pain.

Individual lesions tend to appear in a symmetrical distribution, principally on the dorsal aspect of the phalanges of the fingers (Fig. 20.46) and toes (Fig. 20.47) and on the heels, lower legs, thighs,

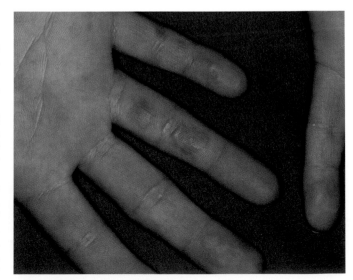

Figure 20.46 Perniosis (chilblains). Edematous red, painful nodules appeared on the fingers after exposure to cold.

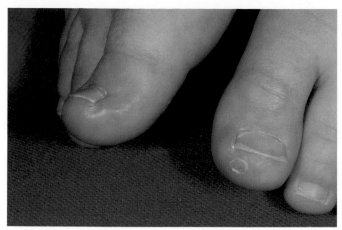

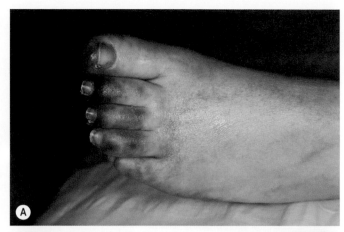

Figure 20.47 Perniosis (chilblains). Note the inflamed nodules on the toes of this adolescent girl. Although nodules resolved, painful nodules continued to develop on an annual basis beginning in January and lasting until April. She was otherwise healthy.

nose, and ears. The course is usually self-limiting and lasts 2 or 3 weeks. In young girls and adolescent women who wear skirts rather than slacks, the calves and shins are common sites of involvement. Chronic perniosis occurs repeatedly during cold weather and disappears during warm weather. Blistering and ulceration occasionally occur and, at times, lesions may heal with residual areas of pigmentation.

Children with more persistent or atypical lesions should have laboratory testing to eliminate possible underlying causes. These include complete blood count, ANA, and cryoglobulin, cryofibrinogen, and cold agglutinin levels (see below). Serum protein electrophoresis levels are usually assessed in affected adults, but the incidence of patients with monoclonal gammopathy is much lower in children. Treatment consists of proper clothing to prevent undue exposure to cold, application of antipruritics, soothing lotions or ointments, and, in severe cases, administration of nifedipine[245,246] or pentoxifylline.[247]

Cold-sensitive Dysproteinemias

The cold-insoluble proteins that precipitate at low temperatures include cryoglobulins, cryofibrinogens, and cold agglutinins. Cryoglobulins are composed of immunoglobulins (see also discussion of cryoglobulinemia and its subtypes, in Ch. 21), often in association with hepatitis C virus RNA.[248] Cryofibrinogenemia involves increased circulating levels of fibrinogens (as well as fibrins and fibrin-split products) that gel in the cold.[249,250] In contrast to cryoglobulins, which may be found in serum samples, cryofibrinogens are consumed in clotting, and thus are only present in plasma samples. Cold agglutinins are antibodies that promote aggregation of erythrocytes with cold exposure, and are most commonly found in pediatric patients with mycoplasmal infection, although association with EBV has also been described.[251] Because cryoproteins may precipitate at a temperature as high as 35°C, the blood sample for testing must be maintained at 37°C until centrifugation. For testing, the sample is chilled to 4°C for 72 h.

The most common manifestation of cold-induced dysproteinemia is palpable purpura that is often retiform (net-like) (see Ch. 21) and can progress to severe vasoocclusion (Fig. 20.48). Most individuals with cold-related occlusion syndromes have circulating cryoglobulins, rather than cryofibrinogens or cold agglutinins. Other manifestations of increased levels of circulating cryoglobulins

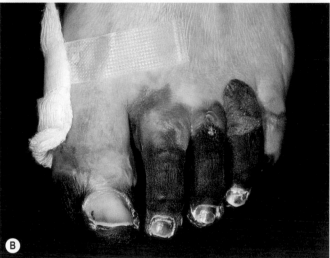

Figure 20.48 Cryoglobulinemia. In this patient, palpable purpura and early vasoocclusion (A) progressed within 24 h to severe vasoocclusion (B), requiring digital amputation.

are urticaria, urticarial vasculitis, cold urticaria, livedo reticularis, pernio, Raynaud phenomenon, acral bullae, and digital ulcerations. In children, cryofibrinogenemia usually occurs as a secondary disorder related to infection.[252] The most common visceral manifestations of cryofibrinogenemia are arthralgias, weakness, neuropathy, and glomerulonephritis. A rare autosomal dominant form has been described in children and is characterized by painful purpura, slow healing of small ulcerations, and pedal edema during the winter season.[253] If cold agglutinins cause clinical problems, the typical manifestation is hemolysis; acrocyanosis, Raynaud phenomenon, livedo reticularis, and necrosis have rarely been described. Identification and treatment of the underlying disorder, as well as cold avoidance, are important.

Cutaneous reactions to heat

Burns are the most common adverse reaction to heat. (Burns and branding injuries are discussed in Ch. 26.) Erythema ab igne rarely occurs in the industrialized world with central heating.

Erythema Ab Igne

Erythema ab igne is an acquired persistent reticulated erythematous and pigmented condition of the skin produced by prolonged or

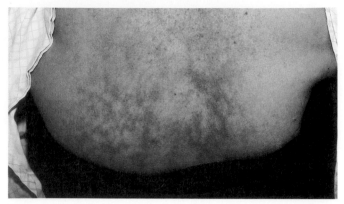

Figure 20.49 Erythema ab igne. Reticulated brown pigmentation on the lower back following prolonged exposure to a heating appliance.

repeated exposure to moderately intense, but not burning, heat. It most commonly occurs from use of heating pads, but has been described after exposure to heat from fireplaces, hot water bottles, radiators, heating elements in cars,[254] and heating blankets in the intensive care unit,[255] and on the thighs from exposure to laptop computers.[256,257]

The disorder is characterized by a mottled appearance of the skin exposed to the heat and eventually is manifested by a reticulated, annular, or gyrate erythema that progresses to a pale-pink to purplish dark-brown color with superficial venular telangiectasia and hyperpigmentation (Fig. 20.49). As in burn scars, squamous cell carcinomas have been reported in plaques of erythema ab igne. When present, these carcinomas tend to be aggressive, with metastases occurring in more than 30% of cases.

Treatment of erythema ab igne consists of protection from further exposure to the offending heat source. Once exposure to heat is discontinued the erythema may fade, but the hyperpigmented changes are frequently permanent.

Scombroid and ciguatera fish poisoning

Scombroid fish poisoning (scombrotoxism) is a clinical syndrome that results from the ingestion of spoiled fish of the Scombroidea family (tuna, mackerel, and bonito) and fish such as bluefish, mahi-mahi, amberjack, herring, sardines, and anchovies.[258,259] The disorder, thought to be related to high levels of histamine and saurine produced when these fish are improperly refrigerated, is characterized by pruritus, a diffuse erythema of the face and upper body, somewhat resembling a sunburn and, at times, giant hive-like lesions that develop within minutes to hours after ingestion of the toxic fish. Symptoms resemble a histamine reaction and frequently include a hot burning sensation rather than pruritus. The conjunctivae are often markedly injected, and many patients have a severe throbbing headache, tachycardia, palpitations, nausea, vomiting, abdominal cramps, diarrhea, dryness and a burning sensation or peppery taste in the mouth, urticaria, angioneurotic edema, oral blistering, hypotension, blurred vision, and asthma-like symptoms. Although superficially resembling an allergic reaction, patients with scombroid fish poisoning can be reassured that they do not have fish allergy and that scombroidosis will not occur when fish are handled properly. Symptoms are generally self-limiting and even if untreated tend to resolve within 8–10 h. Most patients treated with oral antihistamines become asymptomatic within 2 or 3 h.

In contrast to scombroid fish poisoning, *ciguatera fish poisoning* is a common disorder endemic throughout the Caribbean and Indo-Pacific islands, but has been reported in the USA. It is caused by the ingestion of ciguatoxin,[259] which originates from a dinoflagellate (*Gambierdiscus toxicus*). Present in certain fish such as the red snapper, amberjack, and sturgeon fish, ingestion of affected fish (whether cooked, raw, or frozen) may result in this disorder. Clinical symptoms, which usually appear within 12 h but sometimes within minutes after ingestion of ciguatoxin, include abdominal pain, cramping, diarrhea, nausea, vomiting, paresthesias, pain or burning when cold water is touched, arthralgia, myalgia, and, in severe cases, hypotension, shock, respiratory depression, paralysis, coma, and death. The duration of illness averages 8.5 days but may be prolonged. Treatment consists of supportive measures, and intravenous mannitol has been found to be extremely effective, lessening the neurologic and muscular dysfunction of affected patients within minutes of administration.[260]

Sweet's syndrome (acute febrile neutrophilic dermatosis)

Acute febrile neutrophilic dermatosis (Sweet's syndrome) is characterized by raised painful papules, nodules, plaques, or bullae on the limbs, face, and neck, accompanied by fever and leukocytosis.[261] Many children have a history of upper respiratory tract illness 1–3 weeks before the onset of lesions. The disorder has been described in an infant as young as the first weeks of life[262] but only 5% of cases are in children;[263] it is most frequent in women between 35 and 66 years of age.

Although commonly 'idiopathic', 58% of children with Sweet's syndrome have an associated underlying disease, which is usually uncovered by complete history and physical examination, as well as a complete blood count with smear evaluation. Most of these are 'parainflammatory' conditions with infection, particularly upper respiratory infection 1–3 weeks before the eruption. Otitis media, viral meningitis, and human immunodeficiency virus[264] may also occur, with or without immunodeficiency[265] (T-cell deficiency,[266] common variable immunodeficiency,[267] glycogen storage disease with neutropenia, and chronic granulomatous disease[268]). Other associated inflammatory disorders are inflammatory bowel disease, systemic lupus erythematosus,[269,270] chronic multifocal osteomyelitis, vasculitis,[261] and Takayasu arteritis. Approximately 25% of children with Sweet's syndrome have an underlying neoplastic or premalignant disorder (myelogenous leukemia, juvenile myelomonocytic leukemia,[264] myelodysplastic syndrome,[271] acute lymphoblastic leukemia, osteosarcoma, aplastic anemia, or Fanconi anemia[272]). Paraneoplastic Sweet's syndrome more often presents on the face and mucosa. In these cases, the Sweet's syndrome manifested simultaneously with the malignancy, suggesting that the possibility of malignancy must be investigated upon presentation but is unlikely to develop after the initial evaluation. Drugs have been linked to Sweet's syndrome: granulocyte or granulocyte-macrophage colony-stimulating factor,[273] all-transretinoic acid,[274] trimethoprim–sulfamethoxazole, carbamazepine, imatinib, and minocycline, but in each case the patient had an underlying inflammatory or neoplastic disorder.

Patients with acute febrile neutrophilic dermatosis usually have spiking fevers early in the course associated with raised, brightly erythematous, painful papules, plaques, or nodules asymmetrically distributed on the face, neck, and limbs (particularly the upper arms), with sparing of the areas between the upper chest and thighs. Lesions often occur in crops and pathergy is common. Elevated plaques measure 1 cm or more in diameter, are distributed in an asymmetric pattern, and tend to develop partial clearing, resulting in an arcuate configuration as the border of the lesion advances (Fig. 20.50). They are indurated, red to plum-colored, and heal without scarring, often leaving a residual reddish brown color (Fig. 20.51). Larger plaques frequently have a mammillated surface from edema that simulates vesicles, but is firm to palpation.

Leukocytosis ranging from 15 000–20 000 (with 80–90% polymorphonuclear leukocytes) is common and myalgia, polyarthralgia, and polyarthritis of large joints have been reported in 15–25% of patients.[275] The fever precedes the cutaneous eruption by days to weeks in at least 50% of patients. Conjunctivitis and episcleritis may be present. Systemic inflammatory response syndrome with septic shock and multiorgan dysfunction has been associated in one child.[276] Rarely, post-inflammatory slack skin with arterial laxity and

aortic or mitral valve regurgitation has followed Sweet's syndrome;[277,278] these children may develop potentially fatal coronary artery disease.[279,280]

Acute febrile neutrophilic dermatosis generally presents a fairly characteristic clinical picture that can be confirmed by cutaneous biopsy. To establish the diagnosis, it has been suggested that patients must fulfill both major criteria and at least two of the minor criteria (Table 20.10). Biopsy specimens show a dense dermal perivascular infiltration of polymorphonuclear leukocytes, sometimes with nuclear dust, but without vasculitis. A similar histologic picture can be seen in patients with neutrophilic urticarial dermatosis, usually related to underlying systemic lupus erythematosus in pediatric patients,[281] but distinguishable clinically from Sweet's syndrome by urticarial macules or plaques without edema and lasting <24 h.

If untreated, lesions of Sweet's syndrome may extend and persist for up to a year, eventually resolving spontaneously without residual scarring. Patients generally respond to systemic corticosteroids (1–2 mg/kg per day) within a few days. Once the patient responds, the systemic corticosteroids should be tapered gradually over 2–3 months in an effort to prevent recurrences; some patients respond to corticosteroids but flare with withdrawal. Potassium iodide, colchicine, dapsone, methotrexate, cyclosporine and chlorambucil are treatment alternatives.

Bowel-associated dermatosis-arthritis syndrome

Bowel-associated dermatosis-arthritis syndrome (intestinal bypass disease, bowel bypass syndrome) was originally described as a complication of jejunoileal bypass surgery, which is only rarely performed in an adolescent for obesity.[282] However, the disorder has also been described in individuals with gastrointestinal disorders, including inflammatory bowel disease.[283] The disorder is characterized by a flu-like illness (chills, malaise, and myalgia), asymmetric polyarthritis, tenosynovitis, thrombophlebitis, retinal vasculitis, and crops of skin lesions. Lesions are most often seen on the arms and hands and less often on the shoulders and flanks. They are generally asymptomatic or mildly pruritic. Lesions begin as 3–10 mm erythematous macules, which develop into purpuric vesiculopustules that undergo central necrosis and resemble insect bites. Lesions over acral areas may be painful and often mimic the pustulovesicular lesions of gonococcemia; lesions on the shins or ankles, which are generally erythematous, tender nodules, may be mistaken for erythema nodosum.

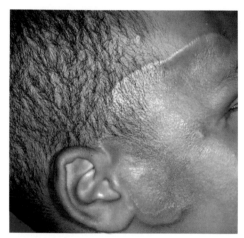

Figure 20.50 Sweet's syndrome. Asymmetric indurated annular plaques.

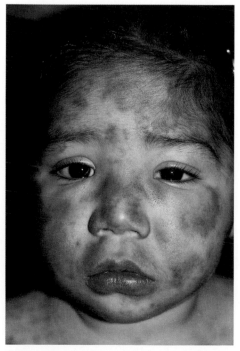

Figure 20.51 Sweet's syndrome. Asymmetrically distributed indurated plum-colored plaques and nodules. (Courtesy of Dr Sarah Chamlin.)

Table 20.10 Major and minor criteria for diagnosis of Sweet's syndrome
Major criteria
Abrupt onset of tender or painful erythematous or violaceous plaques or nodules
Predominantly neutrophilic infiltration of the dermis without leukocytoclastic vasculitis
Minor criteria
Illness preceded by fever or infection
Fever accompanied by arthralgia, conjunctivitis, or underlying malignancy
Leukocytosis >10 000/mm³
Good response to systemic corticosteroids and lack of response to antibiotics

The eruption usually lasts for 2–6 days and recurs at varying intervals for weeks to months. It is thought to result from bacterial overgrowth in blind intestinal loops and production of circulating immune complexes directed against the bacterial peptidoglycans. Biopsies of skin show a massive dermal infiltrate of neutrophils showing leukocytoclasia and occasionally a necrotizing vasculitis; some patients show lobular neutrophilic and septal panniculitis.

Short-term treatment of 10–20 mg/day of prednisone markedly ameliorates the cutaneous and rheumatologic manifestations. Tetracycline, minocycline, metronidazole, clindamycin, sulfisoxazole, and dapsone have been suggested for both acute exacerbations and chronic prophylaxis. Surgical revision is curative.

Hypereosinophilic syndrome

Hypereosinophilic syndrome is a multisystemic disorder characterized by peripheral blood eosinophilia of at least 1500 eosinophils/μL without parasitic or allergic causes. Characteristically, the increase in eosinophils is present for ≥6 months and is associated with infiltration of organs by eosinophils.[284] The condition is seen primarily in middle-aged men, but pediatric patients have been described.[285,286] The pathogenesis of the hypereosinophilic syndrome remains unknown, but many affected individuals have myeloproliferative disorders. The activated eosinophils are thought to cause the end-organ damage.

The manifestations can be variable, and almost any organ system can be involved. Approximately 50% of patients demonstrate cutaneous involvement. Pruritic erythematous or hyperpigmented macules, papules, serpiginous lesions with vesicles, purpuric papules (Fig. 20.52), splinter hemorrhages, nailfold infarcts, urticaria, Wells syndrome (see below), erythema annulare, diffuse erythema, angioedema, livedo reticularis, and nodules, some of which are ulcerated, and mucosal ulcers have been described. These lesions may appear anywhere on the body but are generally present over the trunk and extremities.

Except for the blood and bone marrow involvement, cardiovascular disease is the major cause of morbidity and mortality. The heart often shows restrictive cardiomyopathy and subendocardial fibrosis; myocardial infarction may result.[285] Pulmonary complications (seen in 40% of patients) include interstitial infiltrates, a persistent nonproductive cough, and pleural effusion. Neurologic findings include hemiparesis, dysesthesias or paresthesias, slurred speech, confusion, and, at times, coma. Affected individuals often show hepatosplenomegaly. Hepatic dysfunction and diarrhea, with or without malabsorption, and renal involvement with persistent hematuria and hypouricemia have also been reported.

Recent reclassification of pathogenesis-based subsets of hypereosinophilic syndrome and disease-specific treatment advances has altered the approach to patients. Systemic corticosteroids are the treatment of choice for most pediatric patients, but monoclonal antibody therapy directed against IL-5 is another option[287] and imatinib has revolutionized the therapy for patients with the myeloproliferative form of the hypereosinophilic syndromes.

Wells syndrome

Wells syndrome (eosinophilic cellulitis) occasionally occurs in pediatric patients, including in neonates and young children.[288–291] The condition starts with a prodromal burning sensation or itching and spreads rapidly for 2 or 3 days. Patients most commonly show sudden outbreaks of erythematous, often painful or pruritic, edematous urticarial or cellulitis-like plaques, often with sharp pink or violaceous borders. The morphology of lesions can vary. Although most children show plaque-type Wells lesions, annular granuloma-like lesions, papulovesicular, papulonodular, urticarial, bullous, and fixed drug-like lesions have been described. Lesions most commonly affect the lower limbs, followed in frequency by the upper limbs, trunk, face, scalp and neck. The disorder gradually subsides over 2–8 weeks to be replaced by blue or slate-colored indurated patches that slowly fade. Recurrences are typical. The preceding history of insect bites, parvovirus B19 infection,[292] fungal infections, drug eruptions (particularly penicillin), reactions to vaccinations,[293] or underlying hematologic disease in some patients suggests that Wells syndrome represents a hypersensitivity reaction.

The clinical picture is striking, and the affected areas frequently resemble acute bacterial cellulitis, urticaria, insect bites, or a vesiculobullous contact dermatitis. Biopsy is usually necessary to confirm the diagnosis, and shows diffuse infiltration of eosinophils throughout the dermis with 'flame figures', which can be seen in a variety of disorders of eosinophil activation. Peripheral eosinophilia is common. Although the prognosis of Wells syndrome is generally excellent, and most lesions tend to fade spontaneously, systemic corticosteroids hasten resolution. Dapsone, griseofulvin, minocycline, cyclosporine, and colchicine have sometimes been found to be effective.

Pregnancy and pregnancy-related dermatoses

Pregnant adolescents may show a variety of physiologic changes during their pregnancy and postpartum periods (Table 20.11). In addition to these physiologic changes, a variety of pruritic dermatoses in association with pregnancy have been described. Although controversial, the specific dermatoses of pregnancy have recently been re-classified into pemphigoid gestationis (4.2%); pruritic urticarial papules and plaques of pregnancy (PUPPP) (21.6%); cholestasis of pregnancy (3%); a new category of atopic eruption of pregnancy, which includes eczema during pregnancy (49.7%), prurigo of pregnancy (0.8%), and pruritic folliculitis of pregnancy (0.2%); and miscellaneous dermatoses (20.6%) (Table

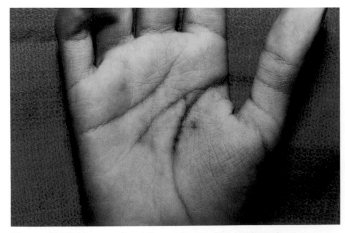

Figure 20.52 Hypereosinophilic syndrome. This patient shows purpuric areas on the palms, but a wide variety of cutaneous manifestations occur in 50% of patients, ranging from pruritic erythematous or hyperpigmented macules and papules to serpiginous lesions with vesicles to purpuric papules, petechiae, and livedo reticularis.

Table 20.11 Most common physiologic changes of pregnancy and the postpartum period

Skin
Striae
Acrochordons
Vascular
Palmar erythema
Hemorrhoids
Varicosities
Edema, non-pitting
Spider angiomas
Pyogenic granulomas
Pigment
Melasma
Linea nigra
Hyperpigmentation of the areolae
Hair
Hirsutism
Postpartum alopecia
Telogen effluvium
Androgenetic alopecia
Nail dystrophy

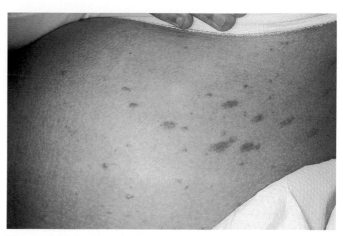

Figure 20.53 Pruritic urticarial papules and plaques of pregnancy (PUPPP). Note the small erythematous papules and urticarial wheals on the distended abdomen of this pregnant adolescent.

Table 20.12 Classification of pruritic dermatoses of pregnancy

Name	Alternate names	Risk to fetus
Pemphigoid gestationis	Herpes gestationis Gestational pemphigoid	Increased risk of prematurity and small-for-gestational age babies
Pruritic urticarial papules and plaques of pregnancy (PUPPP)	Toxic erythema of pregnancy Polymorphic eruption of pregnancy (PEP)	None
Atopic eruption of pregnancy Eczema in pregnancy Prurigo of pregnancy	Prurigo gestationis (of Besnier) Papular dermatitis of pregnancy Early onset prurigo of pregnancy Pruritic folliculitis of pregnancy	None
Cholestasis of pregnancy	Obstetric cholestasis Intrahepatic cholestasis of pregnancy	Increased risk of premature labor, fetal distress, meconium staining, and fetal death

20.12).[294–296] Pustular psoriasis (see Ch. 4) may be triggered by pregnancy as well, and presents during the 3rd trimester with erythematous patches studded with subcorneal pustules. *Pustular psoriasis of pregnancy* (also called impetigo herpetiformis) may lead to stillbirth or neonatal death because of placental insufficiency. Apart from *pemphigoid gestationis*, an intensely pruritic immune-mediated blistering eruption (reviewed in Ch. 13), the cause of pregnancy-related dermatoses is unknown.

Pruritic urticarial papules and plaques of pregnancy (PUPPP, also called polymorphic eruption of pregnancy or PEP) is the most common cutaneous disorder specifically related to pregnancy. Intensely pruritic, the dermatitis occurs late in the 3rd trimester or in the immediate postpartum period. It occurs in approximately 1 in 160 pregnancies and 75% of the time affects a primigravida.[297] The disorder has only once been described in the neonate of an affected mother (in contrast to pemphigoid gestationis).[298] This is a disorder of exclusion, and no diagnostic test is available.

The condition usually begins as 1–2 mm urticarial papules on the abdomen (Fig. 20.53), often within the abdominal striae. These papules soon coalesce to form large erythematous plaques and then spread to involve the abdomen, buttocks, thighs, and, in some cases, the arms and legs. The upper chest, face, palms, soles, and mucous membranes tend to be spared. Although pruritus is frequently extreme and patients are often unable to sleep, excoriations are rare. Topical application of corticosteroids usually provides symptomatic relief; if the condition is severe or unresponsive to topical medication, brief courses of systemic corticosteroids are frequently beneficial.

Intrahepatic cholestasis of pregnancy occurs in 1 in 1500 pregnancies (20% of cases of obstetrical jaundice) and is characterized by intense pruritus. The only skin lesions are excoriations. By definition, affected females have generalized pruritus, without history of exposure to hepatitis or hepatotoxic drugs, with appearance usually during the last trimester of pregnancy and disappearance within 2–4 weeks after delivery. The condition tends to recur during subsequent pregnancies in 65% of affected women, and has been associated with risks to the fetus (Table 20.12). The risk with twin pregnancies is higher and a positive family history is seen in 50% of affected individuals.

Pruritus tends to be worse at night, and on the trunk, palms, and soles. No primary skin lesions are seen. Approximately half of affected patients show jaundice, dark urine, or stools light in color. More severely affected women may have malabsorption, including that of vitamin K. The diagnosis can be confirmed by finding increased serum bile acids, without evidence of viral hepatitis or another explanation. Treatments include rest and a low-fat diet, cholestyramine, oral guar gum (a dietary fiber that lowers bile acid levels), and ursodeoxycholic acid (which can substitute for more toxic bile acids).

Prurigo of pregnancy is a term used to describe a heterogeneous group of disorders that occurs earlier than PUPPP, usually in mid-trimester, and is now included as part of *atopic eruption of pregnancy* (Table 20.12). Cholestasis as a cause of pruritus must be eliminated through finding normal liver function tests. *Pruritic folliculitis of pregnancy*, a subset of prurigo of pregnancy, presents between the fourth and ninth months of pregnancy as a pruritic follicular papular and pustular eruption and generally resolves within a few weeks after delivery. Eczema in pregnancy presents, most commonly during the 2nd trimester, as eczematous patches and plaques that can be generalized. Topical application of corticosteroids or narrow band UVB light have been helpful in the management of this subset of patients.

Autoimmune progesterone dermatitis

This rare disorder most commonly begins at menarche and is thought to represent an autosensitivity reaction to progesterone.[299] It thereafter occurs approximately 3–10 days prior to the onset of menstrual flow and ends approximately 2 days into menses. It may also be seen in individuals on anovulatory hormone therapy and in pregnant women during the 1st trimester of pregnancy. The condition is characterized by urticarial vesiculobullae, papules, pustules, erythema multiforme, and dyshidrotic eczema-like eruptions on the extensor surfaces of the thighs, forearms, hands, and buttocks.[300,301] Rarely, the disorder may manifest with angioedema and laryngeal spasms requiring epinephrine administration.[302]

The diagnosis of autoimmune progesterone dermatitis can be confirmed by an urticarial wheal at the site of intradermal skin test to an aqueous progesterone suspension. Treatment consists of estrogens or tamoxifen. Oophorectomy can be considered for patients unresponsive to other modes of therapy.

Eccrine hidradenitis

Idiopathic palmoplantar hidradenitis occurs suddenly in otherwise healthy children as erythematous painful nodules on the palms and soles. The condition has been linked to vigorous physical activity, excessive sweating, and prolonged exposure to moisture. Lesional biopsies show neutrophilic perieccrine infiltrates, and the lesions are thought to result from mechanical rupture of the eccrine glands. Plantar surfaces are more commonly involved, leading to consideration of erythema nodosum, erythema multiforme, bite reactions, chilblains, cellulitis, and embolic disease. Although episodes recur in up to 50% of children, resolution typically occurs in 1–4 weeks,

especially with rest. Therapy with topical and systemic corticosteroids and nonsteroidal anti-inflammatory medications is not clearly beneficial.

Another form of eccrine hidradenitis is neutrophilic eccrine hidradenitis, a complication of cancer chemotherapy. Neutrophilic eccrine hidradenitis tends to develop 7–14 days after initiating chemotherapy, most commonly cytarabine. The disorder reflects the direct cytotoxicity of chemotherapy to the eccrine glands. Affected children are usually febrile, and the eruption is most commonly characterized by erythematous papules and plaques on the trunk, extremities, and face.

Key References

The complete list of 302 references for this chapter is available online at: **www.expertconsult.com.**
See inside cover for registration details.

Bailey E, Shaker M. An update on childhood urticaria and angioedema. *Curr Opin Pediatr.* 2008;20:425–430.

Berk DR, Bayliss SJ. Neutrophilic dermatoses in children. *Pediatr Dermatol.* 2008;25:509–519.

Caputo R, Marzano AV, Vezzoli P, et al. Wells syndrome in adults and children: a report of 19 cases. *Arch Dermatol.* 2006;142:1157–1161.

Farkas H, Varga L, Szeplaki G, et al. Management of hereditary angioedema in pediatric patients. *Pediatrics.* 2007;120:e713–e722.

Grosber M, Alexandre M, Poszepczynska-Guigne E, et al. Recurrent erythema multiforme in association with recurrent Mycoplasma pneumoniae infections. *J Am Acad Dermatol.* 2007;56:S118–S119.

Hospach T, von den Driesch P, Dannecker GE. Acute febrile neutrophilic dermatosis (Sweet's syndrome) in childhood and adolescence: two new patients and review of the literature on associated diseases. *Eur J Pediatr.* 2009;168:1–9.

Koh MJ, Tay YK. An update on Stevens-Johnson syndrome and toxic epidermal necrolysis in children. *Curr Opin Pediatr.* 2009; 21:505–510.

Schneck J, Fagot JP, Sekula P, et al. Effects of treatments on the mortality of Stevens-Johnson syndrome and toxic epidermal necrolysis: A retrospective study on patients included in the prospective EuroSCAR Study. *J Am Acad Dermatol.* 2008;58:33–40.

Segal AR, Doherty KM, Leggott J, et al. Cutaneous reactions to drugs in children. *Pediatrics.* 2007;120:e1082–e1096.

Shah KN, Honig PJ, Yan AC. 'Urticaria multiforme': a case series and review of acute annular urticarial hypersensitivity syndromes in children. *Pediatrics.* 2007;119:e1177–e1183.

Torrelo A, Hernandez A. Panniculitis in children. *Dermatol Clin.* 2008;26:491–500, vii.

Vasculitic Disorders

21

The term 'vasculitis' refers to inflammation of blood vessels, a finding that can be seen in association with a variety of clinical manifestations, and as either a primary or secondary phenomenon. Along with vessel inflammation, there is deposition of fibrinoid material in vessel walls and the presence of nuclear fragments (nuclear dust) resulting from disintegration of neutrophilic nuclei (karyorrhexis) within the vessel wall and surrounding tissues (hence the terminology 'leukocytoclastic' vasculitis).

The vasculitic disorders are a heterogeneous group of conditions, many of which present with (or eventually result in) cutaneous manifestations. Classification of the vasculitides is difficult, and has most often been based on the gross and microscopic features of the disease process, primarily the vessel size involved (i.e., large, medium-sized, or small). Large-vessel vasculitides, which will not be discussed here, include giant cell (temporal) arteritis and Takayasu arteritis. Medium-sized vasculitides involve predominantly visceral arteries and include two of the most common forms of pediatric vasculitis syndromes, polyarteritis nodosa and Kawasaki disease, both of which will be discussed. The other entities covered in this chapter all represent small-vessel disorders, which tend to involve primarily capillaries and venules. It should be remembered that this classification of vasculitis based on vessel size is imprecise, and overlap in the size of involved vessels is common. A summary classification of pediatric vasculitides is shown in Table 21.1.

Henoch–Schönlein (anaphylactoid) purpura

Henoch–Schönlein purpura (HSP), also known as *anaphylactoid purpura*, is a form of small-vessel vasculitis that occurs primarily in children (especially boys) between 2 and 11 years of age. The classic presentation is a combination of non-thrombocytopenic palpable purpura in dependent areas, arthritis, abdominal pain, and glomerulonephritis. HSP is an inflammatory disorder that has been linked hypothetically to several potential etiologic agents, including group A beta-hemolytic streptococci (GABHS), other bacterial or viral organisms, immunizations, and drugs, although the exact etiology remains unclear.[1] There are reports of patients with co-existing HSP and acute rheumatic fever, highlighting the potential association between GABHS and HSP.[2] *Bartonella henselae* has also been suggested as a potential etiologic infectious agent.[3] Although the nature of the immunologic reaction in HSP is not completely clear, the frequent history of antecedent upper respiratory tract infection preceding the onset of symptoms suggests a hypersensitivity phenomenon resulting in localized or widespread vascular damage. A fairly consistent immunologic observation is the deposition of IgA immune complexes in affected organs (i.e., skin, kidneys) when studied by immunofluorescence. IgA complexes, however, are not a necessary requirement for the development of HSP and their absence should not exclude the diagnosis. Around one-third of patients have elevated serum IgA levels.[4] Several polymorphisms involving cytokines and cell adhesion molecules which modulate inflammatory responses and endothelial cell activation have been observed, and may correlate with disease susceptibility, extent of involvement and/or severity of renal disease.[5]

The clinical picture of HSP is often, but not always, distinctive. Most patients with a rash present with an initial urticarial eruption of macules and papules (Fig. 21.1), which rapidly become purpuric and are distributed primarily on the lower extremities (Figs 21.2–21.4) and buttocks (Fig. 21.5). Lesions may also occur on the upper extremities, trunk, and face, and in some instances, skin lesions may develop in patterns at pressure sites. In some patients, petechiae (Fig. 21.6) or ecchymoses ('bruises') (Fig. 21.7) may predominate over palpable purpuric lesions. The cutaneous eruption is the presenting feature of HSP in 50% of cases.[1] Newer purpuric lesions develop, and may result in a polymorphous appearance. Other skin lesion morphologies, including vesicular or bullous lesions, erosions or ulcers, necrosis, gangrene, and even erythema multiforme-like lesions, may occur.[6,7] Marked edema of the hands, feet, scalp, or face may also be seen, especially in younger patients.[1,8] The disease often consists of a single episode, which may last for several days to weeks, but in some cases recurrent attacks may occur at intervals for weeks to months.

Individual lesions of HSP occur in crops, tend to fade after about 5 days, and eventually are replaced by areas of hyperpigmentation or ecchymoses. Although the differential diagnosis of the skin lesions may include drug reaction, erythema multiforme, or urticaria, the presence of *palpable purpura* (the hallmark of leukocytoclastic vasculitis) will usually clarify the true nature of the disorder. This characteristic finding, created by edema and extravasation of erythrocytes, gives individual lesions their diagnostic palpable and purpuric appearance as well as their non-blanching quality (i.e., individual lesions cannot be blanched when viewed through a glass slide exerting pressure over the surface – a technique called diascopy).

Occasionally the face, mucous membranes of the mouth and nose, and the anogenital regions may show petechiae. In males, vasculitis of the scrotal vessels may lead to acute scrotal swelling, with or without erythema or purpura (Fig. 21.8). Pain may be severe, and this presentation may mimic that of testicular torsion, necessitating ultrasonography and/or radionuclide scans in order to differentiate between these disorders. In one study, roughly 20% of males with HSP had scrotal involvement, and these patients were noted to have an association with headache, edema and elevated C3 levels.[9]

Systemic involvement in HSP, which is seen in up to 80% of cases, most commonly occurs in the kidneys, gastrointestinal tract, and joints. The degree of systemic involvement varies, with joint or gastrointestinal symptoms seen in as many as two-thirds of affected children. Renal disease occurs most frequently, and is the most significant correlate of long-term prognosis.[4]

Table 21.1 Classification of pediatric vasculitides

Predominant vessel size	Disorder
Large	Takayasu arteritis
Medium	Polyarteritis nodosa
	Kawasaki disease
Small	Hypersensitivity vasculitis (cutaneous leukocytoclastic vasculitis)
	Henoch–Schonlein purpura
	Acute hemorrhagic edema of infancy
	Urticarial vasculitis
	Cryoglobulinemic vasculitis
	Erythema elevatum diutinum (primarily adults)
	ANCA-associated:
	Wegener's granulomatosis
	Churg–Strauss syndrome
	Microscopic polyangiitis

ANCA, antineutrophil cytoplasmic antibody.

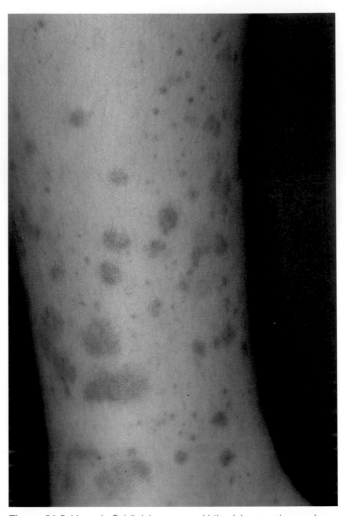

Figure 21.2 Henoch–Schönlein purpura. Urticarial, purpuric papules and plaques on the lower extremity.

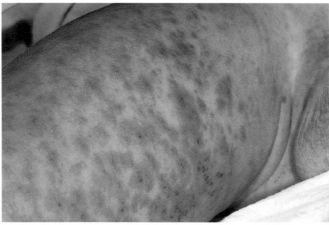

Figure 21.1 Henoch–Schönlein purpura. These early lesions are urticarial in nature. Note associated central erosion/crusting in some of the plaques.

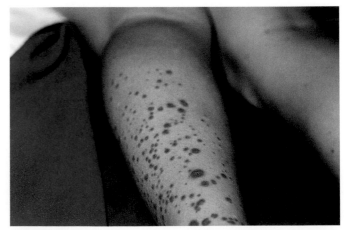

Figure 21.3 Henoch–Schönlein purpura. Palpable purpuric papules and plaques.

The clinical expression of HSP kidney involvement varies, from transient microscopic hematuria to rapidly progressive glomerulonephritis. Glomerulonephritis is seen overall in 40–50% of children with HSP, and is usually transient and benign.[10] The renal lesion in HSP is indistinguishable histopathologically from that of IgA nephropathy (Berger disease), although the latter tends to occur more often in older patients.[1] The renal involvement may not become apparent for several weeks, hence the importance of long-term follow-up for development of this complication. Most often, however, if kidney involvement is going to be seen, it will be found within 3 months of disease onset.[11] Potential correlates of kidney disease in HSP include age over 4 years, persistent purpura, severe abdominal pain, and depressed coagulation factor XIII activity <80%.[11] Initial renal insufficiency appears to be the single best predictor of the further clinical course in children with HSP nephritis.[12]

Gastrointestinal signs and symptoms result from edema and hemorrhage of the bowel wall as a result of vasculitis. They most often include colicky abdominal pain (which may be severe and associated with vomiting), hematochezia, and hematemesis. Vis-

ceral infarction or perforation, pancreatitis, cholecystitis, esophageal involvement, colitis, protein-losing enteropathy, intussusception, hemorrhage, or shock may also be associated. Intussusception, seen in up to 2% of patients, is more common in boys. Since non-HSP-associated intussusception generally occurs in children younger

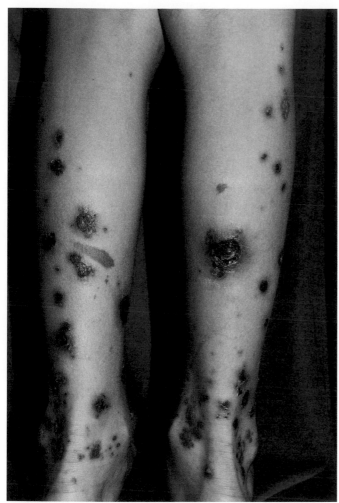

Figure 21.4 Henoch–Schönlein purpura. These purpuric plaques became bullous with subsequent necrosis.

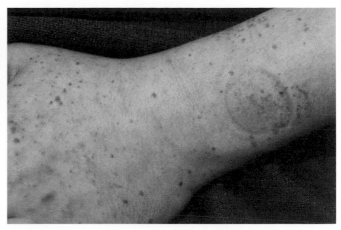

Figure 21.6 Henoch–Schönlein purpura. This patient had small petechial macules of the upper extremities, with larger, more classic purpuric plaques of the buttocks and lower extremities.

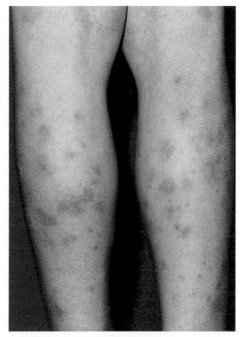

Figure 21.7 Henoch–Schönlein purpura. Occasional patients present with ecchymotic (bruise-like) lesions without classic purpura, as in this 9-year-old male.

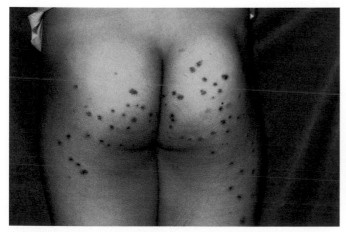

Figure 21.5 Henoch–Schönlein purpura. Palpable purpura of the buttocks, a classic site of involvement in HSP.

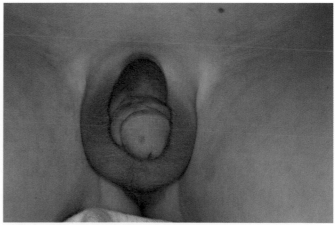

Figure 21.8 Henoch–Schönlein purpura. This patient with HSP developed an acute onset of scrotal pain, with edema and purpuric changes.

than 2 years of age, when intussusception is diagnosed in older children HSP must be strongly considered. Chronic intestinal obstruction with ileal stricture has also been reported, occurring months after resolution of the acute illness.[13]

Joint involvement in HSP is characterized by tender and painful joints with primarily periarticular swelling. True arthritis is less common. Although the ankles and knees are most frequently affected, the elbows, hands, and feet may also be involved. Arthritic symptoms are usually transient and rarely result in permanent deformity.

In addition to the skin, genitourinary and gastrointestinal tracts, and joints, other organ involvement is occasionally seen in HSP. CNS involvement results most commonly in headache, and occasionally behavioral alteration, hyperactivity, intracerebral bleeds, paresis, or seizures.[1,14] Status epilepticus has been rarely reported.[15] Respiratory involvement may range from an asymptomatic pulmonary infiltrate to recurrent episodes of pulmonary hemorrhage. Bleeding diathesis may occasionally occur.

The diagnosis of HSP is seldom difficult when patients present with the classic 'tetrad' of organ involvement (skin, kidneys, gastrointestinal tract, and joints). However, many patients present with only some of these findings, and the differential diagnosis depends on which organ-specific symptoms predominate. The differential diagnosis of palpable purpura may include hypersensitivity vasculitis (usually caused by drug reaction; see Hypersensitivity vasculitis, below), hemorrhagic diathesis (i.e., factor deficiency), or sepsis. In addition, the more 'ecchymotic' lesions of HSP may be mistaken for child abuse,[16] and must be evaluated within the context of the overall clinical presentation. When the diagnosis remains in doubt, histopathologic examination of a skin biopsy specimen is useful in confirming the presence of vasculitis. Direct immunofluorescence revealing IgA immune complexes is highly suggestive of, but not pathognomonic for, HSP. Other laboratory investigations to be considered include serum chemistry profile, blood cell counts, coagulation studies, abdominal radiographic studies, stool guaiac testing, urinalysis, and kidney biopsy.

The overall prognosis for most patients with HSP is excellent, and full recovery without permanent residua is the norm. The disease tends to run its course over 4–6 weeks. In younger children, the disease is generally milder and of shorter duration, with fewer renal and gastrointestinal manifestations and few recurrences. Renal disease is the most important prognostic indicator, and end-stage renal disease may occur in up to 5% of patients with nephritis. Long-term follow-up is indicated in patients with kidney involvement. Recurrent flares of HSP may occur in up to 3% of patients, and in one study had a lag period of 2–26 months following the initial presentation.[17]

Supportive care is sufficient for the majority of patients, and nonsteroidal antiinflammatory agents are useful for significant joint pain. The goals of HSP therapy are to minimize symptoms, decrease short-term morbidities, and prevent chronic renal insufficiency.[18] Systemic corticosteroids have been advocated for patients with severe gastrointestinal, joint, or scrotal involvement, as well as for renal involvement. They are generally not recommended for rash, mild joint pain, or mild abdominal discomfort alone. Various regimens have been recommended for HSP nephritis, including oral methylprednisolone or prednisone, high-dose intravenous pulse methylprednisolone, urokinase, cyclophosphamide, azathioprine, plasma exchange, dipyridamole, and heparin/warfarin.[12,19–23] A meta-analysis revealed that corticosteroids reduced the mean resolution time of abdominal pain, reduced the odds of developing persistent kidney disease, and reduced the odds of both surgical intervention and recurrence.[18]

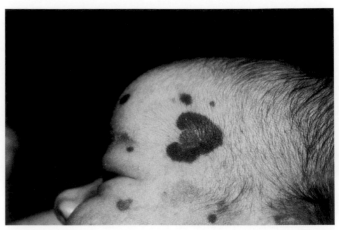

Figure 21.9 Acute hemorrhagic edema of infancy. Medallion-like ('cockade') purpura in a newborn female with congenital onset of the disease.

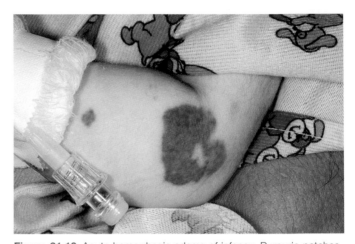

Figure 21.10 Acute hemorrhagic edema of infancy. Purpuric patches with scalloped borders in an infant male with the disorder.

Acute hemorrhagic edema of infancy

Acute hemorrhagic edema of infancy (AHE, acute hemorrhagic edema of childhood, Finkelstein disease) is a form of leukocytoclastic vasculitis characterized by fever, large purpuric skin lesions, and tender edema, and reported most often in infants and children between the ages of 4 months and 3 years. The cutaneous lesions often have a 'cockade' (medallion-like) pattern, with scalloped borders and central clearing (Fig. 21.9). They begin as edematous papules with petechiae and expand centrifugally with coalescence to result in the characteristic clinical pattern (Figs 21.10, 21.11).[24] Facial edema is common. Although the cutaneous eruption may be impressive, the patients are usually otherwise well, and involvement of the gastrointestinal tract, kidneys and joints is uncommon. Intussusception has been rarely observed.[25] The etiology is unclear, although an infectious trigger (i.e., upper respiratory infection, conjunctivitis, pharyngitis, otitis media, or pneumonia) is hypothesized. Prodromal symptoms most often are limited to those of respiratory tract illness or diarrhea.[26]

Skin biopsy in AHE reveals leukocytoclastic vasculitis, similar to HSP. Direct immunofluorescence studies, however, do not consistently reveal IgA deposition, and in up to three-quarters of patients

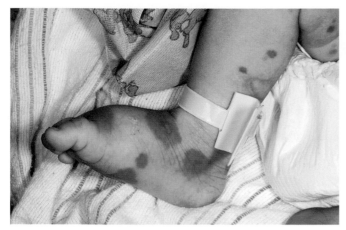

Figure 21.11 Acute hemorrhagic edema of infancy. Multiple purpuric papules and plaques in the same patient shown in Figure 21.10.

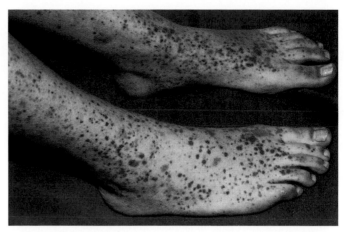

Figure 21.12 Hypersensitivity vasculitis. Multiple purpuric papules in an adolescent female with a drug-induced hypersensitivity vasculitis.

are entirely negative.[24–28] Laboratory findings may include leukocytosis and an elevated erythrocyte sedimentation rate, but hematuria, proteinuria, and hematochezia are usually absent. The course of AHE is marked by a rapid onset with a short benign course followed by complete recovery. No treatment is generally necessary. Although the disorder resembles HSP, controversy exists over whether it represents an infantile form of HSP or whether it is a distinct and unrelated clinical entity. Arguments in favor of the latter include the lack of internal organ involvement, the absence of IgA immune deposits in most patients, and the benign course without a propensity toward recurrences.

Hypersensitivity vasculitis

Hypersensitivity vasculitis (HV, cutaneous small-vessel vasculitis, cutaneous leukocytoclastic vasculitis, cutaneous leukocytoclastic angiitis) is a term used to denote a leukocytoclastic vasculitis involving primarily the skin, and in most cases, secondary to a drug ingestion or infectious process. It is most common in adults, and significantly less common in children, in whom HSP is the most common form of cutaneous vasculitis. Potential infectious etiologies of HV include Streptococci, hepatitis B and C, non-typhoidal *Salmonella* and *Mycobacteria* (both tuberculous and non-tuberculous).[29,30]

The diagnosis of HV is one of exclusion, and other causes of primary cutaneous vasculitis (i.e., HSP, cryoglobulinemic vasculitis) or secondary cutaneous vasculitis (i.e., urticarial vasculitis, connective tissue disorders, malignancy, endocarditis, Behçet disease) must be ruled out. The lesions of HV tend to occur in 'crops' (groups of lesions of similar age) because of simultaneous exposure to the inciting antigen.[31]

Patients with HV most often present with palpable purpura (Fig. 21.12), and less often with urticaria, vesicles, pustules, superficial ulcers, or necrotic lesions. The lesions may be smaller and petechial in appearance in some patients (Fig. 21.13). Skin involvement is most notable in dependent areas, and in areas of trauma or tight-fitting clothing.[32] Symptoms are usually absent, although pain or burning may be present, and systemic involvement is uncommon.

The list of potential drug causes of HV is extensive, and includes multiple classes of antibiotics, non-steroidal antiinflammatory agents, antiepileptic drugs, insulin, propylthiouracil, omeprazole, and oral contraceptives.[32–37] (For a more complete listing of potential drug etiologies, see Ch. 20.) Identification and withdrawal of the offending agent is vital in patients with HV and in those with

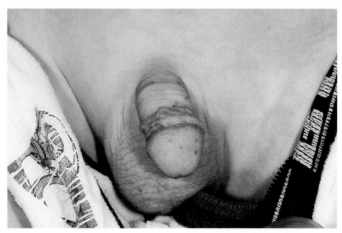

Figure 21.13 Hypersensitivity vasculitis. Petechial macules of the penile shaft, glans penis, and scrotum in a young male with hypersensitivity vasculitis.

skin-limited disease, no other specific therapy is usually necessary. For patients with either severe cutaneous or systemic involvement, therapeutic options include corticosteroids, colchicine, dapsone, or other immunosuppressive agents. The lesions of HV usually resolve over weeks to months, with resultant post-inflammatory hyperpigmentation.

Urticarial vasculitis

Urticarial vasculitis (UV) refers to a type of cutaneous leukocytoclastic vasculitis that presents with urticarial features and is often associated with an underlying systemic disease. In contrast to common urticaria, the lesions of UV are distinct in that they last for >24–48 h, often have a dusky or purpuric appearance, are associated more often with burning than pruritus, and leave post-inflammatory hyperpigmentation after resolution.[31,38] Confirmation of the diagnosis of UV often requires skin biopsy, given the potential overlap with other conditions, especially allergic urticaria.[39] Deposits of immunoglobulins, complement or fibrin may be found around blood vessels in UV in up to 80% of patients.[40]

UV may be idiopathic or associated with other diseases, including autoimmune disorders, infections, drug reactions, or paraneoplastic syndromes. Most patients can be characterized as having either normocomplementemic UV (in which case the majority represent idiopathic UV) or hypocomplementemic UV. Patients with hypocomplementemic UV have a propensity toward more severe multiorgan involvement and systemic disease associations.[31,38,39] The most commonly associated autoimmune disorders are systemic lupus erythematosus (SLE) and Sjogren's syndrome (see Ch. 22). Serum sickness-like reactions to drugs, cryoglobulinemia, and hepatitis C virus infection are also associated in some patients with UV.

Hypocomplementemic Urticarial Vasculitis Syndrome

Hypocomplementemic urticarial vasculitis syndrome (HUVS) is the terminology used to describe patients with UV in association with angioedema and systemic symptoms, most often obstructive pulmonary disease and ocular inflammation (iritis, episcleritis, uveitis). Decreased serum C1q levels are seen in most patients, and autoantibodies against this factor are detectable in the serum.[38] Although antibodies to C1q are also found in some patients with SLE, HUVS now appears to be a unique entity.

The cutaneous lesions of UV are urticarial in nature, favor the trunk and proximal extremities, and often have a purpuric quality (Fig. 21.14). The primary distinguishing features are the persistence of lesions longer than is typical for allergic urticaria (2–6 h), pain or burning, and associated hyperpigmentation as the lesions resolve. If the diagnosis of UV is confirmed, a thorough physical examination and laboratory investigation to assess for associated conditions are indicated. If an underlying disease is identified, specific therapy for that disorder is indicated. There is otherwise no specific therapy for UV. Various therapeutic modalities, including prednisone, hydroxychloroquine, indomethacin, azathioprine, colchicine, methotrexate, cyclophosphamide, cyclosporine, and dapsone have been used, but with an inconsistent response.[32,38–41]

Cryoglobulinemic vasculitis

Cryoglobulins are circulating immunoglobulins that precipitate at temperatures below 37°C, and that may be associated with any of several infectious, autoimmune, or malignant disorders. When these immune complexes deposit in blood vessel walls and activate complement, cryoglobulinemic vasculitis (CV) results. Cryoglobulins have been classified into three types based on the presence or absence of monoclonality and their association with rheumatoid factor. Type I (monoclonal cryoglobulinemia) is a monoclonal antibody and is usually associated with a hematologic malignancy, whereas types II and III are composed of a mixed antibody response, and hence are termed *mixed cryoglobulinemia*. The terminology *essential mixed cryoglobulinemia* is used to describe mixed cryoglobulinemia in the absence of other identified infectious, immunoplastic or neoplastic disorders.[42] The most common infectious disease to be associated with CV is hepatitis C, which is associated with mixed cryoglobulins.[43] In one large series of adults with SLE, cryoglobulins were detected in the sera of 25% of the patients, and was associated with an increased incidence of hepatitis C virus infection.[44] Patients with CV may present with a variety of skin manifestations, including purpura, papules, nodules, skin necrosis, urticaria, livedo reticularis, and bullous or ulcerated lesions.[32] The classic triad of cryoglobulinemic vasculitis is purpura, weakness and arthralgias, along with possible multiorgan involvement.[42] Treatment for CV should be directed toward the underlying systemic disease, when one is identified. A variety of antiinflammatory and immunosuppressive agents have been used in CV with variable success.

Necrotizing vasculitis with granulomas

There are several systemic diseases in which necrotizing vasculitis is seen in association with granulomatous changes, including Wegener's granulomatosis, allergic granulomatosis (Churg–Strauss syndrome), and lymphomatoid granulomatosis. The first two will be discussed in this section. These disorders are primarily seen in adults, but may occasionally occur in children. They are often associated with antineutrophil cytoplasmic antibodies (ANCA), which may play a pathogenic role and, more importantly, are useful in the diagnosis and management of (mainly small vessel) vasculitides.[4] Wegener's granulomatosis and Churg–Strauss syndrome, along with the entity microscopic polyangiitis, have been collectively referred to as *ANCA-associated vasculitides*. Microscopic polyangiitis, which is not discussed in detail here, is characterized by a necrotizing small vessel vasculitis without granuloma formation, and with a similar presentation to Wegener's granulomatosis, with less common involvement of the ear, nose and throat and occasional limitation to the kidneys.[45]

Wegener's granulomatosis

Wegener's granulomatosis (WG) is a necrotizing granulomatous vasculitis involving the upper and lower respiratory tract in association with kidney involvement and variable degrees of vasculitis in other organ systems. Although it is quite rare, among the primary systemic vasculitides in children WG is one of the most common and has an annual incidence of 0.03–3.2 per 100 000 children.[46] Classification criteria for WG have been proposed by the American College of Rheumatology (ACR) and the European League Against Rheumatism/Pediatric Rheumatology European Society (EULAR/PRES).[46]

WG usually presents with constitutional symptoms (malaise, fatigue, fever and weight loss) and symptoms referable to the upper and/or lower respiratory tracts, including cough, rhinorrhea, nasal stuffiness, nasal mucosal erosions or ulcers, earache, or sinusitis. Hemoptysis or pleurisy may be present, and nodular cavitary lesions in the lungs are a characteristic finding on radiographic studies. The

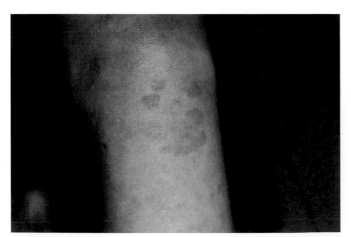

Figure 21.14 Urticarial vasculitis. These urticarial plaques, which had been persistent and had a faint purpuric quality, revealed leukocytoclastic vasculitis on histologic evaluation. The patient was ultimately diagnosed with systemic lupus erythematosus.

nose, nasal sinuses, nasopharynx, glottis, trachea, bronchi, and lungs may all be affected by the necrotizing vasculitis, and subglottic stenosis and nasal deformity may result, the former occurring more commonly in children.[47] Conjunctival injection may be present, as may arthralgias, myalgias and glomerulonephritis, although pediatric disease may present without renal involvement. End-stage renal failure may occasionally result.

Skin involvement occurs in up to 53% of pediatric patients with WG.[47,48] The manifestations are variable, but most commonly consist of palpable purpura. Necrotic papules and plaques (Fig. 21.15), subcutaneous nodules, vesicles, pustules, and ulcers resembling pyoderma gangrenosum may occur. Papulonecrotic lesions may favor the extremities (especially the elbows), but may also occur on the face and scalp.[32] Gingivitis can occur, and presents as spongy, friable, and exuberant tissue with petechiae and preferential involvement of the interdental papillae. Ophthalmologic findings (which may occur in up to 50% of patients) include not only conjunctivitis, but also dacryocystitis, episcleritis, corneoscleral ulceration, retinal artery thrombosis, uveitis, proptosis, cavernous sinus thrombosis, and pseudotumor of the orbits. Pericarditis, endocarditis, and coronary vasculitis have been reported, and peripheral neuropathy and cerebral vasculitis, with or without subarachnoid or intracerebral hemorrhage, have been noted in up to 25% of patients.

The diagnosis of WG is suggested by the clinical presentation and confirmed by tissue biopsy examination in conjunction with laboratory findings. Histologic evaluation of tissues (especially skin, lung, or kidney) reveals the characteristic necrotizing granulomatous vasculitis picture, which is highly suggestive of (but not pathognomonic for) WG within the appropriate clinical context. Up to 80% of patients with WG have positive cytoplasmic-ANCA (c-ANCA) and usually a negative perinuclear-ANCA (p-ANCA) on laboratory testing. In one series of pediatric WG patients, c-ANCA positivity correlated with kidney involvement.[47]

Prior to the advent of cytotoxic agents, WG was nearly always a fatal disease with a mean survival of 5 months. The most commonly used treatment is a combination of immunosuppressive agents, most often glucocorticoids and cyclophosphamide, and occasionally azathioprine.[4,5,46] Less commonly utilized therapies include plasmapheresis, extracorporeal membrane oxygenation, IVIG, mycophenolate mofetil and rituximab. Survival rates have improved with the addition of cytotoxic agents to the corticosteroids, but side-effects and toxicities related to these drugs are a major source of morbidity. The use of methotrexate is advocated by some, and this agent has shown promise both in induction therapy in combination with glucocorticoids and in maintaining remission of the disease after induction with a cyclophosphamide and glucocorticoid regimen.[49,50] Co-trimoxazole is often used for treatment of WG and may have benefit both in the prevention of opportunistic infection and in modifying disease activity.[5,46]

Churg–Strauss Syndrome

Churg–Strauss syndrome (CSS, allergic granulomatosis) is a rare condition characterized by atopic manifestations and a systemic vasculitis. It occurs primarily in males between 30 and 40 years of age, and only rarely in children. A distinguishing feature of CSS-associated asthma compared with typical allergic asthma is the late onset in the former, at a mean age of 35 years.

Patients with CSS often present with a 'prodromal', phase during which time they have allergic rhinitis and asthma, and occasionally sinusitis and nasal polyps. After several years, they develop peripheral eosinophilia, eosinophilic tissue infiltration, worsening of their asthma, gastroenteritis, and diffuse pulmonary infiltrates ('second'

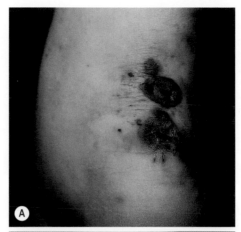

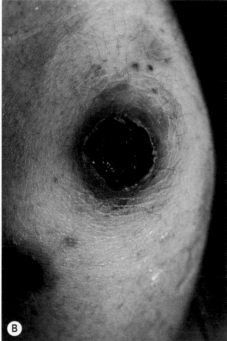

Figure 21.15 Wegener's granulomatosis. Painful, ulcerative, necrotic plaques on the ankle (A) and elbow (B) of a female with Wegener's granulomatosis.

phase). The third, or 'vasculitic' phase presents with fever, weight loss, and widespread vasculitis and inflammation. If left untreated, this phase may result in death. Manifestations may include arthralgias, myositis, peripheral neuropathy, eosinophilic pneumonitis (Loeffler's syndrome), and occasional renal, cardiac, CNS, or ocular involvement. Cardiac involvement occurs in roughly half of the patients, and may include pericarditis, myocarditis and tamponade.[51] Skin involvement may occur in up to 70% of patients, and includes palpable purpura, petechiae, subcutaneous nodules, urticaria, livedo reticularis, and papulonecrotic lesions similar to WG.[32,52] Digital ischemic ulcers and Raynaud phenomenon have also been noted.[53]

The American College of Rheumatology (ACR) criteria for the diagnosis of CSS support the diagnosis when four of the following six criteria are met: asthma, eosinophilia >10%, mononeuropathy/polyneuropathy, non-fixed pulmonary infiltrates, paranasal sinus abnormality, and biopsy containing a blood vessel with extravascular eosinophils.[54] Laboratory studies may be useful, as approximately 70% of adult patients with CSS have a positive ANCA, usually perinuclear with antimyeloperoxidase specificity (MPO-ANCA).[53] However, in distinction to adult patients, pediatric patients with CSS may not be positive for ANCA[51,55] CSS is treated with glucocorticoids, with or without the addition of other immunosuppressive agents (i.e., cyclophosphamide, azathioprine), and the prognosis has traditionally been fairly favorable with a lower mortality rate in comparison to other systemic vasculitides. Combination therapy with other agents, including cyclophosphamide, azathioprine, infliximab or methotrexate, may be useful in some patients. Steroid-dependent asthma, however, is common and may persist even after the vasculitis is in remission.[56] In a large series of children with CSS, more common cardiopulmonary manifestations, less common peripheral neuropathy, and higher mortality were noted when compared with the clinical experience in adults.[55]

Erythema elevatum diutinum

Erythema elevatum diutinum (EED) is an uncommon dermatosis seen most often in middle-aged adults, and characterized by violaceous papules, plaques, and nodules that have a predilection for acral and extensor surfaces. Common locations for the lesions of EED include the elbows, knees, dorsum of the hands and feet, pretibial surfaces, buttocks, and skin overlying the Achilles tendon.[57] The trunk and mucous membranes are usually spared. Histologically, the lesions reveal a leukocytoclastic vasculitis.

EED presents with papules and plaques ranging in size from a few millimeters to several centimeters. They may be yellow and simulate xanthomas, but more often they are violaceous to brown, and less commonly erythema, vesicles, or bullae may be present. The differential diagnosis may include Kaposi sarcoma or bacillary angiomatosis. Although the lesions are typically asymptomatic, they may be tender or painful and may be accompanied by systemic abnormalities such as arthralgias, fever, and malaise. Spontaneous involution may occur after a period of years without scarring, but residual hypo- or hyperpigmentation is common.

The pathogenesis of EED is unknown, although it is believed to be an immune complex-mediated vasculitis. It has been described in association with various conditions, including hematologic malignancies, infections, autoimmune disease, and inflammatory bowel disease.[57,58] Rheumatoid arthritis-associated EED may present with the skin lesions in conjunction with peripheral ulcerative keratitis.[59] In recent years, EED has emerged as an HIV-associated dermatosis.[60] It has been reported in a young woman with juvenile idiopathic arthritis,[61] as well as in a school-aged boy with a history of recurrent streptococcal pharyngotonsillitis, in whom it abated following dapsone therapy and tonsillectomy.[62]

EED tends to run a chronic course and may be persistent or, occasionally, spontaneously resolve. Although topical or intralesional corticosteroids may sometimes be useful, the response to these agents is generally unsatisfactory. Dapsone may be effective, and to many, is considered the treatment of choice, although the lesions often recur upon discontinuation. Surgical excision of large nodules is another therapeutic option.

Polyarteritis nodosa

Polyarteritis nodosa (PAN), also known as periarteritis nodosa, is a relatively uncommon vasculitis in children, characterized by inflammation of medium-sized (and in some cases, small) arteries. Several subtypes of PAN have been identified, and the prognosis is variable and largely dependent upon the extent of associated (extracutaneous) organ involvement. Two variants discussed in this section are 'benign cutaneous PAN' and 'infantile PAN.' The clinical features of pediatric PAN are briefly summarized in Table 21.2.

Patients with PAN often present with constitutional symptoms, including fever, malaise, and arthralgias. Painful skin nodules, purpura, ulcerations, and livedo reticularis (Fig. 21.16) are the most common cutaneous findings. The nodules vary from 0.5 to 1.0 cm, are tender to palpation, and are usually red-purple (Fig. 21.17). They may follow the course of superficial arteries and are especially common around the knee, anterior lower leg, and dorsum of the foot.[32] Healing of the ulcerative skin lesions of PAN may result in

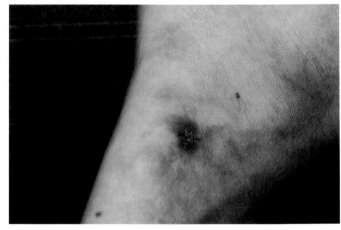

Figure 21.16 Polyarteritis nodosa. Reticulate mottling (livedo reticularis) on the medial foot of a patient with polyarteritis nodosa.

Table 21.2 Clinical features of polyarteritis nodosa in childhood

	Type		
	PAN	iPAN	BCPAN
Presentation	Fever, CS	Fever, severe illness	Fever, CS
Skin findings	Nodules, purpura, ulcers, livedo reticularis	Nodules, gangrene, livedo reticularis	Nodules, ulcers, urticaria, livedo reticularis, gangrene
Extracutaneous involvement	Cardiac, renal, CNS, musculoskeletal, gastrointestinal	Cardiac, renal, CNS, ophthalmologic	Musculoskeletal, occasional peripheral neuropathy
Prognosis	Variable	Poor	Good

PAN, polyarteritis nodosa; iPAN, infantile polyarteritis nodosa; BCPAN, benign cutaneous polyarteritis nodosa; CS, constitutional symptoms; CNS, central nervous system.

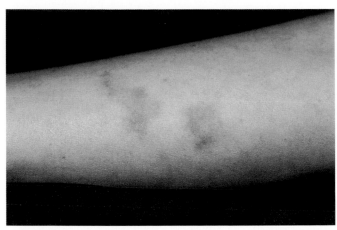

Figure 21.17 Polyarteritis nodosa. These dusky red nodules were firm and tender to palpation.

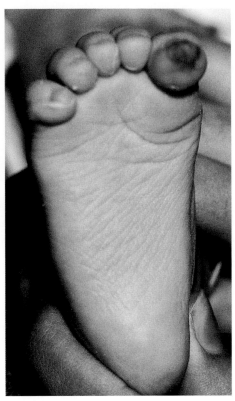

Figure 21.18 Polyarteritis nodosa. This infant with polyarteritis nodosa developed dusky red changes of the toes, followed by necrosis, as a manifestation of peripheral ischemia.

atrophic, ivory-colored, stellate-shaped scars and hyperpigmentation.[31] Other manifestations include abdominal pain, neuropathy, Raynaud phenomenon, and cardiac and renal involvement, which may lead to renovascular hypertension. Myocarditis and coronary artery disease may occasionally result in diagnostic confusion with Kawasaki disease.[63] The lungs are usually spared in patients with PAN. Death, when it occurs, is usually attributable to renal failure, intracranial or intraabdominal hemorrhage, hypertensive heart failure, or myocardial involvement.

Although the cause of PAN is unknown, it is presumed to represent a hypersensitivity-type immune-complex vasculitis, with deposits of IgM, C_3, or both in affected vessel walls.[64] Hepatitis B virus infection is associated in some cases, and group A streptococcal infection has been suggested as another potential infectious etiology. Laboratory findings may reveal anemia, leukocytosis, thrombocytosis, and an elevation of acute phase reactants.[65] Serologic markers may be useful, as patients may have a positive ANCA (usually p-ANCA, although c-ANCA has also been observed). However, serologic studies alone are of limited use in the diagnosis of PAN given their lack of specificity or sensitivity. Skin biopsy is diagnostically valuable, and reveals fibrinoid necrosis and inflammation of arteries in the deep dermis and subcutaneous layer. Direct immunofluorescence studies are variable, occasionally revealing IgM or C_3 deposition. Mutations in the gene for familial Mediterranean fever (FMF), *MEFV*, are found in some pediatric patients with PAN and may represent a susceptibility factor, especially in countries where FMF and FMF carriers are more common.[66]

Infantile Polyarteritis Nodosa

Infantile polyarteritis nodosa characteristically presents in children under 2 years of age as a multiorgan systemic disease, often with signs of heart or renal failure. Some infants with infantile PAN present with a severe acute illness diagnosed only at autopsy by the findings of coronary artery occlusion and vasculitis. Clinical features include coronary arteritis with resultant aneurysms, myocardial infarction, cardiomegaly and congestive heart failure, and renal artery and nervous system involvement, resulting in hypertension, abnormal urinary findings, peripheral ischemia (Fig. 21.18), neuritis, paralysis, and seizures. The prognosis for patients with infantile PAN is poor. Although the small number of reported cases and high rate of mortality of infants with infantile PAN appear to distinguish it from Kawasaki disease, some have suggested that the two disorders may be different manifestations of the same disease process.[67,68]

Benign Cutaneous Polyarteritis Nodosa

Benign cutaneous polyarteritis nodosa (BCPAN) is the terminology used to describe a clinical variant of PAN in which cutaneous lesions predominate and there is no (or very limited) extracutaneous involvement. It is the most common form of PAN in children, and tends to have a chronic course notable for remissions and relapses. The typical skin findings in BCPAN are painful red nodules, especially on the lower extremities and malleoli, with ulcers, urticaria, and livedo reticularis. Peripheral gangrene and autoamputation occur with greater frequency in pediatric patients who have onset of BCPAN in the first decade of life.[69] Constitutional symptoms, arthralgias, and peripheral neuropathy may occur, but visceral involvement is absent. The most notable laboratory aberrations are leukocytosis and elevation of the erythrocyte sedimentation rate.[70] The overall outcome of BCPAN is favorable.

The mainstay of management for PAN is systemic corticosteroids. Cyclophosphamide, dipyridamole, azathioprine, intravenous gamma-globulin, methotrexate, and plasma exchange have also been used.[63,65,71] Refractory disease has been treated with tumor necrosis factor alpha blockade.[72] In patients with skin-limited disease, therapy with aspirin or non-steroidal antiinflammatory agents has also been advocated.[70,73]

Kawasaki disease

Kawasaki disease (KD, acute febrile mucocutaneous lymph node syndrome) is an acute febrile disease of childhood that has become one of the leading causes of acquired heart disease in the world. It was described initially in 1967 by Tomisaku Kawasaki. KD is most prevalent in Japan and its incidence is much higher in Asian-American populations, possibly suggesting a unique genetic susceptibility. Pathologically, KD is a vasculitis involving the small and medium-sized muscular arteries with a predilection for involvement of the main coronary vessels.[74] As mentioned earlier in this chapter, KD may resemble the infantile form of PAN.

The majority of cases of KD occur in children younger than 5 years of age, with a peak incidence in those 2 years and younger. The disease tends to be more common in boys than girls, and the attack rate in siblings (1%) is 10-fold higher than in the general population.[75] The mean age of patients with KD is younger in Japan than in the United States. Regional epidemics of KD have been observed, and the disease may occur year round, although larger numbers occur during the winter and early spring.

The diagnosis of KD may be challenging, and misdiagnosis is common. In fact, missed diagnosis of KD is among the most common malpractice verdicts against child health practitioners.[76] Increasingly, atypical or 'incomplete' presentations of KD are being diagnosed, and tend to be more common in the youngest patients, in whom an extremely high level of suspicion must be maintained.[76] The diagnosis of KD should be considered in any infant with prolonged, unexplained fever. Delays in diagnosis and initiation of therapy may also occur more frequently in older children, who overall have a lower prevalence of disease.[77] In a large prospective study of KD patients, common associated symptoms noted within 10 days before the diagnosis included irritability, vomiting, anorexia, cough, diarrhea, rhinorrhea, weakness, abdominal pain and joint pain.[78]

The diagnostic criteria for KD are listed in Table 21.3. KD should be considered in the differential diagnosis of any infant or child with fever, rash, and red eyes.[75] The fevers in KD are usually of abrupt onset and are quite high (>39.0°C), and the response to antipyretics is usually minimal. The fever usually lasts 1–2 weeks in the absence of treatment, but may last as long as 3–4 weeks.[79] Although the CDC case definition of KD specifies fever persisting for ≥5 days, the diagnosis of KD is in some instances, established before this time when other supporting features are present. The conjunctival injection (Fig. 21.19) is distinctive, with involvement of the bulbar conjunctivae more often than the palpebral conjunctivae, and the absence of exudate. Perilimbal sparing (presenting as a white halo around the iris) is characteristic, and may be useful in differentiating KD eye involvement from other infectious or allergic processes.[75] Irritability is common in children with KD, and may relate to cerebral vasculitis or aseptic meningitis.[80]

Oropharyngeal changes in KD are most notable for dry, red, fissured, and crusted lips (Figs 21.20, 21.21). Hyperemia of the oral

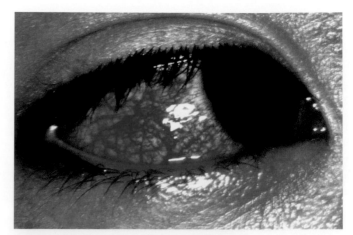

Figure 21.19 Kawasaki disease. Non-exudative, bulbar conjunctival injection.

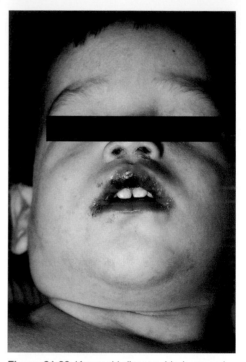

Figure 21.20 Kawasaki disease. Lip hyperemia and crusting with fissures.

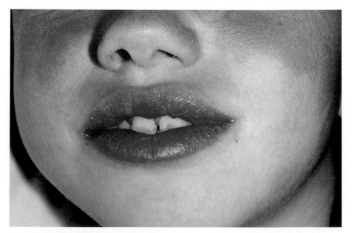

Figure 21.21 Kawasaki disease. Lip hyperemia with mild crusting. Note the associated facial eruption.

Table 21.3 Diagnostic criteria for Kawasaki disease
Fever for 5 days or more,[a] plus at least 4 of the following 5 clinical signs:
Bilateral conjunctival injection
Oral mucous membrane changes: injected pharynx, injected or fissured lips, strawberry tongue
Peripheral extremity changes: erythema or edema (acute), periungual desquamation (convalescent)
Polymorphous rash
Cervical lymphadenopathy (at least 1.5 cm)

[a]In the presence of fever and the other diagnostic criteria for KD, experienced physicians may make the diagnosis before the 5th day of fever.[79]

mucosa, and a red strawberry tongue (Fig. 21.22) (similar to that seen in streptococcal scarlet fever) are also seen. The peripheral extremity changes include non-pitting edema of the dorsal hands (Fig. 21.23) and feet (Fig. 21.24), and erythema of the palms and soles (Fig. 21.25). The edema is characterized by flesh-colored or red-violaceous, brawny swelling, along with fusiform swelling of the digits and taut skin noted on the dorsal surfaces. Patients may complain of pain or refuse to walk. Periungual desquamation (Fig. 21.26) is a later finding, generally seen in the subacute or convalescent stages of KD. It begins at the tips of the digits and, over a period of days to weeks, gradually progresses to involve the fingers, toes, palms, and soles. Recurrent episodes of skin peeling following upper respiratory tract infection may occur in up to 11% of KD patients for several years after their recovery.[81] Transverse linear grooves in the nail plates (Beau's lines, Fig. 21.27) may also be appreciated months into the course of disease.

Cervical lymphadenopathy is the least common feature seen in KD, occurring in approximately 50–75% of patients.[79] When present, it is usually quite obvious on physical examination given the size of the involved node(s). The diagnostic criterion specifies a size of at least 1.5 cm. Some patients with KD present with solely fever and unilateral enlargement of cervical lymph nodes. Generalized lymphadenopathy is not a feature of KD.

The cutaneous eruption of KD is polymorphous, and the majority of patients will have skin manifestations at some point during their illness. The most common presentations are that of a nonspecific, diffuse macular and papular, erythematous eruption (Fig. 21.28) or a diffuse urticarial process (Fig. 21.29). A scarlet fever-like rash with 'sandpapery' papules on a background of erythema and erythema multiforme-like lesions (Fig. 21.30) may also occur. Small pustules

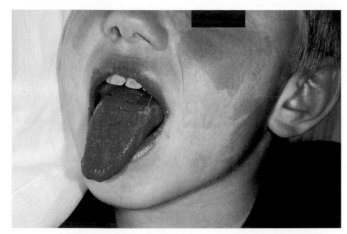

Figure 21.22 Kawasaki disease. Hyperemia of the tongue, with prominent lingual papillae ('red strawberry tongue').

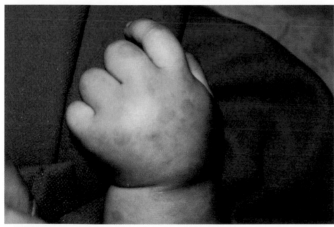

Figure 21.23 Kawasaki disease. Non-pitting edema of the hand in a young male with Kawasaki disease.

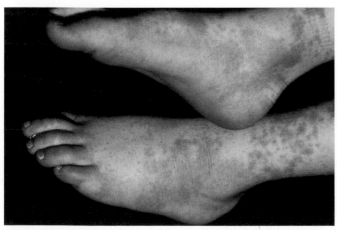

Figure 21.24 Kawasaki disease. Mild edema of the feet accompanied by blanchable, erythematous macules and patches.

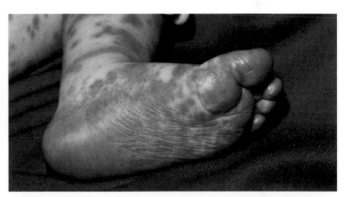

Figure 21.25 Kawasaki disease. Confluent, erythematous patches and plaques of the sole in a young boy with Kawasaki disease.

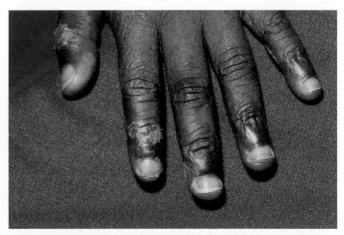

Figure 21.26 Kawasaki disease. Digital and periungual desquamation occurred late in the course of the disease in this boy who had coronary arterial aneurysms.

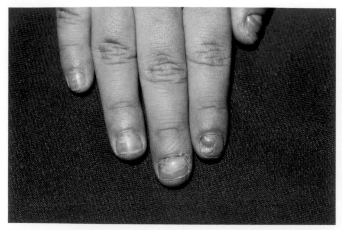

Figure 21.27 Kawasaki disease. Transverse ridges (Beau's lines) and nail plate separation, which may occur several months after treatment for Kawasaki disease.

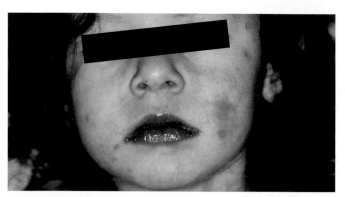

Figure 21.28 Kawasaki disease. This young girl has hyperemic lips with crusting and a diffuse, confluent erythematous skin eruption.

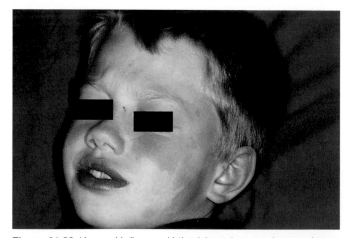

Figure 21.29 Kawasaki disease. Urticarial patches are the prominent skin finding in this patient.

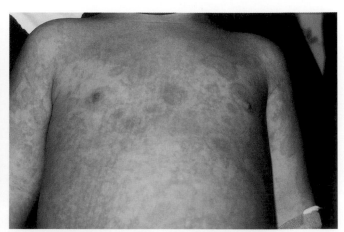

Figure 21.30 Kawasaki disease. This child had a diffuse erythematous eruption, with annular and targetoid (erythema multiforme-like) lesions.

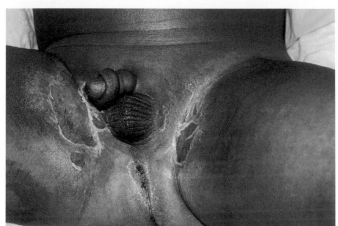

Figure 21.31 Kawasaki disease. The classic perineal eruption of Kawasaki disease is notable for accentuation in folds and desquamation.

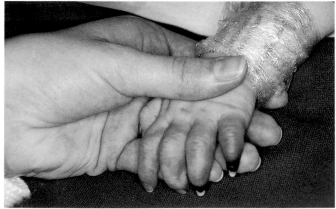

Figure 21.32 Kawasaki disease. Peripheral ischemia with gangrene of the distal digits.

superimposed on urticarial erythema have also been observed.[82] An important finding on skin examination is accentuation of the eruption in fold areas, especially the groin (Fig. 21.31), which is quite common and should increase the practitioner's suspicion for KD in the presence of other suggestive clinical features. This erythematous, desquamating perineal eruption was found to occur in 67% of patients with KD in one series.[83] Erythema, induration, and ulceration at the BCG vaccination site have been described during the course of KD.[84,85] Rarely, severe peripheral ischemia with resultant gangrene may occur (Fig. 21.32).[79] Although the cutaneous eruption of KD is quite polymorphous, vesicles, bullae, and purpura are virtually never seen. The histopathologic features of skin biopsy material from patients with KD are nonspecific.

A psoriasis-like skin eruption, occasionally with a pustular psoriasis appearance, may also be seen in children during the acute or convalescent phases of KD.[86,87] In one series, two of nine patients had a family history of psoriasis, and in all of the patients, the psoriasis resolved with therapy for the KD and did not recur.[86] Whether this observation reflects activation of 'latent' psoriasis in genetically predisposed individuals or a common etiologic agent for both KD and psoriasis is unclear.

The differential diagnosis of children with fever, rash, and red eyes is broad, and in addition to KD includes toxin-mediated bacterial infections (scarlet fever, toxic shock syndrome, staphylococcal scalded skin syndrome), Rocky Mountain spotted fever, viral exanthematous illnesses (i.e., adenovirus, measles, enterovirus), drug reactions (including Stevens–Johnson syndrome and toxic epidermal necrolysis) and a variety of other infectious, inflammatory, or connective tissue disorders. The differentiation of KD from acute adenoviral infection can be challenging. Although the presentations of these two processes can be very similar, two potentially distinguishing features of adenovirus infection are a purulent (versus non-purulent) conjunctivitis and the lack of a perineal accentuation of the rash.[88] A Kawasaki-like syndrome has also been observed in adults infected with human immunodeficiency virus.[89] Since there exists no reliable diagnostic test to confirm KD, the diagnosis continues to rest on clinical vigilance and the overall picture of the patient. Table 21.4 lists some useful clues to the diagnosis of KD.

Recurrent toxin-mediated perineal erythema (RTPE) is a benign, self-limited mucocutaneous disorder which may mimic some aspects of KD. The reported patients presented with perineal erythema, occasional involvement of the axillary and inguinal folds, and occasional desquamation of the fingers and feet.[90] Patients may report a recurrent history of such eruptions, and are generally otherwise well. RTPE is believed to be caused by a unique clinical response to toxins elaborated by streptococci and staphylococci. Some patients have had positive pharyngeal or perianal cultures for group A β-hemolytic streptococcus.[90,91]

Other clinical features of KD include cardiac manifestations, central nervous system and gastrointestinal involvement, extreme irritability, lethargy, urethritis with sterile pyuria, anterior uveitis, musculoskeletal complaints (arthritis and arthralgia), and peripheral gangrene. CNS involvement may include meningeal signs with CSF pleocytosis, cerebral infarction, sensorineural hearing loss, and cranial nerve palsies. Gastrointestinal manifestations include hepatomegaly, hepatitis, gallbladder hydrops, diarrhea, and jaundice. Laboratory findings of KD are listed in Table 21.5.

Cardiac sequelae represent the most serious complications of KD. Cardiac involvement may occur during the acute or later stages of the disease. Early manifestations include pericardial effusions and myocarditis, which may present with tachycardia and gallop rhythm.[74] Congestive heart failure, arrhythmias, and valvular regurgitation (especially mitral) may also occur. The most significant cardiac complication, though, is the development of dilatation or aneurysms of the coronary arteries, which occur in up to 5–10% of patients despite the use of appropriate therapy.[76,92] Changes in the coronary arteries may continue to evolve beyond the acute phase of the illness, but the development of aneurysms more than 8 weeks after the acute illness is quite unusual. Although death due to coronary occlusion has occasionally been noted after apparent recovery from the illness, most deaths occur suddenly between 3 and 8 weeks after the onset of the disease.

The etiology of KD remains a mystery. Hypothetical causes have included infectious agents (via conventional antigen), a toxin-mediated superantigen process, genetic predisposition, and immune activation. In support of an infectious etiology are the fact that KD presents in a similar fashion to some other self-limited exanthematous diseases, the seasonal predilection, the rare occurrence in infants under the age of 6 months (possibly suggesting protective maternal immunity), and the rarity of recurrences.[75] Many agents have been implicated, but none proven definitively, including *Staphylococcus*, *Streptococcus* species, *Candida* species, *Rickettsia* species, herpesviruses, and Gram-negative bacteria.[74,93,94] Superantigen-secreting bacteria such as staphylococci and streptococci, specifically those that stimulate a Vβ2 T-lymphocyte response, have been postulated to be involved in the pathogenesis of KD.[95] IgA plasma cells have been identified in coronary vessel walls, pancreas, kidney, and respiratory tract in patients who succumbed to KD, suggesting entry of the KD etiologic agent through the upper respiratory tract with systemic spread to other organs.[96] The genetic predisposition hypothesis is appealing, given the disproportionately high attack rate among Japanese Americans, but the exact association remains unclear. Polymorphisms in the genes for C-reactive protein and tumor necrosis factor alpha (TNF-α) may be associated with a predisposition towards KD, with single-nucleotide polymorphisms occurring with greater frequencies in KD as compared to control subjects.[97] Research into the pathogenesis of KD has been extensive, but the etiology remains elusive.

Table 21.4 Clinical clues to the diagnosis of Kawasaki disease

Persistent fever for more than 5 days
Fever unresponsive to antipyretics
Extreme irritability inconsolable nature of child
Perilimbal sparing of conjunctival injection
Perineal accentuation of erythematous/desquamating rash
Erythema, induration or ulceration of BCG vaccination site
Sterile pyuria
Increasing ESR in light of clinical improvement/defervescence

BCG, Bacillus Calmette-Guérin; ESR, erythrocyte sedimentation rate.

Table 21.5 Laboratory findings in Kawasaki disease

Finding	Comment
Leukocytosis	Often neutrophilic
Anemia	Normocytic, normochromic
Thrombocytopenia	Associated with severe coronary disease, myocardial infarction
Thrombocytosis	In subacute stage (usually ≥10 days after onset of illness)
Increased ESR	
Increased CRP	
Low albumin	
Abnormal lipids	Decreased HDL, total cholesterol; increased triglycerides, LDL
Increased transaminases, bilirubin	Secondary to gallbladder hydrops
Sterile pyuria	Mild proteinuria occasionally
CSF pleocytosis	Mononuclear

ESR, erythrocyte sedimentation rate; CRP, C-reactive protein; HDL, high-density lipoprotein; LDL, low-density lipoprotein; CSF, cerebrospinal fluid.

Treatment of KD is predicated on the ability to recognize the condition and rapidly render a diagnosis, which in some patients remains a challenge. The ultimate goals of therapy are to reduce inflammation and thus the potential for damage to the arterial wall.[75] The mainstays of therapy for KD are intravenous immunoglobulin (IVIG) and aspirin, which should be initiated within the first 10 days of illness whenever possible.[77] In the USA, IVIG is generally given in one intravenous infusion of 2 g/kg, which was shown to be more effective than the more traditional 4-day course.[98] Issues surrounding IVIG therapy in KD include the expense of the preparation, and the potential transmission of blood-borne pathogens, such as hepatitis C. Such transmission of infectious diseases is extremely rare since institution of the current purification and processing practices in 1994.[76] A subgroup of patients with KD are resistant to IVIG therapy, and seem to be at greatest risk for the development of coronary artery aneurysms and long-term sequelae.[74]

Aspirin is also started concurrently with IVIG, initially at a dosage of 80–100 mg/kg per day until the fever subsides. This high-dose regimen is useful for its anti-inflammatory effect. Low-dose aspirin therapy (3–5 mg/kg per day) is then recommended, primarily for its antiplatelet effect. Unless the echocardiogram detects coronary artery abnormalities, aspirin therapy is discontinued once the laboratory studies normalize, which is usually within 2 months of the onset of disease. Risks of aspirin therapy include hepatitis, hearing loss, and Reye syndrome, the latter of which is mainly of significance in the setting of acute varicella or influenza. Lower doses of aspirin (i.e., 30–50 mg/kg per day) are used in Japan given concerns in that population about potential hepatotoxicity. Suffice it to say that the exact role of aspirin therapy, as well as the risk-to-benefit ratio of high-dose versus low-dose regimens, in patients with KD remains controversial. Other therapies that have been evaluated for KD (and for which there is no current consensus) include corticosteroids, pentoxifylline, and anti-tumor necrosis factor agents. A randomized prospective study failed to show any significant advantages of the addition of intravenous methylprednisolone to conventional primary KD therapy.[99] Infliximab, a chimeric monoclonal antibody to TNF-α, has been used increasingly for IVIG-resistant disease in hospitalized patients in the USA.[100] It was shown in one prospective trial to be both efficacious and safe when compared to a second infusion of IVIG in patients who had received initial IVIG therapy.[101] Steroid pulse therapy may be useful for KD

patients with IVIG-resistant disease and persistent fever, although transient coronary artery dilatation may be noted during this treatment.[102] The optimal therapy for IVIG-resistant patients remains to be determined.

Long-term cardiac follow-up of patients with KD should include an echocardiogram once or twice during the first 2 months after illness onset, with further follow-up depending on the individual patient's coronary artery status. Children whose coronary arteries are normal at 2 months following the diagnosis of KD are considered free of cardiac disease, although several experts consider a history of KD to be a risk factor for the later development of coronary artery disease.[76] Vascular lesions in adult survivors of KD may include coronary artery aneurysms, calcification and stenosis, as well as valvular incompetence and myocardial fibrosis, either focal or diffuse.[103]

Key References

The complete list of 103 references for this chapter is available online at **www.expertconsult.com.**
See inside cover for registration details.

Cabral DA, Uribe AG, Benseler S, et al. Classification, presentation, and initial treatment of Wegener's granulomatosis in childhood. *Arthr Rheum.* 2009;60(11):3413–3424.

Eleftheriou D, Dillon MJ, Brogan PA. Advances in childhood vasculitis. *Curr Opin Rheumatol.* 2009;21:411–418.

Fiore E, Rizzi M, Ragazzi M, et al. Acute hemorrhagic edema of young children (cockade purpura and edema): A case series and systematic review. *J Am Acad Dermatol.* 2008;59:684–695.

Ferri C, Mascia MT. Cryoglobulinemic vasculitis. *Curr Opin Rheumatol.* 2006;18:54–63.

Son MB, Gauvreau K, Ma L, et al. Treatment of Kawasaki disease: Analysis of 27 US pediatric hospitals from 2001 to 2006. *Pediatrics.* 2009;124:1–8.

Weiss PF, Feinstein JA, Luan X, et al. Effects of corticosteroid on Henoch-Schonlein purpura: A systematic review. *Pediatrics.* 2007;120(5):1079–1087.

Wood LE, Rulloh RM. Kawasaki disease in children. *Heart.* 2009;95:787–792.

Zwerina J, Eger G, Englbrecht M, et al. Churg-Strauss syndrome in childhood: A systematic literature review and clinical comparison with adult patients. *Semin Arthritis Rheum.* 2008;39:108–115.

Collagen Vascular Disorders

The connective tissue (collagen vascular, rheumatic) disorders represent a group of diseases characterized by inflammatory changes of the connective tissue in various parts of the body. Of these, juvenile idiopathic arthritis, lupus erythematosus, dermatomyositis, systemic and localized forms of scleroderma, eosinophilic fasciitis, Sjögren syndrome, mixed connective tissue disease, and antiphospholipid antibody syndrome exhibit cutaneous findings that act as specific markers for the individual disorders.

Juvenile idiopathic arthritis

Juvenile idiopathic arthritis (JIA) is a group of seven arthritides of children under the age of 16 years that last longer than 6 weeks and are of unknown cause. JIA encompasses the former term juvenile rheumatoid arthritis, as well as other arthritides in children.[1] These include systemic arthritis (Still's disease), oligoarthritis, rheumatoid factor (RF)-negative polyarthritis, RF-positive polyarticular arthritis, psoriatic arthritis, and enthesitis-related arthritis (Table 22.1).[1,2] Overall, juvenile arthritis has a prevalence of up to 1 : 1000 children under the age of 16 years.[3] Approximately 6% of these children have systemic onset disease, 13% RF-negative polyarticular arthritis, 2% RF-positive polyarticular arthritis, 52% oligoarthritis, 12% enthesitis-related arthritis, 8% psoriatic arthritis (see Ch. 4), and 8% undifferentiated.[4] However, subtype distribution varies among countries; for example, although oligoarthritis is most common in Europe, polyarthritis is more common in New Zealand and India.

RF, usually an IgM antibody against IgG, rarely occurs in children, especially children under 7 years of age, and is associated with greater synovial erosion with a poor prognosis. Antinuclear antibody (ANA) levels (which are positive in 10% of normal children, usually at a level of 1 : 40 to 1 : 80) are most commonly positive in children with oligoarticular disease (40–80%), especially in girls and with uveitis. The different subtypes of JIA are associated with HLA types. Oligoarthritis is associated with HLA-DR8, -DR6, and -DR5, with chronic uveitis in oligoarthritis linked to HLA-DR5. RF-positive polyarticular JIA has been associated with HLA-DR4, whereas RF-negative polyarthritis has been linked to HLA-DR8, -DPw3, and -DQw4. Systemic onset disease has been associated with HLA-DR4, -DR5, and -DR8, and the enthesitis-related arthritis (juvenile spondylitis) with HLA-B27 and a striking familial occurrence.

Of the various forms of JIA other than psoriatic arthritis, systemic onset disease is the only one that has been linked to cutaneous disease. Its underlying pathomechanism with a strong role for the innate immune system, its clinical features, and its poor response to therapies which ameliorate other forms of JIA has led several investigators to classify systemic JIA with autoinflammatory diseases (see Ch. 25), rather than with autoimmune disorders.[5,6] Systemic onset disease affects boys and girls equally.[7] The eruption of systemic onset JIA is usually intermittent, occurring most often when patients have their characteristic daily or twice daily spiking fevers. The fevers generally reach 39 °C or higher, and the children appear acutely ill with exacerbation of joint pain when fevers occur. The characteristic flat to slightly elevated macules or occasionally papules may resemble wheals but are not pruritic. They measure from 2 mm to 6 mm in diameter. Lesions vary from salmon-pink to red and display a characteristic slightly irregular or serpiginous margin. The blanching macules are often evanescent, and frequently subside during periods of remission and a few hours after defervescence. Individual lesions may coalesce to form large plaques 8–9 cm in diameter. The eruption occurs predominantly on the trunk, but often affects the extremities and occasionally the face (Fig. 22.1); it is accentuated by local heat or trauma. Seen in 25–50% of patients, it may precede fevers or visceral involvement by up to 3 years. In some patients the rash occurs during a period of time of only 1 week, in others for a year or more.

Many patients have extra-articular features, particularly hepatosplenomegaly, pleuritis, pericarditis, and lymphadenopathy which may predate the joint manifestations by weeks to rarely years. Some 50% of affected individuals go on to have a mild oligoarticular course with a good prognosis for remission; of the remaining 50%, approximately half will develop a severe, recalcitrant, and destructive progressive polyarticular arthritis. *Macrophage activation syndrome* is a severe, life-threatening complication of systemic onset JIA that may be induced by viral infection or a change in therapy with antiinflammatory medications or stem cell transplantation. Patients show the sudden onset of fever, hemophagocytosis with hepatic dysfunction, disseminated intravascular coagulation, and sometimes encephalopathy, respiratory distress, and renal failure. The disease may present as pancytopenia with a falling ESR level, in contrast to the usual leuko-, granulo- and thrombocytopenia with increased ESR of JIA. Elevated levels of ferritin, lactate dehydrogenase and D-dimers facilitate diagnosis. Early recognition and treatment with high-dose corticosteroids with or without cyclosporine, etoposide, and/or etanercept may be life saving.[8] Other complications of systemic onset JIA are destructive arthritis, secondary amyloidosis, secondary infection, osteoporosis, and growth retardation.

Oligoarticular JIA occurs more often in girls than in boys and peaks between the ages of 2 and 4 years. Children with oligoarticular JIA often limp and show joints that are warm and effused, but not red and hot. In about 50% of cases, the onset is monoarticular with the knee, ankle, or elbow most commonly affected; small joints are usually spared. The acute onset of painful monoarthritis with refusal to bear weight is unlikely to be JIA, and infectious, traumatic, and malignant causes of joint pain should be considered. Approximately 20–30% of children with JIA have uveitis, which occurs most commonly in ANA-positive girls with early onset oligoarthritis.[9,10] The classic picture is a chronic bilateral anterior uveitis, which is usually asymptomatic until substantial damage to intraocular structures occurs, requiring repeated screening examinations. Treatment of the uveitis includes topical corticosteroids, mydriatics, systemic immunosuppressive agents, and surgical management of complications.

Table 22.1 Subtypes of juvenile idiopathic arthritis

Systemic onset arthritis
Definition: Arthritis with or preceded by daily fever of at least 2 weeks' duration plus at least one of the following:
Evanescent, nonfixed erythematous eruption
Generalized lymphadenopathy
Serositis
Hepatosplenomegaly

Oligoarthritis
Definition: Arthritis that affects one to four joints during the first 6 months of disease. Two subtypes occur: (1) persistent oligoarthritis that never affects more than four joints; or (2) extended oligoarthritis that affects a total of five or more joints after the first 6 months of the disease.
Exclusions:
Family history of confirmed psoriasis in at least one 1st- or 2nd-degree relative
Family history of confirmed HLA B-27-associated disease in at least one 1st- or 2nd-degree relative
HLA-B27-positivity in a boy with the onset of arthritis after 8 years of age
Positive RF testing
Presence of systemic onset arthritis as defined above

Polyarthritis (RF-negative)
Definition: Arthritis that affects five or more joints during the first 6 months with RF-negative testing at least twice and at least 3 months apart. Systemic onset JIA must be excluded.

Polyarthritis (RF-positive)
Definition: Arthritis that affects five or more joints during the first 6 months of disease, associated with a positive RF test twice and at least 3 months apart. Systemic onset JIA must be excluded.

Psoriatic arthritis
Definition: Must have arthritis and psoriasis, or arthritis and at least two of the following:
Dactylitis
Nail pitting or onycholysis
Family history of confirmed psoriasis in at least one 1st-degree relative

Enthesitis-related arthritis
Definition: Arthritis and enthesitis, or arthritis or enthesitis and at least two of the following:
Sacroiliac joint tenderness and/or inflammatory spinal pain
HLA-27 positivity
Family history of at least one 1st- or 2nd-degree relative with confirmed HLA-27-associated disease
Anterior uveitis that is usually symptomatic (pain, redness, photophobia)
Onset of arthritis in a boy after the age of 8 years
Systemic onset JIA and confirmed psoriasis in at least one first- or second-degree relative must be excluded.

RF, rheumatoid factor; JIA, juvenile idiopathic arthritis

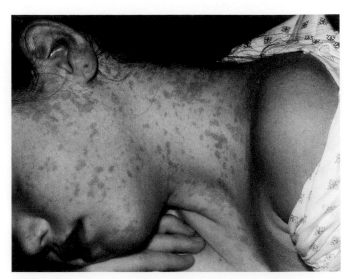

Figure 22.1 Juvenile idiopathic arthritis. Evanescent macular eruption occurred with fever in this girl with systemic onset JIA.

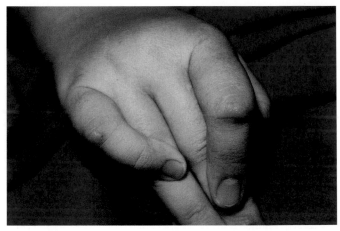

Figure 22.2 Juvenile idiopathic arthritis. Rheumatoid nodules developed on the elbows and dorsal aspects of the fingers in this girl whose JIA was poorly controlled despite systemic immunosuppressive medications.

Polyarthritis usually has an insidious onset, although it may be acute. It can involve both large and small joints (particularly of the hands and feet), and frequently involves the temporomandibular joints and cervical spine. Lymphadenopathy, hepatomegaly, and fevers may occur, although the fevers do not show the daily (quotidian) spikes.

Children with enthesitis-related arthritis have inflamed tendons in addition to arthritis of one or more joints. Most affected individuals are boys over the age of 10 years. Although children rarely show typical ankylosing spondylitis at onset, spondyloarthropathy not uncommonly develops by adulthood.[11] Arthritis associated with inflammatory bowel disease is a subset of this type. Acute anterior uveitis can occur in up to 27% of children, and tends to present as an acutely painful, red, photophobic eye.

Subcutaneous nodules rarely are seen in children with JIA, and occur most commonly in patients with RF-positive polyarthritis, particularly if recalcitrant to therapy. Barely palpable to several centimeters in size, they may be the first presenting sign of juvenile rheumatoid arthritis. Their most common location is near the olecranon process on the ulnar border of the forearm. Less commonly they may occur on the dorsal aspect of the hands (Fig. 22.2), on the knees and ears, and over pressure areas such as the scapulae, sacrum, buttocks, and heels. In the areas of fingers and toes, subcutaneous nodules are only a few millimeters in size. Subcutaneous nodules are firm and non-tender and may be attached to the periarticular capsules of the fingers. They can be easily confused with the subcutaneous form of granuloma annulare. Although more characteristic of patients with SLE, scleroderma, and dermatomyositis, cuticular telangiectases may be seen in children with JIA.

Traditional non-steroidal anti-inflammatory medications (NSAIDs) continue to be the first line of therapy,[12,13] in addition to physical therapy and psychosocial support.[14] NSAIDs that preferentially inhibit the cyclooxygenase-2 (COX-2) enzymes have fewer gastrointestinal adverse effects and may be preferred in some patients. Pseudoporphyria, presenting with tense blisters in photo-distributed sites, has most commonly been associated with the use of naproxen sodium, but has been reported after administration of other NSAIDs as well, including COX-2 inhibitors (see Ch. 19).

Intra-articular injections of corticosteroids are used for children who do not respond to NSAID therapy or as initial therapy for oligoarthritis.[15] Methotrexate is usually the second line of treatment for persistent, active arthritis, but is best initiated early in the disease course. Patients with oligoarticular arthritis tend to respond most favorably.[16,17] Blockade of tumor necrosis factor with biologics (etanercept, infliximab, adalimumab) in combination with methotrexate, is particularly effective for children with polyarticular arthritis.[18] Sulfasalazine has largely been used for enthesitis-related arthritis.

Moderate or high doses of systemic corticosteroids, including pulse intravenous steroids to avoid long-term high-dose treatment, are occasionally used for short periods while awaiting the effects of other medications, but otherwise are usually reserved for patients with systemic onset JIA with severe symptoms not controlled by NSAIDs. Systemic onset JIA responds poorly to non-steroidal anti-inflammatory medications and TNF-α blockers (30% response), but will typically respond to corticosteroids and often to anakinra (anti-IL-1 receptor antagonist),[19] tocilizumab (humanized anti-IL-6 receptor monoclonal antibody),[20] or abatacept (T-cell activating agent/IgG1 fusion protein).[21] As a chronic inflammatory disorder and in relation to usage of systemic corticosteroids, JIA is associated with an increased risk of osteoporosis, which can be countered by treatment with calcium and vitamin D supplementation, bisphosphonates, and calcitonin.[22]

Lupus erythematosus

Lupus erythematosus (LE) is a chronic inflammatory small vessel vasculopathy that affects the skin in the majority of cases and may affect most other organ systems as well. Although the etiology is unknown, reports of familial cases and a high concordance for clinical disease in monozygotic, but not dizygotic, twins suggest a strong genetic component and altered cellular immunity in genetically predisposed individuals as factors in its pathogenesis. Exposure to ultraviolet light is a trigger, not only for cutaneous manifestations, but also for flares of systemic involvement.

Approximately 15–20% of all cases of systemic lupus erythematosus (SLE) occur within the first two decades of life. Of these, 60% occur between the ages of 11 and 15, 35% between 5 and 10 years, and 5% in children younger than 5 years of age. Other than neonatal lupus (see below), the disorder is rarely seen before the age of 3 years. The disorder occurs in a ratio of approximately 1 : 1 to 4 : 1 in prepubertal girls and boys, but the ratio of female to male patients after puberty is 9 : 1.[23] The overall prevalence is 5–10/100 000 children and both increased prevalence and severity is seen in African-American and Hispanic children, especially because of the increased prevalence of nephritis.[24] In comparison with SLE in adults, affected children have more severe disease in general with an increased risk of renal[25] and central nervous system involvement,

as well as hemolytic anemia.[26–28] In one study, 77% of pediatric patients required moderate to high dosages of corticosteroids, compared with 16% of adult patients.[29]

The diagnosis of SLE requires a patient to exhibit at least four criteria of the disorder (see Table 22.2), and four of these criteria are mucocutaneous features: the malar eruption, discoid eruption, photosensitivity (overall 20%)[23] and oral ulcerations.[30] About 80% of patients with SLE have cutaneous involvement at some time, often as the presenting sign of the disorder. The *malar* or *butterfly rash*, although seen in approximately 60% of patients with SLE,[23] is not specific. This erythematous, mildly scaling eruption (Fig. 22.3) often appears over the cheeks and bridge of the nose, resembling the shape of a butterfly. It can be confused with the malar erythema of seborrheic dermatitis, erythematotelangiectatic acne rosacea, parvovirus infection or cutaneous lichenoid graft-versus-host disease;[31] seborrheic dermatitis typically involves the nasolabial fold and shows scaling as well. Brightly erythematous papules and plaques can also be seen on the photo-exposed extremities; when on the dorsal aspect of the hands, the areas overlying joints are typically spared, in contrast to the pattern of juvenile dermatomyositis (Fig. 22.4).

Discoid lesions of LE (*discoid lupus erythematosus*, DLE) are a common early sign of SLE in children,[32,33] occurring more often in

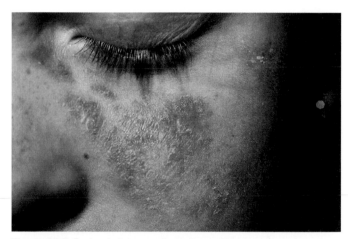

Figure 22.3 Systemic lupus erythematosus. Mild scaling and erythema of the malar rash.

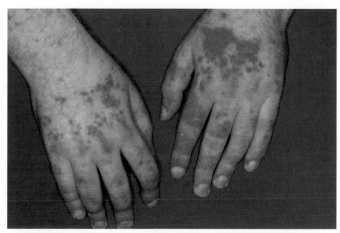

Figure 22.4 Systemic lupus erythematosus. Note periungual telangiectasia, but also the relative sparing of the skin overlying the joints, in contrast to the distribution of Gottron's lesions in juvenile dermatomyositis.

Table 22.2 Criteria for classification of systemic lupus erythematosus

Criterion	Definition
1. Malar rash	Fixed erythema, flat or raised, over the malar eminences (tending to spare the nasolabial folds)
2. Discoid rash	Erythematous plaques with adherent keratotic scaling and follicular plugging; atrophic scarring may occur in old lesions with dyspigmentation
3. Photosensitivity	A cutaneous rash following exposure to sunlight (by history or observation)
4. Oral ulcers	Oral or nasopharyngeal ulceration
5. Arthritis	Nonerosive arthritis (characterized by tenderness, swelling, or effusion) involving two or more peripheral joints
6. Serositis	Pleuritis (history of pleuritic pain or rub heard by a physician, or evidence of pleural effusion) *or* Pericarditis (by electrocardiogram, pericardial rub, or other evidence of pericardial effusion)
7. Renal disorder	Persistent proteinuria >0.5 g/day (≥3 if quantification not performed) *or* Cellular casts
8. Neurologic disorder	Seizures in the absence of offending drugs or known metabolic derangements *or* Psychosis, altered mental status, or peripheral neuropathy
9. Hematologic disorder	Hemolytic anemia with reticulocytosis Leukopenia <4000/mm³ on two or more occasions *or* Thrombocytopenia <100 000/mm³ (in the absence of offending drugs)
10. Immunologic disorder	Anti-DNA antibody to native DNA in abnormal titer *or* Anti-Sm (presence of antibody to Sm nuclear antigen) *or* Antiphospholipid antibodies (IgG or IgM anticardiolipin antibody, lupus anticoagulant, or chronic false-positive serologic test for syphilis, positive for at least 6 months)
11. Antinuclear antibody	An abnormal titer of antinuclear antibody in the absence of drugs known to be associated with 'drug-induced lupus' syndrome

A person is diagnosed as having systemic lupus erythematosus if any four or more of the criteria above are present, serially or simultaneously, during any interval of observation.

association with systemic disease than DLE in adults (approximately 25% vs 5–20% in adults).[34] In 75% of these patients, the DLE lesions are present at the onset of systemic signs, but full criteria for SLE may develop later, mandating serial clinical and serologic evaluations for systemic disease. In one study, 87.5% of patients with DLE and criteria for SLE showed involvement of the skin of more than one body segment, in contrast with 34.6% of children with DLE without SLE.[34] Photosensitivity is seen in 36% without SLE, and ANA titers are 1/160 and above in 19.2% of children without SLE. Individual discoid lesions are well-circumscribed, elevated, indurated red to purplish plaques with adherent scale (Figs 22.5, 22.6) and fine telangiectasia. When untreated or as a sequela, discoid lesions may develop persistent areas of

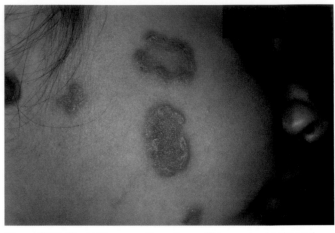

Figure 22.5 Discoid lupus erythematosus. This young girl showed well-circumscribed, elevated, indurated red to purplish annular plaques of discoid lupus.

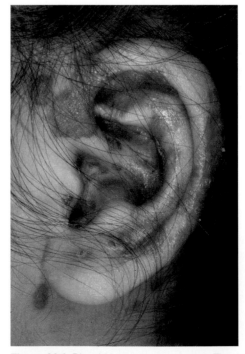

Figure 22.6 Discoid lupus erythematosus. The ear is often involved in children with discoid lupus erythematosus. Note the well-defined plaques of purplish erythema with post-inflammatory hyperpigmentation and focal overlying scaling.

hyperpigmentation or hypopigmentation with atrophy (Fig. 22.7). Discoid lesions can be asymmetrical and are often exacerbated by exposure to ultraviolet light. DLE is most commonly found on the face, frequently with lesions on the ear helices and conchal bowls. Although the face is often the sole site of DLE without SLE, the scalp, arms, legs, hands, fingers, back, chest, or abdomen may also be involved. At times the openings of hair follicles are dilated and plugged by an overlying scale. If the scale is thick enough, it can be lifted off in one piece. The undersurface then reveals follicular projections that resemble carpet tacks, a characteristic sign of LE. Discoid lesions have been described in a linear orientation that follows the lines of Blaschko.[35,36]

Red to purplish urticarial plaques (*lupus erythematosus tumidus*), which are relatively fixed in shape and do not undergo atrophy or scaling, usually occur on the face or other exposed areas of the body as a sign of photosensitivity. Although cutaneous lesions and photosensitivity are of diagnostic and cosmetic significance, photosensitivity reactions have also been known to precipitate fatal exacerbations of the disease. *Subacute cutaneous lupus erythematosus* (SCLE), which represents 10–15% of all cases of LE, only occasionally occurs in pediatric patients, usually in white adolescent girls. The cutaneous lesions of SCLE arise quite suddenly, mainly on the upper trunk, extensor part of the arms, and dorsal aspect of the hands and fingers. The lesions may be annular and may enlarge and merge into psoriasiform or polycyclic lesions with thin and easily detached scales (Fig. 22.8). Ultraviolet light is usually associated with exacerbations, but lesions tend to be non-scarring. Although arthritis and fatigue are common, patients usually only have mild systemic manifestations. The majority of patients with SCLE have anti-Ro (SSA) antibodies. Non-bullous annular lesions that clinically and histologically resemble Sweet's syndrome (see Ch. 20) can also been seen as a manifestation of SLE; biopsy shows unique histologic features called the 'histiocytoid' form of neutrophilic dermatosis.[37]

Livedo reticularis (Fig. 22.9, see also Fig. 12.75), blotchy bluish red discoloration of the skin due to vasospasm, is seen in several collagen vascular disorders, among them SLE, drug-induced SLE, antiphospholipid antibody syndrome, and scleroderma. Aggravated by exposure to cold, the reticulated erythema tends to be persistent and is most commonly found on the lower extremities. Raynaud phenomenon, seen in 10–30% of patients with LE, may precede the onset of SLE by months or years. This phenomenon is described in more detail in the section on systemic scleroderma. Pernio

(chilblains) are tender cyanotic to reddish blue nodular swellings on the fingers or toes of some patients with LE that represent cold-induced chronic vasospasm of digital vessels (see Ch. 20).

Intense inflammation of the fat (*lupus panniculitis, lupus profundus*) occurs in approximately 2% of patients with cutaneous LE, and may be associated with discoid LE, SLE, or, not infrequently, as an isolated disorder.[38] Lesions are seen as firm, often asymptomatic, sharply defined, rubbery dermal and subcutaneous plaques or nodules with a predilection for the scalp, forehead, cheeks, upper arms, breasts, thighs, and buttocks. Although the skin overlying the lesions usually appears normal, it often ulcerates (Fig. 22.10) or becomes depressed. Biopsy shows a perivascular lymphocytic, plasma cell, and histiocytic infiltration in the deep dermis and subcutaneous fat without accompanying fat necrosis. The

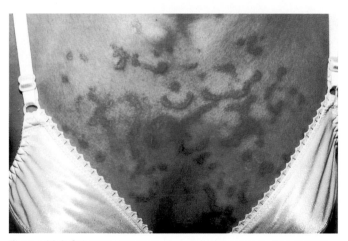

Figure 22.8 Subacute cutaneous lupus erythematosus. The annular and polycyclic erythematous scaling lesions arose suddenly on this adolescent's anterior chest after sun exposure.

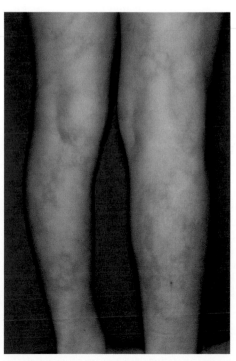

Figure 22.9 Livedo reticularis. Bluish red reticulated discoloration of the lower extremities in a teenager with increased antiphospholipid antibodies.

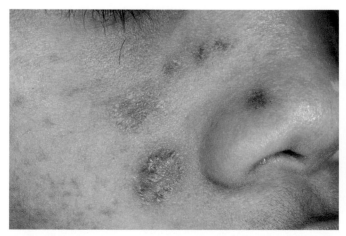

Figure 22.7 Discoid lupus erythematosus. Persistent areas of hyperpigmentation and atrophy in this adolescent patient who showed evidence of associated SLE.

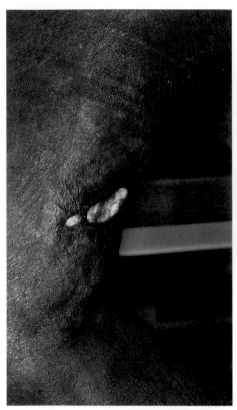

Figure 22.10 Lupus panniculitis. This boy with SLE and lupus panniculitis (lupus profundus) developed tender nodules on the thighs that ulcerated.

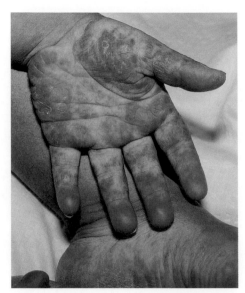

Figure 22.11 Systemic lupus erythematosus. Erythema and papular telangiectasia on the palm and fingers of a child with lupus erythematosus.

panniculitis may be lobular alone or involve both septae and lobules; most specimens show mucin deposition. Direct immunofluorescence often reveals immunoglobulins or C_3 deposits at the basement membrane. Approximately 70% of patients with lupus panniculitis also have typical lesions of DLE and 50% eventually develop systemic involvement or symptoms of SLE such as fever, arthralgia, and lymphadenopathy. Lesions of lupus profundus may persist for years and leave significant disfigurement. Although erythema nodosum (see Ch. 20) may occur in a patient with SLE, lupus panniculitis can often be distinguished by its lack of tenderness, greater chronicity, and lack of predilection for the lower legs. Lupus panniculitis must also be distinguished from subcutaneous lymphoma by histologic features and T-cell rearrangement studies. Inflammatory panniculitis followed by lipoatrophy, likely autoimmune in mechanism but not associated with SLE or dermatomyositis, can involve localized areas, such as the ankles or abdomen.[39] A newly described syndrome features chronic atypical neutrophilic dermatoses, lipodystrophy and elevated temperature (CANDLE syndrome), but affected children do not show an elevated ANA titer or other autoantibodies; the underlying pathomechanism is unclear.[40] These patients tend to show annular violaceous plaques and persistent eyelid swelling, in addition to their progressive lipodystrophy.

Chronic urticaria-like lesions (*urticarial vasculitis*) in children with SLE may be distinguished from classic urticaria by their tendency to persist >24 h and their lesser tendency to be pruritic (see Ch. 21, Fig. 21.14). A manifestation of immune complex deposition, urticarial vasculitis generally occurs in patients demonstrating clinical or serologic evidence of systemic disease activity, especially hypocomplementemia. Biopsy confirms the presence of leukocytoclastic vasculitis. Leukocytoclastic vasculitis can also be seen in

biopsy specimens from purpuric lesions in patients with SLE. These purpuric lesions may ulcerate, leaving significant scarring. Erythema and papular telangiectasia of the palms and fingers (Fig. 22.11), linear telangiectasia of the cuticles and periungual skin (with or without thromboses), periorbital or hand and feet edema,[41] and mucinous papulonodules[42] are other cutaneous features of SLE.

Although bullous or crusted lesions of SLE may simply reflect fragility of skin because of liquefaction degeneration of basal keratinocytes, a distinctive complication of SLE resembles bullous pemphigoid or dermatitis herpetiformis and has been called *bullous* (or *vesiculobullous*) LE (see Ch. 13, Fig. 13.30).[43,44] Indirect immunofluorescence on salt-split skin shows immunoglobulin and C_3 deposits on the dermal side, and immunoblotting shows autoantibodies directed against type VII collagen, as in patients with epidermolysis bullosa acquisita (see Ch. 13). Other forms of immunobullous disorder, such as linear IgA disease, have also been described in association with SLE, emphasizing the need for immunofluorescence testing.[45]

Mucosal membrane lesions (gingivitis, mucosal hemorrhage, erosions, and small ulcerations) are seen in 3% of patients with cutaneous LE and in up to 30% of pediatric patients with the systemic form of the disorder. A silvery whitening of the vermilion border of the lips is highly characteristic, and the lips may show slight thickening, roughness, and redness, with or without superficial ulceration and crusting (Fig. 22.12). The gingival, buccal, and nasal mucosae may also appear red, edematous, friable, and eroded, or may exhibit silvery white changes.

Several forms of alopecia may occur in patients with SLE (overall in about 30% of patients). Scarring alopecia may begin with multiple well-demarcated patches (Fig. 22.13) that exhibit erythema, scaling, telangiectasia, atrophy, and plugging (the classic changes of LE). Patients with SLE may develop hair fragility, especially with acute exacerbations, that leads to hair breakage several millimeters from the roots, resulting in a receding hairline with a short, unruly, broken hairs ('lupus hair'), especially at the temple and forehead. Telogen effluvium and alopecia areata have both been described in patients with SLE (see Ch. 7).

The most common symptoms of SLE at presentation are constitutional (malaise, fever, and weight loss).[23] The arthritis, which

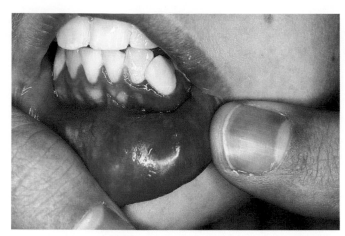

Figure 22.12 Systemic lupus erythematosus. The gingival and buccal mucosae are red, edematous, and eroded, with subtle whitening. Note the roughness and erythema of the lips with the subtle whitening of the vermilion border.

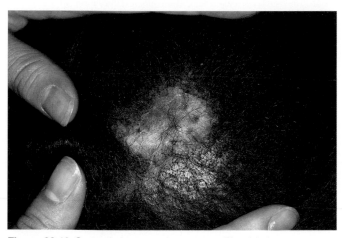

Figure 22.13 Systemic lupus erythematosus. Discoid plaque associated with scarring alopecia of the scalp in a patient with systemic lupus erythematosus.

occurs in up to 79% of pediatric patients,[23,46] is a symmetric polyarthritis involving both small and large joints. It is commonly quite painful (in contrast to the arthritis of JIA), often out of proportion to the clinical findings, and tends to be non-deforming. Approximately 55% of pediatric patients develop renal involvement, most often during the first year of the SLE. Four types of nephritis has been described based on renal biopsy pattern: mesangial lupus nephritis, focal proliferative, diffuse proliferative, and membranous glomerulonephritis. Diffuse proliferative glomerulonephritis occurs most commonly (40–50%), but carries the worst prognosis, often leading to end-stage renal disease in approximately 10–15% of lupus nephritis patients.[47] The presence of anti-dsDNA antibodies and hypocomplementemia is frequently associated with severe renal damage. Pulmonary involvement, particularly pleuritis, occurs in up to 30% of patients. Cardiac manifestations, including pericarditis, myocarditis, vasculitis affecting coronary arteries, and Libman–Sachs endocarditis, occur in approximately 15% of patients. A recently recognized issue, however, is the long-term risk of accelerated atherosclerosis;[47] as a result, the overall survival for SLE has improved for all causes except cardiovascular disease. Individuals with childhood-onset SLE can develop myocardial ischemia as early

as 20–30 years of age. Neuropsychiatric SLE (central nervous system involvement) most commonly features headache, seizures, alterations in mental status, psychosis, and peripheral neuropathy, and is seen in 20–30% of affected children;[48] most show evidence of neuropsychiatric involvement during the first year of the disease, but cognitive dysfunction occurs in almost 25%. Neuroimaging studies may show structural abnormalities, such as infarction; the addition of SPECT scans may show evidence of cerebral vasoconstriction and vasculitis as perfusion abnormalities and allow a diagnosis of lupus psychosis. Lymphadenopathy, although it occurs more commonly in adults, is seen in up to 40% of children with SLE. Ocular findings are seen in 25% of patients (cotton-wool patches, optic neuropathy, perivasculitis, and edema of the optic disk).

The diagnosis of SLE is chiefly clinical and is based on the presence of cutaneous lesions, systemic manifestations, and confirmatory laboratory tests (Table 22.2). Biopsy of cutaneous lesions will confirm the diagnosis and shows: (1) hyperkeratosis with keratotic plugging; (2) epidermal atrophy; (3) liquefactive degeneration of basal cells; and (4) a patchy, chiefly lymphoid cell infiltrate, especially around appendages and vessels.[49] Biopsy of lesional skin in discoid lupus or systemic lupus erythematosus usually shows the deposition of immunoreactants at the epidermal-dermal border (the lupus band test). Sun-exposed areas should be avoided for this biopsy because of the risk of a false-positive lupus band test at sun-exposed sites.

Serologic examination is the most important evaluation for children thought to have SLE, and ANA is the most valuable screening test. The serologic profiles in children with SLE are similar to those of adults, although some authors have reported a slightly increased incidence of positive antibody tests. The ANA test is almost always positive when a human substrate is used (e.g., Hep-2 cells); in contrast, 5–10% of patients with SLE show a negative ANA test when non-human tissues are used for testing. Having a positive ANA does not make a diagnosis of lupus. It can be seen in patients with several other collagen vascular disorders and is present in 5–10% of the normal population.[50] However, an ANA of >1:160 usually suggests an autoimmune disorder. Five patterns of ANA have been described: speckled (the most nonspecific); homogeneous; peripheral or shaggy pattern (most patients with SLE and this pattern have anti-double-stranded (ds; also called native) DNA antibodies); nucleolar pattern (often seen in patients with scleroderma); and centromere pattern (largely associated with CREST or calcinosis, Raynaud, esophageal dysmotility, sclerodactyly, and telangiectasia; see discussion on systemic sclerosis below).

Monitoring of serum complement is a critical test for determining lupus activity. The development of hypocomplementemia frequently signals the onset of renal disease. Total complement activity is monitored by functional hemolytic assay (CH50). Specific complement levels, particularly of C3 and C4, should be routinely checked by single radioimmunodiffusion assay. Not uncommonly, C4 levels may be depressed when C3 is normal, probably because patients with SLE are often missing one or more C4 alleles.[51]

One risk factor for the development of SLE, especially with onset during childhood, is hereditary deficiency of the early complement components, C1 (C1q and less often C1r/s), C4, C2, and C3.[52] Virtually all children with C1q deficiency develop SLE.[53] The SLE that occurs in complete C1- or C4-deficient individuals typically presents early during childhood. C2-deficient individuals tend to have a lower risk and less severe disease with lower titers of antinuclear antibodies, but increased anti-Ro antibodies. Lupus and other autoimmune disorders do not tend to occur in individuals with deficiency of the later components of complement, which instead are associated with an increased risk of developing infections, including neisserial infections. Lupus has also been associated with patients and carriers of chronic granulomatous disease, and in patients with IgA deficiency.

Children who may have lupus should be tested for the presence of anti-dsDNA antibodies, which are found in about 50% of patients with SLE and have been associated with an increased risk of renal disease, particularly if complement levels are low. In contrast, anti-ribosomal P antibodies are inversely associated with renal involvement in juvenile-onset SLE.[26] Anti-single-stranded (ss)DNA antibodies are found in about 70% of patients and are nonspecific. However, complement-fixing anti-ssDNA antibodies are associated with renal disease, even without anti-dsDNA antibodies. Some patients with SLE have antibodies directed against nuclear ribonuclear proteins (nRNPs). Patients with anti-RNP antibodies (30–40%) have a lower risk of renal disease and a better prognosis. Anti-nRNP antibodies and a speckled ANA pattern have also been described in patients with an overlap syndrome of lupus in association with sclerodactyly, esophageal dysmotility, Raynaud phenomenon, and pulmonary disease (also called *mixed connective tissue disease*, see below). The Raynaud phenomenon typically precedes the appearance of other signs and symptoms by several years in affected children. Fever, arthralgia, and myalgia are associated, and patients often have hypergammaglobulinemia, a positive rheumatoid factor, and normal complement levels.[54] The anti-Smith (Sm) antibody is specific for SLE, occurs in 20–35% of patients, and is associated with a higher risk of renal disease. Anti-Ro and anti-La antibodies are less common in children than in adults (except in neonatal lupus, see below) and occur in about 20% (anti-Ro) and 10% (anti-La) of children with SLE; they are associated with the highest risk of photosensitivity. Subacute cutaneous lupus is rare in children, but anti-Ro and anti-La antibodies can also be seen in children with SLE and complement deficiencies or Sjögren syndrome (see Sjögren syndrome).[55] Antiphospholipid antibodies can occur in up to 65% of children with SLE and should be monitored annually; they portend for the development of irreversible organ damage, not just a higher risk of thrombosis.[56]

Other useful laboratory tests include the erythrocyte sedimentation rate as a measure of inflammation; complete blood counts to detect leukopenia, thrombocytopenia, and a Coombs-positive hemolytic anemia; and routine urinalysis with BUN and creatinine levels to detect renal abnormalities. Renal biopsy and serial blood pressure measurements are important tools for managing children with SLE and evidence of renal disease. If a patient with SLE has cytopenia and unexplained fever, the diagnosis of *macrophage activation syndrome* must be considered. The disease is best recognized by hyperferritinemia, and subsequently hypertriglyceridemia and hypofibrinogenemia.[57]

Lupus may be triggered in pediatric patients by drugs, although the features tend to be milder (Table 22.3).[58,59] The occurrence in children is considerably less than in adults, likely reflecting the more limited utilization of medications in children. The cutaneous features of drug-induced lupus can be divided into those of SLE, SCLE, and chronic cutaneous lupus (CCLE or discoid lupus). In drug-induced SLE, the typical cutaneous features of classic SLE are usually absent (e.g., malar rash, discoid lesions, Raynaud phenomenon, mucosal ulcers, alopecia). Rather, photosensitivity, lesions involving the skin vasculature (livedo reticularis, palpable purpura, ulcers, bullae, urticaria and urticaria vasculitis) and erythema nodosum are most often described. The exception is reactions caused by TNF-α antagonists, which may manifest as the malar rash or discoid lesions. The most common cause of drug-induced SLE in pediatric patients is minocycline, primarily used by adolescents with acne (see also Ch. 8). This reactivity to minocycline is specific, and has not been described in patients who are administered tetracycline or doxycycline. Patients usually present with malaise in association with myalgia, arthralgia, or arthritis. Livedo reticularis, antineutrophil antibodies, and elevation of hepatic transaminase levels have been described, but evidence of vasculitis, renal disease, and neurologic involvement are unexpected. Drug-induced lupus from minocycline occurs most commonly in female patients and at an average of 2 years after starting the medication. Affected individuals usually show a symmetric polyarthralgia or polyarthritis involving the small joints of the wrists and hands. Isoniazid, hydralazine, and procainamides may lead to the polyserositis of lupus, but rarely cause cutaneous or renal disease. Drug-induced lupus is usually associated with increased titers of antihistone antibodies, a positive ANA, and often antibodies against ssDNA. Antibodies against dsDNA are usually absent and complement levels tend to be normal. Drug-induced SCLE shows the typical cutaneous features of SCLE, appearing at sun-exposed areas as annular polycyclic or papulosquamous lesions, but the legs are often involved, in contrast to classic SCLE. Disease usually develops 4–20 weeks after initiation of treatment. Among the many drugs that can cause SCLE are two classes often taken by pediatric patients: NSAIDs and anti-fungal medications (terbinafine and griseofulvin).[60,61] Drug-induced chronic cutaneous lupus erythematosus is very rare, and usually results from use of TNF-α antagonists. Treatment is discontinuation of the offending agent and topical application of topical anti-inflammatory medications if needed and systemic corticosteroids if a vasculitis. Cutaneous changes may improve within weeks after drug discontinuation, but complete resolution may be prolonged over several months.

Table 22.3 Features of drug-induced lupus erythematosus

	Skin features	Non-cutaneous signs	Laboratory findings
Drug-induced SLE	Photosensitivity, purpura, erythema nodosum, urticaria and urticarial vasculitis, necrotizing vasculitis. Usually absent: malar rash, discoid lesions, mucosal ulcers, alopecia, Raynaud phenomenon	Fever, arthralgias, myalgias, pericarditis, pleuritis. Usually absent: CNS, renal, pulmonary involvement. Hepatic changes from minocycline	ANA, antihistone antibodies, elevated ESR; may be mild cytopenia
Drug-induced SCLE	Annular polycyclic lesions and/or papulosquamous lesions, including on legs; less commonly, erythema multiforme-like or vesiculobullous lesions, necrotizing vasculitis	Usually no arthritis, serositis, or major organ involvement	ANA, anti-Ro, anti-La
Drug-induced CCLE	Discoid lesions in photosensitive distribution	Usually no other signs	ANA

SLE, systemic lupus erythematosus; SCLE, subacute cutaneous lupus erythematosus; CCLE, chronic cutaneous lupus erythematosus/discoid lupus.

The prognosis for children with SLE has improved dramatically from nearly 100% mortality to a survival rate of >90% because of earlier recognition and earlier and more aggressive therapy.[62,63] The main causes of death in children are renal failure, central nervous system lupus, myocardial infarction, cardiac failure, or infection. Although life expectancy is increased, the sequelae of disease activity and administration of systemic medications cause considerable morbidity in 88% of patients.[64] These include hypertension, growth retardation, chronic pulmonary impairment, premature atherosclerosis, ocular abnormalities, permanent renal damage, neuropsychiatric and neurocognitive impairment, osteoporosis, musculoskeletal damage, and gonadal impairment.

Our knowledge of the pathogenesis of LE has improved substantially, although the molecular basis is still unclear. The final common pathway of end organ damage in children with SLE is activation of the complement pathway and other destructive inflammatory processes after deposition of immune complexes, mediated by polyclonal B-cell activation. Autoantibodies are the hallmark of SLE, and bodies develop from stimulation by specific B-cells of CD4+ helper cells, suggesting that activated B-cells, T helper cells and the cytokines that modulate inflammatory responses are the most appropriate targets for therapy.

The therapy for LE currently depends on the extent of local and systemic involvement.[65-67] Discoid lesions without SLE usually respond to topical antiinflammatory medications and sun protection, but antimalarials and occasionally systemically administered corticosteroids may be needed for control.[68] Avoidance of exposure to sun and unshielded fluorescent light by wearing hats, sun-protective clothing, and appropriate broad-spectrum sunscreens with UVA as well as UVB protection is essential. These include sunscreens with an SPF factor of ≥30 that contain good UVA blockers, such as titanium dioxide, zinc oxide, avobenzone and/or the newer, more photostable UVA organic blockers (see Ch. 19). Cosmetic camouflage is an option for patients with residual dyspigmentation. Topical corticosteroids or calcineurin inhibitors (tacrolimus, pimecrolimus)[69] are effective for most inflamed cutaneous lesions, although relatively potent formulations may be required.

Antimalarial therapy is beneficial for long-term suppression of the disease. When antimalarials are used, the patient should have a pretreatment ophthalmologic examination and serial examinations every 6 months because of the low risk of irreversible retinopathy following long-term use. The average dose of hydroxychloroquine for children is 5–10 mg/kg per day, with a maximal dosage of 400 mg/day. Several months of antimalarial therapy may be required before efficacy is seen. Patients with mild disease and arthralgias without nephritis may respond to nonsteroidal antiinflammatory agents, although gastrointestinal irritation is a risk. Chronic administration of ibuprofen has rarely been associated with increased levels of creatinine and aseptic meningitis. Although aspirin is generally not a treatment of choice for the arthralgias, 1 mg/kg per day is the recommended dosage for individuals with elevated levels of IgG antiphospholipid antibodies.

In patients with more than mild disease, corticosteroids are the mainstay of therapy. In general, children are treated more aggressively than adults, with 97% receiving systemic steroids and 66% other immunosuppressive drugs.[25] High dosages of systemic corticosteroids are usually given until complement and anti-dsDNA antibody levels normalize with improvement noted in the clinical state. High-dose pulsed intravenous methylprednisolone 30 mg/kg dosage is generally administered for significant acute flares. Corticosteroids can then be administered orally and tapered slowly to the lowest possible level that controls the disease. Both alternate day and single morning dose therapy may be effective for maintenance, although alternate day dosing is preferable to lower the risk

of growth retardation. Avascular necrosis occurs more frequently in children than in adults (10–15%) from steroid usage. Children with SLE and immunosuppressive medications are at increased risk of infection, including pneumococcal; unfortunately, the response to administration of pneumococcal vaccination has been poor. Patients should not receive live vaccinations during corticosteroid administration, and placement of a tuberculin test before starting therapy is recommended.

Given the association of chronic use of systemic corticosteroids with adverse effects on major organs (renal, cardiac, neurologic) and the recalcitrance of many patients to steroids alone, other immunosuppressive medications have also been administered to achieve or maintain disease control. The addition of an immunosuppressive agent to the corticosteroid has been shown to be more beneficial for patients with nephritis than the corticosteroid alone and allows a reduction of steroid dosage.[70] Azathioprine and more recently mycophenolate mofetil[71] may reduce disease activity or allow lowering of the steroid dosage. The recommended pediatric dose for azathioprine is 2.5–3.5 mg/kg per day and for mycophenolate mofetil 0.5–3 g/day (600–1200 mg/m^2 per day). Cyclophosphamide use is most commonly reserved for patients with central nervous system disease or severe nephritis. The major potential side-effects of these agents are hemorrhagic cystitis and sterility (cyclophosphamide), hepatitis (azathioprine), and aplastic anemia, infection, and malignancy (both cyclophosphamide and azathioprine). Mycophenolate mofetil has a better side-effect profile. Dapsone is of little value for SLE, but can be quite effective for the bullous lesions in bullous SLE. Autoantibodies and polyclonal B-cell activation are thought to be important in the pathomechanism of SLE; Targeting of specific B cells with rituximab (anti-CD20 chimeric mouse/human monoclonal antibody) has led to improvement in anecdotal reports and small trials, particularly for lupus nephritis and autoimmune cytopenia. Use of higher dosages than used for lymphoma (e.g. 750 mg/m^2 rather than 350 mg/m^2), repeated therapy, and combination therapy (e.g. with cyclophosphamide and corticosteroids) has led to improved efficacy. For end-stage renal disease, dialysis and transplantation are therapeutic options. Autologous stem cell transplantation has been associated with significant morbidity and mortality, as well as high relapse rates in pediatric cases.[65]

Levels of 1, 25-dihydroxy vitamin D and intact parathyroid are significantly lower in children with SLE, especially if overweight.[72] Preventive therapy for osteopenia in pediatric patients with SLE should include high dietary calcium intake, and supplemental calcium and vitamin D (osteocalcin) as needed.[73] Maintenance of a good exercise program and minimizing steroid weight gain are also helpful. Although bisphosphonates are not routinely given in pediatric patients, their use in patients with pathologic fractures secondary to steroid-induced osteoporosis should be considered.

Neonatal lupus erythematosus

Neonatal LE is a unique variant of LE found in infants born to mothers with or who have a tendency for SLE, Sjögren syndrome, or undifferentiated autoimmune syndrome (Table 22.4).[74-76] The occurrence of NLE is not related to titers and is not strictly genetic, based on its discordance in identical twins.[77] Nevertheless, developing the skin manifestations of NLE has been linked to carrying a polymorphism in the TNF-α receptor (-308A; increases TNF-α expression in response to UV light) and the DRB1*03 genotype;[78] a polymorphism in TGF-β (Leu10, associated with increased fibrosis) has been linked to cardiac block.[79] The diagnosis of NLE is most important as a marker for the mother, who is at risk. Approximately

Table 22.4 Neonatal lupus erythematosus
Seen in infants born to mothers with a tendency for systemic lupus erythematosus, rheumatoid arthritis, Sjogren syndrome, or undifferentiated connective tissue disease
May present as lupus-like rash, often in areas of sun exposure: facial erythema, especially periorbitally (raccoon eyes), annular lesions, discoid lesions, atrophic lesions, and/or telangiectasia
Associated with anti-Ro (SSA), anti-La (SSB), and anti-U$_1$RNP (nRNP) antibodies
Congenital atrioventricular heart block in 15–30%

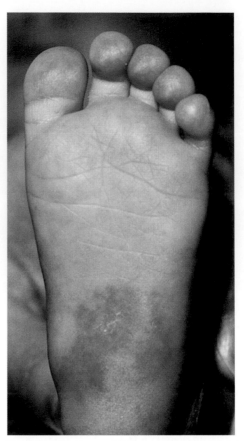

Figure 22.14 Neonatal lupus erythematosus. Cutaneous manifestations of neonatal lupus may occur in areas not exposed to the sun, as shown by this plantar surface eruption in an affected 2-month-old infant.

half of mothers of affected infants are asymptomatic at the time of delivery, and about half of these originally asymptomatic mothers develop SLE, Sjögren syndrome or, most often, undifferentiated autoimmune syndrome within a median of 3 years. In addition, mothers with undifferentiated disease may progress to SLE, Sjögren syndrome, or overlap syndromes.[80] Thus, mothers of affected infants with NLE must be evaluated and followed regularly.

Approximately 50–78% of babies with NLE will show cutaneous manifestations at some point, with onset usually by a few weeks of age.[81] However, up to 23% of affected babies show manifestations at birth, especially the cardiac manifestations and occasionally the cutaneous features.[82] Typically, new lesions do not occur after approximately 3 months of age. Lesions are most commonly localized to sun-exposed areas, particularly on the head and neck, and the extensor surfaces of the arms. Lesions have been described on the vulva, and on the palms and soles in 5% of patients (Fig. 22.14).

A variety of cutaneous manifestations have been described. Annular lesions or periorbital erythema (termed 'raccoon eyes', 'owl eyes', or 'eye-mask') (Figs 22.15, 22.16) should always trigger consideration of the diagnosis in an infant. The annular lesions may be confused with annular erythema of infancy, Sweet syndrome[83] or neonatal dermatophyte infection.[84] Discoid lesions (Fig. 22.17), scaly atrophic macules and patches, and telangiectasia, have also been described. Atrophic lesions may resemble round, ice-pick scars, are often congenital and frequently localize to the temporal areas of the forehead. The telangiectasia may be more petechial or may resemble the reticulated lesions of cutis marmorata telangiectatica congenita.[85] In addition to the cutaneous eruption, mucosal ulcerations have been noted in several affected babies.

NLE is the most frequent cause of congenital heart block. Congenital heart block occurs in 15–30% of affected patients owing to *in utero* inflammation, fibrosis, and calcifications of the atrioventricular node and sometimes the sinoatrial node; 10% of patients with cardiac disease show cardiomyopathy[77,86] Although the cardiomyopathy is usually apparent early, rarely it first manifests several months after birth.[87] Unlike the cutaneous complications of neonatal LE, congenital heart block is usually irreversible. Some infants with first-degree and rarely with second-degree heart block have shown spontaneous resolution during the first few months of life, but the majority of patients progress rapidly to third-degree block, including after birth and two-thirds of infants with heart block require pacemakers.[88] Cardiac disease results in a 20% mortality[89] not only from the heart block, but also congestive heart failure or other associated complications such as transposition of the great vessels, patent ductus arteriosus, septal defects, and endocardial fibroelastosis.

Other systemic complications include liver involvement in 10–26% of patients (generally manifested by hepatomegaly and abnormalities of liver function tests, but occasionally cholestatic disease and liver failure),[77,86] splenomegaly, lymphadenopathy and

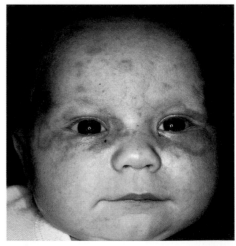

Figure 22.15 Neonatal lupus erythematosus. Raccoon eyes and annular forehead plaques.

hematologic abnormalities in 27% of affected infants, including leukopenia, thrombocytopenia, and anemia (both Coombs positive and Coombs negative). Subclinical evidence of CNS disease has been seen on computerized tomographic scans and ultrasounds,[90] but clinical neurologic features are unusual.[91] Hydrocephalus has recently been described as an uncommon complication, suggesting

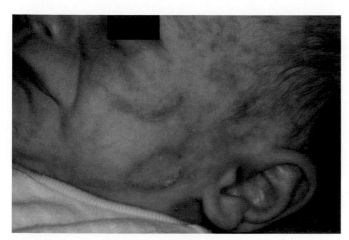

Figure 22.16 Neonatal lupus erythematosus. Annular scaling plaques on the cheeks of this 6-week-old boy. Note the significant cutaneous atrophy of the small circular lesions of the temporal area and the prominent venous pattern.

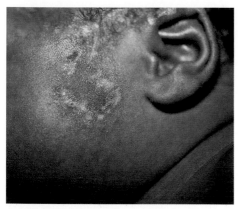

Figure 22.17 Neonatal lupus erythematosus. Annular discoid lesions on the scalp of a 2-month-old infant. His mother first showed signs of systemic lupus erythematosus 1 year after this baby was born.

that imaging studies are appropriate for NLE infants with a head circumference greater than the 95th percentile.[92]

NLE results from the transplacental passage of maternal antibodies.[75] In 95% of cases, these antibodies are anti-Ro (SSA) antibodies, often in association with anti-La (SSB) antibodies. These antibodies have been found at sites of pathology in the epidermis and heart.[93] A subset of infants with neonatal lupus and their mothers have anti-U$_1$RNP (nRNP) antibodies, although cardiac disease is extremely rare in this subset.[94] Infants and mothers may also demonstrate a positive ANA titer and antiphospholipid antibodies.[93] Breast-feeding has not been shown to alter antibody levels nor affect the development of cutaneous lesions.[95]

The anti-Ro antibodies have been shown to be causative for the cardiac block. Anti-Ro (52 kDa) antibodies bind to fetal, but not to adult, cardiac myocytes and selectively injure the conducting system; anti-U$_1$RNP antibodies do not bind to cardiac myocytes. When pregnant mice are injected with anti-Ro/La antibody intraperitoneally the antibody binds to the heart, epidermis, and liver, sites of inflammation in NLE and leads to apoptosis.[96] Mice lacking Ro protein in their tissues (i.e., similar to the functional depletion of Ro protein by antibody attack) develop signs of lupus.[97] Overall, 10–20% of babies of women with anti-Ro ± anti-La antibodies develop cutaneous NLE; 1–2% develop heart block, and 27% laboratory abnormalities.[98]

The diagnosis of neonatal LE is aided by the presence of typical cutaneous lesions, systemic manifestations, and confirmatory laboratory studies (positive anti-Ro, anti-La, or anti-U$_1$RNP antibody tests of the infants and mothers). Because of the possibility of involvement of internal organs, a thorough physical examination, complete blood cell count with platelet count, and liver function tests are often recommended for infants suspected of having neonatal LE. Infants with bradycardia or a murmur deserve an electrocardiogram and echocardiography. If any question regarding the diagnosis remains, cutaneous biopsy of a skin lesion can be performed and will show histopathologic features of LE with injury to the basal epidermal cells as a prominent feature.[99]

Clearance of cutaneous lesions generally occurs by 6–12 months of age, concurrent with the waning of the maternally derived antibodies. In a few patients, however, the cutaneous lesions disappeared within 1 month, and the eruption has lasted up to the age of 26 months. Affected individuals may show residual telangiectasia, dyspigmentation, atrophy, and/or scarring[100,101]; however, most cutaneous lesions clear without sequelae. Appropriate treatment of NLE includes avoidance of sun exposure and treatment of visceral complications, which may necessitate administration of systemic corticosteroid therapy. Low- to mid-potency topical steroids or topical calcineurin inhibitors can be used to treat the cutaneous lesions, but lesions clear spontaneously and the use of topical anti-inflammatory agents has not been shown to affect residua.[101]

Patients with NLE do not show an increased risk of developing lupus and other autoimmune disorders beyond that of their siblings, suggesting that the small increased risk in this group of patients reflects their familial tendency, not the previous occurrence of NLE.[102] Mothers who have had a child with neonatal LE, however, have a 36% overall risk of having a second affected child.[78] The risk of cutaneous manifestations in the second child is 23%, and the risk of cardiac issues almost 13%, six-fold higher than the overall risk congenital heart block in a first affected baby. A mother with a previous baby with NLE involving skin can have a subsequent baby with congenital heart block and vice versa. Fetal echocardiograms (weekly to every other week) between 16 and 26 weeks' gestational age, the peak period of cardiac injury, are recommended for at-risk pregnancies. However, the ability of maternal treatment with fluorinated corticosteroids to prevent the progression towards third degree heart block, which occurs very quickly *in utero* is controversial.[103–105] Given the risks of *in utero* exposure to steroids, their administration prophylactically is not recommended.[106]

Antiphospholipid antibody syndrome

The antiphospholipid antibody syndrome (APS) is an autoimmune thrombotic disorder, characterized by venous and/or arterial thrombosis and the persistence of at least one circulating antiphospholipid (aPL) antibody (found on two or more measures at least 12 weeks apart). aPLs are a heterogeneous group of autoantibodies reactive against either negatively charged phospholipids (e.g. phosphatidyl serine and cardiolipin) or proteins that are complexed with them (e.g. β2 glycoprotein I). Manifestations may range from headache or livedo reticularis to stroke or severe tissue necrosis (Table 22.5). In approximately half of affected pediatric patients, APS syndrome is primary. The disorder can also occur secondarily, most commonly in children with SLE (38% of children overall).[107,108] In a recent report of a registry of 121 affected children, 30% of the patients with SLE and APS initially presented with primary APS, with a mean duration of 1.2 years before the onset of SLE.[107,108] The age of onset is significantly younger in children with primary APS

Table 22.5 Antiphospholipid antibody syndrome in children

Cutaneous and subcutaneous features
    Livedo reticularis
    Raynaud phenomenon
    Palpable purpura/leukocytoclastic vasculitis
    Superficial vein thrombosis
    Deep venous thrombosis with ulceration
    Pyoderma gangrenosum-like ulceration
    Degos-like disease
    Gangrene

Non-cutaneous features[a]
    Thromboses[a]
        Pulmonary thromboembolism, hypertension
        Strokes, transient ischemic attacks
        Transverse myelopathy
        Cerebral venous sinus thrombosis
        Retinal vein thrombosis
        Renal artery thrombosis
    Hematologic abnormalities (38%)
        Evans syndrome
        Thrombocytopenia
        Leukocytopenia
        Autoimmune hemolytic anemia
    Neurologic abnormalities, non-thrombotic (16%)
        Migraine headaches
        Chorea
        Seizures
    Hepatomegaly, enzyme elevation

[a]Venous thromboses occur in 60% of patients; arterial thromboses in 32% (45% of patients with primary APS and 18% with secondary APS); mixed thromboses in 3% of patients; and small vessel thromboses, particularly leading to digital infarctions in 6% of patients.

(8.7 vs 12.7 years), and 45% of tested children have one or more inherited thrombophilic risk factors. These inherited prothrombotic disorders include methylenetetrahydrofolate reductase C677T polymorphism, factor V Leiden, protein S or protein C deficiency, prothrombin G20210A heterozygosity, and antithrombin III deficiency. Antiphospholipid antibodies have been associated with a high risk of miscarriage in pregnant women. In successful pregnancy, transplacental passage of maternal aPL antibodies can rarely lead to neonatal thrombosis,[109] most commonly manifesting as stroke. The risk may be increased in aPL+ neonates by acquired thrombic risk factors, such as central lines, sepsis, prematurity and heart disease, or the hereditary prothrombic diseases mentioned above.

Thrombosis is the major manifestation of antiphospholipid antibody syndrome (Table 22.5), particularly venous thromboses involving the lower extremities. Recurrence of the thrombosis occurs in approximately 20% of children,[107–109] and almost always affects the same type of blood vessel. Recurrences occur most often in children with inadequate anticoagulant therapy and with an underlying inherited thrombophilia. Five percent of children present with life-threatening thrombotic disease involving at least three organ systems over a short period of time ('catastrophic APS') and 7% die, largely due to thrombotic complications.

The most common cutaneous manifestations of APS in children are livedo reticularis and Raynaud phenomenon, each occurring in approximately 6% of affected children. Livedo reticularis is characterized by prominent reticulated cutaneous vasculature, most commonly noted on the lower extremities (Fig. 22.9; see Ch. 12, Fig. 12.75). The clinical triad of livedo reticularis, hypertension, and cerebrovascular disease, or Sneddon syndrome, is linked to antiphospholipid antibodies in individuals and has rarely been described in

children.[110] Other cutaneous and non-cutaneous features of APS are listed in Table 22.5.[111–114]

aPL antibodies in APS are thought to be pathogenic, rather than merely a serological marker. Anticardiolipin, lupus anticoagulant and anti-β2 glycoprotein I antibodies are found in 81%, 72%, and 67% of patients, respectively, without a significant difference between primary and secondary types of APS. Only 33% of pediatric patients have all three aPL subtypes and 48% have two simultaneously, emphasizing the need to evaluate all three antibodies for diagnosis. Of note, having more than one aPL antibody does not increase the risk of thrombosis. ANA and anti-dsDNA antibodies are detected much more commonly in children with secondary APS (86% vs 35% and 59% vs 6%, respectively). Of note, aPL antibodies are commonly found after bacterial and viral infections in children, leading to the imperative that the aPL antibodies persist for at least 12 weeks after initial testing for diagnosis.[107,108]

Despite the established association between antiphospholipid antibodies and thromboses, most individuals with circulating antiphospholipid antibodies do not show evidence of thrombosis. As such, it remains controversial whether to treat individuals prophylactically who show persistently positive antiphospholipid antibody levels but have no history of thromboses. There is currently no evidence to support the routine administration of low-dose aspirin in individuals with IgM or low titers of IgG antibodies; however, anticoagulants (at a minimum 1 mg/kg day of aspirin) should be considered in patients with higher levels of aPL antibodies, especially patients who will be immobilized or undergo surgery. Administration of hydroxychloroquine may be protective against the development of thrombosis in aPL+ children with SLE.[115] In addition, at-risk adolescents should be discouraged from smoking or treatment with estrogen-containing oral contraceptives. Children with antiphospholipid antibodies and thrombosis require anticoagulant therapy, but consideration should be given to their use in very active children and non-compliant adolescents because of the greater risk of hemorrhage. Children with catastrophic APS are treated with intravenous anticoagulation, plasmapheresis and sometimes rituximab.

Degos disease

Degos disease, also known as malignant atrophic papulosis, is an often-fatal disorder characterized by multiple infarcts in the skin and viscera owing to a thrombotic vasculopathy of unknown cause. Altered platelet function or fibrinolysis have been noted in some patients. The condition is particularly rare in children, but has been reported to occur as young as 1 day of age.[116] Typical lesions are asymptomatic 3–10 mm papules with an atrophic, porcelain white center surrounded by an erythematous, telangiectatic border (Fig. 22.18). Lesions may appear in crops and typically involve the trunk and extremities; one adolescent with cutaneous Degos-like lesions has been described with localized unilateral involvement of the abdomen.[117] Biopsy of lesional skin shows a characteristic acellular, ischemic wedge-shaped area of dermis underlying an atrophic but hyperkeratotic epidermis. The gastrointestinal tract[118] and central nervous system[119] are the most commonly affected organs. Although involvement of the GI tract is most typical, of the 25 reported pediatric cases of Degos disease, 56% showed CNS involvement and 48% GI involvement. Acute hematemesis, abdominal pain, dyspepsia, abdominal distension, diarrhea or constipation are signs of GI tract involvement, and patients may develop peritonitis, bowel infection or performation.[120] CNS manifestations include fatal hemorrhagic or ischemic strokes, polyradiculoneuropathy, and nonspecific neurologic symptoms especially headache. In most cases, the

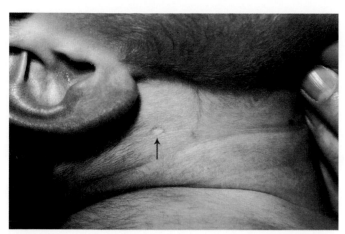

Figure 22.18 Degos disease. Note the atrophic, porcelain white center surrounded by telangiectasia. Note the hypertrichosis in this young boy from administration of prednisolone.

skin lesions precede the occurrence of other manifestations by months to years. Most affected patients die within 2–3 years, particularly from sepsis from peritonitis, central nervous system bleeding, or pleural or pericardial involvement. Approximately 36% of affected children have a more benign course without evidence of systemic involvement,[117] in contrast to 15% of patients of all ages. Familial cases have been described.[121] Degos-like lesions have been described in patients with antiphospholipid antibodies and/or SLE and, less commonly, dermatomyositis,[113] suggesting that Degos disease is a distinctive disease pattern rather than a unique entity.[122] In patients with SLE and dermatomyositis, the lesions tend to be more telangiectatic and show more mucin deposition. Administration of medications that inhibit increased platelet aggregation (especially aspirin and dipyridamole) may be helpful in some cases. Immunosuppression may worsen the skin lesions of Degos disease.

Juvenile dermatomyositis

Juvenile dermatomyositis (JDM) is an inflammatory disorder with an incidence of three per million children per year that primarily affects the skin, striated muscles, and occasionally other internal organs in children as well as adults (Table 22.6).[123–125] In cases in which cutaneous changes are absent, the term *polymyositis* is used. Since the clinical and pathologic features of involved skin and muscles are similar, dermatomyositis and polymyositis are believed to be variants of the same disease process; however, 85–95% of children with an inflammatory myopathy have JDM.[126]

The criteria to make a diagnosis of JDM were originally described in 1975[127] and remain largely the same today, except that electromyographs, which are painful and technically challenging, have largely been replaced by MRI evaluation (Table 22.7). Muscle biopsies, although currently performed to diagnose the disease in only 61% of patients, provide important diagnostic and prognostic information, especially given the recently developed scoring tool,[123] and are critical if the cutaneous features are not typical.

JDM occurs more frequently in girls than boys (2.3 : 1) and shows a bimodal age distribution, with one peak between 2 and 5 years of age and another at 12–13 years of age, giving a mean age of onset of 7 years of age; only 18% of patients with JDM are 4 years of age or under at diagnosis. Approximately 25% of all individuals afflicted with dermatomyositis are younger than 18 years of age at the time of onset. Malignancy is associated with adult dermatomyositis in about 20% of cases, but is rarely paraneoplastic in pediatric

Table 22.6 Clinical features of juvenile dermatomyositis
General
Fever
Lethargy
Adenopathy
Skin, subcutaneous, mucosae
Heliotrope rash
Gottron's papules
Nail fold capillary changes
Malar or facial eruption
Mouth ulcers
Gingival telangiectasia, bleeding gingivae
Skin ulcers
Limb edema
Xerosis of skin, incl. scalp with pruritus
Poikiloderma
Calcinosis
Lipodystrophy
Muscle
Muscle tenderness and myalgias
Muscle weakness
Joints
Arthralgia
Arthritis
Contractures
Gastrointestinal
Dysphagia/dysphonia
Gastrointestinal symptoms, especially pain
Pulmonary
Dyspnea from interstitial lung disease
Cardiac
Murmurs, cardiomegaly, pericarditis
Rarely, myocarditis, conduction abnormalities

Table 22.7 Diagnostic criteria for juvenile dermatomyositis
Progressive symmetrical weakness of the proximal muscles (limb girdle and anterior neck flexors), with or without dysphagia or respiratory weakness
Muscle biopsy evidence of myositis and necrosis
Elevation of muscle-derived serum enzyme levels
Evidence of myopathy on electromyography/magnetic resonance imaging
Typical cutaneous findings of dermatomyositis

A definitive diagnosis of dermatomyositis can be made when specific skin findings and three of the above criteria (excluding the rash) are present; a probable diagnosis of dermatomyositis requires two of the above criteria plus the rash.

patients.[128] In contrast to adults, children tend to have more inflammation and necrosis of muscle, more calcinosis, more small vessel vasculopathy, and a lower mortality.

The immune alterations that drive the small vessel occlusive vasculopathy of JDM are still poorly understood, but recent studies suggest important roles for environmental triggers, immune dysfunction, and specific tissue responses. Although the onset shows seasonality and many children have preceding infectious features, no evidence of an associated infectious agent has been discovered. Maternal microchimerism has also been implicated in causing JDM, and has been noted in 70% of peripheral blood T lymphocytes and 80–100% of muscle tissue samples from patients.[129] The major histocompatibility complex alleles HLAB8, -DQA1*0501, -DQA1*0301, -DRB*0301, and -DPB1*0101 confer increased risk. In addition, several other polymorphic gene loci have been shown to be risk factors.[123] A polymorphic variant of the TNF-α promoter that increases TNF-α expression (-308A), including in response to ultraviolet light, is associated with a higher risk of calcinosis, ulcerations, and disease chronicity.[130,131] Polymorphisms in IL-1 and the IL-1 receptor antagonist also increase the risk of the development of calcinosis and JDM, respectively.[132,133]

The onset of JDM is insidious in approximately 50% of affected children with subtle weakness, anorexia, malaise, abdominal pain, and the gradual development of a rash. In about 30% of children, the onset of the disorder is fulminant, with fever, profound weakness, and severe multisystemic involvement. The remainder have a subacute onset, often with the cutaneous eruption preceding the appearance of constitutional symptoms or evidence of myopathy by 3–6 months, although occasionally by as long as several years. An amyopathic form, characterized by typical cutaneous manifestations without clinical or laboratory evidence of myositis for at least 6 months, affects a minority of children with JDM. A recent literature review suggested that 26% of these children with 'amyopathic JDM' develop evidence of myositis during a mean follow-up period of 3.9 years and the 4% who developed calcinosis all developed myositis, suggesting that children without myositis do not need aggressive immunosuppressive management.[134]

The cutaneous features of JDM may be striking or so minor that they might be easily overlooked. A variety of cutaneous findings maybe noted (Table 22.6). Characteristic cutaneous lesions are inflammatory and telangiectatic, and are found in 75% of affected children at presentation. A purplish red erythema occurs on the face, especially on the eyelids, and is called the 'heliotrope rash' because it matches the color of reddish purple flower of the heliotrope plant (Fig. 22.19). The eruption can also be seen on the upper cheeks, forehead, temples, and ears (Fig. 22.20). Sometimes the facial lesions are very edematous, leading to a periorbital and cheek edema. Often confluent, violaceous telangiectatic erythema with fine scaling may also appear at the hairline of the scalp, nape of the neck, and extensor surfaces of the arms and shoulders, on the elbows and knees (Fig. 22.21), and overlying the knuckles (Gottron's sign). Involvement of the shoulder and center of the upper anterior trunk has been called the 'shawl sign' (Fig. 22.22). The eruption is often accentuated when the affected area is dependent, for example, on the face when the child lowers the face. The distribution of the eruption and the frequent sparing of sun-protected areas suggest photosensitivity; ultraviolet light exposure is known to trigger both cutaneous and muscle signs.

Periungual telangiectasia (Fig. 22.23) is a characteristic feature of JDM and provides a good indication of cutaneous, rather than muscle, disease activity.[135] Viewing the nail fold area through a dermatoscope, ophthalmoscope or otoscope to magnify the area

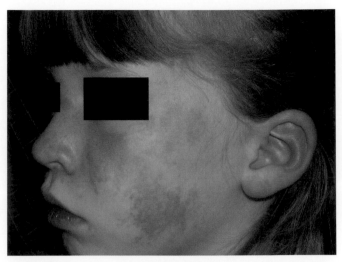

Figure 22.20 Juvenile dermatomyositis. Periorbital and cheek telangiectasia. Note the increased involvement with edema and swelling on the left cheek compared with the right.

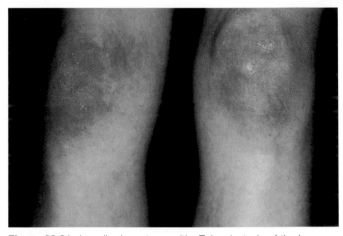

Figure 22.21 Juvenile dermatomyositis. Telangiectasia of the knees (as shown here) and on the elbows can be a subtle but characteristic manifestation.

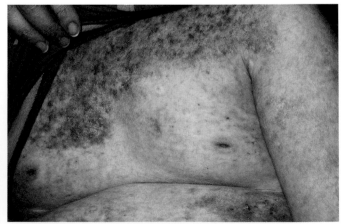

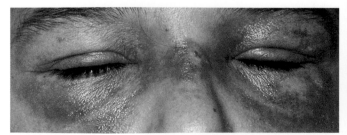

Figure 22.19 Juvenile dermatomyositis. Heliotrope rash of the periorbital areas. Asymmetry of involvement is unusual, but this boy shows more involvement on the left side of the face.

Figure 22.22 Juvenile dermatomyositis. Telangiectasia and atrophy induced by sun exposure in this young girl whose relatively uninvolved area was covered by her bathing suit.

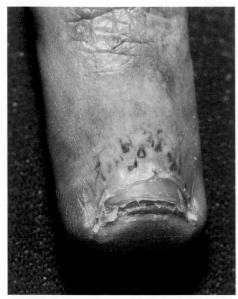

Figure 22.23 Juvenile dermatomyositis. Periungual telangiectasia with cuticular hypertrophy.

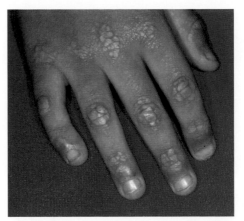

Figure 22.25 Juvenile dermatomyositis. Gottron's papules overlying the joints of the hands.

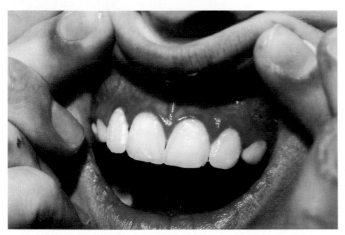

Figure 22.24 Juvenile dermatomyositis. Telangiectasias of the gingivae are commonly associated. Note the periungual telangiectasia as well.

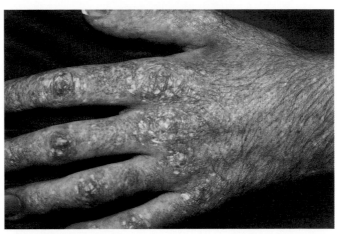

Figure 22.26 Juvenile dermatomyositis. Atrophy telangiectasia and depigmentation are residual signs after clearance of the Gottron's papules in this patient with chronic skin changes.

after local application of mineral oil improves visualization. Nail fold capillary microscopy has shown that the periungual telangiectasia represents bushy capillary loops adjacent to avascular areas, perhaps a form of compensatory neovascularization. Erythema of the cuticle at the base of the nails commonly accompanies the periungual telangiectasia. At times, the cuticles may also be thickened, hyperkeratotic, and irregular, giving an appearance of excessive picking or manicuring. Pitted ulcerations of the fingertips, pressure points such as the elbows, lateral aspects of the trunk, axillae, and lateral ocular canthi are usually seen at presentation or with disease flares.[125] Thought to be a marker of severe disease, these ulcers leave residual atrophic scars. The mucous membranes often show telangiectatic involvement, with erythema of the palate and buccal mucosa, with or without ulceration, and telangiectasia of the gum margin (Fig. 22.24).

A pathognomonic sign of dermatomyositis is Gottron's papule, a violaceous flat-topped lesion over the dorsal interphalangeal joints (Fig. 22.25). Coupled with the facial eruption, these inflammatory lesions on the dorsum of the hand may be misdiagnosed as contact dermatitis. When the papule resolves, atrophy, telangiectasia, and hypopigmentation may persist (Fig. 22.26). Other cutaneous features include palmar erythema and thickening, which is sometimes so severe that the hyperkeratosis, fissuring, and hyperpigmentation have been compared to a 'mechanic's hand'. A more generalized hyperkeratotic disorder that resembles pityriasis rubra pilaris and generalized erythroderma with scaling have also been described.[136,137] Sclerodactyly may be seen in children with overlap syndrome that includes systemic sclerosis. Panniculitis may manifest clinically as tender, indurated plaques and nodules, especially on the arms, thighs, and buttocks; however, panniculitis is often observed in biopsy specimens and is not noted clinically. Limb edema is noted in some patients at presentation, but anasarca is rare and should prompt consideration of nephritic syndrome.[138]

Several cutaneous features of JDM are seen more commonly with disease chronicity. Many children and adolescents with chronic disease have intensely pruritic, xerotic skin that shows poikiloderma (Fig. 22.27), which is the combination of cutaneous atrophy, telangiectasia, and dyspigmentation (see Ch. 11). The scalp is dry, scaling and pruritic as well. Cutaneous calcinosis now develops in 24% of children,[126,139] in contrast to the up to 70% incidence of earlier reports; this decreased incidence of calcinosis can be attributed to both earlier diagnosis and to more aggressive, earlier treatment (see below). Most commonly seen at sites of trauma,

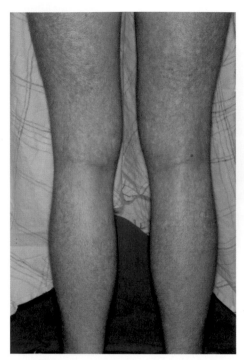

Figure 22.27 Juvenile dermatomyositis. Poikilodermatous changes on the legs, characterized by telangiectasia, atrophy, and reticulated hyperpigmentation.

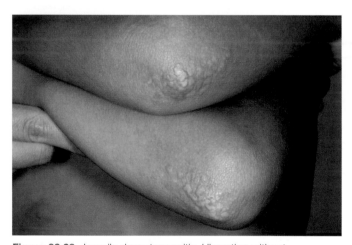

Figure 22.28 Juvenile dermatomyositis. Ulceration without calcifications can also be painful and should not be confused with calcification.

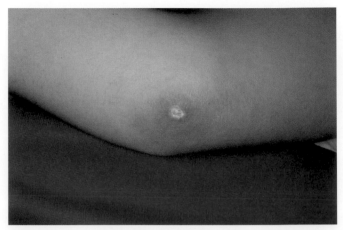

Figure 22.29 Juvenile dermatomyositis. Even a single calcification over a joint may ulcerate and be exquisitely painful.

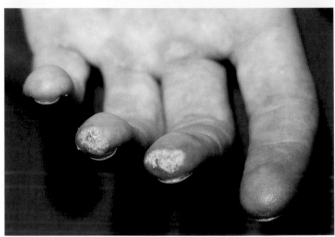

Figure 22.30 Juvenile dermatomyositis. Note calcinosis on the fingertips.

particularly on the buttocks, elbows, knees, and fingers, and around the shoulders, subcutaneous calcium deposits may produce local pain and can be extruded, leading to ulcers, sinuses, or cellulitis (Figs 22.28, 22.29) (see Ch. 23 for other causes of calcinosis). Ulcerations may also appear in children with dermatomyositis without calcifications, especially over joints (Fig. 22.30). Calcifications appear as hard, irregular nodules that may drain a whitish, chalky material through their openings to the surface that resembles gritty toothpaste. The mean time to occurrence of calcinosis after onset is 2.5–3.4 years, although 3% patients have calcinosis at diagnosis,[140] even without evidence of myositis. Sometimes patients have widespread calcification along fascial planes, encasing muscles (universalis form) or even appearing as an exoskeleton on X-ray examination. Contractures have been associated with the calcinosis,

and occur in 17–30% of JDM patients. Lipodystrophy is a common feature in children with chronic disease, especially if poorly controlled and of longer duration, overall occurring in 9.7% of patients[139] (Figs 22.31, 22.32). The lipodystrophy may be generalized or partial and is characterized by a slowly progressive symmetrical loss. The lipodystrophy is associated with insulin resistance and hyperlipidemia, but these cardiac risk factors can be present in chronic patients, even without the lipodystrophy. Acanthosis nigricans has been described in 10% of patients later in the disease course (Fig. 22.33). The insulin resistance correlates with muscle atrophy, pro-inflammatory circulating cytokines and a family history of diabetes, but not with corticosteroid utilization.[141]

The myopathy of JDM affects primarily the proximal groups of muscles, especially the triceps and quadriceps, usually in a symmetric distribution. Muscle tenderness or stiffness is not uncommon, but usually occurs later in the course rather than as a presenting sign. Affected children often complain of great fatigue and are unable to do simple tasks, such as rising, squatting, walking, or reaching. In young children, muscle weakness may manifest as more demanding behavior. Physical therapists may be helpful as assessors of muscle strength, particularly in younger children. Speech may become nasal because of nasopharyngeal muscle weakness, and approximately 10–15% of patients complain of difficulty with swallowing.

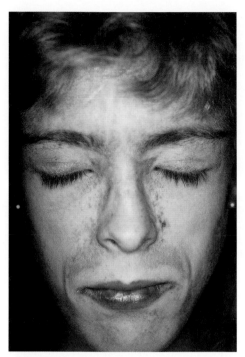

Figure 22.31 Juvenile dermatomyositis. Facial lipoatrophy and persistent telangiectasia in an older adolescent. The onset of her JDM was 8 years earlier; although the myositis has been controlled, she had residual disfiguring cutaneous and subcutaneous manifestations with extensive, problematic calcifications.

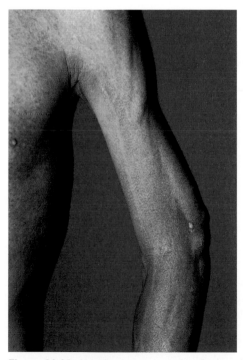

Figure 22.32 Juvenile dermatomyositis. Profound lipoatrophy on the limbs of a young adult with a history since elementary school of JDM.

A non-destructive, generally nondeforming arthritis occurs in approximately half of affected children at some time during the disorder, most commonly an asymptomatic arthritis of the knees; large and small joint polyarthritis has also been described.[140] Vasculopathy of the gastrointestinal tract may lead to ulceration,

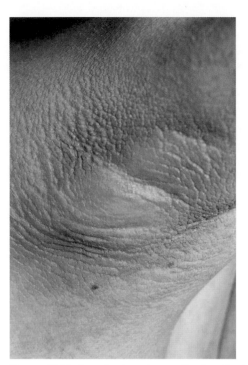

Figure 22.33 Juvenile dermatomyositis. Acanthosis nigricans of the axillary area.

perforation, pneumatosis intestinalis or hemorrhage. D-Xylose absorption has been decreased in patients with JDM, suggesting the decreased absorption of nutrients and medications, including oral corticosteroids, and leading to the suggestion that the disorder be treated with intravenous methylprednisolone for acute cases.[142] Dysphagia from impaired muscle function may lead to esophageal reflux and aspiration pneumonia, requiring intravenous feeding. Children with JDM have occasionally been described with hepatomegaly, cholestasis, or pancreatitis.

The majority of patients with JDM show a reduced ventilatory capacity without respiratory complaints, probably owing to respiratory muscle weakness and poor chest wall compliance. Decreased diffusion capacity and evidence of interstitial lung disease is uncommon, but may present with dyspnea on exertion. Cardiac disease is rare in children with JDM, and mainly involves murmurs and cardiomegaly. Although pericarditis occurs, conduction defects and acute myocarditis are uncommon but severely damaging. Central or peripheral nervous system disease is very rare, in contrast with SLE. Similarly, other than conjunctival vessel tortuosity, eye disease is usually limited to cataracts from administration of systemic corticosteroids. Immunoglobulin A nephropathy has been described, but renal disease is not generally a feature of JDM.[143]

The presence of arthritis, significant dysphagia, renal disease, Raynaud phenomenon, or neuropathy should also prompt consideration of evaluation for overlap disease. Up to 10% of children with JDM show an overlap syndrome with features of SLE, systemic scleroderma, or juvenile idiopathic arthritis.

The diagnosis of JDM is suspected on clinical grounds, based on the typical cutaneous manifestations and evidence of muscle weakness and/or tenderness. Increased levels of muscle enzymes and the demonstration of increased signal intensity on fat-suppressed T2-weighted MRI scans[144] provide evidence of muscle inflammation. The increased signal intensity on MRI scans relates to accumulated extracellular water content. It is indistinguishable from other inflammatory myopathies or rhabdomyolysis, but can be differentiated from muscular dystrophies. Several enzyme levels should be assessed concomitantly (serum aldolase, aspartate aminotransferase, lactic dehydrogenase, and serum creatine phosphokinase levels), because having elevation of just one level is not unusual. In one study, 36% of patients with active disease failed to show an increase in serum creatine phosphokinase. Muscle biopsy of a site shown to be affected by clinical examination or MRI testing can be performed to confirm the presence of perifascicular and perivascular lymphocytic infiltration with atrophy, necrosis, and late fibrosis of the muscle fibers. Skin biopsy is usually not valuable.

Children with active JDM are often lymphopenic, but show a relative increase in the percentage of B cells, as defined by anti-CD19 monoclonal antibody binding. Overall, 70% of children with JDMS have one or more detectable myositis-specific and myositis-associated antibody if full serological testing is performed.[123] The high frequency of myositis –specific antibodies, particularly anti-Jo-1 in adults with DM, in contrast to children, has been a distinguishing feature between adult and pediatric disease. Indeed, anti-Jo-1 antibodies (against histidyl-tRNA synthetase) are found in 2–5% of patients with JDM and anti-Mi-2 antibodies (against a DNA helicase) in ~5%. Recently identified antibodies, however, are found more often in affected children. These include anti-p155/140 or anti-p155, which is detected in 23–29% of children and is linked to more severe cutaneous involvement with generalized lipodystrophy, and anti-p140, which is noted in 13–23% of pediatric patients and associated with calcinosis and contractures.[145] Children with overlap disease may have anti-PM-Scl (5–7%) or anti-U1-RNP (~6%) antibodies. ANA is also present in 60–70% of newly diagnosed children, usually in a coarse speckled pattern.

The course of juvenile dermatomyositis can be monophasic (lasting remission within 1 or 2 years, 37%), chronic (60%), or polyphasic (3%).[146] In a recent report of JDM patients followed into adulthood (median time from diagnosis, 16.8 years), 90% of patients had persistent damage to the skin (77%), muscle (65%) and skeletal (57%) systems.[147] Unfortunately, prediction of disease course has been a challenge, although inadequate treatment is a strong predictor of poor outcome. A shorter duration of untreated disease and a lower JDM skin disease activity score at onset of disease are correlated with a monocyclic course.[135] The presence of persistence skin eruptions (especially Gottron's papules) 3 months after initiation of treatment predicts a longer time to remission, and if Gottron's papules and nail fold capillaroscopy are both abnormal at 6 months after initiation, the outcome is particularly poor.[146] Organ damage 6 months after onset of treatment is also a predictor for poor prognosis.[147] By 36 weeks, persistent nail fold capillary changes, which correlate with skin disease rather than muscle disease, also predict a non-monocyclic disease.[135]

During the active phase of dermatomyositis, children are particularly at risk for sudden, overwhelming Gram-negative sepsis, sometimes masked by corticosteroids. Hospitalization may be advisable in the acute stage, especially if the disease involves palatal-respiratory muscles, to prevent aspiration and to ensure adequate respiration, including by feeding intravenously and using mechanical ventilation if necessary. A high index of suspicion must be maintained for aspiration due to weak palatal-respiratory function or perforation of a viscus, and early aggressive therapy must be instituted when necessary. Nevertheless, the mortality rate, formerly about 30%, generally due to these complications, has been markedly reduced by intervention, and most recently was found to be 3–4%.[126,139]

Most JDM is treated with high-dosage corticosteroid therapy, and many specialists now initiate pulsed intravenous steroids (30 mg/kg or up to 1.5 g), administered every 24–48 h until laboratory values normalize. Usage of pulse steroids, followed by oral corticosteroids or intermittent pulses if needed for continued control, has been shown to decrease the duration of rash, cause less functional impairment, and markedly reduce calcifications in comparison with those children treated with oral corticosteroids only. Side-effects are not increased with pulse steroids and the overall dosage of required corticosteroids tends to be less than that with oral treatment.

Some patients may fail to respond even to very large doses of corticosteroids. Methotrexate is generally the second-line treatment for JDM, when the disease is recalcitrant or corticosteroid usage is problematic. Treatment of severe JDM early in the course with both intravenous methylprednisolone and methotrexate appears to be more useful than with either agent alone,[148] and milder patients have responded to methotrexate (or IVIG) alone.[149] Methotrexate can be administered orally or, preferably, by injection at a dosage of 1 mg/kg per week with a maximum of 40 mg/week. Intravenous gammaglobulin has also been found to be an effective steroid-sparing agent, especially for cutaneous manifestations. Other cytotoxic agents such as azathioprine in dosages of 1–3 mg/kg (up to 200 mg/day) or cyclosporine (5.0 mg/kg per day) may be used in severe life-threatening forms of dermatomyositis, or when the disease cannot be adequately managed with prednisone alone. However, biologics and particularly rituximab are showing promise. Rituximab has been generally well tolerated, with infections and particularly infusion reactions as the main adverse events. Although the onset of action can be slow, the response is good, including with more than one course.[150,151] TNF-α has been implicated in the pathogenesis and severity of JDM, and some patients have shown benefit, especially with administration of infliximab;[152] however, other patients have not responded, particularly with etanercept, or have even worsened on a TNF-α antagonist. Disease that is refractory to immunosuppressants, including rituximab, can be treated successfully with autologous stem cell transplantation.[153]

The response of the cutaneous features of JDM to treatment may not correlate with the response of muscle; skin manifestations may persist for years despite resolution of other signs of disease. Oral antimalarial agents, especially hydroxychloroquine (5 mg/kg per day), have been helpful in controlling the cutaneous manifestations of dermatomyositis. Although the risk of retinopathy in patients receiving long-term hydroxychloroquine use is low, ophthalmic examinations every 6 months are recommended. Topical corticosteroids and calcineurin inhibitors do little to reverse the skin signs of JDM, although topical fluocinolone 0.025% in oil has been helpful with the pruritus of chronic scalp involvement. Counseling about sun protection is critical (see discussion for SLE).

The problematic calcinosis may gradually disappear, but can cause considerable morbidity. Despite the long list of medications that have been used successfully in anecdotal reports in an effort to hasten clearance, no agent has been helpful in the majority of cases. Nevertheless bisphosphonates have led to dramatic improvement in some patients.[154] Surgical procedures may also be useful in selected situations.[155] Occlusive dressings (such as Duoderm) over joint areas, particularly when areas are ulcerated and draining, have promoted healing. Physiotherapy is important for patients with or at risk for contractures to prevent deformity and increase muscle strength; MRI evaluations, myometry, and blood studies did not show increased muscle inflammation after exercise, suggesting that a moderate exercise program is acceptable with active myopathy.[156]

Progressive systemic sclerosis (scleroderma)

Scleroderma (meaning hard skin) can be classified into two major categories, a variety limited to the skin (see Morphea) and the multisystemic disease, systemic scleroderma (progressive systemic sclerosis). Other scleroderma-like disorders include chronic graft-versus-host disease (see Ch. 25), eosinophilic fasciitis, scleroderma from toxins, nephrogenic systemic fibrosis, and sclerodermatous plaques in progeria, Werner syndrome (Ch. 6) and phenylketonuria (Ch. 24). In the neonate, stiff skin syndrome (Ch. 6) can be confused with systemic sclerosis.

Juvenile onset systemic sclerosis (jSSc) features pathologic thickening and tethering of skin, as well as visceral fibrosis, as a result of small vessel vasculopathy. Fewer than 5% of patients with systemic sclerosis have their onset before the age of 16 years. The disorder has a mean age of onset of 8 years, but has been described as young as 0.4 years of age. On average it requires 1–4 years to make the diagnosis because the onset is often insidious.[157] As in adult-onset systemic sclerosis, jSSc predominantly affects females (female: male ratio of 2.1–10.5:1), including in prepubertal patients.[158–161,162] However, jSSc shows many clinical and immunologic features that distinguish it from adult-onset systemic sclerosis.[163,164] The new classification for jSSc was proposed in 2007[165] (Table 22.8) and focuses on symmetrical proximal skin sclerosis/induration being the major criterion for diagnosis. This classification distinguishes jSSc from overlap disease, which is more common in children than in adults (in one large study in 29% of pediatric patients).[166] Diffuse involvement (vs limited cutaneous sclerosis) is seen in 90–100% of patients. In comparison with adults, jSSc has less frequent visceral involvement, but a greater prevalence of arthritis and myositis.[167]

Although morphea and systemic sclerosis may share some of the same pathomechanisms and both show cutaneous sclerosis, they remain different disorders with a tremendous difference in prognosis; only rare cases of morphea have shown any evidence of visceral involvement (see below). The presence of sclerodactyly and/or Raynaud phenomenon should alert the physician to consider a systemic form of scleroderma; overall, Raynaud phenomenon and skin induration are seen in 84% of affected children. Capillary microscopy of the nail folds, performed with an ophthalmoscope, otoscope or dermatoscope after a drop of mineral oil is placed on the nail fold area, may be useful in confirming the diagnosis. Enlarged, dilated nail fold capillaries forming 'giant' or sausage-shaped capillary loops are seen in virtually all children with systemic sclerosis. The dilatation and loss of capillary loops of systemic scleroderma is indistinguishable from that of patients with juvenile dermatomyositis, but is distinct from the nail fold capillary changes seen in SLE and is not seen in patients with isolated Raynaud disease, acrocyanosis, or morphea. The presence of these nail fold capillary changes attests to the endothelial cell damage in systemic sclerosis. Nail changes in which the distal portion of the nail beds adheres to the ventral surface of the nail plate and obliterates the space that normally separates these two structures have also been described. Digital infarcts affect 10–28% of children and calcinosis up to 18%.

Raynaud phenomenon, although extremely uncommon in childhood, is the first sign of systemic sclerosis in 70% of pediatric patients (Fig. 22.34). Precipitated by cold or emotional stress, it is characterized by pallor, cyanosis, and hyperemia with pain, burning, numbness, tingling, swelling, and hyperhidrosis of the affected fingers or toes. Rarely, Raynaud phenomenon affects the nose, lips, cheeks, or ears. This disorder is present in almost all patients with systemic sclerosis, in 10–30% of patients with SLE, in some cases of JDM and mixed connective tissue disease, and in other individuals as a primary disorder. The condition may occur in children as young as 1 year of age.

Primary disease, rather than that associated with an underlying collagen vascular disease, affects 69% of children who show Raynaud phenomenon.[168] In both primary and secondary forms of Raynaud phenomenon, female children predominate (80%). The age of onset, presence of livedo reticularis, and presence of antiphospholipid antibody cannot distinguish secondary from primary disease, but a positive ANA and abnormal capillary pattern correlate strongly with the presence of an underlying disease.[168] Raynaud phenomenon must be differentiated from acrocyanosis, which is common in thin adolescent girls as a purplish discoloration. The discoloration of acrocyanosis tends to affect the toes more than the fingers, to be mottled, and to largely persist with warming. Nail fold capillary changes are absent in acrocyanosis, but distal pulses may be faint.

The hands of most children with progressive systemic sclerosis become shiny, with tapered fingertips and restricted movements (Fig. 22.35). Prior to showing evidence of sclerosis, the hands and

---

Table 22.8 Proposed criteria for diagnosis of systemic sclerosis

Major criterion
 Sclerodactyly

Minor criteria
 Raynaud phenomenon
 Nail fold capillary changes
 Ulcers of the digital tips
 Dysphagia
 Gastroesophageal reflux
 Arrhythmias
 Heart failure
 Pulmonary fibrosis
 Reduced carbon monoxide lung capacity
 Tendon friction rubs
 Arthritis
 Myositis
 Neuropathy
 Carpal tunnel syndrome
 Antinuclear antibodies
 SSc-selective autoantibodies (anti-topoisomerase I, anti-PM-Scl, anti-centromere, etc.)

Requires one major and at least two of the 20 minor criteria to be present. This classification has a specificity of 96% and a sensitivity of 90%. Modified from Zulian 2008.[166]

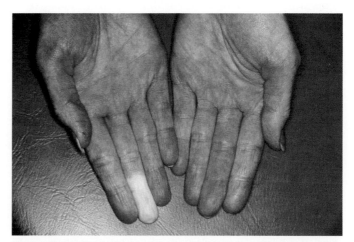

Figure 22.34 Raynaud phenomenon. Note the blue discoloration of the thumbs and fingers with the sharply demarcated white coloration of the distal aspect of the third finger.

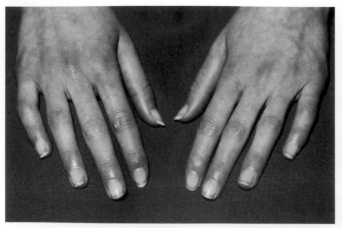

Figure 22.35 Systemic scleroderma. Sclerodactyly with shiny, tight skin of the fingers. Note the small calcification on the index finger.

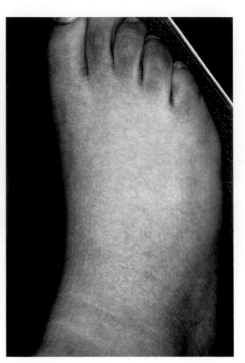

Figure 22.37 Systemic scleroderma. Speckled 'salt and pepper' pigmentation on the foot of a teenage girl with systemic scleroderma.

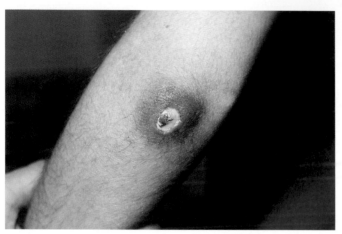

Figure 22.36 Systemic scleroderma. Ulceration overlying a joint.

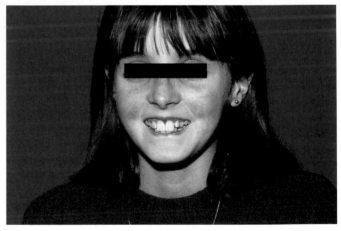

Figure 22.38 Systemic scleroderma. Smooth atrophic skin, pinched nose, and fixed grimace are evident on the face of this adolescent.

feet may be edematous for a few weeks. In addition, telangiectases, calcification (Fig. 22.35), ulceration (Fig. 22.36), and dyspigmentation may be seen. These pigmentary changes may be homogeneously hypopigmented or hyperpigmented, or may have a 'salt and pepper'-like appearance due to retained perifollicular hyperpigmentation in areas of hypopigmentation (Fig. 22.37). The appearance of the face is characteristic. The forehead is smooth and cannot be wrinkled, and atrophy and tightening of the skin give a characteristic appearance due to a fixed stare, pinched nose, prominent teeth, pursed lips, reduced oral aperture, and a perpetual grimace-like facies (Fig. 22.38).

Early scleroderma is often associated with arthralgias and limited joint mobility. Patients often complain initially of weight loss, fatigue, gastrointestinal symptoms, and exertional dyspnea. Muscle weakness is seen in up to 40% of children, and often is associated with evidence of myositis. Overall, gastrointestinal manifestations have been described in up to 75% of children. In addition to the acid reflux[169] and decreased esophageal motility, patients have reported constipation, bloating, discomfort, regurgitation, weight loss, and malabsorption.

Pulmonary disease is a major cause of mortality, and evidence of its presence should be sought. Pulmonary function testing tends to be a sensitive indicator, usually showing restrictive lung disease (54% of children), even if clinically silent.[170] High-resolution computed tomographic (CT) scanning is more sensitive than pulmonary function testing (and certainly than routine chest radiographs). Its use is particularly appropriate for young children who cannot adequately undergo pulmonary function tests, if not for all pediatric patients with scleroderma.[171] Serum levels of KL-6, a mucin-like glycoprotein antigen, are significantly higher in children with systemic sclerosis and pulmonary fibrosis than in patients without interstitial lung disease.[172] Cardiac disease (occurring in 15%) may be secondary to pulmonary hypertension or may be primary (pericarditis, arrhythmia, cardiac failure). Severe cardiomyopathy has been described in children with systemic sclerosis/myositis overlap.[173] Up to 60% of children have shown evidence of renal involvement, usually during the first 3 years of diffuse scleroderma. However, only 5% develop renal failure and 0.7% scleroderma renal crisis. Regular monitoring of blood pressure is critical to identify rapid progression and hypertensive renal crisis. Central nervous system involvement affects only 3% of affected children.

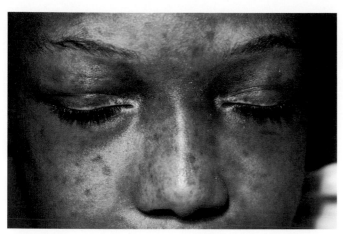

Figure 22.39 CREST syndrome. Telangiectatic mats on the face. This young girl showed sclerodactyly, Raynaud syndrome, and esophageal dysmotility.

Limited cutaneous scleroderma, the CREST syndrome (Fig. 22.39), is quite rare in children. Patients generally have a more slowly progressive form of the disease and have anticentromere antibodies. Although some patients with the CREST syndrome may develop severe pulmonary hypertension, more extensive cutaneous lesions, and visceral involvement, the patients with this subset generally tend to have a relatively benign course.

The diagnosis of systemic scleroderma is easily established when cutaneous sclerosis of the face and hands is present, particularly when it is associated with Raynaud phenomenon, nail fold telangiectasia, and visceral involvement. Symptoms or signs of dysphagia or gastroesophageal reflux help to confirm the diagnosis. Most children with systemic scleroderma have antinuclear antibodies (81–97%), often of the speckled or nucleolar configuration. Antibodies directed against Scl70, a breakdown product of topoisomerase I, correlate with diffuse disease, but not poorer survival in children; these antibodies are found in 28–34% of children with systemic sclerosis. Antibodies against centromeres are rare (7–8%, vs 21–23% in adults), commensurate with the rarity of CREST syndrome in the pediatric population.

The survival rate for jSSc is 89–94% at 5 years, 80–87.4% at 10 years and 74–87.4% at 15 years, considerably better than in adults with SSc.[158,165] Most deaths result from cardiac (most common), pulmonary or renal disease. Treatment of systemic scleroderma in children is challenging and similar to that in adults. Early treatment before the occurrence of the irreversible fibrotic damage to tissue is ideal. General measures include avoidance of factors producing vasospasm (tension, fatigue, stress, cold weather, and smoking in adolescents) and minimizing trauma to the hands. Heated gloves are available and emollients and dressings can be applied to ulcerated cutaneous sites. Calcium channel blockers such as nifedipine or nicardipine, which reduce smooth muscle contraction by reducing the uptake of calcium, are considered first-line therapy for Raynaud phenomenon. Pentoxifylline, which lowers blood viscosity thus increasing blood flow, can also help control the severity of Raynaud phenomenon and digital ulcers. Intravenous infusion of iloprost or other prostanoids are used for severe jSSc-related Raynaud phenomenon and digital ulcers. Physiotherapy is important to limit contractures.

The arthritis may respond to NSAIDs or salicylates. Proton pump inhibitors (e.g., omeprazole and lansoprazole) are the treatment of choice for reflux esophagitis. General measures for treating reflux include elevating the head of the bed, staying upright after eating, a bland diet, and restricting the size of meals. Prokinetic drugs, such as domperidone, may improve motility, and antibiotics administered in rotation may decrease the risk of malabsorption from bacterial overgrowth. Intravenous pulse therapy cyclophosphamide has been recommended at a dosage of $0.5–1$ g/m^2 every 4 weeks for at least 6 months for interstitial lung disease. Good hydration and frequent voiding are important to decrease the risk of cystitis. Endothelin receptor antagonists or phosphodiesterase inhibitors, followed by intravenous infusions of prostacyclin analogues have been used for the pulmonary artery hypertension.[174] Oxygen, antibiotics, and diuretics may also be required for lung disease, especially with congestive heart failure.

Immunosuppression with methotrexate or mycophenolate mofetil have been shown to improve the skin manifestations, and have been particularly useful for children with overlap disorders. Corticosteroids do not appear to help the sclerodermatous process and may trigger renal crisis; however, systemic steroids may be appropriate to treat severe disabling arthritis or myositis. Angiotensin-converting enzyme inhibitors, such as losartan and captopril, are critical in controlling hypertension and stabilizing renal function. The renal disease may require dialysis. Several children who have failed other therapies have been treated with autologous stem cells with improvement in clinical signs and stabilization of pulmonary function.[175,176] New experimental drugs are endothelin receptor antagonists (such as bosentan and sitaxentan) for pulmonary arterial hypertension and digital infarcts, and sildenafil (vasodilator for Raynaud phenomenon).

The pathogenesis of systemic sclerosis involves alterations in the immune system, vasculature, and connective tissue. Cytokine mediators, such as transforming growth factor-beta (TGF-β), platelet-derived growth factor (PDGF) and connective tissue growth factor (CTGF) are particularly important in inducing fibroblast activation and differentiation to myofibroblasts,[177] triggering collagen synthesis. An imbalance between matrix metalloproteinases and tissue inhibitors of matrix metalloproteinases may also play a role. Also of major importance are the presence of autoantibodies and the vasospastic phenomena with endothelial damage that precede digital, pulmonary, and renal fibrosis. New experimental therapies target TGF-β/Smad signaling[178] and PDGF signaling (such as imatinib).[179] Support groups for patients with scleroderma are the Scleroderma Foundation (www.scleroderma.org); the Scleroderma Society (www.sclerodermasociety.co.uk), and the Scleroderma Society of Canada (www.scleroderma.ca).

Eosinophilic fasciitis

Eosinophilic fasciitis (diffuse fasciitis with eosinophilia) is a sclerodermatous disease characterized by diffuse infiltration of the skin of the extremities and trunk without visceral involvement or Raynaud phenomenon (Table 22.9). Seen rarely in children, eosinophilic fasciitis has been reported to evolve into generalized or localized morphea (localized scleroderma) in two-thirds of 21 children carrying the diagnosis in one series[180] and in several case reports,[181,182] suggesting that the disorder is likely to be an acute variant within the spectrum of severe morphea.[183] In contrast to adults with eosinophilic fasciitis, the childhood form shows a female predominance, frequently affects the hands with painless contractures and sclerosis, and is associated with arthritis in only 25% of cases (vs 44% of adults). The hematologic abnormalities that have been noted in adults (aplastic anemia, thrombocytopenic purpura) have not been described in children. However, renal involvement, especially IgA nephropathy, has been noted.

Table 22.9 Eosinophilic fasciitis

Scleroderma-like disease without Raynaud phenomenon or visceral involvement
Painful swelling and induration of skin and subcutaneous tissue
Usually acute onset after trauma, stress, or strenuous physical activity
Cobblestone or puckered appearance; later scleroderma-like skin changes in two-thirds of patients
Eosinophilia and hypergammaglobulinemia common; occasional elevation in ANA or aldolase
Good initial response to systemic corticosteroids

The disorder is characterized by a sudden onset of painful swelling, induration, and scleroderma-like changes of the skin with marked thickening of the subcutaneous fascia. The skin has a cobblestone or puckered appearance with a yellowish or erythematous color. It is indurated, taut, and bound down without pigmentary change. The hands, forearms, feet, and legs are most commonly affected initially, although the disease may progress to the trunk and face. In the majority of patients, onset of the disorder follows trauma or excessive physical exertion. Although systemic changes are usually absent in affected children, patients show transient peripheral eosinophilia early in the disease, hypergammaglobulinemia, and an elevated sedimentation rate. The ANA may be positive during the course, but is usually negative, especially at onset. A deep biopsy, including fascia, is necessary to confirm the diagnosis. Sections show edema and infiltration of the lower subcutis and deep fascia by lymphocytes, plasma cells, and histiocytes. Eosinophils may be detected in early lesions; thick, sclerotic dermis is characteristically seen late in the disorder.

Patients usually show a good initial response to oral or pulse intravenous systemic corticosteroids, sometimes in combination with methotrexate, with resolution of soft tissue induration and correction of laboratory abnormalities.[184] However, gradual progression during one or more years to cutaneous fibrosis and/or painless flexion contractures, especially of the hands and feet, occurs in the majority of affected children.[180] Younger age at onset (<7 years of age) and greater disease severity have been correlated with a higher risk of progression to residual fibrosis. Physiotherapy is important adjunctive therapy. In children who do not respond to systemic corticosteroids, methotrexate, azathioprine, cyclosporine, cyclophosphamide, intravenous immunoglobulin,[185] dapsone,[186] infliximab,[187] rituximab,[188] retinoids, and UVA1 irradiation[183,189] may be considered.

Eosinophilic fasciitis must be distinguished from eosinophilia-myalgia syndrome, which has rarely been described in children.[190] These patients show pronounced eosinophilia with myalgias, especially centrally, and vasculitis of the skin and other organs. Generally, oral ingestion of contaminated L-tryptophan is to blame, although contaminated tryptophan in total parenteral nutrition has also been implicated. The associated myopathy and sometimes elevated muscle enzymes can lead to confusion with an overlap autoimmune syndrome (of scleroderma and dermatomyositis).[184,191]

Nephrogenic systemic fibrosis

Nephrogenic systemic fibrosis (NSF; previously known as nephrogenic fibrosing dermopathy) is has increasingly been recognized as a sclerosing disorder predominantly seen in patients with renal dysfunction who receive gadolinium-based contrast media as part of magnetic resonance imaging testing. First described in 2000,[192] the first pediatric cases were reported in 2003;[193] in total, 10 pediatric cases have been published to date. The signs of NSF may develop 2–75 days after exposure to the gadolinium.[194] Lesions are characterized by indurated papules and plaques, brawny thickening of skin with a *peau d'orange* appearance, and sometimes joint contractures. The extremities, buttocks and trunk are usually involved, and the face is typically spared. Patients usually complain of associated pruritus, burning, and pain. Biopsy sections of skin show widened septae in with subcutaneous tissue with increased collagen and fibroblasts. Calcinosis cutis and perforating collagenosis may be seen concomitantly in biopsy sections. The disorder must be distinguished from scleroderma, scleromyxedema, and scleredema. The FDA warns against the use of all gadolinium agents in patients with glomerular filtration rates (GFR) <30 mL/min and the European guidelines with GFR of 30–60 mL/min.[195] The most successful treatment is renal transplantation or recovery of the acute renal injury to improve renal function. Gadolinium should be avoided or limited in patients at risk.

Scleredema

Scleredema (scleredema adultorum of Buschke) is a rare disorder of diffuse large areas of induration of skin that must be distinguished from scleroderma.[196] The condition most commonly occurs in adult diabetics, but 29% of described cases are in children, half of these during the first decade of life. Although scleredema may begin spontaneously, 65–95% of patients have the onset of their disorder within a few days to 10 weeks after an acute febrile illness. Of these, 58% of the infections are streptococcal; scleredema may also follow infections from influenza, measles, mumps and varicella.[197,198]

The skin changes usually begin suddenly on the neck and then gradually spread to the upper trunk, and occasionally the arms and face, as non-pitting thickening. The abdomen and lower extremities, if involved, tend to show less thickening than the upper half of the body. The texture of skin has been described as brawny or woody, and children with facial involvement may show a mask-like facies. Although affected individuals are usually asymptomatic, some patients display a prodromal period with fever, malaise, and myalgias. In general the condition is benign, although involvement of the skeletal and cardiac muscles has been reported. Tachycardia, arrhythmias, and pericardial effusions have been noted. In addition, the tongue has been involved, making protrusion and mastication difficult. The thickening results from deposition of acid mucopolysaccharide, largely hyaluronic acid, which can easily be detected with colloidal iron or Alcian blue stains of lesional biopsies. The mechanism by which infection triggers scleredema in children is unclear. Therapy is generally unsuccessful, although high-dose intravenous corticosteroids may have been helpful in one affected child.[199] Lesions usually resolve spontaneously within months to 2 years.

Scleredema has rarely been described in a generalized form in sick neonates (sclerema neonatorum) and must be distinguished from subcutaneous fat necrosis of the newborn in this age group (see Ch. 2).

Morphea

Morphea is an autoimmune disorder characterized by localized areas of cutaneous sclerosis. Although sometimes termed 'localized scleroderma', use of the term morphea decreases the potential confusion with systemic sclerosis, or scleroderma, a disorder with significantly greater morbidity.[200,201] Morphea has been divided into a number of different subgroups. In children, linear morphea (or linear scleroderma) is most common (42–65%), followed by the relatively localized plaque type (26–37%); in contrast, the plaque type of morphea is the most common form in adults.[202-204] Linear scleroderma includes the *en coup de sabre* and *Parry–Romberg syndrome* forms, in which facial involvement occurs. Morphea can be a generalized disorder of skin and subcutaneous tissues (*generalized morphea*, ~7%), manifest in *deep morphea* forms (including *morphea profunda*, *subcutaneous morphea* and *disabling pansclerotic morphea* extending from the dermis to the bone) or, very rarely, be *bullous*.

The incidence of localized scleroderma is 0.4–1/100 000 individuals, and more often in Caucasians than other racial groups.[202,203] In children the localized form of scleroderma occurs at least 10 times more often than the systemic form of scleroderma.[170] The disorder occurs primarily in children and young adults with a 2–3 : 1 female-to-male ratio. The mean age in children is 7.3–8.2 years of age,[202,204] but morphea has been described in infants and even neonates. A family history of rheumatic or autoimmune disorders is reported in the 1st- or 2nd-degree relatives of 12–24% of children, but only 2% of relatives have morphea itself.

The unilateral nature of the disorder in most patients and the patterning of lesions have led investigators to hypothesize that affected patients have genetically susceptible cells in this distribution triggered by environmental exposure to develop morphea. Some patterns of morphea seem to follow lines of Blaschko, but others are clearly distinct. Although a link with infection has been postulated, especially based on the similarity of localized scleroderma to erythema migrans and sclerosis of cutaneous lesions of Lyme disease, investigations from North America and more recent studies from Europe have not found *Borrelia burgdorferi* infection by serologic or polymerase chain reaction (PCR) testing.[205] Administration of valproic acid has been thought to trigger morphea in two patients.[206] Trauma has also been postulated to trigger lesions of pediatric morphea, and this possibility is supported by the frequency of activation of morphea when corrective procedures are performed; however, trauma is so common in children that controlled studies would be required to further consider its role.

The onset of plaque-type morphea is insidious and begins with flesh-colored, erythematous or purplish patches that evolve during weeks to months into firm, hyperpigmented or ivory plaques, with or without a surrounding lilac or violaceous inflammatory zone. The ivory plaques may resemble lesions of lichen sclerosus et atrophicus tend to evolve with the development of hyperpigmentation (Fig. 22.40). Morphea may also show localized areas of atrophy and resemble atrophoderma (see Atrophoderma of Pasini and Pierini) (Fig. 22.41). Occasionally, patients may have 1–3 mm papules of morphea (*guttate morphea*). Affected areas, in order of decreasing frequency, are the trunk, neck, extremities, and face. In the plaque type, lesions typically vary from a few centimeters to several inches in diameter; fusion of many plaques may result in the more generalized form of morphea.

Linear lesions (linear scleroderma) generally affect the limbs (occasionally the head or trunk). Their clinical appearance is similar to that of plaque-like forms but the violaceous peripheral ring is inconspicuous or only present at the advancing border. Lesions usually present as broad linear bands of induration with dyspigmentation (both hyperpigmentation and hypopigmentation). Much less commonly a thin linear band of involvement is seen (Fig. 22.42) and must be distinguished from linear atrophoderma of Moulin (see below). Associated atrophy of the skin and underlying subcutaneous tissue leads to a puckered or indented appearance

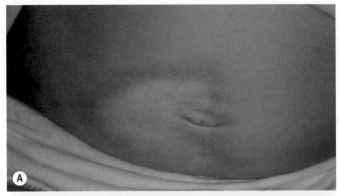

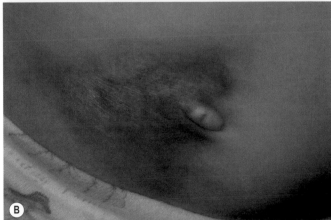

Figure 22.40 Morphea. (A) Ivory-colored, indurated plaque that resembles the lesions of lichen sclerosus et atrophicus. Note the sharp midline demarcation. (B) As this lesion evolves, it becomes intensely hyperpigmented, despite softening.

with prominent veins (Fig. 22.43); atrophy may also affect the underlying muscles, fascia, and bones. Linear scleroderma involving an extremity is associated with a risk of undergrowth, both linear and circumferential, of the affected limb (Fig. 22.44), and involvement of the breast area can lead to undergrowth and severe deformity in female adolescents (Fig. 22.45). Impaired joint mobility and contractures (Fig. 22.46) are additional risks when the sclerodermatous area overlies a joint. Occasionally, roughening of one surface of the long bones underlying a linear area of morphea may be noted. This disorder, termed *melorheostosis*, is characterized radiographically by a picture suggesting that of wax flowing down the side of a candle. Calcinosis is occasionally present in plaques of linear scleroderma, and the underlying muscle may show an interstitial myositis.

Linear scleroderma involving the frontal or frontoparietal region of the scalp (with or without associated facial hemiatrophy) is called *en coup de sabre* (cut of a saber). Although usually unilateral, bilateral cases of en coup de sabre have rarely been described.[207,208] This variant begins with a purplish to brown patch that becomes sclerotic and often progresses to a linear depressed groove. The initial presentation may be confused with a port-wine stain if purplish in color without induration or depression, but pulsed dye laser does not lead to improvement.[209] With loss of subcutaneous tissue, it thus resembles a saber wound or cut on the frontoparietal scalp (Fig. 22.47). The groove may extend downward into the cheek, nose, and upper lip, and, at times, may involve the mouth, gum, chin, or neck. Extension to the scalp or periocular area leads to

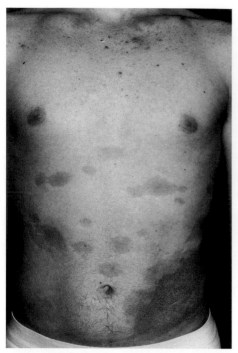

Figure 22.41 Morphea. Atrophodermic patches in a boy with generalized morphea.

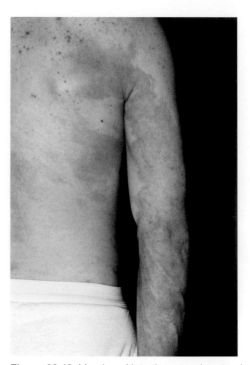

Figure 22.43 Morphea. Note the extensive atrophy with a clear cliff-drop border to the affected area and prominent veins.

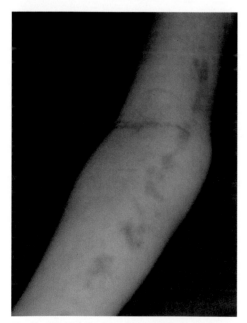

Figure 22.42 Morphea. This distribution of morphea in a thin linear configuration is unusual. This lesion does not show the atrophoderma of 'linear atrophoderma of Moulin', but otherwise looks similar.

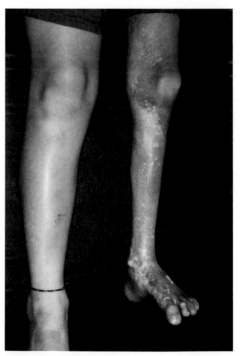

Figure 22.44 Linear scleroderma. Severe circumference and linear hypotrophy of the bone and soft tissue of the affected leg led to gait disturbance and compensatory scoliosis.

associated alopecia of the scalp in a linear distribution (Fig. 22.48) or local loss of eyebrow or eyelashes.

The en coup de sabre variety probably represents a more superficial form of progressive facial hemiatrophy (the Parry–Romberg syndrome), a condition of slowly progressive atrophy of the soft tissue of half of the face with (Fig. 22.49A) or without (Fig. 22.49B) associated dermal sclerosis. Either en coup de sabre or Parry–Romberg syndrome may be accompanied by alopecia, seizures, headaches (including migraine), trigeminal neuralgia, enophthalmos, myopathy of external eye muscles, and atrophy of the ipsilateral half of the upper lip, gum, and tongue. Intracerebral atrophy, white matter hyperintensity, and calcifications may be seen on MRI and CT evaluations of affected patients,[207,210,211] especially in patients with neurologic abnormalities.

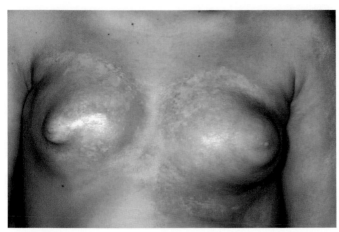

Figure 22.45 This girl with generalized morphea and uncomfortable sclerosis of the chest had resultant undergrowth and deformity of the breasts.

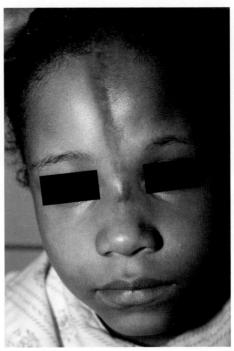

Figure 22.47 En coup de sabre. Extensive soft tissue atrophy in a linear pattern of the forehead and nose. Note the alopecia of the medial brow.

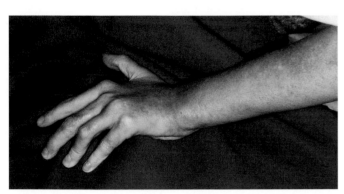

Figure 22.46 Linear scleroderma. Flexion contraction of the hand in a girl with linear scleroderma. This is the extent to which she can straighten her hand.

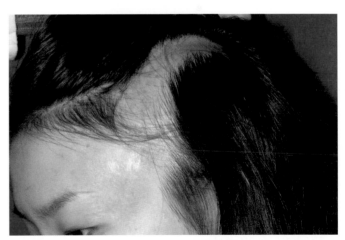

Figure 22.48 En coup de sabre. Note the extension into the scalp, leaving cicatricial alopecia.

Deep morphea feels indurated at a deep level; the skin surface may appear slightly puckered or hyperpigmented, but often appears normal, except in the disabling pansclerotic type. When there is deep as well as superficial involvement and fixation to underlying structures, this disorder has been termed *disabling pansclerotic morphea*. This variant, usually affecting girls from 1 to 14 years, tends to have a relentless disabling course and may produce marked disability in the form of flexion contractures and musculoskeletal atrophy of the extremities. Non-healing ulcers and squamous cell carcinoma may develop at sites of involvement.[212,213]

In most pediatric patients the diagnosis of localized scleroderma is made clinically. However, histologic evaluation of lesional skin shows early inflammation with edema, subsequent sclerosis, and eventual atrophy. The dermis progressively thickens and dermal appendages are lost. In contrast to systemic sclerosis there is more inflammation and more sclerosis of the papillary dermis. Although the development of the cutaneous sclerosis occurs in both morphea and systemic sclerosis, the clinical features and prognosis of these two autoimmune disorders differs. Raynaud phenomenon and nail fold capillary dilation and dropout are seen in systemic sclerosis, but rarely in morphea. The only systemic manifestation seen with some regularity is arthralgias, which occur in 16.9% of affected children[202] and have been described more commonly with linear scleroderma, generalized morphea, and deep morphea. Dysphagia is not uncommon, and ocular (esp. anterior segment inflammation)[214] and renal[215] abnormalities have also been described.

However, the restrictive pulmonary and esophageal complications of systemic sclerosis (see above) very rarely arise in morphea.[202] Children affected with morphea and evidence of systemic sclerosis generally have arthralgia and more extensive skin disease (e.g., extensive linear scleroderma, generalized morphea). Morphea, however, may occur in patients with other collagen vascular disorders as part of an overlap syndrome (4.9%).[203]

Several laboratory tests may be abnormal in individuals with morphea, although to date they do not have significant diagnostic or prognostic value. Erythrocyte sedimentation rate may be increased, especially in children with linear and deep morphea.[204] Eosinophilia is seen in 15% overall, most often in the deep type.[204] ANA positivity, especially speckled and nucleolar patterns, occurs in 30–42% of affected children,[203] and rheumatoid factor is positive

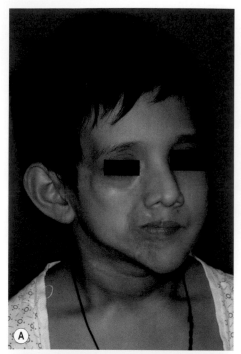

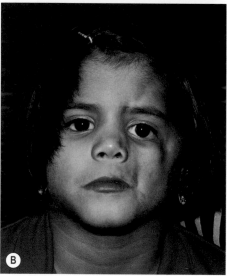

Figure 22.49 Parry–Romberg syndrome. Hemifacial atrophy: (A) with or (B) without induration of the overlying skin. In (A) the superficial sclerosis and atrophy is clearly visible.

subcutaneous fat.[219]; laser Doppler flowmetry has recently been shown to be even more accurate than thermography for discriminating disease activity non-invasively.[220]

Plaque-type morphea lesions tend to improve within 3–5 years, but the residual hypopigmentation, hyperpigmentation, and occasional atrophy may persist indefinitely. Lesions of linear scleroderma tend to last longer, and their associated atrophy and dyspigmentation, especially of the atrophy of the en coup de sabre/facial hemiatrophy variant, usually persists. Sequelae can be serious and range from significant cosmetic impairment to functional disability from joint contractures, limb length discrepancies, loss of skin adnexae, calcinosis in linear lesions, and ocular or central nervous system dysfunction.

Treatment for morphea is difficult and depends on the extent of involvement, activity of the disease, and cosmetic or functional ramifications. Potent topical or intralesional corticosteroid therapy has been reported to hasten resolution of lesions, but this form of therapy is generally unrewarding, can result in localized atrophy, and is not recommended. Topical calcipotriene ointment has been shown to stop the progression of morphea and linear scleroderma when used early in the course and especially when used twice daily under occlusion.[221] This vitamin D_3 derivative does not reverse tissue loss. Calcipotriol-betamethasone dipropionate has recently been found to be helpful.[222] The combination of physiotherapy, massage, warm baths, and exercise are frequently helpful for patients with linear morphea in whom the involvement overlies a joint because of the risk of contractures.

The first-line systemic therapy for disfiguring or disabling morphea/linear scleroderma is the combination of methotrexate and corticosteroids.[223] The systemic corticosteroids are given (either orally or pulse intravenous) for the first 2–3 months and methotrexate 0.3–0.6 mg/kg per week (either orally or intramuscularly) initially and on a continuing basis. More than 90% of children with linear scleroderma show disease improvement.[224,225] and in one trial of 10 patients with localized scleroderma all patients responded to this therapy and skin lesions became inactive.[223] The mean time to response was 3 months, and relapses were seen after the methotrexate was discontinued. Mycophenolate mofetil has more recently been used successfully in individuals who have failed to respond to steroids and methotrexate. In a recent study of 10 patients, all patients treated with 600–1200 mg/m² per day experienced improvement that allowed withdrawal or reduction in steroid and methotrexate within 3–6 months.[226] Oral calcitriol has also led to significant improvement in some children with linear scleroderma.[227] Calcitriol therapy is limited by its risk of excessive urinary excretion of calcium, leading to renal calcium stones. Dietary calcium must be restricted, and serum calcium and phosphorus as well as the calcium/creatinine ratio in a 24-h collection of urine must be monitored. In children, the starting dose is 0.25 µg/day with increases to a maximum of 0.75 µg/day in children and 1.5 µg/day in adolescents.

PUVA (psoralen plus UVA light) has been shown to be efficacious for morphea, but its toxicity restricts its use in children. Medium-dose (70 J/cm²) UVA1 (340–400 nm) significantly reduce the skin thickness of morphea.[228] While UVA1 light has been thought to work best in lighter skin, a recent study suggests good effects as well in darker skin.[229] Twice-daily application of calcipotriol ointment combined with UVA1 phototherapy has led to significant softening and repigmentation of morphea lesions, but it is unclear whether these results are superior to topical calcipotriol or UVA1 therapy alone.[230]

Successful repair of contractures may be performed by release and coverage with grafts.[231] Leg-shortening procedures to the normal leg may be performed after full growth is achieved when the affected

in 16% of patients. Anti-topoisomerase II antibodies have been detected in 76% of patients with localized scleroderma (and 85% in generalized morphea); these antibodies (in contrast to anti-topoisomerase I/Scl 70 antibodies) have been found in 14% of patients with systemic scleroderma and are detectable in <10% of normal children and of children with SLE or JDM.[216] Serum levels of B-cell activating factor (BAFF) are increased in morphea (as well as in systemic sclerosis and systemic lupus erythematosus), but not in autoimmune blistering disorders such as pemphigus or pemphigoid.[217] In addition, anti-matrix metalloproteinase-1 antibodies are markedly increased in about 50% of patients with morphea or systemic sclerosis, suggesting that decreased collagen I degradation may contribute.[218] Thermography is a sensitive new means for evaluating disease activity and risk of further tissue damage, particularly in patients without severe associated atrophy of skin and leg is significantly shortened by linear scleroderma. Orthodontic devices can assist in craniofacial development and minimize the progressive asymmetry of the lower face from Parry–Romberg syndrome.[232] For residual facial lesions with atrophy, transplants of fat, bone, or cartilage and laser to lighten the associated hyperpigmentation have been used.[233]

Lichen sclerosus et atrophicus

Lichen sclerosus et atrophicus (LSA, LS&A) is a disorder primarily of females (85–90%) with a prevalence of >1 in 900 girls. It has its onset before 13 years of age in 10–15% of affected individuals; 70% of these childhood cases occur before 7 years of age, and the condition has been described during the first weeks of life. The mean age at development of symptoms is 5 years with a mean age at diagnosis of 6.7 years.

The eruption of lichen sclerosus et atrophicus is characterized by sharply defined, small, pink to ivory white, slightly raised, flat-topped papules a few millimeters in diameter that aggregate and coalesce into plaques of various sizes (Fig. 22.50). As the condition progresses, atrophy and delling (fine follicular plugs on the surface of macules) may become highly diagnostic features of the disorder. The anogenital region is involved in 75% of affected children. Of those who have involvement elsewhere on the body, up to 42% have anogenital involvement as well. Extragenital lesions are asymptomatic and may begin asymmetrically but eventually become distributed in a symmetrical manner, primarily on the trunk, neck, and extremities.

The Koebner phenomenon has been documented in cases of lichen sclerosus et atrophicus in childhood; lesions may develop in surgical scars or sites of vaccination, and exacerbations of quiescent lesions may occur following local trauma or irritation. Lesions of lichen sclerosus et atrophicus occasionally occur in association with morphea, and it has been suggested that lichen sclerosus et atrophicus is a variant form of morphea with more superficial manifestations.

In females the anogenital lesions frequently tend to surround both the vulvar and perianal regions in an hourglass or figure-of-8 pattern (Fig. 22.51). Lichen sclerosus et atrophicus in children most commonly presents in the genital area in girls with itching (50%), pain, and bleeding from the vulvar and perianal area on urination and particularly defecation, resulting in constipation and urinary symptoms. In studies of girls with vulvar disease or pruritus of the vulvar area, 18% and 11% had lichen sclerosus, respectively.[234,235] A vaginal discharge may precede the vulvar lesions in about 20% of affected girls. Anogenital lesions uncommonly extend to include the skin on the inner aspect of the thighs. In many girls erythema, purpuric areas (Figs 22.52, 22.53), blistering, and excoriations predominate, especially on the labia minora and clitoris.

When seen on the dorsum of the glans penis in males, the disorder has been termed *balanitis xerotica obliterans*. Clinical evidence of lichen sclerosus of the genital area in boys is less common than in girls, but lichen sclerosis has been blamed for 60% of cases of acquired phimosis based on histologic evidence of its presence and is found in biopsy sections of 15% of boys with hypospadias.[236,237]

Occurrence of lichen sclerosus in more than one member of the immediate family is not rare.[238,239] Another autoimmune disease is present as well in up to 15% of patients and 65% have a family history of an autoimmune disorder.

Lichen sclerosus is often misdiagnosed when present in the genital area of girls as irritant dermatitis because of the associated itching and erythema or as sexual abuse owing to the purpura and bleeding. The associated white coloration may lead to confusion with vitiligo or postinflammatory hypopigmentation (Fig. 22.53).

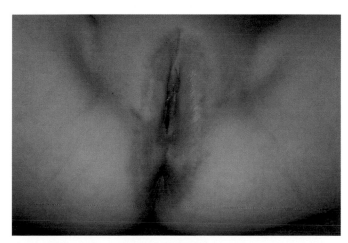

Figure 22.51 Lichen sclerosus et atrophicus. Whitening and atrophy of the labia majora and labia minora is seen in an hourglass configuration involving the anal area as well.

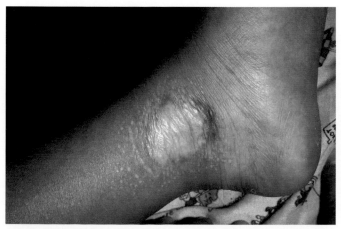

Figure 22.50 Lichen sclerosus et atrophicus. Ivory atrophic plaque in a girl who also showed genital area involvement.

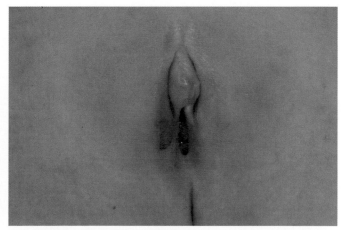

Figure 22.52 Lichen sclerosus et atrophicus. Note the whitening, underlying pink coloration and purpura.

Topical corticosteroids have been the treatment of choice, with ultrapotent topical steroids used more commonly for approximately 6–8 weeks to rapidly alleviate symptoms.[244] In prepubertal boys with phimosis, skin stretching and application of potent topical corticosteroids bid for 6 weeks led to a retractable prepuce, including in 67% of the boys with clinically detectable lichen sclerosus.[237] Topical tacrolimus 0.1% ointment has been used successfully to clear lichen sclerosus in girls, both as initial treatment and to promote continued remission.[245,246] Complete circumcision is the treatment of choice in boys with phimosis; application of topical tacrolimus ointment 0.1% ointment for 3 weeks after therapeutic circumcision led to disease control in all treated boys with lichen sclerosus.[247] Plastic surgery may be required to correct labial fusion or clitoral obliteration from scarring. Treatment of extragenital lichen sclerosus is much more challenging than treatment of genital region disease. Although topical steroids and retinoids are occasionally helpful,[248] ultraviolet A light treatment (especially UVA1) and systemic medication used to treat morphea, such as methotrexate or mycophenolate mofetil (see Morphea, above) may be required.[249,250]

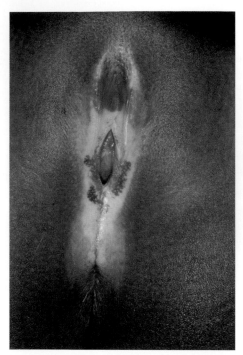

Figure 22.53 Lichen sclerosus et atrophicus. This dark-skinned girl with advanced lichen sclerosis et atrophicus shows sparing of the perianal area (which is unusual) and partial obliteration of the clitoris. Note the associated depigmentation.

The anal pruritus often raises the possibility of pinworm infestation, and the inflammation and discharge should cause one to consider candidiasis or bacterial vulvovaginitis. The associated constipation or dysuria often leads to unnecessary gastrointestinal or urinary tract investigations as well.

Lichen sclerosus has been described in girls with an infantile perianal pyramidal protrusion (see also Ch. 15), a benign tag-like lesion that has been associated with constipation in many patients.[240–242]

Although biopsies of lesional skin show characteristic epidermal atrophy with subepidermal vacuolization, a hyalinized superficial dermis, and a bandlike infiltration of lymphocytes beneath it, the diagnosis of lichen sclerosus is usually made on clinical grounds and confirmatory biopsy is both traumatic and unnecessary. Lichen sclerosus has been reported to improve or disappear at puberty in 60% of affected girls, although a recent study suggested that signs of the disease persisted in the majority of children and adolescents. In the remaining one-third, the condition tends to persist. In females, atrophy of the clitoris and labia minora may occur, with fusion of the latter and stricture of the introitus. In patients in whom improvement has taken place, the disorder may be reactivated years later by trauma, pregnancy, or the administration of anovulatory drugs.

Although vulvar lichen sclerosus et atrophicus in childhood does not predispose to neoplasia, the incidence of lesional squamous cell carcinoma in adult cases has been estimated as 4.4%. Patients with cases persisting beyond puberty or having onset after puberty accordingly should be observed at intervals of 6–12 months for the possibility of leukoplakia or carcinoma. Newly arising nodules, erosions, or ulcers in lesions of lichen sclerosus et atrophicus that persist for more than a few weeks require histologic examination. Development of genital carcinoma has been reported in an adult after clearance of lichen sclerosus during childhood.[243]

Anetoderma

Anetoderma (from the Greek, meaning 'relaxed skin') describes an idiopathic atrophy of the skin characterized by oval lesions of thin, soft, loosely wrinkled, depigmented outpouchings of skin that result from weakening of the connective tissue of the dermis.[251] The disorder may be classified as primary macular anetoderma, which arises from apparently normal skin, or as secondary macular anetoderma, which follows previous inflammatory and infiltrative dermatoses. Some of these dermatoses include lupus erythematosus and other collagen vascular disorders, secondary syphilis, sarcoidosis, leprosy, tuberculosis, urticarial lesions, purpura, lichen planus, acne vulgaris, urticaria pigmentosa, molluscum contagiosum,[252] varicella,[253] juvenile xanthogranuloma,[254] and pilomatricomas.[255,256] A peculiar laxity of the eyelid (blepharosclerosis) may also follow chronic or recurrent dermatitis of the eyelids. When eyelid changes are seen in association with adenoma of the thyroid and progressive enlargement of the lips due to inflammation of the labial salivary glands, the disorder is termed *Ascher's syndrome*.

Based on whether an inflammatory reaction occurred before the appearance of the atrophy, two types of primary macular anetoderma have been described: *anetoderma of Jadassohn–Pellizzari*, in which the atrophic lesions are preceded by inflammation, and *anetoderma of Schweninger–Buzzi*, in which there is no evidence of inflammation. Although the underlying etiopathogenesis of primary anetoderma has not been established, serologic and direct immunofluorescent findings suggest that immunologically mediated mechanisms play a role in the elastolytic process seen in individuals with this disorder.

Anetoderma of Jadassohn–Pellizzari is characterized by crops of round or oval pink 0.5–1 cm macules that develop on the trunk, shoulders, upper arms, thighs, sacral area, and occasionally face or scalp (Fig. 22.54). Usually seen in females in their teens to 30s, and occasionally in children, the anetoderma begins with a sharply defined red spot, which grows peripherally and becomes round or oval and slightly depressed. As the redness disappears, the characteristic atrophic, wrinkled, and pale herniation ensues. The herniation yields on pressure, admitting the finger through the surrounding ring of normal skin. Much like an umbilical hernia, the bulge reappears when the finger is released and at times, fatty tissue may infiltrate the lesions, giving them a more firm, soft tumor-like appearance.

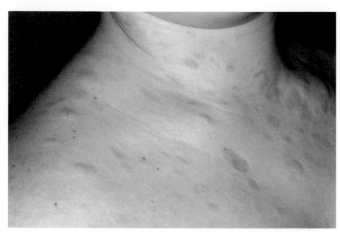

Figure 22.54 Anetoderma. Well-demarcated circles of cutaneous atrophy developed progressively during a 3-year period on the anterior trunk and neck of this young boy. Antiphospholipid antibodies were negative.

Anetoderma of Schweninger–Buzzi is manifested by the sudden appearance of large numbers of bluish-white macules, some of which are protuberant, without any preceding inflammatory eruption. Women are affected more commonly than men. Lesions are generally seen on the trunk, neck, face, shoulders, extremities, and back and range from 10 to 20 mm in diameter. Seen during childhood or adult life, the disease is slowly progressive and new lesions appear one by one or in groups, a few at a time, over a period of years. The essential difference in this form of anetoderma is a lack of inflammation and the relative absence of coalescence of lesions.

Anetoderma has also been described in premature infants after use of gel electrocardiographic electrodes, perhaps because of local hypoxemia from the pressure of the electrodes (see Ch. 2).[257,258] More widespread congenital anetoderma of unclear cause has also been described.[259] Drug-induced anetoderma has been described after administration of penicillamine, particularly in patients with Wilson's disease. Prothrombotic abnormalities and antiphospholipid antibodies have been detected in the majority of patients in more than one investigation, and criteria for the diagnosis of antiphospholipid antibody syndrome have been fulfilled in some patients.[114,260,261] In all forms of macular anetoderma the primary histopathologic feature is the destruction and loss of elastic fibers. No therapy is effective.

Atrophoderma of Pasini and Pierini

Atrophoderma of Pasini and Pierini is a relatively uncommon atrophic disorder of the skin. Of unknown etiology, it may appear at any age (and may be congenital),[262] and usually begins on the trunk during the late teens or early 20s. The atrophy begins as an asymptomatic, slightly erythematous macular lesion on the trunk (particularly the back). Initially there may be a singular lesion, but more often there are multiple lesions, varying from 1 to 12 cm in diameter. Lesions typically develop a slate gray to brown pigmentation within weeks, but hypopigmented and skin-colored lesions of atrophoderma have been described.[263] The atrophic patches extend very slowly with a depressed center and a 'cliff-drop' border. They tend to increase in number for 10 years or more, primarily on the trunk, neck, and proximal extremities, and then generally persist without apparent change. During this period new lesions may occur and old ones slowly enlarge.

Skin biopsy may be helpful to distinguish from other disorders with a more distinct histopathological picture; a rim of clinically normal skin must be included for comparison.[263] Many experts consider atrophoderma to be a subset of morphea (Fig. 22.41).[264] In a series that included 48 children, atrophoderma of Pasini and Pierini was found to be three times more common in females than in males, and encompassed 10% of cases of localized morphea.[265] In 12.5% of the affected children, the atrophodermic area developed induration centrally during a mean follow-up period of 10 years; an additional 12.5% of the children with atrophoderma had separate lesions of morphea in addition to the atrophoderma. European investigators have found antibodies to *B. burgdorferi* in 38% of patients with atrophoderma and stabilization by treatment with antibiotic in 80% of patients in one study;[266] a relationship to *B. burgdorferi* and success with antibody treatment has not been noted in studies in the United States. A linear form of atrophoderma (linear atrophoderma of Moulin) has also been described;[267] this chronic, non-progressive atrophic, band-like lesion can be distinguished from linear scleroderma by its lack of inflammation, induration, or pigmentary change but can lead to significant cosmetic impairment.[268] The course of atrophoderma is benign, and there is no known effective treatment. The disorder remains active for months to years and lesions persist indefinitely, but there are no reports of systemic involvement or complications.

Relapsing polychondritis

Relapsing polychondritis is an uncommon disorder in children characterized by inflammation of cartilage.[269] Most patients have demonstrated circulating antibodies against type II collagen, a component of cartilage, suggesting an autoimmune pathomechanism. This concept is supported by the report of an infant with transient disease born to a woman with the condition.[270] Some patients have, or develop, concomitant collagen vascular disorders, especially lupus erythematosus.[271]

Erythema, swelling, and pain of the ear is the most common manifestation (90%), with typical involvement of the auricle but sparing of the earlobe. With chronic disease, the ear cartilage is destroyed, resulting in a scarred 'cauliflower' ear. Nasal cartilage inflammation occurs in 70% of affected individuals and can eventuate in a saddle nose deformity. Nonerosive arthritis has been described in approximately 80% of patients, particularly involving the sternoclavicular, sternomanubrial, and costochondral joints. Approximately 65% of patients have ocular inflammation (conjunctivitis, episcleritis, uveitis, corneal ulceration, or inflammation of the optic nerve).

The most serious potential feature is respiratory tract involvement.[272] Patients may show hoarseness, dyspnea, cough, wheezing, or anterior neck tenderness with palpation of the trachea. Secondary pulmonary infection, airway collapse, or airway obstruction may ensue. Renal and cardiac manifestations have rarely been described. A variety of dermatologic features have been associated, among them aphthous ulcerations, palpable purpura, panniculitic nodules, pyoderma gangrenosum,[273] livedo reticularis, and neutrophilic disorders of skin, such as Sweet's syndrome.

In children, the most commonly seen disorder to be considered in the differential is oto melalgia ('red ear syndrome'), a condition characterized by erythema, swelling, and pain of the entire ear that does not spare the earlobe. The condition is short-lived, responds to application of ice, and is episodic, rather than persistent (see Ch. 12; Fig. 12.77). 'Red ear syndrome' can be associated with migraines.

The treatment of choice for relapsing polychondritis is systemic corticosteroids (1 mg/ kg per day initially) and NSAIDs. Dapsone

Table 22.10 Sjögren's syndrome

Major clinical features
   Inflammation and chronic enlargement of salivary glands
   Keratoconjunctivitis sicca (dryness and atrophy of cornea and
      conjunctiva)
   Xerostomia (dryness of mouth)
   Fatigue
   May be associated with other autoimmune disorders, especially
      juvenile idiopathic arthritis

Cutaneous features
   Dryness and scaling of skin (with partial or complete loss of
      perspiration)
   Sparse, dry, brittle hair
   Hypergammaglobulinemic purpura (usually lower extremities)
   Raynaud phenomenon

Laboratory abnormalities
   Positive ANA, RF, anti-Ro, anti-La antibodies in majority
   Tests to show decreased tear formation and salivary flow

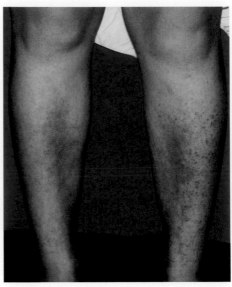

Figure 22.55 Hypergammaglobulinemic purpura. Recurrent episodes of purpuric lesions on the lower extremities left darkly hyperpigmented macules that persisted. Joint pain and high levels of anti-Ro and anti-La antibodies as well as IgG were associated. Administration of hydroxychloroquine eliminated her joint pain and dramatically suppressed her cutaneous flares, leading to gradual fading of the hyperpigmentation.

and methotrexate have been used as steroid-sparing agents.[274] Tracheostomy and/or airway stents may be required for upper respiratory tract involvement.[272] One child responded to oral ingestion of type II collagen as a toleragen.[275]

Sjögren syndrome

Sjögren syndrome is a chronic autoimmune disorder of unknown etiology that is uncommon in children.[276] Characteristic features are keratoconjunctivitis sicca (inflammation of the cornea and the conjunctiva with dryness and atrophy), xerostomia (dryness of the mouth from lack of normal secretion), and enlargement of the salivary and lacrimal glands (as a result of lymphocytic and plasma cell infiltration) (Table 22.10). Sjögren syndrome can occur alone (primary) or in association with virtually any other autoimmune disorder (secondary), although the most common is juvenile idiopathic arthritis. The manifestations of Sjögren syndrome may precede the onset of another autoimmune disorder by years.

In a review of 39 pediatric cases, the female:male ratio in children was >3:1 with a mean age at onset of 8 years.[277] In children the presenting sign is usually parotitis (62.5% versus 13% in adults) with parotid gland enlargement, which may be bilateral.[278,279] Almost 10% of the children; however, presented with an extraglandular manifestation, and 51% experienced at least one extraglandular manifestation during the course of the disease. The most common extraglandular feature was leukopenia (35%) with or without splenomegaly. Arthritis occurred in 15% of children (vs 38.5% of adults). Purpura and intense residual hyperpigmentation, especially on the lower extremities (hypergammaglobulinemic purpura), was the most common cutaneous manifestation (12% of children) (Fig. 22.55). Annular erythema, erythema nodosum, mesangial proliferative glomerulonephritis,[280] and lipodystrophy have also been described.

The most prominent mucosal manifestations are associated with dryness of the gingiva and mucous membranes of the mouth and, at times, the conjunctivae, nose, pharynx, larynx, vagina, and respiratory tract. The tongue may become smooth, red, and dry, and in severe cases there may be difficulty in swallowing dry food. The lips may be cracked, fissured, or ulcerated, particularly at the corners of the mouth; the teeth frequently undergo rapid and severe decay; the eyes may be reddened and moist; and thick, tenacious secretions forming ropy mucous strands in the inner canthi may be noted

(particularly when the patient first arises in the morning). Other ocular manifestations include a burning sensation, as if a foreign body is present in the eye, and inability to produce tears in response to irritants or emotion.

A positive ANA has been seen in 67% of children (versus 92% of adults) and rheumatoid factor in 71%. Positive anti-Ro and/or anti-La antibodies are detected in 73% of children with Sjögren syndrome. Patients may show a decreased stimulated salivary flow rate and positive Schirmer (<5 mm wetting of a strip of filter paper inserted under the lower eyelid) and rose bengal (conjunctival staining) tests of the eyes. Sialography, sonograms, and computed tomographic scans of the parotid glands may show evidence of enlargement and inflammation.

The management of Sjögren's syndrome includes treatment of the dry skin, keratoconjunctivitis, and xerostomia with lubricants, and therapy for the associated collagen vascular disorder if present. Although systemic corticosteroids are capable of reducing the swelling of the salivary glands, they usually do not improve the function of affected glands, and their use is reserved for severely affected patients.

Mixed connective tissue disease

Only 0.6% of all pediatric patients with rheumatologic disease have mixed connective tissue disease (MCTD; overlap syndrome), and MCTD begins before 16 years of age in 23% of individuals with MCTD.[281] Approximately 85% are female, and the earliest age of onset described has been 2 years age (mean onset at 9.5–12 years). The disease is characterized by the combination of clinical features and laboratory data similar to those of systemic lupus erythematosus, scleroderma, dermatomyositis, juvenile idiopathic arthritis, and/or Sjögren disease (Table 22.11). The most common presenting features of pediatric-onset MCTD are fatigue and pain (arthralgias, myalgias) and Raynaud phenomenon (mean, 73% of children).[282]

In one study, myositis was the most common manifestation at onset, with SLE-like features least common.[281] Although some patients with mixed connective tissue disease have deforming arthritis, an evanescent non-erosive, non-deforming polyarthritis similar to that seen in patients with systemic lupus erythematosus is more common.

Approximately two-thirds of children with mixed connective tissue disease have cardiac involvement, including pericarditis, myocarditis, congestive heart failure, and aortic insufficiency; about 10% have clinical evidence of renal disease (more by biopsy evaluation);[283] and about 10% of individuals have neurologic abnormalities (trigeminal sensory neuropathy, 'vascular' headaches, seizures, multiple peripheral neuropathies, and cerebral infarction or hemorrhage). Severe thrombocytopenia appears to be limited to childhood forms, and the incidence of renal and cardiac involvement is higher in children than in adults.[283] However, the course is more slowly progressive, overall shows a lower risk of renal disease and responses to lower doses of steroids than SLE or scleroderma. Progression towards scleroderma can be predicted by changes on capillaroscopy.

The distinguishing laboratory marker for this disease is the demonstration of serum antibody specific for ribonuclear protein (nRNP, U_1RNP), a ribonuclease-sensitive component of extractable nuclear antigen (ENA). In addition, most patients with mixed connective tissue disease have high serum titers of antinuclear antibody in a speckled pattern. Up to 50% of patients show a high titer of rheumatoid factor.

Immunosuppressive medications, particularly systemic corticosteroids, hydroxychloroquine and methotrexate, are most commonly used as therapy. Immunoadsorption onto protein A in combination with low-dose systemic steroids and bosentan led to remission in a recalcitrant patient.[284] Long-lasting remission occurs in only 3% of patients, with most having at least persistent Raynaud disease and a favorable outcome in 82%. Mortality is lower in children than in adults, especially if organ involvement can be detected and treated early.

Table 22.11 Mixed connective tissue disease (Kasukawa's criteria)[281]

Criteria: Must meet all three to be diagnosed with MCTD
Raynaud's and/or swollen fingers or hands
Positive anti-RNP antibody
Must have at least one abnormal finding from two or more of the following disorders: SLE (facial eruption, polyarthritis, serositis, lymphadenopathy, leukopenia, thrombocytopenia); scleroderma (sclerodactyly, pulmonary fibrosis, vital capacity <80% of normal, carbon monoxide diffusion <70% of normal, decreased esophageal motility)

Mucocutaneous features
Alopecia
Heliotrope rash
Hypo- and/or hyperpigmentation
Livedo reticularis
Lupus-like lesions, including malar telangiectasia and/or erythema
Mucosal dryness
Periungual telangiectasia
Photosensitivity
Sclerodactyly

Musculoskeletal features
Arthritis or arthralgia
Proximal muscle weakness
Raynaud phenomenon
Tapered or sausage-shaped fingers

Gastrointestinal features
Abnormal esophageal motility

Cardiac features
Aortic insufficiency
Congestive heart failure
Pericarditis/myocarditis

Pulmonary features
Abnormal pulmonary function tests
Pulmonary fibrosis

Neurologic features
Headache
Peripheral neuropathy
Seizures

Renal features
Glomerulonephritis

Laboratory abnormalities
Elevated anti-RNP titer
Speckled ANA

Key References

Avcin T, Cimaz R, Rozman B. The Ped-APS Registry: the antiphospholipid syndrome in childhood. *Lupus*. 2009;18:894–899.

Christen-Zaech S, Hakim MD, Afsar FS, et al. Pediatric morphea (localized scleroderma): review of 136 patients. *J Am Acad Dermatol*. 2008;59:385–396.

Hiraki LT, Benseler SM, Tyrrell PN, et al. Clinical and laboratory characteristics and long-term outcome of pediatric systemic lupus erythematosus: a longitudinal study. *J Pediatr*. 2008;152:550–556.

Izmirly PM, Llanos C, Lee LA, et al. Cutaneous manifestations of neonatal lupus and risk of subsequent congenital heart block. *Arthritis Rheum*. 2010;62:1153–1157.

Martini G, Foeldvari I, Russo R, et al. Systemic sclerosis in childhood: clinical and immunologic features of 153 patients in an international database. *Arthritis Rheum*. 2006;54:3971–3978.

Mier RJ, Shishov M, Higgins GC, et al. Pediatric-onset mixed connective tissue disease. *Rheum Dis Clin North Am*. 2005;31:483–496, vii.

Ravelli A, Trail L, Ferrari C, et al. Long-term outcome and prognostic factors of juvenile dermatomyositis: a multinational, multicenter study of 490 patients. *Arthritis Care Res (Hoboken)*. 2010;62:63–72.

Wedderburn LR, Rider LG. Juvenile dermatomyositis: new developments in pathogenesis, assessment and treatment. *Best Pract Res Clin Rheumatol*. 2009;23:665–678.

Zulian F, Athreya BH, Laxer R, et al. Juvenile localized scleroderma: clinical and epidemiological features in 750 children. An international study. *Rheumatology (Oxford)*. 2006;45:614–620.

Zulian F. Systemic sclerosis and localized scleroderma in childhood. *Rheum Dis Clin North Am*. 2008;34:239–255; ix.

23 Endocrine Disorders and the Skin

Endocrinologic diseases frequently display cutaneous features that may provide diagnostic clues, and patients with these disorders may be more susceptible to a variety of mucocutaneous problems. Some of these conditions and their therapy, where applicable, are reviewed here. A thorough discussion of all endocrine disorders and their treatment is beyond the scope of this chapter.

Thyroid disorders

Patients with hyper- or hypothyroidism may present with a variety of skin findings. In some cases, associated hair or nail defects may also be seen. Some of these findings are related to the imbalance in thyroid hormone, which may play a role in skin homeostasis via its influence on proteoglycan synthesis, epidermal differentiation, hair formation and sebum production.[1]

Hyperthyroidism

Table 23.1 summarizes the various cutaneous changes that may be seen in hyperthyroidism. This disorder is most often caused by an autoimmune thyroid disease, Graves disease. It may also be associated with a hyperfunctioning thyroid nodule, thyroid multinodular goiters, non-Graves thyroiditis, excessive thyroxine intake or hypersecretion of thyroid stimulating hormone (TSH). Cutaneous features occur most commonly in association with Graves disease, and these manifestations may more often be due to autoimmune mediation rather than direct effects of thyroid hormones.[2]

The clinical features of hyperthyroidism include nervousness, emotional lability, tachycardia and palpitation, heat intolerance, weakness, fatigue, tremors, hyperactivity, increased appetite, weight loss, increased systolic and pulse pressure, accelerated growth, sleep disturbances, school problems, vomiting, diarrhea and, occasionally, exophthalmos. An enlarged thyroid gland is often present. Specific findings that suggest Graves disease include thyroid ophthalmopathy, pretibial myxedema, and acropachy. The ophthalmopathy is secondary to periorbital deposition of glycosaminoglycans, and may present with proptosis, ocular paralysis, or lid lag.

Pretibial myxedema

Pretibial myxedema (PTM, also known as thyroid dermopathy) is manifested as plaques on the anterior tibial surfaces, and is related to localized accumulation of acid mucopolysaccharides. Other locations of involvement are occasionally reported. The majority of patients with PTM have ophthalmopathy.[3,4] The onset of PTM usually follows the diagnosis of hyperthyroidism. Examination reveals non-pitting edema, nodules, and plaques, with pink to yellow-brown discoloration. The overlying epidermis is thin with a waxy and sometimes translucent quality. Hypertrichosis with dilated hair follicles and a 'peau d'orange' appearance may be noted. Polypoid or elephantiasis forms occur less commonly.[3] While the pretibial surfaces are most commonly involved, other areas including the face, scalp, extremities and trunk may reveal similar changes. The differential diagnosis may include cellulitis, trauma, erythema nodosum, or other mucinoses, and PTM can be confirmed by tissue examination of skin biopsy material in conjunction with laboratory findings. Histologic evaluation may reveal mucin deposition and reduced elastic fibers.

Thyroid acropachy

Thyroid acropachy is more common in adults with hyperthyroidism and only occasionally occurs in children, and classically presents as the triad of digital clubbing, soft tissue swelling and periosteal changes. Examination reveals thickening of the soft tissues over the distal extremities and (secondary to diaphyseal periosteal proliferation) of the distal bones. Drumstick-like clubbing, enlargement of the hands and feet, and radiographic changes (fluffy, spiculated, or homogeneous subperiosteal thickening with new bone formation) may be seen. Associated extremity and joint pain may be reported, and nail clubbing may also be seen. Thyroid acropachy is an indicator of severity of thyroid ophthalmopathy and dermopathy.[5]

Less specific cutaneous changes in hyperthyroidism include skin that is warm, velvety, moist, and smooth. Hair may be fine and thin. Facial flushing, increased sweating (particularly of the palms and soles), and palmar erythema are common, especially in the advanced state of the disease, called *thyrotoxicosis*. The nails grow rapidly, are shiny, and may reveal onycholysis (separation or loosening of the nail plate from the nail bed) with distal upward curvature (Plummer's nails). Koilonychia (spoon-shaped nails, Fig. 23.1) and clubbing may also be noted. Chronic urticaria and generalized pruritus are uncommon manifestations of thyrotoxicosis, and chronic active hyperthyroidism can be complicated by Addison disease-like hyperpigmentation. However, the hyperpigmentation of hyperthyroidism is distributed differently, primarily on the shins (Fig. 23.2), posterior feet, and nail beds.[6] Patients with hyperthyroidism may also have an increased incidence of alopecia areata and/or vitiligo.[7,8] Gynecomastia may be present in males, and may be caused by increased conversion of testosterone to estradiol. *Scleromyxedema*, a condition marked by white-yellow papules, weight loss, monoclonal gammopathy, esophageal dysmotility, myopathy, and Raynaud phenomenon, has also been reported in patients (mainly adults) with hyperthyroidism.[9]

Hypothyroidism

Table 23.2 summarizes the various mucocutaneous changes that may be seen in hypothyroidism. Hypothyroidism in pediatric patients may be congenital or acquired. Clinical features of congenital hypothyroidism are shown in Table 23.3. Symptoms may be subtle in both forms of hypothyroidism, but decreased linear growth is an important indicator of both types of disease. Hypothermia, lethargy, and poor feeding are all characteristic of

Table 23.1 Cutaneous manifestations of hyperthyroidism
Warm, velvety, moist, smooth skin
Thin, fine hair; diffuse non-scarring alopecia
Hyperpigmentation (especially of palmar creases, soles, gingivae, buccal mucosa)
Facial flushing
Palmar erythema
Increased sweating
Nail changes (onycholysis, curvature, koilonychia, clubbing, yellow nails)
Pretibial myxedema
Periorbital edema
Chronic urticaria
Generalized pruritus
Thyroid acropachy (clubbing)
Increased incidence of vitiligo, alopecia areata
Gynecomastia (in men)

Table 23.2 Mucocutaneous manifestations of hypothyroidism
Dry, coarse, pale, cool skin
Dull, brittle hair with thinning
Cutis marmorata
Generalized myxedema (especially hands, feet, periorbital)
Carotenoderma
Nail changes (ridged, brittle, grow slowly)
Lateral eyebrow alopecia
Hypertrichosis (back and shoulders usually)
Easy bruising
Ichthyosis
Eruptive or tuberous xanthomas
Livedo reticularis
Periorbital edema
Dermatitis herpetiformis (has been reported with Hashimoto's thyroiditis, atrophic variant)
Protuberant lips
Macroglossia

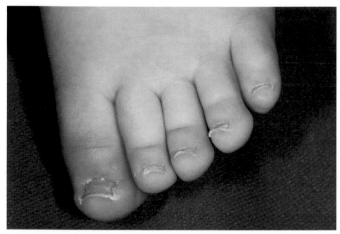

Figure 23.1 Koilonychia. These 'spoon shaped nails' may occur in disease states (such as hyperthyroidism) or as a normal variant in young children, as in this infant.

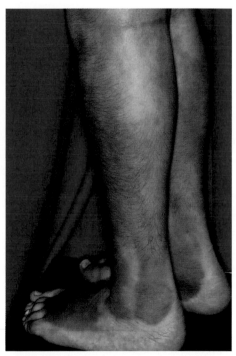

Figure 23.2 Hyperpigmentation of hyperthyroidism. Diffuse hyperpigmentation of the lower extremities was present in this young Hispanic female with Grave's disease.

congenital disease, which is most often diagnosed on routine newborn screening examinations. Children with acquired hypothyroidism tend to be quiet and well behaved, and as a result often receive high grades in school.

Congenital hypothyroidism may develop as a result of agenesis or dysgenesis of the thyroid gland (the most common cause); defective synthesis of thyroid hormone caused by an enzymatic defect; the presence of antithyroid antibodies in a pregnant mother; the lack of maternal iodine during pregnancy (endemic goiter); or the ingestion of antithyroid medications such as propylthiouracil or methimazole by a pregnant woman being treated for thyrotoxicosis. Iodine toxicity from iodine-containing skin antiseptic solutions has been implicated as a potential cause of transient hypothyroidism in newborn infants, although recent studies refute this association.[10,11] Acquired hypothyroidism in children younger than 5 or 6 years of age may be caused by a delayed failure of thyroid remnants (with thyroid dysgenesis); by inborn defects of thyroid hormone synthesis; by ingestion of antithyroid agents; by thyroidectomy or ablation following radiation; or by chronic thyroiditis or hypothalamic-pituitary disease. After the age of 5 or 6 years, although the same etiologies may be involved, chronic lymphocytic thyroiditis

(Hashimoto's thyroiditis) is the most common cause. Although iodine deficiency is the most common cause of hypothyroidism worldwide, it is uncommon in the USA.

Cutaneous features of hypothyroidism are a reflection of the hypometabolic state with reduced body temperature and reflex vasoconstriction. Patients often have dry, coarse, pale, and cool skin. Cutis marmorata (physiologic mottling) may be prominent. Hypohidrosis may lead to acquired palmoplantar keratoderma.[9] Myxedema may occur in hypothyroidism, again as a result of

Table 23.3 Clinical features of congenital hypothyroidism
Puffy (myxedematous) facies
Sallow complexion
Wide anterior fontanelle and sutures
Macroglossia and thick lips
Hypertelorism, depressed nasal bridge
Coarse, brittle hair
Hoarse cry
Translucent ('alabaster') ears
Umbilical hernia and abdominal distention
Heart murmur
Hypotonia and slow reflexes
Short stubby fingers and broad hands
Short lower extremities
Scalp seborrhea, purpura
Prolonged relaxation phase of tendon reflexes
Cold, mottled, or jaundiced skin
Sluggishness and inactivity
Delayed motor development, mental retardation
Lack of coordination and ataxia
Poor weight gain, stunted growth
Subnormal body temperature, poor circulation and intolerance to cold
Delayed/defective dentition
Myxedema (some cases)

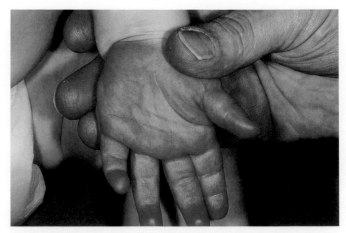

Figure 23.3 Carotenemia. This yellow-orange skin coloration (carotenoderma) is especially prominent on the palms and soles. It may be seen in association with disease states (i.e., hypothyroidism) or with high intake of β-carotene-containing foods, such as prepared baby foods containing orange vegetables, as in this healthy infant.

mucopolysaccharide deposition in skin. It most commonly occurs in the hands, feet and periorbital locations, and may also be deposited in the tongue, giving rise to macroglossia. Generalized puffiness may be present, and the skin may take on a yellow hue as a result of carotenemia (Fig. 23.3). The hair is dull and brittle, and nails are ridged, brittle, and grow very slowly. Patients may have a dull, expressionless facies. Hypertrichosis of the back and shoulders may be seen, and alopecia may involve the lateral portions of the eyebrows. A collodion baby with concomitant congenital hypothyroidism has been reported.[12]

Parathyroid disorders

Disorders of the parathyroid glands (hyperparathyroidism and hypoparathyroidism) may affect the skin in various ways and often present with cutaneous features that can assist the primary or consulting physician in diagnosis and management. Although primary parathyroid disease is uncommon in children, these glands play a major role in the regulation of calcium and phosphorus metabolism, and associated abnormalities manifest distinctive clinical patterns. Parathyroid hormone (PTH) is one of the two main calciotropic hormones (the other one being calcitriol); these hormones regulate phosphate and calcium homeostasis.

Hyperparathyroidism

Primary hyperparathyroidism, one of the least common endocrine disorders of infancy and childhood, is rarely diagnosed in children younger than 16 years of age. When seen, it is usually due to a familial, genetically determined hyperplasia of the parathyroid, which may present as an isolated hyperparathyroidism or as the hyperparathyroidism-jaw tumor syndrome, in which case ossifying tumors of the maxilla or mandible are present.[13] A malignant neoplasm of the parathyroid, or an association with some other disease such as is seen in patients with multiple endocrine adenomatosis (multiple endocrine neoplasia; see below) or chronic renal insufficiency may also result in hyperparathyroidism.[14,15]

The majority of cases of hyperparathyroidism are sporadic, most often being caused by a single adenoma in the parathyroid gland. The clinical features of hyperparathyroidism include systemic effects of hypercalcemia: failure to thrive, muscular weakness, lethargy, anorexia, vomiting, fever, headache, constipation, weight loss, polydipsia, polyuria, mental retardation, metastatic calcification, and, with marked hypercalcemia, stupor or death. Of these, metastatic calcification is the most common cutaneous manifestation, and in patients with sporadic hyperparathyroidism, this may be the only cutaneous finding. Hypercalcemia may also produce an ophthalmologic finding known as *band keratopathy*, which is the result of calcium and phosphate deposition beneath Bowman's capsule. Band keratopathy appears as a superficial corneal opacity resembling frosted or ground glass in a band-like configuration with white flecks or 'holes' in the band resulting in a 'Swiss cheese'-like appearance. It is not specific for hyperparathyroidism, but may also be seen as a manifestation of hypercalcemia secondary to vitamin D intoxication, uremia, or sarcoidosis. It is not commonly found in patients with hyperparathyroidism when serum phosphorus levels are low and glomerular function is maintained.

Patients with chronic renal failure may experience several types of cutaneous manifestations. The skin of the uremic patient may be pruritic, dry, scaly, sallow, and hyperpigmented; the sallow appearance is partially due to anemia, and the hyperpigmentation appears to be the result of decreased renal clearance of melanocyte-stimulating hormone (MSH). Hyperparathyroidism secondary to chronic renal failure results from impaired synthesis of 1,25-dihydroxyvitamin D_3, which leads to hypocalcemia from impaired intestinal calcium absorption and, ultimately, increased levels of parathyroid hormone. Hyperphosphatemia may result in a high serum calcium phosphate product and produce secondary calcification of the skin. This *calcinosis cutis* (see also Ch. 9) manifests as hard calcium deposits in skin and subcutaneous tissues, especially in periarticular locations. These lesions may resolve spontaneously with correction of the serum calcium and phosphate levels. In addition to being seen in hyperparathyroidism, it may also be noted in association with paraneoplastic hypercalcemia, milk alkali syndrome, sarcoidosis and hypervitaminosis D.

When the calcification is more progressive and involves blood vessels, ischemic necrosis of skin and soft tissues occurs and is termed *calciphylaxis*. This rare (especially in children) and life-threatening condition results from vascular calcification and is most commonly reported in patients with end-stage renal disease. Clinically, it is manifested as ecchymotic or infarcted areas of skin, bullous lesions, and plaques of calcinosis with periodic extrusion of calcium. Lesions of pediatric calciphylaxis are most commonly noted on the upper and lower extremities.[16] They are very painful, and mortality related to gangrene and sepsis is high. Extensive calcification in the heart and lungs may result in cardiorespiratory failure.[17] Parathyroidectomy is often, but not always, useful in this setting.[18–20] Histologically, calciphylaxis shows calcification of the walls of small- and medium-sized blood vessels in the dermis and subcuticular regions.

The diagnosis of hyperparathyroidism is established by consistent elevations of total serum calcium above 12 mg/dL, the reduction of serum phosphorus concentrations below 4 mg/dL, and elevated levels of parathyroid hormone. High alkaline phosphatase levels usually indicate bone disease. This complication of hyperparathyroidism may be demonstrated radiographically by generalized demineralization of bones, destructive changes at the growing ends of long bones, subperiosteal erosions (particularly in the phalanges, metacarpals, and lateral portions of the clavicles), and in more advanced disease, generalized rarefaction, cysts, tumors, fractures, and deformities. Radiographs of the abdomen may reveal renal calculi or nephrocalcinosis, and ultrasonography and radioisotope scanning can confirm the diagnosis of primary hyperparathyroidism associated with an isolated parathyroid adenoma. In infants with parathyroid hyperplasia, cupping and fraying at the ends of long bones and ribs may suggest rickets, and severe demineralization and pathologic fractures are common.

Hypoparathyroidism/DiGeorge Syndrome

Hypoparathyroidism is characterized by hypocalcemia and inappropriate response of the parathyroid glands or, less often, with elevated PTH levels and lack of response to the hormone (*pseudohypoparathyroidism*; see below). In childhood, hypoparathyroidism may develop as a congenital idiopathic disorder, but usually appears in the neonatal period or in later infancy or childhood, or as an acute condition following inadvertent removal or damage of the parathyroid glands during thyroid surgery. Congenital hypoparathyroidism may occur alone, may be seen as an autoimmune disorder where it may occur alone or with other endocrine disorders, or may be a hereditary condition associated with an increased familial incidence of other endocrinologic disorders (Addison disease, pernicious anemia, and Hashimoto's thyroiditis), candidiasis, and/or vitiligo. When associated with hypoplasia of the thymus and immunologic defects, the condition is known as DiGeorge syndrome (see below).

Idiopathic or congenital hypoparathyroidism usually is first manifested by tetany or seizures and, in 25–50% of patients, ectodermal defects. The skin of affected individuals is rough, dry, thick, and scaly; the hair and eyebrows are sparse; and the nails are short and thin with brittleness, crumbling, or longitudinal grooving. When hypoparathyroidism occurs during tooth development, pitting, ridging, absence of dental enamel, and absence or hypoplasia of the permanent teeth may result. Extensive calcification of skin and subcutaneous tissues has been reported in an infant with congenital primary hypoparathyroidism, although this is exceedingly rare.[21] Other clinical manifestations include convulsions, carpopedal

spasm, muscle cramps and twitching, numbness or tingling of the extremities, laryngo- or bronchospasm, exfoliative dermatitis, mental retardation, chronic diarrhea (especially in infants), photophobia, keratoconjunctivitis, blepharospasm, and cataracts. Mucocutaneous candidiasis is seen as a complication in 15% of patients with idiopathic hypoparathyroidism. Electrocardiography may reveal prolongation of the QT interval, and head imaging may show calcifications of the basal ganglia.[13] The combination of candidiasis, endocrinopathy, and ectodermal dysplasia has been termed APECED (*a*utoimmune *p*olyendocrinopathy, *c*andidiasis and *e*ctodermal *d*ystrophy) as well as *autoimmune polyglandular syndrome*, and is discussed in more detail below (see also Ch. 17).

The cutaneous manifestations of hypoparathyroidism associated with surgical removal or injury of the parathyroid glands differ from those seen in patients with idiopathic or congenital hypoparathyroidism. These include thinning or loss of hair, the development of horizontal grooves (Beau's lines) in the nails, or a complete loss of nails following episodes of tetany (these abnormalities revert to normal when hypocalcemia is controlled). Hyperpigmentation (predominantly on the face and distal extremities) may resemble melasma, pellagra, or Addison disease and also may occur in cases of post-thyroidectomy hypoparathyroidism. Although cutaneous calcification has been noted, this complication is relatively uncommon.

DiGeorge syndrome is a T cell deficiency disorder that develops as a result of faulty embryologic development of the thymus and the parathyroid glands (a congenital malformation of the third and fourth pharyngeal pouches and the surrounding arches). The classic triad consists of cardiac malformation, hypocalcemia, and T cell immunodeficiency. Defects of the great vessels may include truncus arteriosus, interrupted aortic arch, double aortic arch, or aberrant subclavian artery. Oral candidiasis is an almost constant finding in patients with this disorder, and overwhelming fungal, viral, or bacterial infection usually leads to death early in infancy. Hypocalcemia and tetany may occur at an early age, and other features include chronic diarrhea, interstitial pneumonia, failure to thrive, micrognathia, hypertelorism, low-set ears, bifid uvula, shortened philtrum, bowed mouth, chronic purulent rhinitis, mental retardation, calcification of the central nervous system, and nephrocalcinosis.[22]

DiGeorge syndrome is associated with a deletion in the long arm of chromosome 22, and is also referred to as a 'chromosome 22q11.2 deletion syndrome' or velo-cardio-facial syndrome.[23] Approximately half of DiGeorge syndrome patients are hemizygous for 22q11, and they have occasionally been found to have overlapping deletions in the 10p13/14 boundary.[24,25] These patients are at increased risk for developing psychiatric disorders, with one in four developing schizophrenia and one in six developing major depressive disorders.[26] Other reported psychiatric morbidities include attention-deficit/hyperactivity disorder, oppositional defiant disorder, and anxiety disorders.[27] When the immunodeficiency is severe, thymic or bone marrow transplantation should be considered.[28]

Pseudohypoparathyroidism/Albright's Hereditary Osteodystrophy

Pseudohypoparathyroidism (PHP) is a hereditary disorder in which there is decreased target tissue responsiveness in the receptor tissues, particularly the kidneys and skeletal system, to parathyroid hormone (rather than a true deficiency). PHP is subclassified into types Ia, Ib, Ic, and type II. Albright's hereditary osteodystrophy (AHO) refers to the clinical constellation of physical features, including short stature, obesity, brachydactyly and ectopic ossification.[29]

Pseudopseudohypoparathyroidism (PPHP) is a term used to describe individuals with AHO who have normal end-organ responsiveness to parathyroid hormone. These patients do not develop hypocalcemia and tetany. PHPIa, PHPIc and PPHP all result from heterozygous deactivating mutations in the *GNAS1* gene, and presence of genetic imprinting may lead to quite diverse clinical phenotypes.[29,30]

Patients with PHP have hypocalcemia, hyperphosphatemia, and elevated serum levels of parathyroid hormone. Hypothyroidism secondary to TSH resistance may be seen in PHPIa. Ectopic calcification is common, and intracranial lesions usually involve the basal ganglia and occasionally other regions. Calcinosis cutis may occur, and presents with multiple small papules, plaques, or nodules with a predilection for the scalp, hands and feet, periarticular regions, and chest wall.[31] Soft tissue ossification (osteoma cutis) may be present at birth or develop during infancy or childhood (Fig. 23.4), and is often a presenting feature of the disease, along with hypothyroidism. The subcutaneous calcifications or ossifications may occasionally present very early in life (even by 2 weeks of age), and in those patients may be vital to early recognition and diagnosis of PHP.[32] Dermal or subcutaneous hypoplasia may occasionally be noted in areas of cutaneous calcification.[33]

The characteristic features of AHO include short stature, obesity, and characteristic facial features, including round face, flat nasal bridge, and a short neck. Brachymetaphalangism refers to shortening of the fourth and fifth metacarpals, and may be recognized by knuckle dimples when the patient makes a clenched fist.[31] In addition, the fourth and fifth fingers and toes may appear shortened (Fig. 23.5).[34] Plain radiography may confirm this feature when the clinical findings are subtle. Mental retardation may be present, and may be less common with aggressive and early treatment for the hypocalcemia.

Disorders of the adrenal glands

Adrenal gland dysfunction may result in a variety of systemic effects with various cutaneous manifestations. Those of particular interest to the pediatrician, dermatologist, and pediatric dermatologist are Addison disease, Cushing syndrome, and the adrenogenital syndrome (discussed under Disorders of Androgen Excess).

Addison Disease

Addison disease (primary adrenocortical insufficiency) is caused by the absence of glucocorticoids and mineralocorticoids, and characterized by weakness, anorexia, weight loss, hypotension, decreased serum sodium and chloride, increased serum potassium, hypoglycemia and hyperpigmentation of the skin and mucous membranes. Sporadic and recurrent 'flu-like' episodes may provide a clinical clue to the diagnosis, especially in the setting of pigmentary alterations.[35] Hyperpigmentation in Addison disease is the result of increased production of proopiomelanocortin, which is cleaved to form melanocyte stimulating hormone (MSH) and adrenocorticotropic hormone (ACTH).[36] This overproduction in the pituitary gland occurs as a compensatory phenomenon associated with decreased cortisol production by the adrenal glands. The hyperpigmentation of Addison disease occurs in the setting of primary adrenocortical failure, as opposed to secondary adrenal insufficiency in which case ACTH levels are low and mineralocorticoid production remains relatively intact.[37]

The pigmentation of Addison disease is most intense in the flexures, at sites of pressure and friction, in the creases of the palms and soles (Fig. 23.6), in the nails, in sun-exposed areas, and in normally hyperpigmented areas such as the genitalia and areolae. Pigmentation of the conjunctivae and vaginal mucous membranes is common, and pigmentary changes of the oral mucosae (Fig. 23.7) include spotty or streaked blue-black to brown hyperpigmentation of the gingivae, tongue, hard palate, and buccal mucosa. In addition, increased pigmentation may be noted in existing nevi.[38] The pigmentation may in some children be quite diffuse.[35] Labial pigmentation and longitudinal pigmentary streaks of the fingernails, similar to Laugier–Hunziker syndrome, have been observed.[39] As the pigmentation may in some cases be subtle, comparison of the

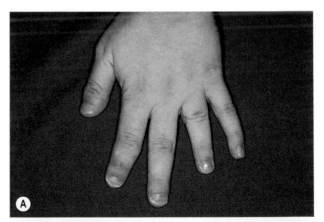

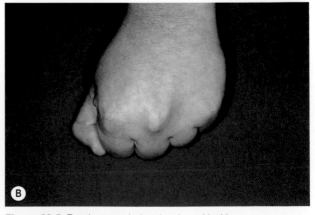

Figure 23.5 Brachymetaphalangism in a girl with pseudohypoparathyroidism, with shortened 4th and 5th metacarpals (A), and the 'knuckle, knuckle, dimple, dimple sign' when she makes a fist (B). (Reprinted with permission from Schachner and Hansen 2003).[34]

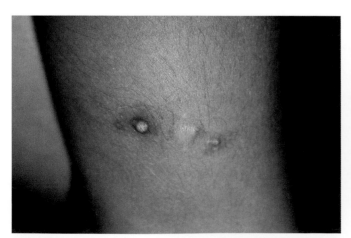

Figure 23.4 Osteoma cutis. These rock-hard papulonodules revealed ectopic ossification microscopically.

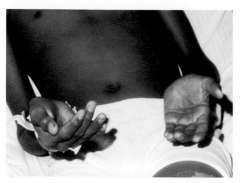

Figure 23.6 Hyperpigmentation of Addison disease. Increased pigmentation of the palmar creases in this male with Addison disease. (Courtesy Anne Lucky, MD.)

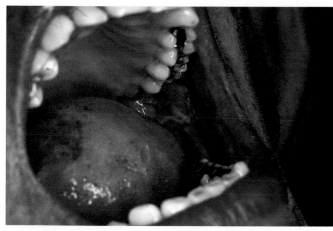

Figure 23.7 Oral mucosa pigmentation of Addison disease. Note hyperpigmentation of the tongue and buccal mucosa in this patient with Addison disease.

Table 23.4 Cutaneous features of Cushing syndrome
Facial plethora and telangiectasias
Hirsutism, fine lanugo hair growth
Violaceous striae (especially over the abdomen, flanks and upper arms)
Acne
Bruising
Poor wound healing
Skin atrophy
Thin, translucent skin
Hyperpigmentation (seen only in ACTH-dependent form)
Acanthosis nigricans
Frequent fungal infections (i.e., tinea corporis, pityriasis versicolor, candidiasis)
Male-pattern alopecia (in females)

patient to other family members may be useful in highlighting the clinical findings.[37] Primary adrenal insufficiency without hyperpigmentation has been reported, and may result in a delay in the diagnosis of Addison disease.[40] Loss of body hair may be another cutaneous finding in this disorder.

The diagnosis of chronic adrenocortical insufficiency is suggested by the clinical features and confirmed by serum electrolyte studies and cortisol level determinations following stimulation by ACTH (the ACTH-stimulation test). A morning serum cortisol ('AM cortisol') level is a convenient and simple test, but may be insensitive as a screening tool.[37] There are multiple potential causes of Addison disease, including adrenal dysgenesis, diseases resulting in adrenal destruction, or impaired steroidogenesis. Although the majority of cases of Addison disease in the past century were attributed to tuberculosis, autoimmune disease currently accounts for most cases presenting outside of the newborn period.[41] Autoimmune polyglandular syndrome types 1 and 2 may both present with this disorder as one component. The frequency of Addison disease is elevated in vitiligo probands and their 1st-degree relatives.[42] When these two disorders occur concurrently, patients may have a striking presentation of hypo- and hyperpigmentation.

Cushing Syndrome

Cushing syndrome is a disorder caused by long-term glucocorticoid excess, which may be due to a variety of different etiologies. It is divided into ACTH-dependent types (including pituitary-dependent *Cushing disease*, ectopic ACTH syndrome, and adrenal hyperplasia) and non-ACTH-dependent types (including adrenal adenoma, adrenal carcinoma, and adrenal hyperplasia).[43] The most common form is pituitary-dependent bilateral adrenal hyperplasia, termed Cushing disease. Endogenous Cushing syndrome is fairly uncommon in children, and the lack of classic features of hypercortisolism in pediatric patients may delay diagnosis and treatment. In all patients with Cushing syndrome, there is loss of diurnal variation of ACTH and cortisol secretion, which leads to sustained hypercortisolism.[44] Growth retardation to complete growth arrest is the hallmark of the disease in children and growing adolescents.[45] Cushing syndrome may also result from the systemic administration of exogenous glucocorticoids (including oral, parenteral or, rarely, topical) or ACTH, and should be suspected by the findings of suppressed ACTH and cortisol with no response to corticotropin-releasing hormone (CRH) or ACTH, respectively.[43] Cushing syndrome has occurred following intralesional corticosteroid injections for keloids in a child.[46] The authors have observed Cushing syndrome in a few children following topical application of ultrapotent corticosteroids for extensive alopecia areata/totalis and severe atopic dermatitis.

The clinical findings in Cushing syndrome are multiple and usually suggest the presence of hypercortisolism. Non-cutaneous signs and symptoms include truncal obesity, growth retardation, diabetes or glucose intolerance, gonadal dysfunction, hypertension, muscle weakness, fatigue, mood disorders, sleep disturbances, menstrual irregularities, osteoporosis, delayed or accelerated bone age, edema, polydipsia, polyuria, and fungal infections.[43,47]

The cutaneous features of Cushing syndrome are listed in Table 23.4. Addison disease-like pigmentation (particularly on the face and neck) has been noted in 6–10% of patients, and is seen primarily in the ACTH-dependent forms of the disease. Other skin findings include a characteristic plethoric 'moon' facies, with telangiectasias over the cheeks; increased fine lanugo hair on the face and extremities; purplish striae (stretch marks, see below) at points of tension such as the lower abdomen, flanks, thighs, buttocks, upper arms, and breasts; fragility of dermal blood vessels with an increased tendency toward bruising at sites of minimal trauma; poor wound healing; and steroid acne. The latter usually presents as red papules or small pustules distributed primarily on the upper trunk (Fig. 23.8), arms, neck, and to a lesser degree, the face. There is a tendency to develop cutaneous fungal infections (i.e., tinea corporis, onychomycosis, candidiasis, pityriasis versicolor), and disseminated mycobacterial infection has been reported.[48] Patients

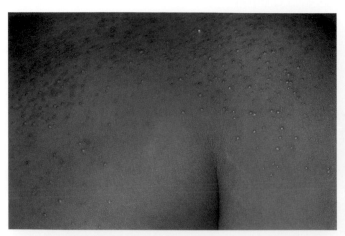

Figure 23.8 Steroid acne. Erythematous papules and papulopustules on the chest and upper arms.

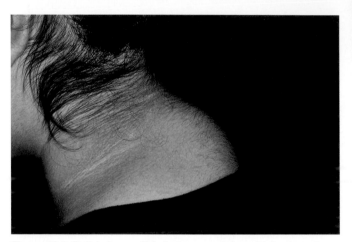

Figure 23.9 Buffalo hump. This finding, consisting of fatty deposits over the posterior neck and upper back, may be associated with either endogenous or exogenous Cushing syndrome.

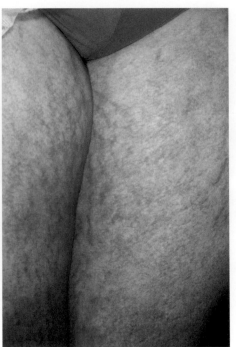

Figure 23.10 Striae distensae. These early lesions appear as pink, linear depressions in the skin.

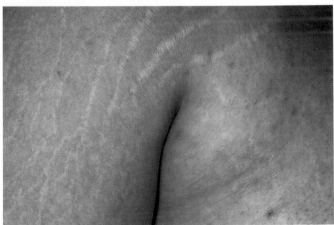

Figure 23.11 Striae distensae. These older lesions appear as flesh-colored, linear, atrophic bands.

with Cushing syndrome classically have fatty deposits over the back of the neck, termed the 'buffalo hump' (Fig. 23.9).

Cushing syndrome is diagnosed based on suspicious clinical findings and the results of laboratory testing. A 24-h urinary free cortisol is a widely used assay for diagnosing hypercortisolism, and has a very high specificity and sensitivity.[43,44] Other diagnostic studies include plasma cortisol measurement (limited by diurnal variation), low-dose dexamethasone suppression test (excellent sensitivity but requires overnight hospitalization), high-dose dexamethasone suppression test, ACTH measurement (useful for discriminating between ACTH-dependent and -independent forms), late night salivary cortisol measurement, inferior petrosal sinus sampling, and the CRH stimulation test.[44,49,50] Radiographic imaging is also useful for assessing for pituitary tumors. The treatment for Cushing syndrome depends on the etiology. With the exception of striae, the cutaneous effects of Cushing syndrome most often completely heal following successful therapy.[51]

Striae distensae (stretch marks), mentioned earlier, are linear depressions of the skin that are initially pink (Fig. 23.10) or purple and later become more flesh-colored, translucent, and atrophic (Fig. 23.11). They are most commonly seen in areas subject to stretching such as the lower back, buttocks, thighs, breasts, abdomen, and shoulders. Striae may develop physiologically in up to 35% of girls and 15% of boys between the ages of 9 and 16 years. Causes of

striae include stretching exercises, rapid growth, obesity, adolescence, pregnancy, Cushing syndrome, and prolonged use of systemic or potent topical corticosteroids. They may be seen in patients with anorexia nervosa, mainly the restrictive (vs the bulimic) form.[52] They can occasionally be mistaken for non-accidental injury or physical abuse.[53] Although the precise cause of striae is unknown, their formation appears to be related to stress-induced rupture of connective tissue, alteration of collagen and elastin, and dermal scarring in which glucocorticoids suppress fibroblastic activity and newly synthesized collagen fills the gaps between ruptured collagen fibers.[54] Elastic fibers are fine in early lesions and thickened in older lesions of striae.[55] Treatment of striae is challenging, and most therapies are generally unsatisfactory. Many of the lesions that occur during adolescence tend to become less noticeable with time. It has been suggested that topical tretinoin cream may be helpful for some patients, although the results are mixed. Other topical agents reportedly effective in some patients include glycolic and trichloroacetic acid peels and topical hyaluronic acid preparations.[56] More recently, the flashlamp-pumped pulsed dye laser has been used for treating these lesions, but data suggest that this modality should be reserved for patients with the more fair skin phenotypes (types II to IV).[57–59] Other treatment modalities that have been reported for striae include intense pulsed light, excimer laser, copper-bromide laser, fractional photothermolysis and microdermabrasion.[56,60,61]

Disorders of androgen excess

Patients with androgen excess may initially present with a variety of skin-related conditions, including hirsutism, acne, and alopecia. Hyperandrogenism may be related to benign or malignant ovarian, testicular, or adrenal tumors, functional overproduction of androgens by the adrenal glands or ovaries, or exogenous androgens. The clinical findings of hyperandrogenism may vary depending upon the pubertal development of the child, and these are summarized in Table 23.5. The two disorders to be discussed in this section are congenital adrenal hyperplasia and polycystic ovary syndrome.

Congenital Adrenal Hyperplasia

Congenital adrenal hyperplasia (CAH, also known as adrenogenital syndrome) is a term used to describe a constellation of diseases characterized by impaired steroid metabolism in the adrenal cortex. The most common cause of CAH is 21-hydroxylase deficiency, and other enzymes that may be defective include 11 β-hydroxylase and 3 β-hydroxysteroid dehydrogenase.[62] 21-hydroxylase deficiency occurs in about 1 : 10 000–1 : 15 000 live births worldwide.[63] It is inherited in an autosomal recessive fashion, and the gene (CYP21A2) is located in the HLA class III region on the short arm of chromosome 6p.[64,65] Owing to the defect in cortisol synthesis, the adrenal cortex in these disorders is stimulated by corticotropin and overproduction of cortisol precursors occurs, some of which are diverted toward synthesis of sex hormones. This androgen excess leads to clinical signs of hyperandrogenism, and concomitant aldosterone

Table 23.5 Clinical features of hyperandrogenism
Pre-pubertal
Precocious sexual development:
Sex appropriate (males)
Sex inappropriate (females)
Rapid linear growth
Accelerated bone age
Axillary and pubic hair development
Acne
Hirsutism
Neonate:
Hyperpigmentation of the genitalia
Ambiguous genitalia
Post-pubertal
Acne
Hirsutism
Androgenetic alopecia
Amenorrhea or irregular menses
Infertility
Other virilizing signs (deep voice, increased muscle mass, male habitus)
Early cardiovascular disease

deficiency may result in salt-wasting, failure to thrive, hypovolemia, and, in some cases, shock.[66]

One of the most classic presenting features of female children with CAH (21-hydroxylase deficiency) is ambiguous genitalia. Due to exposure to high systemic levels of adrenal androgens during gestation, affected girls are born with a large clitoris, rugated and partially fused labia majora, and a common urogenital sinus in place of a separate urethra and vagina.[66] The degree of virilization is variable, and may range from simple clitoromegaly to the appearance of a penile urethra. In severe forms, important features in distinguishing the virilized female genitalia from true male genitalia include the absence of testicles and the presence of normal internal sex organs.[67] Affected boys generally have no obvious physical signs of the disorder, although subtle hyperpigmentation and/or penile enlargement may be present. Some forms of CAH, such as 17 α-hydroxylase/17,20-lyase deficiency, may result in ambiguous or female-appearing external genitalia in males, identical to the androgen insensitivity syndrome.[68]

In patients who are not treated or in whom therapy is inadequate, long-term exposure to these androgens results in rapid somatic growth, advanced skeletal age, and premature development of secondary sexual characteristics, including development of pubic and axillary hair, clitoral growth, and penile growth in males. Although linear growth may be accelerated during childhood, these patients often ultimately have short stature, due to premature epiphyseal closure. Centrally mediated precocious puberty may occur. Hirsutism is a common feature in patients with non-classic (partial) 21-hydroxylase deficiency, and when menstrual irregularity and acne also occur, the presentation may simulate that of polycystic ovary syndrome (see below). Patients with non-classic CAH do not have ambiguous genitalia at birth, and usually present with premature adrenarche and advanced bone age later in life.

Abnormalities of reproductive function are common in CAH, and infertility is frequently present. Affected males have fewer problems with reproductive function. Salt wasting is seen in up to 75% of patients with classic 21-hydroxylase deficiency, due to decreased synthesis of aldosterone. These patients are prone to hyponatremia, hyperkalemia, hypovolemia, dehydration, and shock. Hyperpigmentation, most notably of skin creases and the genitalia, may occur as an early sign of adrenal insufficiency. Classic 21-hydroxylase deficiency is diagnosed by the finding of markedly elevated levels of serum 17-hydroxyprogesterone, the main substrate for the enzyme. The cosyntropin (corticotropin) stimulation test is useful for differentiating this disorder from other steroidogenic enzyme defects. Molecular-based genetic testing is available for CAH, and prenatal diagnosis is possible using chorionic villus and amniotic fluid cells for DNA analysis.[69] Management consists of glucocorticoid and mineralocorticoid replacement, supplemental sodium chloride, and surgical management of ambiguous genitalia, which is generally recommended between 2 and 6 months of life.[66]

Polycystic Ovary Syndrome

Polycystic ovary syndrome (PCOS, Stein–Leventhal syndrome) is the most frequent androgen disorder of ovarian function,[70] and among the most common endocrine disorders in women.[71] PCOS patients have increased androgen production and disordered gonadotropin secretion, resulting in amenorrhea or severe oligomenorrhea, increased testosterone levels, and enlarged polycystic ovaries on ultrasound examination. Women with PCOS also have metabolic derangements related to insulin resistance, and an increased risk of type 2 diabetes mellitus. The hormonal dysregulation seen in PCOS usually begins during adolescence.[72] The pathophysiology of PCOS is multifactorial, and it has been found to cluster in families with a history of PCOS, non-insulin dependent diabetes mellitus, cardiovascular disease and breast cancer.[73] Two sets of diagnostic criteria have been utilized, including the 1990 National Institutes of Health criteria (which requires chronic anovulation plus clinical or biochemical signs of hyperandrogenism) and the 2003 Rotterdam criteria (which requires two or more of chronic anovulation, clinical or biochemical signs of hyperandrogenism and polycystic ovaries).[74]

Hirsutism and acne vulgaris are the most common manifestations of PCOS, and in fact, the leading cause of hirsutism in adolescence is PCOS (also see Ch. 7).[75] Hair growth occurs in androgen-dependent areas, including the face, neck (Fig. 23.12), chest, back, and lower abdomen. It may be less noticeable in adolescents (given their shorter duration of hyperandrogenism), and is less common in some ethnic backgrounds, i.e. Asians.[72] Acne is a common finding, and in one study of 119 women with acne but without menstrual disorders, obesity or hirsutism, PCOS was found on ultrasound in 45%.[76] These findings suggest that PCOS is common in women with acne, even in the absence of other suggestive clinical findings.

Acanthosis nigricans (see below) is another common cutaneous finding in patients with PCOS. It presents with hyperpigmented, velvety plaques of the neck folds, axillae, and other intertriginous areas. Acanthosis nigricans is a marker for insulin resistance, although the latter appears to be only one factor leading to its development.[77] Other important components of PCOS include menstrual irregularity and obesity. Anovulation frequently occurs, although women with PCOS can ovulate spontaneously. Secondary amenorrhea, oligomenorrhea, and dysfunctional uterine bleeding may all occur, and delayed menarche may be seen in girls.[78] Adolescent females with oligomenorrhea secondary to PCOS may be difficult to distinguish from those with physiologic anovulation. Obesity is frequently present, with a centripetal weight distribution and increased waist-to-hip ratio of >0.85.[78] Some patients with PCOS display a metabolic pattern of atherogenic lipid profile, glucose intolerance, and increased fasting insulin level, with an increased incidence of type 2 diabetes and cardiovascular disease.[70] Studies of adult women with type 2 diabetes mellitus show a prevalence of PCOS higher than that reported in the general population.[79]

The clinical presentation of PCOS and its associated features have overlap with other entities described in the literature. The association of hyperandrogenism, insulin resistance and acanthosis nigricans has been called *HAIR-AN syndrome*. Although the potential causes of hyperandrogenism in this syndrome are multiple, PCOS may be present in many patients. It is possible that the etiology of insulin resistance (and resultant hyperinsulinemia) could produce both polycystic ovaries and hyperandrogenism.[80] *Syndrome X* is a term that has been used to describe a systemic disease notable for hyperinsulinemia and hyperandrogenism. More recently, *metabolic syndrome* has been the terminology used to describe patients with abdominal obesity, dyslipidemia, glucose intolerance and, often, PCOS.[81] These patients are also prone to hypertension, hyperuricemia, fatty liver disease, chronic inflammation, endothelial dysfunction, and coagulopathy.[81] Importantly, there is a threefold increase in the risk of coronary heart disease and stroke.

The diagnosis of PCOS is suggested by the clinical features of hyperandrogenism and prolonged menstrual irregularity, and confirmed by finding elevated serum androgens and excluding other potential causes. The ultrasound finding of polycystic changes is common, but such changes may also be seen in normally menstruating adolescents or in other conditions, and hence ultrasonography is not a primary diagnostic modality. In addition, some adolescents with PCOS may not have polycystic ovaries. Screening for glucose intolerance and diabetes mellitus should be performed in all patients with PCOS, as should fasting lipid levels.

Treatments for the condition are primarily directed at symptoms, and include hormonal regulation, weight reduction, and treatment for hirsutism and acne. The use of insulin-sensitizing drugs may be effective for anovulation and may benefit the associated metabolic derangements.[82] Options for treatment of hirsutism include mechanical hair removal (i.e., plucking, waxing, shaving, chemical depilatories, and laser therapy), topical inhibitors of ornithine decarboxylase (eflornithine), oral contraceptive agents, antiandrogen therapies (i.e., spironolactone, flutamide), and gonadotropin-releasing hormone agonists.

Gonadal dysgenesis/Turner syndrome

Gonadal dysgenesis, or Turner syndrome (TS), is a condition characterized by short stature and ovarian dysgenesis. Patients are females with either a missing X chromosome (45 XO) or an abnormality of one of the X chromosomes. It occurs in 1 in 2000 to 1 in 5000 female live births.[83] Genomic imprinting, whereby allelic genes or chromosomes are expressed differently depending on the parent of origin, has been implicated in TS in whom up to 80% of patients have retained the maternal X chromosome.[84] In addition to short stature and ovarian failure, patients with TS may have lymphatic abnormalities, skeletal abnormalities (micrognathia, broad 'shield' chest, kyphoscoliosis, Madelung deformity), hearing and cardiac defects, renal abnormalities, and endocrinopathies (most notably involving the thyroid and glucose metabolism). Characteristic physical findings also include a low posterior hairline, cubitus valgus, unusual rotation of the ears, downward displacement of the lateral canthus, epicanthal folds, inverted or hypoplastic nipples, and shortened fourth and fifth metacarpals and metatarsals. Learning deficits occur in the majority of patients with TS, and psychiatric conditions may be more common.

Abnormalities of the lymphatic system include cystic hygroma (macrocystic lymphatic malformation) which, when occurring *in utero*, may result in neck webbing or pterygium colli (Fig. 23.13). Transient lymphedema of the distal extremities, mainly the hands and the feet, may occur and nail dysplasia may be seen as a result of intrauterine peripheral lymphedema.[85] This lymphedema usually

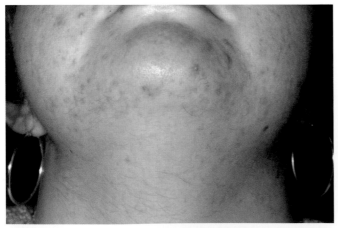

Figure 23.12 Hirsutism. The hair growth in this adolescent female with polycystic ovary syndrome occurs in androgen-dependent areas, and is accompanied by acne.

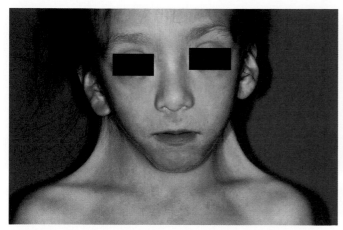

Figure 23.13 Pterygium colli in Turner syndrome. This neck webbing is likely the result of in utero cystic hygroma.

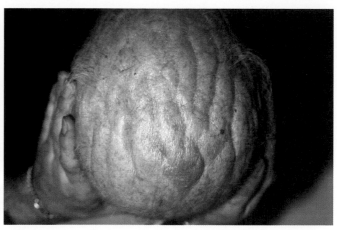

Figure 23.15 Cutis verticis gyrata. This coarse furrowing of the skin on the scalp may be associated with hyperpituitarism or as part of a disorder called pachydermoperiostosis.

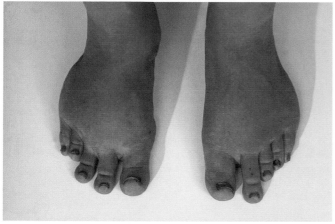

Figure 23.14 Nail changes in Turner syndrome. Note the hypoplastic, hyperconvex toenails and hypoplasia of the fourth and fifth metatarsals in this girl with gonadal dysgenesis. (Reprinted with permission from Schachner and Hansen 2003).[34]

resolves by 2 years of age. Deep furrows of the scalp, similar to what has been termed cutis verticis gyrata, may also be the result of preceding lymphedema.[86]

The nails in patients with TS are characteristic, revealing hypoplasia and hyperconvexity (Fig. 23.14).[34] Increased numbers of melanocytic nevi are commonly noted, although clinical atypia is not necessarily more prominent.[87] Despite the increased numbers of melanocytic nevi, there appears to be a lower-than-expected incidence of malignant melanoma in TS patients, possibly reflecting the relationship between sex hormones and melanoma development.[88,89] Multiple pilomatricomas, including giant lesions, have been reported in girls with TS.[90,91]

Pituitary disorders

Hyperpituitarism

The pituitary, an endocrine organ located in a bony cavity (the sella turcica) at the brain base, is divided into anterior and posterior portions. Both portions secrete a variety of hormones under the influence of the hypothalamus. These hormones include growth hormone (GH), thyroid stimulating hormone (TSH), adrenocorticotropic hormone (ACTH), luteinizing hormone (LH),

follicle-stimulating hormone (FSH), prolactin, antidiuretic hormone (ADH, vasopressin) and oxytocin. Skin manifestations of hyperpituitarism include those related to excess GH, glucocorticoids (see Cushing Syndrome, above), and prolactin (not discussed here). Most growth hormone-secreting pituitary tumors are eosinophilic adenomas. Excessive secretion of GH by pituitary gland tumors produces gigantism in children whose epiphyses have not yet closed and acromegaly in individuals whose normal bone growth has ceased. *Acromegaly* is rare in children, but transitional acromegalic features at times may be seen in affected adolescents. Soft tissue overgrowth of the hands, feet, face, and nasal tip occur. Patients may have a large furrowed tongue, thick lips, lantern jaw, broad spade-like hands with squatty fingers, hypertrichosis, and hyperpigmentation in a pattern similar to that observed in patients with Addison disease. Although the cause of the hypertrichosis is not well understood, the hyperpigmentation is related to increased secretion of MSH. Other cutaneous manifestations of acromegaly include excessive sweating, oily skin, acrochordons (skin tags), heel pad thickening, eyelid swelling, and acanthosis nigricans.[92] Early non-cutaneous complaints in patients with acromegaly may include headache, visual disturbances, weakness and paresthesias, and impaired glucose tolerance may be present.[93]

Cutis verticis gyrata (coarse furrowing of the skin on the posterior aspect of the neck and the vertex of the scalp, Fig. 23.15) is caused by an increase in dermal collagen; as a result, excessive skin buckles and forms furrows and ridges that resemble gyri of the cerebral cortex (hence the terminology). In addition to being an occasional manifestation of hyperpituitarism, cutis verticis gyrata may occasionally occur as a primary disorder without other associated abnormalities. It may also be seen as part of a disorder called *pachydermoperiostosis*, which is manifested by thickening of the skin of the face and scalp, clubbing of the fingers, and periostosis of the long bones. Severe progressive arthritis has rarely been reported in association with this syndrome.[94]

Hypopituitarism

Pituitary insufficiency (hypopituitarism) refers to a group of disorders resulting from a deficiency in secretion of one or more hormones derived from the pituitary gland. These include idiopathic hypopituitarism (panhypopituitarism, Simmond's disease); Sheehan's syndrome (pituitary deficiency usually arising as a result of hemorrhage or infarct); pituitary tumors (especially craniopharyngioma, Langerhans cell histiocytosis); autoimmune disorders; trauma; infections (i.e., tuberculosis); congenital abnormalities; or ablation of the pituitary gland by surgery or radiation used for the treatment of local tumors. Systemic manifestations of hypopituitarism may include those related to mineralocorticoid and glucocorticoid deficiencies (see Addison disease, above), hypothyroidism, growth hormone and gonadotropin deficiency, and diabetes insipidus secondary to ADH deficiency.

The most obvious skin manifestations of pituitary insufficiency are pallor, secondary to anemia and decreased cutaneous blood flow, and a predisposition toward sunburn with decreased ability to tan (due to a decrease in melanin pigmentation secondary to diminished or absent secretion of MSH). Other features (and proposed causes) include smooth, fine skin (GH deficiency) or myxedematous, coarse, dry skin (hypothyroidism and GH deficiency). The face may be slightly puffy and pale or yellowish (secondary to carotenoderma from hypothyroidism). Hair is thin and sparse with alopecia (hypothyroidism and androgen deficiency), and the nails grow slowly. Adolescent males may have a smooth scrotum with absence of hair and rugae (androgen deficiency).[95] Gonadotropin deficiency may result in loss of axillary, pubic, and body hair and micropenis in males.

Multiple endocrine neoplasia syndromes

The multiple endocrine neoplasia (MEN) syndromes are familial disorders characterized by benign and malignant tumors of multiple endocrine glands. Cutaneous manifestations may also be found in these disorders. The clinical manifestations of MEN syndromes are inconsistent and reflect the variable involvement of hormone-producing tissues. These disorders are inherited in an autosomal dominant fashion. The endocrine and cutaneous manifestations of the MEN syndromes are summarized in Table 23.6.

MEN I (Werner syndrome) is characterized by tumors of the parathyroid glands, endocrine pancreas, and anterior pituitary. Thyroid and adrenal gland tumors may also be seen, as may foregut carcinoid tumors.[96] Clinical manifestations may be related to

primary hyperparathyroidism, gastrinoma, tumors secreting neuroendocrine peptides and prolactinomas. There is an increased risk of malignant endocrine tumors, including parathyroid, thymic, bronchial (carcinoid), and enteropancreatic neuroendocrine tumors.[97] The gene for MEN I (*MEN1*) has been identified at llql3, and genetic testing is available.[97,98] This gene encodes a protein called menin, which functions as a tumor suppressor protein, and in whose absence cellular replication, hyperplasia and tumorigenesis are increased.

Cutaneous manifestations of MEN I include lipomas, angiofibromas, collagenomas, confetti-like hypopigmented macules, and gingival papules.[96] Café-au-lait macules may also occur, although not in the high numbers usually associated with neurofibromatosis. The multiple facial angiofibromas are clinically and histologically indistinguishable from those that occur in the setting of tuberous sclerosis, although they tend to present later in life in MEN I, usually during the 3rd or 4th decade.[96,99] In addition, they may involve the upper lip and vermilion border. Nonetheless, facial angiofibromas, which were once felt to be pathognomonic for tuberous sclerosis (and traditionally referred to as 'adenoma sebaceum'), can no longer be considered a specific marker for that disorder. Collagenomas, which are hamartomas of connective tissue, tend to be more discrete and papular in MEN I than the histologically similar lesions ('shagreen patch') seen in patients with tuberous sclerosis.[96] Protuberant collagenomas have been reported, with rapid growth following surgery to remove an endocrine tumor.[100] Melanoma may occur with increased frequency in patients with MEN I.[101]

MEN II (MEN IIA or Sipple syndrome) is a rare autosomal dominant disorder due to a point mutation in the *RET* protooncogene. Clinical findings include medullary thyroid carcinoma, pheochromocytoma, and parathyroid hyperplasia. Cutaneous manifestations are not a significant feature of MEN IIA. The one that has received the most attention is lichen amyloidosis, which presents as multiple infiltrated papules overlying a well-demarcated plaque, especially on the upper back.[102] These lesions often begin with intense pruritus, with the subsequent development of brown-colored papules on the skin[103] and the histologic finding of amorphous material in the papillary dermis which stains as amyloid.[104,105]

MEN III (MEN IIB, mucosal neuroma syndrome) is characterized by medullary thyroid carcinoma, pheochromocytoma, ganglioneuromatosis, a Marfanoid body habitus, and occasional parathyroid hyperplasia. Medullary thyroid carcinoma is the initial presentation in most patients with MEN III (as well as those with MEN IIA), and remains the major cause of morbidity.[106] This disorder is also caused by an activation mutation in the *RET* protooncogene.

Mucocutaneous manifestations of MEN III include multiple mucosal neuromas, which are often present by the preschool years. These ganglioneuromas involve the anterolateral tongue and lips, and may also be located on the conjunctiva and eyelids.[107,108] Lip involvement results in diffusely enlarged lips with a fleshy, bubbled appearance. The upper lip is usually more involved than the lower. The tongue lesions are usually limited to the anterior third of the surface and appear as pink-white, somewhat translucent papules and nodules (Fig. 23.16). They may be congenital or noted during the first few years of life, and are an important feature as they may be the initial marker of the syndrome. Although multiple mucosal neuromas are nearly pathognomonic for this disorder, they may rarely occur without other clinical, biochemical, or molecular evidence of MEN III.[109] Multiple lesions of lichen nitidus have also been observed.[110]

Ocular involvement may involve the limbus of the conjunctivae and the eyelids, in which case it results in thickening of the lid margin and distortion or displacement of the eyelashes (Fig. 23.17). Nasal, laryngeal, and gingival neuromas may also be present, and

Table 23.6 Endocrine and mucocutaneous manifestations of MEN syndromes

Syndrome	Endocrine[a]	Mucocutaneous
MEN I	Parathyroid	Angiofibromas
	Anterior pituitary	Collagenomas
	Endocrine pancreas	Hypopigmentation
	Thyroid	Gingival papules
	Adrenal glands	Lipomas
		Café-au-lait macules
		Melanoma
MEN II (IIA)	Thyroid	Lichen amyloidosis
	Parathyroid	
	Pheochromocytoma	
MEN III (IIB)	Thyroid	Mucosal neuromas
	Parathyroid	Café-au-lait macules
	Pheochromocytoma	Lichen nitidus

MEN, multiple endocrine neoplasia.
[a]May be hyperplasia, benign tumors, malignant tumors.

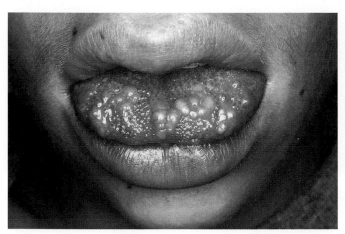

Figure 23.16 Mucosal neuromas in multiple endocrine neoplasia III. Characteristic lingual neuromas and protuberant fleshy lips are present in this 16-year-old male with mucosal neuroma syndrome.

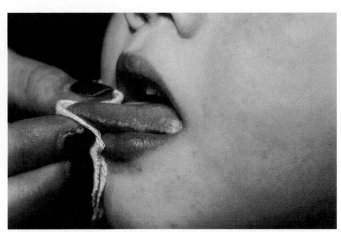

Figure 23.18 Oral candidiasis. White plaques of the lateral tongue (thrush) in a young female with chronic mucocutaneous candidiasis and diabetes mellitus.

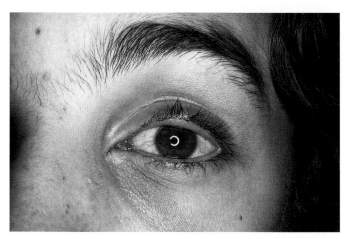

Figure 23.17 Eyelid changes in multiple endocrine neoplasia III. Neuromas of the eyelid margins result in thickening of the I margins and displacement of the lashes.

skin lesions are occasionally seen. Café-au-lait macules may also be a cutaneous component of the syndrome. Intestinal ganglioneuromatosis is another feature of MEN III, presenting with intermittent intestinal obstruction, gas formation, diarrhea, and failure to thrive.[107] Musculoskeletal features of Marfan syndrome are common, including tall stature, elongated limbs, pes cavum, and pectus excavatum, but cardiac or ocular abnormalities typical of that disorder are absent.

Genetic testing for *RET* gene mutations should be performed early in life for individuals with a known family history of MEN IIA or III. In primary relatives of medullary thyroid carcinoma-affected patients with no identified *RET* mutation, linkage analysis and biochemical testing for MEN should be performed. Total thyroidectomy is recommended for all patients at risk.[107]

Autoimmune polyglandular syndromes

Autoimmune polyglandular syndromes (APS) are a group of disorders in which multiple endocrine and non-endocrine defects occur together. The best characterized of these syndromes is APS1, also

known as *autoimmune polyendocrinopathy-candidiasis-ectodermal dystrophy (APECED) syndrome*. This autosomal recessive condition is defined by the presence of two of three conditions:

1. Adrenocortical failure (Addison disease)
2. Hypoparathyroidism
3. Mucocutaneous candidiasis.[111]

It occurs with increased frequency in Finnish, Iranian, Jewish, and Sardinian populations.[112] APS2 is characterized by Addison disease, thyroiditis, and/or diabetes mellitus, whereas APS3 is the association of diabetes mellitus, pernicious anemia, alopecia, and vitiligo.

The symptoms of APS1 frequently begin in childhood. In addition to hypoparathyroidism and adrenal failure, other associations may include insulin-dependent diabetes mellitus, gonadal failure, autoimmune thyroiditis, chronic active hepatitis, malabsorption, and parietal cell atrophy.[113,114] Autoimmune hepatitis may occur and can be one of the presenting features.[115] Candidiasis is seen in nearly all patients, and in the majority of patients, it appears first before the endocrinologic manifestations.[116,117] Oral candidiasis (thrush, Fig. 23.18) tends to be chronic, and has a peak incidence during the first 2 years of life.[118] Candidal infection may also take the form of angular cheilitis (perlèche), hyperplastic or atrophic oral candidiasis, candidal esophagitis, diaper or perianal candidiasis, scalp infection, intertrigo, or nail infection. These changes, taken together, are also referred to as *chronic mucocutaneous candidiasis* (see also Ch. 17). When chronic candidal infection occurs in the esophagus or larynx, stricture formation may result. Nail involvement leads to thickening (Fig. 23.19), brittleness and discoloration, with associated inflammation of the periungual areas (paronychia). Many postpubertal female patients may experience candidal vulvovaginitis.[118] Generalized candidiasis in these patients is rare, but serious lung infection may occasionally occur.

Alopecia areata occurs in around one-third of patients with APS1,[114] often presents in childhood, and may progress to alopecia universalis. It tends to begin around the peripubertal years. Vitiligo occurs in some patients and is quite variable in extent. The most consistent cutaneous features are those representing ectodermal dystrophy. APS1 patients frequently have enamel hypoplasia of permanent teeth, and nail dystrophy with pitting affects around half of the patients.[118] They are more prone to dental caries, abscesses and tooth loss.[119]

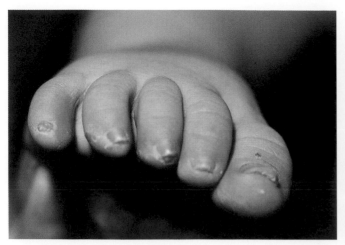

Figure 23.19 Candida onychodystrophy. Nail thickening, subungual debris, and culture positivity for *Candida albicans* were present in this young girl with chronic mucocutaneous candidiasis and endocrinopathy.

The gene for APS1 has been cloned and is termed *AIRE*, for 'autoimmune regulator.' The AIRE protein is localized to the short arm of chromosome 21, and may act as a transcriptional regulator.[112,113] Mutations in *AIRE* result in impaired clonal deletion of self-reactive thymocytes, which may subsequently attack a variety of host organs.[120]

McCune–Albright syndrome

The McCune–Albright syndrome (MAS) is defined clinically as the triad of fibrous dysplasia of bones (polyostotic fibrous dysplasia), patchy cutaneous pigmentation, and various endocrinopathies, most notably precocious puberty. Other associated endocrine disorders include pituitary adenomas (secreting growth hormone), hyperthyroid goiters, and adrenal hyperplasia.[121] The endocrinopathies of MAS are all characterized by autonomous excessive hyperfunction of hormonally responsive cells, which respond to signals through activation of the adenylate cyclase system.[122] Activating mutations in the guanine nucleotide-binding (G) protein gene *GNAS1*, which encodes a subunit of the G protein that stimulates adenylate cyclase, have been identified in MAS patients.[123] A postzygotic somatic mutation leads to a mosaic distribution of cells bearing the defect.[121] As mentioned earlier in this chapter, germline *inactivating* mutations of this same gene are present in patients with Albright hereditary osteodystrophy (pseudohypoparathyroidism).

The pigmentary lesions of MAS, which are seen in approximately 50% of patients, present as one or more café-au-lait macules or patches with a distinct distribution pattern: they rarely extend beyond the midline, and the majority are on the same side of the body as the skeletal lesions.[123] The most common sites of involvement are the buttocks and lumbosacral regions, and lesions may follow the lines of Blaschko. These café-au-lait lesions have irregularly ragged or serrated borders (Fig. 23.20), which are described as resembling the 'coast of Maine', in contrast to the café-au-lait spots of neurofibromatosis, where the smooth borders are said to resemble the 'coast of California'. They are usually present early in life and frequently are the first sign of this disorder. Diffuse scalp alopecia with histologic features of fibrous dysplasia has been reported.[124]

Fibrous dysplasia is a rare bone disorder which results in bone pain, fractures, bony deformity and, occasionally, neurologic

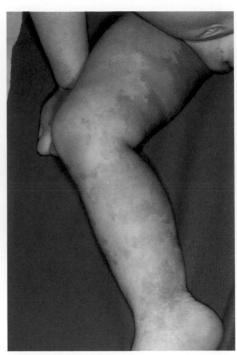

Figure 23.20 Café-au-lait lesions in McCune–Albright syndrome. Well-demarcated tan patches with a ragged border involved the labia majora, thigh, leg, and foot in this 18-month-old female.

compression. It occurs most often as a bone-limited process, and <5% of patients have concomitant endocrine dysfunction.[125] Most patients with MAS have either solitary or multiple fibrous dysplasia lesions of bone, which tend to develop during the first decade. Although any bone can be involved, the femur and pelvis are most common, and progressive deformity with fractures may occur. Radiographic studies reveal lytic lesions with scalloped borders and a 'ground glass' pattern. Computed tomographic imaging or bone biopsy may be required to confirm the diagnosis in questionable cases. Precocious puberty is a common initial manifestation in girls with MAS, and is recognized by the development of secondary sexual characteristics prior to 9 years of age.[123]

Disorders associated with diabetes

Diabetes mellitus is a common, chronic disease, and up to 30% of diabetics may have some form of cutaneous disorder. Some skin findings are clearly associated with diabetes, such as necrobiosis lipoidica diabeticorum, diabetic dermopathy, diabetic bullae, and the syndrome of limited joint mobility and waxy skin, which are nearly diagnostic.[126] For others, the exact association between the skin disorder and diabetes is uncertain, and for many, pathogenesis remains unproven. Table 23.7 lists some potential cutaneous associations with diabetes mellitus. A select number of these disorders will be discussed here. The glucagonoma syndrome, which may be associated with mild diabetes mellitus and cutaneous manifestations, is discussed separately in the next section.

Necrobiosis Lipoidica Diabeticorum

Necrobiosis lipoidica diabeticorum (NLD) is a fairly distinct clinical entity that, although not the most common, is the best recognized cutaneous marker of diabetes.[126] It may be seen outside of the

Table 23.7 Some cutaneous associations with diabetes mellitus
Established or probable association
Necrobiosis lipoidica diabeticorum (NLD)
Diabetic dermopathy
Diabetic bullae
Acanthosis nigricans
Scleredema diabeticorum
Limited joint mobility and waxy skin syndrome
Partial lipodystrophy
Malignant otitis externa
Neuropathic leg ulcers
Perforating disorders
Eruptive xanthomas
Hemochromatosis
Carotenemia
Pruritus
Xerosis and anhidrosis
Yellow nails, koilonychia
Increased susceptibility to infections:
Candida albicans
Staphylococcus aureus
Group A β-hemolytic streptococcus
Pseudomonas aeruginosa
Dermatophytes (tinea pedis, onychomycosis)
Corynebacterium minutissimum (erythrasma)
Possible association
Disseminated granuloma annulare
Vitiligo

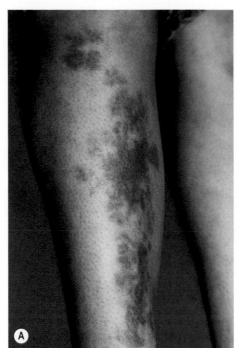

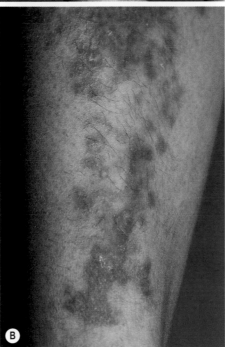

Figure 23.21 Necrobiosis lipoidica diabeticorum. Waxy, yellow-brown plaques (A) were present in this young girl with diabetes mellitus, with subtle atrophy present on closer inspection (B).

setting of diabetes mellitus, although up to three-quarters of patients with NLD have or will have diabetes; among diabetics, it occurs in <1% of patients.[127,128] NLD is predominantly seen in females and has an average age of onset of 34 years.[126,129] However, it may occur in children and its presence may suggest a higher risk for diabetic nephropathy and retinopathy.[130] In up to one-third of patients with NLD, these cutaneous lesions may precede the diagnosis of diabetes by up to several years.

Lesions of NLD typically occur in the pretibial areas and are usually asymptomatic. They present as slowly enlarging, irregularly bordered, red to yellow-brown plaques (Fig. 23.21). The center often becomes atrophic and more yellow, and there may be superficial telangiectasias, especially later in the course. Older lesions may be primarily brown in color. Multiple lesions are usually present, and ulceration may occur in up to one-third of NLD patients. Skin biopsy can be useful for diagnosis, revealing degeneration of collagen with inflammation and granuloma formation. However, it is preferable to avoid surgical procedures in this location in diabetics when possible. The diagnosis is usually strongly suggested in the presence of sharply demarcated, waxy plaques with a red or violaceous border on the anterior tibial surfaces of a diabetic patient. The cause of NLD is unclear, but may relate to microangiopathy, endarteritis, vasculitis, or delayed hypersensitivity.

The treatment of NLD is challenging, and there is no established 'gold standard' of care as the clinical response to various treatments is quite variable. When there is no ulceration and lesions are relatively asymptomatic, watchful waiting and protection from injury is appropriate.[88] The influence of strict diabetic control on the lesions of NLD is controversial. Many have suggested that glucose control has no effect on the appearance or clinical course of NLD, whereas others support the opposite hypothesis.[89,127,131] Cosmetic cover-ups are useful for patients in whom the appearance of lesions is bothersome. Active therapy of lesions has included topical and intralesional corticosteroids, aspirin, dipyridamole, pentoxifylline, systemic corticosteroids, chloroquine, topical tretinoin, hyperbaric oxygen, and topical psoralen plus ultraviolet A (PUVA) therapy.[129,132–136] Local corticosteroid products should be used with caution since they may contribute to further atrophy or ulceration. Antiplatelet therapy with aspirin is reportedly quite effective and well tolerated, although this observation has not been confirmed by randomized clinical trials.[131] Pulsed-dye laser has been used and may benefit the telangiectatic and erythematous components.[137] Ulcerated lesions of NLD are treated with local wound care, semipermeable wound dressings, and topical or systemic antibiotics. Surgical excision with split-thickness skin grafting may be useful.[138]

Diabetic Dermopathy

Diabetic dermopathy (DD, spotted leg syndrome, shin spots) is the most common cutaneous marker for diabetes mellitus. It is considered by some to be a pathognomonic sign of diabetes.[139] DD is seen most often in older diabetics, and only occasionally in children. It presents as multiple, well-circumscribed, brown macules and patches, with a tendency toward bilateral involvement of the pretibial surfaces. The lesions often become atrophic and take on the appearance of scars. They are occasionally scaly, and measure from several millimeters up to 2 cm. Lesions of DD may occasionally occur on the scalp, forearms, or trunk, but the pretibial surfaces are the most common site of involvement in the majority of patients. The etiology of these lesions is unclear, but some have suggested that their presence may be a clinical sign of an increased likelihood of retinopathy, nephropathy, and neuropathy.[140] It may also be associated with large-vessel (i.e., coronary artery) disease.[139]

Lesions of DD are in large part uninfluenced by treatment. Since the condition is asymptomatic, it requires no therapy aside from protection from trauma and supportive wound care should lesions become inflamed or infected. Although lesions may resolve spontaneously, others may appear individually or in asymmetric crops.[129]

Diabetic Bullae

Diabetic bullae are an uncommon association with diabetes, and present as spontaneously arising large blisters with a predilection for the distal extremities. Diabetic bullae are felt to be a distinct marker for diabetes. The most common location for these bullae is the dorsal and lateral surfaces of the lower legs and feet (Fig. 23.22). Occasionally, patients may have lesions on the hands or forearms.[126] They range in size from <1 to several centimeters. There is usually no history of trauma, and the lesions usually have no surrounding erythema. These lesions are generally asymptomatic, and healing occurs over several weeks with supportive wound care. They often heal without scarring, although in some patients, atrophy and scarring typical of dystrophic epidermolysis bullosa may result.[129,141]

Acanthosis Nigricans

Acanthosis nigricans (AN) is a symmetric cutaneous eruption consisting of brown, velvety plaques that involve primarily the skin folds. It may be associated with several different clinical settings, including obesity, insulin resistance, various syndromes, malignancy, and medications, as well as occurring as 'benign' and mixed types.[142] Table 23.8 summarizes the various clinical associations with AN. The discussion here will focus primarily on AN associated with obesity, insulin resistance, and diabetes.

AN presents as dark brown, velvety thickening of the skin involving the axillae (Fig. 23.23) and the neck, especially the posterior and lateral neck folds (Fig. 23.24). The initial change is hyperpigmentation, followed by eventual thickening with intensification of skin markings.[143] In addition to the characteristic areas of involvement, there may be verrucous hyperkeratosis of the knuckles (Fig. 23.25), genitalia, perineum, face, thighs, breasts, and flexural regions of the elbows and knees. Occasionally, the eruption of AN may become generalized,[144,145] and mucosal involvement may occur, manifested as thickening and papillomatosis of eyelids,

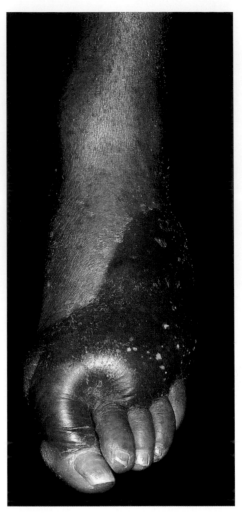

Figure 23.22 Diabetic bullae. These large, painless, tense bullae may occur in the setting of diabetes mellitus, often with no history of preceding trauma.

conjunctivae, lips, and the oral mucosa. The differential diagnosis of AN may include epidermal nevi, lichen simplex chronicus, post-inflammatory hyperpigmentation, erythrasma, and endocrine disorders with hyperpigmentation (Addison disease).

Hyperinsulinemia appears to predispose individuals to AN, and patients with inactivating insulin receptor mutations often have severe involvement.[146] Children with AN often have greater body weight and body fat mass, greater basal and glucose-stimulated insulin levels during oral glucose tolerance testing, and lower insulin sensitivity. Importantly, after adjusting for body fat mass and age, the differences in glucose metabolism and insulin studies were less significant in some studies, suggesting that increased body mass index should still suggest the possibility of hyperinsulinemia whether or not AN is present.[146] However, other studies have disputed this finding, showing that AN is associated with hyperinsulinemia and impaired glucose metabolism independent of body mass index.[147,148] Among African-Americans, AN is strongly associated with obesity and insulin resistance, and identifies a subset with a much higher prevalence of non-insulin-dependent diabetes mellitus (NIDDM) than is present in African-Americans in the general population.[149] AN is associated with obesity in every ethnic group, but occurs with greatest frequency (within the obese population) in Native Americans, followed by African Americans, Hispanics, and

Table 23.8 Clinical associations with/variants of acanthosis nigricans

Association	Comments
'Benign'	Form of epidermal nevus; may be autosomal dominant; associated with multiple nevi
Obesity	Most common type; insulin resistance common; increased incidence of type II diabetes mellitus
Malignancy	Usually adults, rarely observed in children; sudden onset and rapid spread; especially abdominal adenocarcinoma
Syndromes	Multiple syndrome associations, including Bloom, Crouzon, Prader–Willi, Lawrence–Seip, PCOS, Beare–Stevenson; also lupus erythematosus, dermatomyositis, scleroderma
Medications	Niacin, corticosteroids, oral contraceptives, diethylstilbestrol, others
Acral type	Dorsal hands, fingers, feet
Unilateral type	Unilateral distribution or 'nevoid'; may persist unchanged or progress to bilateral involvement
Mixed type	Two of the above types occurring together

PCOS, polycystic ovary syndrome. (Adapted from Schwartz 1994).[142]

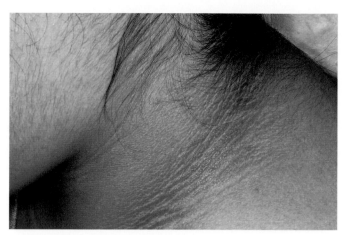

Figure 23.24 Acanthosis nigricans. Velvety hyperpigmentation is present on the lateral and posterior neck folds of this obese teenaged female.

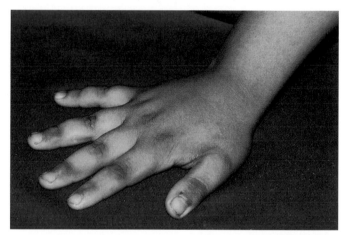

Figure 23.25 Acanthosis nigricans. Hyperpigmentation with verrucous changes may occasionally occur overlying the knuckles.

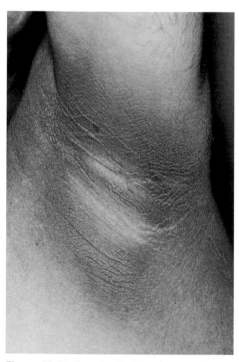

Figure 23.23 Acanthosis nigricans. Velvety hyperpigmentation involves the axillae in this patient.

Caucasians.[150] It should be considered a clinical surrogate for laboratory-determined hyperinsulinemia, and indicates a high risk for NIDDM.[150,151] As mentioned earlier in this chapter, AN and insulin resistance may also be associated with hyperandrogenism as part of the HAIR-AN syndrome, which may also have as a feature polycystic ovary syndrome.

The pathogenesis of AN is unclear. In patients with hyperinsulinemia, insulin may bind to insulin-like growth factor receptors in the epidermis, resulting in papillomatosis (thickening with folding). There are no successful therapies for AN, and the primary focus should be on treatment for the underlying condition. In obesity-associated disease, weight reduction itself seems to reduce the findings of AN. Topical or oral retinoids may benefit some patients, and lactic acid-containing emollients (i.e., LactiCare, AmLactin, Lac-Hydrin) or other keratolytic agents (salicylic acid, urea) may also be useful.

Confluent and reticulated papillomatosis

Confluent and reticulated papillomatosis (CARP) of Gougerot and Carteaud is briefly discussed here because of its clinical overlap with acanthosis nigricans. CARP is a rare disorder characterized by hyperpigmented papules confluent in the center and reticulated at the periphery. They have a characteristic distribution, involving the intermammary region (Fig. 23.26) most commonly, as well as the epigastric area (Fig. 23.27) and upper back. Less commonly, the neck, face, and shoulders may be involved. The differential diagnosis may include AN and tinea versicolor. This disorder is seen

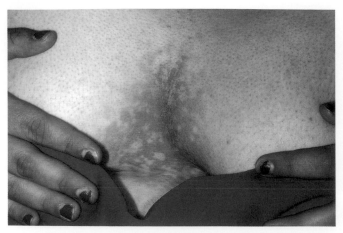

Figure 23.26 Confluent and reticulated papillomatosis. Hyperpigmented papules and plaques, with a reticulate appearance around the periphery, involving the intermammary region.

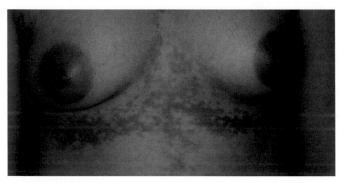

Figure 23.27 Confluent and reticulated papillomatosis. Reticulate tan papules, patches and plaques involving the epigastrium, inframammary areas and sternum.

primarily in adolescents and young adults, and females are involved twice as often as males.

The cause of CARP remains unknown, although there are several speculative theories. An association with insulin resistance has been hypothesized, and the condition has been reported in patients with concomitant AN, obesity, and hyperinsulinemia.[152] However, in most patients, no such association exists. An abnormal host immune response to *Pityrosporum orbiculare* (*Malassezzia furfur*) has also been suggested, given clinical resemblance to tinea versicolor and the occasional response of patients to treatment with topical or oral antifungal agents, although this association remains controversial.[153,154] Potassium hydroxide examinations on skin scrapings for fungal elements are negative in the majority of patients.[155]

Treatment of CARP is often, but not always, successful. A significant proportion of patients seem to respond to minocycline or doxycycline,[156–159] although the mechanism of action is unclear. Minocycline in conjunction with a topical lactic acid-containing emollient is often useful. Other reported therapies, of variable effectiveness, include topical selenium sulfide shampoo, oral or topical retinoids, oral and topical antifungal agents, topical vitamin D analogues, topical salicylic acid, and topical urea.

Scleredema diabeticorum

Scleredema (see also Ch. 22) is a rare disorder characterized by diffuse and symmetric induration of the skin. There are two forms: scleredema of Buschke (which tends to occur following upper respiratory infection, especially streptococcal) and the diabetes-associated form. Scleredema diabeticorum occurs most often in middle aged, obese men, although it has been reported in childhood and even in a congenital form.[160] The most common sites are the neck and upper back, but eventual extension to other areas may occur, including the face, scalp, chest, and arms. The skin in affected areas is firm and indurated without pitting, and cannot be wrinkled or pressed into folds.[126] The surface appears taut and shiny, with loss of normal surface markings. Scleredema is painless, but may be uncomfortable for patients given the textural changes and limitation of movement. Occasionally, involvement of the tongue, pharynx, and esophagus may result in dysarthria and dysphagia. Rare associations include pleural, pericardial, or peritoneal effusion, skeletal muscle dysfunction, and paraproteinemia. Histologic evaluation of biopsy tissue characteristically reveals collagen bundles separated by mucin deposits. The course of scleredema diabeticorum is variable. It may improve with control of the diabetes,[161] although this is inconsistent; in some patients, it persists for many years. Therapy is challenging and the results are often disappointing.

The glucagonoma syndrome

Patients with glucagon-secreting, pancreatic islet α-cell tumors may have a distinctive dermatosis termed *necrolytic migratory erythema* (NME). The glucagonoma syndrome is characterized by the triad of this cutaneous eruption, a glucagon-secreting tumor, and diabetes mellitus.[162] Weight loss, anemia, and stomatitis are common. Patients with this syndrome are generally middle-aged to elderly, with only rare reports of affected adolescents or young adults.

The cutaneous findings of NME are a hallmark of this syndrome. These skin changes may be present for several years before the diagnosis of glucagonoma is made. Characteristic features include erythema that most often begins in the groin, perineum, and buttocks, with eventual extension to the extremities and perioral areas. The erythematous lesions develop into well-demarcated, annular plaques with scaling, vesicles, and bullae. Erosions and pustules may develop (the latter occasionally studding the periphery of the plaques), and crusting is common. Induration, psoriasiform changes, lichenification, and bronze pigmentation may occur. The skin lesions of NME evolve sequentially from erythema to blistering to crusting to resolution, and are characterized by a pattern of spontaneous remissions and exacerbations.[162] Secondary superinfection with *Staphylococcus aureus* or *Candida* (especially at perineal sites) is common. Patients often appear ill and may have venous thromboses and alopecia. The average 5-year survival rate is <50%.[163] The differential diagnosis of NME may include several nutritional deficiency-related dermatoses, staphylococcal scalded skin syndrome, psoriasis, and toxic epidermal necrolysis.

The diagnosis of NME is suggested by the histologic finding of necrosis of the upper layers of the epidermis. The diagnosis of glucagonoma syndrome is confirmed by finding an elevated serum glucagon level or identifying the neuroendocrine tumor radiographically or histologically. Complete surgical resection of the tumor, when feasible, is the treatment of choice and is usually associated with complete to near-complete resolution of the cutaneous eruption.

Key References

The complete list of 163 references for this chapter is available online at **www.expertconsult.com.**
See inside cover for registration details.

Antal Z, Zhou P. Congenital adrenal hyperplasia: Diagnosis, evaluation and management. *Pediatr Rev.* 2009;30:e49–e57.

Brickman WJ, Huang J, Silverman BL, Metzger BE. Acanthosis nigricans identifies youth at high risk for metabolic abnormalities. *J Pediatr.* 2010;156:87–92.

Davidovici BB, Orion E, Wolf R. Cutaneous manifestations of pituitary gland diseases. *Clin Dermatol.* 2008;26:288–295.

Doshi DN, Blyumin ML, Kimball AB. Cutaneous manifestations of thyroid disease. *Clin Dermatol.* 2008;26:283–287.

Elsaie ML, Baumann LS, Elsaaiee LT. Striae distensae (stretch marks) and different modalities of therapy: An update. *Dermatol Surg.* 2009;35:563–573.

Faiyaz-Ul-Haque M, Bin-Abbas B, Al-Abdullatif A, et al. Novel and recurrent mutations in the AIRE gene of autoimmune polyendocrinopathy syndrome type I (APS1) patients. *Clin Genet.* 2009;76(5):431–440.

Nieman LK, Turner ML. Addison's disease. *Clin Dermatol.* 2006;24:276–280.

Yii MF, Lim DE, Luo X, et al. Polycystic ovarian syndrome in adolescence. *Gynecol Endocrinol.* 2009;25(10):634–639.

Inborn Errors of Metabolism

The inborn disorders of metabolism are a group of primarily autosomal recessive hereditary disorders that result in metabolic and clinical defects. (More comprehensive discussion of some of these topics is covered elsewhere: disorders of tyrosine metabolism (Richner–Hanhart syndrome), Gaucher syndrome, and multiple sulfatase deficiency are mentioned in Ch. 5; Menkes syndrome in Ch. 7; alkaptonuria in Ch. 11; Fabry disease and fucosidosis in Ch. 12; and Hartnup disease in Ch. 19.) Most developed countries have instituted comprehensive screening programs during the first week of life that allow detection of many of these defects, among them biotinidase deficiency, aminoacidopathies, urea cycle defects, and organic acid disorders.[1]

Phenylketonuria

Phenylketonuria (phenylpyruvic oligophrenia; PKU) is an autosomal recessive disorder of amino acid metabolism characterized by mental retardation, diffuse hypopigmentation, seizures, dermatitis, and photosensitivity (Table 24.1).[2-4] The classic form is caused by a deficiency of phenylalanine hydroxylase or its cofactor, tetrahydrobiopterin. Its incidence has been estimated to be 1 in 10 000 births. Because of mandatory screening in the neonatal period, the disorder is detected early in developed countries, and the clinical features do not appear if early dietary control is achieved. Screening is achieved by a variety of different tests ranging from a semiquantitative bacterial inhibition assay (Guthrie test) to mass spectrometry assays. If missed in the neonatal period by screening, the diagnosis depends on the demonstration of elevated serum levels of phenylalanine (20 mg/dL or higher, 10–50 times that of normal), normal or elevated levels of plasma tyrosine (normal is approximately 1 mg/dL), or elevated urinary levels of phenylpyruvic acid. The latter can be detected by a characteristic green or blue color that results when a few drops of urine are added to a 10% solution of ferric chloride. The normal phenylalanine : tyrosine ratio is 1 : 1; in PKU it is >3 : 1. The observed pigmentary dilution is thought to result from the inhibitory effect of phenylalanine on tyrosinase.

Most commonly seen in individuals of northern European ancestry, 90% of affected individuals are blond, blue eyed, and fair skinned, given the important role of phenylalanine and its derivative tyrosine in pigment formation. A peculiar musty odor, attributable to decomposition products (phenylacetic acid or phenylacetaldehyde) in the urine and sweat, and early intractable vomiting are characteristic. Infants appear to be normal at birth and, if untreated, develop manifestations of delayed intellectual development sometime between 4 and 24 months of age. Seizures, hyperactivity, hypertonicity, hyperreflexia, a peculiar gait, speech delay, and self-destructive behavior have been described. Skeletal changes include microcephaly, short stature, pes planus, and syndactyly. The dermatitis appears in 10–50% of untreated patients and resembles atopic dermatitis; sclerodermoid changes of the proximal extremities, sparing the hands and feet, may present during the first 2 years of life.[5,6] These changes regress with appropriate treatment.

Management consists of a diet low in phenylalanine content starting at as early an age as possible. This can be initiated by the use of formula from which most of the phenylalanine has been removed or a synthetic amino acid preparation devoid of phenylalanine. Restriction of phenylalanine leads to reversal of the seizures, dermatitis, and pigmentary dilution, but the effect on intellectual function depends on the age at which therapy is initiated. Little benefit on intellectual function can be achieved if therapy is initiated after 2.5 years of age, and optimal benefit is achieved if initiated by 2 months of age. It should be remembered that phenylalanine is high in many foods, and is a metabolite of the sweetener aspartame. Children and adolescents with PKU who achieve dietary control early in life are well adjusted and have an excellent quality of life.[7]

Although there is some controversy about continuation of phenylalanine restriction in later childhood and adults, lack of dietary control during the 1st trimester of pregnancy of affected mothers (> 600 µM or 10 mg/dL phenylalanine) has led to cardiac defects in 15% of offspring, particularly coarctation of the aorta and hypoplastic left heart.[8] Optimal levels during pregnancy of 120–360 µM/L are recommended. Some patients maintain low levels of phenylalanine as adults without dietary manipulation.

Disorders of tyrosine metabolism

Clinical disorders of tyrosine metabolism include neonatal tyrosinemia, tyrosinemia I, and tyrosinemia II (the Richner–Hanhart syndrome). Of these, only the Richner–Hanhart syndrome exhibits cutaneous manifestations, and is described in Chapter 5. These include palmoplantar keratoderma with painful erosions and photophobia with corneal erosions.

Homocystinuria

Homocystinuria is an autosomal recessive disorder of methionine metabolism that results from an absence or deficiency of cystathionine β-synthase, the pyridoxine-dependent hepatic enzyme that catalyzes the formation of cystathionine from homocystine and serine.[9] Based on biochemical testing, the disorder is most common in Ireland (1 in 65 000 births) and has a worldwide incidence of 1 in 344 000.[10] However, a recent study in Norway using genotyping showed an estimated birth prevalence of 1 in 6400.[11]

The disorder affects predominantly the eyes, central nervous system, blood vessels, and bones (Table 24.1). Subluxation of the ocular lenses (ectopia lentis) occurs in 82% of patients by 15 years of age,[12] and is usually present by 10 years of age. Developmental delay is evident during infancy and most untreated patients develop seizures and significant retardation. Bony abnormalities include a

Table 24.1 Errors of protein metabolism

Disorder	Inheritance	Defect	Clinical features	Diagnosis	Treatment
Phenylketonuria	AR	Phenylalanine hydroxylase	90% are blond, blue-eyed, and fair skinned; musty odor; sclerodermatous plaques; eczematous dermatitis; photosensitivity; retardation; microcephaly; short stature	Guthrie test, ferric chloride test	Low phenylalanine diet
Homocystinuria	AR	Cystathionine synthetase	Ectopia lentis, myopia, arachnodactyly, seizures, mental retardation, cerebrovascular accidents, sparse light or blond easily friable hair, malar flush, wide-pored facies, livedoid rash, 'Charlie Chaplin-like' gait and 'rocker-bottom' feet	Cyanide nitroprusside test	Low methionine diet with pyridoxine (vitamin B6)
Alkaptonuria (ochronosis)	AR	Homogentisic acid oxidase	Dark urine; blue to brownish-black pigment on nose, malar region, sclerae, ears, axillae, genitalia; staining of clothing ('beads of ink' perspiration); arthritis; contractures; rupture of Achilles tendon; mitral and aortic valvulitis and/or calcific aortic stenosis	Ferric cyanide reduction	Nitisinone
Trimethylaminuria	AR	Flavin mono-oxygenase type 3	Odor of rotting fish	Trimethylamine in urine	Dietary avoidance of choline
Wilson disease (hepatolenticular degeneration)	AR	ATP7B; ceruloplasmin metabolism	Kayser-Fleischer rings, hyperpigmentation, azure lunulae, neurologic and liver dysfunction	Aminoaciduria, decreased ceruloplasmin	Chelating agents (BAL, versenate, or D-penicillamine)
Lesch–Nyhan syndrome	X-LR	HPRT deficiency	Mental retardation, spastic cerebral palsy, choreoathetosis, self-mutilation	Increased uric acid, orange uric acid crystals in diaper	Allopurinol

AR, autosomal recessive; BAL, British Anti-Lewisite or dimercaprol; HPRT, hypoxanthine-guanine phosphoribosyl transferase; X-LR, X-linked recessive.

body habitus similar to that seen in Marfan syndrome (see Ch. 6), and generalized osteoporosis, which is seen radiographically in 50% of affected individuals by 15 years of age. Platyspondylia (congenital flattening of the vertebral bodies) and hollowing out of the vertebral bodies by pressure of the vertebral disks are also seen radiographically, and kyphoscoliosis, pectus carinatum, and genu valgum are common. Some patients have rocker-bottom feet and most have a shuffling toe-out 'Charlie Chaplin-like' gait. Megaloblastic anemia has also been described.[13]

The vascular complications can be life threatening; the chance of a vascular event during childhood is 25–30% and increases to 50% by 30 years of age. These include pulmonary embolism, myocardial infarction, transient ischemic attacks, cerebrovascular accidents, abdominal aortic aneurysm, and venous thromboses. Cutaneous features include sparse, light or blond, coarse hair that can darken and become softer with treatment; a malar flush; coarse, wide pores on facial skin; and a reticulated livedoid vasculopathy (cutis reticulata) on the face and extremities.

The presence of homocystinuria is suggested by the clinical features and can be confirmed by a urinary cyanide or sodium nitroprusside testing (turns a beet-red color) and by amino acid chromatography of the serum and urine. The presence of homocystine in the urine establishes the diagnosis. In the blood, homocysteine and methionine are elevated, while cysteine levels are

decreased. Unfortunately, there are no neonatal manifestations of homocystinuria and not all newborns with this disorder have increased blood methionine levels.

In at least 50% of patients, the disease is pyridoxine-responsive and can be controlled with the combination of pyridoxine (vitamin B6; 250–500 mg/day), folic acid, and vitamin B12 (cobalamin). For those who do not respond to vitamins alone, a methionine-restricted, cystine-supplemented diet is required as well.[14] Betaine, a methyl donor that remethylates homocysteine to methionine, has been used as an adjunct to treatment, especially in patients who do not respond to vitamin therapy. As with phenylketonuria, early institution of therapy dramatically reduces the risk of complications.

Trimethylaminuria

Trimethylaminuria (the fish odor syndrome) is a metabolic disorder in which accumulation of trimethylamine in the sweat and urine gives rise to an unpleasant 'rotting fish' odor to the skin, sweat, and urine. There are no visible cutaneous changes. The disorder results from mutations in the flavin-containing monooxygenase type 3 (FM03) gene.[15] The liver is unable to convert the trimethylamine generated in the intestinal tract by bacterial degradation of choline- and lecithin-containing foods such as saltwater fish and seafood, egg yolk, liver, kidney, soy beans, meat, broccoli, cauliflower, cabbage, brussel sprouts, wheat germ, milk (from wheat-fed cows), and yeast to the nonodorous oxide metabolite.[16] The psychosocial effects of the condition can be devastating, including disruption of schooling, clinical depression, and attempted suicide. Treatment is best accomplished by avoidance and limitation of choline-containing foods,[14,17] although administration of metronidazole has also led to a clinical and biochemical response.[18]

Wilson disease (hepatolenticular degeneration)

Wilson disease is an autosomal recessive disorder that results from mutations in *ATP7B*, which encodes a copper-transporting ATPase. Deficiency leads to an inability to synthesize normal amounts of ceruloplasmin.[19,20] Patients show abnormal hepatic excretion of copper and toxic accumulations of copper in the liver, brain, and other organs. The clinical triad that results consists of progressive neurologic dysfunction, hepatic cirrhosis, and pathognomonic pigmentation of the corneal margins (Kayser–Fleischer ring) (Table 24.1).

The disorder can be detected as early as 4 years of age but usually manifests during adolescence. The clinical signs at presentation can be quite varied. Although initial signs of the disorder are often neurologic (intention tremors, dysarthria, ataxia, incoordination, personality changes, psychiatric problems, and worsening school performance and handwriting), signs of liver insufficiency (jaundice, ascites, hepatomegaly, hematemesis, and cutaneous spider angiomas) are present at onset in 40–50% of affected individuals.[21]

Kayser–Fleischer rings are seen as dense golden brown or greenish brown pigmentation localized near the limbus of the cornea. Occurring in about 95% of patients with this disorder and best visualized by side lighting and slit-lamp examination, this discoloration is produced by the deposition of copper in Descemet's membrane at the periphery of the cornea. Kayser–Fleischer rings may also be seen in other copper overload states such as primary cirrhosis, intrahepatic cholestasis of childhood (Byler syndrome), and chronic active hepatitis.

Xerosis has been described in 45.7% of affected children.[22] Hyperpigmentation of the anterior lower legs or the genital region has been described and may be misinterpreted as Addison's disease. Blue or azure lunulae of the nails have been reported in individuals with this disorder, but also have been observed in normal individuals as a complication of phenolphthalein or quinacrine ingestion, and in argyria. White discoloration of the nails has also been noted.[22] In addition, patients may manifest a vague greenish discoloration on the skin of the face, neck, and genitalia, and hyperpigmentation due to increased melanin deposition, particularly on the anterior aspects of the lower legs and on the genitalia. No increase in copper or iron is seen in cutaneous biopsy specimens.

Hepatolenticular degeneration is a progressive disease and, if untreated, is inevitably fatal. Death usually results from infection, hepatic disease, or liver failure. Treatment depends on removal of accumulated copper depositions in the body. Chelating agents such as D-penicillamine or trientine (triethylene tetramine dihydrochloride)[23] and zinc acetate (25–50 mg three times a day) are helpful. Since discontinuation of therapy can result in rapid deterioration, treatment is life-long. Penicillamine can produce allergic or toxic reactions, fever, cutaneous rashes, leukopenia, thrombocytopenia, elastosis perforans serpiginosa[24] (see Ch. 6; Fig. 6.12), and other

dermal disorders[25] and immunobullous skin disease;[26] since penicillamine inhibits pyridoxine-dependent enzymes, patients should also be given daily supplements of pyridoxine (12.5–25.0 mg/day). In an effort to minimize copper deposition, patients should be encouraged to limit their ingestion of copper-rich foods such as liver, nuts, chocolate, cocoa, mushrooms, brain, shellfish, dried foods, and broccoli. Liver transplantation can be lifesaving for patients with hepatic failure.[27,28]

Lesch–Nyhan syndrome

Lesch–Nyhan syndrome, an X-linked recessive disorder of purine metabolism, is characterized by mental retardation, choreoathetoid movements, and self-mutilation.[29] The condition is caused by a deficiency of hypoxanthine-guanine phosphoribosyl transferase (HPRT),[30] which leads to an overproduction of uric acid and the clinical features associated with this disorder (Table 24.1). Patients appear normal at birth and may develop normally for 6–8 months. The first recognizable sign of the disease is often orange uric acid crystals (resembling grains of sand) in the diaper or as hematuria during the early months of life.

The onset of cerebral manifestations may be subtle, with difficulty in sitting or standing without help, involuntary movements, dystonia, spasticity, and increased deep tendon reflexes. Although mental retardation may vary in degree it usually is severe, and abnormal behavior remains a striking characteristic of the disease. The main clinical feature of this disorder is a loss of tissue about the mouth or fingers that occurs, not because of an inability to feel pain, but as a result of the child's habit of compulsive self-destructive biting of these areas. In time, without adequate restraints, all of the lower lip accessible to the teeth may be chewed away. The face, fingers, and wrists may also be mutilated, and since young children frequently bite others, caution should be exercised when handling children with this disorder. Other destructive behaviors include head banging, extension of arms when being wheeled through doorways, tipping of wheelchairs, eye-poking, fingers in wheelchair spokes, and rubbing behaviors. Other manifestations of hyperuricemia, such as tophaceous deposits, nephropathy, and gouty arthritis, occur later.

Not to be confused with familial dysautonomia (Riley–Day) and congenital insensitivity to pain with anhidrosis (see Ch. 8), other conditions characterized by biting and self-mutilating behavior, Lesch–Nyhan syndrome can be confirmed by the clinical presentation and laboratory demonstration of increased levels of uric acid in the blood and urine.[31] Heterozygous females are asymptomatic. Management includes the use of allopurinol (in dosages of 100–300 mg/day in divided doses) in an effort to control uric acid levels. Physical restraints (hand bandages and elbow splints) may be used to help control the self-mutilating behavior of patients.[29] Lip biting may require extraction of deciduous teeth, but permanent teeth should be spared, since lip biting usually diminishes with age.

Dermatitis from nutritional abnormalities

Acrodermatitis Enteropathica

Acrodermatitis enteropathica is an autosomal recessive disorder that generally appears in early infancy and is characterized by a triad of acral and periorificial skin lesions (vesiculobullous, pustular, and eczematous), diarrhea, and alopecia (Table 24.2).[32,33] The condition first becomes manifest days to weeks after birth if bottle-fed and

Table 24.2 Genetic and acquired nutritional disorders

Disorder	Cause	Features	Evaluation	Therapy
Zinc deficiency	Acrodermatitis enteropathica Decreased zinc in breast milk Malabsorption Zinc-poor IV hyperalimentation	Periorificial dermatitis, stomatitis, glossitis, alopecia, irritability, diarrhea, failure to thrive, candidal infection, photophobia	Zinc levels, serum alkaline phosphatase; zinc levels in maternal breast milk	Zinc supplementation
Biotin deficiency	Holocarboxylase deficiency Biotinidase deficiency Malabsorption Ingestion of egg whites Biotin-poor IV hyperalimentation	Periorificial dermatitis, conjunctivitis, blepharitis, alopecia, candidal infections, metabolic acidosis, vomiting, lethargy, developmental delay, seizures, ataxia, optic atrophy, hearing loss	Urinary organic acids, plasma ammonia and lactate, serum biotin, specific enzyme activity	Biotin supplementation
Deficiency of vitamin B_{12} or isoleucine from restrictive diets	Organic acidurias Citrullinemia Maple syrup urine disease Methylmalonic acidemia Propionic acidemia	Periorificial dermatitis, alopecia, candidal infections, metabolic acidosis, vomiting, failure to thrive, lethargy, developmental delay, hypotonia, pancytopenia	Urinary organic acids; plasma ammonia and glycine levels, plasma isoleucine levels	Dietary manipulation (results from effects of low-protein diet; some respond to vitamin B_{12} supplementation)
Cystic fibrosis	Deficiency of cystic fibrosis transmembrane conductance regulator (CFTR)	Periorificial and truncal dermatitis, occasionally alopecia, failure to thrive, diarrhea, irritability, edema	Sweat test, serum albumin, gene analysis, mutational analysis of *CFTR* gene	Pancreatic enzymes, vitamin and zinc supplementation
Essential fatty acid deficiency	Inadequate dietary intake	Generalized scaling with underlying erythema, intertriginous erosions, alopecia, decreased pigmentation of hair, failure to thrive, thrombocytopenia and anemia	Plasma linoleic, linolenic, arachidonic and icosatrienoic acid levels; check for other deficiencies	Supplementation of essential fatty acids
Kwashiorkor	Inadequate protein; often infants taken off milk protein for allergies or dietary fads without adequate replacement	Superficial desquamation with erosion (flaky paint), edema with moon facies and pallor, hyperpigmentation and hypopigmentation, ecchymoses, sparse, dry lusterless hair with decreased pigmentation and 'flag sign', cheilitis, dry mucosae, irritability and failure to thrive, irritability and apathy, secondary skin infections, diarrhea, hepatomegaly	Serum albumin, good dietary history	Slow supplementation with protein, correction of electrolyte imbalances

shortly after weaning if breast-fed. The disorder results from mutations in *SLC39A*, which encodes an intestinal zinc transporter ZIP4.[34]

The basic cutaneous lesion of acrodermatitis enteropathica is an erythematosus, scaling, crusted, psoriasiform, eczematous or vesiculobullous eruption (Fig. 2.25). Lesions tend to be localized around the body orifices (mouth, nose, ears, eyes, and perineum) (Fig. 24.1) and symmetrically located on the buttocks (Fig. 24.2) and extensor surface of major joints (elbows, knees, hands, and feet), the scalp, and the fingers and toes (hence the term acrodermatitis). On the face, the eroded and crusted peribuccal plaques may appear impetiginized, and secondary infection with *Candida albicans* is common. When the fingers and toes are involved there is marked

erythema and swelling of the paronychial tissues, often with subsequent nail deformity. If unrecognized or untreated, acrodermatitis enteropathica follows an intermittent but relentlessly progressive course and, as a consequence of general disability, infection, or both, frequently ends in death.

Typically, infants with acrodermatitis enteropathica are listless, anorexic, and apathetic. Many infants show frequent crying, irritability, and restlessness. Tissue wasting is present with an associated failure to thrive. During periods of exacerbation, frothy, bulky, foul-smelling diarrheal stools are present. Other findings include conjunctivitis, photophobia, stomatitis, perlèche, nail dystrophy, recurring candidal or bacterial infection, and alopecia of the scalp, eyelashes, and/or eyebrows.[35] Children suffering from this disorder

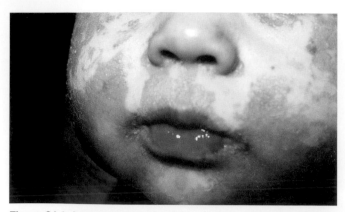

Figure 24.1 Acrodermatitis enteropathica. Moist, sharply marginated psoriasiform plaques around the mouth, nose, and eyes of an infant.

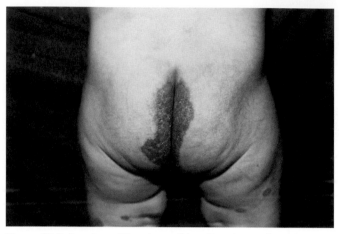

Figure 24.2 Acrodermatitis enteropathica. Sharply marginated psoriasiform plaques of the perianal area and buttock.

exhibit a striking uniformity of appearance, mainly because of the alopecia and periorificial lesions.

In addition to the classic inherited disease, zinc deficiency with signs mimicking acrodermatitis enteropathica may also occur in babies who are breast-fed.[36] This abnormality results from inadequate secretion of zinc in maternal milk. Maternal mutations in *SLC30A2* (ZnT-2), which encodes a protein required for zinc secretion, have been found.[37] Zinc deficiency with clinical manifestations may also be seen in individuals receiving long-term parenteral nutrition with inadequate zinc supplementation, patients who have had intestinal bypass procedures, premature infants with low zinc storage (particularly those fed exclusively with human milk), as a complication of Crohn's disease,[38] in infants with HIV infection and diarrhea (causing inadequate absorption of zinc), in patients with *cystic fibrosis* with poor zinc absorption,[39,40] chronic alcoholics or patients with anorexia nervosa,[41] in individuals on zinc-deficient vegetarian diets, and in patients with low pancreatic enzyme levels resulting in poor intestinal absorption of zinc.[42] In babies with cystic fibrosis, the manifestations of zinc deficiency typically are noted at 3–5 months of age, before any evidence of pulmonary disease. The low serum albumin level and abnormal sweat test can confirm the diagnosis.

The diagnosis of acrodermatitis enteropathica is based on the clinical features and low serum zinc levels (50 μg/dL or lower). It should be noted, however, that zinc contamination of glass tubes and rubber stoppers often occurs; blood samples should be collected in acid-washed sterile plastic tubes with the use of acid-washed plastic syringes. Low serum alkaline phosphatase levels (even when the serum zinc level is normal), low serum lipid levels, and defective chemotaxis may be found. Skin biopsy is not diagnostic, but may be useful in some patients. Zinc levels can also be measured in maternal milk.

Zinc sulfate supplementation is provided at 5–10 mg/kg per day, which usually provides approximately 1–2 mg/kg per day elemental zinc, although the dosage may differ to provide sufficient elemental zinc if other formulations are used. When given in divided doses two or three times a day, improvement in temperament and decrease in irritability can generally be noted within 1 or 2 days; the appetite improves in a few days, and diarrhea and skin lesions begin to respond within 2 or 3 days after the initiation of therapy. Hair growth begins after 2–3 weeks of therapy, and increase in the growth of the infant generally occurs within approximately 2 weeks. After the patient's condition appears to be stabilized, zinc levels should be monitored at periodic (6-month) intervals, followed by the adjustment of supplemental zinc to the lowest effective dosage schedule. Since foods may have an effect on the absorption of zinc, zinc supplementation should be administered 1 or 2 h before meals. Zinc supplementation can cause gastrointestinal upset (nausea, vomiting, gastric hemorrhage); zinc gluconate tends to cause fewer gastrointestinal problems. Less zinc supplementation may be required for acquired or dietary zinc deficiency. In infants who have zinc deficiency as a result of defective maternal mammary zinc secretion, zinc supplementation can be discontinued after weaning.

Disorders that resemble acrodermatitis enteropathica

Biotin deficiency/organic acid disorders

A dermatitis resembling acrodermatitis enteropathica, often in association with alopecia and changes in hair texture, has been described in patients with *biotin deficiency* and in certain *organic acid disorders*.[43,44] The cutaneous features resembling acrodermatitis enteropathica have been described in methylmalonic academia,[45] propionic academia,[45] glutaric aciduria type I,[46] maple syrup urine disease,[47] ornithine transcarbamylase deficiency,[48] and citrullinemia[49] because of dietary restriction and deficiency of amino acids, especially isoleucine (Fig. 24.3).[50,51] Acrodermatitis enteropathica-like eruptions have also been reported in children with Hartnup disease (see Ch. 19).[52,53]

Biotin, part of the vitamin B complex, is required for the function of four carboxylase enzymes[42]:

1. 3-Methyl crotonyl-CoA carboxylase, essential for the catabolism of leucine
2. Propionyl CoA carboxylase, essential for the catabolism of isoleucine, threonine, valine, and methionine
3. Pyruvic acid carboxylase, required for the gluconeogenesis and regulation of carbohydrate metabolism
4. Acetyl CoA carboxylase, an enzyme of long-chain fatty acid synthesis that contains biotin.

Biotin deficiency may be induced by a biotin-deficient diet: a diet in which patients ingest large quantities of raw egg white (which contains the protein avidin that binds to biotin, thus preventing its absorption in the intestine) and/or prolonged parenteral nutrition to which biotin has not been added (Table 24.2). The resulting deficiency is manifested by anorexia, lassitude, a pale tongue, grayish pallor of the skin, atrophy of the lingual papillae, hair loss, anemia, muscle pains, dryness of the skin, and a scaly dermatitis,

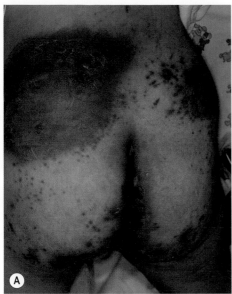

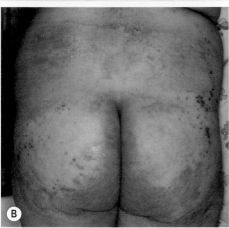

Figure 24.3 Methylmalonic acidemia. This patient developed the typical erosive and desquamative eruption while on a restricted diet (A); isoleucine deficiency was discovered and the eruption cleared within a week when isoleucine was added to the diet (B).

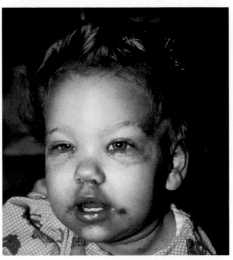

Figure 24.4 Biotin deficiency. Scaly periorificial dermatitis in a child with biotin-responsive carboxylase deficiency.[58]

all of which disappear following biotin administration or by cooking, boiling, or steaming of egg white (which causes avidin to lose its biotin-binding capacity). Decreased biotin levels have also been noted in patients administered anticonvulsants (phenytoin, carbamazepine), and may result in seborrheic dermatitis and alopecia.[54,55]

Several autosomal recessive disorders may manifest as an acrodermatitis enteropathica-like eruption because they require biotin as a cofactor. Cheilitis and diffuse erythema with erosions and desquamation are features of methylmalonic acidemia before therapeutic amino acid restriction.[56] Inherited biotin deficiency also occurs in two forms of multiple carboxylase deficiency, one of which presents acutely during the neonatal period (neonatal form) and the other during early infancy (juvenile form).[57] These disorders occur in up to 1:40 000 births. Both forms usually show a sharply marginated, brightly erythematous scaling eruption of the periorificial areas, scalp, eyebrows, and eyelashes (Fig. 24.4). Alopecia can manifest as hair thinning or total alopecia. Secondary candidiasis is not uncommon.[59] The neonatal form, which results from deficiency of holocarboxylase synthetase, appears in the first few weeks of life with metabolic acidosis, ketosis, and, rarely, the cutaneous

manifestations. Patients show feeding and breathing difficulties, seizures, hypotonia, and lethargy; without early diagnosis and treatment, they usually die. The juvenile form of the disorder, which first manifests at 2 months of age or older, is the result of deficiency of biotinidase, which is required for recycling of endogenous biotin. Patients have low levels of biotin in the blood and urine and impaired biotin absorption and/or transport. In addition to the cutaneous features, the juvenile form is characterized by seizures (especially myoclonic spasms that respond partially to anticonvulsants), hyperventilation or apnea, recurrent infections (including candidal skin infections), keratoconjunctivitis, ataxia, hypotonia, glossitis, and life threatening acidosis and massive ketosis. More than 50% of patients whose disease is not recognized early have hearing loss that does not improve with biotin therapy.

The diagnosis of biotin deficiency can be established by a decreased concentration of plasma biotin. Deficiencies of biotinidase or holocarboxylase synthetase also show an increase in the urinary metabolites 3-hydroxyisovaleric acid, 3-methylcrotonylglycine, 3-hydroxypropionic acid, methylcitric acid, and lactic acid. Biotin deficiency can be treated by intravenous multivitamins containing 60 μg of biotin or by the oral administration of 5–10 mg of biotin daily. Higher concentrations of biotin may be required for holocarboxylase synthetase deficiency.[60] Skin and neurologic signs tend to improve within a few weeks, although neurologic dysfunction can be permanent if treatment is delayed.

Kwashiorkor

Kwashiorkor is a severe form of protein deficiency in which edema, hypoalbuminemia, and dermatosis predominate. Seen primarily in underdeveloped countries, several cases of kwashiorkor have been described in developed countries as well.[61,62] Cases in developed countries have been described because of nutritional ignorance, food allergen avoidance, food fads, and child abuse.[63] Particularly common is the substitution of rice 'milk', which has only a miniscule content of protein and is not a milk substitute. In children with chronic protein and caloric malnutrition, particularly from Africa, signs usually present during the second or third year of life with the onset of weaning from breast-feeding. In contrast, patients in developed countries most commonly show features during the first year of life with a rapid onset of edema. Kwashiorkor has also been described with malabsorption, including infantile Crohn's disease[64] and cystic fibrosis.[65]

The clinical picture consists of a blanching erythema with an overlying reddish-brown scale that shows a sharply marginated raised edge. This edge resembles paint that is lifting up and about to peel off, leading to the term 'flaky paint dermatosis' (Figs 24.5, 24.6). In contrast to lesions of pellagra, the dermatosis seldom appears on areas exposed to sunlight and tends to spare the feet and dorsal areas of the hands. Photosensitivity, purpura, and excessive bruisability may also be present. Other associated features include changes in mental behavior, anorexia, apathy, irritability, growth retardation, and fatty infiltration of the liver with hypoproteinemia. As a result of the hypoalbuminemia, affected children show edema of the face ('moon facies') (Fig. 24.7), feet, and abdomen (potbelly appearance).

In mild cases the cutaneous eruption is associated with a superficial desquamation; in severe cases there are large areas of erosion.

As the disease progresses, the entire cutaneous surface develops a reddish or coffee-colored hue. Other associated features include circumoral pallor, loss of pigmentation (especially after minor trauma), and depigmentation of the hair. In darker haired children the hair color can change to a reddish-brown hue or even gray or straw color (Fig. 24.8). The dyschromia with hypopigmentation has

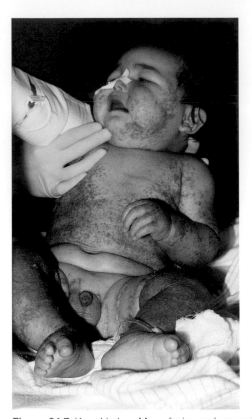

Figure 24.7 Kwashiorkor. Moon facies and generalized dermatosis.

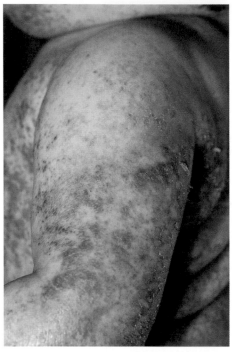

Figure 24.5 Kwashiorkor. Sharply marginated raised edge of reddish-brown scaling ('flaky paint dermatosis') on the arm of an infant with severe hypoalbuminemia from dietary deficiency.

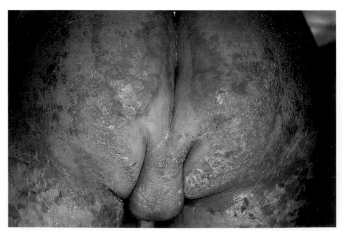

Figure 24.6 Kwashiorkor. Note the brown peeling 'flaky paint' appearance of the posterior aspect of the upper thighs.

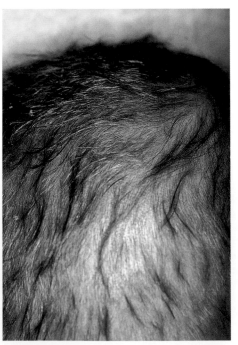

Figure 24.8 Kwashiorkor. The hair often loses its coloration and may become gray or straw-colored.

been attributed to deficiency of tyrosine, which is critical for melanin synthesis. When periods of malnutrition alternate with intervals of adequate dietary intake, alternating bands of light and dark color (the flag sign) are produced in the hair.

The condition may be difficult to distinguish from acrodermatitis enteropathica and, in fact, children may have concomitant zinc deficiency as well. The hypoalbuminemia and edema are helpful signs to distinguish kwashiorkor from acrodermatitis enteropathica and other disorders of nutritional deficiency. Children with marasmus have both protein and caloric deficiency. They appear emaciated (vs the edematous appearance of children with kwashiorkor), have dry, scaling skin that may show follicular hyperkeratosis, and often have thin, sparse hair.

Children afflicted with kwashiorkor are extremely ill, and if they are not treated, the mortality rate can be 30% or more, primarily resulting from infection (impairment of immunity) and electrolyte imbalance with diarrhea. In underdeveloped countries where the disorder is common, breast-feeding should be continued for as long as possible to prevent the protein malnutrition. Treatment of affected individuals with gradual administration of a high-protein diet, vitamin supplementation, and correction of dehydration and electrolyte imbalance leads to resolution of the clinical abnormalities.

Essential fatty acid deficiency

Essential fatty acid deficiency (EFA) can also be manifested by periorificial dermatitis and a generalized xerotic or eczematous dermatitis (Table 24.2).[66] Failure to thrive, alopecia with lightly colored hair, and thrombocytopenia are other signs that may occur. The condition usually occurs in patients receiving parenteral nutrition without lipid supplementation and in association with severe fat malabsorption from gastrointestinal disorders or surgery of the gastrointestinal tract. EFA has also been described in patients with cystic fibrosis, anorexia nervosa, and acrodermatitis enteropathica. Decreased plasma levels of linoleic, linolenic, arachidonic, and icosatrienoic acid, as well as an icosatrienoic: arachidonic acid ratio of >0.4 confirms the diagnosis. The treatment consists of oral or parenteral fat emulsions. If these cannot be administered, topical application of 2–3 mg/kg soybean or safflower oil may be sufficient to restore plasma levels of linoleic acids, but may not maintain stores in the liver or other tissues.[67]

The hyperlipidemias

The hyperlipidemias (hyperlipoproteinemias) represent a group of metabolic diseases characterized by persistent elevation of plasma cholesterol levels, triglyceride levels, or both. Since plasma lipids circulate in the form of high-molecular-weight complexes bound to protein, the term *hyperlipidemia* also indicates an elevation of lipoproteins, hence justification for the term *hyperlipoproteinemia* for this group of disorders. The dermatologic manifestation is the xanthoma, which may also be seen in metabolic disorders with normal levels of lipids (sitosterolemia and cerebrotendinous xanthomatosis) and disorders with deficiencies in high-density lipoproteins. Xanthomas can provide a clue that a child has a serious lipid abnormality and is at risk for other abnormalities, particularly vascular disease.

Lipid levels can be assayed in blood samples taken after a 12-hour overnight fast. Plasma lipoproteins differ significantly in electrostatic charges, thus permitting their separation by electrophoretic mobility techniques into four major fractions: chylomicrons and β-, pre-β-, and α-lipoproteins. By means of ultracentrifugation it is also possible to separate the plasma lipoproteins into four major groups: chylomicrons and very low density (VLDL; which includes the pre-β

mobility lipoproteins), low density (LDL, which is the β-mobility lipoprotein), and high density (HDL; which is α-mobility lipoprotein), which correlate well with those separated by electrophoresis. Triglycerides are the major core lipids of chylomicrons and VLDLs. Cholesterol esters predominate in the core of LDLs, HDLs, remnants of VLDLs (also known as intermediate-density lipoproteins or IDLs), and chylomicrons. Apolipoproteins mediate the binding of lipoproteins to their receptors in target organs as well as activate enzymes that metabolize lipoproteins (Table 24.3). The levels of lipoproteins allow classification of the familial hyperlipidemias into five groups, designated as hyperlipoproteinemias I through V (Frederickson classification system), each with its own specific clinicopathologic, prognostic, and therapeutic features (Tables 24.4, 24.5, see below). Of these, types I and II most commonly present during childhood.

Lipoproteins can be synthesized from dietary intake or made endogenously in the liver. Dietary triglycerides are degraded by pancreatic lipase and bile acids to fatty acids and monoglycerides, but are repackaged after intestinal absorption with cholesterol esters to form the central core of a chylomicron. This core is surrounded by free cholesterol, phospholipids, and apolipoproteins (Table 24.3). In the circulation, this triglyceride core is hydrolyzed by lipoprotein lipase (LPL), leaving a chylomicron remnant of predominantly cholesterol ester and releasing fatty acids to peripheral tissues; LPL is activated by apolipoprotein C-II and requires hormones such as insulin. The endogenous pathway of lipid synthesis begins in the liver with the formation of VLDLs from hepatic triglycerides and circulating free fatty acids.

Xanthomas are lipid-containing papules, plaques, nodules, or tumors that may be found anywhere on the skin and mucous membranes.[68,69] Although the mechanism of their formation is not completely understood, it appears that serum lipids infiltrate the tissues where they are phagocytized by macrophages to form lipid-laden foam cells. They are then deposited, particularly in areas subjected to stress and pressure. Depending on their morphology, anatomic location, and mode of development, xanthomas can be categorized as *plane, eruptive* or *papuloeruptive, tendinous,* or *tuberous.* Recognition of these types of lesions, in addition to biochemical testing and physical examination, provides clues to possible metabolic abnormalities and diagnosis of specific metabolic diseases. Of note,

Table 24.3 Apolipoproteins and their function

Apolipoprotein	Association with lipoprotein	Function
ApoA-1	HDL, chylomicrons	Main protein of HDL; activates lecithin:cholesterol acyltransferase
ApoB-48	Chylomicrons	Only in chylomicrons; ApoB-100 without LDL receptor-binding domain
ApoB-100	LDL, VLDL	Main protein of LDL; binds to LDL receptor
ApoC-II	HDL, VLDL, chylomicrons	Activates lipoprotein lipase
ApoE$_2$, E$_3$, E$_4$	HDL, VLDL, chylomicron remnants	Binds to LDL receptor

Table 24.4 Laboratory findings in lipid disorders

Disorder and inheritance	Cholesterol	Triglycerides	VLDL	Chylomicrons	LDL	HDL	Cause
Type I HL/AR	↑	↑↑↑	↑	↑	↓	↓↓↓	Lipoprotein lipase deficiency Dysfunctional ApoC-II
Type II HL/AD	↑	NI(IIa); ↑ (IIb)	↑ (IIb)	NI	↓	↓	LDL receptor defect Dysfunctional ApoB-100
Type III HL/AR	↑	↑	↑	↑	↓	NI	ApoE abnormalities
Type IV HL/AD	↑	NI ↑	↑	NI	↓	↓↓	Renal disease, diabetes
Type V HL/AR	↑	↑↑↑	↑	↑	↓	↓↓↓	Similar to ApoC-II deficiency

AD, autosomal dominant; AR, autosomal recessive; ↑, increased; ↓, decreased; HL, hyperlipoproteinemia; NI, normal.

juvenile xanthogranuloma (JXG; see Ch. 10), the most common xanthomatous skin lesion seen in children, does not have an association with systemic hyperlipidemias or other metabolic abnormalities.

Plane (planar) xanthomas

Plane (planar) xanthomas are soft, yellow to orange or brownish yellow macules to slightly elevated plaques (Fig. 24.9). They are generally seen on the face, sides of the neck, upper trunk, buttocks, elbows, and knees, but may occur anywhere on the body and have a marked predilection for surgical or acne scars and the palmar creases. The most frequently seen plane xanthomas are *xanthelasmas*, which occur on or near the eyelids and are rarely seen in children or adolescents. Xanthelasmas in pediatric patients, in contrast with those in adults, are almost always associated with an underlying lipid abnormality. Intertriginous plane xanthomas, as in the antecubital fossae or the web spaces of the fingers, are usually associated with homozygous familial hypercholesterolemia.[58] Plane xanthomas of the palmar creases (xanthoma striatum palmare) suggest the diagnosis of dysbetalipoproteinemia, especially when the child also has tuberous xanthomas. Plane xanthomas also occur in children with cholestasis from biliary atresia or primary biliary cirrhosis (Table 24.6), because of the accumulation of circulating unesterified cholesterol, and in patients with an underlying monoclonal gammopathy, such as in Castleman disease.

Eruptive (papuloeruptive) xanthomas

Eruptive (papuloeruptive) xanthomas appear in crops of multiple 1–4 mm red to yellow-orange papules (Fig. 24.10), often surrounded by an erythematous base. Although they may involve the trunk and oral mucosa, they have a predilection for sites subjected to pressure or trauma, particularly the extensor surfaces of the arms, legs, and buttocks. Papuloeruptive xanthomas are almost always associated with hypertriglyceridemia (often to levels of >3000 mg/dL). They can result from deficiency of lipoprotein lipase activity (as in patients with lipoprotein lipase deficiency (type I hyperlipoproteinemia), dysfunctional apolipoprotein C-II, or impaired insulin activity), or from overproduction by the liver of triglyceride-rich lipoproteins (as in endogenous familial hypertriglyceridemia (type IV hyperlipoproteinemia) or the elevations of both chylomicrons and VLDLs of type V hyperlipoproteinemia). Environmental factors and underlying diseases can also significantly elevate triglyceride levels. Among these are obesity, alcohol abuse, diabetes mellitus, nephrotic syndrome, and therapy with estrogens or retinoids (Table 24.6). The mechanism for retinoid-induced hypertriglyceridemia is by elevation of hepatic VLDL production.

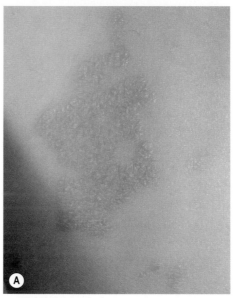

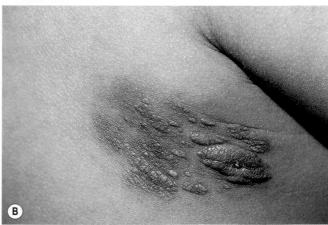

Figure 24.9 Xanthomas in hyperlipidemia. Plane xanthomas with somewhat different appearances in a boy (A) and an unrelated girl (B) with homozygous type II hyperlipoproteinemia.

Tendinous xanthomas

Tendinous xanthomas are skin-colored or yellowish, smooth, freely movable subcutaneous nodules and tumors. They have a predilection for the extensor tendons of the elbows, knees, heels (Fig.

Table 24.5 Clinical findings in disorders of lipids

Disorder	Xanthomas	Cardiovascular	Gastrointestinal	Neurologic	Ophthalmologic	Other findings
Type I HL	Eruptive Tendinous Xanthelasmas	None	Acute abdomen Hepatosplenomegaly Pancreatitis	None	Lipemia retinalis	Diabetes Lipemic plasma
Type II HL	Planar, esp. intertriginous Tendinous Tuberous	Generalized atherosclerosis	None	None	Arcus cornea	None
Type III HL	Planar, esp. palmar Tuberous	Atherosclerosis	None	None	None	Abnormal glucose tolerance Hyperuricemia
Type IV HL	Eruptive Tuberous	Atherosclerosis	Acute abdomen Hepatosplenomegaly Pancreatitis	None	Lipemia retinalis	Obesity
Type V HL	Eruptive Tuberous	Atherosclerosis	Acute abdomen Hepatosplenomegaly Pancreatitis	None	Lipemia retinalis	Obesity Hyperinsulinemia
Tangier	Macular rash; foam cells in biopsies	Atherosclerosis	Acute abdomen; hepatosplenomegaly	Peripheral neuropathy	Corneal infiltration	Enlarged orange tonsils; lymphadenopathy
Apolipoprotein A–I and C–III deficiency	Planar and tendon xanthomas; foam cells in biopsies	Atherosclerosis	Normal	Normal	Corneal clouding	None
HDL deficiency with planar xanthomas	Planar xanthomas; foam cells in biopsies	Atherosclerosis	Hepatomegaly	Normal	Corneal opacity	None

HL, hyperlipoproteinemia.

Table 24.6 Potential causes of secondary hyperlipidemia in pediatric patients

Endocrine
  Anorexia nervosa
  Diabetes mellitus
  Hypopituitarism
  Hypothyroidism
  Lipodystrophy
  Pregnancy

Hepatic
  Cholestasis
    Biliary atresia
    Biliary cirrhosis
  Hepatitis

Renal
  Chronic renal failure
  Hemolytic-uremic syndrome
  Nephrotic syndrome

Storage disease
  Cystine storage disease
  Gaucher disease
  Glycogen storage disease
  Neimann–Pick disease
  Tay–Sachs disease

Medications
  Alcohol
  Anabolic steroids
  Highly active antiretroviral therapy
  Oral contraceptives
  Corticosteroids
  Retinoids

Others
  Burns
  Klinefelter syndrome
  Progeria
  Werner syndrome

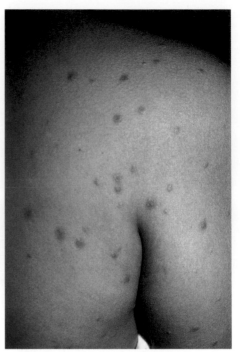

Figure 24.10 Xanthomas in hyperlipidemia. Eruptive xanthomas in a boy with nephritic syndrome. More commonly eruptive xanthomas are grouped. Biopsy confirmed the diagnosis of xanthoma.

24.11), hands, and feet. These non-tender, firm nodules measure 1 cm or more in diameter. They usually are seen or palpated on the Achilles tendon and the tendons on the dorsal aspect of the hands. They are most commonly seen in either heterozygotes or homozygotes with familial hypercholesterolemia (type II hyperlipidemia), but may also be seen in individuals with familial defective apolipoprotein B-100, cerebrotendinous xanthomatosis, and sitosterolemia.

Tuberous (tuberoeruptive) xanthomas

Tuberous (tuberoeruptive) xanthomas are large, firm, nodular, sessile or pedunculated, flesh-colored or yellowish to red xanthomas (Fig. 24.12). They occur on the palms and extensor surfaces subject to stress or trauma, particularly the elbows, knees, hands, and buttocks. Located in the dermis and subcutaneous layers, they can enlarge to 5 cm or more in diameter and, in contrast to tendon xanthomas, are not attached to underlying structures. These lesions are found in patients with hypercholesterolemia, particularly with familial hypercholesterolemia (type II hyperlipoproteinemia), hepatic cholestasis, or dysbetalipoproteinemia (type III hyperlipoproteinemia). Some 80% of individuals with dysbetalipoproteinemia have tuberous xanthomas. Tuberous xanthomas are also found in sitosterolemia (see below).[70]

Other xanthomas

Other xanthomas, not part of the hyperlipoproteinemia spectrum, include *xanthoma disseminatum*, an uncommon clinical entity characterized by red-yellow or mahogany-colored papular and nodular lesions with a predilection for the flexural creases (see Ch. 10), and *verruciform xanthomas*, a rare disorder manifested by solitary 0.2–2.0-cm verrucous papillary or flat to lichenoid, gray to reddish-pink, sessile, occasionally pedunculated lesions most commonly seen on the oral mucosa and lips and occasionally on the penis, scrotum, vulva, groin, digits, nostrils, and areas of epidermal hyperplasia such as in CHILD syndrome (see Ch. 5) or epidermolysis bullosa (see Ch. 13).

The five major types of hyperlipoproteinemias are summarized in Tables 24.4 and 24.5. *Type I hyperlipoproteinemia* (*Bürger–Grütz disease, familial lipoprotein lipase deficiency, familial hyperchylomicronemia syndrome*) is usually discovered accidentally because of lactescence (manifested by a creamy or chocolate appearance of whole blood) in a child with bouts of abdominal pain, which may be caused by lipid accumulations in the liver and spleen, splenic infarct, or pancreatitis. The risk of atherosclerosis is not increased in this form. About two-thirds of children with type I disease have eruptive xanthomas, primarily localized to the buttocks, shoulders and extensor surfaces of the extremities.[71] Eruptive xanthomas occur when the serum triglyceride level exceeds ~2000 mg/dL. The disorder results from LPL or apolipoprotein C-II deficiency, or due to the presence of an LPL inhibitor. Increased levels of chylomicrons can also be found in familial hypertriglyceridemia or in patients with diabetes, hypothyroidism, or therapy with retinoids, glucocorticoids or estrogens.

Type II hyperlipoproteinemia (*familial hypercholesterolemia*) is the most common and best understood disorder of the lipoprotein disorders in pediatric patients.[72,73] Heterozygotes (1:200–1:500 individuals) have plasma concentrations of total cholesterol and

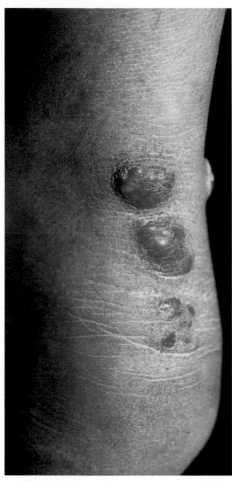

Figure 24.11 Xanthomas in hyperlipidemia. Tendinous xanthomas in adolescent with type II hyperlipoproteinemia.

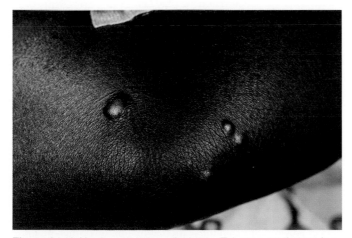

Figure 24.12 Xanthomas in hyperlipidemia. Tuberous xanthomas in a boy with biliary atresia.

LDL cholesterol that are increased by two- to three-fold.[74] Homozygotes have levels five to six times normal values from birth to early childhood. Children with homozygous disease may have planar xanthomas at birth or by the first decade (including intertriginous xanthomas), and tendon and tuberous xanthomas by 15 years of age.[75,76] Rarely, tuberous xanthomas are the first manifestation.[77] Arcus cornea (lipid deposits around the edge of the cornea), angina pectoris and myocardial infarction often present during the second decade. Carotid plaque has been noted as early as 4 years of age[78] and coronary artery bypass or aortic valve replacement may be required during childhood.[79–81] Ten to 15% of heterozygous individuals develop tendon xanthomas during the second decade of life, particularly involving the Achilles tendon and the extensor tendons of the hands, but only rarely show angina pectoris during late teenage years. Approximately 5% of families have a mutation in ApoB-100 (Table 24.3), and lack tendon xanthomas.

Type III hyperlipoproteinemia (dysbetalipoproteinemia; broad beta disease) is usually first diagnosed in adulthood. Most affected individuals are homozygotes for the ApoE2 allele, which is seen in 1 : 100 individuals; clinical expression is thought to be triggered by environmental factors, such as hormonal abnormalities, obesity, or medications, since only 1 : 2000 individuals are known to have the disorder. Some 75% of patients have plane xanthomas of the palms and/or tuberous xanthomas. *Type IV disease (endogenous familial hypertriglyceridemia)* is usually not seen before the age of 20 years, although it may appear in children with renal disease or in diabetics who have become ketotic. *Type V disease (familial hyperchylomicronemia with hyperprebetalipoproteinemia or occasionally ApoC-II deficiency)* occasionally presents in preadolescent children. Patients are usually obese and present with acute abdominal pain. Eruptive xanthomas are most common. Diabetes, glycogen storage disease, ingestion of contraceptives, and alcohol abuse may trigger manifestations.

Treatment of hyperlipidemias is type-specific, but may include dietary modification, statins (HMG-CoA reductase inhibitors), cholesterol lowering agents (nicotinamide, cholestyramine, fibrates), and/or ezetimibe (selectively inhibits the absorption of cholesterol). Successful therapy can lead to dramatic shrinkage or clearance of xanthomas.

Alagille Disease

Hyperlipidemia with hypercholesterolemia and xanthomas is also a feature of *Alagille syndrome (arteriohepatic dysplasia, Watson–Alagille syndrome)*,[82,83] an autosomal dominant disorder caused by mutations in Jagged 1, which encodes a ligand for the Notch receptor and is critical for determination of cell fates in early development.[84] The most characteristic feature is congenital intrahepatic biliary hypoplasia with cholestasis and pruritus. Most patients show an unusual facies with a prominent forehead, hypertelorism, eyes deeply set in orbits, atrophy of the iris, a pointed, bulbous, or saddle-shaped nose, and a sharply pointed chin, even in relatives without other features.[85] Other features may include vertebral anomalies, cardiovascular disease (generally pulmonic stenosis or aneurysms), renal abnormalities, hypogonadism, and physical and mental retardation.[86] The xanthomas have been described in approximately 30% of affected children, may appear as early as the first year of life, and are associated with high cholesterol levels.[83] The xanthomas are most often tuberous and often widespread, especially over extensor surfaces and fold areas. They may form confluent plaques, especially on the elbows and knees. Secondary eczematization is not uncommon, given the intense pruritus from cholestasis. A porphyria cutanea tarda-like photosensitivity has rarely been described.[87] Death prior to 5 years of age due to cardiac failure, renal failure, or both has occurred, but the prognosis of children with Alagille syndrome is generally better than that of patients with congenital biliary atresia, in whom survival to 2 years of age is unusual. Transplantation and other means to lower cholesterol result in clearance of the xanthomas.[83]

Sitosterolemia

Individuals with this autosomal recessive disorder have markedly elevated plasma levels of plant sterols and often have increased cholesterol levels owing to mutations in two adjacent sterol ATP-binding cassette transporters, *ABCG5* (encoding sterolin-1) or *ABCG8* (encoding sterolin-2).[88] These proteins are thought to prevent dietary non-cholesterol sterols from being retained by the body and for cholesterol excretion into bile. Affected children show tuberous and tendinous xanthomas during the first decade of life, as well as arthritis, premature vascular disease with a high risk of fatal cardiac events during teenage years, and sometimes hemolysis and thrombocytopenia.[70,89,90] Treatment with ezetimibe, which inhibits cholesterol absorption, reduces the plasma concentrations of plant sterols in patients.[91] The combination of ezetimibe and cholestyramine has also been used successfully to clear the xanthomas.[92,93]

Cerebrotendinous Xanthomatosis

Cerebrotendinous xanthomatosis is an autosomal recessive disorder caused by mutations in CYP27A1 (sterol 27-hydroxylase).[94] As a result, large amounts of cholestanol, the 5-α-dihydro derivative of cholesterol, accumulate in virtually every tissue, leading to tendinous xanthomas, juvenile cataracts, diarrhea, and atherosclerosis.[95] Neurologic signs include dementia, psychiatric disturbances, seizures, progressive paresthesias, retardation, and cerebellar problems.[96] Replacement therapy with chenodeoxycholic acid (750 mg/day) reduces cholestanol synthesis and concentrations. If started early enough (the neurologic manifestations can be seen during infancy), therapy improves neurologic function and clears the xanthomas.[94]

Deficiencies in HDL

Low levels of HDL cholesterol are most commonly seen in disorders of triglyceride metabolism, but may occur in the presence of otherwise normal levels of lipids and be associated with xanthomas. These disorders are Tangier disease, apolipoprotein A-I and C-III deficiency, and HDL deficiency with planar xanthomas (with decreased levels of ApoC-III).

Tangier Disease

Tangier disease (familial high-density lipoprotein deficiency) is an autosomal recessive disorder characterized by hypocholesterolemia (50–125 mg/dL), an almost complete absence of plasma HDL, and massive deposition of cholesterol esters in tissues. The disorder results from homozygous mutations in the ATP-binding cassette (ABC1) transport protein, which mediates the efflux of cellular cholesterol to the HDL particle in plasma for transport to the liver.[97,98] Triglyceride levels may be normal or slightly elevated (150–250 mg/dL) and plasma ApoA-I levels are <3% of normal. The disorder frequently manifests during childhood. The tonsils are enlarged and show distinctive alternating bands of red, orange, or yellowish white striations overlying the normal red mucosa. Lipid deposits in the skin and other organs may be accompanied by a persistent maculopapular eruption over the trunk and abdomen, hepatosplenomegaly, lymph node enlargement, infiltration of the cornea in adults, and alterations in the intestinal and rectal mucosa. Several patients have had recurrent peripheral neuropathy.

The mucopolysaccharidoses

The mucopolysaccharidoses are inherited disorders of lysosomal hydrolases that catabolize glycosaminoglycans (GAG), sulfated components of connective tissue.[99] As a result, dermatan sulfate, heparin sulfate, and/or keratan sulfate accumulate within cells and are excreted in excess amounts in the urine. First described by Hunter in 1917 (and labeled 'gargoylism' in 1936), these disorders can now be divided into at least seven subtypes that share clinical features, mode of inheritance, and nature of the accumulated mucopolysaccharide. Affected individuals are normal in appearance at birth but, as with all lysosomal storage disorders, progressively show features with advancing age, beginning during infancy. Patients with any of the mucopolysaccharidoses can show hypertrichosis, especially over the back and extremities, and thickened, roughened, taut inelastic skin, especially over the fingers due to the accumulation of GAG. Only individuals with Hunter syndrome (MPS type II or iduronate-2-sulfatase deficiency) have specific cutaneous features (papulonodules), although extensive, persistent Mongolian spots have rarely been described in children with Hunter[100] and Hurler[101,102] syndromes.

The disorders tend to present because of dysmorphic features or psychological and learning difficulties, or as severe bony dysplasia. Considerable heterogeneity within subgroups has been described. Urinary screening tests for GAG should be followed by specific enzyme assays. Hunter syndrome (MPS II) is an X-linked recessive disorder; all others are autosomal recessive. Hurler syndrome, or MPS I, is presented as the prototype mucopolysaccharidosis; Hunter syndrome is also discussed in detail because it is the one form of mucopolysaccharidosis that shows a distinctive cutaneous feature, dermal papules and nodules. Table 24.7 summarizes the clinical and biochemical features of all of the mucopolysaccharidoses.

Hurler syndrome

Hurler syndrome (mucopolysaccharidosis I-H, MPS I in McKusick's original classification) is the most common of this group of disorders.[103,104] Seen in approximately 1 in 100 000 births, it appears in the first year of life. MPS I is a particularly grave disorder, with death occurring in almost all cases before the age of 10 years, usually from cardiac failure or respiratory infection.

Patients are usually diagnosed toward the end of the first year of life because of their facial features. Many have umbilical and inguinal hernias at presentation and recurrent respiratory infections prior to diagnosis. Cardinal features of the Hurler syndrome include coarsening of facial features (Fig. 24.13); macrocephaly with frontal bulging; premature closure of the sutures with hyperostosis, frequently leading to a scaphocephalic skull; flattened nasal bridge with a saddle-shaped appearance; hypertelorism; protuberant tongue; short neck; protuberant abdomen due to hepatic and splenic enlargement; deformity of the chest; shortness of the spine; laxity of the abdominal wall with inguinal and umbilical hernias; broad hands with stubby fingers; a claw hand due to stiffening of the phalangeal joints (Fig. 24.14); limitation of extensibility of the joints; severe, progressive mental retardation; and marked retardation of growth. Although most affected infants are normal or above normal in length during the first year of life, the growth rate starts to decrease by 2 years of age. By age 3, almost all patients are below the third percentile for stature. Clouding of the cornea develops in all patients with Hurler syndrome, and is best seen by side-lighting of the cornea; if severe visual loss occurs, however, it is usually related to retinal involvement. Deafness is almost always a feature, and cardiac involvement may range from severe early life-threatening cardiomyopathy to progressive valve disease. Approximately 40% of affected individuals have hydrocephalus, and a large head

Table 24.7 The mucopolysaccharidoses (MPS)

Disorder	Inheritance	Enzyme	Storage	Clinical features
MPS I-H Hurler	AR	α-Iduronidase	DS, HS	Severe retardation, corneal clouding, hepatosplenomegaly, chondrodystrophic dwarfism, generalized Mongolian spots; early death.
MPS I-S Scheie	AR			Bone and joint involvement, retinopathy, corneal clouding, sometimes cardiac abnormalities. Normal intelligence.
MPS II Hunter	X-LR	Iduronate 2-sulfatase	DS, HS	Cutaneous papules and nodules on scapula, posterior axillae, thigh, buttocks, atypical retinitis pigmentosa. Normal cornea.
MPS III Sanfilippo	AR	Several subtypes[a]	HS	Aggressive behavior, severe neurologic involvement, mild somatic changes.
MPS IV Morquio	AR	A: Galactose-6-sulfatase B: β-galactosidase	KS	Striking dwarfism but not dysmorphic, corneal opacity, severe osteoporosis, extreme short stature, atlantoaxial dislocation leads to chronic cervical myelopathy and progressive paresis. Restrictive respiratory disease usually leads to death. Normal intelligence.
MPS VI Maroteaux-Lamy	AR	Galactosamine-4-sulfatase	DS	Dwarfism, severe corneal, and bony lesions. Cardiac involvement, respiratory obstruction. Normal intelligence.
MPS VII Sly	AR	β-glucuronidase	HS, DS	Often born with hydrops fetalis. Severe Hurler-like phenotype if survive.
MPS IX	AR	Hyaluronidase	HA	One patient. Short stature, periarticular soft tissue masses.

[a]A: heparan N-sulfatase; B: N-acetylglucosaminidase; C: acetyl-CoA:glucosamine N-acetyltransferase; D: N-acetylglucosamine-6-sulfatase.
AR, autosomal recessive; DS, dermatan sulfate; HA, hyaluronic acid; HS, heparan sulfate; KS, keratan sulfate; X-LR, X-linked recessive.

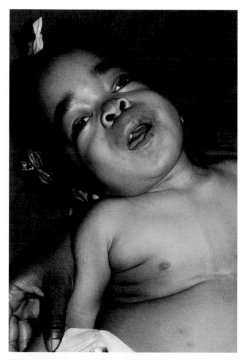

Figure 24.13 Hurler syndrome. Coarse facial features, macrocephaly, scaphocephalic skull, flattened nasal bridge, hypertelorism, short neck, chest deformity, and protuberant abdomen in a girl with Hurler syndrome (mucopolysaccharidosis I).

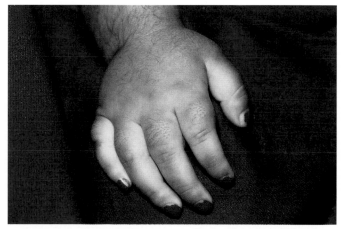

Figure 24.14 Hurler syndrome. Broad hands with stubby fingers and limited joint extension. Note the hypertrichosis.

circumference, even without hydrocephalus, is often noted. Dysplasia of the odontoid process increases the risk of atlantoaxial subluxation and acute spinal cord damage. Upper respiratory tract obstruction and sleep apnea related to the large tongue and midfacial hypoplasia may require corrective surgery. MPS I is the most common metabolic disorder associated with generalized Mongolian spots during the first decade of life.[101,105]

There is a wide range of heterogeneity in severity and manifestations of Hurler syndrome. At the other end of the spectrum is Scheie syndrome (MPS I-S, formerly MPS V), which also results from mutations in the gene encoding (alpha)-L-iduronidase. Patients with Scheie syndrome have normal intelligence and may have a normal lifespan, with predominantly bone and joint problems. Carpal tunnel syndrome occurs commonly and corneal transplantation may be considered for corneal clouding (assuming lack of concurrent retinopathy as a cause of visual loss). Cardiac valvular insufficiency may develop and require surgery.

Hunter syndrome

Hunter syndrome (mucopolysaccharidosis II, MPS II) is distinguished from Hurler syndrome by an X-linked recessive inheritance, longer survival, lack of corneal clouding, the characteristic papulonodules, and the different biochemical defect. Mental retardation progresses at a slower rate and humping of the lumbar area (gibbus) does not occur. Progressive deafness is a feature of 50% of patients, which can impair speech development. A mild form of MPS II (type IIB) may show only mild skeletal abnormalities, and skin lesions may be the presenting feature.[106]

The distinctive cutaneous changes are found in the minority of affected boys. They consist of firm flesh-colored to ivory-white papules and nodules that often coalesce to form ridges or a reticular pattern in symmetrical areas between the angles of the scapulae and posterior axillary lines, the pectoral ridges, the nape of the neck, buttocks (Fig. 24.15), and/or the lateral aspects of the upper arms and thighs. They appear before age 10 and can spontaneously disappear.

Palliative therapy for the hydrocephalus and joint stiffness and pain are appropriate, but surgical correction of the skeletal or cardiac abnormalities is not, given the limited life expectancy. Hematopoietic stem cell transplantation have been beneficial for some patients with MPS I-H, especially when used before 18 months of age, and in some individuals with MPS H.[107,108] Organomegaly and cardiomyopathy may resolve, and neurocognitive

Table 24.8 Other storage disorders with cutaneous manifestations during childhood

Disorder	Inheritance	Enzyme	Cutaneous features	Clinical features
Aspartylglycosaminuria	AR	Aspartylglycosaminidase	Angiokeratomas	Speech delay, otitis media, behavioral change resembling MPS III
Fabry	X-LR	α-Galactosidase	Angiokeratomas, hypohidrosis	Acroparesthesias, progressive renal disease (see Ch. 12)
Farber lipogranulomatosis	AR	Ceramidase	Painful subcutaneous nodules, especially over joints	Hydrops fetalis, chronic pulmonary disease with granulomatous infiltration of the lungs, hepatosplenomegaly neurodegeneration; granulomatous infiltration of the mucosae with hoarse cry, recurrent vomiting, dysphagia
Fucosidosis	AR	α-Fucosidase	Angiokeratomas, sweating abnormalities, purple nail bands	Neurodegeneration, dysostosis, respiratory infections, hepatosplenomegaly, growth retardation, resembles MPS (see Ch. 12)
Galactosialidosis	AR	Defective protective protein/cathepsin A; proteolysis of both β-galactosidase and neuraminidase	Angiokeratomas	Hydrops fetalis, skeletal abnormalities, myoclonus, cherry-red macular spots, ataxia, mild mental retardation
Gaucher, type II	AR	β-Glucocerebrosidase	Collodion baby	Severe neurologic involvement, marked hepatosplenomegaly (see Ch. 5)
GM1 gangliosidosis	AR	β-Galactosidase	Angiokeratomas, extensive Mongolian spots	Dysostosis multiplex, hepatosplenomegaly, early neurologic degeneration, corneal clouding
Mannosidosis	AR	α-Mannosidase	Angiokeratomas	Middle ear and respiratory infections; may have mild learning difficulties to severe MPS I-like phenotype and seizures
Multiple sulfatase deficiency	AR	Post-translational processing of multiple sulfatases	Ichthyosis (recessive X-linked)	Hepatosplenomegaly, dysostosis, progressive neurologic deterioration (see Ch. 5)
Mucolipidosis I (sialidosis type II)	AR	Neuraminidase I	Angiokeratomas	MPS I phenotype; dysostoses multiplex, progressive retardation
Mucolipidosis II (I-cell disease)	AR	Transferase[a]	Malar telangiectasia, puffy eyelids, prominent periorbital veins; thick, rigid skin	MPS I phenotype; gingival hypertrophy, dysostosis multiplex, stiff joints, respiratory tract infections, cardiac failure
Salla disease (infantile sialic acid storage)	AR	Sialic acid transporter	Hypopigmentation	Hydrops fetalis, recurrent infections, failure to thrive, dysostosis multiplex, cardiac disease, coarse facies, learning disabilities
Schindler	AR	α-N-Acetylgalactosaminidase	Angiokeratomas	Variable; may have myoclonus, spasticity, progressive dementia

AR, autosomal recessive; X-LR, X-linked recessive; MPS, mucopolysaccharidosis.

[a]UDP-N-acetylglucosamine:lysosomal enzyme N-acetylglucosaminyl-1-phosphotransferase.

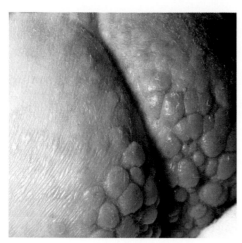

Figure 24.15 Hunter syndrome. Distinctive, firm, flesh-colored papules and nodules on the buttocks (a cutaneous marker of Hunter syndrome or MPS II).

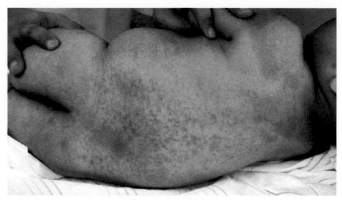

Figure 24.16 GM1 gangliosidosis. Extensive Mongolian spots in an infant with GM1 gangliosidosis (Courtesy of Denise Metry, MD; Reprinted with permission from Archives of Dermatology.[56])

development progresses nicely after transplantation. Although the coarse facies and long bones grow better, the vertebral bodies are not improved, and marked spinal deformity can develop. Enzyme replacement therapy (ERT) with α-L-iduronidase (laronidase) has resulted in significant improvement in respiratory obstruction, hepatomegaly, and joint mobility in patients with MPS I.[103,109] ERT with idursulfase, recombinant lysosomal iduronate-2-sulfatase, has also been noted to improve the skin texture, as well as the hepatosplenomegaly, bronchitis and physical activity of Hunter syndrome.[110] However, ERT cannot pass the blood-brain barrier to improve neurocognitive function.[109,111–113] The combination of ERT and transplantation may benefit patients with more severe manifestations.[103]

Other storage disorders

Several other storage disorders may show cutaneous features, most commonly angiokeratoma. Among these are the mucolipidoses (sialidosis II or mucolipidosis I and mucolipidosis II), the sphingolipidoses (Fabry disease, Farber lipogranulomatosis, Gaucher disease, GM1 gangliosidosis Fig. 24.16), and multiple sulfatase deficiency), and other storage disorders of carbohydrate metabolism (aspartylglycosaminuria, fucosidosis, galactosialidosis, α-mannosidosis, Salla disease, and Schindler disease).[114–120] The features of these storage disorders, their cutaneous manifestation(s), and their underlying causes are summarized in Table 24.8. (Fabry disease and fucosidosis are discussed in more detail in Chapter 12.)

The neonatal form of Gaucher disease, type II, may present as a collodion baby, whereas multiple sulfatase deficiency (mucosulfatidosis) is phenotypically identical to recessive X-linked ichthyosis (see Ch. 5). All of these conditions are inherited in an autosomal recessive fashion, except for Fabry disease, which is X-linked recessive.

Key References

 The complete list of 120 references for this chapter is available online at: **www.expertconsult.com.**
See inside cover for registration details.

Ashrafi MR, Shabanian R, Mohammadi M, et al. Extensive Mongolian spots: a clinical sign merits special attention. *Pediatr Neurol.* 2006; 34:143–145.

Choh SA, Choh NA, Rasool A, et al. Homozygous familial hypercholesterolemia. *J Pediatr Endocrinol Metab.* 2009;22:573–575.

Gehrig KA, Dinulos JG. Acrodermatitis due to nutritional deficiency. *Curr Opin Pediatr.* 2010;22:107–112.

Heath ML, Sidbury R. Cutaneous manifestations of nutritional deficiency. *Curr Opin Pediatr.* 2006;18:417–422.

Muenzer J, Wraith JE, Clarke LA. Mucopolysaccharidosis I: management and treatment guidelines. *Pediatrics.* 2009;123:19–29.

O'Regan GM, Canny G, Irvine AD. 'Peeling paint' dermatitis as a presenting sign of cystic fibrosis. *J Cyst Fibros.* 2006;5:257–259.

Ozturk Y. Acrodermatitis enteropathica-like syndrome secondary to branched-chain amino acid deficiency in inborn errors of metabolism. *Pediatr Dermatol.* 2008;25:415.

Seyhan M, Erdem T, Selimoglu MA, et al. Dermatological signs in Wilson's disease. *Pediatr Int.* 2009;51:395–398.

25 Skin Signs of Other Systemic Diseases

Primary immunodeficiency disorders

Recurrent infections, including those involving the skin, raise the possibility that a child has an immune deficiency. The most common cause of immunodeficiency in children is acquired immunodeficiency because of HIV infection (see Ch. 15). Less frequently, children with evidence of an immunodeficiency have an inherited disorder.[1-5] Genetic immunodeficiency disorders may show a variety of cutaneous abnormalities, some of which are unique and characteristic of the disorder and others, such as dermatitis, are shared by other immunodeficiencies and other disorders.

Some of these immunodeficiencies are discussed elsewhere because of their manifestations. Wiskott–Aldrich syndrome and hyperimmunoglobulinemia E syndrome are discussed in Chapter 3, owing to the frequent presence of dermatitis. Chediak–Higashi and Griscelli syndromes, the silvery hair syndromes associated with immunodeficiency, are reviewed in Chapter 11 with the disorders of pigmentation. The telangiectasias that allow ataxia-telangiectasia to be distinguished from other forms of ataxia, are described in Chapter 12. Complement deficiencies are mentioned in Chapter 14 because individuals with a deficiency of a late complement component have an increased risk of neisserial infection, in Chapter 20 because hereditary angioedema (HAE) can be confused with angioedema, and in Chapter 22 because deficiency of the early components of complement may lead to a lupus-like disorder. Given its characteristic recurrent and recalcitrant candidal infections, chronic mucocutaneous candidiasis is reviewed in Chapter 17.

Signs that should raise the suspicion of acquired or hereditary immunodeficiency are listed in Table 25.1. Screening laboratory tests for a patient with recurrent cutaneous infections suspected of having an immunodeficiency are suggested in Table 25.2.

Immunoglobulin Deficiencies

Children with deficiencies of immunoglobulins primarily manifest bacterial infections beginning at 3–6 months of age as the transplacentally derived maternal immunoglobulins wane.[6,7] In general, the treatment of hypogammaglobulinemia is antibody replacement by intravenous infusions of immune serum globulin and vigorous antibiotic therapy.[8]

The most common immunoglobulin deficiency is *selective IgA deficiency*, found in 1 in 500 individuals, of which 10–15% show clinical manifestations. About 5% of patients with IgA deficiency have mutations in *TACI*, which encodes a TNF receptor family member. B cells in individuals with *TACI* mutations have impaired isotype switching and do not produce IgA and often IgG in response to TACI ligand. The most common features are sinopulmonary bacterial infections and *Giardia* gastroenteritis. Approximately one-third of patients with clinical manifestations develop autoimmune disorders, some of which involve the skin. These include an atopic-like dermatitis, lupus erythematosus, vitiligo, recurrent candidal infections, lipodystrophy, and idiopathic thrombocytopenic purpura. Other manifestations of allergy, including asthma, cow's milk allergy, and allergic rhinoconjunctivitis, are frequently described. In addition to their decreased levels of IgA, almost half of the affected individuals also have serum anti-IgA antibodies. Because of this high frequency of anti-IgA antibodies, immune serum globulin or blood products with IgA-bearing lymphocytes are contraindicated to prevent fatal anaphylactic reactions.

IgA deficiency may transition into (and is seen with increased frequency in families with) *combined variable immunodeficiency (CVID)*,[9] a heterogeneous group of disorders with decreased immunoglobulin levels (IgG, IgA and sometimes IgM) and variable functional T cell abnormalities.[10-13] Patients with CVID most commonly show pyodermas, extensive warts, widespread dermatophyte infections, and dermatitis. They are predisposed to pyogenic infections of the upper and lower respiratory tract, as well as gastrointestinal infections, particularly due to *Giardia*. Non-caseating granulomas of the lungs, liver, spleen, and/or skin have been described and are not associated with microorganisms. Individuals with CVID have an increased risk of autoimmune diseases, including vitiligo (Fig. 25.1), alopecia areata, and vasculitis. The incidence of lymphoma is increased 400-fold, and of cancer overall 8- to 13-fold. CVID is primarily a disorder of adults, with the mean age of onset 23–28 years; however, 25% of cases are diagnosed before 21 years of age, with a peak incidence in children aged 5–10 years and a minimum age of 4 years used to exclude patients with other primary immunodeficiency disorders.[14] Death in patients with CVID usually results from infection, respiratory insufficiency, or neoplasia.

Most cases of panhypogammaglobulinemia in children represent *X-linked hypogammaglobulinemia* (also called X-linked agammaglobulinemia), a disorder due to mutations in *Btk*, which encodes a tyrosine kinase that regulates the conversion of pre-B cells to B cells that are able to differentiate and produce immunoglobulins.[15] Less commonly pediatric patients may have a transient form during infancy with early failure to thrive, protracted diarrhea, sinopulmonary infections, pyodermas, and cutaneous abscesses, but with reversal when immunoglobulin is produced at 18–30 months of age. Approximately 10% have an autosomal recessive form of panhypogammaglobulinemia.

Boys with X-linked hypogammaglobulinemia develop recurrent bacterial infections in the first year of life and have an increased susceptibility to hepatitis B and enteroviral infections. Furuncles and cellulitis are the most common infections. An atopic-like dermatitis is common, and noninfectious cutaneous granulomas have been described. There is an increased predisposition to the development of pyoderma gangrenosum, which has been recently linked to Warthin–Starry positive *Helicobacter bilis* infection; although difficult to grow, the *Helicobacter* organisms are detectable by PCR and electrospray ionization time-of-flight mass spectrometry.[16] A small percentage of patients develop a dermatomyositis-like disorder with

Table 25.1 Signs of immunodeficiency

History of infections
    Increased frequency, severity and duration
    Unusual manifestations
    Unusual infecting agents
    Chronic infections, incomplete clearing
    Poor response to appropriate agents
    Severe viral infections
    Recurrent osteomyelitis

Failure to thrive

Diarrhea, vomiting, malabsorption

Clues to specific types of immunodeficiency
    Hematologic abnormalities (e.g., Wiskott–Aldrich syndrome)
    Arthritis (e.g., Wiskott-Aldrich syndrome or early complement deficiency)
    Paucity of lymph nodes (e.g., SCID), or lymphadenopathy (e.g., CGD)
    Hepatosplenomegaly (e.g., CGD, Omenn syndrome, or Wiskott–Aldrich syndrome)
    Poor wound healing (e.g., leukocyte adhesion deficiency)
    Silvery hair (e.g., Chediak–Higashi or Griscelli syndromes)

CGD, chronic granulomatous disease; SCID, severe combined immunodeficiency.

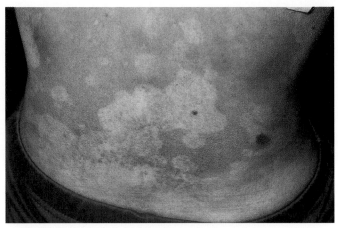

Figure 25.1 Common variable immunodeficiency (CVID). Individuals with CVID or IgA deficiency have an increased incidence of autoimmune disorders, as evidenced in this adolescent with CVID and vitiligo.

Table 25.2 Screening laboratory testing for the child with recurrent infections

Test	Primary immunodeficiency
Complete blood count with differential, platelet count and examination of smear	Giant leukocyte granules (Chédiak–Higashi) Thrombocytopenia (Wiskott–Aldrich) Leukocytosis (chronic granulomatous disease and leukocyte adhesion deficiency)
Quantitative immunoglobulins	Selective IgA deficiency Transient hypogammaglobulinemia X-linked hypogammaglobulinemia Hypogammaglobulinemia with hyper-IgM Common variable immunodeficiency Wiskott-Aldrich syndrome Hyperimmunoglobulin E
Flow cytometry (T and B cells)	Severe combined immunodeficiency Leukocyte adhesion defect (CD18 deficiency) Chronic granulomatous disease

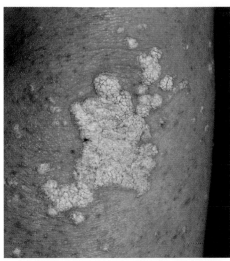

Figure 25.2 Hyperimmunoglobulinemia (HIM) syndrome. Extensive warts are a frequently observed cutaneous manifestation of boys with this form of immunodeficiency.

slowly progressive neurologic involvement, usually related to echoviral meningoencephalitis. Up to 6% of patients develop lymphomas.

Patients with *X-linked hypogammaglobulinemia with hyper-IgM* (HIM) syndrome tend to have deficiencies of IgA, IgE, and IgG with neutropenia, but increased levels of IgM and isohemagglutinins.[17] Rather than a primary B-cell defect, affected individuals have a primary T-cell defect. Cross-linking of CD40 on B cells induces switching of immunoglobulin classes from IgM to IgG, IgA, or IgE. Mutations in X-linked HIM lead to a dysfunction of the ligand for CD40 (CD40L). B cells from patients with HIM express functional CD40, but the T cells express the defective CD40 ligand and cannot bind CD40.[18,19] Three other forms of HIM are autosomal recessive;

these result from mutations in: (1) deficiency of CD40 itself; (2) activation-induced cytidine deaminase (AICD), or (3) uracil-N-glycosylase (UNG),[20] the latter two being signaling components downstream of the CD40 receptor that are critical to B-cell differentiation and class switching. A rare form of X-linked immunodeficiency, sometimes associated with hyper-IgM, is associated with hypohidrotic ectodermal dysplasia (see Ch. 7), and has been linked to mutations in the *NEMO* gene, the same gene that is mutated in incontinentia pigmenti (see Ch. 11). Patients with HIM often present during infancy with pyodermas, bacterial sinopulmonary, and gastrointestinal infections; hepatosplenomegaly cervical adenitis, autoimmune disorders (especially thyroiditis, and hemolytic anemia),[21] and an increased risk of lymphoma. Numerous, widespread warts (Fig. 25.2), and oral and perianal area ulcerations are additional features.[22] Extensive warts are also a feature of WHIM syndrome (warts, hypogammaglobulinemia, infections, and myelokathexis), which results from mutations in the chemokine receptor CXCR4.[23]

X-linked lymphoproliferative disease is characterized by an abnormal response to Epstein-Barr virus infection due to mutations in

SH2DIA, which encodes SAP (signaling lymphocytic activation molecule (SLAM)-associated protein), a critical protein for cytotoxic T-cell function.[24,25] Affected boys are healthy until they first develop infectious mononucleosis during childhood or adolescence. Fever, pharyngitis, maculopapular rash, lymphadenopathy hepatosplenomegaly, purpura, and jaundice are the typical features. The virus stimulates a rapidly progressive B-cell lymphoma, often with superimposed bacterial sepsis, which leads to death in 70% of affected boys.

Chronic Granulomatous Disease

Chronic granulomatous disease (CGD) is a group of disorders characterized by severe recurrent infections due to an inability of phagocytic leukocytes to generate oxidative metabolites and activate neutrophil granule elastase and cathepsin G, thus blocking the killing of intracellular bacteria and fungi.[26,27] In all forms of CGD the function of the nicotinamide dinucleotide phosphate (NADPH) oxidase complex is reduced. Affecting boys in 90% of cases, the disorder usually presents with recurrent pneumonias, hepatosplenomegaly, and lymphadenopathy. Patients develop granulomas, primarily of the lungs, liver, skin, and genitourinary and gastrointestinal tracts, as an abnormal immune response.[28–32]

The most common form of CGD is X-linked recessive and results from mutations in the membrane-bound component of NADPH oxidase gp91^{phox} (phox is short for phagocyte oxidase). Autosomal recessive forms (30% of patients) are due to mutations in other components of phagocyte NADPH oxidase, p22^{phox} and the cytoplasmic components p47^{phox} and p67^{phox}.

The skin, lungs, and perianal area are most often the sites of infection. Early lesions are usually cutaneous staphylococcal pyodermas and abscesses of the face and perianal area, not uncommonly associated with purulent dermatitis and regional lymphadenopathy. Seborrheic dermatitis, Sweet's syndrome, scalp folliculitis, perioral and intraoral ulcerations that resemble aphthous stomatitis, and lupus-like eruptions have also been described. In addition to affected individuals, female carriers of gp91^{phox} mutations may show aphthous stomatitis and lupus-like eruptions.[33,34]

The organisms associated with CGD are usually *Staphylococcus aureus* and opportunistic Gram-negative bacteria, including *Serratia*,[35] *Klebsiella*, *Pseudomonas*, and *Escherichia coli*. These organisms all require oxidative metabolism for intracellular killing. Other organisms that may cause infection in patients with CGD with increased frequency are *Aspergillus*, *Candida*, *Cryptococcus*, and *Nocardia*. Bronchopneumonia and suppurative lymphadenitis are the most prevalent noncutaneous infections, and respond to appropriate antibacterial therapy and, in some cases, surgical drainage. The extracutaneous organs most frequently involved in CGD are the lymph nodes, lungs, liver, spleen, and gastrointestinal tract (Table 25.3).

Patients with CGD frequently show leukocytosis, anemia, elevated erythrocyte sedimentation rate, and hypergammaglobulinemia. Skin tests for delayed hypersensitivity, phagocytosis, and chemotaxis are normal. Carrier and affected patients are often detected by quantitative dihydrorhodamine flow cytometry,[36] and the nitroblue tetrazolium (NBT) screening assay is now rarely performed (in which the oxidized yellow form of NBT is reduced to a blue formazan precipitate). Ferricytochrome C reduction assay is a quantitative assay that shows absence of the respiratory burst. Immunoblots can detect the selective loss of membrane phagocyte oxidase components. However, mutations that lead to deficiency of gp91^{phox} or p22^{phox} cannot be differentiated by immunoblotting, since both are components of cytochrome b$_{558}$ and the entire cytochrome is absent if one is deficient; gene sequencing is required to confirm the mutation in gp91^{phox} or p22^{phox}.

Table 25.3 Signs and symptoms in patients with chronic granulomatous disease

Seen in >50% of patients
Lymphadenopathy, lymphadenitis
Hepatosplenomegaly
Bronchopneumonia
Failure to thrive
Seen in ≥25% of patients
Persistent diarrhea
Pleuritis or empyema
Septicemia or meningitis
Hepatic or perihepatic abscess
Osteomyelitis
Seen in <25% of patients
Perianal abscess
Periorificial dermatitis
Aphthous stomatitis
Conjunctivitis
Lung abscess
Peritonitis
Obstructive granulomas

Antibiotic treatment of infection with surgical intervention as needed, and prophylactic trimethoprim-sulfamethoxazole and itraconazole therapy[37] have been used in most affected individuals.[38] Short courses of systemic corticosteroids have been helpful for patients with obstructive visceral granulomas. Stem cell therapy has led to reversal of the immunodeficiency in severe cases.[39]

Leukocyte Adhesion Deficiencies

The leukocyte adhesion deficiencies (LAD) are a group of three autosomal recessive disorders that affect the ability of neutrophils, cytolytic T lymphocytes, and monocytes to be mobilized into extravascular sites of inflammation.[40] In most affected individuals (LAD1), mutations in CD18 occur, leading to deficiency or dysfunction of the β$_2$ subunit of integrins. The principal ligand for these integrins is ICAM-1, which participates actively in neutrophil and monocyte chemotaxis and phagocytosis. More than 75% of patients with severe disease die by 5 years of age; more than half of the patients with moderate deficiency die between the ages of 10 and 30 years.

Patients with LAD have frequent skin infections (especially facial cellulitis and perianal infection), mucositis, and otitis. Poor wound healing is characteristic, and leads to paper-thin or dysplastic cutaneous scars. Minor skin wounds may become large ulcerations that resemble pyoderma gangrenosum (Fig. 25.3), especially if secondarily infected. Periodontitis is a typical feature and, if severe, may lead to loss of teeth. Bacterial and fungal infections may be life threatening. Delayed separation of the umbilical cord is a frequent historic clue to the diagnosis. Affected individuals have a 5- to 20-fold increase in peripheral blood leukocytes.

A second form of LAD (type 2) is an autosomal recessive disorder due to mutations in *FUCT1*. *FUCT1* encodes a GFP-fucose transporter that is required for formation of sialyl-Lewis X, a ligand for selectins on the surface of neutrophils.[41] In addition to their elevated leukocyte counts and recurrent bacterial infections, patients have short stature, a distinctive facies, and developmental delay. A third type of LAD, which features a bleeding tendency, is caused by a mutation in FERMT3, which encodes kindlin-3, and prevents activation of β1, β2, and β3 integrins.[42] Dermal hematopoiesis, leading to the 'blueberry muffin' presentation, has been described in affected infants and children.[43]

Therapy of the soft tissue infections includes antimicrobial agents and, as appropriate, debridement of wounds. Scrupulous dental hygiene reduces the severity of the periodontitis. Death usually occurs by 2 years of age in patients with severe LAD unless successful bone marrow transplantation or cord blood transplantation is performed.[44] Oral fucose has been helpful for some patients with LAD2.

Severe Combined Immunodeficiency

Severe combined immunodeficiency (SCID) is a group of disorders with similar clinical manifestations and immune dysfunction, but

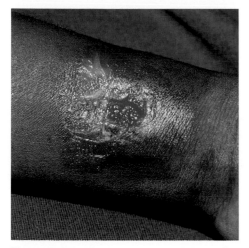

Figure 25.3 Leukocyte adhesion deficiency. Small wounds can lead to large ulcerations that may resemble pyoderma gangrenosum. The ulceration on this boy's leg, initiated by a scratch from his sister, eventually extended to several centimeters in diameter and required a graft. (Reprinted with permission from Schachner LA and Hansen R, eds. Pediatric dermatology, London: Churchill Livingstone; 1995).

different biochemical, cellular, and molecular features (Table 25.4).[45–48] Overall, 75% of affected patients are boys. The majority of cases are autosomal recessive. Approximately 46% have the X-linked recessive form due to mutations in gene that encodes γ_c, which leads to an absence of T and natural killer (NK) cells but normal B-cell numbers.[49] This γ_c chain is a component of several interleukin receptors and is critical for T- and NK-cell function. Mutations in adenosine deaminase lead to the second most common form of SCID. Accumulation of adenosine when its deaminase is missing is toxic to lymphocytes. Omenn syndrome usually results from deficiency of RAG (recombination activating gene) proteins, which mediate the DNA double strand breaks that allow V(D)J (variable/diversity/joining) recombination and immunoglobulin diversity.[50–52]

Infants may present with a generalized seborrheic-like dermatosis, a morbilliform eruption, or exfoliative erythroderma with alopecia. Extensive cutaneous inflammation is a characteristic of 98% of infants with Omenn syndrome, a subset of SCID with reticuloendothelial cell proliferation. Patients with Omenn syndrome typically show hepatosplenomegaly (88%), lymphadenopathy (80%), alopecia (57%), eosinophilia, and a high serum IgE level.[50] Oral and genital ulcers are characteristic of defects in patients with an *Artemis* mutation, especially in Athabaskan-speaking American Indian children.[53]

Acute graft-versus-host disease (GVHD) from maternal cell engraftment or non-irradiated transfusions should also be considered in an infant with an extensive cutaneous eruption[54] (see later discussion). Biopsy will allow differentiation. A more chronic form of GVHD (often with the acute form *in utero*) may also present as lesions that resemble lichen planus, lamellar ichthyosis, or scleroderma (see below).

Recurrent infections, diarrhea, and failure to thrive are apparent by 3–6 months of age. The most common early infections are candidal infections and pneumonia due to bacteria, viruses, or *Pneumocystis jiroveci*.

Patients with SCID usually lack tonsillar buds, thymus, and palpable lymphoid tissue, despite recurrent infections. Nearly all

Table 25.4 Classification of severe combined immunodeficiency

Disorder	Gene location	Gene	Diagnostic tests	Cells
Adenosine deaminase (ADA) deficiency[a]	20q12–13	*Adenosine deaminase*	Red cell ADA levels and metabolites	T⁻/B⁻/NK⁻
Artemis deficiency	10p13	*Artemis*	Defects in V(D)J recombination; increased sensitivity to radiation	TB⁻NK⁺
CD45 deficiency	1q31–32	CD45	CD45 expression	T⁻B⁺NK
IL-7 receptor deficiency	5p13	IL-7 receptor α	IL-7 receptor α expression	T⁻/B⁺/NK⁺
JAK3 deficiency	19p13	*JAK3*	*JAK3* expression/signaling	T⁻L/B⁺/NK⁻
MHC class II deficiency	16p13	*CIITA*	HLA-DR expression	T⁺/B⁺/NK⁺
	1q21	*RFX5*		
	13q13	*RFXAP*		
Purine nucleoside phosphorylase (PNP) deficiency	14q11	Purine nucleoside phosphorylase	Red cell PNP levels and metabolites	T⁻/B⁻/NK⁻
Recombinase activating gene (RAG) deficiency, Omenn's syndrome	11p13	*RAG1* and *RAG2*	Defects in V(D)J recombination; T- and B- cell clonal analysis	T⁻/B⁻/NK⁺
T cell receptor deficiency	11q23	*CD3g*	*CD3* expression	T⁻/B⁺/NK⁺
X-linked SCID[a]	Xq13	Common γ chain	γ_c expression by FACS	T⁻/B⁺/NK⁻
ZAP70 deficiency	2q12	*ZAP-70*	*ZAP-70* expression	T⁻/B⁺/NK⁻

[a]Most common forms.
(Adapted from Schachner LA and Hansen RC, eds. Pediatric dermatology, New York: Mosby; 2003).

patients with SCID have a profound deficiency of T lymphocytes and a low absolute lymphocyte count. Patients are further classified by the results of fluorescent activated cell sorter (FACS) analysis into those with B lymphocytes (T⁻/B⁺ SCID) and those without B lymphocytes (T⁻/B⁻ SCID). Further subclassification can be made according to the presence or absence of NK cells (Table 25.4). The specific diagnosis is confirmed primarily by direct gene analysis and flow cytometric analysis of peripheral blood mononuclear cells with antibodies directed against specific proteins missing from the cell surface, such as JAK3 or γ_c. The natural outcome for SCID is poor, and most patients die by 2 years of age without intervention. Early diagnosis of SCID is critical, preferably before the administration of live vaccines or non-irradiated blood products, which has led to the initiation of perinatal screening in some states. Hematopoietic stem cell transplantation in infants is the treatment of choice, and leads to survival of 95% of infants if performed in the first 3 months of age.[55,56]

Graft-versus-host disease

The *host-versus-graft reaction* occurs when a graft or transplant (skin, heart, or kidney) is placed in a normal individual and the host's circulating immune cells react against the foreign tissue, causing graft or transplanted tissue destruction. In *graft-versus-host disease* (GVHD) the reverse happens.[57] The inflammation from conditioning regimens is thought to activate host antigen presenting cells and chemokines that recruit donor leukocytes into host target organs.[58] Activated donor T cells stimulate dendritic cells, leading to further T cell stimulation and expansion and culminating in target organ apoptosis and dysfunction. GVHD most frequently occurs in children with malignancy, suppressed by radiation and chemotherapy, who receive hematopoietic stem cell transplantation or in immunodeficient children who receive non-irradiated blood products. The risk of both acute and chronic GVHD is greater in males who receive female donor cells because of responses to H-Y minor histocompatibility antigens.[59] It has been estimated that moderate to severe GVHD occurs in 10–50% of patients given an allogeneic transplant from an HLA-identical donor and much more commonly in patients given a transplant from a partially matched family donor or an unrelated volunteer.[60] *In utero* GVHD may occur in immunodeficient babies exposed to maternal antigens.[54] GVHD rarely occurs in solid organ transplant recipients.

The response to the host can be early (acute) or late (chronic). Acute GVHD develops during the first few months (usually 2–4 weeks) and usually involves the skin, gastrointestinal tract, and liver.[61] Patients who receive autologous transplants may have a mild cutaneous form of acute GVHD that occurs 1–3 weeks after transplantation and resolves spontaneously. Reactions to transfusions often occur 7–10 days after the transfusion.[62] The most common cutaneous manifestation of acute GVHD is erythematous macules and maculopapules that often begin on the ears, face, neck, palms, and soles and then become generalized (Figs 25.4–25.6). The rash may become confluent and desquamate. Severe acute GVHD may resemble exfoliative erythroderma or toxic epidermal necrolysis. Patients with acute GVHD may complain of nausea or crampy abdominal pain, and have watery or bloody diarrhea, hepatomegaly, and hepatic function abnormalities. Many patients are anorexic and have fever.

Milder forms of acute GVHD may be difficult to distinguish from an infection (especially viral) or drug reaction. Abnormalities seen in biopsy specimens reflect the clinical severity of the cutaneous manifestations, and range from nonspecific changes to basal keratinocyte vacuolization with scattered necrotic keratinocytes

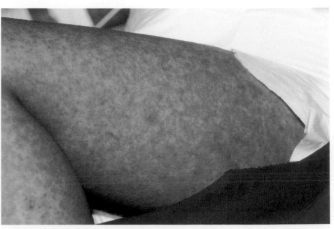

Figure 25.4 Acute GVHD. Erythematous macules were first noted on the ears, palms, and soles on this girl approximately 3 weeks after transplantation, and rapidly generalized.

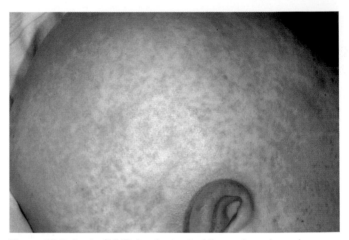

Figure 25.5 Acute GVHD. Involvement of the scalp and ears is common.

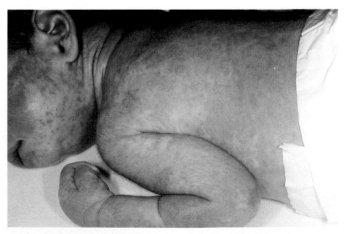

Figure 25.6 Acute GVHD. Almost confluent eruption of erythematous macules and papules in an immunodeficient neonate treated with extracorporeal membrane oxygenation (ECMO) and transfusion of non-irradiated blood.

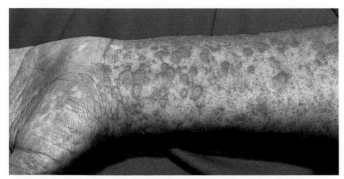

Figure 25.7 Chronic GVHD, lichenoid. After bone marrow transplantation, this boy had acute GVHD and subsequently developed cutaneous scaling papules and plaques typical of lichen planus.

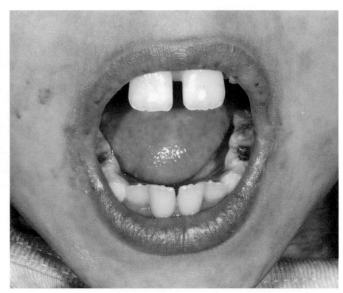

Figure 25.8 Chronic GVHD, lichenoid. Note the white coloration on the lips and tongue of this girl with early chronic GVHD.

surrounded by lymphocytes (the characteristic 'satellite cell necrosis') to severe epidermal necrosis. As such, biopsies are not helpful for patients with milder disease and do not tend to affect treatment decisions.[65] Laboratory tests may show eosinophilia and elevation of bilirubin and hepatic transaminase levels.

Chronic GVHD occurs in 6% (matched sibling cord blood) to 65% (matched unrelated donor peripheral blood stem cell transplants) of pediatric patients. It typically presents 6–18 months after allogeneic stem cell transplantation. Patients may have previous acute GVHD that resolves or progresses directly into chronic GVHD, or may have no history of preceding acute GVHD. A newly proposed diagnosis and scoring system uses clinical and histopathologic signs of presentation, rather than time of onset since transplantation (formerly ≥100 days), and divides chronic GVHD into mild, moderate, and severe.[63] Chronic GVHD often resembles autoimmune disorders and, in contrast to acute GVHD, can affect virtually any organ, leading to significant morbidity with decreased quality of life and overall survival.[64] Decreased survival of chronic GVHD has been associated with thrombocytopenia, progressive onset, extensive cutaneous involvement, gastrointestinal involvement and a low Karnofsky performance status at diagnosis.[65]

Chronic GVHD often manifests with generalized cutaneous involvement.[65] Early lesions may resemble lichen planus with flat-topped violaceous papules and plaques (including mucosal changes of lichen planus) (Figs 25.7, 25.8) (see Ch. 4). Lichenoid lesions may be localized to Blaschko's lines or to the site of previous *Herpes zoster* infection.[66] Some patients with chronic GVHD manifest acquired ichthyosis that resembles ichthyosis vulgaris (Fig. 25.9) or lichen sclerosus (Fig. 25.10). Later changes of chronic GVHD include generalized xerosis, patchy hypo- and hyperpigmentation (Fig. 25.11), progressive poikiloderma, sclerodermatous changes[67,68] with joint contracture and ulcerations (mean onset 529 days after transplant in one study[69]) (Figs 25.12, 25.13), cicatricial alopecia (Fig. 25.14), and nail dystrophy resembling that of dyskeratosis congenita (see Ch. 7, Fig. 7.59).[70] Affected individuals may have dry eyes (as in Sjögren syndrome, see Ch. 22) and desquamative esophagitis with stricture formation. Weight loss can result from dysphagia and mucositis. Other manifestations are chronic diarrhea, hepatomegaly, lymphadenopathy myositis, arthritis, pleural and pericardial effusions, and pulmonary fibrosis.

Patients with chronic GVHD show evidence of immune dysfunction and have recurrent infections. The majority of patients with chronic GVHD have eosinophilia and hypergammaglobulinemia. Many have thrombocytopenia and increased titers of a wide variety of autoimmune antibodies, especially ANA.[65] Liver function testing may show evidence of cholestasis. Pulmonary function tests are

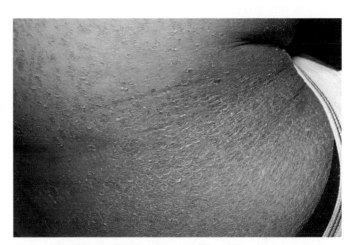

Figure 25.9 Chronic GVHD, ichthyotic. The ichthyotic changes of chronic GVHD resemble those of ichthyosis vulgaris.

abnormal in approximately 50% of patients and chest radiographs may reveal interstitial fibrosis. Biopsies of skin lesions show changes consistent with the clinical picture. For example, patients with lichenoid lesions have the histologic changes of lichen planus (see Ch. 4), often with satellite cell necrosis. Patients with sclerosis tend to show band-like inflammation at the dermal-epidermal junction and dermal sclerosis with obliteration of adnexae. Direct immunofluorescence analysis of skin specimens often shows the linear deposition of immunoreactants at the dermal-epidermal junction.

The mortality of GVHD ranges from 12% for mild acute GVHD to 55% for severe acute GVHD, usually because of infection.[71] The mortality of chronic GVHD is 25%, usually from infection, hepatic failure, and malnutrition. Having acute GVHD is a major risk factor for development of chronic GVHD (11-fold increased risk), emphasizing the importance of preventing acute GVHD. Other risk factors are an unrelated or mismatched donor, possibly the use of peripheral blood stem cells, older age of donor or recipient, use of total body irradiation, male recipient with a female donor, and malignant disease.[72] Two techniques for the prevention of GVHD have

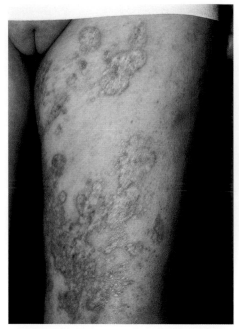

Figure 25.10 Chronic GVHD. The changes of chronic GVHD can resemble those of other autoimmune skin disorders. In this case, the cutaneous plaques resembled those of lichen sclerosus et atrophicus.

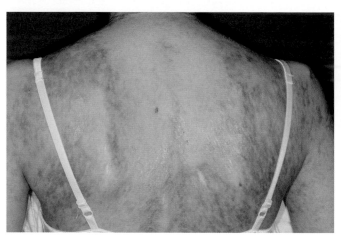

Figure 25.11 Chronic GVHD. Hypo- and hyperpigmented scaling, indurated plaques in a generalized distribution, seen here on her back.

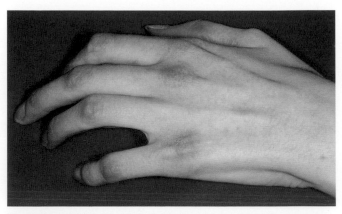

Figure 25.12 Chronic GVHD. Sclerodactyly and subtle telangiectasia overlying knuckles, as seen in patients with systemic scleroderma and juvenile dermatomyositis

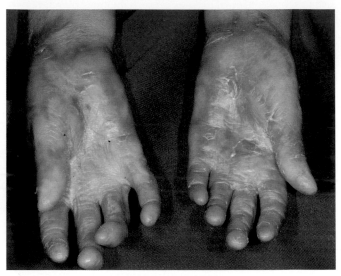

Figure 25.13 Chronic GVHD. Sclerodactyly and generalized scaling were noted at birth in this girl with immunodeficiency and *in utero* GVHD. Her skin softened considerably with high dosages of thalidomide.

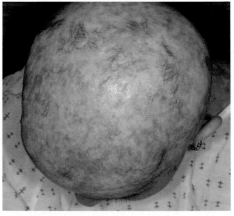

Figure 25.14 Chronic GVHD. Note the extensive alopecia of the scalp with dyschromia and numerous sclerodermatous plaques. In this girl, the dyschromia and sclerodermatous plaques were generalized in distribution as well.

been used: elimination of immunoreactive T cells from the transplanted tissue prior to transfer; and immunosuppressive medications during the first 100–180 days after transplantation. The former approach may decrease the success of engraftment and increase the risk of relapse of leukemia. Combination therapy of tacrolimus (less commonly cyclosporine) and methotrexate decreases the risk of development of acute GVHD, but does not decrease the incidence of chronic GVHD or increase survival after allogeneic transplantation. Prophylaxis against GVHD most commonly involves tacrolimus (FK506). Environmental isolation, bowel rest through hyperalimentation, irradiation of blood products, and prevention of infection are other protective measures.

If grade II-IV acute GVHD develops, the first-line therapy is continuing prophylactic immunosuppression and adding methylprednisolone 2–2.5 mg/kg per day. Patients who fail to respond to corticosteroid alone after 5–7 days can be treated with salvage therapy, such as mycophenolate mofetil,[73–75] anti-thymocyte

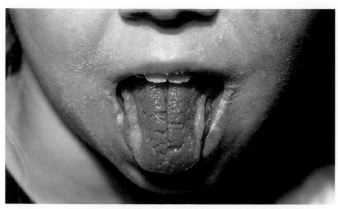

Figure 25.15 Melkersson–Rosenthal syndrome. Scrotal tongue.

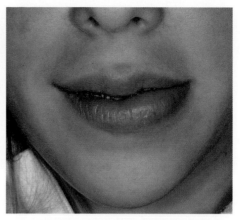

Figure 25.16 Melkersson–Rosenthal syndrome. Granulomatous infiltration limited to the lip(s) is called cheilitis granulomatosa.

globulin, humanized chimeric monoclonal antibodies (anti-T cell, anti-TNF-α, and anti-IL-2),[76] sirolimus (rapamycin),[77–79] extracorporeal photopheresis,[80–83] pentostatin[84,85] and mesenchymal stem cells.[61,86] Responses in general are poor if initial steroid treatment is not successful, and the risk of infection is high.

Similar regimens have been used to treat chronic GVHD, although there is no proven standard, with prednisone and calcineurin inhibitors most commonly used for first-line therapy.[65] The mean duration of therapy for patients with chronic GVHD is 3 years, with about half of the patients able to discontinue therapy 5 years after transplantation. Rituximab has been tried for chronic GVHD,[87] and imatinib mesylate has received increasing attention for sclerodermatous chronic GVHD,[88–91] given the presence in many patients of autoantibodies to platelet-derived growth factor receptor.[92,93] Overall, the 5-year survival is 50% for those who respond to therapy for GVHD and 30% for those with no or an incomplete response. Mucocutaneous manifestations of GVHD may also benefit from administration of thalidomide, acitretin, application of topical tacrolimus, or treatments with narrowband ultraviolet B light, psoralen plus ultraviolet A light, or UVA1 light.[94–98] Supportive intervention for chronic GVHD includes supplemental nutrition (usually parenteral), scrupulous care of wounds, physical therapy to prevent joint contractures and disability, artificial tears, cutaneous emollients and sunscreens, and prophylaxis against Pneumocystis infection with trimethoprim-sulfamethoxazole.

Melkersson–Rosenthal syndrome

Melkersson–Rosenthal syndrome, when fully manifested, is characterized by a triad of recurrent facial paralysis, face and lip swelling (macrocheilitis), and a furrowed or 'scrotal' tongue (lingua plicata) (Fig. 25.15).[99] The complete triad, however, is unusual.[100] Facial swelling is most common (93% of patients), and the edema of the lips is noted in 66% of affected individuals. Furrowing of the tongue and facial palsy have each been reported to occur in approximately 30% of patients. When the condition is limited to the lips, it is called *cheilitis granulomatosa* (granulomatous cheilitis) (Fig. 25.16).

No prodrome warns of attacks, and patients experience no associated erythema, pain, or pruritus. The swelling can increase the size of the lip by two- to three-fold, leading to chapping from exposure of the mucosa. Both lips may be involved, and the swelling may be bilateral or unilateral. In addition to the swelling of the lips and other oral mucosal structures, the eyelids may be swollen. The attacks usually disappear within days or weeks but frequently tend to persist after several recurrences. Facial palsy usually occurs on the side of the facial swelling and tends to resolve spontaneously.[101]

The cause is unknown. Attacks usually start during adolescence with paralysis of a facial nerve, repeated severe headaches, and edema of the circumoral tissue of the upper lip or cheeks and occasionally edema of the gingivae, sublingual area, and lower lip. The edema is usually asymmetrical, but the whole face may be involved. Associated signs include hyperhidrosis, loss of taste, and visual impairment. Biopsy specimens show noncaseating granulomas in an edematous stroma that may be indistinguishable from the granulomas of Crohn's disease (see below) and from infections, especially mycobacterial.[102]

Intralesional injections of triamcinolone or systemic administration of corticosteroids can control the facial and mucosal swelling; intermittent application of topical clobetasol gel may also lead to improvement. Minocycline, with or without corticosteroids, and sometimes macrolides have also been helpful.[103–105] Other therapies include dapsone, clofazimine, and TNF-α inhibitors, particularly infliximab.[106–108] Wedge resection of the inner lip should be reserved for patients who fail to respond to other options.

Crohn's disease

Crohn's disease is a granulomatous disorder of the intestinal tract that usually has its onset between 15 and 30 years of age, but has been described in young children.[109,110] Approximately one-third of pediatric patients have small intestinal disease, one-third ileocolitis, and one-third colitis, with total colitis more common than segmental or isolated proctitis.[110] Growth failure,[111,112] delayed pubertal development, and osteopenia[113] are important complications of Crohn's disease.

The pathogenesis of Crohn's disease is complex. The disorder is thought to occur in genetically predisposed individuals when the intestinal mucosal immune function is altered by exogenous agents, such as infectious organisms, or host factors, such as intestinal barrier function, vascular supply, or stress.[114] The disorder occurs two- to fourfold more often in Ashkenazi Jews, and has been linked to certain HLA alleles (DR3, DQ2, DR103), as well as to mutant alleles of *NOD2/CARD15*. The *CARD15* protein senses bacterial peptidoglycan and regulates NF-κB signaling[115,116] (see the discussion of Blau syndrome, below).

Skin manifestations may occur before, concomitantly, or after other evidence of disease. Perianal skin tags are found in 75–80% of patients with Crohn's disease (Fig. 25.17), and occur before gastrointestinal manifestations in 25% of patients. In addition to tags, skin and mucosal findings have been noted in 22–44% of

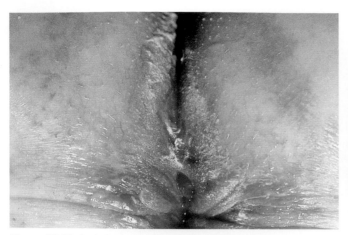

Figure 25.17 Crohn's disease. Perianal tags are an early manifestation and seen in most affected children.

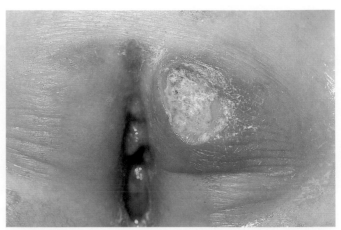

Figure 25.18 Crohn's disease. Pyoderma gangrenosum on the vulva of an affected girl. Pyoderma gangrenosum is more commonly seen in individuals with ulcerative colitis than in those with Crohn's disease.

Table 25.5 Mucocutaneous manifestations of Crohn's disease

	Specific	Nonspecific
Cutaneous	Metastatic Crohn's disease	Erythema nodosum Pyoderma gangrenosum Polyarteritis nodosa Erythema multiforme Vasculitis
Anogenital	Perianal fissures and tags Sinus tracts Labial or scrotal edema	
Oral	Orofacial granulomatosis Cobblestoning Mucosal tags	Aphthous stomatitis Angular cheilitis

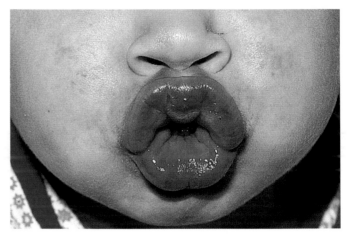

Figure 25.19 Crohn's disease. Note the infiltration of the lips, which showed noncaseating granulomas in biopsy sections.

patients (Table 25.5), and occur more often in patients with colonic versus small intestinal disease. Several mucocutaneous manifestations of Crohn's disease also are features of ulcerative colitis. Erythema nodosum (see Ch. 20) occurs in up to 15% of patients with Crohn's disease and has been shown to correlate with the presence of arthritis.[117] Pyoderma gangrenosum occurs less frequently in Crohn's disease[118] (approximately 1% of patients) (Fig. 25.18) than in ulcerative colitis (up to 5% of pediatric patients), occasionally precedes the development of bowel symptoms, and has a course unrelated to the activity of the bowel disease. Oral aphthous ulcers have been described in >50% of pediatric patients with Crohn's disease.[119] Pyostomatitis vegetans, erythematous pustular lesions associated with erosions and ulcerations, is considered a marker for inflammatory bowel disease. Cutaneous changes related to nutritional deficits (particularly acrodermatitis enteropathica due to zinc deficiency) can occur as well.

Other mucocutaneous manifestations are more specific for Crohn's disease.[110] Cobblestoning of the buccal mucosa is seen in up to 20% of affected individuals. Painless swelling of the lips, resembling cheilitis granulomatosis (see above), may be the initial presentation of Crohn's disease in a child or adolescent and may precede the gastrointestinal symptoms by several years (Fig. 25.19).[120–124] Similarly, the vulva may show erythema, swelling and fissuring,[125,126] and the scrotum and penis may be swollen and erythematous.[127,128] Perianal lesions may extend onto the adjacent perineum, abdomen, or buttocks with fissures and sinus tracts are

common.[129] Nasal perforation has been described.[130] Abdominal surgical sites may also be loci for cutaneous involvement. Biopsy provides the clue to diagnosis, although the noncaseating granulomas resemble those of Melkersson–Rosenthal/cheilitis granulomatosa and sarcoidosis. Special stains (periodic acid-Schiff, Ziehl–Nielsen and Gram) are important to consider infectious causes of granulomas. These granulomatous lesions of the lips and anogenital area are considered 'contiguous' Crohn's because of their proximity to the gastrointestinal tract. Granulomatous lesions elsewhere are considered 'metastatic' cutaneous Crohn's disease.[131,132] These lesions typically are dusky red swollen/indurated plaques, most commonly found on the genital region of children, lower extremities, abdomen, or trunk; lesions less commonly show no erythema or are ulcerating.[133]

Barium contrast studies are particularly important for investigating small bowel disease, but endoscopy and colonoscopy are important tools for upper and lower bowel disease, respectively. Initial treatment involves administration of systemic corticosteroids and aminosalicylates, with the early addition of azathioprine or 6-mercaptopurine as steroid-sparing alternatives for maintenance therapy.[134] Tumor necrosis factor-α inhibitors (etanercept, adalimumab and infliximab) are very helpful as well and reduces the need for surgery.[135–139] The development of psoriasis in patients with Crohn's disease, even when treated with TNF-α inhibitors, has been

Table 25.6 Common features of sarcoidosis in older versus younger children	
Older children and adolescents	**Preschool-aged children**
Fever, weight loss	Low-grade fever
Skin lesions	Polyarthritis
Cough, dyspnea	Skin lesions
Lymphadenopathy	Uveitis
Hepatomegaly	Parotid gland enlargement
Splenomegaly	Lymphadenopathy, especially
Arrhythmias	peripheral
Congestive heart failure	
Renal stones (hypercalciuria)	
Uveitis	
Facial paralysis	

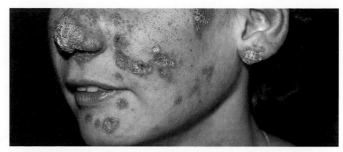

Figure 25.20 Sarcoidosis. The lupus pernio form of sarcoidosis shows infiltrated violaceous plaques on the nose, cheeks, and ears. This girl presented with hoarseness owing to her laryngeal involvement with sarcoidosis, and was left with severe scarring after treatment.

described.[140,141] Colectomy in Crohn's disease does not prevent recurrence and should be used selectively.[142,143] Oral metronidazole has been used for metastatic Crohn's disease;[144,145] intralesional or topical applications of potent topical corticosteroids or tacrolimus have helped to clear the ulcerations of pyoderma gangrenosum (see below).

Sarcoidosis

Sarcoidosis is a systemic granulomatous disorder of unknown etiology with CD4+ Th1 cell and monocyte activation, leading to hypergammaglobulinemia, sarcoidal granulomas, predominantly affecting the lungs, eyes, skin, and reticuloendothelial system, and ultimately fibrosis. The condition presents most frequently in young adults between the ages of 20 and 40 years. In pediatric patients, it is most commonly seen in adolescents between 9 and 15 years of age, in which manifestations resemble those of adult patients. However, sarcoidosis rarely occurs in preschool children as well[146,147] (Table 25.6). In US series of pediatric sarcoidosis, 7–28% of younger children are African-American, while 72–81% are African-Americans among older children.[148]

Sarcoidosis in Older Children and Adolescents

Adolescents and older children may present with fever and weight loss. Cutaneous involvement occurs in approximately 25% of patients.[149] Several specific and nonspecific lesions have been described, although no lesion is pathognomonic.[150] Most typical are yellow-brown to red flat-topped papules, infiltrated plaques, and nodules that show an apple jelly color when diascopy (pressure applied with a glass slide) is performed, a characteristic sign of granulomas. Scaling is sometimes associated. These granulomatous lesions are most commonly localized to the face, and an annular configuration of lesions around the nares, lips, and eyelids is highly characteristic, although any site, including the mucosae, palms, and soles may be involved. Lesions often occur in areas of trauma or scarification. Other cutaneous manifestations of sarcoidosis include subcutaneous, often painful nodules (*Darier–Roussy* sarcoidosis), ichthyosis (*ichthyosiform sarcoid*, usually most prominent on the lower extremities), generalized erythroderma with scaling, and hypopigmentation. More than 20% of affected children have erythema nodosum (see Ch. 20), which is often manifested at onset,

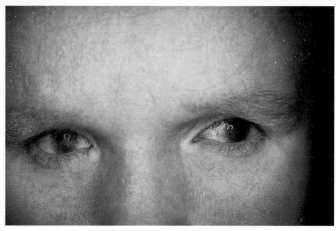

Figure 25.21 Sarcoidosis. Uveitis in a teenager with sarcoidosis since early childhood. She had ichthyosiform scaling overlying granulomatous papules and arthritis.

is a good prognostic sign[148] and usually portends clearance of the adenopathy. The combination of erythema nodosum, bilateral hilar adenopathy, uveitis, and fever has been called *Lofgren syndrome*. *Lupus pernio* is a variant of sarcoidosis in which soft infiltrated violaceous plaques are located on the nose, cheeks, ears, forehead, and on the dorsal aspects of the hands, fingers, and toes (Fig. 25.20). This variant can cause significant scarring and deformity, and is a marker for upper respiratory involvement, including of the larynx.

The lung is the most commonly involved site in older children and adolescents, as in adults. A dry, hacking cough is the most common complaint, but patients may have dyspnea and develop parenchymal lung disease. Lymphadenopathy may be generalized, but typically involves the hilar nodes and is symmetrical. More than 90% show an abnormal chest X-ray at onset. Clinical evidence of liver involvement is detected in approximately one-third of patients, although more than half show granulomas when the liver is biopsied. Splenic enlargement has been associated with extensive visceral fibrosis and a poor prognosis. Granulomatous infiltration of the heart may lead to arrhythmias and of the lung to congestive heart failure. Some patients with renal involvement will show hypercalciuria, renal stones, and ultimately renal failure from excessive production of 1,25-dihydroxyvitamin D_3, with or without hypercalcemia; calciphylaxis has also been reported in association with end-stage renal disease, manifesting as painful violaceous plaques, retiform purpura or subcutaneous nodules, which can progress to non-healing ulcers and cutaneous gangrene.[151]

Overall, up to 50% of pediatric patients have eye involvement, particularly anterior segment uveitis (Fig. 25.21). Conjunctival granulomas are often seen on biopsy and lacrimal gland inflammation is not uncommon. Chorioretinitis, keratitis, and glaucoma may occur as well, resulting in blindness. Neurologic manifestations are associated with a poorer prognosis, and overall affect 5–10% of older patients, most commonly facial nerve paralysis. The combination of uveitis, facial nerve palsy, parotid gland enlargement, and fever has been called *uveoparotid fever* or *Heerfordt syndrome*. Lytic lesions of the distal bones rarely occur and are asymptomatic.

Sarcoidosis in Preschool Children

Preschool-age children with sarcoidosis differ from older children, adolescents, and adults in that they tend to have polyarthritis and severe uveitis (frequently suggesting a diagnosis of juvenile idiopathic arthritis),[152] cutaneous manifestations, and a conspicuous absence of pulmonary abnormalities.[153,154] The majority of cutaneous lesions in this age group consist of asymptomatic generalized eczematous or infiltrated plaques and papules, which may leave small pitted scars. Relapses and remission are common. Children may also have ichthyosiform changes, lichenoid papules,[155,156] or erythematous patches. Arthralgias, low-grade fever, and abdominal pain are the most frequent symptoms in children with sarcoidosis. More than half of affected children have arthritis with non-painful swelling and boggy synovial thickening of the wrists and fingers. In contrast to the arthritis of juvenile idiopathic arthritis, range of motion is usually not reduced. The most common radiographic finding in children is that of bilateral hilar lymph node enlargement, with or without detectable lung changes; any symptoms referable to the lungs are usually mild. Ocular involvement is extremely common in children, especially granulomatous anterior uveitis, although keratitis, retinitis, glaucoma, and involvement of the eyelids and lacrimal glands may also occur. Partial or total blindness occurs in a relatively high percentage of children with sarcoidosis who have ocular involvement. Most other signs of sarcoidosis in adults are rare in children. Parotid gland enlargement and peripheral adenopathy, however, are common. Hepatic, splenic, pulmonary, and cardiac involvement, although clinically underappreciated, are frequently seen at autopsy.

Sarcoidosis must also be distinguished from infectious granulomatous conditions, particularly mycobacterial and fungal, but cultures and special stains of biopsy sections are negative. In young children, sarcoidosis (Table 25.6) is difficult to distinguish from *Blau syndrome* (Table 25.7), an autosomal dominant autoinflammatory disorder characterized by generalized erythematous papules (Figs 25.22, 25.23) and plaques, iritis,[157] arthritis, synovial cysts overlying the ankle and wrist joints, and camptodactyly (usually congenital flexion contracture of a finger).[158] Onset of manifestations is usually during the first years of life. The classic triad of skin eruption, arthritis and recurrent uveitis is only found in 42% of patients with Blau syndrome,[159,160] with cutaneous features the most common manifestation.[161] Of those with ocular involvement, 50% develop cataracts and about one-third secondary glaucoma. The susceptibility gene for Blau syndrome, also known as familial granulomatous arthritis, is *caspase recruitment domain (CARD)15* (also known as *NOD2*). Mutations in *CARD15* lead to constitutive activation of nuclear factor-κB signaling. Mutations in *CARD15* have not been found in older individuals with sarcoidosis;[162] however, the majority of children with early-onset sarcoidosis (but not all) have Blau syndrome with mutations in *CARD15*.[163] Mutations in *CARD15/NOD2* have also been associated with the development of Crohn's disease (see earlier section), but mutations that increase the susceptibility to Crohn's disease are in regions of the *CARD15/NOD2* gene different than those that predispose to Blau syndrome.[164,165] The cutaneous granulomatous papules may respond to chronic administration of erythromycin, but may leave tiny atrophic macules. Methotrexate and TNF-α inhibitors are most often used for extracutaneous manifestations, and thalidomide has also been reported to be effective.[166]

There is no single reliable test for sarcoidosis. Since the clinical picture may be mimicked by other diseases, histologic confirmation is advisable. In typical lesions, the characteristic histopathologic finding consists of islands of large, pale-staining epithelioid cells containing few if any giant cells intermingled with histiocytes and lymphocytes. Thorough evaluation also includes ophthalmologic examination with slit-lamp testing, chest radiographs (with chest computed tomography (CT) scanning if needed), pulmonary function testing, electrocardiogram, and 24-h urine calcium measurements. Many affected patients have hyperglobulinemia, especially African-Americans. Patients may show hypercalcemia (7–24% and usually transient), leukopenia, eosinophilia (>50% of children),

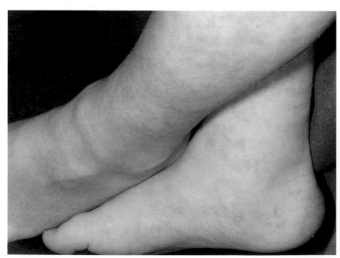

Figure 25.22 Blau syndrome. Discrete, erythematous papules were present in a generalized distribution in this young boy with arthralgias. Biopsy showed non-caseating granulomas.

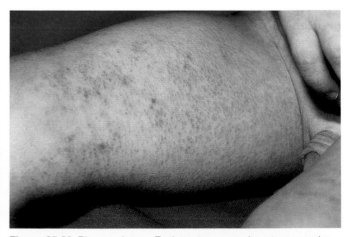

Figure 25.23 Blau syndrome. Erythematous granulomatous papules on the thigh of a 5-year-old boy with a *CARD15* mutation. Note the pitted scars on the thigh, left after clearance of previous lesions. Recent evidence suggests that most young patients with sarcoidosis have mutations in *CARD15* and thus have Blau syndrome.

and usually an increased erythrocyte sedimentation rate. The Kveim test, which involves development of sarcoidal granulomas at the site of an intradermal injection of a 10% suspension of human sarcoidal tissue, is not approved by the Food and Drug Administration and is no longer performed. The angiotensin-converting enzyme (ACE) level is often elevated, but may be increased in other granulomatous disorders as well and has a 40% false negative rate. Cutaneous anergy is common, but children should be tested for reactivity to tuberculin.

The natural course of sarcoidosis in childhood is insidious and the condition often regresses completely after many years, especially in those with an acute onset. Chronic, progressive sarcoidosis has a poorer prognosis and rarely involutes. Features that portend a worse prognosis include chronicity; lupus pernio; symptoms lasting longer than 6 months; black race; involvement of more than three organ systems; and later stage pulmonary disease.[167] The overall mortality is 1–5%.

Corticosteroids (1 mg/kg per day initially with tapering as possible) can suppress the acute manifestations of the disorder. However, given the hazards of prolonged systemic corticosteroid therapy and the frequent spontaneous resolution of sarcoidosis, the administration of systemic corticosteroids is best reserved for rapidly progressive, disfiguring skin lesions, ocular disease, and significant visceral abnormalities (persistent hypercalcemia; joint involvement; lesions of the nasal, laryngeal, and bronchial mucosa; severe, debilitating, or rapidly progressing lung disease; central nervous system lesions; persistent facial palsy; myocardial involvement; and hypersplenism). Methotrexate is the most commonly used steroid-sparing systemic agent for pediatric sarcoidosis, and mycophenolate mofetil and TNF-α inhibitors (particularly infliximab) have also been used successfully.[168] Ophthalmic steroid preparations may be used adjunctively for eye disease. NSAIDs can be used for the arthritis, and hydroxychloroquine and allopurinol have been used successfully for skin lesions.

Autoinflammatory disorders

The autoinflammatory disorders are a group of monogenic inherited disorders characterized by intermittent or fluctuating degrees of inflammation, particularly of the abdomen, skin, and joints, without evidence of high-titer autoantibodies or antigen-specific T cells (Table 25.7). One group of autoinflammatory disorders, *inflammasomopathies*, result from abnormalities of the inflammasome; the inflammasome is a macromolecular complex that senses microbial products and endogenous 'danger signals' to activate caspase-1 and ultimately IL-1β, key steps in the innate immune response. Some of these are intrinsic defects of the inflammasome, such as the *cryopyrinopathies* (defective cryopyrin: familial cold autoinflammatory syndrome, Muckle-Wells syndrome and neonatal onset multisystemic inflammatory disorder). Others result from abnormalities or deficits in proteins that interact directly or indirectly with the inflammasome, such as pyrin (*hereditary periodic fever syndromes*) and PSTPIP1 (*PAPA syndrome*). The *hereditary periodic fever syndromes* (familial Mediterranean fever, mevalonate kinase deficiency and TNF receptor-associated periodic syndrome) show recurrent episodes of fever, often in association with a cutaneous eruption, serositis (peritonitis, pleuritis), arthritis and lymphadenopathy. Progressive amyloidosis of the liver and kidneys has been reported in association with several types of periodic fever syndromes and may be life threatening.

The *pyogenic* autoinflammatory disorders include PAPA, PFAPA and SAPHO (see Ch. 8) syndromes and deficiency of the interleukin-1 receptor antagonist (DIRA); they feature neutrophilic infiltration,

with clinical features including pyogenic arthritis, aphthous ulcerations, pyoderma gangrenosum-like lesions, and pustular skin eruptions. Autoinflammatory disorders such as Crohn's disease and Blau syndrome (discussed above under sarcoidosis) are related to sequence variations in *NOD2/CARD15*, which plays a central role in the NF-κB activation response to microbial products. Among other disorders considered autoinflammatory are Behçet's syndrome and systemic onset juvenile idiopathic arthritis (see Ch. 22).[169–172]

Hereditary Periodic Fever Syndromes

Familial Mediterranean fever

Familial Mediterranean fever (FMF, benign paroxysmal peritonitis, familial paroxysmal polyserositis, familial recurrent polyserositis, Armenian disease) is the prototype of the hereditary autoinflammatory disorders.[173,174] An autosomal recessive disorder, FMF results from mutations in *MEFV* (Mediterranean fever gene), which encodes pyrin (or marenostrin).[175] Pyrin is thought to act as an antiinflammatory molecule of polymorphonuclear leukocytes and cytokine-activated monocytes. The disorder is most frequently seen in individuals of Arabic, Turkish, or non-Ashkenazi Jewish descent, in which the gene is carried in one of five persons.

The acute attacks of high fever and serositis (peritonitis, pleuritis, and synovitis, with abdominal, chest, and articular pain) begin during the 1st decade in 67% of cases and by the 2nd decade in 90%. The erysipelas- or cellulitis-like lesions, the most frequent cutaneous manifestations, occur in almost 10% of patients (Fig. 25.24).[176] Of importance, these painful, warm, swollen erythematous well-defined plaques can occur in children without a history of fevers, although acute phase reactants are increased.[177] Both the skin signs and the arthritis may be precipitated by trauma. Other cutaneous manifestations include urticaria, erythematous papules, vesicles, bullae, and subcutaneous nodules histologically resembling periarteritis nodosa or vasculitis. Skin lesions usually appear on the calves, around the ankles, and on the dorsal aspects of the feet.

Usually a single organ is affected during an attack. Attacks last from a few hours to 4 days and recur throughout life with variable periodicity. Asymptomatic intervals may last as long as several years. Although symptoms of the monoarticular joint inflammation persist longer than episodes of peritonitis, sometimes for several months, chronic residual manifestations are rare.

Amyloidosis occurs in about 25% of untreated patients and causes death in 90% of individuals affected with amyloid-induced renal dysfunction before the age of 40. The risk of developing amyloidosis is a function of the duration between disease onset and diagnosis, and of the frequency of episodes of chest pain, arthritis, and erysipelas-like erythema.[178]

The diagnosis of familial Mediterranean fever is dependent on clinical features and, as needed, genetic testing. Colchicine (1–2.5 mg/kg per day) prevents the recurrence of attacks and the amyloidosis;[179,180] once daily usage may be as effective and safe as two to three divided daily doses.[181] Anakinra (directed against interleukin-1), interferon-alpha, corticosteroids, and cyclophosphamide have been used in rare patients who are unresponsive to colchicine.[182,183]

TNF receptor-associated periodic syndrome

TNF receptor-associated periodic syndrome (TRAPS) is an autosomal dominant disorder caused by mutations in the p55 tumor necrosis factor receptor (TNFR1), encoded by *TNFRSF1A*[184] or defects in shedding of the receptor.[185] The febrile attacks tend to last longer than those of FMF, at least 5 days and sometimes up to 3

Table 25.7 Autoinflammatory disorders

Disorder	Inheritance	Gene defect	Gene product	Associated features
Granulomatous				
Blau syndrome	AD	NOD2/CARD15	CARD15	Onset usually <5 years old granulomatous dermatitis, uveitis, synovitis Good response to TNF inhibitors
Periodic fevers				
Familial Mediterranean fever	AR	MEFV	Pyrin (marenostrin)	Recurrent fever of short duration (24–48 h) Serositis with abdominal pain, pleuritis; erysipelas-like eruption in minority of patients; pericarditis, scrotal swelling, splenomegaly. High risk of renal amyloidosis if untreated Good response to colchicine, sometimes IL-1 blockade
TNF receptor-associated periodic syndrome (TRAPS)	AD	TNFRSF1A	P55 TNF receptor	Recurrent fevers that are prolonged (1–3 weeks) Serositis, rash, conjunctivitis, periorbital edema, arthritis. Moderate incidence of renal amyloidosis Response to TNF- and IL-1 blockade
Mevalonate kinase deficiency (MVK; Hyper-IgD syndrome; HIDS)	AR	MVK	Mevalonate kinase	Early onset (usually 1st year) Periodic fever lasting 4–5 days Rash (>90%), abdominal pain with vomiting and diarrhea, arthritis; headache, hepatosplenomegaly, cervical adenopathy, leukocytosis, high levels of IgD Response to steroids Often improves by adulthood Amyloidosis rare
Cryopyrinopathies				
Familial cold auto-inflammatory syndrome (familial cold urticaria)	AD	CIAS1	Cryopyrin	Cold-induced nonpruritic urticaria, arthritis, fever and chills, leukocytosis
Muckle–Wells syndrome	AD	C/AS1	Cryopyrin	Recurrent urticaria, sensorineural hearing loss, amyloidosis
Neonatal onset multisystem disease (NOMID)[a]	AD	CIAS1	Cryopyrin	Neonatal onset urticaria, chronic aseptic meningitis, arthropathy and bone deformities, fever, ocular changes and hearing loss
Pyogenic				
PAPA syndrome	AD	PSTPIP1/C2BP1	PSTPIP1/C2BP1	Pyogenic (sterile, destructive) arthritis, pyoderma gangrenosum, acne, myositis
PFAPA syndrome	Unknown	Unknown	Unknown	Periodic fevers, aphthous stomatitis, pharyngitis, and cervical adenitis. Malaise, headache
Majeed's syndrome	AR	LPIN2	Lipin-2	Multifocal osteomyelitis, congenital dyserythropoietic anemia, inflammatory dermatosis
Deficiency of the interleukin-1 receptor antagonist (DIRA)	AR	IL1RN	IL-1 receptor antagonist	Fetal distress, joint swelling with periosteal inflammation, severe osteopenia, lytic bone lesions, respiratory involvement, thromboses, aphthae, pyoderma gangrenosum, pustulosis

[a]Also called chronic infantile neurologic cutaneous and articular (CINCA) syndrome.

Note: Amyloidosis is unusual in Blau, HIDS, PAPA and PFAPA syndromes.

weeks;[186] they usually have no periodicity, despite the name. Manifestations usually begin during childhood, and >75% of patients have cutaneous involvement.[187] Most typical is the erythematous swollen plaque with indistinct margins that is warm and tender to palpation. It is most commonly located on the extremities, where it begins distally and migrates proximally during the attack. This pseudocellulitis is accompanied by painful myalgias in virtually all patients, which may precede the appearance of cutaneous signs.

Generalized serpiginous plaques and annular erythematosus patches have also been described. In addition to severe abdominal pain, thoracic and scrotal pain, arthralgias and occasionally arthritis, orbital edema, and conjunctivitis are frequent complaints. In adults, fevers are less common. Amyloid deposition, especially in the kidneys and liver, is described in 14–25% of individuals with TRAPS.

The diagnosis of TRAPS can be confirmed by gene testing. Corticosteroids are the most effective treatment, but daily administration

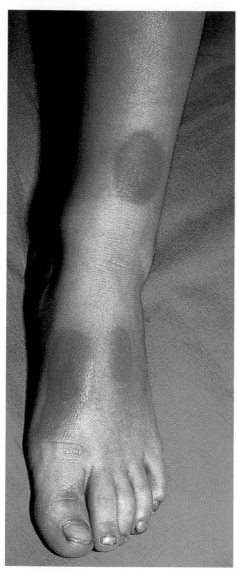

Figure 25.24 Familial Mediterranean fever. Erythematous nodules on the dorsal aspect of the foot and pretibial area of an affected child. (Courtesy of James E. Rasmussen, MD; reprinted from Hurwitz S. The skin and systemic disease in children. Chicago: Year Book Medical Publishers; 1985.)

Figure 25.25 Deficiency of interleukin-1 receptor antagonist (DIRA). This Puerto Rican boy with failure to thrive and multifocal lytic lesions of bone showed numerous plaques of erythematous pustules.

The disorder results from mutations in *MVK*, which encodes mevalonate kinase.[192,193] Deficiency of this kinase leads to accumulation of isoprenoid compounds, which are proinflammatory.[194] Complete deficiency of mevalonate kinase (vs the 1–8% residual activity in MKD) results in mevalonic aciduria, which is associated with growth and mental retardation, and morphologic abnormalities, in addition to recurrent fevers, rash, lymphadenopathy, and inflammation of the joints and gastrointestinal tract. Definitive diagnosis of HIDS cannot rely on the demonstration of high levels of IgD, as this has now been shown in some patients with FMF and TRAPS, but rather depends on finding evidence of mevalonate kinase deficiency or mevalonic aciduria.

Fevers respond dramatically to steroids, but the frequent recurrence of fevers makes steroid therapy untenable. Colchicine, NSAIDs, and thalidomide have not been helpful for affected individuals. However, some patients respond to TNF inhibitors or anakinra.[195,196] In addition, administration of simvastatin improves inflammatory attacks; simvastatin inhibits 3-hydroxy-3-methylglutaryl-coenzyme A (HMG-CoA) reductase, which precedes mevalonate kinase in the isoprenoid pathway.[197]

The Cryopyrinopathies: Familial Cold Autoinflammatory, Muckle–Wells, and CINCA/NOMID Syndromes

Although originally described as separate disorders, these three autosomal dominant syndromes are now known to be caused by mutations in the gene *NLRP3/CIAS1* (cold-induced autoinflammatory syndrome).[198] This gene encodes a protein called cryopyrin (or NALP3) which forms a complex that activation caspase 1. Caspase 1 cleaves the inactive interleukin (IL)-1β to the active form of IL-1β. The mutations that result in the different syndromes are largely distinct.

Recurrent urticarial-like eruptions are common to all three syndromes. In familial cold autoinflammatory syndrome (FCAS, familial cold urticaria), the mildest condition of the group, the urticaria is delayed in its onset, usually a few hours after exposure to cold, and persists for <24 h. Fever, conjunctivitis, and arthritis are also seen in association. Muckle–Wells syndrome is an autosomal dominant disorder in which the urticaria is associated with sensorineural

has been required; TNF-α inhibitors, such as etanercept, are effective in some patients,[188] and more recently anakinra has been shown to lead to long-term efficacy.[189]

Periodic fever associated with mevalonate kinase deficiency

Periodic fever associated with mevalonate kinase deficiency (MKD) is an autosomal recessive disorder that presents during infancy, often during the first year of life. Focal signs occur in more than two-thirds of affected individuals, and include abdominal pain, diarrhea, vomiting, headache, painful cervical lymphadenopathy hepatosplenomegaly non-destructive arthritis, and skin rash. The high serum level of IgD distinguishes this periodic fever, also called familial hyperimmunoglobulinemia D and periodic fever syndrome or HIDS, from familial Mediterranean fever.[190] More than 90% of patients show the cutaneous eruption of erythematous maculopapules or papules. Inflammatory attacks typically last approximately a week and recur every 4–8 weeks. Renal deposition of amyloid is rare.[191]

deafness and renal amyloidosis. Conjunctivitis and occasionally arthritis have been described in association.

Chronic infantile neurological cutaneous and articular (CINCA) or neonatal onset multisystemic inflammatory disease (NOMID) syndrome typically presents as nonpruritic urticarial erythema during the first week of life. About 50% of patients have cryopyrin mutations. The urticarial rash usually begins on the extremities and tends to migrate, even during examination. It has a waxing and waning course, but never tends to resolve entirely.[199] Arthralgias and arthritis develop early during the first weeks of life, and are thereafter persistent, leading to disabling destructive arthropathy during infancy. Bony deformities, especially of the knees, are characteristic, with distinctive radiographic findings of patellar and long bone ossification with overgrowth. Chronic aseptic meningitis has been associated with headaches in older children, and patients may have seizures, spasticity, and motor defects. Some affected children have developed brain atrophy during the neonatal period, which has been linked to developmental delay and retardation. Papillitis with optic atrophy and anterior uveitis are the most common ocular manifestations, with a mean age of onset of 4.5 years; severe visual loss occurs in 26% of patients with ocular disease.[200] Bilateral sensorineural progressive hearing loss is commonly associated as well. Most patients show a typical angelic facies with frontal bossing, a saddleback nose and midfacial hypoplasia. Lymphadenopathy, splenomegaly, increased ESR, eosinophilia, leukocytosis, and hyperglobulinemia are features of chronic inflammation. Early death has been linked to infection, vasculitis, and amyloidosis.

Although colchicine has helped the arthropathy of Muckle–Wells syndrome, and etanercept and systemic steroids have been helpful in patients with CINCA/NOMID syndrome,[201] treatment was challenging before the more recent availability of IL-1 inhibitors. Several patients with Muckle–Wells[202] syndrome and CINCA/NOMID[203] have shown rapid resolution of clinical evidence of inflammation with anakinra, an inhibitor of interleukin-1β. Newer IL-1 inhibitors that have a longer duration of action (such as canakinumab) show great promise.[204,205]

Deficiency of the interleukin-1 receptor antagonist

Deficiency of the interleukin-1 receptor antagonist (DIRA) is a recently described autosomal recessive disorder[206,207] in which IL-1 activity is markedly increased because of deficiency of an antagonist that also binds to the IL-1 receptor and prevents IL-1 activity.[208] Affected infants and young children show fetal distress, joint swelling with periosteal inflammation, severe osteopenia with lytic bone lesions, respiratory involvement, thrombotic episodes, oral mucosal and cutaneous pyoderma gangrenosum-like ulcerations, and a localized to generalized pustular eruption that resembles pustular psoriasis (Fig. 25.25). Administration of anakinra (2 mg/ kg per day) dramatically reverses the inflammatory manifestations, whereas other systemic immunomodulators have largely failed to cause improvement. DIRA must be distinguished from Majeed syndrome, an autosomal recessive disorder that also features chronic recurrent multifocal osteomyelitis and an inflammatory dermatosis that can vary from a Sweet syndrome-like eruption to chronic pustulosis, but Majeed syndrome features congenital dyserythropoietic anemia and results from mutations in LPIN2, encoding lipin-2.[209]

Pyogenic Sterile Arthritis, Pyoderma Gangrenosum, Acne (PAPA) Syndrome

This autosomal dominant disorder is characterized by pyoderma-gangrenosum-like ulcerative lesions, usually in the second decade of life, severe cystic acne, and episodes of inflammatory arthritis that lead to significant joint destruction.[210] The pyoderma gangrenosum lesions are usually seen on the leg, and sterile abscesses have been described at sites of parenteral injections. Affected family members may show some features of the disorder, but not others. Mutations occur in PSTPIP1/CD2BP1, which encodes a protein that interacts with pyrin.[211] PAPA syndrome is treated with oral corticosteroids, and marked improvement has been noted with TNF inhibitors and anti-IL-1 treatment.[171]

Periodic Fever, Aphthous Stomatitis, Pharyngitis, and Cervical Adenitis (PFAPA) Syndrome

PFAPA syndrome (or Marshall's syndrome) is a periodic fever syndrome that usually occurs in children under 5 years of age. Affected children present with a mean of 4–5 days of fever >39°C, which recurs regularly every 3–8 weeks. Pharyngitis has been described in almost 90% of patients, cervical adenitis in 62% and stomatitis in 38–71%.[212–214] Attacks of mild abdominal pain, vomiting, headache, and malaise are common.

Other inflammatory disorders with fever, including infectious disorders, must be considered. The fever tends to be poorly responsive to acetaminophen or ibuprofen. Short courses (one or two doses) of corticosteroids can be highly effective in controlling symptoms, but may shorten the duration of remission.[215] Cimetidine and tonsillectomy have been advocated as well.[213,216] Episodes tend to occur less frequently or disappear with advancing age, without any long-term sequelae.

Pyoderma gangrenosum

Pyoderma gangrenosum is a severe, chronic, inflammatory disorder of the skin characterized by a painful sloughing ulceration with purulent or vegetative base and an elevated dusky blue or reddish purple undermined border surrounded by a rim of inflammation (Figs 25.18, 25.26).[217] The lesion usually begins as a tender papulopustule or erythematous nodule that undergoes necrosis and ulcerates. The ulceration heals with cribriform scarring (Fig. 25.27). Lesions in older children and adolescents (as in adults) are most often found on the lower extremities (especially the anterior tibial surface), but can be seen anywhere on the body, including mucosal and peristomal sites.[218] The head, airway, and anogenital areas are more common sites of involvement in infants and younger children.[219,220] Pustular, bullous, and superficial variants have been described. The bullous form may be difficult to distinguish from bullous Sweet's syndrome (see Ch. 20). The diagnosis is based on clinical features. Biopsy findings are nonspecific, but special stains and cultures of biopsy specimens may help to distinguish pyoderma gangrenosum from other disorders, including vasculitis and infectious causes of ulceration.

Although virtually always described in adults, 4% of cases have occurred in infants and children.[221,222] Pathergy (the development of lesions at sites of minor trauma), which occurs in 20% of patients with this disorder, maybe more common in childhood cases; in a recent report, an abused child developed pyoderma gangrenosum at multiple sites of physical abuse.[223] Although the disorder may occur without associated disease, including in siblings,[224] it usually develops in pediatric patients with any of a variety of systemic disorders. Most common in children is inflammatory bowel disease (especially ulcerative colitis; see Crohn's above), but immunodeficiency (especially HIV infection and leukocyte adhesion defect[225]), hematologic disorders (especially leukemia),[226,227] Takayasu's disease,[228,229] and rheumatic disorders (especially juvenile idiopathic arthritis, systemic lupus erythematosus, and in association with

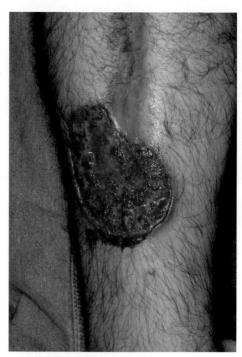

Figure 25.26 Pyoderma gangrenosum. Painful leg ulceration with an inflamed, undermined border. Note the pustule distal to the ulceration, often the earliest sign of a new site of involvement. The most common underlying condition in affected children is inflammatory bowel disease, although no underlying abnormality may be discovered.

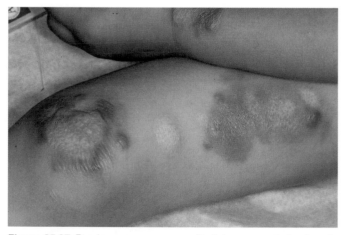

Figure 25.27 Pyoderma gangrenosum. Partial response to treatment with cyclosporine. Note the persistent inflammation and evidence of healing ulcerations with residual cribriform scarring. The pyoderma gangrenosum healed fully and remained quiescent while administered etanercept, but this young boy developed Takayasu's disease several years after onset of the pyoderma gangrenosum, despite ongoing inhibition of TNF-α activity.

anti-phospholipid antibodies)[230,231] have all been reported. Pyoderma gangrenosum can also be seen during adolescence in patients with PAPA syndrome, chronic recurrent multifocal osteomyelitis,[232] and SAPHO syndrome (synovitis, acne, pustulosis, hyperostosis, osteitis).[233] In children with the onset during infancy, Takayasu's disease is the most common association, and may occur years after the onset of the pyoderma gangrenosum.

Treatment of pyoderma gangrenosum involves use of systemic and topical antiinflammatory medications to promote wound healing and decrease pain, as well as a vigorous attempt to control the underlying disease. Debridement and other mechanical trauma may worsen the ulcerations and should be avoided. Systemic corticosteroids are usually the initial drug of choice. Cyclosporin or systemic tacrolimus,[234] TNF-α inhibitors (etanercept, adalimumab, infliximab),[235-239] dapsone, clofazimine, mycophenolate mofetil, and intravenous immunoglobulin[240] have been used successfully as steroid-sparing agents. Topical tacrolimus ointment applied a few times daily has improved ulcer healing;[241] intralesional steroid injections may be appropriate for adolescents.

Behçet syndrome

Behçet syndrome is a chronic multisystemic autoinflammatory disease characterized by recurrent oral and genital ulcerations and inflammatory disease of the eye.[242] Although onset in infants as young as 2 months of age has been noted, Behçet syndrome usually begins in patients between 10 and 45 years of age and has a predilection for males. Approximately 17% of cases begin before 17 years of age.[243] In general, the disease is less severe and more delayed in its full manifestation in pediatric patients.[244] Behçet syndrome has also been described in infants born to mothers with the disease. This form of the disorder, neonatal Behçet syndrome, is characterized by aphthous stomatitis and skin phenomena and generally disappears spontaneously by the time the infants reach the age of 6 months; rarely, affected neonates have severe, life-threatening complications.[245,246]

The pathomechanism for Behçet disease is not understood, although the majority of patients in several studies carry HLA-B51 alleles.[247] Some 15–45% of children have an affected family member, in contrast to 8% of adults.[243,248] The deposition of immunoreactants around blood vessels induced by cutaneous trauma appears to play a role.[249]

Cutaneous and oral lesions are the most common clinical features of pediatric Behçet disease.[250,248,251] Oral lesions, noted at some point in the course of virtually every affected child, are the initial manifestation in 60–80% of pediatric patients. The ulcerations begin as erythema and, within 1–2 days, become superficial erosions that range from smaller ulcerations, indistinguishable from aphthous stomatitis, to deeply punched-out necrotic ulcers on the lips, buccal mucosa, tongue (Fig. 25.28), and gingivae. They tend to appear in crops, have regular sharp edges, and vary from a few millimeters to a centimeter in diameter. The ulcer base is covered with a yellowish gray exudate, and the margin is surrounded by a red halo. Oral lesions generally persist for 7–14 days, heal without scarring, and recur at intervals varying from weeks to months. Features of Behçet syndrome and relapsing polychondritis have also been described as the *MAGIC syndrome* (mouth *and* genital ulcers with inflamed cartilage).

Genital ulcerations are seen in 60–80% of patients with Behçet syndrome, but are found less often in pediatric patients than in adults. They are found on the scrotum or base of the penis in males and the vulva and vagina of females (Fig. 25.29). They are similar in appearance to the oral ulcerations, but less painful and may be overlooked. Perianal ulcerations are less common, but have been noted more often in children than in adults (up to 30%) (Fig. 25.30). Genital ulcerations are usually deeper than oral ulcerations and may scar. As with oral ulcerations, they remit in 1–2 weeks and tend to recur.

Cutaneous lesions of Behçet syndrome present a varied picture. Seen in approximately 80% of affected children, they consist of folliculitis, papules, vesicles, pustules, pyoderma, acneiform lesions, furuncles, abscesses, ulcerations, erythema nodosum-like lesions,

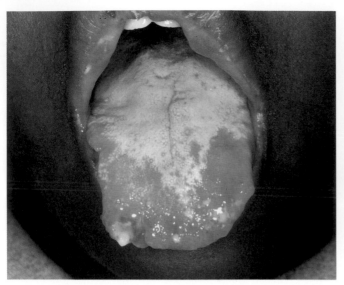

Figure 25.28 Behçet syndrome. Large oral ulceration of the tongue and buccal mucosae.

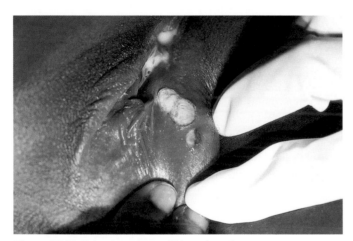

Figure 25.29 Behçet syndrome. Vulvar ulcerations.

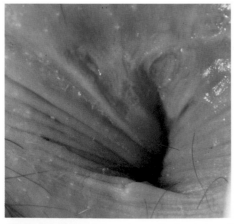

Figure 25.30 Behçet syndrome. Perianal ulcerations, shown here at the superior aspect.

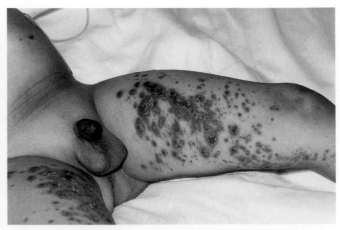

Figure 25.31 Behçet syndrome. Palpable purpura on the inner thighs and glans penis of this boy with Behçet syndrome. Superficial ulcerations were also noted on the penile shaft. Biopsy of affected areas showed leukocytoclastic vasculitis.

and palpable purpura (Fig. 25.31). Pathergy (the formation of an ulceration at an area of trauma, skin prick, or venipuncture) is typical.

Ocular lesions, seen in approximately 50% of affected children, are less common than in adults, but associated with a worse prognosis. Conjunctivitis and photophobia may be early ocular findings. Bilateral panuveitis is the most common manifestation (more than 80% of children with eye findings),[252] although posterior uveitis is found more often than anterior uveitis. Retinal vasculitis and retinitis occur in the majority of children with ocular features, and cataracts, maculopathy and optic atrophy have been described.

Fever and constitutional symptoms are variable. Musculoskeletal complaints, especially arthralgia and arthritis, are found in up to 75% of affected children. Gastrointestinal complaints are more common in children than in adults. They range from vague abdominal pain (up to 50%) and anorexia to diarrhea and hemorrhagic colitis. Central nervous system involvement, often the most severe prognostic feature of this disorder, is seen in 20–50% of patients. Renal involvement, an uncommon complication, may be seen with a spectrum ranging from asymptomatic abnormalities detected on urinalysis to a rapidly progressive glomerulonephritis and nephrosis. Other unusual findings in children include recurrent thrombophlebitis, pericarditis, orchitis, and epididymitis.

The diagnosis of Behçet syndrome in a patient with the full triad of oral and genital ulcers and ocular inflammation is not difficult. Two or more major criteria (oral, genital, ocular, or cutaneous involvement) or a combination of major and minor criteria (vascular, neurologic, musculoskeletal, or intestinal); however, allow diagnosis. Although pathergy is common and a helpful criterion to the diagnosis, it may also be seen in children with pyoderma gangrenosum, leukemia, and bowel bypass syndrome (see Ch. 20); a negative pathergy test does not rule out the diagnosis. Biopsy is usually not helpful.

Treatment of the aphthous ulcers with potent topical or intralesional corticosteroids, topical application of tacrolimus, oral rinses with elixir of diphenhydramine, or application of 2% viscous lidocaine can give symptomatic relief. For mucocutaneous ulcerations, colchicine is often helpful. Therapy is begun with a dosage of 0.6 mg twice daily for the first week. If the patient has no nausea, vomiting, or diarrhea, the dosage can be increased to three times a day, but colchicine is poorly tolerated by most pediatric patients. Thalidomide 50–100 mg once weekly to once daily has also led to improvement, but its use is limited by constipation, fatigue, and

Table 25.8 Cutaneous signs of anorexia nervosa and bulimia nervosa
Xerosis
Generalized pruritus
Loss of subcutaneous fat
Carotenemia
Acne
Petechiae and purpura
Edema, especially pretibial and pedal
Calluses on the dorsum of the hand (Russell's sign)
Other self-inflicted injuries
Poor wound healing
Pellagra
Scurvy
Seborrheic dermatitis

Acral changes
   Periungual erythema
   Acrocyanosis
   Acral coldness
   Perniosis

Oral changes
   Cheilitis/perlèche
   Aphthous stomatitis
   Gum recession
   Enamel erosion and dental caries

Hair changes
   Telogen effluvium
   Increased lanugo-like body hair
   Dry hair

Brittle, dystrophic nails
Enlarged parotid and salivary glands (full cheeks despite malnutrition)

peripheral neuropathy, which may be irreversible. Dapsone can also be helpful, especially in children with recurrent oral ulcerations. In severe cases, corticosteroids, alone or in combination with immunosuppressive agents such as methotrexate, cyclosporine, cyclophosphamide, chlorambucil, or azathioprine, currently appear to be the treatment of choice. Inhibitors of tumor necrosis factor-α[253–255] and IL-1[256] have also been used successfully. The overall mortality of Behçet disease in children is 3%; death usually results from large vessel vasculopathy (aneurysm, thrombosis), intestinal perforation, central nervous system involvement, or a complication of therapy.

Anorexia nervosa and bulimia

Anorexia nervosa and bulimia nervosa are severe disorders associated with potentially serious medical complications (Table 25.8).[257,258] Anorexia nervosa occurs in up to 3% of pubertal females and, less commonly in prepubertal females or males. In both disorders, patients have an intense preoccupation with food and irrational concern about gaining weight. Bulimic patients tend to binge eat and attempt to lose weight by vomiting and abusing laxatives, diuretics, diet pills, or emetics. The cutaneous features, which reflect endocrinologic changes and malnutrition, usually occur when the body mass index drops to <16 kg/m². [259,260] Affected individuals often show self-induced lesions as well, particularly the characteristic superficial ulcerations and hyperpigmented calluses or scars on the dorsal aspect of the second and third fingers (Russell's sign), the result of repeated abrasion of the skin against the maxillary incisors during forced emesis. Other emesis-associated complications include recurrent sore throats, hoarse voice, and dental erosions. Because of the potential severity of these disorders, it is important that physicians recognize the early signs and symptoms, particularly in view of the fact that patients tend to deny their illness or minimize the severity of their symptoms. The cutaneous manifestations are reversible when weight is gained. Many patients respond well to the combination of antidepressant and cognitive-behavioral therapy.

Key References

The complete list of 260 references for this chapter is available online at: **www.expertconsult.com.**
See inside cover for registration details.

Auletta JJ, Cooke KR. Bone marrow transplantation: new approaches to immunosuppression and management of acute graft-versus-host disease. *Curr Opin Pediatr.* 2009;21:30–38.

Baird K, Cooke K, Schultz KR. Chronic graft-versus-host disease (GVHD) in children. *Pediatr Clin North Am.* 2010;57:297–322.

Dinarello CA. Interleukin-1beta and the autoinflammatory diseases. *N Engl J Med.* 2009;360:2467–2470.

Dinauer MC. Disorders of neutrophil function: an overview. *Methods Mol Biol.* 2007;412:489–504.

Farasat S, Aksentijevich I, Toro JR. Autoinflammatory diseases: clinical and genetic advances. *Arch Dermatol.* 2008;144:392–402.

Gattorno M, Federici S, Pelagatti MA, et al. Diagnosis and management of autoinflammatory diseases in childhood. *J Clin Immunol.* 2008;28(Suppl 1):S73–S83.

Notarangelo LD, Fischer A, Geha RS, et al. International Union of Immunological Societies Expert Committee on Primary Immunodeficiencies: Primary immunodeficiencies. *J Allergy Clin Immunol.* 2009;124:1161–1178.

Ratzinger G, Sepp N, Vogetseder W, Tilg H. Cheilitis granulomatosa and Melkersson-Rosenthal syndrome: evaluation of gastrointestinal involvement and therapeutic regimens in a series of 14 patients. *J Eur Acad Dermatol Venereol.* 2007;21:1065–1070.

Shetty AK, Gedalia A. Childhood sarcoidosis: A rare but fascinating disorder. *Pediatr Rheumatol Online J.* 2008;6:16.

Strumia R. Dermatologic signs in patients with eating disorders. *Am J Clin Dermatol.* 2005;6:165–173.

Wollina U. Pyoderma gangrenosum – a review. *Orphanet J Rare Dis.* 2007;2:19.

Abuse and Factitial Disorders

Child abuse

Child abuse is a broad term used to describe a spectrum of non-accidental trauma inflicted upon children. Kempe et al. are generally credited with emphasizing the prevalence and importance of this entity, when they coined the term 'battered child syndrome' in 1962.[1] This 'syndrome' has subsequently been expanded to include an array of childhood abuses, including physical abuse, sexual abuse, and neglect. Child abuse continues to be one of the most significant causes of childhood morbidity and mortality in the USA.[2] In one 10-year study of medical records submitted to the National Pediatric Trauma Registry, child abuse accounted for 10.6% of all blunt trauma to patients under 5 years of age.[2] Abused children tend to be younger, with the highest incidence seen in those under 3 years of age. High-risk groups include children with a history of prematurity, physical handicap, and behavioral problems. Factors which appear to be associated with an increased risk of abuse are summarized in Table 26.1.[3-5] Up to 75% of abuse may be missed in the acute care setting due to failure of recognition by medical professionals, and this may lead to lost opportunities to intervene.[6]

Various abusive patterns may be evident in families where abuse is an issue. These include parents who were the victims of abuse themselves, parents with emotional disturbances, stressful crises within the family unit (i.e., loss of job or financial distress), and lack of a close support network for the family (Table 26.1).[7] Recognition of abuse is vital, as the trauma tends to be repeated (an abused child has up to a 50% chance of being abused again), and the risk of future injury or death is high. Instances in which there is a delay in reporting the injury, in which the degree and type of injury are at variance with the history offered, or in which the parents are evasive or vague as to the cause of injury are all suspicious and should lead to consideration for an abuse investigation. In evaluating the child with possible abuse, a detailed history is the most important component of the assessment.[8] Vital details include the alleged mechanism of the injury, developmental history of the child, past medical history (especially of any disorders that may mimic abuse, such as coagulopathy or skin disorders), history of prior injuries, social history, and family history. A complete physical examination should be performed, and should include high-quality photography of cutaneous lesions.

Although abused children may exhibit multiple abnormalities on physical and radiographic examination, this section will focus primarily on the cutaneous stigmata.

Physical Abuse

Non-accidental injuries in children may take many forms, and often the skin reveals pathologic findings. Cutaneous trauma may be seen in the form of ecchymoses, burns, lacerations, bite marks, abrasions, underlying hematomas, pigmentary changes, and scars.

Ecchymoses (bruises) are the most common type of skin injury seen in abused children. Lesions on the hands and face, adult human bites, and lesions on the cheeks, mouth, lips, lower back, buttocks, or inner thighs are particularly suspect. Ecchymoses in various different stages of healing are more suggestive of abuse. Ecchymoses on padded areas (buttocks, torso, face, and genitalia) or uncommonly injured areas (earlobe, neck, lip, philtrum) are more concerning for possible abuse.[3] In a study of discriminating bruising characteristics in abused children, characteristics that were more predictive of abuse included bruising on the torso, ear (Fig. 26.1) or neck (in a child ≤4 years of age, termed the 'TEN region') and bruising in any region in an infant <4 months of age.[6] Abuse-associated bruising should be differentiated from accidental bruising, which is more common in ambulatory children, and occurs most commonly over bony prominences such as the forehead and shins.[3] Any bruising in the non-cruising infant under 9 months of age should raise significant suspicion for abuse. There are many potential mimics and non-abuse-related causes of ecchymoses, including Mongolian spots, hypersensitivity vasculitis (i.e. Henoch–Schonlein purpura or acute hemorrhagic edema of infancy), Ehlers–Danlos syndrome, vascular malformations, infantile hemangiomas, inks or dyes, and bleeding disorders.

The configurations of lesions in battered children are morphologically similar to the items or methods used to inflict the trauma, and may be useful in the abuse investigation. Multiple evenly spaced markings (Fig. 26.2) or curvilinear loops and arcuate lesions (Figs 26.3, 26.4), as may be induced by lashing with a doubled-over belt or electric cord, are typical of these trauma-induced lesions. They are usually ecchymotic, but they may also present as abrasions, lacerations, or hyperpigmentation.

Belt buckle imprints (ecchymotic or hyperpigmented) may result from intentional trauma with these items. Adjacent, small ecchymotic macules (Fig. 26.5) are typical of pinch marks. Shackles on the wrists, ankles, or neck leave easily identifiable rings, which are red if fresh and hyperpigmented if longstanding. Ligature marks on the neck or extremities and grab or slap marks (fingertip bruises, Fig. 26.6) on the shoulders, hands, or legs are particularly suspicious and highly suggestive of deliberate trauma. Slapping injuries result in linear bruising, which outlines the blunt objects (fingers) because of the breakage of superficial skin capillaries. Çao gio ('coining') and cupping, Asian customs believed to treat a variety of ailments, may be confused with ecchymotic lesions of abuse and must be appropriately recognized (see below).

Burns are a very common type of injury seen in abused children, and result from thermal injury to the skin and subcutaneous tissues. Burns can also be electrical, chemical or radiant in nature. Thermal burns may be inflicted with cigarettes, matches, scalding liquid, or other heated objects and are frequently mistaken for lesions of impetigo. Cigarette burns present as 8–10 mm, deep, round crusted ulcers that heal with scars and pigmentary changes (Figs 26.7, 26.8). Although they may be accidental, multiple lesions with deeper involvement and significant scarring are highly indicative of abuse,

Table 26.1 Factors associated with an increased risk of child abuse

Child	Parent	Both
Prematurity	Partner violence within the family	Neighborhood factors
Mental retardation	History of past abuse or neglect	Crime
Disability	Substance abuse	Poor recreational activities
Congenital anomalies	Mental illness	Poverty
Clinging	Unemployment	Poor parent–child relationships
Excessive or inconsolable crying	Lack of external support	Substandard housing
Expectations inconsistent with normal child development	African-American child in single-parent household	Poor impulse control
Toilet training or toilet accidents (pre-schoolers)	Adolescent in age	Rely on children for emotional support

Adapted from Swerdlin et al. (2007);[3] Peck and Priolo-Kapel (2002);[4] Dubowitz and Bennett (2007).[5]

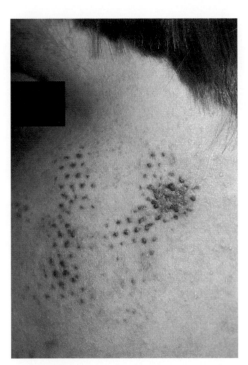

Figure 26.2 Child abuse. The evenly spaced nature of these markings should arouse suspicion for an outside source of these skin findings.

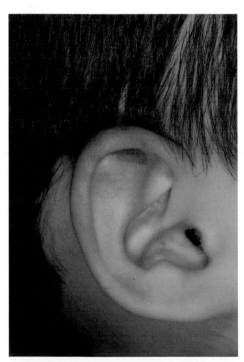

Figure 26.1 Child abuse. Ecchymoses in certain locations, like this lesion noted on the superior ear, are more suggestive on non-accidental trauma. Of ear ecchymoses, the most concerning location for abuse-associated bruising is the earlobe.

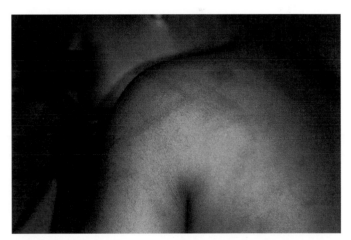

Figure 26.3 Child abuse. These multiple, overlapping, linear and hyperpigmented patches were the result of post-inflammatory changes at sites of whipping.

as this pattern is usually suggestive of prolonged contact. The differential diagnosis of cigarette burns includes ecthyma, cellulitis, herpes, and bullous impetigo.

Branding injuries occur after prolonged contact with a heated object, and they may take on the shape of the object used to inflict them. Burns inflicted with a hot iron (Figs 26.9, 26.10) reveal differing pigmentary changes between the heated metal surface and the steam vent openings. Figures 26.11 and 26.12 demonstrate burns inflicted by a heated metal spoon, with the shape of the spoon readily visible in the resultant skin markings. Dunking scald injuries are most commonly seen in infants and toddlers, and present with a characteristic 'stocking and glove' distribution on the extremities, or with 'doughnut-type sparing', which occurs when the child's buttocks are held against the cooler tub or basin.[7] These patients present with erythema and blistering indicative of a 2nd-degree burn. It should be remembered that children will not stay in contact with a hot surface or scalding hot water. They normally test the heat of the water and step into the bath with one foot at a time. Accordingly, symmetrical burns on the feet, the

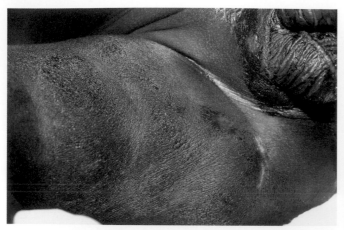

Figure 26.4 Child abuse. These burns, the result of intentional contact with a hot wire, presented as curvilinear erosions.

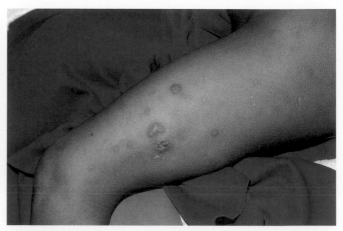

Figure 26.7 Cigarette burns. This patient has evidence of fresh lesions (erythematous eroded plaque) and older lesions, in the forms of hyperpigmentation and scars.

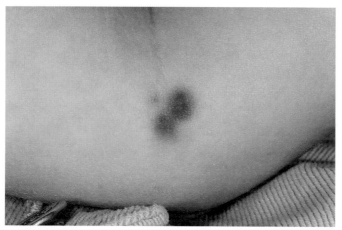

Figure 26.5 Child abuse. Adjacent, ecchymotic macules are typical of pinch marks.

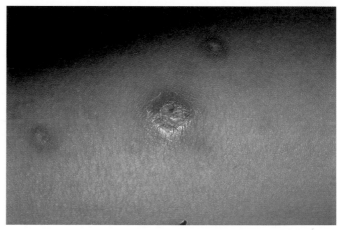

Figure 26.8 Cigarette burns. These burns demonstrate the classic abuse finding of lesions in various stages of healing.

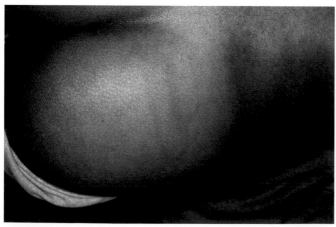

Figure 26.6 Child abuse. Fingertip bruises present as hyperpigmented patches in the shape of fingers, at sites of excessive slapping or spanking.

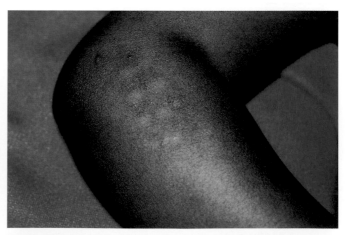

Figure 26.9 Iron burn. This hyperpigmented patch is studded with evenly spaced, normally pigmented regions, which correlate with sites of steam vent openings.

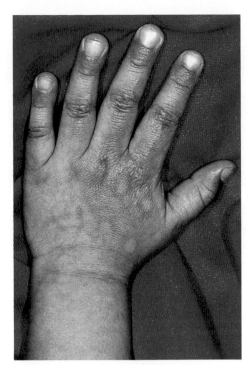

Figure 26.10 Iron burn. This child's hand reveals the classic hyperpigmentation with evenly spaced macules of sparing, which occur at sites of steam vent openings.

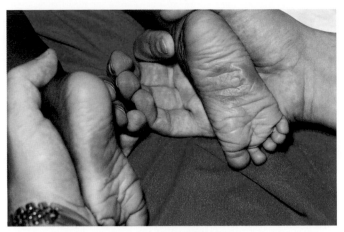

Figure 26.12 Child abuse. The same infant as that shown in Figure 26.11 had these blistering burns on the plantar surfaces. They were inflicted with a heated metal spoon.

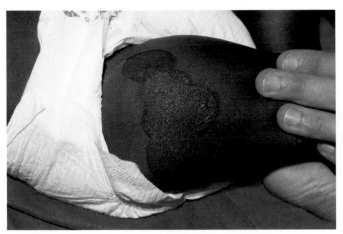

Figure 26.11 Child abuse. This infant had burns inflicted with a heated, metal spoon. Note the overlapping, oval-shaped patches of pigmentation and crusting.

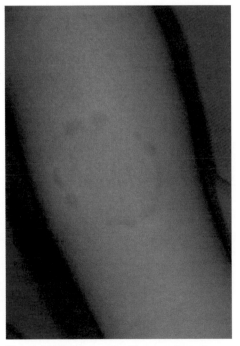

Figure 26.13 Bite marks. These erythematous, petechial macules and papules revealed a dental arch width of 2.5 cm, more consistent with a child's bite. There were no other clinical features of (or concerns for) child abuse in this 2-year-old female.

buttocks, or the hands require careful investigation and evaluation. Stun gun injuries have been observed in the setting of physical abuse, and present as evenly spaced (4–5 cm apart), erythematous to hypopigmented papules and macules, usually occurring in multiples.[9]

Bite marks are another pathognomonic sign of non-accidental trauma. The human bite is differentiated easily from the dog bite by the contusing and crushing characteristics of the latter; dog bites rip and tear the flesh. It is important to distinguish adult from child bite marks, since the former is more likely to be seen in an abusive setting. Adult bites are characterized by a dental arch width >4 cm[3], whereas the markings of a child's bite tend to be significantly narrower (Fig. 26.13). The discovery of one bite mark necessitates a thorough examination of the child's entire body for further evidence of bites or other findings of abuse.[10] Traumatic alopecia may occur when the parent pulls the child's hair, since the hair provides a readily-accessible 'handle' that can be used to grab or jerk at the child. The resultant alopecia is an irregularly bordered area that may reveal hemorrhage, hair breakage, and scalp tenderness.

Oral injuries are another common feature in abused children. Findings may include tears of the labial or lingual frenulum, caused by a blow to the mouth, forced feeding, or forced oral sex.[10] Other manifestations include burns or lacerations of the gingivae, tongue, or palate from overly hot food or utensils. Teeth may also be involved, including fracture, displacement, or avulsion.

A difficult situation arises when the physician observes recent skin injuries in the child who does not present for trauma. In one large series, 76% of children between 9 months and 17 years of age seen in a clinic for a reason other than trauma were found to have at least one recent skin injury. Injuries were more prevalent in the summer (in regions with a temperate climate) and were most frequently observed on the shins and knees.[11] The authors offered certain unusual characteristics that may suggest a greater risk of physical abuse (or bleeding disorder), and these include uncommon location, >15 injuries, bruises in a child <9 months of age, numerous injuries elsewhere than the lower limbs, numerous injuries in cold seasons in a temperate climate, and injuries other than bruises, abrasions, or scratches.[11] In another series of infants aged 6–12 months, bruises were noted to be generally limited to the face, head, or shins, and there was a direct correlation between the number of bruises and increases in mobility.[12] In this group, the prevalence rate of bruises was 12%, and they were most often solitary.

Sexual Abuse

Sexual abuse has been defined in many ways, including 'any exploitative sexual activity between a child and an adult' or 'any sexual activity that a child cannot comprehend or give consent to, or that violates the law' or 'when a child is engaged in sexual activities that he/she cannot comprehend, for which he/she is developmentally unprepared and cannot give consent, and/or that violates the law or social taboos of society'.[7,13,14] Some studies have suggested that 1% of children experience some form of sexual abuse each year.[14] It is important to realize that boys may be the victims of sexual abuse as well as girls, although the former tend to be less likely to disclose abuse, and thus it is likely underreported, underrecognized, and undertreated.[15] Adolescents are the perpetrators in up to 20% of reported cases of sexual abuse, and while women may be perpetrators, these allegations are significantly less likely than those involving males.[14] Up to one-fifth of adolescents who regularly use the internet have been solicited by strangers for sex through the internet.

The perpetrator of childhood sexual abuse is often well known, or related, to the victim. Activities involved in sexual abuse may include oral-genital, genital, or anal contact by or to the child, as well as non-physical abuses such as voyeurism, exhibitionism, or involvement of the child in pornography.[14] Sexual abuse should be differentiated from 'sexual play' or age-appropriate exploratory behavior. The child who has been sexually abused may present with a variety of features, including behavioral changes, school difficulties, regression, depression, eating disturbance, sexual acting-out, symptoms referable to the genitourinary or gastrointestinal tracts, pregnancy, various somatic complaints, or a sexually transmitted disease.[13]

Mucocutaneous findings suggestive of sexual abuse are listed in Table 26.2. However, it should be noted that many children who have been sexually abused in the past may have a relatively normal physical examination. Many prepubescent patients seen in emergency departments for a sexual abuse evaluation have not experienced recent abuse, in distinction to adolescents, who often present after the acute assault.[16] A normal anogenital examination, therefore, does not preclude prior sexual abuse. The physical examination should be most focused on areas involved in sexual activity, including the mouth, breasts, genitals, perineum, buttocks, and anus. In females, a more thorough examination of the medial

Table 26.2 Mucocutaneous findings in childhood sexual abuse

Finding	Comment
Hymenal changes	Attenuated hymenal tissue, disruption of hymenal contour; acute laceration or ecchymosis
Anal area changes	Boys and girls; changes in anal tone, hematomas, abrasions, lacerations; scarring, skin tags; and dilation
Fossa navicularis scarring	
Posterior fourchette scarring	
Inner thigh changes	Abrasions, ecchymosis (concerning, but not diagnostic)
Labia minora changes	Scarring or tears (concerning, but not diagnostic)
Other genital injuries	Circumferential injuries to penile shaft or glans penis
Oral injuries or diseases	Unexplained erythema or petechiae of the palate; oral or perioral gonorrhea or syphilis (pathognomonic for sexual abuse in the prepubertal child)

Table 26.3 Implications of STDs and clinical findings for the diagnosis of childhood sexual abuse

STD or finding	Implication for abuse	Suggested action
Gonorrhea[a]	Diagnostic	Report
Syphilis[a]	Diagnostic	Report
HIV infection[a,b]	Diagnostic	Report
Chlamydia[a]	Diagnostic	Report
Trichomoniasis	Highly suspicious	Report
Anogenital warts[a,c]	Suspicious	Report
Genital herpes[d]	Suspicious	Report
Bacterial vaginosis	Inconclusive	Clinical follow-up
Presence of sperm, semen or acid phosphatase	Diagnostic	Report
Pregnancy	Diagnostic	Report

STD, sexually transmitted disease. [a]If not perinatally acquired. [b]If not transfusion acquired. [c]Not uncommonly transmitted via benign mode; see discussion in Ch. 15. [d]Unless due to autoinoculation.

(Adapted from Swerdlin et al. 2007[3] and Kellogg et al. 2005).[14]

thighs, labia majora and minora, clitoris, urethra, hymen and hymenal opening, fossa navicularis, and posterior fourchette should be included.[14] In males, the thighs, penis, and scrotum should be closely examined.

Examinations for sexually transmitted diseases (STDs) should be performed when indicated. Factors to be considered include the possibility of oral, genital, or rectal contact and the child's symptomatology. Table 26.3 summarizes the implications of various STDs and clinical findings for reporting childhood sexual abuse. Anogenital warts, which may be sexually transmitted in children, are often the result of benign, non-sexual transmission, especially in infants and young toddlers (see Ch. 15). Non-sexual modes of transmission include perinatal transmission, autoinoculation (child with common warts spreads them via skin-to-skin contact to his/her own anogenital region), heteroinoculation (caregiver with common warts spreads them via skin-to-skin contact to anogenital region of child), and possibly indirect spread from fomites. Importantly, molluscum contagiosum lesions involving the anogenital region in children are nearly always a result of benign transmission or autoinoculation, and should not be considered as indicative of childhood sexual abuse. The details of the evaluation, treatment, and reporting of childhood sexual abuse are beyond the scope of this chapter, but are well documented elsewhere.

Neglect

Neglect may be either physical, emotional, or both. The former results when a parent or caretaker fails to provide necessities of life, such as food, appropriate supervision shelter, clothing, or medical care.[7] General findings in the neglected child may include lack of immunizations, poor nutrition and growth, and developmental or behavioral problems. Potential cutaneous findings include poor hygiene, untreated injuries, infections, and infestations. Severe or extensive sunburns (Fig. 26.14) may be a sign of parental neglect, although several conditions and medications may make children more sensitive to ultraviolet light. It is important to bear these in mind whenever the possibility of neglect or abuse is being considered.

Physical neglect may also present as dental neglect, which is defined as the 'willful failure of parent or guardian to seek and follow through with treatment necessary to ensure a level of oral health essential for adequate function and freedom from pain and infection'.[17] Findings may include dental caries, periodontal disease (Fig. 26.15), and other oral conditions. When left untreated, these conditions can lead to significant pain, infection, and loss of function.[17]

Factitial skin disorders

Factitial skin disorders are a group of disorders characterized by self-inflicted lesions or artifacts on the skin. The individual cases vary in terms of the visible lesions and the underlying motive that causes the patient to act. These disorders may be associated with a variety of psychopathologic conditions, and co-management with a psychologist or psychiatrist is often necessary. Factitial skin disorders fall under the rubric of psychodermatologic conditions or psychocutaneous disorders, although these two classifications also include dermatologic conditions with secondary psychiatric sequelae (i.e., alopecia areata or albinism), and dermatologic conditions that may be aggravated by psychologic factors (i.e., acne, atopic dermatitis, psoriasis).[18] Diagnosis of factitial skin disorders is often delayed, and management is challenging, requiring the development of a therapeutic alliance between the physician and patient, and treatment of any underlying psychiatric comorbid conditions. The diagnosis of factitial skin disorders largely remains a diagnosis of exclusion.[19] Treatment often requires a multidisciplinary approach, which may include the pediatrician, dermatologist, psychologist, and/or psychiatrist.

Factitious Dermatitis/Dermatitis Artefacta

Factitious dermatitis is caused by a conscious or subconscious behavior driven in response to internal psychologic stressors, and not associated with secondary gain.[19] Dermatitis artefacta (DA), in distinction, is a disorder in which the skin is the purposeful target of self-inflicted injuries. In DA, the patient creates the lesions on the skin in order to satisfy a psychological need (of which he or she is often not consciously aware), and in the pursuit of secondary gain.[19,20] There appears to be the need to satisfy an internal emotional necessity – the need to be cared for.[21,22] The desired gain may be obvious or may not be readily evident. DA occurs predominantly among women, with a wide range in the quoted ratios of women to men, from 3:1 to 20:1.[21] It may have its onset at any time, although it most commonly occurs in teenagers and young adults. Several comorbid conditions may be present, including borderline personality disorder, disorders of impulse control, depression, anxiety, obsessive-compulsive disorder, and psychotic disorders.[18,20,22,23] It may also result from a transient maladaptive response to a recent psychosocial stressor(s). A past and/or current history of sexual abuse is common.[21,24] Patients with DA often have a close connection (either personally or through a close family member) with the healthcare field, and many have an 'encyclopedic' grasp of medical knowledge and/or terminology.

DA has a variety of presentation patterns. Importantly, the cutaneous features are often only one facet of the entire picture, as these

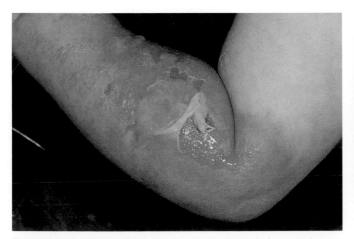

Figure 26.14 Neglect. This toddler came to the clinic for a routine eczema follow-up, and was noted to have this blistering sunburn.

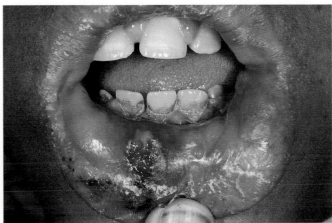

Figure 26.15 Neglect. Dental neglect in this young boy presented as dental caries, periodontal disease, and aphthous ulcerations of the labial surfaces. This lesion was also culture-positive for herpes simplex virus.

patients frequently have involvement of other organ systems and have visited numerous medical specialists for other bizarre or unexplained symptoms. The skin lesions themselves may consist of purpura, excoriations, abrasions, crusting, necrosis, blisters, ulcers, erythema, nodules, or scarring. The lesions usually lack features of recognizable dermatoses. Notable features often include linearity, geometric arrangements, and sharp demarcation from the surrounding normal skin. The face, upper trunk, and upper extremities are the sites most often involved, and there is notable sparing of areas outside of the patients' reach (i.e., the middle back). There is often a prominence on one side, depending on the handedness of the patient. The lips may also be involved, presenting usually as persistent bleeding and crusting.[25] The lesions are often fully formed, and all in a similar stage of development. This inability of the patient to give details of evolutionary change has been termed 'hollow history' and is quite typical of DA.[20,21,26] Reported modes of injury include rubbing, scratching, picking, cutting, gouging, pinching, puncturing, biting, sucking, applying suction, applying heat, dye or caustic substances, and injecting caustic materials or bodily secretions.[18,20] The differential diagnosis may be broad, and depends on the nature of the inflicted injury. A clue to the diagnosis of DA is indifference or lack of concern on the part of the patient, who will often deny pain or discomfort despite the impressive physical findings.[19]

Factitious purpura, which is a form of mechanical purpura, may result in a detailed, lengthy investigation for other medical causes before the diagnosis is entertained. Patients may be entirely unaware that they are causing the skin lesions. A common form of factitious purpura is that caused by sucking air from a drinking glass placed over the chin and lower lip, resulting in a well-demarcated, circular area of purpura (Fig. 26.16).[27] Other forms may be caused by a variety of instruments or objects, with the purpuric lesions corresponding to the patterns of those objects. Figures 26.17–26.29 depict some various presentations of dermatitis artefacta.

Malingering may present with lesions similar to DA, but in this setting the patient self-inflicts injury consciously, often with a secondary gain. These patients may exhibit 'la belle indifférence', which refers to an apparent lack of frustration, despite the recurrent nature of their symptomatology.

Neurotic (psychogenic) excoriations are lesions self-inflicted by patients who have an irresistible urge to manipulate their skin.[22] It is often related to mood disorders, anxiety disorder, drug abuse or obsessive-compulsive disorder.[28] The cycle of neurotic excoriations may begin with a true physical stimulus, such as pruritus, or a skin lesion or irregularity, such as an acne papule. The latter is referred to as *acne excoriée des jeunes filles*, and occurs when even mild acne lesions (especially those on the forehead) are squeezed or excoriated (Fig. 26.30). This behavior may result in permanent scarring, and although some patients may fulfill diagnostic criteria for

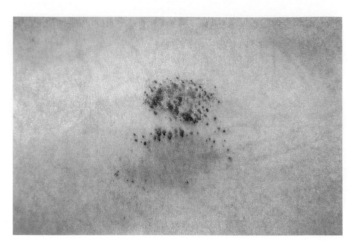

Figure 26.17 Dermatitis artefacta. Well-demarcated abrasions and hyperpigmentation in a 10-year-old male.

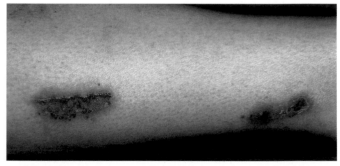

Figure 26.18 Dermatitis artefacta. Sharply-demarcated, eroded, erythematous plaques from chronic rubbing.

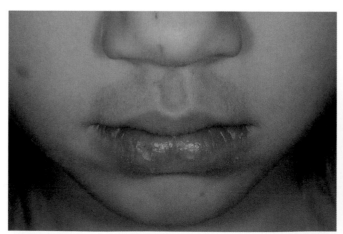

Figure 26.16 Suction purpura. This well-demarcated, petechial patch over the upper lip and philtrum area arose after this young girl repeatedly sucked air from a cup placed over her lips and upper chin.

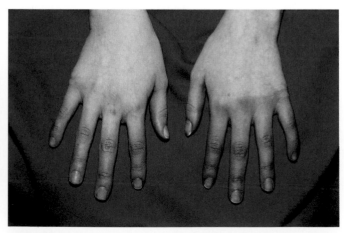

Figure 26.19 Dermatitis artefacta. This localized discoloration of the hand had been caused by intentional exposure to fabric dye.

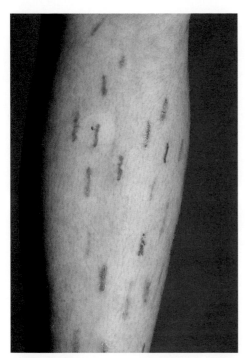

Figure 26.20 Dermatitis artefacta. These evenly spaced, linear, hemorrhagic markings were self-induced.

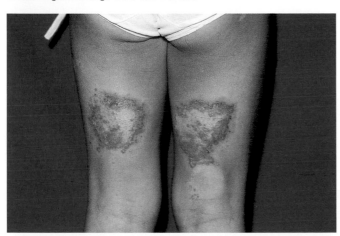

Figure 26.21 Dermatitis artefacta. This patient with underlying atopic dermatitis had acute worsening in these areas, which ultimately were found to be self-inflicted.

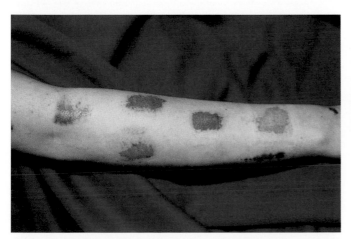

Figure 26.22 Dermatitis artefacta. These well-demarcated erosions are notable for their even spacing and sharp, linear borders.

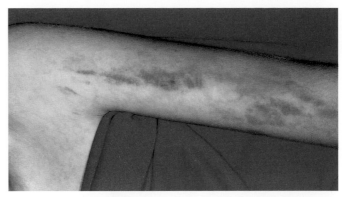

Figure 26.23 Dermatitis artefacta. Linear purpura is a common finding in factitial skin disease.

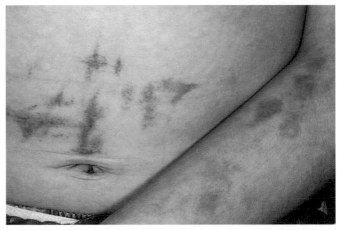

Figure 26.24 Dermatitis artefacta. These linear and stellate, purpuric patches were present in the same patient shown in Figure 26.23. Note the associated resolving purpuric areas located on the arm.

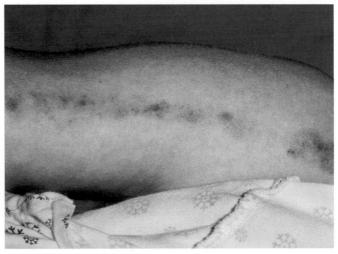

Figure 26.25 Dermatitis artefacta. Linear purpura was present on both arms of this school-age boy.

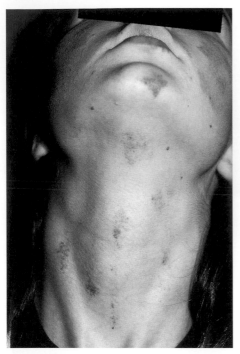

Figure 26.26 Dermatitis artefacta. Irregularly shaped purpuric patches of the neck and face.

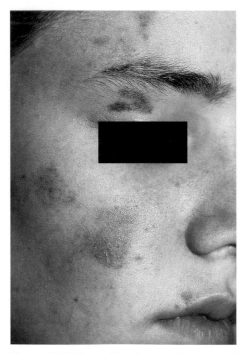

Figure 26.27 Dermatitis artefacta. Purpuric patches with geometric and linear borders in the same patient shown in Figure 26.26.

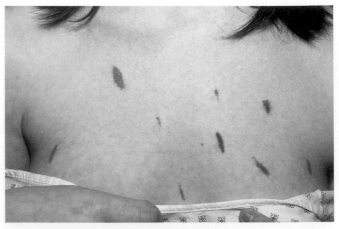

Figure 26.28 Dermatitis artefacta. Well-demarcated, linear purpuric macules.

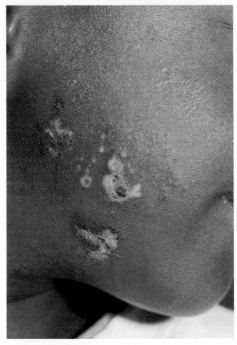

Figure 26.29 Dermatitis artefacta. These eroded and scarred plaques reveal irregular borders consistent with self-manipulation.

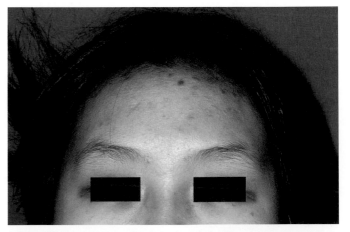

Figure 26.30 Acne excoriée. Acne papules with erosions, scarring, and hyperpigmentation are typical of this condition.

obsessive-compulsive disorder, many do not. Patients with neurotic excoriations usually acknowledge the behavior, and may have any of several comorbid conditions, including obsessive-compulsive disorder, a personality disorder, anxiety, or depression. The picking activity is performed most often with the fingernails, although some patients may use an auxiliary tool, such as the point of a knife.[20] The resultant skin lesions reveal erythema, erosions, weeping, crusting (Fig. 26.31), pigmentation, or scarring. There is often a notable sparing of the upper lateral back areas.

Prurigo nodularis (PN) is a condition characterized by firm papules and nodules with pruritus. It most typically presents with discrete, 2–10 mm firm lichenified, hyperkeratotic papules which may reveal some central excoriation or crusting (Fig. 26.32). Common locations include the extremities and the upper and lower back, often

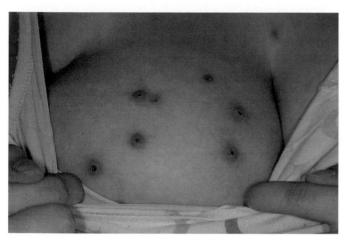

Figure 26.31 Neurotic excoriation. This adolescent female acknowledged her repeated picking and scratching, which resulted in these erythematous, eroded and crusted papules on her bilateral breasts.

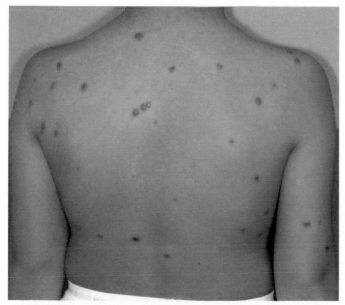

Figure 26.32 Prurigo nodularis. This boy had numerous, discrete, lichenified firm papules on his upper and lower back, forearms and lower extremities. Note the zone of sparing over the middle back, an area which was difficult for him to reach.

with a zone of sparing noted in the middle back, which is a difficult location for the patient to reach. The cause of PN is unknown. It has been seen in a variety of settings, including bite reactions, atopic dermatitis (see Fig. 3.14), allergic contact dermatitis, folliculitis, psychosocial disorders, thyroid disease, malignancy, iron-deficiency anemia, kidney failure, gluten sensitivity, obstructive biliary disease and infections (including hepatitis, HIV and mycobacteria).[29,30] If generalized pruritus is reported by the patient, a laboratory investigation (including blood counts, kidney and liver function tests, and thyroid and parathyroid screening) may be warranted.[30] Skin biopsy may be useful if infection is included in the differential diagnosis. Treatment for PN is notoriously difficult, and may include topical corticosteroids or calcineurin inhibitors (i.e. tacrolimus and pimecrolimus), topical capsaicin, ultraviolet phototherapy and antihistamines. In severe cases, systemic agents such as cyclosporine, thalidomide, naltrexone and etretinate have been used.[29,30] Psychological intervention is frequently necessary.

Delusions of Parasitosis

A delusional disorder is characterized by adherence to a possible, yet implausible, belief for which there is no supportive objective evidence.[31] Monosymptomatic hypochondriacal psychosis (MHP) is characterized by a delusional ideation that revolves around one concern, in contrast to schizophrenia, in which case patients have multifunctional deficits in mental functioning.[32] The most common type of MHP with dermatologic relevance is delusions of parasitosis. This disorder, also known as delusional infestation, is characterized by the conviction of an individual that he or she is infested with parasites, in the absence of any objective evidence. Patients with this disorder, most often older adult females, complain of having the sensation of crawling, burrowing, and biting insects or worms on their skin. They may resort to self-mutilation in an attempt to remove the offending arthropods.

Patients with delusions of parasitosis often attend the clinic with spurious samples of the 'parasite' which, when microscopically examined, turns out to be lint, skin cells, scabs, or other debris. Skin findings may include excoriations, lichenification, pigmentary alteration, and scarring. Treatment of the disorder is challenging, with the antipsychotic medication pimozide being the most often utilized pharmacologic agent. Prior to therapy, however, exclusion of true skin disorders (i.e., scabies, dermatitis herpetiformis, or insect bite reactions) should be considered.[33]

Morgellons disease is a term that initially began to surface in 2002, and whose name was taken from the label, given in 1674 in France by Sir Thomas Browne, to children who presented with hair-like skin extrusions and sensations of movement.[34] This terminology provides an alternative to the decades-old nomenclature of delusions of parasitosis, although many consider the two disorders to be part of the same spectrum.[35–38] Patients with Morgellons disease complain of cutaneous dysesthesias, resulting in skin manipulations in an effort to extract the 'organisms' or foreign materials. They may experience itching or crawling sensations, and many report the sense that bugs or worms are stinging or biting them. The examination findings may include excoriations, ulcers, lichenification and prurigo nodules. Patients with Morgellons disease, much like those with delusions of parasitosis, may bring samples or debris in bottles, jars or bags to the appointment. Examination of these contents often reveals lint, hair, debris, fuzz, dead skin, material fibers or bugs.[36] Management of the condition is difficult, and includes establishing good rapport, excluding skin or other organic conditions, consideration for the use of psychotropic medications, and treatment of secondary skin infection, when necessary. Long-term antibiotic therapy has reportedly been useful.[37,39] Collaborative care with a psychiatrist or a psychodermatology clinic is strongly encouraged for both Morgellons disease and patients with delusions of parasitosis.

Obsessive-Compulsive Disorders

Obsessive-compulsive disorder (OCD) is characterized by the presence of obsessions (recurrent thoughts or images experienced as intrusive or senseless) or compulsions (repetitive, intentional behaviors performed to diminish discomfort or future harm, and felt to be unreasonable or excessive).[40] The essential feature required for diagnosis in the *Diagnostic and Statistical Manual of Mental Disorders [DSM] IV* is that the obsessions or compulsions are severe enough to be time consuming or cause impairment in relationships, employment, school, or social activities.

The expression of OCD may take the form of a dermatologic disorder. Entities that may fall into this spectrum are listed in Table 26.4. Clinical features that may suggest an OCD-related spectrum disorder include a heightened concern for cleanliness, fear of contamination, excessive worry about life-threatening or sexually transmitted diseases, inappropriate concerns about body odor, and worries regarding an unattractive appearance or hair loss.[18,41]

OCD often begins in childhood or early adulthood, and most patients have a waxing and waning course. Comorbid conditions are common, including depression and anxiety disorders. Childhood OCD may be associated with Tourette's syndrome, tics, family history of OCD, developmental delay, and hyperactivity.[42] The most common cutaneous presentations are trichotillomania (Ch. 7), onychophagia, and acne excoriée (Ch. 8).[41] Importantly, patients with pediatric OCD experience chronicity and intractability of the disorder, despite multiple interventions.[43]

Body dysmorphic disorder (BDD) is defined as preoccupation with an imagined defect in appearance. BDD, which falls into the OCD spectrum of disorders, may present with dermatologic symptoms or concerns. These include concerns about an unattractive appearance, acne scarring, hair loss, early skin aging, hirsutism, greasy skin, body odor, or blushing.[41,44] Patients with BDD may spend many hours a day worrying about their obsession and visually inspecting the 'abnormality', which may impact on social and professional functioning.

Treatment of OCD spectrum disorders includes both behavioral and pharmacologic therapies, most notably the serotonin reuptake inhibitors.

Psychogenic Purpura/Gardner–Diamond Syndrome

Psychogenic purpura (autoerythrocyte sensitization syndrome, Gardner–Diamond syndrome) is a rare disorder characterized by recurrent episodes of painful ecchymoses (Fig. 26.33) in various locations. The patients are most often young adult females with emotional disturbances, and the lesions frequently occur after trauma, surgery, or severe emotional stress.[45,46] The individual lesions resolve over 2 weeks. Psychiatric associations include depression, OCD, hypochondriasis, hysterical and borderline personality disorders and anxiety.[45-47] Gardner and Diamond, in 1955, suggested that the disorder was associated with autosensitization of patients to their own blood.[48] Traditionally, the diagnosis was confirmed by intradermal injection of the patient's own erythrocytes, which may result in reproduction of the clinical lesions.

The skin lesions of Gardner–Diamond syndrome are often consistent with a factitial dermatosis, given their purpuric nature, irregular distribution, peculiar morphology, and erratic onset. However, confirmation of a self-inflicted process is often difficult, if not impossible. During the prodromal stage, nonspecific symptoms such as malaise and fatigue may be reported. The skin lesions develop rapidly following sensations of burning and stinging, and evolve over 1 or 2 days from erythematous to ecchymotic. They resolve over 7–10 days. Associated findings, such as hematuria, epistaxis or menorrhagia, are occasionally noted. Histologic evaluation of skin biopsy samples reveals nonspecific features, including perivascular inflammation (without frank vasculitis), erythrocyte extravasation and pigment deposition.[49] Avoidance of confrontation with the patient, establishment of rapport, and psychiatric evaluation and therapy are indicated. Psychotropic medications and hypnotherapy have occasionally been utilized.[49]

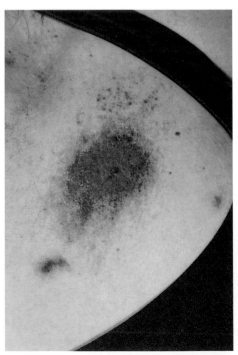

Figure 26.33 Psychogenic purpura. This young female, with a history of anxiety disorder, complained of recurrent, spontaneous ecchymoses. Examination revealed ecchymotic patches with superimposed abrasions.

Table 26.4 OCD and some possibly associated dermatologic conditions

Disorder	Chapter no. for details
Acne excoriée	8
Body dysmorphic disorder	Current
Irritant dermatitis (hand-washing)	3
Lichen simplex chronicus	3
Lip-licker's dermatitis	3
Neurotic (psychogenic) excoriations	Current
Onychophagia	7
Prurigo nodularis	3
Trichotillomania	7

OCD, obsessive-compulsive disorder.

Munchausen Syndrome and Munchausen Syndrome by Proxy

Munchausen syndrome is a form of factitious disorder characterized by dramatic presentations with factitious complaints, exaggerated lying, and 'physician shopping'. Patients have recurrent feigned symptoms, and often have borderline or antisocial personality types. Munchausen syndrome by proxy (MSBP, also known as pediatric symptom falsification) occurs when a parent or caregiver creates an illness in a child. It is a form of child abuse inflicted most often by the mother. The stereotype of a MSBP mother is one who works in the healthcare field, is estranged from the child's father, is quite friendly with the medical staff, and seems relatively unconcerned when the physician is unable to render a diagnosis.[50] The perpetrators are often quite familiar with medical terminology and diseases, and usually have pathologic attachments to their children.[51] A history of working in a daycare setting is also common.[50] There are four criteria for MSBP: medical illness in a child is fabricated by a parent; the child is brought for repeated medical evaluation or treatment and often undergoes multiple medical procedures; the perpetrator denies the actions; and acute symptoms and signs resolve when the child and caregiver are separated.[26] Two circumstances should be present for this diagnosis to be confirmed: harm or potential harm to the child involving medical care, and a caregiver who is causing it to happen.[52]

There are a variety of clinical symptoms or features that may be seen in the child victim of MSBP. These include infant apnea, factitious coagulopathy, failure to thrive, hypoglycemia, abnormal urinalysis, seizures and other neurologic symptoms, cyanosis, vomiting and diarrhea, sepsis, lethargy, behavior problems, fever, electrolyte abnormalities, and bone and joint problems.[26,50-53] The dermatologic aspects of MSBP may invariably be referred to as 'factitious dermatitis by proxy' or 'dermatitis artefacta by proxy'. Skin findings have been reported in 3–9% of cases of MSBP.[53] These lesions may present with any of the morphologies discussed earlier for factitious dermatitis/dermatitis artefacta.

The diagnosis of MSBP may be made by inclusion or by exclusion. The former is rendered when there is unquestionable evidence of commission, such as capturing the act during covert videotape surveillance in the hospital setting.[54] Some experts believe that such video surveillance is required in order to make a definitive and timely diagnosis in most cases of MSBP.[50] When used, adequate safeguards including continuous surveillance and an agreed-upon plan of action must exist in order to prevent further injury to the child.[52] A diagnosis of exclusion is rendered when all other possible explanations for the child's condition have been considered and excluded.[54] Consultation with all colleagues who have cared for the child, and a 'separation test', in which the child is demonstrated to be free of disease outside the care of the mother, are useful.[55] Child protective services should be involved, and the perpetrator referred to a professional with significant experience in MSBP. Long-term morbidity or permanent disability is common in survivors.

Cutaneous mimickers of abuse and factitial disorders

Although child abuse or factitial disorders should always be considered in the child with unusual skin marks or injuries, there are several potential mimickers that must be kept in mind. These are summarized in Table 26.5.[56,57]

There are a number of folk remedies that may be confused with abuse, given the trauma-induced skin lesions that result from these practices. With the increasing influx of Asian immigrants entering the USA, such traditional Oriental medicine methods are being practiced with increasing frequency. The philosophy of Oriental medicine is to achieve a state of balance and equilibrium, including proper flow of energies within 'channels' or 'meridians'.[58] The goal of traditional folk remedies is to facilitate this energy balance. It is important for the pediatric practitioner to be familiar with these culturally based therapies, which include coining, cupping, moxibustion, blood letting, and warm needle acupuncture.[58,59] The former three entities will be briefly discussed here.

'Coining' is also known as coin rubbing, skin scraping, spooning, or *çao gio*. It is an ancient Vietnamese folk remedy performed by applying heated, mentholated oil to the back, chest, and shoulders, and then vigorously rubbing a coin on selected parts of the body in order to produce linear petechiae or ecchymoses (Fig. 26.34).[60] Other items that may be used include a spoon, comb, or edge of a jar cap. Whereas a coin is traditionally used by the Vietnamese, a spoon is commonly the instrument used by the Chinese, in which case the practice is referred to as *quat sha*.[61] Those who utilize coining believe it to be useful for a variety of complaints, including headache, fever, pain, and inflammation. Although serious injury is rare, minor and even major burns (resulting from ignition of the oil in the skin) have been reported.[60]

Cupping is an ancient technique dating back to the fourth century BC in Egypt.[62] It is practiced in the USA most often by Russian immigrants, but is also utilized by Asian and Mexican–American culture (where it is referred to as *ventosas*).[61] It is used to relieve such symptoms as abdominal pain, abscesses, stroke paralysis, fever, congestion, and poor appetite. With this remedy, a cup or jar is immediately placed on the skin after a cotton-ball soaked with alcohol has been ignited within the cup to create a suction vacuum. The procedure results in circular ecchymotic lesions (Figs 26.35, 26.36).

Moxibustion is another folk remedy utilized primarily in Asian cultures for a variety of complaints, including enuresis, behavioral disorders, asthma, and pain.[58,61] It has also been utilized for correction of breech presentation[63] and for treatment of tennis elbow.[64] In moxibustion, the moxa herb (*Artemisia vulgaris*) is rolled into a cone or cigar, ignited, and placed on the appropriate body part (either directly or indirectly with a medium separating the moxa from the skin). It is allowed to burn to the point of pain, and the resulting skin lesions vary from transient redness to second degree burns, which may scar. As with all folk remedies, these lesions may be confused with intentional child abuse.

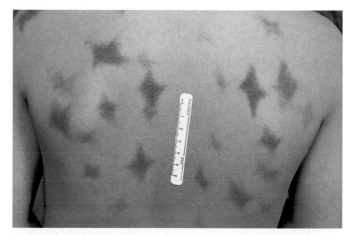

Figure 26.34 Coining. These linear and stellate purpuric patches were caused by the vigorous rubbing of a coin on the skin, termed coining, or *çao gio*. (Courtesy of Jean Hlady, MD.)

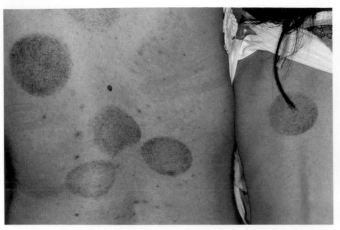

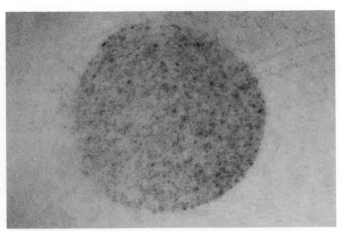

Figure 26.35 Cupping. This 7-year-old girl (right), who presented to clinic for an unrelated skin complaint, was noted to have this round, ecchymotic lesion on her back. Examination of her mother (left) revealed multiple such lesions, which were being induced by cupping in hopes of treating her rheumatoid arthritis. The family performed the procedure on the girl at her request.

Figure 26.36 Cupping. Close-up of the ecchymotic lesion seen in the girl patient in Figure 26.35.

Table 26.5 Potential mimickers of abuse or factitial disorders

Disorder	Chapter/comment
Accidental burns	Various, including enuresis blanket, acetic acid, objects heated by sun (i.e., bike seats, car upholstery)
Anal fissures	Most commonly associated with constipation, passage of hard stools; however, occasionally associated with sexual abuse
Autoimmune bullous disease	Ch. 13; i.e., vulvar pemphigoid, linear IgA bullous disease of childhood
Behçet syndrome	Ch. 25
Berloque dermatitis	Ch. 19; phototoxic reaction to fragrance products
Bullous impetigo	Ch. 14; may be confused for cigarette burns
Crohn's disease	Ch. 25; may present with perianal erythema, fissures, skin tags, bleeding, scarring, swelling
Ecthyma	Ch. 14; confused with cigarette burns; usually caused by GABHS
Ehlers–Danlos syndrome	Ch. 6; may have poor wound healing, frequent scarring, easy bruising
Enlarged hymenal opening	Important reassuring features include intact hymenal tissue at posterior rim, lack of laceration/deep notching/bruising/bleeding[56]
Epidermal nevus	Ch. 9; perianal lesions may be confused with anogenital condylomata[57]
Epidermolysis bullosa	Ch. 13; especially dominant dystrophic or simplex varieties
Fixed drug eruption	Ch. 20
Folk remedies	(Current chapter; see text)
Hematologic disorders	Various, including hemophilia, von Willebrand disease, leukemia, ITR vasculitis
Incontinentia pigmenti	Ch. 11; vesicular and pigmentary lesions with bizarre patterning
Labial adhesions	
Lichen sclerosus et atrophicus	Ch. 22; genital variant confused with sexual abuse; may be bullous
Mongolian spots	Ch. 11
Netherton syndrome	Ch. 5; dermatitis, ichthyosis, failure to thrive, and alopecia may be confused for abuse
Nevus of Ota or Ito	Ch. 11
Normal bruising	Most commonly children 2–5 years; consider distribution, developmental status, history
Osteogenesis imperfecta	Ch. 6; frequent fractures, osteoporosis, short stature, frontal bossing, blue sclerae
Perianal pyramidal protrusion	Ch. 15
Perianal streptococcal dermatitis	Ch. 14
Phytophotodermatitis	Ch. 19; phototoxic reaction to psoralens (lemons, limes, celery, parsley, dill)
Vaginal foreign body	May result in vaginal discharge, bleeding
Xeroderma pigmentosum	Ch. 19; severe sunburn may be confused with neglect

GABHS, group A beta-hemolytic streptococci; ITP, idiopathic thrombocytopenic purpura.

Key References

Dubowitz H, Bennett S. Physical abuse and neglect of children. *Lancet.* 2007;369:1891–1899.

Harvey WT. Morgellons disease. *J Am Acad Dermatol.* 2007;705–706.

Kellogg N and the American Academy of Pediatrics Committee on Child Abuse and Neglect. The evaluation of sexual abuse in children. *Pediatrics.* 2005;116(2):506–512.

Peck MD, Priolo-Kapel D. Child abuse by burning: A review of the literature and an algorithm for medical investigations. *J Trauma.* 2002;53:1013–1022.

Pierce MC, Kaczor K, Aldridge S, et al. Bruising characteristics discriminating physical child abuse from accidental trauma. *Pediatrics.* 2010;125(1):67–74.

Shah KN, Fried RG. Factitial dermatoses in children. *Curr Opin Pediatr.* 2006;18:403–409.

Stirling J and the Committee on Child Abuse and Neglect. Beyond Munchausen syndrome by proxy: Identification and treatment of child abuse in the medical setting. *Pediatrics.* 2007;119(5): 1026–1030.

Swerdlin A, Berkowitz C, Craft N. Cutaneous signs of child abuse. *J Am Acad Dermatol.* 2007;57:371–392.

Index

Page numbers followed by "f" indicate figures, "t" indicate tables, and "b" indicate boxes.

A

abacavir, AIDS, 369
abatacept, juvenile idiopathic arthritis, 499
abdominal zoster, 354
abscess, 2t–7t
  scalp, in newborns, 13f
Absidia spp., 414
Acanthamoeba spp., and AIDS, 368t
acanthosis, 77
acanthosis nigricans
  diabetes mellitus, 542–544, 543f–544f, 543t
  juvenile dermatomyositis, 513f
  polycystic ovary syndrome, 536
acanthosis nigricans type of epidermal nevi, 195
ACE inhibitors
  side-effects
    angioedema, 455t
    telogen effluvium, 147t
acetaminophen
  side-effects
    fixed drug eruption, 455t
    Stevens-Johnson syndrome, 455t
acetyl CoA carboxylase, 550
N-acetylglucosamine, melasma, 262
Achard-Thiers syndrome, 157
acitretin
  graft-versus-host disease, 569
  ichthyosis, 106–107
  psoriasis, 78t, 80
acne
  androgen access, 168t, 178
  with facial edema, 179
  infantile, 176–178, 177f
  polycystic ovary syndrome, 536
  pomade, 9, 178
  steroid, 534f
acne conglobata, 179
acne cosmetica, 178
acne excoriée, 178–179, 179f, 586–589, 588f
  obsessive-compulsive disorders, 590t
acne fulminans, 169, 170f
acne inversa, 180–181, 181f
acne keloidalis, 146, 146f
acne keloidalis nuchae, 9
acne neonatorum, 16, 16f, 176–178, 177f
acne rosacea, 178
acne vulgaris, 167–176
  androgen access, 168t
  comedones, 167, 168f–169f
  dyspigmentation, 170f
  inflammatory, 169f
  lesions associated with, 168t
  microcomedones, 167
  nodulocystic, 9, 169f

pathogenesis, 167, 168f
post-acne erythema, 170f
Propionibacterium acnes, 167
scarring, 170f
treatment, 171–176, 171f, 172t, 174t, 176t–177t
acneiform drug reactions, 455t
acneiform lesions, 7
acquired immunodeficiency syndrome *see* AIDS
acquired raised bands of infancy, 27, 27f
acridine dyes, photosensitivity, 442–443
acro-dermato-ungual-lacrimal-tooth (ADULT) syndrome, 140t, 141
acrochordon, 537
  newborns, 23
acrodermatitis chronica atrophicans, 345
acrodermatitis enteropathica, 548–550, 549t, 569–570
  clinical features, 550f
  diaper area, 17t, 22, 22f
  differential diagnosis, 46
  disorders resembling, 549t, 550–553
  nail matrix arrest, 159t
acrodynia, 264
acrogeria, and elastosis perforans serpiginosa, 124
acrokeratosis verruciformis of Hopf *see* Darier disease
acromegaly, 537
acropustulosis of infancy, 17t, 19, 19f
  differential diagnosis, 77t
acrycyanosis, 11
ACTH
  causing hypertrichosis, 155t
  stimulation test, 533
actinic lichen planus, 89t
actinic prurigo, 440–441, 440f
Actinomadura spp., 409
Actinomyces spp., noma, 330
Actinomyces israelii, 341
actinomycosis, 341
acute febrile neutrophilic dermatosis *see* Sweet's syndrome
acute generalized exanthematous pustulosis, 469
  clinical features, 469f
acute hemorrhagic edema of infancy, 484t, 486–487, 486f–487f
acute HIV infection syndrome, 368
acute intermittent porphyria, 448t–449t, 451
acute necrotizing gingivitis, 355
acyclovir
  atopic dermatitis, 51
  herpes gladiatorum, 352
  herpes zoster, 354t
  HSV infection, 349t

neonatal HSV, 32
varicella, 373
adactyly, 125
adalimumab
  Crohn's disease, 570–571
  juvenile idiopathic arthritis, 499
  psoriasis, 80
  pyoderma gangrenosum, 577
Adams-Oliver syndrome, 25, 295–296
adapalene, acne vulgaris, 172t
Addison disease, 532–533, 533f
  and mucocutaneous candidiasis, 408
adenoma sebaceum, 204, 244–245, 245f, 538
adenosine deaminase deficiency, 565t
adhesive tape dermatitis, 69, 69f
adrenal gland disorders, 532–535
  Addison disease, 532–533, 533f
  Cushing syndrome, 533–535, 533t, 534f
adrenogenital syndrome, 535
aeroallergens, 48
African-Americans, 9
Aicardi-Goutieres syndrome, 476
AIDS, 367–369
  demodicidosis in, 368t
  diagnosis, 369
  drug-induced eruptions, 368t
  metabolic disturbances, 369
  mucocutaneous manifestations, 368t
  and syphilis, 368t
  treatment, 369
ALA dehydratase porphyria, 448t–449t, 451
alafacept, psoriasis, 80
Alagille disease, 557
albendazole
  cutaneous larva migrans, 433
  side-effects, telogen effluvium, 147t
albinism, 8–9, 197
  oculocutaneous, 238–240, 238t, 239f
Albright's hereditary osteodystrophy, 215, 531–532
alclometasone dipropionate, atopic dermatitis, 49t
Alezzandrini syndrome, 238
alkaptonuria, 263, 546, 547t
allergic contact dermatitis, 61–70, 63t
  adhesive tape, 69, 69f
  clothing, 69–70
  Compositae, 70
  cosmetics and topical medications, 68–69
  diagnosis, 62, 63t
    patch testing, 62–64, 64t
  differential diagnosis, 45
  distribution, 63t
  metals/metal salts, 63t, 66–67
    see also individual metals
  Rhus dermatitis, 1, 62, 64–66, 65f–66f
  shoe dermatitis, 67–68, 68f